Contemporary Issues in Bioethics

CONTEMPORARY ISSUES IN BIOETHICS

THIRD EDITION

Edited by

Tom L. Beauchamp & LeRoy Walters

Kennedy Institute of Ethics and Department of Philosophy

Georgetown University

Wadsworth Publishing Company
Belmont, California
A Division of Wadsworth, Inc.

Philosophy Editor: Kenneth King
Production Editor: Leland Moss
Managing Designer: Andrew H. Ogus
Print Buyer: Barbara Britton
Compositor: TypeLink, Inc.
Copy Editor: René Lynch
Editorial Assistant: Michelle Palacio
Cover: Andrew H. Ogus

Printed in the United States of America   34

1 2 3 4 5 6 7 8 9 10–93 92 91 90 89

Library of Congress Cataloging-in-Publication Data

Contemporary issues in bioethics.

   Includes bibliographies.
   1. Medical ethics.   I. Beauchamp, Tom L.   II. Walters,
LeRoy.
R724.C67   1989   174′.2   88-27914
ISBN 0-534-10182-8

CONTENTS

PART III Life and Death

PREFACE

The objective of this anthology is to make students aware of complex situations in biology and medicine that require moral reflection, judgment, or decision, while at the same time revealing how such moral thinking can be accomplished. The essays have been chosen on the basis of their clarity of conceptual and ethical reflection, their teachability, and their significance for current controversies. Whenever possible, the essays have been arranged in a debate-like format: Divergent viewpoints have been juxtaposed, so that the reader may explore the strengths and weaknesses of alternative positions on an issue. Each chapter of readings is preceded by an editor's introduction, which sets the essays in context and surveys the major arguments on the chapter topic. At the end of each chapter we have recommended readings and have listed bibliographical resources that contain numerous additional citations.

This third edition of *Contemporary Issues in Bioethics* continues the focus in previous editions on moral perplexities generated by the biomedical fields. The second edition published in 1982 involved massive changes in the selections, and this third edition is as different from the second as the second was from the first. The chapter on ethical theory has been thoroughly revised and includes new sub-sections under the section "Ethics, Law, and Public Policy." Each of the remaining chapter introductions has been revised, and often expanded. A new structure of Parts organizes the volume, and we have added new chapters on "Bioethics as a Field of Ethics" and "Frontiers in Biology and Medicine." Other new material has been added on the topics of hospital ethics committees, conflicts of obligations, committee review of research, new technologies, screening for AIDS, and for-profit health care. In all, 71 essays are new, whereas 26 essays are carried over into this edition. However, many familiar landmarks remain. We have retained most of the chapter topics from the second edition and most of the major divisions in those chapters.

We have received many helpful suggestions for improving this anthology. It is impossible to recognize them all, but special thanks should be given to a talented research staff that has assisted us for two years in the collecting of materials and evaluation of them. Three graduate students, Eric Meslin, David DeGrazia, and Jeffrey Kahn, provided invaluable assistance and advice in this process. They repeatedly forced us to make our selections more pertinent and the introductions more readable for students. Superb assistance was also provided through our university offices, where for several months drafts were faithfully prepared in what must have seemed an endless flow of editing, rewriting, and proofing. We are especially indebted for this assistance to Denise Brooks and Michael Stanley. We also thank Elissa Felder, Tanja Hens, Perry Zizzi, Michael Smith, Charles Tung, and Tammee Thompson for technical assistance that improved the accuracy and detail of every chapter.

We also wish to thank Leland Moss for expertly overseeing the production of this book, and Kenneth King of Wadsworth for his helpful editorial advice. Reviewers Oliva Blanchette, Boston College; Alister Brown, formerly of the University of British Columbia–Vancouver; Russell Hittinger, formerly of St. Louis University; and Douglas C. Long, University of North Carolina–Chapel Hill all provided helpful comments.

We have been generously supported in this edition by a grant awarded by the Biomedical Research Support Grant Program, Division of Research Resources, National Institutes of Health (BRSG SO7 RR 0713616). We also acknowledge with appreciation the support provided by the Kennedy Institute's library and information retrieval systems, which kept us in touch with the most important literature and reduced the burdens of library research.

In particular, we thank Doris Goldstein, Frances Abramson, Mary Coutts, Marlene Johnson, Lucinda Fitch, Tamar Joy Kahn, Patricia McCarrick, Sue Meinke, and Cecily Orr. And again we acknowledge the backing provided by the Kennedy Institute of Ethics and its Director, Dr. Edmund Pellegrino.

Finally, we are grateful to our spouses, Ruth R. Faden and the late Jane M. Walters, for their constant encouragement, support, and love.

Tom L. Beauchamp
LeRoy Walters
Kennedy Institute of Ethics
and Philosophy Department
Georgetown University

1.
Ethical Theory and Bioethics

The moral problems discussed in this book have emerged from professional practice in the fields of clinical medicine, biomedical research, nursing, and in some cases the social and behavioral sciences. The goal of this first chapter is to provide a basis in ethical theory sufficient for reading and criticizing the essays in the later chapters. This chapter focuses on ethical theory and refrains from exploring the history and nature of bioethics—two topics considered in Chapter 2.

FUNDAMENTAL PROBLEMS

THE STUDY OF MORALITY

The study of morality requires a look at moral practices as well as the theory that underlies those practices. In this chapter we will not only study morality in medicine and research but the nature and justification of morality generally.

Some Basic Definitions. The terms "ethical theory" and "moral philosophy" refer to philosophical reflection on the nature and place of morality. The purpose of theory is to introduce clarity, substance, and precision of argument into the domain of morality. The term "morality," by contrast, is used to refer to traditions of belief about right and wrong human conduct. Morality is a social institution with a history and a code of learnable rules. Like political constitutions and languages, morality exists before we are instructed in its relevant rules, and thus it has a trans-individual status as a body of guidelines for action. Individuals do not create their morality by making their own rules, and morality cannot be purely a personal policy or code, because it is by nature a social code.

We learn the requirements of morality as we grow up. We learn moral rules alongside other important social rules, which is one reason it later becomes difficult to distinguish the two. For example, we are constantly reminded in our early years that we must observe social rules such as saying "Please" when we want something and "Thank you" when we receive it. We are taught these rules of etiquette and many more specific ones, such as "A judge is addressed as 'judge.'" We are also taught rules of prudence, including "Don't touch a hot stove," as well as rules of drawing, housekeeping, dressing, and the like.

But the whole of these rules does not amount to morality. Morality enters the picture only when certain things ought or ought not to be done because of their deep social importance in the ways they affect the interests of other people. We first learn maxims such as "It is better to give than to receive" and "Respect the rights of others." These are elementary instructions in morality; they express what society expects of us and everyone in terms of taking the interests of other people into account. We thus learn about moral instructions and expectations, and gradually we come to understand morality as a set of principles about doing good, avoiding harm, respecting others, and observing the rules of justice.

Following this analysis, the terms "ethical" and "moral" are to be understood in this introduction as identical in meaning, and "ethics" will be used as a general term referring to *both* morality and ethical theory. Moral philosophy, ethical theory, and philosophical ethics are terms that will be reserved for philosophical theories, including philosophical reflection on social morality. Although popular discussions of moral problems use moral language, they seldom invoke ethical theory and its techniques.

Four Approaches to the Study of Ethics. Morality can be studied and developed in a variety of ways, only some of which can be correctly called "ethical theory." In particular, four ways of either studying moral beliefs or doing moral philosophy have been prominent in the literature of ethics. Two of these approaches presumably describe and analyze morality without taking moral positions, and these approaches are therefore called "nonnormative"; two other approaches do involve taking moral positions and involve appeal to ethical theory. These four approaches can be summarized as follows:

A. *Nonnormative approaches*
   1. Descriptive ethics
   2. Metaethics
B. *Normative approaches*
   3. General normative ethics
   4. Applied normative ethics

It would be a mistake to regard these categories as expressing rigid, sharply differentiated approaches. They are often undertaken jointly, and they overlap in goal and content. Nonetheless, when understood as broad polar contrasts exemplifying models of inquiry, these distinctions are important.

First among the two nonnormative fields of inquiry into morality is descriptive ethics, or the factual description and explanation of moral behavior and beliefs. Anthropologists, sociologists, and historians who study moral behavior employ this approach when they explore how moral attitudes, codes, and beliefs differ from person to person and from society to society. We often find these descriptions in novels about foreign lands in long-ago times. These works dwell in great detail on sexual practices, codes of honor, and rules governing permissible killing in a society. A more commonplace example is the sociological study of biomedical research involving human subjects and the standards of informed consent used in performing the research. Although philosophers do not generally engage in descriptive ethics in their work, some have combined descriptive ethics with philosophical ethics—for example, by analyzing the ethical practices of American Indian tribes or researching Nazi experimentation during World War II.

A second nonnormative field, metaethics, involves analysis of the meanings of central terms in ethics, such as "right," "obligation," "good," "virtue," and "responsibility." The proper analysis of the term "morality" and the distinction between the moral and the nonmoral are typical examples of metaethical problems. Crucial terms in medical ethics, including "informed consent," "person," and "access" to health care, can be given the same kind of careful conceptual attention, as they are in various chapters in this volume. (Descriptive ethics and metaethics may not be the only forms of nonnormative inquiry. In recent years there has been an active discussion of the biological bases of moral behavior and the ways in which humans do and do not differ from animals. This form of inquiry is obviously different from the study of attitudes, codes, or beliefs.)

General normative ethics attempts to formulate and defend basic principles and virtues governing the moral life. Ideally, any ethical theory will provide a whole system of moral principles or virtues and reasons for adopting them, and will defend claims about the range of their applicability. In the course of this chapter the most prominent of these theories will be examined in detail, as will the principles of respect for autonomy, justice, and beneficence—three principles that have often played a major role in these theories.

The principles used in general normative ethics are often applied to specific moral problems, including abortion, widespread hunger, racial and sexual discrimination, and research involving human subjects. This use of ethical theory is referred to as "applied ethics." Philosophical treatment of medical ethics, engineering ethics, journalistic ethics, jurisprudence, and business ethics all involve an application of general ethical principles to moral problems that arise in these professions. Substantially the same general ethical principles apply to problems across these professional fields and in areas beyond professional ethics as well. One might appeal to principles of justice, for example, in order to illuminate and resolve issues of taxation, health care distribution, criminal punishment, and reverse discrimination. Similarly, principles of veracity (truthfulness) apply to debates about secrecy and deception in international politics, misleading advertisements in business ethics, balanced reporting in journalistic ethics, and the disclosure of the nature and extent of an illness to a patient in medical ethics.

Applied ethics is the main approach found in the readings in this volume. It has been employed in recent years in contexts of public policy and professional ethics, where an interdisciplinary approach is required. Usually this approach is used to reason about moral dilemmas, but the attempt to resolve these dilemmas also may lead to moral disagreement.

MORAL DILEMMAS AND DISAGREEMENTS

In the teaching of ethics in professional schools, moral problems are often examined through case studies, because these cases vividly display dilemmas that require students to identify the moral principles at issue and to confront problems of disagreement. We can approximate this same method in order to look at moral dilemmas and disagreements.

Moral Dilemmas. In a case presented in Chapter 8, two judges became entangled in apparent moral disagreement when confronted with a murder trial. A woman named Tarasoff had been killed by a man who previously had confided to a psychiatrist his intention to kill her as soon as she returned home from a summer vacation. Owing to obligations of confidentiality between patient and physician, a psychologist and a consulting psychiatrist did not report the threat to the woman or to her family, though they did make one unsuccessful attempt to commit the man to a mental hospital.

One judge held that the therapist could not escape liability, saying that, "When a therapist determines, or pursuant to the standards of his profession should determine, that his patient presents a serious danger of violence to another, he incurs an obligation to use reasonable care to protect the intended victim against such danger." Notification of police and direct warnings to the family were mentioned as possible instances of due care. The judge argued that, although medical confidentiality must generally be observed by physicians, it was overridden in this particular case by an obligation to the possible victim and to the "public interest in safety from violent assault."

In the minority opinion, a second judge stated his firm disagreement. He argued that a patient's rights are violated when rules of confidentiality are not observed, that psychiatric treatment would be frustrated by nonobservance, and that patients would subsequently lose confidence in psychiatrists and would fail to provide full disclosures. He also suggested that violent assaults would actually increase because mentally ill persons would be discouraged from seeking psychiatric aid.[1]

The Tarasoff case is an instance of a moral dilemma, because strong moral reasons support the rival conclusions of the two judges. The most difficult and recalcitrant moral controversies that we shall encounter in this volume generally have at least some dilemmatic features. They involve what Guido Calabresi has called "tragic choices." Everyone who has been faced with a difficult decision—such as whether to have an abortion, to have a pet "put to sleep," or to commit a member of one's family to a mental institution—knows through deep anguish what is meant by a personal dilemma. These dilemmas occur whenever good reasons for mutually exclusive alternatives can be cited; if any one set of reasons is acted upon, outcomes desirable in some respects but undesirable in others will result. Here an agent morally ought to do one thing and also morally ought to do another thing, but the agent is precluded by circumstances from doing both. Although the moral reasons behind each alternative are good reasons, neither set of reasons clearly outweighs the other. Parties on both sides of dilemmatic disagreements thus can *correctly* present moral principles in support of their competing conclusions. Most moral dilemmas present a need to balance rival, ideal claims in untidy circumstances.

One possible response to the problem of moral dilemmas and disputes is that we do not have and are not likely ever to have a single ethical theory or a single method for resolving disagreements. In any pluralistic culture there may be many sources of moral value and consequently a pluralism of moral points of view on many issues: bluffing in business deals, providing national health insurance to all citizens, involuntarily committing the mentally disturbed, civil disobedience, and so on. If this response is correct, it is obvious why there seem to be intractable moral controversies both inside and outside professional philosophy. On the other hand, there may be ways out of at least some dilemmas and disputes, as we shall now see.

The Resolution of Moral Disagreements. Can we hope—in light of complex dilemmas and other sources of dispute—to resolve moral disagreements? Probably no single set of considerations will prove consistently reliable as a means of ending disagreement and controversy (and resolutions of cross-cultural conflicts will always be especially elusive). Nonetheless, several methods for dealing constructively with moral disagreements have been employed in the past, and each deserves recognition as a method of easing and perhaps settling controversies. These methods can at least help us manage dilemmas, even if no entirely satisfactory resolution emerges.

1. *Obtaining Objective Information.* First, many moral disagreements can be at least partially resolved by obtaining factual information concerning points of moral controversy. It has often been uncritically assumed that moral disputes are (by definition) produced solely by differences over moral principles or their application, and not by a lack of information. This assumption is overly simplistic, however, because disputes over what morally ought or ought not to be done often have nonmoral elements as central ingredients. For example, debates about the allocation of health dollars to preventive and educational measures (see Chapter 11) have often bogged down over factual issues of whether specific measures actually function to prevent illness and promote health.

In some cases new information has made possible a move toward negotiation and resolution of disagreements. New scientific information about the alleged dangers involved in certain kinds of scientific research, for instance, have turned public controversies regarding the risks of science and the rights of scientific researchers in unanticipated directions. In one recent controversy over recombinant DNA research, it had been feared that the research might create an organism of pathogenic capability that known antibodies would be unable to combat and that could produce widespread contagion. Accusations of unjustifiable and immoral research were heard in the corridors of certain universities and congressional hearing rooms, although the researchers contended that the risks were minimal. New scientific information from risk-assessment studies indicating that the research was less dangerous than had been feared had a dramatic effect on the moral and political controversy about the justifiability of the risks to society presented by this scientific research.

Controversies about saccharin, toxic substances in the workplace, IQ research, fluoridation, and the swine-flu vaccine, among others, have been similarly laced with issues of both values and facts. Current controversies over whether there should be compulsory screening for AIDS often turn critically on factual claims about how HIV (human immunodeficiency virus) is transmitted, how much can be learned by screening, how many persons are threatened, whether health education campaigns can successfully teach safe sex practices, and the like. Related moral problems about whether nurses and other health professionals have a role obligation to feed, ambulate, or otherwise administer to an AIDS patient may also be resolvable only by recourse to the facts about AIDS transmission.

The arguments used by disagreeing parties in these cases *may* turn on some dispute about liberty or justice and therefore *may* be primarily moral, but they may also rest on purely factual disagreements. New information may have only a limited bearing on the resolution of some of these controversies, whereas in others it may have a direct and almost overpowering influence. The problem is that rarely, if ever, is all the information obtained that would be sufficient to settle these factual matters.

2. *Providing Definitional Clarity.* Second, controversies have been settled by reaching conceptual or definitional agreement over the language used by disputing parties. In some cases stipulation of a definition or a clear explanation of what is meant by a term may prove sufficient, but in other cases agreement cannot be so conveniently achieved. Controversies over the morality of euthanasia, for example, are often needlessly entangled because disputing parties use different senses of the term and have much invested in their particular definitions. For example, it may be that one party equates euthanasia with mercy killing and another party equates it with voluntarily elected natural death. Some even hold that euthanasia is by definition nonvoluntary mercy killing. Any resulting moral controversy over "euthanasia" is ensnared in terminological problems (see Chapter 6), rendering it doubtful that the parties are discussing the same problem.

There is no common point of discussion and disagreement in many cases, because the parties are addressing different issues as a result of their different conceptual assumptions. Under these conditions it cannot reasonably be expected that the issues can be pushed forward. Although conceptual agreement provides no guarantee that a dispute will be settled, it should at least facilitate discussion of the issues. For this reason, many essays in this volume dwell at some length on issues of conceptual analysis. This is especially true of Chapters 3 and 4, where the difficult concepts of person, health, and disease are treated.

3. *Adopting a Code.* Third, resolution of moral problems can be facilitated if disputing parties can come to agreement on a common set of moral principles. If this method requires a complete shift from one starkly different moral point of view to another, agreement will rarely if ever be achieved. Differences that divide persons at the level of their most cherished principles are deep divisions, and conversions are infrequent. Various forms of discussion and negotiation can, however, lead to the adoption of a new or changed moral framework that can serve as a common basis for discussion.

For example, a recent national commission appointed to study ethical issues in research involving human subjects unanimously adopted a common framework of moral principles, which provided the general background for deliberations about particular problems.

Commissioners developed a framework of three moral principles: respect for persons, beneficence, and justice. These principles were analyzed in detail in the light of contemporary philosophical ethics and were then applied to a wide range of moral problems that confronted the commission.[2] This common framework of moral principles facilitated discussion of the controversies they addressed and led to many agreements that might otherwise have been impossible.

Virtually every professional association has a code of ethics, and the precise reason for their existence is to give guidance in a circumstance of uncertainty or dispute. This body of rules includes codes of medical and nursing ethics and codes of research ethics, which apply to all persons in the relevant professional roles in the practice of medicine, nursing, and research. These codes are very general and cannot be expected to cover every possible case, but agreed-upon general principles do provide an important beginning.

4. *Using Examples and Counterexamples.* Fourth, resolution of moral controversies can be aided by a method of example and opposed counterexample. Cases or examples favorable to one point of view are brought forward, and counterexamples to these cases are thrown up by a second person against the examples and claims of the first. The long-standing debate over truth telling in medicine is a typical case. (See Chapter 8.) Personal experience and empirical research have provided a set of examples (anecdotes and empirical evidence) about the consequences of telling the truth and not telling the truth to seriously ill patients. Argument often proceeds by citing relevant cases and then presenting alternative cases (counterexamples) that support a different approach, on grounds that the counterexample shows the superiority of the second approach. This use of example and counterexample serves as a format for weighing the strength of conflicting approaches and policies.

This form of debate occurred when the national commission mentioned in the preceding section came to consider the level of risk that can justifiably be permitted in scientific research involving children as subjects where no therapeutic benefit is offered to the child. On the basis of principles of acceptable risk used in their own previous deliberations, commissioners were at first inclined to accept the view that only low-risk or "minimal-risk" procedures could be justified in the case of children (where "minimal risk" refers analogically to the level of risk present in standard medical examinations of patients). Many examples were put forward of unnecessary risk presented to children in research. However, examples from the history of medicine were cited that revealed how certain significant diagnostic, therapeutic, and preventive advances in medicine would have been unlikely, or at least retarded, unless procedures that posed a higher level of risk had been employed. Counterexamples of overzealous researchers who placed children at too much risk were then thrown up against these examples, and the debate continued at the level of counterexample for several months.

Eventually a majority of commissioners abandoned their original view that nontherapeutic research involving more than minimal risk was unjustified. Instead, the majority accepted the position that a higher level of risk can be justified by the benefits provided to other children, as when a group of terminally ill children becomes the subject of research in the hope that something will be learned about their disease that can be applied to other children. Once a consensus on this particular issue crystallized, resolution was quickly achieved on the entire moral controversy about the involvement of children as research subjects (although two commissioners never agreed).

5. *Analyzing Arguments.* Fifth and finally, one of the most important methods of philosophical inquiry, that of exposing the inadequacies, gaps, fallacies, and unexpected

consequences of an argument, can also be brought to bear on moral disagreements. If an argument is inconsistent, for example, pointing out the inconsistency will change the argument and shift the focus of discussion. There are, in addition, many more subtle ways of attacking an argument than pointing to straightforward inconsistencies. For example, in Chapters 4 and 5 below there are discussions of the nature of "persons," and these discussions are carried into later chapters dealing with problems of abortion, fetal rights, and the definition of death. Some writers on these topics have not appreciated that their arguments about persons—used, for example, to discuss fetuses and those who are irreversibly comatose—were so broad that they carried important but unnoticed implications for both infants and animals. Their arguments implicitly provided reasons they had not noticed for denying rights to infants (rights that adults have), or for granting (or denying) the same rights to fetuses that infants have, and in some cases for granting (or denying) the same rights to animals that infants have.

It may, of course, be correct to hold that infants have fewer rights than adults, or that fetuses and animals should be granted the same rights as infants (see Chapter 9 on "Research with Human and Animal Subjects"). The point is that if a moral argument leads to conclusions that a proponent is not prepared to defend and did not previously anticipate, part of the argument will have to be changed, and this process may reduce the distance between the parties who are disagreeing. This style of argument is often supplemented by one or more of the other four ways of reducing moral disagreement. Much of the work published in philosophical journals takes these forms of attacking arguments, using counterexamples, and proposing alternative frameworks of principles.

Some moral disagreements may not be resolvable by any of the five means discussed. We need not claim that moral disagreements can always be resolved, or even that every rational person must accept the same method for approaching such problems. There is always a possibility of ultimate disagreement. However, if something is to be done about problems of justification in contexts of disagreement, a resolution is more likely to occur if the methods outlined in this section are used. These strategies will often be found in the articles included in this anthology.

RELATIVISM AND OBJECTIVITY IN ETHICS

The fact of moral disagreement raises questions about whether there can be correct or objective moral judgments. Cultural differences and individual disagreements among friends over issues like abortion, euthanasia, and the right to health care have led many to doubt the possibility that there are correct and objective positions in morals. This doubt is fed by popular aphorisms asserting that morality is more properly a matter of taste than reason, that it is ultimately arbitrary what one believes, and that there is no neutral standpoint from which to view disagreements.

Tension between the belief that morality is purely a matter of personal or social convention and the belief that it has an objective grounding leads to issues of relativism in morals. Moral relativism is no newcomer to the scene of moral philosophy. Ancient thinkers were as perplexed by cultural and individual differences as moderns, as is evidenced by Plato's famous battle with a relativism popular in his day. Nevertheless, it was easier in former times to ignore cultural differences than it is today, because there was once greater uniformity within cultures, as well as less commerce between them. The contrast between ancient Athens and modern Manhattan is evident, and any contemporary pluralistic culture is saturated with individuality of belief and lifestyle. At the same time, we tend to reject the claim that this diversity compels us to tolerate racism, social caste systems, sexism, genocide, and a wide variety of inequalities of treatment that we deeply believe to be morally wrong but find sanctioned either in our own culture or in others. Which view, then, is correct?

Cultural Relativism.   Relativists defend their position by appeal to anthropological data indicating that moral rightness and wrongness vary from place to place and that there are no absolute or universal moral standards that could apply to all persons at all times. They add that rightness is contingent on cultural beliefs and that the concepts of rightness and wrongness are therefore meaningless apart from the specific contexts in which they arise. The claim is that patterns of culture can only be understood as unique wholes and that moral beliefs about normal behavior are thus closely connected in a culture to other cultural characteristics, such as language and fundamental political institutions. Studies show, they maintain, that what is deemed worthy of moral approval or disapproval in one society varies, both in detail and as a whole pattern, from moral standards in other societies.

This form of relativism has plagued moral philosophy, and many philosophical arguments have been advanced in criticism of it. Among the best-known criticisms is that there is a universal structure of human nature, or at least a universal set of human needs, which leads to the adoption of similar or perhaps identical principles in all cultures. This factual argument rests at least partially on empirical claims about what actually is believed across different cultures.

More important than this empirical thesis is the argument that although cultural or individual beliefs vary, it does not follow that people fundamentally disagree about ultimate moral standards. Two cultures may agree about an ultimate principle of morality yet disagree about *how to apply* the principle in a particular situation or practice. For example, if personal payments for special services are common in one culture and punishable as bribery in another, then it is undeniable that these customs are different, but it does not follow that the moral principles underlying the customs are relative. One culture may exhibit the belief that practices of grease payments produce a social good by eliminating government interference and lowering the salaries paid to functionaries, while the people of another culture may believe that the overall social good is best promoted by eliminating all special favors. Both justifications rest on an appraisal of the overall social good, but the people of the two cultures apply this principle in disparate, indeed apparently competing ways.

This possibility indicates that a basic or fundamental conflict between cultural values can only occur if apparent cultural disagreements about proper principles or rules occur at the level of ultimate moral principles. Otherwise, the apparent disagreements can be understood in terms of, and perhaps be arbitrated by, appeal to deeper shared values. If a moral conflict were truly fundamental, then the conflict could not be removed even if there were perfect agreement about the facts of a case, about the concepts involved, and about background beliefs.

Those opposed to relativism need not, however, rely on this argument alone. Suppose that certain persons or cultures *do not* agree on an ultimate principle so that their ultimate moral norms are in fact culturally relative. It does not follow from this disagreement that there is no ultimate norm or set of norms in which everyone *ought* to believe. To see this point, consider an analogy to religious disagreement: From the fact that people have incompatible religious or atheistic beliefs, it does not follow that there is no single correct set of religious or atheistic propositions. Given current anthropological data, one might be *skeptical* that there could be a compelling argument in favor of one system of religion or morality. But nothing more than skepticism seems justified by the facts adduced by anthropology, and nothing more than this skepticism would be justified if fundamental conflicts of belief were discovered. Skepticism of course presents serious philosophical issues, but alone it does not support relativism; and skepticism leaves ethical theory free to try to determine which is the best set of moral beliefs.

Normative Relativism. Cultural relativists might reasonably be said to hold that "What is right at one place or time may be wrong at another." This statement is ambiguous, however, and can be interpreted as a second form of relativism. Some relativists interpret "What is right at one place or time may be wrong at another" to mean *it is right* in one context to act in a way that *it is wrong* to act in another. This thesis is normative, because it makes a value judgment; it delineates *which standards or norms determine right and wrong behavior.* One form of this normative relativism asserts that one ought to do what one's society determines to be right (a group or social form of normative relativism), and a second form holds that one ought to do what one personally believes is right (an individual form of normative relativism).

This normative position has sometimes crudely been translated as "Anything is right or wrong whenever some individual or some group judges that it is right or wrong." However, less crude formulations of the position can be given, and more or less plausible examples can be adduced. One can hold the slightly more sophisticated view, for example, that in order to be right something must be conscientiously and not merely customarily believed. Alternatively, it might be formulated as the view that whatever is believed is right if it is part of a well-formed traditional moral code of rules in a society—for example, a medical code of ethics developed by a professional society.

The evident inconsistency of this form of relativism with many of our most cherished moral beliefs is one major reason to be doubtful of it. For example, no general theory of normative relativism is likely to convince us that we must tolerate *all* acts of others, although that is exactly the commitment of this theory. At least some moral views seem relatively enlightened, no matter how great the variability of beliefs; the idea that practices such as slavery cannot be evaluated across cultures by some common standard seems patently unacceptable. It is one thing to suggest that these practices might be *excused*, still another to suggest that they are *right*. But how can normative relativism be refuted, if it can?

First, recall our earlier discussion (pages 1–2 above) that morality is concerned with practices of right and wrong transmitted within cultures from one generation to another. The terms of social life are set by these practices, whose rules are pervasively acknowledged and shared in that culture. Within the culture, then, there is a significant measure of moral objectivity, because morality by its nature does not exist through a person's individual judgment. Individuals cannot create it by stipulation or correctly call a personal policy a morality. Such moral individualism would be as dubious as anarchism in politics and law, and none of us readily accepts a declaration by another person that his or her political and legal beliefs are validly determined by himself or herself alone.

It is, of course, true that some moral codes and practices must be formulated within social institutions and will be modified over time. But this fact does not mean that moral rules can be created without regard for the prevailing morality or be invented like the latest technology. For example, a hospital corporation cannot develop its professional ethics from whole cloth. No hospital chain can draw up a code that brushes aside the need for confidentiality of patient information, or that permits surgeons to proceed without adequate consents from patients; and a physician cannot make up his or her individual "code" of medical ethics. Room for invention or alteration in morality is thus restricted by the broader understanding of morality in the culture. Rules cannot be *moral* standards or beliefs simply because they are so labeled. If relativism means they can be so invented or labeled, then relativism is mistaken.

However, it must be acknowledged that this particular defense of objectivity in morals is not transcultural and so does not refute *cultural* forms of relativism. This argument only supplies strong reasons for doubt about *individual* relativism. Can an equally strong reason be given for rejecting cultural forms? One plausible answer is that cultural relativism is not definitively refutable but may nonetheless be a theory of morality that deserves to be discarded in living the moral life.

One argument to this conclusion appeals to the unacceptable consequences of accepting any form of cultural relativism, especially if relativism has the effect of preventing serious reflection on and resolution of moral problems. Consider this analogy: If a husband and a wife have a serious disagreement over whether to allow a handicapped newborn to die, they place different values on the life of the infant and they may have very different views of family life and of their relationship. Their problem will not vanish simply by declaring that their views about children are relative to their different views about the value of fetal life, family life, and spousal relationships. Their problem is in pressing need of resolution, and among reasonable persons resolution will come only through hard thinking and perhaps considerable negotiation and compromise—the time-honored way of handling problems through diplomatic channels, for example.

Similarly with pressing moral problems—even if extraordinarily different viewpoints prevail a resolution is still needed, and there is no reason to think it is not possible by appeal to some range of shared values. From this perspective, trans-individual moral reflection is in order *even if relativism is entirely true.* When two parties argue about some serious, divisive, and contested moral issue—killing animals or withholding information from contracting parties, for example—we tend to think that some genuinely fair and justified compromise may be reached, or perhaps we remain uncertain while anticipating the emergence of the best argument.

We seldom infer from the mere fact of a conflict between beliefs that there is no way to establish one view as correct or as better argued than the other—or certainly that there is no ground for compromise. The more absurd the position advanced by one party, the more convinced we become that some views being defended are mistaken or require supplementation. We are seldom tempted to conclude that there could not be any correct ethical perspective or any reasonable negotiation that might resolve disputes among reasonable persons. One use of ethical theory is to provide a structured approach to moral reasoning that enables us to work on these problems. This use entails a rejection of normative relativism and questions the need for any form of commitment to relativism.

MORAL JUSTIFICATION

According to some definitions introduced above, *morality* consists of social norms of behavior, whereas *ethical theory* consists of the philosophical reasons for—or against—a set of reflections about morality. Usually the latter effort centers on *justification*. Philosophers seek to justify a system of standards or some moral point of view on the basis of carefully analyzed and defended theories and principles, including respect for autonomy, distributive justice, and beneficence—some of the principles commonly employed in contemporary moral philosophy.

Questions of justification are matters of immediate practical significance, and at the same time they are related to the most theoretical dimensions of philosophy. A good case can be made that philosophy in general, in all of its fields, is primarily concerned with the criticism and justification of positions or points of view—whether the subject matter under discussion is religion, science, law, education, mathematics, or some other field. Similarly, a good case can be made that the central questions in ethics are those of justification. But what is required in order to justify a moral point of view?

Moral judgments are justified by giving reasons for them. Not all reasons, however, are good reasons, and not all good reasons are sufficient for justification. For example, a good reason for involuntarily committing certain mentally ill persons to institutions is that they present a clear and present danger to other persons. Many believe that this reason is also sufficient to justify various practices of involuntary commitment. By contrast, a reason for commitment that is sometimes offered as a good reason, but which many people (including Thomas Szasz in an essay in this volume) consider a bad reason (because it involves a deprivation of liberty), is that some mentally ill persons are dangerous to themselves.

If someone holds that commitment on grounds of danger to self is a good reason and is solely sufficient to justify commitment, that person should be able to give some account of why this reason is good and sufficient. That is, the person should be able to give further justifying reasons for the belief that the reason offered is good and sufficient. The person might refer, for example, to the dire consequences for the mentally ill that will occur if someone fails to intervene. The person might also invoke certain principles about the moral importance of caring for the needs of the mentally ill. In short, the person is expected to give a set of reasons that amounts to an argued defense of his or her perspective on the issues. These appeals are usually either to moral principles or to consequences of actions, and they form the heart of justification.

There are also different levels on which justification proceeds. Consider first the different kinds of discourse involved in moral reasoning and argument. A moral *judgment* expresses a decision, verdict, or conclusion about a particular action or character trait. Moral *rules* are general guides governing actions of a certain kind; they assert what ought (or ought not) to be done in a range of particular cases. Moral *principles* are more general and more fundamental than rules and serve (at least in some systems of ethics) as the justifying reasons for accepting rules. A simple example of a moral rule is "It is wrong to deceive patients," but the principle of respect for autonomy (as discussed below) may be the basis of several moral rules of the deception-is-wrong variety. Finally, ethical *theories* are bodies of principles and rules that are more or less systematically related.

The different kinds of moral discourse can also be developed as a theory of levels of justification.[3] Judgments about what ought to be done can be viewed as justified (that is, good and sufficient independent reasons for the judgments given) by rules, which in turn are justified by principles, which then are justified by ethical theories (these theories are discussed in the following section). This structure of levels can be diagrammed as follows (where the arrow indicates the direction of justification, the particular or less general moral assertion being justified by appeal to the more general):

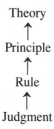

Theory

↑

Principle

↑

Rule

↑

Judgment

Many justifications found in this volume either conform to or can be reconstructed to conform to this diagram. Consider again, for example, the Tarasoff case. One argument and justification used by the psychiatrist (the defendant) and indeed by one of the judges can be diagrammed as follows:

Consequential theory (perhaps utilitarianism)

↑

Principle of autonomy

↑

Rule of confidentiality of a physician's information

↑

Judgment that the psychiatrist's confidential information
should remain confidential (undisclosed to others)

The particular judgment made by the psychiatrist (and one judge) that confidential information should remain undisclosed in this case is shown in this diagram to be justified in terms of a rule of confidentiality, which in turn is justified in terms of a more general principle of respect for autonomy, which is then justified by a more general theory that recognizes the importance of consequentialist appeals. (Of course, more than one rule or principle may be invoked at these levels in the attempt to justify a judgment.)

This discussion of justification and argument implicitly raises the question of the best justifying reasons and theories—and thus takes us to the topic of classical ethical theories.

CLASSICAL ETHICAL THEORIES

If there is to be a meaningful ethics in the cultures of medicine and research, practitioners in these fields must be able to implement standards that are more than loose abstractions. We need both an acceptable *theory* for bioethics and a way to make the theory institutionalized in *practice*. Matters of practice and professional responsibility are largely the subjects of later, more applied chapters in this book. At present we are not concerned with a theory of practice but rather with the theories that underlie practice.

A structured normative ethical theory is a system of principles used to determine moral obligations. Modern ethical theory has come to be classified in terms of two general types: deontological and utilitarian. In almost every chapter in this volume at least one author defends some utilitarian-based or deontological-based conclusion.

Some professionals do not see the need for abstract theory or for any revisions of prevailing practices that might flow from a theory. They find present moral conventions and rules comfortable and adequate. However, others are concerned about relating ethical theory to practice and take the competing view that traditional or operative standards are often incomplete, poorly understood, and inconsistent—as well as suffering from the lack of a uniform theory that would make the body of rules consistent and coherent. Those who take this viewpoint are inclined to revise or possibly set aside present practices, and they often look to some system of ethical theory to provide a basis for revisions.

In light of this controversy, we should be prepared not only to understand ethical theory but also to make some assessment of its value for bioethics.

UTILITARIAN THEORIES

Utilitarianism is rooted in the thesis that an action or practice is right (when compared to any alternative action or practice) if it leads to the greatest possible balance of good consequences or to the least possible balance of bad consequences in the world as a whole.

In taking this perspective, utilitarians invite us to consider the larger objective or function of morality as a social institution, where "morality" is understood to include our shared rules of justice and other principles of the moral life. The point of the institution of morality, they insist, is to promote human welfare by minimizing harms and maximizing benefits: There would be no point at all in having moral codes and understandings unless they served this purpose.

Utilitarians thus see moral rules as the means to the fulfillment of individual needs as  well as to the achievement of broad social goals. A good example of this way of thinking is found in Chapter 9, which is partly devoted to ethical issues of research involving human subjects. Some authors in this chapter see both the purpose of biomedical research and the purpose of rules that constrain the involvement of humans as the minimization of harm (in the form of injury and disease) and the maximization of benefits (health benefits, in particular).

Mill's Utilitarianism. In both utilitarianism and deontology there are classic works of such enduring influence and excellence that they form the basis for development of the theory. The major exposition of utilitarianism has generally been regarded as that of John Stuart Mill in his book *Utilitarianism* (1863). In this work Mill discusses two foundations of utilitarianism: (1) a normative foundation in the principle of utility, and (2) a psychological foundation in human nature. He proposes the principle of utility, or the Greatest Happiness Principle, as the foundation of morals: "Actions are right in proportion as they tend to promote happiness, wrong as they tend to produce the reverse of happiness, i.e., pleasure or absence of pain." Pleasure and freedom from pain, Mill argues, are alone desirable as ends; all desirable things (which are numerous) are therefore desirable either for the pleasure inherent in them, or as means to the promotion of pleasure and the prevention of pain.

Mill's second foundation of utilitarianism derives from his belief that most and perhaps all persons have a basic desire for unity and harmony with their fellow human beings. Whereas Mill's utilitarian predecessor, Jeremy Bentham, had tried to justify the principle of utility by claiming that it is in our self-interest to promote everyone's interest, Mill appeals to social feelings of mankind for his justification. Just as we feel horror at crimes, he says, so we have a basic moral sensitivity to the needs of others. His view seems to be that the purpose of morality is at once to tap natural human sympathies so as to benefit others while at the same time controlling unsympathetic attitudes that cause harm to others. The principle of utility is conceived as the best means to these basic human goals.

For Mill and many other utilitarians, moral theory is grounded in a theory of the general goals of life, which they conceive as the pursuit of pleasure and the avoidance of pain. The production of pleasure and pain assumes moral and not merely personal significance when the consequences of our actions affect the pleasurable or painful states of others. Moral rules and moral and legal institutions, as they see it, must be grounded in a general theory of value, and morally good actions are alone determined by these final values.

Utilitarians, as we shall now see, have not always agreed on these goals and values, but one main task for any utilitarian is to provide an acceptable theory that explains which things are intrinsically good and why they are so. Additionally, there is a question of whose goals are to count in a utilitarian calculation. For example, when discussing the morality of biomedical research, are the pains of *animals* to count (a topic taken up in Chapter 9); and in considering euthanasia for defective newborns, are the interests of *fetuses* and *newborns* to count, and if so, by what utilitarian criteria (a topic considered in Chapters 4 and 5)?

The Theory of Value. Within utilitarian theories of value, a major distinction is drawn between hedonistic and pluralistic utilitarians. Bentham and Mill are hedonistic, because they conceive utility entirely in terms of pleasure. In effect, they argue that the good life is constituted by happiness, which is equivalent to pleasure (though they do not argue that the word "good" means happiness or pleasure in ordinary language). All good things are valuable only as means to the production of pleasure or the avoidance of pain. Hedonistic utilitarianism, then, holds that acts or practices which maximize pleasure are right actions.

Pluralistic utilitarian philosophers, by contrast, believe that no single goal or state constitutes the good and that many values besides happiness possess intrinsic worth—for example, the values of friendship, knowledge, love, devotion, health, and beauty. Those who subscribe to this pluralistic approach prefer to interpret the principle of utility as demanding that the rightness or wrongness of an action be assessed in terms of the total range of intrinsic values ultimately produced by the action, not in terms of pleasure alone. The greatest aggregate good, then, must be determined by considering multiple intrinsic goods. Several essays in this volume appear to interpret health as such an intrinsic good and suggest a utilitarian scheme for the public distribution of this good.

Mill went to considerable lengths to clarify his use of the term "happiness." He insisted that happiness does not refer merely to "pleasurable excitement" but rather encompasses a realistic appraisal of the pleasurable moments afforded in life, whether they take the form of tranquillity or passion. Mill and Bentham both believed that pleasure and the freedom from pain could at least in rough ways be measured and compared, and Bentham argued that pleasure and pain could be measured by using a hedonic calculus. To determine the moral value of an action, he maintained, one must add up the total happiness to be produced, subtract the pains involved, and then determine the balance, which expresses the moral value of the act. Thus, a person literally is able, in Bentham's scheme, to calculate what ought morally to be done.

Many philosophers have objected to this quantification, arguing that it either is impossible or too complicated to be practical for determining what we ought to do in daily life. Whatever the merits of this objection, Mill and Bentham realized that it is unrealistic in our daily practical affairs to pause and rationally calculate in detail on every occasion where choices must be made. They maintained that we must rely heavily on our common sense, our habits, and our past experience. For example, most people know that too-frequent use of x-ray examinations is dangerous and that utility is maximized by prudent utilization of such tests. But our knowledge of the consequences of x-rays over time is limited, and predictions are risky when those involved try to formulate hospital policies and legislation to protect against such dangers. Mill and Bentham agreed that we can only ask reasonable predictability and choice in these cases—not perfect predictability and error-free calculations.

Both the hedonistic and the pluralistic approaches have nonetheless seemed to some recent philosophers relatively problematic for purposes of objectively aggregating widely different interests in order to determine where maximal value, and therefore right action, lies. Many utilitarians therefore depart from Mill and interpret the good as that which is *subjectively* desired or wanted; the satisfaction of desires or wants is seen as the goal of our moral actions. This third approach is based on individual preferences, and utility is analyzed in terms of an individual's actual preferences, not in terms of intrinsically valuable experiences or states of affairs. To maximize an individual's utility is to maximize what he or she has chosen or would choose from the available alternatives. To maximize the utility of those persons affected by an action or policy is to maximize the utility of the aggregate group. This theory, too, plays a role in some articles in this anthology—especially those centered on health policy (Chapter 12) and the allocation of resources (Chapter 11).

This preference-based utilitarian approach to value has been viewed by many as superior to its predecessors, but it is not trouble free as a general theory of morals. A major theoretical problem arises when individuals have morally unacceptable preferences. For example, a person's strong sexual preference may be to rape young children, but this preference is morally intolerable and society therefore denounces it. Utilitarianism based purely on subjective preferences will be a satisfactory moral theory only if a range of *acceptable and unacceptable* preferences can be formulated. This task has proved difficult in theory, and an attempt to limit or discount actual preferences may be inconsistent with a pure preference approach.

Nonetheless, some plausible replies to this objection are open to utilitarians. First, since most people are not perverse and do have morally acceptable (albeit sometimes odd) values, some utilitarians believe they are justified in proceeding under the assumption that the preference approach is not fatally marred by a speculative problem. As Mill noted, any moral theory whatever may lead to unsatisfactory outcomes if one assumes universal idiocy. Second, because "perverse" desires have been determined on the basis of past experience to subvert the objectives of utilitarianism by creating conditions productive of unhappiness, the perverse desires (preferences) could never be permitted to count as goods but only as evils. We could discount preferences to rape children not only because they obstruct the preferences of children and their parents but because, more generally, these preferences eventuate in a great deal of unhappiness to society. Preferences that serve merely to frustrate the preferences of others are thus ruled out by the goal of utilitarianism. As Mill himself argued, the cultivation of certain kinds of desires is built into the "ideal" of utilitarianism.

Still, even if most persons are not perverse and if the ideals of utilitarianism are well entrenched in society, some rational agents may have preferences that are immoral or unjust, and a major problem for utilitarian theory is that it may stand in need of a supplementary criterion of value in addition to mere preference. (Many critics have suggested that at least a principle of justice must supplement the principle of utility.)

Act and Rule Utilitarianism. A significant dispute has arisen among utilitarians over whether the principle of utility is to be applied to *particular acts* in particular circumstances or to *rules of conduct* that determine which acts are right and wrong. For the rule utilitarian, actions are justified by appeal to rules such as "Don't deceive" and "Don't break promises." These rules, in turn, are justified by appeal to the principle of utility. An act utilitarian simply justifies actions directly by appeal to the principle of utility.

Act utilitarianism is often characterized as a "direct" or "extreme" theory because the act utilitarian directly asks, "What good and evil consequences will result directly from this action in this circumstance?"—not "What good and evil consequences will result generally from this sort of action?" In this formulation, the right act is the one that has the greatest utility in the circumstances. This approach seems natural because utilitarianism aims at maximizing value, and the most direct means to this goal would seem to be that of maximizing value on every single occasion. This position does not demand, however, that every single time we act we must determine what should be done without any reference to general guidelines. We learn from past experience, and the act utilitarian does permit summary rules of thumb. The act utilitarian regards rules such as "You ought to tell the truth to patients" as useful but not as unbreakable rules. These rules may legitimately be abandoned if an action would lead to the greatest good for the greatest number in a particular case.

Consider the following case, which occurred in the state of Kansas and which anticipates some issues about euthanasia encountered in Chapter 6. An elderly woman lay ill and dying. Her suffering came to be too much for either her or her faithful husband of fifty-four years to endure, so she requested that he kill her. Stricken with grief and unable to bring himself to perform the act, the husband hired another man to kill his wife. An act utilitarian might reason that in this case hiring another to kill the woman was justified, although in general we would not permit physicians, for example, to engage in a practice of this sort. After all, only this woman and her husband were directly affected, and relief of her pain was the main issue. It would be unfortunate, the act utilitarian might reason, if our "rules" against killing failed to allow for selective killings in extenuating circumstances, because it is extremely difficult to generalize from case to case. The jury, as it turned out, convicted the husband of murder, and he was sentenced to twenty-five years in prison. An act utilitarian might maintain that the rigid application of rules of criminal justice inevitably leads to injustices and that rule utilitarianism cannot escape this consequence of a rule-based position.

Many philosophers object vigorously to act utilitarianism, charging its exponents with basing morality on mere expediency. On act-utilitarian grounds, they say, it is desirable for a physician to kill babies with many kinds of birth defects, since the death of the child would relieve the family and society of a great burden and inconvenience and thus in some respects would lead to the greatest good for the greatest number. Many opponents of act utilitarianism have thus argued that strict rules, which cannot be set aside for the sake of convenience, must be maintained. Many of these apparently desirable rules can be justified by the principle of utility, so utilitarianism need not be abandoned if act utilitarianism is judged unworthy.

Rule utilitarians pick up on this point and hold that rules have a central position in morality and cannot be compromised by the demands of particular situations. Compromise would threaten the effectiveness of the rules; effectiveness is judged by determining that the observance of a given rule would, in theory, maximize social utility better than would any possible substitute rule (or having no rule). The rule utilitarian believes that this position is capable of escaping counterexamples and objections to act utilitarianism such as the one about defective newborns mentioned above, because rules are not subject to change by the demands of individual circumstances. Utilitarian rules are, in theory, firm and protective of all classes of individuals, just as human rights (as we will later see) rigidly protect all individuals regardless of social convenience and momentary need.

Still, it is necessary to ask whether rule-utilitarian theories can escape the criticisms they acknowledge as tarnishing act utilitarianism. Dilemmas often arise that involve conflicts among moral rules—for example, rules of confidentiality conflict with rules protecting individual welfare, as in the Tarasoff case found in Chapter 8. Many believe a pregnant woman's rights can conflict with the rights of a fetus, as discussed in Chapter 5. If the moral life were so ordered that we always knew which rules and rights should receive priority, there would be no serious problem for moral theory. Yet a ranking of rules seems clearly impossible, and in a pluralistic society there are many rules that some persons accept and others reject. Even if everyone agreed on the same rules and on their interpretation, in one situation it might be better to break a confidence in order to protect someone, and in another circumstance it might be better to keep the information confidential.

Mill briefly considered this problem. He held that the principle of utility should itself decide in any given circumstance which rule is to take priority. However, if this solution is accepted by rule utilitarians, then their theory must rely directly, on at least some occasions, on the principle of utility to decide in particular situations which action is preferable to which alternative action in the absence of a governing rule. If whole sets of utility-based rules or statements of rights cannot determine whether a woman who has become pregnant because of rape is justified in seeking an abortion, how is rule utilitarianism to be distinguished from act utilitarianism? And do all the same criticisms and counterexamples that rule utilitarians (and others) bring against act utilitarians apply to rule utilitarianism itself?

The rule utilitarian can reply to this criticism by asserting that a sense of relative weight and importance should be built directly into moral rules, at least insofar as possible. For example, the rule utilitarian might argue that rules prohibiting the active killing of newborn babies are of such vital social significance (as a result of their social utility) that they can never be overridden by appeal to rules that allow parents the freedom to make fundamental choices for their children.

Rule utilitarians should and do acknowledge that weights cannot be so definitely formulated and built into principles that irresolvable conflicts among rules will never arise. What they need not concede is that this problem is unique to rule utilitarianism. Every moral theory has practical limitations in cases of conflict. This is a general problem with the moral life itself, the rule utilitarian will argue, and thus not unique to a particular theory. It will nonetheless be possible to distinguish theories that require strict observance of rules from those, such as act utilitarianism, that do not. This form of rule utilitarian argument emerges in Chapter 6, where the adequacy of present rules governing killing (and whether the basis is in utility) is discussed. (See the first four essays in that chapter in particular.)

Criticisms of Utilitarianism. Two criticisms of utilitarianism are of major importance for our purposes in this volume. The first centers on the suggestion that goods can be measured and comparatively weighed. Because utility is to be maximized, one who makes a utilitarian choice must be in a position to compare the different possible utilities of an action. But can units of happiness or some other utilitarian value be measured and compared so as to determine the best among alternatives? In deciding how to allocate resources, for example, how is a state legislature to compare the value of a good screening program for AIDS or for genetic disease with the value of regular medical examinations at publicly funded clinics—or any of these with public health education? It is difficult for individuals to rank their own preferences, and still more difficult to compare one person's preferences with the preferences of others. Yet a comparison is required if the utility of everyone affected by the actions is to be maximized.

The utilitarian reply to these criticisms is that we make rough and ready comparisons of values every day. For example, we decide to go on a picnic rather than have an office party because we think one activity will be more pleasurable or will satisfy more members of a group than the other. Physicians commonly recommend courses of treatment or nontreatment to families based on judgments of pain avoidance and family welfare. It is easy to overestimate the demands of utilitarianism and the precision with which its exponents have thought it could be employed. Accurate measurements of others' goods or preferences can seldom be provided because of limited knowledge and time. In everyday affairs—including medical practice, hospital administration, or legislative decision making—prior knowledge about the consequences of our actions is severely limited. What is important, morally speaking, is that a person conscientiously attempts to determine the most favorable action, and then with equal seriousness attempts to perform that action.

A second criticism is that utilitarianism can lead to injustices, especially to unjust social distributions. The argument may be expressed as follows: The action that produces the greatest balance of value for the greatest number of people often will benefit one group of persons at the expense of another. Such "balancing" may bring about unjustified harm or disvalue to a minority. An ethical theory requiring that the rights of individuals be surrendered in the interests of the majority seems plainly deficient; if a fair opportunity is denied the minority or the sick, the theory that underwrites this denial is unjust. Many political philosophers and legal theorists have argued that documents on the order of the Bill of Rights in the United States Constitution contain a set of fixed rules not subject to utilitarian balancing. These rights rigidly protect citizens from invasions in the name of the public good. Several writers in Chapter 11 accuse utilitarianism of this difficulty in their approach to the allocation of scarce health care resources.

One contemporary example of this problem comes from the use of cost/benefit analysis in health policy. According to cost/benefit models, an evaluation of all benefits and costs of a potential program or action must be made in order to determine which among alternative programs or actions is to be recommended. These costs and benefits can include both economic and noneconomic factors. Opponents of utilitarianism and cost/benefit analysis argue as follows: At least some cost/benefit analyses will reveal that a particular government program or new technology will prove highly beneficial to some members of society at a "justifiable" financial cost, yet the costs of providing this benefit might function to deny basic medical or welfare services to the most disadvantaged members of society. These critics suggest that the disadvantaged ought to be subsidized as a matter of justice, either in terms of health services or financial awards—no matter what cost/benefit analyses reveal. Planning efforts employing cost/benefit analyses that cut out minority interests are morally pernicious, they say, because they fail to account for considerations of distributive justice.

In the last opinion he wrote for the Supreme Court (in July 1986), former Chief Justice Warren Burger affirmed an earlier opinion in the following words: "The fact that a given law or procedure is efficient, convenient and useful in facilitating functions of government, standing alone, will not save it if it is contrary to the Constitution. Convenience and efficiency are not the primary objectives—or the hallmarks—of democratic government."[4] Burger's criticism captures the essence of what many have argued against utilitarianism: that it fails to account for basic principles that in justice cannot be modified in the name of efficiency, productivity, and convenience.

A utilitarian reply to these objections is that we should not always follow the dictates of single, short-range cost/benefit calculations. For example, suppose that a new diagnostic device significantly increased health benefits for the wealthy, who alone could afford it, but exposed operators of the equipment to near-fatal doses of radiation. A rule utilitarian would agree that it would be immoral to use this equipment, even if statistical calculations indicated a highly favorable overall cost/benefit equation: many lives saved and only a few technicians lost. The rule utilitarian bases this reply on a framework of moral rules that follows from the general program of moral philosophy governing rule-utilitarian thinking. The point is that considerations of social utility and the basic rules of justice determined by those considerations set a limit on the risk of harm that can be permitted, under utilitarian theory, on the basis of short-range cost/benefit calculations.

This utilitarian reply rests on two strategies of argument. First, utilitarians insist that *all* the entailed costs and benefits must be considered. In the case of the sick and dying, for example, costs include protests from advocates of the poor and minorities, impairment to social ideals, further alienation of the poor from the government and public officials, and the like. Second, rule-utilitarian analyses emphatically deny that single cost/benefit determinations ought to be accepted. These utilitarian analyses propose that general rules of justice (justified by broad considerations of utility) ought to constrain particular actions or uses of cost/benefit analysis in all cases. They also claim that the criticisms regarding possible denial of services to the disadvantaged as a result of cost/benefit analyses are short-sighted, because they focus on injustices that might be done through a superficial, short-term application of the principle of utility. If one takes a long-range view, rule utilitarians argue, one will see that utility never eventuates in overall unjust outcomes.

DEONTOLOGICAL THEORIES

We have seen that utilitarianism conceives the moral life in terms of intrinsic value and the means to produce this value. Deontologists, by contrast, argue that moral standards exist independently of utilitarian ends and that the moral life should not be conceived in terms of means and ends. (The Greek word *deon*, or binding obligation, is the source of the term "deontology.") An act or rule is right, in the view of a deontologist, insofar as it satisfies the demands of some overriding principle(s) of obligation.

Deontologists urge us to consider that actions are morally wrong not because of their consequences but because the action type—the class of which the actions are instances—involves a moral violation. Because of the wide diversity in these theories it is hard to find the unity, but the following two conditions are close to the heart of deontological theories. First, the *justification* of principles and actions is not entirely by appeal to the consequences of adopting the principles or performing the actions. Second, some principles must be followed or actions performed irrespective of the consequences. Thus, there are not only justificatory grounds of obligation that are independent of the production of good consequences, but these grounds are at least sometimes sufficient to defeat the consequences no matter what the consequences are.

A radical deontologist will argue that consequences are irrelevant to moral evaluations: An act is right if and only if it conforms to an overriding moral obligation and wrong if and only if it violates the overriding moral duty or principle. Many deontological theories are not so radical, however, holding that moral rightness is only in part independent of utilitarian conceptions of goodness. The fairness of distribution, keeping a personal promise, repaying a debt, and abiding by a contract would be right, according to these theories, whether or not utility was maximized.

Deontologists believe that our duties to others are manifold and diverse, some springing from special relationships that utilitarians unjustifiably ignore. These relationships include, for example, those of parent and child, physician and patient, and employer and employee. Physicians have obligations to their patients that they do not have to other individuals, no matter the utilitarian outcome of treating their patients and not treating others. Children incur special obligations to their parents, and vice versa; parents have a moral obligation to oversee and support the health and welfare needs of their children that they do not have in regard to other children in their neighborhood. This is not to suggest that utilitarians denigrate or downgrade these relationships. They do not. The point is that deontologists do not believe that these relationships can be justified on consequentialist grounds.

Deontologists also believe that utilitarians give too little consideration to the performance of acts in the past that create obligations in the present. If a person has promised something or has entered into a contract, he or she is bound to the terms of the agreement, no matter what the consequences of keeping it are. If one person harms another, the person who inflicted the injury is bound to compensate the injured one, whether the compensation serves utilitarian goals or not.

As an example of differences in utilitarian and deontological thinking, consider a survey conducted by researchers K. Ann Coleman Stolurow and Dale W. Moeller.[5] Stolurow and Moeller were interested in the frequency with which x-rays are routinely used as part of dental checkups. They conducted a telephone survey of dental offices in the Boston area and found that in 95 percent of the offices surveyed x-ray procedures are customarily ordered in connection with the initial investigation of new patients, and that in nearly half of those offices the procedures employed involve full-mouth x-rays. To obtain accurate information, these researchers misrepresented themselves over the telephone as new residents in the Boston area inquiring about available dental services, and they asked a series of specific questions that followed a prepared written survey instrument, wholly undisclosed to the dentists or their offices. This misrepresentation apparently contributed significantly to the accuracy of the results, because the data obtained showed a frequency of dental x-ray use far greater than that reported by an earlier study in which the researchers did not conceal their purposes.

This use of deception raises ethical issues of whether the researchers violated the moral rights of the participants or unjustifiably invaded privacy. Many act utilitarians would likely consider this study justifiable: There are public benefits of obtaining accurate information about dental x-rays. The information, for instance, might form the basis on which the American Dental Association would refocus its ongoing efforts to reduce unnecessary x-ray exposure, from lessening dosage levels to cutting down on the frequency of exposure. One also might draw an analogy with consumer surveys, noting that the survey seeks to evaluate a contractual service between providers and customers. The utilitarian could then argue that the terms of the contract give potential customers grounds to know accurate information about the service, and that this customer interest overrides conflicting rights of dental office owners and employees. A deontologist, by contrast, may find indefensible the deception and invasion of privacy essential to the conduct of the study. In any event, the deontologist will not frame the moral problem exclusively in terms of a weighing of consequences.

Since deontologists believe that moral standards are independent of utilitarian ends, what is the source of these standards and how is moral obligation based on these standards? Throughout the history of philosophy deontologists have identified starkly different ultimate principles of obligation as the final moral standards. Although these many different views cannot be surveyed here, it is possible to briefly distinguish several different grounds to which they have appealed. Perhaps the best known deontological account is the divine command theory. The will of God is the ultimate standard in this account, and an action or action type is right or wrong if and only if commanded or forbidden by God. Other deontologists hold that some actions or action types are naturally right or wrong, good or evil, requiring no reason having to do with religion, politics, or social organization.

Finally, some deontologists appeal to a social contract reached under conditions of absolute fairness as the source of moral obligation. The ultimate principle of obligation is action in accordance with moral rules fairly derived from a situation of mutual agreement. Many writers in this volume appeal to the recent work of John Rawls on the topic of justice, and Rawls is one representative of the social contract point of view. (Rawls's theories of deontology are discussed below in pages 25–26 and again in the introduction to Chapter 11 and in several essays in that chapter.)

Types of Deontological Theory. Just as there are act and rule utilitarians, there are also act and rule deontologists. Act deontologists hold that the individual in any given situation must grasp immediately what ought to be done without relying on rules. Because each situation is potentially unique, and so not subsumable under general rules, particular and changing features of moral experience must determine right action. For example, one might argue that only conscience, intuition, or religious faith can in the end determine what ought to be done, because when these conflict with rules the rules must be overridden.

These theories have not made a strong appeal in contemporary ethics, but rule deontology continues to be influential. According to this theory, types of acts are right or wrong because of their conformity or nonconformity to one or more principles or rules. These guides are more significant than mere rules of thumb based on past experience, and they are valid independently of their general tendency to promote good consequences. A rule-deontological theory may envisage only one supreme principle—a monistic theory—or many principles—a pluralistic theory. Monistic deontological theories generally maintain that one fundamental principle provides the source from which other more specific moral rules can be derived. A simple theory of this description is that all moral rules and duties ultimately derive from the golden rule, which states that you should treat others as you would wish to be treated yourself. Pluralistic deontologists, by contrast, affirm two or more irreducible moral principles.

Rule deontology seems to have made a greater appeal than act deontology for several reasons. First, rules facilitate decision making. We often have no opportunity or time to think through the steps from basic principles to conclusions. Second, act theories present problems for cooperation and trust. Lawyers, physicians, teachers, and even our friends would not be bound by any firm moral obligations, and a recognition of this fact would stand to diminish our trust that they will live up to their normal obligations. Third, act deontologists reduce moral rules—for example, "Do not deceive"—to mere rules of thumb approximating the nonmoral rule "Have a medical checkup once a year." These rules obviously give wide latitude to individual discretion in moral judgment.

Rule deontologists find this view unsatisfactory as an account of moral rules, which they see as more binding than optional rules of thumb. Rules that prohibit murder, rape, torture, and cruelty, for example, cannot simply be set aside on any given occasion in the way "Wash your hair once a day" or "Have a medical checkup once a year" can be set aside. Codes of medical and nursing ethics similarly set limits on the way human subjects may be involved in biomedical research. These limits are not optional ones that can be set aside by individual discretion. (See, for example, the introduction to Chapter 9, which discusses such rules as necessary conditions of morally justified research.)

The Assessment of Motives. Deontologists commonly insist on the importance of the motives and the character of human actors, apart from the consequences planned or produced by the agent. A utilitarian will agree that motives are critical to our assessment of persons but will insist that right motives are determined exclusively by the intention to produce the best possible consequences. Deontologists tend to regard this form of assessment as too restricted in scope, because they see certain kinds of motives as morally superior.

Especially important is the agent's motivational structure in performing an action. A person who does not harm others should not only have a disposition to act nonmalevolently but should also have *a morally appropriate form of motivation and attitude.* The person should have a moral concern about not harming others, not simply the motive to act in accordance with a rule of obligation. Any person can perform a morally right action, but there is more to our moral assessment than the mere rightness of what was done. Imagine that a person faithfully performs his or her obligation but hates having to do so, regrets that others benefit from those acts, and in general sees morality as a burdensome constraint. This person is dutiful but lacks the proper moral motivation and for that reason is far from morally commendable.

If one does what is morally right simply because one is scared, because one derives pleasure from doing that kind of act, because one is selfish, or because the action is in one's own interest, then there is nothing morally praiseworthy about the action, and the motivation behind the action may be condemnable. For example—to take up a subject found in Chapter 8—if a physician tells the truth to a patient only because the physician fears a malpractice suit if he or she tells a lie and not because of a concern about the patient's feelings or because of a belief in the moral importance of patient autonomy and truth telling, then this person acts rightly but deserves no moral credit.

Kant's Ethical Theory. The single most widely studied deontological theory is the rule-oriented theory developed by Immanuel Kant, who believes that an act is morally praiseworthy only if done neither for self-interested reasons nor as the result of a natural disposition, but rather from *duty*. That is, the person's motive for acting must be a recognition of the act as resting on duty. It is not good enough, in Kant's view, that one merely performs the morally correct action, because one could perform one's duty for self-interested reasons having nothing to do with morality. For example, if an employer discloses a health hazard to an employee only because he or she fears a lawsuit, and not because of a belief in the importance of truth telling, then this employer acts rightly but deserves no moral credit for the action.

Kant tries to establish the ultimate basis for the validity of moral rules in pure reason, not in intuition, conscience, or utility. Morality, he contends, provides a rational framework of principles and rules that constrain and guide everyone, without regard to their personal goals and interests. Moral rules apply universally, and any rule qualifies as universally acceptable only if it cannot be rationally rejected. The ultimate basis of morality, then, rests on principles of reason that all rational agents possess.

Kant thinks all considerations of utility and self-interest secondary, because the moral worth of an agent's action depends exclusively on the moral acceptability of the rule on the basis of which the person is acting—or, as Kant prefers to say, moral acceptability depends on the rule that determines the agent's will. An action has moral worth only when performed by an agent who possesses what Kant calls a good will, and a person has a good will only if moral duty based on a universally valid rule is the sole motive for the action.

When a person behaves according to binding moral rules valid for everyone, Kant considers that person to have an autonomous will. Kant compares autonomy with what he calls heteronomy—the determination of the will by persons or conditions other than oneself. Autonomy of the will is present when one knowingly governs oneself in accordance with universally valid moral principles. His concept of autonomy, however, does not simply imply personal liberty of action in accordance with a plan chosen by oneself. (For contrasting views, see the discussion of the principle of respect for autonomy later in this chapter.) Under "heteronomy" Kant includes many kinds of coercive determinations of human conduct.

The difference between governance of oneself by moral obligation and governance by coercive force is critical to Kant's moral theory. Coerced acts such as being raped at knifepoint are obviously heteronomously produced, but Kant also holds that actions done from personal desire, impulse, or inclination are heteronomous. For example, refraining from theft merely out of fear of being caught is an instance of heteronomy. Actions that are autonomous and morally right, by contrast, are based on moral principles that we accept (but have the freedom to reject).

It is easy to misunderstand this argument. To say that an agent "accepts" a moral principle does not mean either that the principle is merely subjective or that each individual must wholly create (author or originate) his or her own moral principles. Kant holds only that each individual must will the acceptance of the moral principles to be acted upon. A person's autonomy consists in the ability to govern himself or herself according to these moral principles. Moreover, Kant urges, moral relationships between persons are contingent on mutual respect for autonomy by all the parties involved. Kant develops this notion into a fundamental moral demand that persons be treated as ends in themselves and never solely as means to the ends of others. This principle is invoked repeatedly by many authors in this volume.

Kant's supreme principle, also called "the moral law," is expressed in several ways in his writings. In what appears to be his favored formulation, the principle is stated as follows: "I ought never to act except in such a way that I can also will that my maxim should become a universal law." This Kantian principle has often been compared to the golden rule, but Kant calls it the "categorical imperative." He gives several examples of moral maxims that are made imperative by this fundamental principle: "Help others in distress"; "Do not commit suicide"; and "Work to develop your abilities." The categorical imperative is categorical, he argues, because it admits of no exceptions and is absolutely binding. It is imperative because it gives instruction about how one must act.

Kant clarifies this basic moral law—the condition of morality, in his view—by drawing a distinction between a categorical imperative and a hypothetical imperative. A hypothetical imperative takes the form "If I want to achieve such and such an end, then I must do so and so." These prescriptions—so reminiscent of utilitarian thinking—tell us what we must do, provided that we already have certain desires, interests, or goals. An example would be "If you want to regain your health, then you must take this medication," or "If you want to improve infant mortality rates, then you must improve your hospital facilities." These imperatives are obviously not commanded for their own sake; they are commanded only as means to an end that has already been willed or accepted. Hypothetical imperatives are not moral imperatives in Kant's philosophy because moral imperatives tell us what must be done independently of our goals or desires.

As the above formulation suggests, Kant emphasizes the notion of "rule as universal law." Rules that determine duty are made correct by their universality, that is, the fact that they apply consistently to everyone. This criterion of universality offers some worthwhile lessons for bioethics. Some of the clearest cases of immoral behavior involve a person trying to make a unique exception of himself or herself purely for personal reasons. Obviously this conduct could not be made universal, or else the rules presupposed by the idea of "being an exception" would be destroyed. If carried out consistently by others, this conduct would violate the rules presupposed by the system of morality, thereby rendering the system inconsistent—that is, having inconsistent rules of operation.

Kant's view is that wrongful practices, including invasion of privacy, theft, cheating, and bribes, are "contradictory"; that is, they are not consistent with what they presuppose. Consider cases of promising, information disclosure, and lying—as found in Chapter 8 in this volume. If one were consistently to recommend the rule "Lie when it works to your advantage," our conventional practices of truth telling would be inconsistent with such a rule of behavior. The universalization of rules that allow lying would entitle everyone to lie to you, just as you could lie to them. In this event, one could never tell if a person were telling the truth or lying. Such a rule would thus be inconsistent with the practice of truth telling it presupposes. Similarly, fraud in research is inconsistent with the practice of publishing the truth. How could one cheat in research if there were no criteria that assumed honesty? All such practices are inconsistent with a rule or practice that they presuppose.

As noted earlier, Kant states his categorical imperative in another and distinctly different formulation (which many interpreters take to be a wholly different principle). This form is probably more widely quoted and endorsed in contemporary philosophy than the first form, and certainly it is more frequently invoked in bioethics. Kant's later formulation stipulates that "One must act to treat every person as an end and never as a means only." This imperative insists that one must treat persons as having their own autonomously established goals and that one must never treat them solely as the means to one's own personal goals.

It has been widely stated in contemporary textbooks that Kant is arguing categorically that we can never treat another as a means to our ends. This interpretation, however, misrepresents his views. He argues only that we must not treat another *exclusively* as a means to our own ends. When adult human research subjects are asked to volunteer to test new drugs, for example, they are treated as a means to someone else's ends (perhaps society's ends), but they are not exclusively used for others' purposes, because they do not become mere servants or objects. Their consent legitimates using them as means to the end of research. (This assertion is somewhat controversial, however, as the readings in Chapters 9 and 10 reveal.)

Kant's imperative demands only that persons in such situations be treated with the respect and moral dignity to which all persons are entitled at all times, including the times when they are used as means to the ends of others. To treat persons merely as means, strictly speaking, is to disregard their personhood by exploiting or otherwise using them without regard to their own thoughts, interests, and needs. It involves a failure to acknowledge that every person has a worth and dignity equal to that of every other person.

As appealing as his ethical theory may be, Kant has often been criticized on grounds that he leaves unresolved how duty is to be determined when two or more different duties are in conflict. This criticism is similar to the one directed at rule utilitarians. For example, if one rule demands truth telling to patients while another rule demands the protection of patients from unnecessary harm, what ought to be done in a situation where the disclosure of a piece of information requested by the patient will bring him or her significant harm—perhaps a heart attack or the end of a treasured marriage? The categorical imperative seems to give no advice to someone with this dilemma; it seems, in fact, to demand that both relevant duties be fulfilled. As mentioned above, it may be that no ethical theory can resolve this problem. But Kant's philosophy not only seems unable to help; it apparently obliges moral agents to perform two or more actions when only one *can* be performed. And this is an outcome that he himself declared no moral theory can allow and remain viable.

Ross's Theory.   W. D. Ross, a prominent twentieth-century British philosopher, developed a deontological theory intended to assist in resolving this problem of a conflict of duties. Ross's views are based on an account of what he calls prima facie duties, which he contrasts with actual duties. A prima facie duty is a duty that is always to be acted upon unless it conflicts on a particular occasion with an equal or stronger duty. A prima facie duty, then, is always right and binding, all other things being equal; it is conditional on not being overridden or outweighed by competing moral demands. One's actual duty, by contrast, is determined by an examination of the respective weights of competing prima facie duties.

Ross writes as if there were two ways to determine respective weights. First, one duty might be a stricter prima facie duty. For example, not killing seems a stricter duty than not deceiving. When these two prima facie rules conflict, the stricter will rightly prevail. Second, if two rules are equally strict, duty is determined by the balance of rightness over wrongness as determined in the circumstance.

Ross argues that there are several basic rules of moral duty, and that they do not derive from either the principle of utility or Kant's categorical imperative. For example, our promises create duties of fidelity, wrongful actions create duties of reparation, and the generous gifts of our friends create duties of gratitude. Ross defends several additional duties, such as duties of self-improvement, nonmaleficence, beneficence, and justice. Unlike Kant's system and the utilitarian system, Ross's list of duties is not based on any overarching principle. He defends it simply as a reflection of our ordinary moral conventions and beliefs.

The idea that moral principles are absolute values has had a long but troubled history. Both utilitarians and Kantians have defended their basic rule (the principle of utility and the categorical imperative) as absolute, but this claim to absoluteness has been widely challenged. For Ross's reasons, among others, many moral philosophers have with increasing frequency come to regard duties and rights not as unbending standards but rather as strong prima facie moral demands that may be validly overridden in circumstances of competition with other moral claims. The hope to be able to arrange moral principles in a hierarchical order that avoids conflict has waned with the rise of the idea of all principles as prima facie.

Although Ross admits that neither he nor any moral philosopher has been able to present a system of moral rules free of conflicts and exceptions, he argues that this implication of the theory is no more of a problem for him than for anyone else, Kant included, because the complexity of the moral life simply makes an exception-free hierarchy of rules and principles impossible. The Ross-inspired trend in recent moral theory to believe that many different moral principles—for example, utility, justice, and respect for persons—are equally weighted in abstraction from particular circumstances has proven particularly controversial, however. This is because many philosophers believe that some principle—be it of respect for autonomy or utility or justice—is more basic or has greater weight than other principles. This problem of how to value or weight different moral principles remains unresolved in contemporary moral theory.

Rawls's Theory. In recent years a book in the Kantian tradition has enjoyed a wide audience in deontological ethics. John Rawls's *A Theory of Justice* (1971) presents a deontological theory as a direct challenge to utilitarianism on grounds of social justice. Rawls's basic objection to utilitarianism is that social distributions produced by maximizing utility could entail violations of basic individual liberties and rights that ought to be guaranteed. Utilitarianism, which is concerned with total satisfaction in a society, is indifferent as to the distribution of satisfactions among individuals. This indifference would, in Rawls's view, permit the infringement of some people's rights and liberties if the infringement genuinely promised to produce a proportionately greater utility for others.

Rawls therefore sets as his task the development of an alternative ethical theory capable of sustaining nonutilitarian principles of justice. Rawls turns for this purpose to a hypothetical social contract procedure that is strongly indebted to what he calls the "Kantian conception of equality." According to this social contract account, valid principles of justice are those to which we would all agree if we could freely and impartially consider the social situation from a standpoint (the "original position") outside any actual society.

Impartiality is guaranteed in this situation by a conceptual device Rawls calls the "veil of ignorance." This notion stipulates that, in the original position, each person is (at least momentarily) ignorant of all his or her particular fortuitous characteristics. For example, the person's sex, race, IQ, family background, and special talents or handicaps are unrevealed in this hypothetical circumstance.

The veil of ignorance prevents people from promoting principles of justice biased toward their own combinations of talents and characteristics. Rawls argues that under these conditions, people would unanimously agree on two fundamental principles of justice. The first requires that each person be permitted the maximum amount of equal basic liberty compatible with a similar liberty for others. The second stipulates that once this equal basic liberty is assured, inequalities in social primary goods (for example, income, rights, and opportunities) are to be allowed only if they benefit everyone and only if everyone has fair equality of opportunity. Rawls considers social institutions to be just if and only if they are in conformity with these two basic principles.

Rawls's theory makes equality a basic characteristic of the original position from which the social contract is forged. Equality is built into that hypothetical position in the form of a free and equal bargain among all parties, where there is equal ignorance of all individual characteristics and advantages that persons have or will have in their daily lives. Furthermore, people behind this veil of ignorance would choose to make the equal possession of basic liberties the first commitment of their social institutions. Nevertheless, Rawls rejects radical egalitarianism, arguing that equal distribution cannot be justified as the sole moral principle. If inequalities were to be introduced that rendered everyone better off by comparison to initial equality, these inequalities would be desirable—as long as they were consistent with equal liberty and fair opportunity. More particularly, if these inequalities work to enhance the position of the most disadvantaged persons in society, then it would be self-defeating for the least advantaged or anyone else to seek to prohibit the inequalities. Rawls thus rejects radical egalitarianism in favor of his second principle of justice.

The first part of his second principle is called the "difference principle." This principle permits inequalities of distribution as long as they are consistent with equal liberty and fair opportunity. Rawls formulates this principle more precisely so that such inequalities are justifiable only if they most enhance the position of the "representative least advantaged" person—that is, a hypothetical individual particularly unfortunate in the distribution of fortuitous characteristics or social advantages. Formulated in this way, the difference principle could allow, for instance, extraordinary economic rewards to entrepreneurs if the resulting economic stimulation were to produce improved job opportunities and working conditions for the least advantaged members of society. A strong egalitarian flavor is retained, however, in that such inequalities would be permissible only if it could be demonstrated that they worked to the greatest advantage of those who were worse off.

The difference principle rests on the view that because inequalities of birth, historical circumstance, and natural endowment are undeserved, society should correct them by improving the unequal situation of naturally disadvantaged members. This is a deontologically based demand that Rawls believes fundamental to moral life in society. (Rawls's theory of justice and its implications for distributions in society are further discussed in the introduction to Chapter 11.)

Criticisms of Deontological Theories.   Although some arguments against deontological theories have been woven into the preceding discussion, there are two additional criticisms expressed in contemporary philosophy that require examination, together with responses that deontologists might offer to these criticisms.

Deontological theories vary in the consideration they give to the consequences of actions. Kant, as we have seen, asserts that actions are determined to be right or wrong independent of particular consequences, whereas Ross admits that consequences are relevant, although not the only consideration. An important utilitarian criticism is that deontologists covertly appeal to consequences in order to demonstrate the rightness of actions. John Stuart Mill, for example, argues that Kant's theory does not avoid appeal to the consequences of an action in determining whether it is right or wrong.

According to Mill's interpretation of Kant, the categorical imperative demands that an action be morally prohibited if "the consequences of [its] universal adoption would be such as no one would choose to incur." Kant fails "almost grotesquely," as Mill puts it, to show that any form of formal contradiction or certification of a moral rule appears when we universalize rules of conduct. Mill argues that Kant's theory relies on a covert appeal to the utilitarian principle that if the consequences of the universal performance of a certain type of action can be shown to be undesirable overall, then that sort of action is wrong.

One possible defense of Kant against these charges is the following: It is inaccurate to say that Kant urges us to disregard consequences, or even that he believes an action is morally right (or wrong) without regard to its consequences. Kant holds only that the features of an action making it right are not dependent upon any particular outcome; he never advises that we disregard consequences entirely. The consequences of an action often cannot be separated from the *nature* of the action itself, and so they too must be considered when an agent universalizes the action in order to determine whether it is permissible. Kant occasionally overstates his views by too strongly condemning consequential reasoning, but his writings indicate that he was more willing to consider the consequences as an integral part of the universalization process.

A second criticism is centered on pluralistic deontological theories. The contention is that pluralistic theories lack unity, coherence, and systematic organization. Critics suggest that whereas the principle of utility tells us what makes right actions right on all occasions, thinkers such as Ross merely provide a disconnected list of diverse right-making considerations. If one takes the basic task of philosophical ethics to be that of providing ultimate principles specifying good and sufficient reasons for our moral judgments, then pluralistic deontological theories fail. They tend to retreat, critics say, into an intuitionist theory, where we either intuit on given occasions which obligation is the stronger or else must remain uncertain as to where obligation lies.

Ross was himself concerned about this problem and acknowledged that his catalogue of duties is unsystematic and probably incomplete. His response to those who criticize deontologists for this alleged shortcoming follows the lines of his general criticisms of Kant's appeal to a single categorical imperative. He argues that critics are forcing an "architectonic" of "hastily reached simplicity" on ethics. Although his critics maintain that his views lack systematic unity, he sees this untidiness as an ineradicable feature of the moral life. Untidiness and complexity may be unfortunate features of morality, but if they are nonetheless true characterizations, his theory of morality can hardly be faulted for taking account of them.

It is also open to deontologists to argue that their theories are no worse off than utilitarian theories in this regard. Rule utilitarians have an extremely general principle of obligation based on certain views about goodness, from which a number of competing rules of obligation are derived. These rules are not given systematic unity in utilitarian theories (beyond their derivation from the principle of utility itself). Deontologists could point out that the general demand to act on the most stringent prima facie obligation is a rule that provides all the cohesion and unity that can reasonably be expected. They might conclude that this principle overrides all other principles on every occasion, and that this measure of systematic unity is all that one needs or could hope to find.

MAJOR ETHICAL PRINCIPLES

How are we to determine, in light of the preceding theories and analysis of justification, whether a particular action is morally acceptable? Understandably, this question is complex, and there is no way to answer it with confident finality. But this much seems reasonable to assume: If a particular act is wrong, then it will have certain similarities, certain shared features, with other wrong actions; conversely, if a particular act is morally required, it will share similar features with other actions that are morally required. Philosophers who have tried to develop a general normative theory of right and wrong have, of course, tried to discover what these shared features are. Often they are formulated as principles that hold across a range of cases.

Theories of the two general sorts just discussed have been used by moral philosophers to support derivative moral principles (and rules—such as the one stating that it is right to keep our promises and wrong to break them). Not all these principles are needed for or even applicable to a discussion of any particular moral problem—for example, the morality of suicide. But in order to take a reasoned approach to the range of problems in bioethics, we need principles that permit us to take a consistent position on specific and related issues.

Although it is neither possible nor necessary to outline a full ethical theory in this volume, three moral principles are needed as a framework of principles for bioethics: respect for autonomy, beneficence, and justice. These three principles should not be construed as jointly forming a complete moral system, but they should be sufficiently comprehensive to provide an analytical framework through which we can reason about problems in bioethics. But let us see what these principles are before discussing questions of adequacy.

RESPECT FOR AUTONOMY

Respect for autonomy is one of the most frequently mentioned moral principles in the literature of bioethics, where it is conceived as a principle rooted in the liberal Western tradition of the importance of individual freedom and choice, both for political life and for personal development. "Autonomy" and "respect for autonomy" are terms loosely associated with several ideas, such as privacy, voluntariness, self-mastery, choosing freely, the freedom to choose, choosing one's own moral position, and accepting responsibility for one's choices.

Historically, the word "autonomy" is a legacy from ancient Greece, where *autos* (self) and *nomos* (rule or law) were joined to refer to political self-governance in the city-state. In moral philosophy personal autonomy has come to refer to personal self-governance: personal rule of the self by adequate understanding while remaining free from controlling interferences by others and from personal limitations that prevent choice. "Autonomy," so understood, has been analyzed in terms of freedom from external constraint and the presence of critical internal capacities integral to self-governance.

It is one thing to be autonomous and another to be *respected* as autonomous. Many issues in bioethics concern failures to respect autonomy, ranging from manipulative underdisclosure of pertinent information to nonrecognition of a refusal of medical interventions. To respect an autonomous agent is to recognize with due appreciation that person's capacities and perspective, including his or her right to hold certain views, to make certain choices, and to take certain actions based on personal values and beliefs. Such respect has historically been connected to the idea that persons possess an intrinsic value independent of special circumstances that confer value. As expressed in Kantian ethics, autonomous persons are ends in themselves, determining their own destiny, and are not to be treated merely as means to the ends of others. Thus, the burden of moral justification rests on those who would restrict or prevent a person's exercise of autonomy.

The moral demand that we respect the autonomy of persons can be formulated as a *principle of respect for autonomy*: *Autonomy of action should not be subjected to controlling constraint by others.* The principle provides the justificatory basis for the right to make autonomous decisions, which in turn takes the form of specific autonomy-related rights. For example, in the debate over whether autonomous, informed patients have the right to refuse self-regarding, life-sustaining medical interventions, the principle of respect for autonomy suggests a morally appropriate response. But the principle covers even simple exchanges in the medical world, such as listening carefully to patients' questions, answering the questions in the detail respectfulness would demand, and not treating patients in a patronizing fashion.

To respect the autonomy of such self-determining agents is to recognize them as *entitled* to determine their own destiny, with due regard to their considered evaluations and view of the world. They must be accorded the moral right to have their own opinions and to act upon them (as long as those actions produce no moral violation). Thus, in evaluating the self-regarding actions of others, we are obligated to respect them as persons with the same right to their judgments as we possess to our own, and they in turn are obligated to treat us in the same way.

Medical and nursing codes have begun in recent years to include rules that are based on this principle. For example, the first principle of the American Nurses' Association *Code* reads as follows: ''The fundamental principle of nursing practice is respect for the inherent dignity and worth of every client. Nurses are morally obligated to respect human existence and the individuality of all persons who are the recipients of nursing actions. . . . Truth telling and the process of reaching informed choice underlie the exercise of self-determination, which is basic to respect for persons. Clients should be as fully involved as possible in the planning and implementation of their own health care.''[6]

The controversial problems with the noble-sounding principle of respect for autonomy, as with all moral principles, arise when we must determine precise limits on its application and how to handle situations when it conflicts with other moral principles such as beneficence and justice. The best known problems of conflict involve overriding refusals of treatment by patients—as in Jehovah's Witnesses' refusals of blood transfusions. Some persons cannot act with substantial autonomy because they are immature, incapacitated, ignorant, or coerced. A person of diminished autonomy is highly dependent on others, less than self-reliant, and in at least some respect incapable of choosing a plan on the basis of controlled deliberations.

Many controversies involve questions about the conditions under which a person's right to autonomous expression demands actions by others and also questions about the restrictions society may rightfully place on choices by patients or subjects when these choices conflict with other values. If choices might endanger the public health, potentially harm a fetus, or involve a scarce resource for which a patient cannot pay, it may be justifiable to restrict exercises of autonomy severely, perhaps by state intervention. If restriction is in order, the justification will rest on some competing moral principle such as beneficence or justice. This issue of *balancing* the demands made by conflicting moral principles was discussed above and can now be seen to apply to each of these principles.

BENEFICENCE

The welfare of the patient is the goal of health care and also of what is often called "therapeutic research." This welfare objective is medicine's context and justification: Clinical therapies are aimed at the promotion of health by cure or prevention of disease. This value of benefiting the person has long been treated as a foundational value—and sometimes as *the* foundational value—in medical ethics.

Among the most quoted principles in the history of codes of medical ethics is the maxim *primum non nocere*—"above all, do no harm." This principle was present in nursing codes as early as Florence Nightingale's *Pledge for Nurses*. The current ANA *Code* demands that the nurse's "primary commitment" as a professional is to protect the patient from harm and to promote the patient's welfare.

Other duties in medicine, nursing, public health, and research are expressed in terms of a *more positive* obligation to come to the assistance of those in need of treatment or in danger of injury. In the International Code of Nursing Ethics, for example, it is said that "[T]he nurse shares with other citizens the responsibility for initiating and supporting action to meet the health and social needs of the public."[7] Various sections of the Principles of Medical Ethics of the American Medical Association express a virtually identical point of view.[8]

The range of duties requiring abstention from harm and positive assistance may be conveniently clustered under the single heading of the principle of beneficence. The term "beneficence" has a broad set of meanings, including the doing of good and the active promotion of good, kindness, and charity. But in the present context the obligation of beneficence has a narrower meaning. In its most general form, the principle of beneficence requires us to abstain from injuring others and to help others further their important and legitimate interests, largely by preventing or removing possible harms.[9] Presumably such acts are required when they can be performed with minimal risk to the actors—not under all circumstances of risk.

According to William Frankena, this principle can be expressed as including the following four elements: (1) One ought not to inflict evil or harm (a principle of nonmaleficence). (2) One ought to prevent evil or harm. (3) One ought to remove evil or harm. (4) One ought to do or promote good.[10] Frankena suggests that the fourth element may not be an obligation at all (being an act of benevolence that is over and above obligation) and contends that these elements appear in a hierarchical arrangement so that the first takes precedence over the second, the second over the third, and the third over the fourth.

There are philosophical reasons for separating passive nonmaleficence (as expressed in 1) and active beneficence (as expressed in 2–4). Ordinary moral discourse expresses the view that certain duties not to injure others are more compelling than duties to benefit them. For example, we do not consider it justifiable to kill a dying patient in order to use the patient's organs to save two others. Similarly, the obligation not to injure a patient by abandonment seems to many stronger than the obligation to prevent injury to a patient who has been abandoned by another (under the assumption that both are moral duties).

Despite the attractiveness of this hierarchical ordering rule, it is not firmly sanctioned by either morality or ethical theory. The obligation expressed in (1) may not *always* outweigh those expressed in (2)–(4). For example, the harm inflicted in (1) may be negligible or trivial, while the harm to be prevented in (2) may be substantial. For instance, saving a person's life by a blood transfusion justifies the inflicted harm of venipuncture on the blood donor. One of the motivations for separating nonmaleficence from beneficence is that they themselves conflict when one must *either* avoid harm *or* bring aid. In such cases, one needs a decision rule to prefer one alternative to another. But if the weights of the two principles can vary, as they can, there can be no mechanical decision rule asserting that one obligation must always outweigh the other.

Such problems lead us to unify the moral demands that we should benefit and not injure others under a single principle of beneficence, taking care to distinguish, as necessary, between strong and weak requirements of this principle. The strength of these requirements corresponds only in some cases to the ordering of (1)–(4). In its general form, then, the principle of beneficence requires us to abstain from intentionally injuring others and to further the important and legitimate interests of others, largely by preventing or removing possible harms.

One of the most vexing problems in ethical theory is the extent to which the principle of beneficence generates *general moral duties* that are incumbent on everyone—not because of a professional role but because morality makes a general demand of beneficence. Any analysis of beneficence in the broad sense delineated above potentially demands severe sacrifice and extreme generosity in the moral life—for example, giving a kidney for transplantation or donating bone marrow. As a result, some philosophers have argued that this form of beneficent action is virtuous and a moral *ideal*, but not an obligation. From this perspective, the positive benefiting of others is based on professional obligations or personal ideals that are supererogatory rather than obligatory: We are not *required* by the general canons of morality to promote the good of persons, even if we are in a position to do so and the action is morally *justified*.

Several proposals have been offered in moral philosophy to resolve this problem by showing that beneficence *is* a principle of obligation, but these theoretical ventures are extraneous to our concerns here. The scope or range of acts required by the obligation of beneficence is an undecided issue, and perhaps an undecidable one. Fortunately, our arguments do not depend on its resolution. That we are morally obligated on *some* occasions to assist others—at least in professional roles such as nursing, medicine, and research—is hardly a matter of moral controversy. Beneficent acts are demanded by the roles involved in fiduciary relationships between health care professionals and patients, lawyers and clients, researchers and subjects (at least in therapeutic research), bankers and customers, and so on.

We will treat the basic roles and concepts that give substance to the principle of beneficence in medicine as follows: The positive benefits the physician and nurse are obligated to seek is the alleviation of disease and injury, if there is a reasonable hope of cure. The harms to be prevented, removed, or minimized are the pain, suffering, and disability of injury and disease. In addition, the physician and nurse are of course enjoined from *doing* harm if interventions inflict unnecessary pain and suffering on patients.

In therapeutic research, the benefits and harms presented to subjects are similar—the cure, removal, or prevention of pain, suffering, disability, and disease. In nontherapeutic research, the subjects' interests are less at center stage, because the positive benefit sought by the scientist is new knowledge. Often (but not necessarily) this knowledge is desired because it is expected to contribute to the resolution of important medical or social problems. Therapeutic and nontherapeutic research thus differ in the kinds of benefits each hopes to achieve. Although in both there is an equally strong imperative to avoid harming the subject, therapeutic research may legitimately present increased potential for harms if they are balanced by a commensurate possibility of benefits to the subject.

Those engaged in both medical practice and research know that risks of harm presented by interventions must constantly be weighed against possible benefits for patients, subjects, or the public interest. The physician or nurse who professes to "do no harm" is not pledging never to cause harm but rather to strive to create a positive balance of goods over inflicted harms. This is recognized in the Nuremberg Code, which enjoins: "The degree of risk to be taken should never exceed that determined by the humanitarian importance of the problem to be solved by the experiment." Such a balancing principle is essential to any sound moral system: Beneficence assumes an obligation to weigh and balance benefits against harms, benefits against alternative benefits, and harms against alternative harms. When a life is at stake, it may be justified to take high risks of harm and death.

Health care professionals and research investigators often disagree over how to weigh and balance the various factors, and there may be no objective evidence that dictates one course rather than another. In clinical contexts, this balancing can also present situations in which health care professionals and patients differ in their assessments of the professional's obligations. In some cases, benefit to another is involved—as, for example, when a pregnant woman refuses a physician's recommendation of fetal surgery. In other cases the refusal may be exclusively self-regarding. Some health care professionals will accept a patient's refusal as valid, whereas others are inclined to ignore the fact that an informed consent to treatment has not been given, and so try to "benefit" the patient through a medical intervention.

This problem of whether to override the decisions of patients in order to benefit them or prevent harm to them is one dimension of the problem of medical paternalism, in which a parental-like decision by a professional overrides an autonomous decision of a patient. This problem of paternalism is treated in detail later in this introduction in the section on Law, Authority, and Autonomy. It is shown there how the problem of paternalism is generated by a conflict between principles of respect for autonomy and beneficence, each of which can be and has been conceived by different parties as the overriding principle in cases of conflict. This conflict between the demands of beneficence and respect for autonomy underlies a broad range of controversies in this volume.

JUSTICE

Every civilized society is a cooperative venture structured by moral, legal, and cultural principles that define the terms of social cooperation. Beneficence and respect for autonomy are principles in this fabric of social order, but *justice* has been the subject of more treatises on the terms of social cooperation than any other principle.

A person has been treated in accordance with the principle of justice if treated according to what is fair, due, or owed. For example, if equal political rights are due all citizens, then justice is done when those rights are accorded. Any denial of a good, service, or piece of information to which a person has a right or entitlement based in justice is an injustice. It is also an injustice to place an undue burden on the exercise of a right—for example, to make a piece of information owed to a person unreasonably difficult to obtain.

The more restricted expression "distributive justice" refers to the proper distribution of social benefits and burdens. Usually it refers to the distribution of primary social goods, such as economic goods and fundamental political rights. But social burdens must also be considered. Paying taxes and being drafted into the armed services to fight a war are distributed burdens; Medicare checks and grants to do research are distributed benefits. Recent literature on distributive justice has tended to focus on considerations of fair economic distribution, especially unjust distributions in the form of inequalities of income between different classes of persons and unfair tax burdens on certain classes. But there are many problems of distributive justice besides issues about income and wealth, including the issues raised in prominent contemporary debates over health care distribution, as discussed in Chapter 11.

The notion of justice has been analyzed in different ways in rival theories. But common to all theories of justice is this minimal principle: Like cases should be treated alike—or, to use the language of equality, equals ought to be treated equally and unequals unequally. This elementary principle is referred to as the formal principle of justice, or sometimes as the formal principle of equality—formal because it states no particular respects in which people ought to be treated. It merely asserts that whatever respects are under consideration, if persons are equal in those respects, they should be treated alike. Thus, the formal principle of justice does not tell us how to determine equality or proportion in these matters, and it therefore lacks substance as a specified guide to conduct. Because in any group of persons there will be many respects in which they are both similar and different, this account of equality must be understood as "equality in relevant respects."

Because this formal principle leaves space for differences in the interpretation of how justice applies to particular situations, philosophers have developed diverse theories of justice. These theories attempt to be more specific than the formal principle by elaborating how people are to be compared and what it means to give people their due. Philosophers attempt to achieve the needed precision and specificity by developing material principles of justice—so called because they put material content into a theory of justice. Each material principle of justice identifies a relevant property on the basis of which burdens and benefits should be distributed.

The following is a sample list of major candidates for the position of valid principles of distributive justice (though longer lists have been proposed): 1. To each person an equal share. 2. To each person according to individual need. 3. To each person according to acquisition in a free market. 4. To each person according to individual effort. 5. To each person according to societal contribution. 6. To each person according to merit. There is no obvious barrier to acceptance of more than one of these principles, and some theories of justice accept all six as valid. Most societies use several in the belief that different rules are appropriate to different situations.

Egalitarian theories of justice emphasize equal access to primary goods, libertarian theories emphasize rights to social and economic liberty, and utilitarian theories emphasize a mixed use of such criteria so that public and private utility are maximized. The utilitarian theory follows the main lines of the explanation of utilitarianism above, and thus economic justice is viewed as one among a number of problems concerning how to maximize value. The ideal economic distribution, utilitarians argue, is any arrangement that would have this maximizing effect.

Egalitarianism is the theory that individual differences are not significant in an account of social justice. Distributions of burdens and benefits in a society are just to the extent they are equal, and deviations from equality in distribution are unjust. Most egalitarian accounts of justice are guardedly formulated, so that only *some* basic equalities among individuals take priority over their differences. In recent years an egalitarian theory discussed above in the section on deontological theories has enjoyed wide currency: John Rawls's *A Theory of Justice*. This book has as its central contention that we should distribute all economic goods and services equally except in those cases in which an unequal distribution would actually work to everyone's advantage, or at least would benefit the worst off in society. Rawls considers social institutions to be just if and only if they conform to his two principles of justice (see page 26 above).

The libertarian theory is sharply opposed to egalitarianism. What makes libertarian theories *libertarian* is the priority afforded to distinctive processes, procedures, or mechanisms for ensuring that liberty rights are recognized in economic practice—typically the rules and procedures governing social liberty and economic acquisition and exchange in free-market systems. Because free choice is the pivotal goal, libertarians place a premium on the principle of respect for autonomy. In some libertarian systems, this principle is the sole basic moral principle, and there thus are no unique principles of justice. We will see in Chapter 11 that many philosophers believe that this approach is fundamentally wrong because economic value is generated through an essentially communal process that our health policies must reflect if justice is to be done.

Libertarian theorists, however, explicitly reject the conclusion that egalitarian patterns of distribution represent a normative ideal. People may be equal in a host of morally significant respects (for example, entitled to equal treatment under the law and equally valued as ends in themselves), but the libertarian contends that it would be a basic violation of *justice* to regard people as deserving of equal economic returns. In particular, people are seen as having a fundamental right to own and dispense with the products of their labor as they choose, even if exercise of this right leads to large inequalities of wealth in society. Equality and utility principles, from this libertarian perspective, sacrifice basic liberty rights to the larger public interest by coercively extracting financial resources through taxation.

These theories of justice all capture some of our intuitive convictions about justice, and each exhibits strengths as a theory of justice. Perhaps, then, there are several equally valid, or at least equally defensible, theories of justice and just taxation. This situation of competing and apparently viable theories has led some writers to note that there seem to be severe limits to philosophy's capacity to resolve public-policy issues through theories of distributive justice. They believe these theories are simply unsuited for public-policy formulation. The final section of this chapter looks at possible ways in which moral reasoning might assist in the formulation of public policy, whether by appeal to justice or to some other analytical framework.

ETHICS, LAW, AND PUBLIC POLICY

Most moral principles are already embedded in public morality and public policies, generally in a vague and underanalyzed form. But if they are already there, how can philosophical development of these principles assist us in the enormously complicated task of creating law and public policy?

ETHICS AND PUBLIC AFFAIRS

There are at least two ways in which applied ethics often overlaps with, and provides foundations for, law and public policy. First, there are conceptual problems that require careful explication in order that people communicate clearly and efficiently. What is meant in various contexts when crucial terms are used, such as "liberty," "fair distribution," "competence," "rights," "paternalism," "responsibility," and "coercion by law"? At stake is not whether and how justice or liberty should be ensured or what rights and responsibilities should be granted to what persons. The point of conceptual analysis of these fundamental terms is to be as clear and precise as possible without begging any substantive moral issue. The importance of such conceptual clarification became obvious in the discussion of moral disagreement.

Second, normative problems require equally careful attention, in order that we determine what ought to be done in law and social policy. Here, philosophers must abandon the neutrality about issues involved in conceptual clarification, for they are engaged in that controversial world of human affairs where there are conflicting interests, goals, and ideals. Their objective should be to formulate and apply general principles that can be fairly used to guide public policy. For example, a theory of human rights might be developed that determines which rights all persons have and a theory of justice that explains how goods should be distributed in society without regard to the special interest of any person or class of persons.

Many articles in this volume are concerned with the use of ethical theory for the formulation of public affairs. Joel Feinberg has made a suggestive comment about how the problems raised in these essays might *ideally* be viewed:

It is convenient to think of these problems as questions for some hypothetical and abstract political body. An answer to the question of when liberty should be limited or how wealth ideally should be distributed, for example, could be used to guide not only moralists, but also legislators and judges toward reasonable decisions in particular cases where interests, rules, or the liberties of different parties appear to conflict. . . . We must think of an ideal legislator as somewhat abstracted from the full legislative context, in that he is free to appeal directly to the public interest unencumbered by the need to please voters, to make "deals" with colleagues, or any other merely "political" considerations. . . . The principles of the ideal legislator . . . are still of the first practical importance, since they provide a target for our aspirations and a standard for judging our successes and failures.[11]

However, an ideal approach is not always one on the basis of which it is possible to formulate a public policy. A "public policy" is composed of a set of normative guidelines intended for *practice*. Moral principles will have to be adapted to real-world problems of efficiency, cultural pluralism, political procedures, uncertainty about risk, noncompliance by patients, and the like. The principles provide only the background for policy, whereas the policy itself requires empirical data and information drawn from relevant fields of medicine, biology, law, psychology, and so on, and the rules it contains cannot be identical with the rules of an ethical theory. The abstract principles of ethical theory cannot by their nature contain enough specific information or advice to suffice. There will thus have to be some mediating rules that transform the theory into a practical strategy and set of guidelines.[12]

Public policies relevant to bioethics serve the purposes of regulation and the allocation and distribution of social benefits and social burdens. In this book we will consider policies pertaining to euthanasia, ethics committees mandated for hospitals, the nature and scope of abortion regulation, public allocations for health care, regulation of risk in the workplace, protection of animal and human subjects of research, legislative definitions of death, liability for failures of disclosure and confidentiality, policies to control developments in genetics, and a host of other problems of ethics and public policy.

A specific example of ethics at work in the formulation of public policy is found in the work of the National Commission for the Protection of Human Subjects of Biomedical and Behavioral Research, which was established in 1974 by a federal law. Its mandate was to develop ethical guidelines for the conduct of research involving human subjects and to make recommendations to the Department of Health and Human Services (DHHS). To discharge its duties, the commission studied the nature and extent of various forms of research, its purposes, the ethical issues surrounding the research, present federal regulations, and the views of representatives of professional societies and federal agencies. The commission engaged in extensive deliberations on these subjects in public, a process in which persons from various fields of ethics were as intimately involved as the representatives of any other discipline.

Subsequent government regulations regarding research (issued by DHHS) were developed on the basis of work provided by the commission. These public laws show the imprint of the commission in virtually every clause. These regulations cannot be regarded as exclusively ethical in orientation, but much distinctive philosophical material is found in the commission documents, and ethical analysis provided the framework for its deliberations and recommendations. The commission also issued one exclusively philosophical volume, which sets forth the moral framework that underlies the various policy recommendations it made. It is among the best examples of the use of moral frameworks for actual (not merely theoretical or programmatic) policy development and of a philosophical publication issued through a government-sponsored body.

MORALITY AND LAW

Public policy such as that developed by the commission often has the force of law, and the "morality" of many actions that have a public impact is often gauged by whether the law prohibits that form of conduct. This takes us to the need to analyze the connections between morality and law.

Most of the chapters in this book contain selections from case law (judge-made law expressed in court decisions). Often selections in the chapters will mention actual or proposed statutory law (federal and state statutes and their accompanying administrative regulations). Law in these forms has brought a string of important bioethical issues before the public. Case law, in particular, has established influential precedents that provide material for reflection on both legal and moral obligations. Yet it is vital to distinguish *moral* evaluation from *legal* evaluation. Issues of legal liability, costs to the system, practicability within the litigation process, and questions of compensation may demand that legal requirements be different from moral requirements.

Despite an important intersection between morals and law, the law is not the repository of our moral standards and values, even when the law is directly concerned with moral problems. A law-abiding person is not necessarily morally sensitive or virtuous, and from the fact that something is legally acceptable, it does not follow that it is morally acceptable. Numerous failures to fulfill promises do not involve legal violations of contract but may nonetheless involve serious moral violations. Questions are raised in later chapters about the morality of many actions in medicine and research—such as the proper form of interaction with patients and the morality of abortion—although such actions are not illegal.

Issues of law and morality are commonly treated in public debate as if the only matter of abiding concern worthy of public scrutiny is whether a person has conformed to or violated the law. One problem with this approach is what often forms its bottom line: The conduct is judged *acceptable* in general because (1) there is no legal violation and (2) there ought not to be any new legal standard enacted that would hold the person liable. Ignored is the fact that the acceptability of the conduct may be inappropriate and condemnable by the standards of morality.

Law and morality should therefore be kept distinct. The two often brush in close contact—as in the legal cases in many of the following chapters—because they share concerns over matters of basic social importance. Principles, duties, and criteria of evidence are often shared by morality and law, and laws may be shaped by moral principles and established to protect moral interests. Law, in certain respects, is our agency for translating morality into explicit social guidelines and practices. But these generalizations about the intersection of law and morality could also be applied to religion, economics, politics, and many overlapping disciplines and areas of conduct, all of which should be kept as separate as possible from morality.

It is often not a straightforward move from a judgment that an act of a certain type is morally right (or wrong) to a judgment that a law promoting or prohibiting the act is morally right (or wrong). Factors such as the deprivation of liberty and the cost of enforcement must be considered. For example, one can consistently hold that abortion is morally wrong without holding that the law should prohibit it. The judgment that an act is morally acceptable also does not imply that the law should permit it. For example, the moral position that various forms of euthanasia are morally justified is consistent with the thesis that the government should legally prohibit these forms of euthanasia, on grounds that it would not be possible to control potential abuses.

Bioethics in the United States is currently involved in an entangled, complex, and mutually stimulating relationship with law. The law often appeals to moral duties and rights, places sanctions on violators, and in general strengthens the social importance of moral beliefs. Nevertheless, the law rightly backs away from attempting to legislate against everything that is morally wrong. In recent years the judges have been searching in their opinions for extra-legal mechanisms such as peer review, committees, codes of ethics, and self-regulatory procedural mechanisms that will limit the involvement of the law and escape involvement by legislatures, regulatory agencies, and the courts. As the courts and legislatures become more pressed for time, it seems inevitable that procedures to protect ethical interests that are outside the reach of the law will assume greater significance.

LEGAL AND MORAL RIGHTS

Much of the modern ethical discussion that we shall encounter throughout this volume turns on ideas about rights, and many public-policy issues concern rights or attempts to secure rights. Our political tradition itself has developed from a conception of natural rights. However, until the seventeenth and eighteenth centuries, problems of social and political philosophy were rarely discussed in terms of rights, perhaps because duties to lord, king, state, church, and God had been the dominant focus of political and ethical theory. New political views were introduced at this point in history, including the notion of universal natural rights. Thus, historically, the notion of natural (or human) rights emerged from a need to check the sovereign power of states. Rights quickly came to be understood as powerful assertions of claims that demand respect and status.

There are substantial differences between moral and legal rights, because legal systems do not formally require reference to moral systems for their understanding or grounding, nor do moral systems formally require reference to legal systems. One may have a legal right to do something patently immoral, or have a moral right without any corresponding legal guarantee. Legal rights are derived from political constitutions, legislative enactments, case law, and the executive orders of the highest state official. Moral rights, by contrast, exist independently of and form a basis for criticizing or justifying legal rights. Finally, legal rights can be eliminated simply by lawful amendments to political constitutions, or by a coup d'etat, but moral rights cannot be eroded or banished by political votes, powers, or amendments.

Yet the idea that certain moral rights exist prior to and independent of social conventions and laws has led philosophers to speculate about the nature and source of rights. Some carefully drawn distinctions regarding the nature and types of moral rights have emerged in ethical theory, and it will prove useful to examine some of these distinctions.

Prima Facie and Absolute Rights. Prima facie duties were discussed earlier, in the section on deontological theories. It was noted there that moral philosophers generally regard duties not as absolute but rather as strong moral demands that may be validly overridden by more stringent competing demands in circumstances of competition. This competition occurs in the case of rights as well. Here the problem is whether rights may be overridden by competing rights. It has often been assumed, owing perhaps to political statements about fundamental human rights, that rights are absolute. Yet there appear to be many counterexamples to the thesis that they are absolute.

For example, it is sometimes assumed that the right to life is absolute, irrespective of competing claims or social conditions. This thesis is controversial, however, as evidenced by common moral judgments about capital punishment, international agreements about killing in war, and beliefs about the justifiability of killing in self-defense. Most writers in ethics agree that we have only a right not to have our life taken without sufficient justification. Although there is disagreement about which conditions are sufficient for taking another's life, most agree that some conditions—for example, self-defense—can be specified. The right to life and all rights, according to this ethical thesis, are not absolute: Any right can be legitimately exercised and can create duties on others only when the right has an overriding status.

Negative and Positive Rights. Philosophers have often drawn a distinction between positive and negative rights. A right to well-being—generally the right to receive goods and services—is a positive right, and a right to liberty—generally a right not to be interfered with—is a negative right. The right to liberty is a negative right because no one has to do anything to honor it. Presumably all that must be done to honor negative rights is to leave people alone. The same is not true with respect to positive rights. To honor those rights someone has to provide something. For example, if a person has a human right to well-being and is starving, then someone has an obligation to provide that person with food.

This distinction between positive and negative rights has led those who would include a right to well-being on the list of human rights to argue that the obligation to provide for positive rights falls on the state. Others, however, wish to limit the power of the state to regulate our affairs, and they see only the protection of negative rights as the prerogative and responsibility of state officials. This important distinction between positive and negative rights is analyzed in the introduction to Chapter 11, under the subject of the right to health care, which is a positive right (if it exists).

Because general negative rights are rights of noninterference, their direct connection to liberal individualism is apparent, with its typical emphasis on freedom from government and protection of zones of privacy. Because general positive rights require that all members of the community yield some of their resources to advance the welfare of others by providing social goods and services, there is a natural connection in theories that emphasize general positive rights to a communitarianism or sense of "the commons" that limits the scope of individualism. To generalize the point: The broader the scope of positive rights in a theory, the more likely that theory is to emphasize a scheme of social justice that confers positive rights to redistributions of resources (as we see in Chapter 6).

Accordingly, a moral system composed of a powerful set of general negative obligations and rights is antithetical to a moral system composed of a powerful set of general positive obligations and rights, just as a strong individualism is opposed to a strong communitarianism. Rights of privacy and the pursuit of one's autonomous projects will inevitably conflict with obligations to assist or provide resources for others. Many of the conflicts that we encounter throughout this book spring from these basic differences over the existence and scope of negative and positive rights and obligations—especially regarding the number, types, and weight of *positive* rights and obligations.

LAW, AUTHORITY, AND AUTONOMY

Various autonomy rights are often said to be fundamental rights, but no right is strong enough to entail a right to unrestricted exercises of autonomy in the public life. The notion of "acceptable liberty" refers to actions in which people ought to be free to engage. Although it would be difficult to determine a set of right and wrong exercises of autonomy, some valid restrictions on our liberty are appropriate. But which ones?

Liberty-Limiting Principles. Various "moral" principles have been advanced in the attempt to establish valid grounds for the limitation of autonomy. The following four "liberty-limiting principles" have been defended and have played a significant role in recent philosophical controversies:

1. *The Harm Principle:* A person's liberty is justifiably restricted to prevent harm to others caused by that person.
2. *The Principle of Paternalism:* A person's liberty is justifiably restricted to prevent harm to self caused by that person.
3. *The Principle of Legal Moralism:* A person's liberty is justifiably restricted to prevent that person's immoral behavior.
4. *The Offense Principle:* A person's liberty is justifiably restricted to prevent offense to others caused by that person.

Each of these four principles represents an attempt to balance liberty and other values. Although different people differently assess the weight of certain values in this balancing process, the harm principle is universally accepted as a valid liberty-limiting principle (despite certain unclarities that surround the notion of a harm). However, much controversy surrounds the other three liberty-limiting principles, and their general validity is widely doubted.

Only one of these supplementary principles is pertinent to a number of the controversies that arise in this volume: paternalism. Here the central problem is whether this form of justification for a restriction of liberty may ever validly be invoked, and, if so, how the principle that stands behind this judgment is to be formulated. In order to answer this question, we must look more closely at the nature of paternalism.

Paternalism. The word "paternalism" loosely refers to treating individuals in the way that a parent treats his or her child. But in ethical theory the word is more narrowly used to apply to treatment that restricts individual autonomy: Paternalism is the intentional limitation of the autonomy of one person by another, where the person who limits autonomy appeals exclusively to grounds of beneficence for the person whose autonomy is limited. The essence of paternalism is an overriding of the principle of respect for autonomy on grounds of the principle of beneficence.

Several writers have argued that paternalism is pervasively present in modern society; many actions, rules, and laws are commonly justified by appeal to a paternalistic principle. Examples in medicine include court orders for blood transfusions when patients have refused them, involuntary commitment to institutions for treatment, intervention to stop "rational" suicides, resuscitating patients who have asked not to be resuscitated, withholding medical information that patients have requested, denial of an innovative therapy to someone who wishes to try it, and some government efforts to promote health. Other health-related examples include laws requiring motorcyclists to wear helmets and motorists to wear seat belts and the regulations of governmental agencies such as the Food and Drug

Administration that prevent people from purchasing possibly harmful or inefficacious drugs and chemicals. In all cases the motivation is the beneficent promotion of health and welfare.

In the case of medical paternalism, it is often said that the patient-physician relationship is essentially paternalistic. This view is held because patients can be so ill that their judgments or voluntary abilities are significantly affected, or because they may be incapable of grasping important information about their case, thus being in no position to reach carefully reasoned decisions about their medical treatment. The paternalism of the medical profession has been under attack in recent years, especially by defenders of the autonomy rights of patients. The latter hold that physicians intervene too often and assume too much control over their patients' choices. Many recent philosophical, legal, and medical writings have reflected this harsh judgment of the profession.

Philosophers and lawyers have tended to support the view that the autonomy of patients is the decisive factor in the patient-physician relationship and that interventions can be valid only when patients are in some measure unable to make voluntary choices or to perform voluntary actions. Physicians too have increasingly criticized authoritarianism in their profession. A recent draft of principles of ethics of the American Medical Association asserted that "paternalism by the profession is no longer appropriate."

Any careful proponent of a principle of paternalism will specify precisely which goods and needs deserve paternalistic protection and the conditions under which intervention is warranted. In most recent formulations, it has been argued that one is justified in interfering with a person's liberty only if the interference protects the person against his or her own actions where those actions are extremely and unreasonably risky (for example, refusing a life-saving therapy in nonterminal situations) or are potentially dangerous and irreversible in effect (as some drugs and surgery are). According to this position, paternalism is justified if and only if the evils prevented from occurring to the person are greater than the evils (if any) caused by interference with his or her liberty and if it can be universally justified, under relevantly similar circumstances, always to treat persons in this way.

This fairly moderate formulation of paternalism still leaves many resolutely opposed to all possible uses of this principle. Their arguments against paternalism invariably turn on some defense of the importance of the principle of respect for autonomy, and we will many times encounter such appeals in this volume—especially as applied to rightful state intervention in order to benefit patients or subjects without their authorization.

One major source of the difference between supporters and opponents of paternalism rests on the emphasis each places on capabilities for autonomous action by patients making "choices." Supporters of paternalism tend to cite examples of persons of diminished or compromised capacity, for example, persons lingering on kidney dialysis, chronic alcoholics, compulsive smokers, and seriously depressed suicidal patients. Opponents of paternalism cite examples of persons who are capable of autonomous choice but have been socially restricted in exercising their capacities. Examples of this group include those involuntarily committed to institutions largely because of eccentric behavior, prisoners not permitted to volunteer for risky research, and those who might rationally elect to refuse treatment in life-threatening circumstances. One critical element of this controversy thus concerns the quality of consent or refusal by the persons whose autonomy might be restricted by such policies.

Many articles reproduced in this volume deal with public policies that involve such substantive moral issues as liberty and liberty-limiting principles, and legal versus moral rights. These policies affect not only doctor and patient, lawyer and client, researcher and subject—they affect every individual in society.

CONCLUSION

This chapter has surveyed some central themes in philosophical discussions of ethical theory. This form of theory should not be expected to be solely sufficient to resolve the many problems in medical practice and research discussed in this volume. Some controversies are largely factual, and, as seen in the next two chapters, some controversies are more conceptual than moral. Practical wisdom and sound judgment are also indispensable allies of theory. Moral philosophy can yield well-constructed arguments and criticisms that advance our understanding, but the person of sound judgment is of no less value than the person of sound theory. Moral dilemmas require a balancing of competing claims in untidy circumstances, and this effort requires every resource we can marshal.

T.L.B.

NOTES

1. *Tarasoff* v. *Regents of the University of California*, California Supreme Court (17 California Reports, 3d Series, 425. Decided July 1, 1976). Reprinted in Chapter 8.

2. These principles and their analysis by the National Commission for the Protection of Human Subjects of Biomedical and Behavioral Research have been published as *The Belmont Report: Ethical Principles and Guidelines for the Protection of Human Subjects of Research* (Washington, D.C.: U.S. Government Printing Office, DHEW Publication, 1978).

3. For a more developed discussion of levels of justification, see Tom L. Beauchamp and James F. Childress, *Principles of Biomedical Ethics*, 3rd edition (New York: Oxford University Press, 1989), Chap. 1.

4. See Al Kamen, "Budget Law Rejected by High Court," *Washington Post*, July 8, 1986, p. 1.

5. K. Ann Coleman Stolurow and Dale W. Moeller, "Dental X-Ray Use in Boston," *American Journal of Public Health* 69 (July 1979), 709–710.

6. American Nurses' Association, *Code for Nurses with Interpretive Statements* (Kansas City, Mo.: ANA, 1985), pp. 2–3.

7. 1953 and 1973 International Codes of Nursing Ethics of the International Council of Nurses.

8. Section 10 of the 1977 Principles of Medical Ethics of the American Medical Association.

9. The conditions for X's having an obligation of beneficence to Y have been plausibly analyzed by Eric D'Arcy as follows. X has a duty of beneficence to Y if and only if: (1) Y is at risk of significant loss or damage; (2) X's action is necessary to prevent loss or damage; (3) X's action would probably prevent loss or damage; (4) X's own losses or damages would probably be minimal or negligible; (5) Benefit to Y will probably outweigh the harm to X. Eric D'Arcy, *Human Acts: An Essay in Their Moral Evaluation* (Oxford: Clarendon Press, 1963), pp. 56–57.

10. William Frankena, *Ethics*, 2nd edition (Englewood Cliffs, N.J.: Prentice-Hall, 1973), p. 47.

11. Joel Feinberg, *Social Philosophy* (Englewood Cliffs, N.J.: Prentice-Hall, 1973), pp. 2–3.

12. Dennis Thompson, "Philosophy and Policy," *Philosophy and Public Affairs* 14 (Spring 1985), 205–218.

SUGGESTED READINGS FOR CHAPTER 1

MORALITY AND MORAL PHILOSOPHY

Frankena, William K. *Ethics*. 2nd edition. Englewood Cliffs, N.J.: Prentice-Hall, 1973.

Gowans, Christopher W., ed. *Moral Dilemmas*. New York: Oxford University Press, 1987.

MacIntyre, Alasdair. *A Short History of Ethics*. New York: Macmillan, 1966.

Mackie, John. *Ethics: Inventing Right and Wrong*. Harmondsworth, Eng.: Penguin Books Ltd., 1977.

Rachels, James. *The Elements of Moral Philosophy*. New York: Random House, 1986.

Regan, Tom, ed. *Matters of Life and Death*. 2nd edition. New York: Random House, 1986.

Singer, Peter. *Practical Ethics*. New York: Cambridge University Press, 1979.

RELATIVISM AND DISAGREEMENT

Brandt, Richard B. "Ethical Relativism." In Edwards, Paul, ed. *Encyclopedia of Philosophy*. New York: Macmillan, 1967. Vol. 3, pp. 75–78.

Fishkin, James S. *Beyond Subjective Morality*. New Haven: Yale University Press, 1984.

Glover, Jonathan. *Causing Death and Saving Lives*. New York: Penguin Books, 1977. Chap. 2.

Krausz, Michael, and Meiland, Jack W., eds. *Relativism: Cognitive and Moral*. Notre Dame, Ind.: University of Notre Dame Press, 1982.

Ladd, John, ed. *Ethical Relativism*. Belmont, Calif.: Wadsworth Publishing Company, 1973.

Rachels, James. "Can Ethics Provide Answers?" *Hastings Center Report* 10 (June 1980), 32–40.

Wong, David B. *Moral Relativity*. Berkeley, Calif.: University of California Press, 1984.

JUSTIFICATION

Beauchamp, Tom L. *Philosophical Ethics*. New York: McGraw-Hill, 1982. Chaps. 9 and 10.

Brandt, R. B. *A Theory of the Good and the Right*. Oxford: Clarendon Press, 1979. Chaps. 10–12.

Griffiths, A. Phillips. "Ultimate Moral Principles: Their Justification." In Edwards, Paul, ed. *Encyclopedia of Philosophy*. New York: Macmillan, 1967. Vol. 8, pp. 177–182.

Pennock, J. Roland, and Chapman, John W., eds. *NOMOS XXVIII: Justification*. New York: New York University Press, 1986.

Williams, Bernard. *Ethics and the Limits of Philosophy*. Cambridge, Mass.: Harvard University Press, 1985.

UTILITARIANISM

Bentham, Jeremy. *Introduction to the Principles of Morals and Legislation* (1789), W. Harrison, ed., with *A Fragment on Government*. Oxford: Hafner Press, 1948.

Frey, R. G., ed. *Utility and Rights*. Minneapolis, Minn.: University of Minnesota Press, 1984.

Gorovitz, Samuel, ed. *Mill: Utilitarianism, with Critical Essays*. New York: Bobbs-Merrill, 1971.

Hare, R. M. *Moral Thinking: Its Levels, Method and Point*. Oxford: Clarendon Press, 1981.

Mill, John Stuart. *On Liberty*. London: J. W. Parker, 1863. (Widely reprinted.)

Scheffler, Samuel, ed. *Consequentialism and Its Critics*. Oxford: Oxford University Press, 1988.

Sen, Amartya. *On Ethics and Economics*. Oxford: Basil Blackwell, 1987.

————, and Williams, Bernard, eds. *Utilitarianism and Beyond*. Cambridge: Cambridge University Press, 1982.

DEONTOLOGY

Donagan, Alan. *The Theory of Morality*. Chicago: University of Chicago Press, 1977.

Kant, Immanuel. *Foundations of the Metaphysics of Morals*. Lewis White Beck, trans. Indianapolis, Ind.: Bobbs-Merrill, 1959.

Nell, Onora. *Acting on Principle, an Essay on Kantian Ethics*. New York and London: Columbia University Press, 1975.

Rawls, John. *A Theory of Justice*. Cambridge, Mass.: Harvard University Press, 1971.

Ross, William D. *The Right and the Good*. Oxford: Oxford University Press, 1930.

MORAL PRINCIPLES

Beauchamp, Tom L., and Childress, James F. *Principles of Biomedical Ethics*. 3rd edition. New York: Oxford University Press, 1989. Chaps. 3–6.

Callahan, Daniel. "Autonomy: A Moral Good, Not a Moral Obsession." *Hastings Center Report* 14 (October 1984), 40–42.

Dworkin, Gerald. "Autonomy and Behavior Control." *Hastings Center Report* 6 (February 1976), 23–28.

Engelhardt, H. Tristram, Jr. *The Foundations of Bioethics*. New York: Oxford University Press, 1986.

Feinberg, Joel. *Harm to Self, The Moral Limits of Criminal Law*. Vol. 3. New York: Oxford University Press, 1986.

Jonsen, Albert. "Do No Harm: Axiom of Medical Ethics." In Spicker, Stuart F., and Engelhardt, H. Tristram, Jr., eds. *Philosophical Medical Ethics: Its Nature and Significance*. Boston: D. Reidel, 1977, pp. 27–41.

Mack, Eric, ed. *Positive and Negative Duties*. Tulane Studies in Philosophy. New Orleans, La.: Tulane University, 1985.

Pellegrino, Edmund, and Thomasma, David. *For the Patient's Good: The Restoration of Beneficence in Health Care*. New York: Oxford University Press, 1988.

Shelp, Earl E., ed. *Justice and Health Care*. Boston: D. Reidel, 1981.

Sterba, James, ed. *Justice: Alternative Political Perspectives*. Belmont, Calif.: Wadsworth Publishing Company, 1980.

Toulmin, Stephen. "The Tyranny of Principles." *Hastings Center Report* 11 (December 1981), 31–39.

Veatch, Robert M. *A Theory of Medical Ethics*. New York: Basic Books, 1981.

ETHICS AND PUBLIC POLICY

Areen, Judith, et al. *Law, Science, and Medicine*. Mineola, N.Y.: Foundation Press, 1984. Supplementary volume, 1987.

Brock, Dan W. "Truth or Consequences: The Role of Philosophers in Policy-Making." *Ethics* 97 (July 1987), 786–791.

Thompson, Dennis. "Philosophy and Policy." *Philosophy and Public Affairs* 14 (Spring 1985), 205–218.

Weisbard, Alan J. "The Role of Philosophers in the Public Policy Process." *Ethics* 97 (July 1987), 776–785.

MORALITY AND LAW

Dworkin, Ronald. *Taking Rights Seriously*. Cambridge, Mass.: Harvard University Press, 1977.

———. *A Matter of Principle*. Cambridge, Mass.: Harvard University Press, 1985.

Feinberg, Joel. "Rights: Systematic Analysis." In Reich, Warren T., ed. *Encyclopedia of Bioethics*. New York: Free Press, 1978. Vol. 4., pp. 1507–1511.

———. *The Moral Limits of the Criminal Law*. 4 vols. New York: Oxford University Press, 1984–1987.

Lyons, David. *Ethics and the Rule of Law*. Cambridge: Cambridge University Press, 1984.

Waldron, Jeremy, ed. *Nonsense upon Stilts*. London: Methuen, 1987.

LIBERTY, AUTHORITY, AND PATERNALISM

Bayles, Michael D. *Principles of Legislation: The Uses of Political Authority*. Detroit: Wayne State University Press, 1978.

Beauchamp, Tom L., and McCullough, Laurence B. *Medical Ethics*. Englewood Cliffs, N.J.: Prentice-Hall, 1984. Chap. 4.

Buchanan, A. "Medical Paternalism." *Philosophy and Public Affairs* 7 (1978), 370–390.

Childress, James. *Who Should Decide?: Paternalism in Health Care*. New York: Oxford University Press, 1982.

De George, Richard T. *The Nature and Limits of Authority*. Lawrence, Kans.: University Press of Kansas, 1985.

Dworkin, Gerald. "Paternalism." *The Monist* 56 (1972), 64–84.

Sartorius, Rolf, ed. *Paternalism*. Minneapolis: University of Minnesota Press, 1983.

BIBLIOGRAPHIES

Goldstein, Doris Mueller. *Bioethics: A Guide to Information Sources*. Detroit: Gale Research Company, 1982. See under "Ethics" and "Bioethics."

Lineback, Richard H., ed. *Philosopher's Index*. Vols. 1– . Bowling Green, Ohio: Philosophy Documentation Center, Bowling Green State University. Issued quarterly. See under "Autonomy," "Bioethics," "Coercion," "Consequentialism," "Distributive Justice," "Duty," "Egalitarianism," "Equality," "Ethics," "Fairness," "Human Rights," "Justice," "Kant," "Law," "Medical Ethics," "Mill," "Moral(s)," "Morality," "Natural Rights," "Normative Ethics," "Obligations," "Paternalism," "Principles," "Public Policy," "Rawls," "Reasoning," "Respect," "Rights," "Situations," and "Utilitarianism."

2.
Bioethics as a Field of Ethics

INTRODUCTION

Bioethics emerged as a discrete area of intellectual inquiry in the late 1960s and early 1970s. The publication of Paul Ramsey's book, *The Patient as Person*, in 1970 serves as a convenient reference point for intensified academic, professional, and public interest in this interdisciplinary field.

No new field arises without building on antecedent discussions and disciplines. Bioethics is no exception to this rule. Within the Western intellectual tradition, discussions of professional ethics for physicians go back at least to the time of Hippocrates. As nursing became a profession in the 1800s, creative leaders like Florence Nightingale laid the foundations for the later codes of nursing ethics. However, the development of ethical standards by and for professionals is only part of the total picture. Influential philosophers and theologians—such as Plato, Aristotle, Augustine, and Thomas Aquinas—discussed problems like personhood, abortion, and euthanasia even before the advent of advanced medical technology. Over many centuries the major Western religious traditions, especially Judaism and Roman Catholicism, developed rather elaborate sets of rules and an impressive literature of case analysis on moral questions like those treated in this book. The law, both in its domestic and international modes, has increasingly been called upon to wrestle with topics like human experimentation, reproductive technologies, and the prolongation of life. Bioethics as it has emerged in the last three decades of the twentieth century draws upon this earlier moral experience and intellectual labor.

Why did bioethics emerge precisely when it did? There is no simple answer to this important question. New biomedical technologies and procedures were surely one important factor. The respirator, the dialysis machine, cardiac transplantation, and the contraceptive pill raised new questions about death, resource allocation, and reproduction. But the social upheavals of the 1960s also played a pivotal role in the emergence of bioethics. It is no accident that popular concern about bioethical questions developed close on the heels of the U.S. civil rights movement and anti-Vietnam War protests. Traditional ethical standards and structures of authority were being called into question in numerous social spheres. Public and professional consciousness about research ethics can be traced in part to a different set of circumstances, one that began with the Nazi medical atrocities and that led, via courageous articles by Henry Beecher in 1966, to the development of elaborate review procedures for research involving human subjects. Further, the economic substructure for bioethics should not be overlooked. As a fraction of the U.S. gross national product, health care has grown from a modest 5.9 percent in 1960 to a hefty 10.9 percent in 1986.[1] In other industrialized nations, health care generally accounts for between 6 percent and 9 percent of the gross domestic product.[2] It is likely that any sphere of economic activity this substantial will continue to be a major focus for ethical discussion and debate.

In his essay in this chapter Stephen Toulmin relates bioethics to Anglo-Saxon moral philosophy in the early twentieth century. According to Toulmin, the direct engagement of moral philosophers with concrete cases and issues in medicine and biomedical research helped to rescue ethics from the abstract irrelevance into which much of the field had fallen.

Danner Clouser provides an encyclopedic map of bioethics. He clearly regards the new field as an *application* of themes and categories from traditional moral philosophy to a specific sphere of human activity. In contrast, Tristram Engelhardt outlines a more ambitious program for bioethics, one that envisions bioethics as the core discipline in a radical reconstruction of metaphysics, ethics, and political philosophy.

L.W.

NOTES

1. U.S. Health Care Financing Administration, Division of National Statistics, Office of the Actuary, "National Health Care Expenditures, 1986–2000," *Health Care Financing Review* 8 (4):1–36; Summer 1987.

2. Organization for Economic Cooperation and Development, *Measuring Health Care, 1960–1983* (Paris: OECD, 1985), 29, 156.

STEPHEN TOULMIN

How Medicine Saved the Life of Ethics

During the first 60 years or so of the twentieth century, two things characterized the discussion of ethical issues in the United States, and to some extent other English-speaking countries also. On the one hand, the theoretical analyses of moral philosophers concentrated on questions of so-called metaethics. Most professional philosophers assumed that their proper business was not to take sides on substantive ethical questions but rather to consider in a more formal way what *kinds* of issues and judgments are properly classified as moral in the first place. On the other hand, in less academic circles, ethical debates repeatedly ran into stalemate. A hard-line group of dogmatists, who appealed either to a code of universal rules or to the authority of a religious system or teacher, confronted a rival group of relativists and subjectivists, who found in the anthropological and psychological diversity of human attitudes evidence to justify a corresponding diversity in moral convictions and feelings.[1]

For those who sought some "rational" way of set-

From *Perspectives in Biology and Medicine* 25 (4): 736–750, Summer 1973. Reprinted with permission of the author and publisher, The University of Chicago Press.

tling ethical disagreements, there developed a period of frustration and perplexity.[2] Faced with the spectacle of rival camps taking up sharply opposed ethical positions (e.g., toward premarital sex or anti-Semitism), they turned in vain to the philosophers for guidance. Hoping for intelligent and perceptive comments on the actual substance of such issues, they were offered only analytical classifications, which sought to locate the realm of moral issues, not to decide them.

Two novel factors contributed to this standoff by making the issue of subjectivity an active and urgent one. For a start, developments in psychology—not least, the public impact of the new psychoanalytic movement—focused attention on the role of feelings in our experience and so reinforced the suspicion that moral opinions have to do more with our emotional reactions to that experience than with our actions in it [3]. So, those opinions came to appear less matters of reason than matters of taste, falling under the old tag, *quot homines, tot sententiae* [as many opinions as there are human beings]. This view of ethics was strengthened by the arguments of the ethnographers and anthropologists, who emphasized the differences to be found between the practices and attitudes of different peoples rather than the common core of problems, institutions, and patterns of life that they share. To cap it all, the anthropologist Edward Westermarck took over Albert Einstein's term "relativity" from physics and discussed the moral implications of anthropology under the title of *Ethical Relativity* [4].

Between them, the new twentieth-century behavioral and social sciences were widely regarded as supporting subjectivist and relativist positions in ethics; this in turn provoked a counterinsistence on the universal and unconditional character of moral principles; and so a battle was joined which could have no satisfactory outcome. For, in case of substantive disagreement, the absolutists had no further reasons to offer for their positions: all they could do was shout more insistently or bring up heavier theological guns. In return, the relativists could only turn away and shrug their shoulders. The final answers to ethical problems thus came, on one side, from unquestioned principles and authoritative commands; on the other, from variable and diverse wishes, feelings, or attitudes; and no agreed procedure for settling disagreements by reasonable argument was acceptable to both sides.

How did the fresh attention that philosophers began paying to the ethics of medicine, beginning around 1960, move the ethical debate beyond this standoff? It did so in four different ways. In place of the earlier concern with attitudes, feelings, and wishes, it substituted a new preoccupation with situations, needs, and interests; it required writers on applied ethics to go beyond the discussion of general principles and rules to a more scrupulous analysis of the particular kinds of "cases" in which they find their application; it redirected that analysis to the professional enterprises within which so many human tasks and duties typically arise; and, finally, it pointed philosophers back to the ideas of "equity," "reasonableness," and "human relationships," which played central roles in the *Ethics* of Aristotle but subsequently dropped out of sight [5, esp. 5.10.1136b30–1137b32]. Here, these four points may be considered in turn.

THE OBJECTIVITY OF INTERESTS

The topics that preoccupied psychologists and anthropologists alike during the first half of the twentieth century were foreign to the concerns of physicians, and they tended to distract attention from those shared features of human nature which define the physiological aspects of human medicine and so help to determine the associated ethical demands. To begin with, the novel anthropological discoveries that exerted most charm over the general public were those customs, or modes of behavior, which appeared odd, unexpected, or even bizarre, as compared with the normal patterns of life familiar in modern industrial societies. The distinctive features of unfamiliar cultures (rain dances, witch doctors, initiation ceremonies, taboos, and the like) captured the imaginations of general readers far more powerfully than those which manifested the common heritage of humanity: the universal need to eat and drink, the shared interest in tending wounds and injuries, and so on. Theoretically, likewise, field anthropologists focused primarily on the differences among cultures, leaving the universals of social structure to the sister science of sociology. In their eyes, the essential thing was to explain the modes of life and activity typical of any culture in terms appropriate to that particular culture, not in terms brought in from outside with the anthropologist's own cultural baggage.

As a result, the whole field of medicine was something of a stumbling block to anthropology. If one studied the procedures employed in handling cases of tuberculosis among, say, pygmies in the Kalahari Desert, it might well turn out that they did not recognize this affliction as being, by Western standards, a true "disease." In that case it might—anthropologically speaking—be inappropriate to comment on their procedures in medical terms at all. On the contrary, witch doctoring must be appraised in "ethnomedical" terms, by standards adapted to the conception of witch doctoring current inside the culture in question.

For those who were concerned with the internal systematicity of a given culture, this might be an acceptable method. In adopting it, however, one was obliged to set aside some of the basic presuppositions of the modern Western (and international) profession of medicine: notably, the assumption that human beings in all cultures share, in most respects, common bodily frames and physiological functions. While the epidemiology of, say, heart disease may in some respects be significantly affected by such cultural factors as diet, the evils of heart disease speak no particular language, and to that extent the efficacy of different procedures for dealing with that condition can be appraised in transcultural terms.

So, the *cross*-cultural study of epidemiology and kindred subjects—what may be called "comparative medicine"—has to be distinguished sharply from the *intra*cultural study of "ethnomedicine." The latter is concerned with the attitudes, customs, and feelings current within exotic cultures in the face of those afflictions that we ourselves know to be diseases, whether or not the people concerned so perceive them. The former, by contrast, is concerned with the treatments available in different countries or cultures, regardless of the special attitudes, customs, or feelings that may cluster around those conditions locally, in one place or another. Fieldworkers from the World Health Organization, for instance, are concerned with comparative medicine and are not deterred from investigating the links between, say, eye disease and polluted water supplies just because members of the affected community do not recognize these links. The central subject matter of medicine thus comprises those objective, universal conditions, afflictions, and needs that can affect human beings in *every* culture, as contrasted with those relative, subjective conditions, complaints, and wishes that are topics for anthropological study in *any given* culture.

Now we are in a position to see how needlessly moral philosophers thrust themselves into the arms of the "ethical relativists" when they adopted anthropology as their example and foundation. An ethics built around cultural differences quickly became an ethics of local attitudes. The same fate overtook those philosophers who sought their example and foundation in the new ideas of early twentieth-century psychology. For they were quickly led into seeing ethical disagreements between one human being and another as rooted in their personal responses to and feelings about the topics in debate; as a result, questions about the soundness of rival moral views were submerged by questions about their origins.

Contrast, for instance, the statement, "She regards premarital sex as wrong *because* her own straitlaced upbringing left her jealous of, and censorious toward, today's less puritanical young"—which offers us a psychological account of the causes by which the ethical view in question was supposedly generated—with the statement, "She regards it as wrong *because* of the unhappiness which the current wave of teenage pregnancies is creating for mothers and offspring alike"—which states the interests with which the view is concerned and the reasons by which it is supported. Modeling ethics on psychology thus once again diverts attention from genuine interests and focuses them instead on labile, personal feelings.

The new attention to applied ethics (particularly medical ethics) has done much to dispel the miasma of subjectivity that was cast around ethics as a result of its association with anthropology and psychology. At least within broad limits, an ethics of "needs" and "interests" is objective and generalizable in a way that an ethics of "wishes" and "attitudes" cannot be. Stated crudely, the question of whether one person's actions put another person's health at risk is normally a question of ascertainable fact, to which there is a straightforward "yes" or "no" answer, not a question of fashion, custom, or taste, about which (as the saying goes) "there is no arguing." This being so, the objections to that person's actions can be presented and discussed in "objective" terms. So, proper attention to the example of medicine has helped to pave the way for a reintroduction of "objective" standards of good and harm and for a return to methods of practical reasoning about moral issues that are not available to either the dogmatists or the relativists.

THE IMPORTANCE OF CASES

One writer who was already contributing to the renewed discussion of applied ethics as early as the 1950s was Joseph Fletcher of the University of Virginia, who has recently been the object of harsh criticism from more dogmatic thinkers for introducing the phrase "situation ethics."[3] To judge from his critics' tone, you might think that he was the spokesman for laxity and amorality, whereas he belongs, in fact, to a very respectable line of Protestant (specifically, Episcopalian) moral theologians. A main influence on him in his youth was Bishop Kenneth Kirk, whose book on *Conscience and Its Problems*, published in 1927 [9], was one of the few systematic works by an early twentieth-century Protestant theologian to employ the "case method" more usually associated with the Catholic casuists. Via Kirk, Fletcher thus became an inheritor of the older Evangelical tradition of Frederick Dennison Maurice.[4]

Like his predecessors in the consideration of "cases of conscience," Kirk was less concerned to discuss conduct in terms of abstract rules and principles than he was to address in concrete detail the moral quandaries in which real people actually find themselves. Like his distinguished predecessors—from Aristotle and Hermagoras to Boethius, Aquinas, and the seventeenth-century Jesuits—he understood very well the force of the old maxim, "circumstances alter cases." As that maxim indicates, we can understand fully what is at stake in any human situation and how it creates moral problems for the agents involved in it only if we know the precise circumstances "both of the agent and of the act": if we lack that knowledge, we are in no position to say anything of substance about the situation, and all our appeals to general rules and principles will be mere hot air. So, in retrospect, Joseph Fletcher's introduction of the phrase "situation ethics" can be viewed as one further chapter in a history of "the ethics of *cases*," as contrasted with "the ethics of *rules and principles*"; this is another area in which the ethics of medicine has recently given philosophers some useful pointers for the analysis of moral issues.

Let me here mention one of these, which comes out of my own personal experience. From 1975 to 1978 I worked as a consultant and staff member with the National Commission for the Protection of Human Subjects of Biomedical and Behavioral Research, based in Washington, D.C.; I was struck by the extent to which the commissioners were able to reach agreement in making recommendations about ethical issues of great complexity and delicacy.[5] If the earlier theorists had been right, and ethical considerations really depended on variable cultural attitudes or labile personal feelings, one would have expected 11 people of such different backgrounds as the members of the commission to be far more divided over such moral questions than they ever proved to be in actual fact. Even on such thorny subjects as research involving prisoners, mental patients, and human fetuses, it did not take the commissioners long to identify the crucial issues that they needed to address, and, after patient analysis of these issues, any residual differences of opinion were rarely more than marginal, with different commissioners inclined to be somewhat more conservative, or somewhat more liberal, in their recommendations. Never, as I recall, did their deliberations end in deadlock, with supporters of rival principles locking horns and refusing to budge. The problems that had to be argued through at length arose, not on the level of the principles themselves, but at the point of applying them: when difficult moral balances had to be struck between, for example, the general claims of medical discovery and its future beneficiaries and the present welfare or autonomy of individual research subjects.

How was the commission's consensus possible? It rested precisely on this last feature of their agenda: namely, its close concentration on specific types of problematic cases. Faced with "hard cases," they inquired what particular conflicts of claim or interest

were exemplified in them, and they usually ended by balancing off those claims in very similar ways. Only when the individual members of the commission went on to explain their own particular "reasons" for supporting the general consensus did they begin to go seriously different ways. For, then, commissioners from different backgrounds and faiths "justified" their votes by appealing to general views and abstract principles which differed far more deeply than their opinions about particular substantive questions. Instead of "deducing" their opinions about particular cases from general principles that could lend strength and conviction to those specific opinions, they showed a far greater certitude about particular cases than they ever achieved about general matters.

This outcome of the commission's work should not come as any great surprise to physicians who have reflected deeply about the nature of clinical judgment in medicine. In traditional case morality, as in medical practice, the first indispensable step is to assemble a rich enough "case history." Until that has been done, the wise physician will suspend judgment. If he is too quick to let theoretical considerations influence his clinical analysis, they may prejudice the collection of a full and accurate case record and so distract him from what later turn out to have been crucial clues. Nor would this outcome have been any surprise to Aristotle, either. Ethics and clinical medicine are both prime examples of the concrete fields of thought and reasoning in which (as he insisted) the theoretical rigor of geometrical argument is unattainable: fields in which we should above all strive to be *reasonable* rather than insisting on a kind of *exactness* that "the nature of the case" does not allow [5, 1.3.1094b12–27].

This same understanding of the differences between practical and theoretical reasoning was taken over by Aquinas, who built it into his own account of "natural law" and "case morality," and so it became part of the established teaching of Catholic moral theologians. As such, it was in harmony with the pastoral practices of the confessional [12, D.3, Q.5, A.2, Solutio]. Thus, Aquinas's own version of the fundamental maxim was framed as an injunction to the confessor—"like a prudent physician"—to take into account *peccatoris circumstantiae atque peccati*, that is, "the circumstances both of the sinner and of the sin." Later, however, the alleged readiness of confessors to soften their judgments in the light of irrelevant "circumstances" exposed them to criticism. In particular, the seventeenth-century French Jesuits were attacked by their Jansenist coreligionists on the ground that they "made allowances" in favor of rich and high-born penitents that they denied to those who were less well favored. And, when the Jansenist Arnauld was brought before an ecclesiastical court on a charge of heterodoxy, his friend Pascal launched a vigorous counterattack on the Jesuit casuists of his time by publishing the series of anonymous *Lettres provinciales* which from that time on gave "casuistry" its unsavory reputation.[6]

Looking back, however, we may wonder how far this reputation was really justified. No doubt, a venal priest could corrupt the confessional by showing undue favor to penitents of wealth or power: for example, by fabricating specious "extenuating circumstances" to excuse conduct that was basically inexcusable. But we have no reliable way of knowing how often this really happened, and the mere possibility of such corruption does nothing to change the original point—namely, that practical decisions in ethics can never be made by appeal to "self-evident principles" alone and rest rather on a clinical appreciation of the significant details characteristic of particular cases. No doubt, we are free to use the word "casuistry"—like the parallel words "wizardry" and "sophistry"—to refer to "the *dishonest* use of the casuist's (or the clinician's) arts,"[7] but that does no more to discredit the honest use of "case morality" than it does the honest use of case methods in clinical medicine.

By taking one step further, indeed, we may view the problems of clinical medicine and the problems of applied ethics as two varieties of a common species. Defined in purely general terms, such ethical categories as "cruelty" and "kindness," "laziness" and "conscientiousness," have a certain abstract, truistical quality: before they can acquire any specific relevance, we have to identify some *actual* person, or piece of conduct, as "kind" or "cruel," "conscientious" or "lazy," and there is often disagreement even about that preliminary step. Similarly, in medicine: if described in general terms alone, diseases too are "abstract entities," and they acquire a practical relevance only for those who have learned the diagnostic art of identifying real-life cases as being cases of one disease rather than another.

In its form (if not entirely in its point) the *art* of practical judgment in ethics thus resembles the art of clinical diagnosis and prescription. In both fields, theoretical generalities are helpful to us only up to a point, and their actual application to particular cases demands, also, a human capacity to recognize the slight but significant features that mark off, say, a "case" of minor muscular strain from a life-threatening disease or a "case" of decent reticence from one of cowardly silence. Once brought to the bedside, so to say, applied ethics and clinical medicine use just the same Aristotelean kinds of "practical reasoning," and a correct choice of therapeutic procedure in medicine is the *right* treatment to pursue, not just as a matter of medical technique but for ethical reasons also.

"MY STATION AND ITS DUTIES"

In the last decades of the nineteenth century, F. H. Bradley of Oxford University expounded an ethical position that placed "duties" in the center of the philosophical picture, and the recent concern of moral philosophers with applied ethics (most specifically, medical ethics) has given them a new insight into his arguments also. It was a mistake (Bradley argued) to discuss moral obligations purely in universalistic terms, as though nobody was subject to moral claims unless they applied to everybody—unless we could, according to the Kantian formula, "will them to become universal laws." On the contrary, different people are subject to different moral claims, depending on where they "stand" toward the other people with whom they have to deal, for example, their families, colleagues, and fellow citizens [13].

For Bradley, that is to say, the central consideration in practical ethics was the agent's standing, status, or station. He himself preferred to use the last of these three words (i.e., "station"), and this led his liberal contemporaries to undervalue his arguments. They suspected him of subscribing to the conservative sentiments of the old couplet, "God bless the Squire and his relations,/And keep us in our proper stations"—that is, the stations to which "it *has pleased* [rather than *shall please*] God to call us." Yet this was an unfortunate response since, as we now realize, Bradley was drawing attention to points of real importance. As the modern discussion of medical ethics has taught us, professional affiliations and concerns play a significant part in shaping a physician's obligations and commitments, and this insight has stimulated detailed discussions both about professionalism in general and, more specifically, about the relevance of "the physician/patient relationship" to the medical practitioner's duties and obligations.[8]

Once embarked on, the subject of professionalism has proved to be rich and fruitful. It has led, for instance, to a renewed interest in Max Weber's sociological analysis of vocation (*Beruf*) and bureaucracy, and this in turn has had implications of two kinds for the ethics of the professions. For, on the one hand, the manner in which professionals perceive their position as providers of services influences both their sense of calling and also the obligations which they acknowledge on that account. And, on the other hand, the professionalization of medicine, law, and similar activities has exposed practitioners to new conflicts of interest between, for example, the individual physician's duties to a patient and his loyalty to the profession, as when his conduct is criticized as "unprofessional" for harming, not his clients, but rather his colleagues.

In recent years, as a result, moral philosophers have begun to look specifically and in greater detail at the situations within which ethical problems typically arise and to pay closer attention to the human relationships that are embodied in those situations. In ethics, as elsewhere, the tradition of radical individualism for too long encouraged people to overlook the "mediating structures" and "intermediate institutions" (family, profession, voluntary associations, etc.) which stand between the individual agent and the larger scale context of his actions. So, in political theory, the obligation of the individual toward the state was seen as the only problem worth focusing on; meanwhile, in moral theory, the differences of status (or station) which in practice expose us to different sets of obligations (or duties) were ignored in favor of a theory of justice (or rights) that deliberately concealed these differences behind a "veil of ignorance."[9]

On this alternative view, the only just—even, properly speaking, the only moral—obligations are those that apply to us all equally, regardless of our standing. By undertaking the tasks of a profession, an agent will no doubt accept certain special duties, but so it will be for us all. The obligation to perform those duties is "just" or "moral" only because it exemplifies more general and universalizable obligations of trust, which require us to do what we have undertaken to do. So, any exclusive emphasis on the universal aspects of morality can end by distracting attention from just those things which the student of applied ethics finds most absorbing—namely, the specific tasks and obligations that any profession lays on its practitioners.

Most recently, Alasdair MacIntyre has pursued these considerations further in his new book, *After Virtue* [16]. MacIntyre argues that the public discussion of ethical issues has fallen into a kind of Babel, which largely springs from our losing any sense of the ways in which *community* creates obligations for us. One thing that can help restore that lost sense of community is the recognition that, at the present time, our professional commitments have taken on many of the roles that our communal commitments used to play. Even people who find moral philosophy generally unintelligible usually acknowledge and respect the specific ethical demands associated with their own professions or jobs, and this offers us some kind of a foundation on which to begin reconstructing our view of ethics. For it reminds us that we are in no position to fashion individual lives for ourselves, purely *as individuals*. Rather, we find ourselves born into communities in which the available ways of acting are largely laid out in advance: in which human activity takes on different *Lebensformen*, or "forms of life" (of which the professions are one special case), and our obligations are shaped by the requirements of those forms.

In this respect, the lives and obligations of professionals are no different from those of their lay brethren. Professional obligations arise out of the enterprises of the professions in just the same kinds of way that other general moral obligations arise out of our shared forms of life; if we are at odds about the *theory* of ethics, that is because we have misunderstood the basis which ethics has in our actual *practice*. Once again, in other words, it was medicine—as the first profession to which philosophers paid close attention during the new phase of "applied ethics" that opened during the 1960s—that set the example which was required in order to revive some important, and neglected, lines of argument within moral philosophy itself.

EQUITY AND INTIMACY

Two final themes have also attracted special attention as a result of the new interaction between medicine and philosophy. Both themes were presented in clear enough terms by Aristotle in the *Nicomachean Ethics*. But, as so often happens, the full force of Aristotle's concepts and arguments was overlooked by subsequent generations of philosophers, who came to ethics with very different preoccupations. Aristotle's own Greek terms for these notions are *epieikeia* and *philia*, which are commonly translated as "reasonableness" and "friendship," but I shall argue here that they correspond more closely to the modern terms, "equity" and "personal relationship" [5].

Modern readers sometimes have difficulty with the style of Aristotle's *Ethics* and lose patience with the book, because they suspect the author of evading philosophical questions that they have their own reasons for regarding as central. Suppose, for instance, that we go to Aristotle's text in the hope of finding some account of the things that mark off "right" from "wrong": if we attempt to press this question, Aristotle will always slip out of our grasp. What makes one course of action better than another? We can answer that question, he replies, only if we first consider what kind of a person the agent is and what relationships he stands in toward the other people who are involved in his actions; he sets about explaining why the kinds of relationship, and the kinds of conduct, that are possible as between "large-spirited human beings" who share the same social standing are simply not possible as between, say, master and servant, or parent and child [5].

The bond of *philia* between free and equal friends is of one kind, that between father and son of another kind, that between master and slave of a third, and there is no common scale in which we can measure the corresponding kinds of conduct. By emphasizing this point, Aristotle draws attention to an important point about the manner in which "actions" are classified, even before we say anything ethical about them. Within two different relationships the very same deeds, or the very same words, may—from the ethical point of view—represent quite different *acts* or *actions*. Words that would be a perfectly proper command from an officer to an enlisted man, or a straightforward order from a master to a servant, might be a humiliation if uttered by a father to a son, or an insult if exchanged between friends. A judge may likewise have a positive duty to say, from the bench, things that he would never dream of saying in a situation where he was no longer acting *ex officio*, while a physician may have occasion, and even be obliged, to do things to a patient in the course of a medical consultation that he would never be permitted to do in any other context.

It is easy to let oneself be distracted by Aristotle's use of "the master-slave relationship" to illustrate the differences between different kinds of *philia*. But the points that he wishes to emphasize have nothing to do with slavery as such, and they hold good equally well if applied instead to our old friend, "the physician-patient relationship." For, surely, the very deed or utterance by Dr. A toward Mrs. B which would be a routine inquiry or examination within a strictly professional "physician-patient relationship"—for example, during a gynecological consultation—might be grounds for a claim of assault if performed outside that protected context. The *philia* (or relationship) between them will be quite different in the two situations, and, on this account, the "circumstances" do indeed "alter cases" in ways that are directly reflected in the demands of professional ethics.

With this as background, we can turn to Aristotle's ideas about *epieikeia* ("reasonableness" or "equity"). As to this notion, Aristotle pioneered the general doctrine that principles never settle ethical issues by themselves: that is, that we can grasp the moral force of principles only by studying the ways in which they are applied to, and within, particular situations. The need for such a practical approach is most obvious, in judicial practice, in the exercise of "equitable jurisdiction," where the courts are required to decide cases by appeal, not to specific, well-defined laws or statutes, but to general considerations of fairness, of "maxims of equity." In these situations, the courts do not have the benefit of carefully drawn rules, which have been formulated with the specific aim that they should be precise and self-explanatory: rather, they are guided by rough proverbial mottoes—phrases about "clean hands" and the like. The questions at issue in such cases are, in other words, very broad questions—for example, about what would be *just* or *reasonable* as between two or more individuals when all the available facts about their respective situations have been taken into account [17–19]. Similar patterns of situations and arguments are, of course, to be found in everyday ethics also, and the Aristotelean idea of *epieikeia* is a direct intellectual ancestor of a central notion (still referred to as "epikeia") in the Roman Catholic traditions of moral theology and pastoral care [11].

In ethics and law alike, the two ideas of *philia* ("friendship" or "relationship") and *epieikeia* (or "equity") are closely connected. The expectations that we place on people's lines of conduct will differ markedly depending on who is affected and what relationships the parties stand in toward one another. Far from regarding it as "fair" or "just" to deal with everybody in a precisely *equal* fashion, as the "veil of ignorance" might suggest, we consider it perfectly *equitable*, or *reasonable*, to show some degree of partiality, or favor, in dealing with close friends and relatives whose special needs and concerns we understand. What father, for instance, does not have an eye to his children's individual personalities and tastes?

And, apart from downright "favoritism," who would regard such differences of treatment as unjust? Nor, surely, can it be morally offensive to discriminate, within reason, between close friends and distant acquaintances, colleagues and business rivals, neighbors and strangers? We are who we are: we stand in the human relationships we do, and our specific moral duties and obligations can be discussed in practice *only* at the point at which these questions of personal standing and relationship have been recognized and taken into the account.

CONCLUSION

From the mid-nineteenth century on, then, British and American moral philosophers treated ethics as a field for general theoretical inquiries and paid little attention to issues of application or particular types of cases. The philosopher who did most to inaugurate this new phase was Henry Sidgwick, and, from an autobiographical note, we know that he was reacting against the work of his contemporary, William Whewell [20, 21]. Whewell had written a textbook for use by undergraduates at Cambridge University that resembled in many respects a traditional manual of casuistics, containing separate sections on the ethics of promises or contracts, family and community, benevolence, and so on [22]. For his part, Sidgwick found Whewell's discussion too messy: there must be some way of introducing into the subject the kinds of rigor, order, and certainty associated with, for example, mathematical reasoning. So, ignoring all of Aristotle's cautions about the differences between the practical modes of reasoning appropriate to ethics and the formal modes appropriate to mathematics, he set out to expound the theoretical principles (or "methods") of ethics in a systematic form.

By the early twentieth century, the new program for moral philosophy had been narrowed down still further, so initiating the era of "metaethics." The philosopher's task was no longer to organize our moral beliefs into comprehensive systems: that would have meant *taking sides* over substantive issues. Rather, it was his duty to stand back from the fray and hold the ring while partisans of different views argued out their differences in accordance with the general rules for the conduct of "rational debate," or the expression of "moral attitudes," as defined in *metaethical* terms. And this was still the general state of affairs in Anglo-American moral philosophy in the late 1950s and the early 1960s, when public attention began to turn to questions of medical ethics. By this time, the central concerns of the philosophers had become so abstract and general—above all, so definitional or analytical—that they had, in effect, lost all touch with the concrete and particular issues that arise in actual practice, whether in medicine or elsewhere.

Once this demand for intelligent discussion of the ethical problems of medical practice and research obliged them to pay fresh attention to applied ethics, however, philosophers found their subject "coming alive again" under their hands. But, now it was no longer a field for academic, theoretical, even mandarin investigation alone. Instead, it had to be debated in practical, concrete, even political terms, and before long moral philosophers (or, as they barbarously began to be called, "ethicists")[10] found that they were as liable as the economists to be called on to write "op ed" pieces for the *New York Times*, or to testify before congressional committees.

Have philosophers wholly risen to this new occasion? Have they done enough to modify their previous methods of analysis to meet these new practical needs? About those questions there can still be several opinions. Certainly, it would be foolhardy to claim that the discussion of "bioethics" has reached a definitive form, or to rule out the possibility that novel methods will earn a place in the field in the years ahead. At this very moment, indeed, the style of current discussion appears to be shifting away from attempts to relate problematic cases to general theories—whether those of Kant, Rawls, or the utilitarians—to a more direct analysis of the practical cases themselves, using methods more like those of traditional "case morality." (See, e.g., the discussion in a recent issue of the *Hastings Center Report* of the moral issues that are liable to arise in cases of sex-change surgery [23, pp. 8–13].)

Whatever the future may bring, however, these 20 years of interaction with medicine, law, and the other professions have had spectacular and irreversible effects on the methods and content of philosophical ethics. By reintroducing into ethical debate the vexed topics raised by *particular cases*, they have obliged philosophers to address once again the Aristotelean problems of *practical reasoning*, which had been on the sidelines for too long. In this sense, we may indeed say that, during the last 20 years, medicine has "saved the life of ethics," and that it has given back to ethics a seriousness and human relevance which it had seemed—at least, in the writings of the interwar years—to have lost for good.

NOTES

1. For a further exploration of the standoff, see [1].

2. It was, in fact, just this problem which presented itself to me when I wrote my doctoral dissertation [2].

3. Just how much of a pioneer Joseph Fletcher was in opening up the modern discussion of the ethics of medicine is clear from the early publication date (1954) of his first publications on this subject [6–8].

4. It was Albert Jonsen who drew my attention to the work of Kenneth Kirk and his great forerunner, the mid-nineteenth-century Evangelical teacher, F. D. Maurice [10]. For further discussion consult A. R. Jonsen [11].

5. The work of the national commission generated a whole series of government publications—mainly reports and recommendations on the ethical aspects of research involving research subjects from specially "vulnerable" groups having diminished autonomy, such as young children and prisoners. I have written a fuller discussion of the commission's work for a forthcoming Hastings Center book on the "closure" of disputes about matters of technical policy. As a member of the commission, A. R. Jonsen was also struck by the casuistical character of its work, and this led to the research project of which this paper is one product.

6. The *Lettres provinciales* were published periodically, and anonymously, in 1656–57, but it did not take long for their authorship to be discovered, and they have remained perhaps the best-known documents on the subject of "case reasoning" in ethics. The intellectual relationship between the vigorous attack on the laxity of the Jesuits' case morality contained in the *Lettres* and the larger program of seventeenth-century philosophy deserves closer study than it has yet received.

7. For the word "casuistry," see the entry in the complete *Oxford English Dictionary*, which revealingly points out how many English nouns ending in "ry" (e.g., "Sophistry," "wizardry," and "Popery") are dyslogistic. It seems to be no accident that the earliest use of the word "casuistry" cited in the *OED* dates only from 1725—i.e., after Pascal's attack on the Jesuit casuists. This helps to explain, and confirm, the current derogatory tone of the word.

8. See Bledstein's discussion [14, p. 107] of the nineteenth-century confusion between codes of ethics and codes of etiquette within such professional societies as the American Medical Association.

9. I borrow this phrase a trifle unfairly from John Rawls [15], but I have argued at greater length in [1] that *any* unbalanced emphasis on "universality" divorced from "equity" is a recipe for the ethics of relations between strangers and leaves untouched those important issues that arise between people who are linked by more complex relationships.

10. Once again, the *Oxford English Dictionary* has a point to make. It includes the word "ethicist" but leaves it without the dignity of a definition, beyond the bare etymology, "ethics + ist."

REFERENCES

1. Toulmin, S. The tyranny of principles, *Hastings Cent. Rep.* 11:6, 1981.

2. Toulmin, S. *The Place of Reason in Ethics*. Cambridge: Cambridge Univ. Press, 1949.

3. Stevenson, C. L. *Ethics and Language*. New Haven, Conn.: Yale Univ. Press, 1944.

4. Westermarck, E. *Ethical Relativity*. New York: Harcourt Brace, 1932.

5. Aristotle, *Nicomachean Ethics*.

6. Fletcher, J. *Morals and Medicine*. Princeton, N.J.: Princeton Univ. Press, 1954.

7. Fletcher, J. *Situation Ethics*. Philadelphia: Westminster, 1966.

8. Fletcher, J. *Humanhood*. Buffalo, N.Y.: Prometheus, 1979.

9. Kirk, K. *Conscience and Its Problems*, 1927.

10. Maurice, F. *Conscience: Lectures on Casuistry Delivered in the University of Cambridge*. London, 1872.

11. Jonsen, A. R. Can an ethicist be a consultant? In *Frontiers in Medical Ethics*, edited by A. Abernathy. Cambridge: Bollingen, 1980.

12. Aquinas, Thomas. *Commentarium Libro Tertio Sententiarum*.

13. Bradley, F. *Ethical Studies*. London, 1876.

14. Bledstein, B. *The Culture of Professionalism*. New York: Norton, 1976.

15. Rawls, J. *A Theory of Justice*. Cambridge, Mass.: Harvard Univ. Press, 1971.

16. MacIntyre, A. *After Virtue*. South Bend, Ind.: Notre Dame Univ. Press, 1981.

17. Davis, K. *Discretionary Justice*. Urbana: Univ. Illinois Press, 1969.

18. Newman, R. *Equity and Law*. Dobbs Ferry, N.Y.: Oceana, 1961.

19. Hamburger, M. *Morals and Law: The Growth of Aristotle's Legal Theory*. New Haven, Conn.: Yale Univ. Press, 1951.

20. Sidgwick, H. *The Methods of Ethics*, Introduction to 6th ed. London and New York: Macmillan, 1901.

21. Schneewind, J. *Sidgwick's Ethics and Victorian Moral Philosophy*. Oxford and New York: Oxford Univ. Press, 1977.

22. Whewell, W. *The Elements of Morality*, 4th ed. Cambridge: Bell, 1864.

23. Marriage, morality and sex change surgery: four traditions in case ethics. *Hastings Cent. Rep.*, August 1981.

K. DANNER CLOUSER

Bioethics

INTRODUCTION

An Encyclopedia of Bioethics—or of Psychology or Religion or any special field of knowledge—need not have an entry on the very title of the work itself. The present encyclopedia is an extensive, almost exhaustive, collection of those issues and topics thought to be part of or directly relevant to bioethics. Yet beyond the scope of all these articles perhaps some questions will remain for the inquisitive reader—such questions as: How is bioethics related to ethics? Where does medical ethics fit in? Does bioethics have special problems or special principles? Is bioethics related to scientific facts in a way ordinary ethics is not? These, and related questions, will constitute the focus of this [article].

It would be inappropriate at this point to define "bioethics" in the sense of setting limits to what should and should not count as bioethics. Rather this article, in dealing with the questions mentioned, will aim at provoking reflection on the nature of bioethics. Such reflection is not necessary for "doing" bioethics, that is, for understanding or working through issues within bioethics. It is intended for the inquisitive who are seeking a conceptual grasp of the field itself—an overview of what it is up to and of its relations with other, but similar, concerns. This article will be a guided tour through some of the questions, tensions, alternatives, and arguments that surround the concept of bioethics but would not necessarily arise in the course of pursuing issues *within* bioethics.

Fitting the object of our focus into its natural landscape is a helpful first step. The varieties of factors giving rise to concerns labeled "bioethics" have

involved two main factors: increased capability and knowledge. Being capable of something (keeping a dying patient alive, discovering fetal characteristics before birth, transplanting body organs, etc.) forces the question, "Ought we to do it?"—a question irrelevant to practice so long as we are not capable of doing it. Increased knowledge, insofar as it discovers unforeseen consequences of our actions (spray cans and the ozone layer, nuclear energy plants and perinatal development, etc.), forces moral decisions we had not anticipated. Moreover, increased capability and knowledge can bring more benefits, which in turn raises the problem of their fair distribution. This mixture is then ignited by a general, culturewide emphasis on individual rights. Additionally, increased knowledge has led to specialization, producing "the expert" into whose hands we have entrusted everything. He alone, we thought, had the necessary competence. Supposedly these were just technical, factual matters that we had relinquished to the expert. The economist, the highway engineer, the energy expert, the diplomat, the financial wizard, the doctor—they all knew best. But we eventually came to realize that *values*, unbeknownst even to the experts, were being unwittingly employed in ostensibly factual equations. The resultant decisions greatly affect our quality of life.

The preceding paragraph is merely a reminder of the context that has given emphasis to a discipline called "bioethics." It is mentioned only to reinforce our seeing bioethics as a natural response to new dilemmas, increased knowledge, and threatened rights—rather than as at bottom a new discovery of basic principles or derivations therefrom. Also, in putting bioethics into perspective, we are reminded that it is part of a general move toward ferreting out values that had been camouflaged by factuality and

Reprinted with permission of the publisher from Warren T. Reich, ed., *Encyclopedia of Bioethics* (New York: Free Press, 1978), pp. 115–161.

clarifying rights to which we had been blinded by the glare of the unquestioned "common good." All this ties in with the position that, by and large, will be taken in this article—namely, that bioethics is not a new set of principles or maneuvers, but the same old ethics being applied to a particular realm of concerns. . . .

A FIRST APPROXIMATION: MEDICAL ETHICS

The issues will be more manageable if we approach "bioethics" by first examining the more limited case of medical ethics. It is a particular instance of the same position that will be taken with respect to bioethics. The basic point can be made and questioned in this more limited arena, and then expanded to the sphere of bioethics. (It should be noted that the distinction between "moral" and "ethical" will not be rigorously adhered to in this article.)

Medical ethics is a special kind of ethics only insofar as it relates to a particular realm of facts and concerns and not because it embodies or appeals to some special moral principles or methodology. It is applied ethics. It consists of the same moral principles and rules that we would appeal to, and argue for, in ordinary circumstances. It is just that in medical ethics these familiar moral rules are being applied to situations peculiar to the medical world. We have only to scratch the surface of medical ethics and we break through to the issues of "standard" ethics as we have always known them. Of course, understanding the facts, distinctions, relationships, and concepts of the world of medicine in order to apply these "ordinary" moral rules is an immense task. But it is precisely that task which primarily comprises medical ethics.

"Do not kill" is a moral rule. It would not be this rule itself that would be challenged or justified within medical ethics. Nor would medical ethics as such be concerned with articulating and defending criteria for exceptions to the rule. Rather medical ethics prepares the ground for the constructions of ordinary ethics. Is withdrawing lifesaving therapy an instance of killing? Is the refusal to initiate a life-support system an instance of killing? Are we killing one when we give the limited lifesaving facilities to another instead? We are not questioning whether we should kill or not; we accept that "ordinary" moral rule. What we are questioning is whether, in these special and difficult situations, our action is appropriately labeled "killing." If we decided these were instances of killing, we would probably take the next step: deliberating whether they

were justifiable exceptions to the moral rule, "Do not kill." In considering the nature of exceptions and their justification, we would in effect be back in "ordinary" ethics. But in examining the medical details for distinctions, relationships, implications, and the like in order to apply the criteria for exceptions, we would be doing medical ethics. That is, we are preparing the ground for the "application" of ethics.

We might see the same points with issues less weighty than that of killing. For example, "Do not deceive" is a moral rule of ordinary ethics (or so it might be argued). But what constitutes deceiving in the medical realm? This again calls for a careful understanding of what goes on in that realm and perhaps for subtle distinctions and conceptual analyses in order to determine when deceiving is really taking place. And, again, intimate knowledge of these particulars would be important in determining when exceptions to the rule are justified.

This clean distinction between ethics, on the one hand, and the world of medicine, on the other, smudges a bit upon closer inspection, though not enough to invalidate the basic point. Two factors are responsible for blurring the demarcation. First, in what has been called "preparing the ground" (i.e., classifying, drawing distinctions, sorting out causes and effects, uncovering implicit values in the medical realm) there may very well be an ethics-laden element. How one views ethics—its point, methods, justification, etc.— may influence how one prepares the factual and conceptual ground to receive the moral rules. There could conceivably be a prejudice in arranging the data for moral deliberation—a familiar phenomenon whenever data and theory are wed.

Second, problems arise within medicine as a result of unusual capabilities and circumstances that were not in view as morality was forged. These in turn put pressure on ethics to answer questions for which it was not designed or to refashion itself in order to answer those questions. If refashioning occurred in the face of these special circumstances, would not the result be what is truly medical ethics and not simply ordinary ethics applied to special circumstances? Very likely, but it is not at all clear that such refashioning has been necessary. However, it is a possibility to which the reader should remain alert. The situation seems analogous to that of the implied rights and powers of the Constitution. Do these implications, having been drawn out and articulated to meet special circumstances, really comprise a new constitution, or are they simply applications of the "old" Constitution to new circumstances?

CHALLENGES TO THIS VIEW OF MEDICAL ETHICS

Before going on to expand the limited case of medical ethics to the more general instance of bioethics, there are questions that ought to be posed concerning the preceding view of medical ethics.

PROLIFERATION OF KINDS OF ETHICS

A sort of *reductio ad absurdum* might go like this: If every area where ethics is applied gets its own name, we will have a proliferation of "kinds" of ethics beyond compare. There will be "baker ethics," "banker ethics," "barber ethics," "bartender ethics," "bicycler ethics," and on and on.

But this does not seem to be a good argument against the view presented, simply because what purports to be *absurdum* is not so absurd after all. All the different realms of activity do in fact have ethical concerns. (Indeed, physicians frequently wonder why *they* are singled out for ethical emphasis instead of car mechanics and myriad others!) What sounds silly, of course, is that each would have its own name. That we do not in fact have separate names for the infinite variety of activities where ethics is applicable can be explained in other ways. Most of these activities are more easily understood, present few conceptual difficulties, do not encounter unique situations that strain ordinary ethics, and are not intimately and deeply involved with human life, death, and well-being. Hence they are not highlighted with names of their own. Notice that some instances of naming ethics for particular areas of concern do not strike us as odd at all: "environmental ethics," "business ethics," "legal ethics," "political ethics." The labels both express and reinforce any focus on concerns that hold for us considerable importance, interest, and complexity.

Actually the *reductio ad absurdum* could be turned on the very position it purports to be defending, namely, that medical ethics is a special kind of ethics, with its own principles, rules, and methods. By extension this might suggest that every area of concern and activity has its own ethical principles—butcher, baker, candlestick maker, and everybody else. This would make a farce of ethics, which at the very least should be the same for all of us. . . .

TRADITIONAL MEANING OF MEDICAL ETHICS

The last challenge is an appeal to what has been traditionally meant by "medical ethics." This has included an extensive range of admonitions varying with culture, time, and type of medicine, and dealing with demeanor, rebates for referrals, decorum in consultations, soliciting another's patient, rumor mongering about other doctors, advertising, and endless other behavioral possibilities within medicine. There is no denying that this is largely what has been known in the past as "medical ethics." But does this traditional view of medical ethics invalidate the view of medical ethics taken in this article? The answer is probably that it partly does and partly does not. That is, traditional medical ethics is such a conglomeration of things that some aspects fall in nicely with the view espoused here, and some do not. But staking claim to the term "medical ethics" is not the goal; understanding is. What follows is an attempt to sort out several strands within traditional medical ethics and to put them in perspective from an ethical point of view. The upshot will be that one strand supports the espoused view, another is consistent with it, and a third is irrelevant to it.

The strand that confirms the view expressed here is that which is attentive to the harm that can be done others. Urging the physicians to keep confidences, to comfort patients when therapy is no longer effective, and not to insult one another might be seen as a translation of general morality into the medical context. These, and many such rules, can be seen as tailoring the general rules of morality, which are binding on us all, to specific situations within medicine. The object, as in general morality, is (very roughly) to avoid causing harm to individuals and to the community at large (e.g., by a general breakdown of trust). . . .

A great deal of medical ethics can be seen as an effort to decide and make explicit what these duties are or should be for physicians. Of course, there is nothing universal about the particulars arrived at, and they fluctuate according to different society structures, differing views of medicine, health, and cure, and different capabilities. The important thing is that they be explicit so that society knows what to expect and that they be consistent with the other moral rules. Indeed, many of the delineated duties are best seen simply as rational social arrangements. However lofty and solemn they may sound, they are at bottom a spelling out of "promises," shaped by abilities, needs, traditions, and expectations. They could be quite other than they are and still be good, so long as they made explicit what could be expected by patients. This interpretation fits nicely with our tendency to refer to these matters as medical "etiquette" rather than "morals." That tendency bespeaks our realization that these matters are of a different order from morality. . . .

[Another] strand distinguishable in codes of medical ethics seems not to be concerned with ethics, according to the position taken in this article. The strictures, "Keep heads clear and hands steady," "Be humble," and "Give respect and gratitude to teachers" sound like tactical advice. Rather than admonishing one not to cause this or that kind of harm, these sayings are recommending how one's life might be enriched and how one might even promote happiness in others. In the ethical view assumed (rightly or wrongly) in this article, these statements are more a "guide to life" than morality; but it is important to observe that other views of ethics might regard them as pertaining to the essence of morality.

In this category one might also place those admonitions that are really self-serving—which protect the physician and his guild and which promote medicine as a profession. These elements are best regarded as strategical advice. Examples are here being avoided because they are individually open to a variety of interpretations, and this is not the place to argue for one or another interpretation, but only to establish this classification. An instance would be the restriction against advertising: Though it seems primarily self-serving, a case might be made for its protecting the public.

Because "medical ethics" has meant such a variety of things, and because our ethical concerns with medicine often lead us beyond issues of medicine narrowly defined, another term might be useful. "Bioethics" is a good candidate. This term offers the advantage (1) of suggesting a much wider concern than simply rules of behavior for a particular guild, and (2) of connoting more broadly both the ethics and the science–technology out of which the issues grow.

BIOETHICS

The plan has been to examine medical ethics prior to dealing with "bioethics." One reason for this approach was that the same stance would be taken with respect to both, namely, that both are instances of ordinary morality applied to new areas of concern. Another reason was the expectation that, if medical ethics is understood as a more particularized case of ethical concern, the expansion to the more general case of bioethics will be easier. Furthermore, the variables unique to each are thereby kept separate, facilitating clarity.

The proposition that "medical ethics" is basically just ordinary ethics applied to the realm of medicine may be vague, but is not very surprising. On the other hand, it may seem more surprising to say that bioethics is just ordinary ethics applied to the "bio-realm," yet that is what will be held, if only to force the relevant issues into the open.

"Bio-realm" obviously designates a much more inclusive universe of concerns than does "medical realm." The impetus for ethical reflection in areas connected with the biological sciences seems to have been biology's startling capabilities, both actual and projected, and the consequent implications for humankind. Though capabilities in the physical sciences and in technology have had similar disconcerting implications and have generated some ethical and societal reflections, it seems to have been recent biomedical developments that have precipitated the major ethical concerns which we group under "bioethics." The ripeness of the times for moral sensitivities was no doubt a contributing factor; civil rights, environmental issues, and population problems were high in the general consciousness. In any case, "bioethics" became the focal point, and subsequently many science-technology-society issues became its concern. This has resulted in a conglomeration that almost defies characterization. The field is more likely defined de facto in terms of its issues than by any shared essence or scientific perspective. (It should be noted that there is an issue of values-in-science that is not being raised in this article. It concerns whether and how value judgments encroach on science, influencing—according to some—the problem selection, observation, reasoning processes, and drawing of conclusions. These values are as frequently aesthetic, political, and social as ethical, and the matter has a literature of its own that predates the recent emphasis on bioethics.)

Assuming that bioethics is just ordinary ethics applied to a specialized area of concern, it becomes a matter of interest to determine whether problems arise in this special area that *in principle* are not amenable to traditional ethics. Whether or not they do cannot be settled here, but identifying and examining the pressures and tensions can be instructive. What is at issue is whether this new field of bioethics will have to develop new ethical principles (not just "derived rules" as discussed earlier) in order to deal with the problems confronting it. What follows should be seen as challenges to traditional ethics, brought on by new developments in the biological sciences. Their success as challenges will not be decided here, inasmuch as that would require a depth study of traditional ethics far beyond the scope of this article. Furthermore, the challenges themselves are too new to have their full complications and implications drawn and assessed. Nevertheless, what follows should elicit some underlying issues and suggest to the reader still other possible challenges.

CONCERNING WHAT IS "NATURALLY GIVEN"

The basic point of this challenge can be quickly seen, though it is not at all clear that it can be sustained under careful scrutiny. It is this: The "naturally given" seems, rightly or wrongly, to influence moral considerations, generally by constituting the inviolable starting point, the point of departure for ethical deliberations. Now, if we are able to tamper biologically with the very framework within which ethical deliberations make sense, then it would seem that more basic ethical principles must be formulated to guide us in how and what may be tampered with. But this point needs considerable elaboration. It is helpful to look at this from the perspectives of individual ethics and social ethics.

Individual Ethics. In individual ethics, when two people encounter each other, the "natural" makeup of each constitutes the given, the point of departure for moral behavior. The preferences, aversions, anger, temperament, etc., of each must be worked with and around by the other. These characteristics constitute the inviolable sphere of the self and the zone of privacy, and, in effect, litigation takes place among these givens. Each person tries not to harm the other unduly, given the other's temperament, aversions, and such characteristics. But what if these personal characteristics could be changed, either before birth, during childhood, or now? What if we could cause a person to have less of a temper or preferences that would coin-

cide with ours? As it is now, we start with complete persons as given—as completed units that barter, bargain, give and take, fashioning a symbiotic relationship that may restrain or require certain behavior but leaves the basic units or persons intact. However, with new capabilities we could perhaps alter "that" person before we even encounter him as a person.

What would guide our decision as to whether and how we would change this other? Currently, we are guided by rationality, that is, by those principles of behavior we can both agree on, being willing to follow them and have them followed with respect to us. But what criteria could we use if we were involved in changing the very makeup of the other? One answer might be: only with the consent of the other. If so, there is no challenge to standard ethics. Once again it is treating the whole person that confronts us as a given; it is not really altering that given until *after* the encounter, and then with that person's permission.

Changing a person without his consent is certainly wrong, and ordinary ethics would find it so. But we can make our problem tougher by casting doubt on the quality of consent (that the "consenter" is not really informed, that he is not in the right frame of mind, etc.). That is, reasons can of course be found for doing something against someone's expressed desire whether the act would be clearly a harm or a benefit. But even this does not necessarily force us beyond the ken of ordinary ethics, inasmuch as it is similar to problems we have had all along.

Tampering with personality characteristics prior to birth may push the problem further. There would be no ethical difficulty correcting a physical defect known to be painful or disabling to the eventual person. But what would justify changing—or refusing to change—the emotions, attitudes, or capabilities of the eventual person? The issue is no longer one of simply avoiding the causing of evil (a principle we would expect all rational beings to advocate) or even one of preventing evil. Rather this has to do with creating a good, and hence it is beyond the scope of ethics (as assumed in this article), which is essentially an avoidance of evils. Here we would not just be avoiding the causing of an evil to some given; we would be *creating* the given. Whereas we might expect universal agreement on what evils to proscribe, rational persons can and do differ widely on what things are good. Hence the problem: What criteria could be appealed to in the cases of whether and how to tamper with the endowments of eventual persons? On an individual basis there seem to be no guidelines and no possibility of there ever being any. It seems that guidelines could be framed only in terms of social goals. So the temptation would be to allow the "natural lottery" to continue; the randomness seems more fair in the absence of universal agreement on what would constitute a good person.

There may be promise of finding relevant ethical guidelines embedded in our raising children, which is, in a sense, creating the eventual person. Yet raising children is also largely fashioned by social goals rather than by ethical imperatives. That is, in molding children we go far beyond merely what morality requires. Furthermore, in raising children as distinguished from juggling genes, it is generally assumed that our influence is not irreversible. If so, this would be a morally significant difference between the two.

Social Ethics. New capabilities of altering what is "naturally given" might raise problems in the area of social ethics as well. The matter of just distribution may come up in a way it never has before. Perhaps society will no longer be willing to rely on the "natural lottery" of talents, dispositions, capabilities, etc., if these variables could be "evened" up before birth. It might be argued that justice would require an equal distribution of talent if that should become possible. Is some new principle of justice required? Or would it simply call for a decision as to the general social desirability of having so many similar and equal characteristics and talents? Yet, if these characteristics make a difference in the advantages one has in society, justice may well require us to make the characteristics equal. (Of course, the most likely solution would be not to make them all alike, but to stop allowing these characteristics to make a difference in one's obtaining rewards and status in society!)

It may be that this problem is no different from any other problem of justice. That is, we have believed justice required an evening up of talents and opportunities, insofar as this is possible with special training. Perhaps there is no difference in principle between balancing the disparities before and after birth. This does not make figuring the moral policy any easier, but it would indicate that it was the same old problem we have always had, and not something peculiar to new technological capabilities.

However, there are slight differences between the tampering before birth and the compensating endeavors after birth, and perhaps someone could argue that the differences are morally relevant. Before birth the mutation of talents, dispositions, and abilities is "arti-ficial," that is, it is induced. After birth it takes some effort of that person to overcome his shortcomings; opportunity would be equal, but results would vary with the effort put forth, which seems intuitively fairer than "magically" making them all equal *in utero*.

Another difference between the two cases which might be seen as morally relevant is the matter of consent. Initiating change after birth at least might have some form of consent from the person himself or from his duly determined proxy.

Similarly some might see a morally relevant difference in the implicit employment of a standard or norm in the case following birth. Justice has seemed to require that corrective help be available to those who fall short in mental, physical, or dispositional ability. But to do this, what is "normal" in each category must be established. Then the obligation is to bring them up to normal, though there seems to be no obligation to help the already normal to rise above normal (or, at least, the below normal seem to have priority on the resources for improvement). Presumably, with the before-birth case, the magical equalizing injections would maximize each attribute rather than recognize norms. But it is not clear how this could be seen as a morally relevant difference of the before-birth case, such that it presents a challenge different in kind from the case following birth. There may be a question as to whether justice requires equal magical potions (and consequently unequal results) or unequal potions (in order to obtain equal results). But that is a frequent dilemma of justice. Furthermore, the post-partum case is probably *more* difficult, since it involves priorities (e.g., Which should be first, the neediest or the most promising?).

Perhaps the issue of distribution deserves further comment. Does the "new biology" (recent biomedical discoveries and technology, current and envisioned) in any sense challenge the "old" concepts of justice such that new basic principles must be articulated? This might be thought to be so in the case of our current practices of awarding certain benefits according to accomplishments and abilities. If those accomplishments and abilities which justified the awards were *themselves* induced by biologic tampering, then by what criteria would we determine who was to receive the benefits of biologic tampering? In short, if we can "artificially" create those merits in virtue of which certain benefits are bestowed, then how do we decide who should receive this merit-making magic? (Shapiro.)

Yet it is not clear that this is different in principle from the ordinary problems of distributive justice. Education and training given to everyone equally have become the basis for subsequent rewards. Of course, it might be argued that natural ability and effort are what is being rewarded. But even in the case of biologic tampering, effort would be relevant. So in any case it is not obvious that the "new biology" presses on us any problem of just distribution that we have not had in principle all along. Whether to award goods on the basis of effort, worth, need, or desert continues to be a basic question. These operate within the context of social ideology, which no doubt helps determine what gets emphasized. And if biotechnology enabled us to make everyone the same in all admirable respects (courage, ability, endurance, etc.) it would be arguments from boredom or versatility in evolution or some such social ideal that would lead us to distribute the goods differently.

THE SCOPE OF MORALITY

Another conceivable challenge might be voiced: Do the new developments in biological knowledge and technology expose as inadequate the compass of traditional ethics? Specifically, can traditional ethics handle obligations and rights in borderline cases (fetuses, the severely retarded, the totally senile) or among those living things normally outside the sphere of morality (animals, plants, streams)? The thrust of the challenge is that because of increased knowledge, new capabilities and the resultant heightened sensitivities, we now see that rights must exist where traditional ethics had never envisioned them.

This cannot be done with the precision one would like. The concept of rights is a huge area. Furthermore, the variety of views on rights is compatible with a variety of ethical theories. But what can be done here is to sketch the general kind of reflection that might be stimulated by "the new biology" with respect to the inadequacy of the "old morality," and then to sketch a reply, arguing that no changes are necessitated, provided we understand rights in a certain way.

There has been a general raising of consciousness concerning the world around us. The intimate interrelationship of humankind with the environment, the interdependence of all living things, and the cumulative effect of any disruption of this balance are matters keenly impressed on us of late. Much of this results from the explosion of knowledge, particularly in the biological fields. It coincides as well with social and political movements that direct attention to environment, conservation, and appropriate lifestyles. The upshot has been pressure to reconsider the scope of moral rights and obligations, specifically whether they should be extended to include plants and animals. It is not enough, the argument goes, to have laws protecting trees and animals from various abuses; rather, we must think of them as having rights of their own, because this alone will give the necessary edge to their defenses, shifting the burden of proof to the proper contestant. With the prima facie right to noninterference anchored firmly in the living thing itself, the challenger would have to show why he should be allowed to harm it, rather than the "defendant's" having to show why not. In short, we would assume that one could not infringe on a tree or an animal without producing adequate reasons, instead of our assuming that these things may be freely infringed upon unless there are adequate reasons to the contrary.

Sensitivity to the plight of animals is not new, but there is a recent surge of concern that appears to be part of the general bioethics movement. Perhaps it is the great empathy for the voiceless oppressed (fetuses and minorities), perhaps it is increased awareness of all suffering, or perhaps it is the scientific eroding of essential differences between man and some animals, but whatever it is, it is being expressed in an effort to include animals within the moral realm (Regan and Singer).

The move to protect the environment is well known. What is not so well known is the possibility and need that elements of the environment have basic rights. One author argues thoroughly and convincingly that natural objects (such as trees and streams) have rights to life and health (Stone). Without the "discovery" of such rights, the abuse of these natural objects can be stopped only if detrimental effects to a human's health or livelihood can be shown. However, if a natural object's right to life and health were acknowledged, evidence of possible harm simply to it would suffice for enjoining the abuse. Stone argues that no amount of rules or laws protecting the object in question are ever equivalent to acknowledging *the right* of that object to health and life. The right has connotations, force, and presumption never embodied completely in a set of rules.

The preceding considerations, though only roughly sketched, may represent a thrust that will significantly alter traditional ethics in scope, if not in substance. These basic intuitions appear to put a stress on the framework of ethics which may force a change whereby bioethics will be essentially different from ethics. However, there are other ways of understanding the matter that, if correct, would obviate the need for basic revision. What follows is one such possibility. Like all else in this article, it is not a detailed argument, though it is a hint of one. Its role here is to suggest that the situation does not necessarily require a new ethics but that the old, adequately understood, can apply to the developing new circumstances.

The suggestion to be made could be called the concept of "bestowed rights." It builds on what is taken to be the purpose of morality, which in turn establishes the scope of morality. If an essential characteristic of a rational person is that he will avoid harm to himself (unless he has a reason not to), then we would expect that the community of rational persons would work to articulate and advocate a morality. That is, they would attempt to formulate rules and procedures to which they could all subscribe in order to settle their differences and otherwise avoid a life that would be "poor, nasty, brutish and short." Thus the rational person's instigating incentive for formulating and advocating moral rules is the avoiding of harm to himself and to others he cares about. As such, morality is a kind of agreement for mutual benefit, and rationality (avoiding of harm to oneself) is the foundation (Gert). Rationality may not compel one to be moral, but it would compel one to urge that *others* be moral. Furthermore, many things and ideas might motivate one to be moral, other than simply avoiding harm to oneself. It is just that avoidance of harm is the one motivation we can count on all rational persons sharing. This motivation has a purchase on those who can be responsible for their actions and who can realize that they are able to harm others and that others can harm them. All others unable to be gripped by this sanction are outside the community of moral agents.

This however does not mean that all others—the senile, the severely retarded, infants, fetuses, the insane—are without rights, but it does mean that the source of their rights is quite different. This is where the "bestowed right" becomes relevant. Those excluded from the moral community by virtue of their inability to act and plan responsibly and their inability to appreciate the force of the sanction at the base of morality are still significant members of society. The moral community has an interest in protecting them:

We ourselves might one day be in their position; we may have an emotional attachment to them; many of us have a "natural sympathy" with all forms of life; we could all become brutalized and consequently suffer if we failed to respect these other lives. Therefore, rights are bestowed on beings outside the community of moral agents. These are extremely important rights, though their foundation is different from those within (Clouser, 1976; Green). This interpretation seems to be more realistic with respect to where *in fact* the sanctions lie and would help arguments for and against rights to focus on the appropriate grounds.

Fetuses, animals, and trees cannot act responsibly or express their interests and desires, nor can they threaten us with retaliation. There is no basis for them to "claim" rights. On the other hand, it would be terribly shortsighted of us not to ascribe rights to them, or bestow rights on them, to avoid long-range harm to ourselves. When neither their interest, nor desire, nor consent can be solicited, what other argument (other than the long-range good of humankind) could ultimately be made for infringing on what would be a basic right of any of these nonrational beings? The point is that no matter what we postulate as to the "basic rights" of these nonrational beings, our ultimate criterion for honoring the rights will be in terms of the long-range good of humankind.

The point of all this has not been the argument itself, but rather to show that bioethics is not necessarily a new ethics: It might still be seen as the old ethics being applied to new circumstances.

OTHER POSSIBLE CHALLENGES

The matter of obligations to future generations is almost always included in any listing of bioethical issues, and yet it is not clearly a new issue. It is in fact a good example of what is probably the heart of bioethics, namely, an old issue that is exacerbated by new discoveries. For a long time we have been able to affect subsequent generations, but only recently have we been able to do it and realize it so vividly. So it is not new and different in principle, though its resolution may be more urgent. All attempts to deal with it have been attempts to draw out the implications of traditional morality, for example, by pointing out that the nature of obligation is always future oriented, or that the nature of a rule is timeless, or that from a moral perspective (whether that of the "ideal observer," the "rational man," or those "behind the veil of ignorance") all persons who are or ever will be must be regarded as contemporaneous.

In short, bioethics would seem to be the response of traditional ethics to particular stresses and urgencies that have emerged by virtue of new discoveries and technology. Ethics is pressed, not to find new principles or foundations, but to squeeze out all the relevant implications from the ones it already has. This, of course, does not solve every problem nor even necessarily narrow down the options significantly. Even after the ethical criteria are met, many alternatives may remain, thus requiring criteria other than morality for settling on a single line of action (Clouser, 1975).

This general theme is encountered time and again. The hackneyed example of the respirator, or of any life-extending apparatus, makes the same point. With new technology we are forced to make certain decisions with a regularity and urgency we had not faced before. This does not call for new ethical principles, but new applications of the old. Our concern for not harming a person and for honoring his wishes remains the same; we ponder only how to express it in these particular circumstances.

A similar case is the prevalent matter of behavior control. We have always been able to control some behavior, but new techniques make such control easier, quicker, and more certain, and have made moral clarity on the issue immensely more urgent. Again, the basic admonition not to interfere with a person's freedom without his consent still stands. But the new circumstances and capabilities drive us to more precision on what constitutes freedom, autonomy, and consent, in order to apply the basic rule. Sometimes it is clear that interference with freedom leads to even greater freedom (e.g., compulsory education); sometimes it is not clear whether meaningful consent is being given (e.g., Does the person *really* know the consequences and alternatives?); sometimes it is not clear whether the "real" self is speaking (e.g., the person before or after the mood-elevator, the shock treatment, or the hemodialysis). Furthermore, much of the concern (as is fairly typical of bioethical issues) has not been over *whether* to restrict the use of these new technologies, but *how*. That is, it is often clear when it is moral and when it is immoral to use these techniques of behavior control, but the problem comes in formulating a general policy that can make and incorporate the distinctions and subtleties necessary to capitalize on the worthy uses without risking the misuses.

BIOETHICS, SCIENCE, AND PUBLIC POLICY

The position taken in this [article] has been that the revelations and capabilities mediated by science create an urgency for moral guidance but do not require a new morality, revised in its basic principles. What is required is analysis of the new circumstances and their pivotal concepts, so that the applications and implications of the "old" morality might be clearly seen. Additionally, ethics itself may be pressed to yield clarity and distinctions it had not heretofore manifested. But it would be odd to call this a "new" morality. We are more likely to see it as a further uncovering, exploration, and articulation of the old, simply because we think of morality as applying to all persons at all places and times. Morality is not invented or legislated; at most it is "discovered," that is, it is an unpacking, explication, and articulation of our deepest intuitions about what we ought and ought not to do. Of course new "derived rules" . . . will emerge, as certain lines of action are discovered to lead to certain results that conflict with basic moral rules. It is in this role that the empirical sciences become very important. Spelling out the cause-and-effect relationships makes clearer where restraints should be imposed, so as to be in accord with the basic moral rules. The facts of sociology, biology, psychology, medicine, and other sciences are crucial in determining the outcome of various acts and policies, apart from which their morality generally cannot be judged. Analyses of pivotal concepts within these sciences (whether done by philosophers or scientists) are also crucial in determining morality: Has a person's "freedom" in fact been curtailed? Is he appropriately labeled "sick"? Was he acting "freely"? Can he really be said to have been "deceived"? And with this kind of conceptual analysis and figuring of consequences lies most of the work of bioethics. The remainder lies with probing the foundations of ethics for implications that relate more exactly to the novel predicaments characteristic of "the new biology."

Bioethics appears to have no essence that would mark it off. Rather it seems to be individuated by a de facto list of issues, extended and interrelated by "family resemblances." The initial set of dilemmas was no doubt introduced by biological discoveries, real and foretold. But we gradually became familiar with a wider list of issues: genetic engineering (cloning, in vitro fertilization, eugenics, etc.), allocation of limited health resources, obligations to future generations, environmental health and pollution, population control, abortion, euthanasia, behavior control (behavior modification, drugs, psychosurgery), human experimentation, organ transplantation, etc. By no means were all these forced on us by new discoveries; most have been around for a long time. Historical and sociological factors in addition to the moral urgency of new knowledge and capabilities contributed greatly to the coagulation of issues distinguishing itself from ordinary ethics. The result has been a considerable focusing on a set of issues, marked by urgency and importance.

Consequently, a common thread joining all the issues is hard to find. Invariably an article or book dealing with bioethics will mention quickly the "new biology" and the "new technology," and then immediately cite examples, namely, an enumeration of those issues which simply as a matter of fact are labeled "bioethics." Yet the conglomeration is not completely haphazard: Business ethics is not included, nor is economic ethics, nor diplomatic ethics. On the other hand, it is difficult to articulate a common essence that unifies the conglomerate. The core and impetus of the de facto list was no doubt concern over the technology of control of man's body, mind, and quality of life. The more such dramatic possibilities were highlighted and the more we became attuned to the issues, we began seeing similar, albeit less dramatic, instances all around us: Not only does the psychosurgeon alter our person, but so do parents, educators, and social systems; not only does the neonatologist determine quality of life, but so does the Highway Commission. Until we saw the grosser possibilities we were not sensitive to the subtler forces already at work. And thus the list grew. Perhaps an original criterion was that the issue have an obvious biological component, which affects coming into or going out of life, the nature of a person, or the quality of life. This of course directly or indirectly included almost everything. And so it must, to extend from the economics of feeding the world to paternalism in the doctor–patient relationship, from cultural determinations of illness and death to a tree's claim of a right to life! Adding to this the relevant data from law, sociology, psychology, biology, philosophy, theology, and other fields results in a vast network of issues categorized roughly as "bioethics." The aim of it all

should not be lost in the vastness: to decide how humankind ought to act in the biomedical realm affecting birth, death, human nature, and the quality of life.

In this context, and as a concluding observation, the matter of public policy should be put in perspective. Much of what is compressed under the umbrella of "bioethics" is really concerned with public policy—that is, with the legislation, policies, and guidelines that should be enacted with respect to all these issues. It is helpful to see this as distinct from ethics per se. Though many views of ethics exist (and this is not the place to thrash out the differences) the assumption of this article has been, very roughly, that ethics concerns those prohibitions all rational persons would urge everyone to obey in an effort to avoid those evils on which they all agree. Specifically, disregarding these prohibitions in order to "promote good" would be regarded as immoral (unless, of course, they met criteria for justifiable exceptions).

However, on a societal level the matter is different. It is not a matter of one individual's deciding on his own how to treat another. Rather, if there is a democratically arrived at consensus that a certain good must be promoted (say, education or welfare), though it means causing some harm (taxation and some loss of freedom), it is morally acceptable. It is at this level that much of what is called "bioethics" is taking place. Whereas individual morality is primarily a system of restraints, society-wide policy is on a level where promotion of goods is a moral option. Here the question becomes "What goods ought to be promoted?" or, contrariwise, "Which goods ought to be restrained (e.g., scientific research)?" Priorities, values, and goods are at center stage, where they must be weighed, balanced, and compared. The sciences and humanities are highly relevant in analyzing and prognosticating and in otherwise assisting a pluralistic society to settle on goods to be promoted. This level and direction of discussion account for a large portion of what comes to be called "bioethics," although, on the ethical theory assumed in this article, it is not really ethics so much as value theory and political theory.

But there is a still higher level at which significant bioethical analysis is done. When a society promotes various goods, inevitably some moral rules are broken with respect to some individuals (depriving them of something, a sacrifice necessary to support the "common good"). Which rules are broken with respect to whom becomes an important consideration in determining the justifiability of the goals or goods fixed upon. This determination is the jurisdiction of justice, the ethics pertaining to the societal level. And insofar as this has to do with the distribution of benefits and burdens relating to biomedical issues, it is a crucial part of bioethics.

BIBLIOGRAPHY

Blackstone, William T., ed. *Philosophy and Environmental Crisis.* Athens: University of Georgia Press, 1971.

Broadie, Alexander, and Pybus, Elizabeth M. "Kant's Treatment of Animals." *Philosophy* 49 (1974): 375–382.

Callahan, Daniel. "Bioethics as a Discipline." *The Hastings Center Studies* 1, no. 1 (1973), pp. 66–73.

Clouser, K. Danner. "Bioethics: Some Reflections and Exhortations." *Monist* 60, no. 1 (1977), pp. 47–61. This issue is devoted to bioethics.

———. "Medical Ethics: Some Uses, Abuses and Limitations." *New England Journal of Medicine* 293 (1975): 384–387.

———. "Some Things Medical Ethics Is Not." *Journal of the American Medical Association* 223 (1973): 787–789.

———. "What Is Medical Ethics?" *Annals of Internal Medicine* 80 (1974): 657–660.

Feinberg, Joel. "The Rights of Animals and Unborn Generations." Blackstone, *Philosophy and Environmental Crisis*, pp. 43–68.

Fox, Renée C. "Ethical and Existential Developments in Contemporaneous American Medicine: Their Implications for Culture and Society." *Milbank Memorial Fund Quarterly* 52 (1974): 445–483. Bibliography.

Gert, Bernard. *The Moral Rules: A New Rational Foundation for Morality.* New York: Harper & Row, 1970.

Green, Ronald M. "Conferred Rights and the Fetus." *Journal of Religious Ethics* 2, no. 1 (1974), pp. 55–75.

Hardin, Garrett; Storr, Anthony; Leiss, William; and Shepard, Paul. "Rights: Human and Nonhuman." *The North American Review*, Winter 1974, pp. 14–42. A collection of papers.

Kass, Leon R. "The New Biology: What Price Relieving Man's Estate?" *Science* 174 (1971): 779–788.

King, Lester Snow. "Development of Medical Ethics." *New England Journal of Medicine* 258 (1958): 480–486.

Passmore, John. "The Treatment of Animals." *Journal of the History of Ideas* 36 (1975): 195–218.

Regan, Tom, and Singer, Peter, eds. *Animal Rights and Human Obligations.* Englewood Cliffs, N.J.: Prentice-Hall, 1976.

Shapiro, Michael H. "Who Merits Merit? Problems in Distributive Justice and Utility Posed by the New Biology." *Southern California Law Review* 48 (1974): 318–370.

Singer, Peter. *Animal Liberation: A New Ethics for Our Treatment of Animals.* New York: New York Review, Random House, 1975.

Stone, Christopher D. "Should Trees Have Standing?—Toward Legal Rights for Natural Objects." *Southern California Law Review* 45 (1972): 450–501.

Veatch, Robert M. "Medical Ethics: Professional or Universal?" *Harvard Theological Review* 65 (1972): 531–559.

H. TRISTRAM ENGELHARDT, JR.

The Emergence of a Secular Bioethics

BIOETHICS AND THE CRISIS IN VALUES

Bioethical questions arise against the backdrop of a moral crisis that is closely tied to a series of losses of both ethical and ontological conviction in the West. When Martin Luther nailed his ninety-five theses to All Saints' Church in Wittenberg on Halloween in 1517, he marked a new era for the West, and the crumbling of the presumed possibility of a uniformity of moral viewpoint. One could no longer hope to live in a society that could aspire to a single moral viewpoint governed by a single supreme moral authority. In little over a century this would lead to the Thirty Years' War. The Pax Westphalica that followed in 1648 signaled the unlikelihood of ever cementing Europe in one Christian vision. And while the religious roots of ethical and metaphysical consensus were fragmenting, progress in the sciences undermined established understandings of man's place in the cosmos. When the first copy of Nicolaus Copernicus's *De revolutionibus orbium coelestium* was placed on his deathbed on May 24, 1543, a bequest was made to a shift in ideas that was to become the metaphor for dramatic and extensive changes in world views. This Copernican revolution was one of the many changes in ideas that would leave us devoid of a sense of absolute or final perspective: man was to cease to be the center of the cosmos, and the established Christian view of the cosmos was to be overturned.

As the religious synthesis weakened, the Enlightenment hope arose that reason alone (through philosophy) could disclose the character of the good life and the general canons of moral probity. As Alasdair MacIntyre and others have shown, this hope has proven

vain.[1] Rather than philosophy being able to fill the void left by the collapse of the hegemony of Christian thought in the West, competing philosophies and philosopical ethics have become ever more academic and therefore ever more removed from practical cultural needs. This [essay] is thus set against a background of considerable skepticism. One must wonder to what extent a moral viewpoint can be elaborated and justified outside a nest of supporting premises fashioned by a particular religious or other cultural tradition.

The discussion of issues in bioethics now transpires within the compass of secular pluralist societies. That such societies are secular is in part the result of recent historical forces that have led to the major institutions of most democracies no longer being associated in a significant fashion with an established church, even where vestiges may remain. Such societies are pluralistic in encompassing a wide divergence of moral sentiments and beliefs. Such divergence has likely always been present, however hidden. Europe of the Middle Ages, though nominally Catholic, included significant populations of Jews, in addition to heretics and some agnostics. In order to fashion a society that is not pluralist, one quite likely must settle for a society on a very small scale, probably not exceeding the compass of a Greek city-state. Whenever one considers a society of greater scope, or for that matter a society that has not voluntarily assembled around a full, willing, and complete submission to a particular moral or ideological perspective, one will have a pluralism of moral beliefs. It is this ever-present inclination to diversity of opinions that makes the single heretic so to be feared. In this [essay] I will talk of peaceable secular pluralist societies so as to indicate societies including a diversity of moral viewpoints, and enjoying in addition a freedom of moral opinion without the fear of repression. "Peaceable secular" is

Reprinted by permission of the publisher from *The Foundations of Bioethics* (New York: Oxford University Press, 1986), pp. 3–16.

best interpreted broadly to indicate the absence of any particular religious or moral orthodoxy imposed by force. I place among the religions of the world, at least by metaphor, such Christian heresies as Marxism. The problem is how to fashion an ethic for biomedical problems that can speak with rational authority across the great diversity of moral viewpoints. This problem is especially acute given the collapse of many of the traditional certainties.

Philosophical reflections have been directed to health care because of (1) major and rapid technological changes that have created pressures to reexamine the underlying assumptions of established practices (e.g., the advent of transplantation contributed to interests in a brain-oriented definition of death);[2] (2) rising health care costs, which have occasioned questions about the allocation of resources; (3) the frankly pluralistic context in which health care is now delivered (e.g., physicians and nurses can no longer presuppose that they share a view in common with their patients, or with each other, or that the conduct of their practice will be framed within acknowledged Judeo-Christian assumptions); and (4) the expansion of publicly recognized rights of self-determination (e.g., the 1965 Supreme Court ruling in *Griswold v. Connecticut*, holding unconstitutional laws forbidding the distribution of contraceptives to married couples).[3] If these changes render the answers of the past suspect, and if there is no accepted or imposed orthodoxy to provide answers, both answers and a conceptual framework must be fashioned anew.

The history of bioethics over the last two decades has been the story of the development of a secular ethic. Initially, individuals working from within particular religious traditions held the center of bioethical discussions. However, this focus was replaced by analyses that span traditions, including particular secular traditions. As a result, a special secular tradition that attempts to frame answers in terms of no particular tradition, but rather in ways open to rational individuals as such, has emerged. Bioethics is an element of a secular culture and the great-grandchild of the Enlightenment. Because the 1980s have been marked in Iran, the United States, and elsewhere by attempts to return to traditional values and the certainties of religious beliefs, one must wonder what this augurs for bioethics in this special secular sense. However, because the world does not appear on the brink of embracing a

particular orthodoxy, and if an orthodoxy is not imposed, as say in Iran or the Soviet Union, bioethics will inevitably develop as a secular fabric of rationality in an era of uncertainty. That is, the existence of open peaceable discussion among divergent groups, such as atheists, Catholics, Jews, Protestants, Marxists, heterosexuals and homosexuals, about public policy issues bearing on health care, will press unavoidably for a neutral common language. Bioethics is developing as the lingua franca of a world concerned with health care, but not possessing a common ethical viewpoint.

It is not hyperbolic to claim that health care and the biomedical sciences are playing a central role in a major cultural change. For instance, in the last hundred years, the United States has gone from a paternalistic view of patients' rights, a free enterprise system of health care delivery, and the legal proscription of abortion and contraception on request, to enforcing rights to free and informed consent, providing health care as a part of a federal welfare system, and legalizing abortion and contraception. These changes constitute a major cultural development, which is the outcome of an interplay between technology and culture.

Changes in technology and the acquisition of new knowledge have contributed ideas that have shaped our appreciation of the human condition. For example, the development of an evolutionary understanding of human origins has made neo-Aristotelian notions of natural and unnatural acts difficult to credit, at least in secular terms. How, for example, could one hold on nonreligious grounds that homosexuality is unnatural if human nature is the product of evolutionary processes that may even have developed genes for homosexuality, given the advantages of the trait in certain circumstances?[4] In any event, the outcomes of evolution would be without intrinsic normative force. Evolution is, after all, a morally blind process that has at best adapted us to environments in which we no longer live. A better knowledge of human origins has implications for arguments in bioethics, if in no other way, through undercutting the rhetorical force of certain kinds of arguments in ethics. Further, the technological developments of the biomedical sciences have themselves influenced the understanding of moral issues. The wide availability of effective contraception has suggested the feasibility of lifestyles that were more difficult in the past (e.g., women being fully sexually active and controlling reproduction, while participating fully in demanding occupations), and offered new areas of possible responsibility (e.g., the obligation to avoid the birth of seriously defective children, as suggested in *Curlender v. Bio-Science Laboratories*).[5]

Bioethics, unlike many codes of ethics, tends not to be national or parochial, because these developments in health care and in the biomedical sciences are tied generally to the development of industrial societies. Though bioethics is a major focus of Western society, that society itself is ever less parochial, and embraces not only North America and Europe, but societies such as Japan and Taiwan as well. Western health care and its problems are no longer solely Western problems. As it addresses this wide range of societies and their difficulties with "Western" biomedicine, bioethics draws on a tradition of the West that in fact attempts to step outside the constraints of particular cultures, including Western culture itself, by giving reasons and arguments anyone should accept. In this sense, bioethics is a general attempt in secular ethics. Although specific problems surely are tied to the particular health care systems of particular cultures, throughout the world the number of areas of common concern is growing. In every country, for example, a contraceptive ethos is in place, and amniocentesis and abortion are available nearly everywhere. The result has been a need to reconsider sexual and reproductive mores. The general availability of expensive life-sustaining technology has made the use of extraordinary care an issue for at least a few in every country. And every nation faces choices regarding the allocation of its resources to health care endeavors. In short, elements of Western culture are international, bound to the character of industrial or industrializing society. These give a common cast to health care and its problems, and evoke international interest in bioethics. In the latter part of the twentieth century, one finds bioethics spanning national boundaries as well as religious and political groups.

BIOETHICS: TAKING IDEAS SERIOUSLY AND REEXAMINING CULTURAL ASSUMPTIONS

As an undertaking in philosophy, bioethics is an attempt to clarify concepts and to search for conceptual presuppositions. It is an intellectual endeavor. But one must recognize that intellectual undertakings have concrete roots that touch us in our everyday lives. For example, the widespread use of IUDs (intrauterine devices) for contraception, with few of the users feel-

ing any guilt in the matter, presumes that: (1) people do not find such a practice unnatural, or if they do, they judge that state of affairs to be of little or no moral consequence, and (2) people do not find the wastage of zygotes that do not implant as a result of the use of IUDs to involve the taking of the lives of persons, or if they do, they judge the circumstances to have no serious moral significance in that context. When one then wishes to know whether one ought to use an IUD, one will likely be pressed to clarify such views. One will need to examine concepts of unnatural actions and their moral implications, if any. One will need to draw distinctions between human biological and human personal life. Such are intellectual undertakings, philosophical endeavors. However, they spring from practical interests, in this case choosing an acceptable means to avoid an unwanted pregnancy.

One has no intellectual problems, no philosophical problems, if one does not worry about giving reasons. However, not attending to reasons and the implications of choices would mean eschewing conversations about moral matters with oneself as well as with others. It would involve acting without concern for consequences. As soon as one wonders whether certain choices are better and how one can tell, the intellectual endeavor is joined. As one attempts to justify actions to others, or to persuade others that their actions are wrong, the intellectual undertaking assumes social dimensions. Such social dimensions exist as soon as one tries to justify one's choices as a patient, physician, or nurse, to another patient, physician, or nurse, or to society in general. The endeavors of health care are public concerns that lead to philosophical questions. This work is written on this premise: bioethics springs naturally from the concerns of patients, physicians, and nurses.

The questions addressed by bioethics are not restricted to the province of physicians, but concern nurses, other health care professionals, patients, and laymen. The term *bioethics* in fact encompasses issues that fall outside health care ethics in the strict sense of an exploration of the *moral* issues raised by health care and the biomedical sciences. Issues concerning *non-moral* values regarding what ought to be treated (e.g., signaling a state of affairs as pathological, as physiologically or psychologically abnormal), and ontological issues concerning when persons begin and cease (e.g., questions about the point at which fetuses should be acknowledged as persons), are also customarily gathered within the compass of bioethics (bioethics in a broad sense).

These issues have a breadth that transcends particular professional boundaries because the differences among the various health care professions primarily represent differences in economic advantages, status, and power within health care institutions and practices.[6] As a result, I will not use the term *health care* in the narrow sense (i.e., as the preservation or promotion of health) that contrasts with the narrow sense of *medical care* (the treatment of disease). Instead I will favor the broad sense of health care that includes a collection of somewhat competing professions (e.g., doctors of medicine, doctors of osteopathy, nurses, dentists, occupational therapists, physician assistants, clinical psychologists) with differing but overlapping interests, who face a common set of puzzles regarding the rights and obligations of professionals, patients, and societies concerning health care. In this [essay] I will not attempt to draw a systematic distinction or set of distinctions between medical care and health care; both are so intimately intertwined, and both terms possess strategic ambiguities. These professions are involved in a set of general cultural unclarities. They share in a set of uncertainties that transcend their particular professional boundaries.

Bioethics, in addressing these uncertainties, is philosophy engaged in one of its central tasks: aiding a culture to clarify its views of reality and of values. Philosophy done well is a culture examining its own conceptual and value presumptions. It is through applying the language of bioethics that health care understands its place in a culture, and the culture comprehends the significance of health care practices and the biomedical sciences it sustains. Bioethics plays a central role in the mutual intellectual adaptation of culture and biomedical technology. This is not simply an isolated, academic endeavor. However, to be much use it must be an academic endeavor in the sense of providing disciplined analyses. Insofar as one asks an intellectual question, one seeks more than consciousness raising, emotional refreshment, or a chance to exchange ideas over a drink. One strives to get ideas clearer because it is important to decide how one ought to resolve the disputes occasioned by the health care arts and sciences. Because they bear on life, death, and the quality of life, one must with care

and discipline attend to drawing conceptual distinctions. For example, deciding when human life ends signals the difference between describing the removal of a heart from a body as murder or as harvesting an organ. Such conceptual niceties (i.e., what is the difference between human biological and human personal life) carry practical weight. Finally, such tasks of intellectual clarification have merit, even when they do not lead to the definitive resolution of a problem. Greater clarity about a problem is better than more confusion, even when final answers are elusive. Philosophical progress is usually incremental: cautious steps forward, not final steps into the light. On this point, it is worth noting that it is frequently difficult to know in advance where such reflection will lead. One often discovers, with chagrin, that one's most heartfelt convictions are indefensible prejudices.

This is apparent on a large scale when one observes changes in public policy due to conceptual refinements. Though at the beginning of this century, for example, it was easy to hold a whole-body-oriented definition of death, that is no longer the case. In fact, now the very contrary holds: a living body with a completely dead brain is most easily seen as no longer a person. This shift occurred over time, following major advances in our understanding of our bodies. One might think of the initial lay reflections concerning cardiac transplants and the possible influence of the donor's heart on the recipient's personality.[7] There was over time a change in the understanding of what it meant to be alive, embodied in this world.[8] One was moving from a whole-body-oriented definition of life and death to a brain-oriented definition. One was as well drawing distinctions between principles of organic life and principles of personhood, of existing as a person in this world.[9] These changes in ontological view influenced bioethical reflections, which in turn have shaped our general understandings of ourselves. Bioethics is a philosophical undertaking that springs naturally from the delivery of health care and the development of the biomedical sciences in social contexts marked by pluralism and rapid technological change, but without an imposed orthodoxy. Bioethics is the disciplined puzzling of people attempting to understand the significance of birth, copulation, illness, and death, especially as these are touched on by health care and the biomedical sciences. Such reflections lead to changes in established cultural views and practices. Bioethics is a central element of a culture's self-understanding and self-transformation.

Since any particular culture is likely to contain a cluster of somewhat contrary, if not actually contradictory, presumptions, one is brought to sketch a rational, consistent account insofar as one is looking for rational, consistent answers. This will require one to be a geographer of concepts and values, analyzing and criticizing the advantages and disadvantages of alternative projections and mappings of concepts and values. Such an undertaking is philosophical; it is not one of empirical anthropology or sociology. It is an attempt to resolve an intellectual quandary: "How can I consistently understand what is right conduct in the health care professions and in the biomedical sciences, and justify it to others?" It is not the attempt to decide what people usually hold about right conduct in a particular society, nor is it an attempt to determine what viewpoint would be most credible to most people. Rather, it is an endeavor to look at reasons and to determine what reasons should be credited by impartial, unprejudiced, nonculturally biased reasoners, whose only interests are in the consistency and force of rational argument. Though no such culturally unprejudiced viewpoint can be fully achieved, the goal of its achievement can serve as a guiding ideal, suggesting a direction to proceed in attempting to clarify one's ideas on a subject. This approach, even when it cannot produce final answers (and, though, as we will see, it cannot ground a concrete ethic), can at least make progress by providing some tentative answers, and by suggesting why some resolutions of moral questions are better than others in terms of consistency, scope, and strength of possible rational justifications.

This intellectual approach to a set of very important questions (e.g., Do we declare this patient dead now? May we morally expend these funds ŏn good Scotch whiskey, rather than on treating the hypertension of indigent populations?) is ultimately unavoidable. One can decide to choose to one's best advantage, using whatever means are available, and think no further. Or one can appeal to intuitions, to one's conscience, to what feels right, and let that suffice. In either case, one rejects morality as a peaceable bond among persons. In the first case, one is not concerned with others as either moral objects or subjects. In the second case, the matrix for possible moral action with others is irrational, surd, and inexplicable for those who do not share the same moral intuitions. One simply affirms one's feelings and holds those who disagree to be wrong, in that they fail to have the grace of one's own

true insights. In either case, there is no bond through which to fashion the moral community, if one means by that a community founded on mutual respect, not force. However, insofar as one is concerned to have a justification that can appeal to other reasonable individuals, one enters into a fabric of ideas and justifications. As soon as one makes a choice, as a decision one would seek to justify, that choice and the actions it supports fit into a geography of ideas that requires philosophical or ethical analysis to provide orientation and justification. (E.g., "I am going to declare that patient dead, because his entire brain is dead." Why is that sufficient ground? "Because being a person requires at least a minimal level of sentience, and the capacities for sentience are supported by the brain.")

In justifying biomedical decisions, one is embedded in a matrix of conceptual and value presuppositions. Making a biomedical decision involves bioethics. The health professions are practiced within a terrain of concepts and values that presupposes particular relations between concepts and values for which philosophers function as the geographers. This is both a forward, as well as a humble, claim. On the one hand, philosophy cannot pull conceptual rabbits out of hats. Philosophers cannot disclose something on the terrain of ideas and values that was not already there, at least implicitly as an element of human reality. Philosophers can call attention to neglected features, forgotten relationships, and unforeseen contradictions. Philosophers can aid in better mapping and in critically evaluating the conceptual and value commitments involved in particular actions and choices.

This should signal certain obvious points about the role of bioethics and of books on bioethics. First, bioethics is not to be understood as a surrogate religion that will convert the evil from the errors of their ways. It will not likely render the uncaring humane, though in some cases it might (some portrayals of ideas capture the imagination and motivate action). Nor is bioethics a basis for a genre of moral counseling that would provide unique answers to particular questions. Such directive counseling is usually beyond its scope, though in some restricted areas bioethics may indeed serve this function. Its role usually will be to provide moral guidance in the sense of giving instruction regarding the likely character of the moral world and the moral significance of choices in biomedicine. This last function, the primary function of bioethics, is a central goal of the humanities generally: to provide an understanding of the human condition through a disciplined examination of the ideas, values, and images that frame the significance of the human world and guide human practices, here those of health care. As an undertaking of men and women, not a deliverance of the gods, its conclusions are likely to be, and probably in most cases will be, tentative.

SECULAR VERSUS RELIGIOUS BIOETHICS

There are numerous competing secular views of the good life and of the canons of moral probity. These are grounded in particular traditions and in particular moral senses. Unless I indicate otherwise, when I speak of secular bioethics, I mean bioethics in the first sense, as the attempt to find those understandings that can be justified across particular moral communities, traditions, and ideologies, including not only particular religious communities, but particular secular communities of thought as well. If one attempts to chart the conceptual and value commitments of individuals in approaching and resolving biomedical problems— simply as rational individuals without the special illumination of some divine grace—one will find a world view that is secular, though not antireligious. Indeed, as this work will argue, the peaceable context of a neutral secular understanding provides the circumstances within which religious views and special secular traditions can be embraced and pursued in security. A general secular bioethics must function as the logic of a pluralism, as the means for the peaceable negotiation of moral intuitions.

Secular bioethics as the provision of a neutral framework to address moral problems in biomedicine is a peaceable solution to the problems of delivering health care, when physicians, nurses, patients, and individuals generally, hold a diversity of moral views. If one is not to embark on an inquisitorial quest of imposing by force or coercion a religiously or metaphysically grounded view of moral probity, or even a *particular* secular tradition, then one will need to content oneself with a general moral framework that lacks such moorings. Without such moorings, there may be a consequent loss of societal certainties. The deliverances of bioethics will often be weaker than a religious thinker, or a partisan of a particular secular moral viewpoint, might wish. Secular bioethics reflec-

tions may not support all the moral restraints that religious individuals or partisans of a particular ideology may want. As this [essay] will show, there will be few serious general secular moral objections to abortion on request. A secular bioethics is unlikely to develop convincing arguments for forbidding many actions that our Western Christian societies have taken to be morally wrong, such as "unnatural sexual activities," suicide, or the active euthanasia of severely defective newborns. In addition, secular bioethics will usually qualify its answers, leaving vexing areas of uncertainty. This will not be out of a pursuit of a minimalist ethics, such as Daniel Callahan has criticized,[10] but rather out of a recognition of the limitations of secular reasoning. These conclusions about the capacities of bioethics will require changes in public policy. If a secular society does not possess general rational arguments to show that certain actions are wrong, the moral authority to enforce such prohibitions weakens. Though this [essay] is not [an essay] in law and medicine and does not pretend to give legal advice, it will offer moral and philosophical reassessments of much of law and public policy in medicine.

Threats to traditional certainties may make an imposed orthodoxy appear attractive. There may seem to be greater security for one's beliefs (if one has the good luck of having the same beliefs as the moral oppressors) through suppressing discussion of the fundamental intellectual foundations of the good life and of the canons of moral probity. In the absence of such an imposed orthodoxy, one sees unveiled the faltering attempts of men and women to come to terms with the task of fashioning an account of the moral life. If one is accustomed to the sure answers of a religiously grounded ethics, a general secular bioethics may occasion frustration when one is forced into lengthy chains of reasoning, and disappointment when final answers are not forthcoming.

With all its defects, however, a secular bioethics has numerous virtues. It promises the possibility of providing a context for health care that can encompass in toleration health care givers and receivers with diverse moral perspectives. Believers should also recognize that a secular bioethics can provide the peaceable neutral framework through which they can reach out to others beyond their own particular religious tradition and convert through witness and example, even if not through force. A secular bioethics is also a check against the temptation to flee to false prophets of private intuition for answers that are best achieved through careful analyses sustained by communities of inquiring individuals. It recalls one to the reality of modern medical practice in a pluralist context. Its failings must be seen in the light of the human condition: secular bioethics is framed by men and women, not gods and goddesses. Those with religious persuasions should know that grace makes plain what religion cannot discern. The grace of conversion is not the force of coercion, but rather a divine gift.

The distinctions drawn in this [essay] between a general secular morality and the moralities of particular moral communities are related to the traditional distinction between what unaided reason can establish and what revelation can teach.[11] Unsupplemented by some special source of knowledge, our understandings of morality and of the ultimate purpose of our lives must remain impoverished.[12] Most of the traditional questions of Western metaphysics concerning the significance of human existence will go at least partially unanswered.[13] The differences between the conclusions in this [essay] and those offered by traditional natural law theory, such as that of St. Thomas Aquinas, will lie in the limitations of reason that this [essay] acknowledges.[14] If one cannot establish through reason alone the great body of Judeo-Christian precepts, there will be, as we shall see, a sharp contrast between secular ethics and the ethics of particular moral communities that rely on special traditions or special revelations. The gulf between church and state will widen, and one will find oneself living a moral life within two complementary but distinct moral perspectives.

Apart from any arguments in principle on behalf of this view of toleration (which arguments will indeed be given in this [essay]), one might ask under what circumstances there could ever be a peaceable union of the peoples of the earth, save through acquiescing in the policy that persons may do with themselves and consenting others whatever they wish, despite what others might think and feel in the matter. The risk to humanity from war and brutal repression in the name of religious and ideological rectitude far outweighs the harms likely to come from tolerating such evils as self-determination, abortion, and infanticide. Perpetual peace in the absence of repression will likely come, if ever, when we are willing to endure the choices persons make with themselves, consenting others, and their private resources. . . . Here it is enough to underscore that the purchase price of such peace is toleration of personal tragedy—the toleration of deviant life-styles, if they are peaceable, and the acceptance of the tragedies that persons experience as the result of their own free choices. To hope to be discharged from such payments is to aspire to the life of the gods, which aspiration is surely to be punished by the plagues that follow hubris.

This gulf and the tensions it engenders characterize the contemporary moral predicament. As we shall see, they are the result of the respect owed to persons, the limits of reason, and the limits on the authority to use force. The purchase price of freedom is tragedy and diversity. It is tragedy because individuals in their freedom will choose in ways that others find to be ill-considered and harmful. Such choices will lead to an untidy diversity of competing moral viewpoints, often making common actions in many areas impossible. Because one is obliged to tolerate such tragedy and diversity, the moral life becomes an ambiguous undertaking. One must often tolerate on moral grounds that which one must condemn on moral grounds. For example, as the reader shall see, there are limits on the public authority to use force in order to compel charity.[15] However, the reader should understand that the author holds just as strongly that charity is central to the good moral life and is one of the proper responses to a universe blind to human sufferings, where persons are often deaf to the needs of others. Such tolerance has not been traditional in many societies of the West. St. Thomas Aquinas recommends that the stubborn or relapsing heretic be exterminated from the world by death.[16] We will need to learn to be tolerant, even about issues less important than the salvation of immortal souls. We will need to eschew contemporary versions of the *writ de haeretico comburendo* (i.e., the writ for the burning of a heretic).

The conclusions in this [essay] are at times perturbing and upsetting. The reader should be advised that the author also was often disturbed by many of the conclusions. The unbiased analysis of settled moral viewpoints has the danger of undermining cherished moral sentiments—or at least of showing that they must be recognized as a part of a community's special moral commitments and not amenable to general rational justification. Then, of course, it would be too much to hope that all of one's culture's mores could find general rational justification. Philosophical analysis is a form of intellectual adventure. One may perhaps arrive at viewpoints one would not have anticipated.

NOTES

1. Alasdair MacIntyre, *After Virtue* (Notre Dame, Ind.: University of Notre Dame Press, 1981).

2. Ad Hoc Committee of the Harvard Medical School to Examine the Definition of Brain Death, "A Definition of Irreversible Coma," *Journal of the American Medical Association* 205 (Aug. 1968): 336–40.

3. Griswold v. Connecticut, 381 U.S. 479, 85 S.Ct. 1678. 14 L.Ed.2d 510 (1965). Similar constitutional protection was extended to the right of unmarried individuals to have access to contraception in Eisenstadt v. Baird, 405 U.S. 438, 92 S.Ct. 1029, 31 L.Ed.2d 349 (1972).

4. It is interesting to note that some individuals have provided arguments to support the notion that homosexuality evolved because it maximized inclusive fitness. For such an argument, see Robert Trivers, "Parent-Offspring Conflict," *American Zoologist* 14 (1974): 249–64.

5. Curlender v. Bio-Science Laboratories and Automated Laboratory Sciences, 165 Cal. Rptr. 477 (Ct. App. 2nd Dist. Div. 1, 1980). I cite this case to illustrate a moral point, even though the decision has since been overturned by a California law (Cal. Cir. Code, sec. 43.6 [1982]), as well as there being a contrary ruling in Turpin v. Sortini, 119 Cal. App. 3rd 690 (1981).

6. H. T. Engelhardt, Jr., "Physicians, Patients, Health Care Institutions—and the People in Between: Nurses," in A. H. Bishop and J. R. Scudder (eds.), *Caring, Curing, Coping: Nurse, Physician, Patient Relationships* (University, Ala.: University of Alabama Press, in press).

7. See, for example, Kenneth Vaux, "A Year of Heart Transplants: An Ethical Valuation," *Postgraduate Medicine* 45 (Jan. 1969): 201–5. Irving S. Wright, "A New Challenge to Ethical Codes: Heart Transplants," *Journal of Religion and Health* 8 (1969): 226–41. Patricia MacMillian, "But My Heart Belongs to Me . . . ," *Nursing Times* 76 (April 1980): 677.

8. For a study of the development of concepts of the cerebral localization of mental capacities, see Robert Young, *Mind, Brain, and Adaptation in the Nineteenth Century* (Oxford: Clarendon Press, 1970); S. F. Spicker and H. T. Engelhardt, Jr. (eds.), *Philosophical Dimensions of the Neuro-Medical Sciences* (Dordrecht: Reidel, 1976).

9. H. Tristram Engelhardt, Jr., "Defining Death: A Philosophical Problem for Medicine and Law," *American Review of Respiratory Diseases* 112 (Nov. 1975): 587–90. Though, as I shall argue in this [essay], the brain-oriented definition of death is best understood as the recognition of the brain as the sponsor of consciousness, there have been attempts to avoid this recognition. See, for example, the President's Commission for the Study of Ethical Problems in Medicine and Biomedical and Behavioral Research, *Defining Death* (Washington, D.C.: U.S. Government Printing Office, 1981), esp. pp. 31–43.

10. Daniel Callahan, "Minimalist Ethics," *Hastings Center Report* 11 (Oct. 1981): 19–25.

11. Classically, there was a distinction made between what can be concluded by natural reason, by reason unaided by grace and revelation, and what can be known through revelation. As St. Thomas stated, "It was therefore necessary that, besides the philosophical disciplines investigated by reason, there should be a sacred doctrine by way of revelation." *Summa Theologica* I, art. 1, *The Basic Writings of Saint Thomas Aquinas*, Anton C. Pegis (ed.), vol. 1 (New York: Random House, 1945), p. 6.

12. Here one must include not only grace and revelation but also special moral traditions and moral senses.

13. Metaphysics in the West has classically included natural theology and discussions on the immortality of the soul. One might think here of the three questions of Kant: "1. What can I know? 2. What ought I to do? 3. What may I hope?" *Critique of Pure Reason* A805 = B833. Norman Kemp Smith (trans.), *Immanuel Kant's Critique of Pure Reason* (London: Macmillan, 1964), p. 635. I, following Kant, consider the limits of our ability to answer such questions.

14. The Roman Catholic Church contends that on the basis of natural reason one can demonstrate the existence of God and the immorality of contraception.

15. One should note that Jesus is reported to have said, "If thou wilt be perfect, go and sell that thou hast, and give to the poor, and thou shalt have treasure in heaven . . ." (Matthew 19:21). There is no evidence that he said, "If you would be perfect, establish a progressive redistributive tax system." Being committed to aiding the poor is not equivalent to being committed to using state force to compel others to be beneficent.

16. St. Thomas Aquinas, *Summa Theologica* II, Q. IX, art. iii–iv. In this regard St. Thomas was reflecting the general ethos of the time. The Fourth Lateran Council, for instance, granted the same indulgences to those who exterminated heretics at home as to those who went to the Holy Land. "Catholici vero qui, crucis assumpto charactere, ad haereticorum exterminium se accinxerint, illa gaudeant indulgentia, illoque sancto privilegio sint muniti, quod accedentibus in Terrae sanctae subsidium conceditur," "Concilium Lateranese IV" [1215], *Conciliorum Oecumenicorum Decreta* (Basil: Herder, 1962), *Constitutiones* 3, p. 210.

SUGGESTED READINGS FOR CHAPTER 2

Caplan, Arthur L. "Can Applied Ethics Be Effective in Health Care and Should It Strive to Be?" *Ethics* 93 (January 1983), 311–319.

Fox, Renée C., and Swazey, Judith P. "Medical Morality Is Not Bioethics—Medical Ethics in China and the United States." *Perspectives in Biology and Medicine* 27 (Spring 1984), 336–360.

Gorovitz, Samuel. "Baiting Bioethics." *Ethics* 96 (January 1986), 356–374.

Jonsen, Albert, and Toulmin, Stephen. *The Abuse of Casuistry: A History of Moral Reasoning.* Berkeley, Calif.: University of California Press, 1988.

McCullough, Laurence B. "Methodological Concerns in Bioethics." *Journal of Medicine and Philosophy* 11 (February 1986), 17–37.

Shelp, Earl E., ed. *Theology and Bioethics: Exploring the Foundations and Frontiers.* Boston: D. Reidel, 1985.

BIBLIOGRAPHIES

Coutts, Mary Carrington. *Basic Resources in Bioethics.* Washington, D.C.: Kennedy Institute of Ethics, Georgetown University, June 1988.

Goldstein, Doris Mueller. *Bioethics: A Guide to Information Sources.* Detroit: Gale Research Company, 1982. See under "Bioethics."

Lineback, Richard H., ed. *Philosopher's Index.* Vols. 1– . Bowling Green, Ohio: Bowling Green State University. Issued quarterly. See under "Bioethics," "Ethics," "Health," and "Medical Ethics."

Walters, LeRoy, and Kahn, Tamar Joy, eds. *Bibliography of Bioethics.* Vols. 1– . Issued annually. Washington, D.C.: Kennedy Institute of Ethics, Georgetown University. See under "Bioethics," "Medical Ethics," and "Nursing Ethics." (The information contained in the annual *Bibliography of Bioethics* can also be retrieved from BIOETHICSLINE, an on-line database of the National Library of Medicine.)

Part II

CONCEPTUAL FOUNDATIONS

3.
Concepts of Health and Disease

Medical science, we often say, is dedicated to the treatment and prevention of disease and to the maintenance of health. But precisely what is disease? And what constitutes health? To ask these questions is to ask not only how disease and health are to be understood but also how they are to be distinguished from other human conditions, such as misery and ecstasy or failure and achievement. The questions "What is health?" and "What is disease?" are requests for comprehensive definitions or conceptual explications of health and disease. However, we also will look beyond conceptual analysis in this chapter in order to probe the implications definitions have for medical care and health policy. These implications give the issues their urgency and direct relevance to ethics and policy. For example, under the Mental Health Act in Great Britain, people can be excused from working, excused from keeping contractual obligations, and protected from punishment, depending on whether or not they have been classified as mentally diseased. And whether they are to be so classified is a matter of the particular categories of disease accepted under the act.[1]

The implications of definitions of health and disease include the conditions under which social allocations are appropriate either to promote "health" or to prevent "disease," the conditions under which health care services can legitimately be used to promote health or control disease, the conditions under which social deviants and the mentally ill should be treated as sick and in need of help, and the nature of illnesses that should be covered by health insurance programs. Our conception of health care *needs* will generally follow the lines of our conception of *health*. The broader the conception of health, the broader the potential list of needs. In a broad conception of health, for example, persons will need adequate exercise, freedom from stress, nutrition, shelter, sanitation, pollution-free environments, rehabilitative services, preventive services, and social services. But should our conception of health be broad enough to embrace this list of needs?

THE DEFINITION OF HEALTH
An influential example in this chapter of the broadest possible definition of "health" is the World Health Organization (WHO) definition: "Health is a state of complete physical, mental, and social well-being and not merely the absence of disease or infirmity." This definition presents an idealized conception of well-being and proper human functioning that medicine should approximate insofar as possible when it aims to restore, promote, or preserve health. Everyone will in some respects fall short of this ideal, and thus medicine and public health will be conceived as having an endless variety of tasks for improving health. The latitude covers physical conditions, mental conditions, and social conditions. Presumably it covers a mental state such as happiness, so that anyone who does not have complete happiness is in some dimension not healthy. In principle *any* deficiency in function or well-being is a health deficiency. Thus, not being in shape to play basketball,

being socially inhibited, and having a low I.Q. can all be described as problems of inadequate health.

This idealized approach to the definition of health has important implications not only for our understanding of the goals of medicine but for public health and public policy as well. If the goal of health care is the maintenance and restoration of all aspects of our potential for well-being, then the scope of medical practice and health policy legitimately includes areas such as social deviancy, sexual inadequacy, and personal difficulties in adapting to new environments. Private and public health policies, such as health insurance coverage, would then be adjusted to this WHO understanding of health. Although we might be able to distinguish *medical* goals from *health* goals, a broad definition of "health" makes it increasingly difficult to determine which aspects of health are appropriately medical. Some critics of the WHO definition believe that it leaves us conceptually unable to distinguish where to call a halt to the legitimate concerns of medicine and public health.

A narrower class of definitions excludes the social dimension altogether, while retaining the physical and mental. Daniel Callahan is tempted by this approach in his essay in this chapter, but he ultimately accepts a third and even more restrictive definition of health as "a state of physical well-being . . . without significant impairment of function." The approach taken by Callahan has the weight of tradition behind it, since in both the history of medicine and the history of philosophy (especially in the works of Plato, Aristotle, and Descartes) a mind-body dualism predominates, and health has primarily been viewed as physical well-being. But this traditional support is not in itself a decisive criterion. Several authors in this chapter and elsewhere have argued that only in recent years have plausible reasons emerged for extending the scope of the concept beyond the body and a biomedical model. Freud's extension of the traditional concepts of health and disease into the mental world are, they note, relatively recent by comparison to the history of medicine and its probing of bodily health. (See Ruth Macklin's essay on this point.)

Another approach to the definition of health is to treat health as the absence of impairments to person that are caused by disease and illness. On this view, health is the absence of disease and illness, and the medical domain is determined by the objective of eliminating and controlling disease and illness. This possibility takes us to the second definitional quest: the definitions of disease and illness.

THE DEFINITION OF DISEASE

Controversies over the definition of disease have a rather different focus than those over the issues about health. One central issue is whether the term "disease" (and "illness," if different) refers to conditions objectively in nature or whether diseases are social constructions that are determined (wholly or partially) by our positive or negative evaluations—or whether some third alternative is correct. According to the objectivist or nonnormativist conception, disease is a value-free concept and is definable in terms of an objective condition in nature. According to the normativist conception, by contrast, disease is not a value-free concept, and those who use the concept do not make a purely objective judgment. The normativist thesis is bluntly exhibited in the following example and conclusion offered by Peter Sedgwick:

The blight that strikes at corn or at potatoes is a human intervention, for if man wished to cultivate parasites (rather than potatoes or corn) there would be no blight, but simply the necessary foddering of the parasite-crop. . . . Outside the significances that man voluntarily attaches to certain conditions, *there are not illnesses or diseases in nature.*[2]

This normative theory of disease has drawn a number of critics. In this chapter Christopher Boorse argues for a naturalist theory of the objectivity of "disease" and the normativeness of "illness." Boorse maintains that health and disease are objective concepts and that both may be defined in terms of the natural functioning typical of a biological species. Health is the absence of disease, and diseases are deviations from the natural or typical functioning in the organizational structure of a species. A natural function is here understood as a causal function in the species that is goal directed.

To explicate the notion of health, Boorse offers an analogy to the mechanical condition of an automobile: It is in perfect condition when it conforms in all respects to the designer's specifications. Likewise in a biological species, perfect health is the condition of perfect functioning toward natural goals of survival and reproduction; and disease is a departure from natural functional organization in an organ or aspect of the biological system. A person's health, then, is determined by the extent to which the person properly functions as a member of the species *homo sapiens*. But for all species, the normal function determines the natural and the natural determines the healthy. Judgments of what is healthy and diseased, Boorse maintains, are value neutral. These judgments are matters of natural science, not matters of social evaluation.

Boorse is therefore particularly opposed to normativist theses such as the one developed by H. Tristram Engelhardt, Jr., who propounds his views in this chapter by analyzing the history of medical views of masturbation. Engelhardt believes that disease is a deviation from a social norm rather than a biological norm. He offers some historical backing for this thesis by pointing to medical descriptions of masturbation as a disease. To show the evaluative underpinnings of disease categories, he points to a period in which drape-tomania, the disease that drove slaves to run away, was considered a medical problem.

Engelhardt and others have argued against Boorse's objectivist theory by trying to show that *any* nontypical functioning in a species must on that theory be a disease—an outcome they take to be absurd. Thus, if someone has an overabundance of muscle that is atypical of the species, the person is diseased. This exchange raises the question whether species-typical functioning is necessarily a *statistical* concept, which is the common interpretation of Boorse's position (see Ruse, for example); that is, are we to understand atypical functioning purely in terms of statistical deviation from normal or average functioning? An argument that has been used in reply to the normativist objection is that the concept of disease is not statistical because it derives from a biological theory of the design of the organism—much as we determine an automobile's deviation not by a statistical deviation but rather by its departure from the engineer's design. From this perspective, the biomedical sciences describe the natural functions in species, and health and disease are to be gauged against the standards developed in these objective, empirical sciences. Psychopathology no less than the other medical sciences is an attempt to determine species-typical functional organizations and departures from them. It is simply that we know much less at the present time about species-typical mental functioning.

The waters of this controversy are tested in this chapter in two essays by Michael Ruse and Arthur Caplan. Ruse questions whether either a normativist or a nonnormativist can provide a convincing answer to the question, "Is someone ill if he or she is sexually attracted to members of one's own sex rather than members of the opposite sex?" Ruse finds it a difficult question to answer by use of any available theory of health and disease. He tries to show that under the different, available scientific theories and philosophical models of disease, we get different answers to the "homosexuality as sickness" question. Thus, he finds theoretical reasons why there exists a whole set of mutually inconsistent answers to this question, each backed by scientific and philosophical premises.

Caplan raises still another controversial issue, which can be described as the "aging as sickness" question. The aging process seems a normal, natural process, and medical texts typically do not discuss the process as a disease. Caplan believes, however, that disease in medicine is to be defined in terms of pathological change of just the sort typical of the aging process. He mounts an argument to show that there are five general criteria of the conditions under which a bodily state or process is a disease. By his criteria, aging has all the properties of a disease.

As Caplan notes, these issues about homosexuality and aging by no means exhaust the range of controversies over which human states count as diseases. Similar controversies that are not frivolous (in the way masturbation and drapetomania are) have arisen, for example, about pregnancy and menopause. On various criteria we might also challenge whether "nervous disorders" or astigmatism really are diseases. These problems tend to show that we are not as clear on the nature of health and disease as we sometimes think— perhaps because they are very complicated notions. It may also be that there are reasons external to the medical sciences, such as moral and political issues, that lead us to label something a disease that we otherwise might not so label. Discussion of this problem has been especially intense around the concept of mental health and disease.

MENTAL HEALTH AND DISEASE

The search for an adequate conceptual analysis of mental health and mental illness has, by almost everyone's account, been beset with more difficulties and has attracted more competing theories than in any other area of the health sciences. The same problems about normality and abnormality haunt these discussions, but they are magnified in both importance and complexity. Diagnostic manuals in psychiatry are indicative of the problem. They range over a vast territory of different human conditions, and many of the diagnostic categories included are controversial within the profession. Different theories of disease are at work in psychiatry, and some psychiatrists even reject the concept of a "disease entity" as irrelevant to their classifications of patients.

One could in principle avoid these problems of definition by deciding that "health" and "disease" should be defined as Callahan suggests, as exclusively concerned with physical well-being. One could then claim that psychiatric designations are either inherently evaluative or stretched beyond the bounds of normal objectivity when used in expressions such as "mental health" and "social disease." A related aspect of this dimension of the problem is whether it is possible to delineate a definition of mental disease that differentiates it from physical disease. If a mental disease is nothing but a form of physical disease, then there is nothing unique in the idea of either mental health or mental disease. However, it has proved very difficult to specify nonphysical criteria of mental disease that do not include more forms of human action than seem diseased. This has been a special problem in criminal justice, where theories of mental illness have often been used to show that criminal behavior is really the result of mental defects. The concept of "behavioral disorders" has sometimes been so broadly described that many kinds of social and political deviancy would have to be classified as mental disorders.

These problems are explored in the final two readings, by Thomas Szasz and Ruth Macklin. Szasz, a psychiatrist, denies the existence of mental illness or mental disease. Mental illness has been invented rather than discovered, he thinks, and psychiatry is a pseudomedical enterprise rather than a medical science. He argues that historically the idea in psychiatry was always to bring mental diseases under the medical model of physical disease, but it has never been successfully done because the behavioral dysfunctions treated in psychiatry do not fit the medical model. All forms of illness and disease are necessarily bodily, in his analysis; that is, they are deviations from an anatomical criterion. Criteria of mental illness, by contrast, are both culture-bound and normative. These judgments of behavior necessarily incorporate a moral viewpoint, and therefore judgments of so-called mental illness, including judgments of insanity and madness, are moral judgments masked in the language of "psychiatric diagnoses." It is not surprising, then, that various groups of psychiatrists have in the past diagnosed liars, communists, revolutionaries, killers, addicts, delinquents, racists, those who engage in masturbation, and so on as insane. Thus Szasz holds that we have no obligations to give assistance to those with "psychiatric illness pain"—including those who are suicidal, depressed, and the like—unless they specifically request our assistance. Otherwise a psychiatrist is merely a paternalist intervening without authority in people's liberty.

Szasz regards these and all pure judgments of "mental illness" in psychiatry as mythical, dangerous, and without intellectual foundation. He does allow, however, for the possibility that some of the behavior classified as psychiatric may be the result of specific forms of brain disease, such as tumors, that are manifested as behavioral dysfunctions. These are properly medical problems and properly categorized as diseases, but only because they are biological problems. He also insists that it is the brain dysfunction and not the behavioral dysfunction that is the disease. One of the problems for Szasz is thus to develop criteria that will differentiate in diagnosis between a biological and a behavioral criterion—a major problem, inasmuch as the tumor or chemical balance may be undetected and yet the behavioral pattern obviously deviant and dangerous to the person.

This problem and several others are explored in the essay by Ruth Macklin. She points out that Szasz does not operate with a clear definition of terms like illness, disease, and sickness and is not even clear on the nature of the "error" made by psychiatrists in labeling disorders "illnesses." Sometimes he seems to say it is a logical error, at others a linguistic mistake, and at others a matter of mistaken scientific theory. She also criticizes his judgments that one is not ill when no physico-chemical cause of a specific disorder has been discovered and that there is a clear line to be drawn between physical and mental illness.

Whatever the final outcome of this debate over mental disease, it does raise important questions about legitimate judgments in psychiatry. Almost everyone is agreed that at various times in the history of psychiatry there have been gross abuses of the model of psychiatric disease and that it has been difficult to bring psychiatry under a medical model. The question remains: Is it possible to have a medical psychiatry that is not intrinsically involved in making moral judgments of human behavior?

TYPES OF DEFINITION

There are at least four different ways to define or analyze terms, and these should be distinguished by evaluating the various attempts in this chapter to define "health" and "disease." Since many other terms will be the subjects of definitional investigation in this book (prominent ones include "personhood," "life," "informed consent," "confidentiality," "privacy," "justice," "death," "euthanasia," "behavior control," and "insanity"), the discussion below is of the *general* nature of these four types of definition.

1. *Descriptive definitions* attempt to report the usage of terms as they are typically or ordinarily employed. All good dictionary definitions have this aim, because they inform us how the words of a particular language actually are used by those who speak the language. If there are different meanings or uses of the same term, the dictionary will distinguish them. Sometimes dictionary definitions do little more than offer a synonym for the word

being defined. The better-formulated definitions, however, explicate the common meaning of terms by specifying the conditions that must hold for the word to apply correctly. Such definitions are either true or false, because they are either correct or incorrect reports of common usage. For example, Boorse seems to believe that his analysis of disease eventuates in descriptive definitions of health and disease.

2. *Stipulative definitions* stipulate meanings instead of reporting actual usage. Usually the stipulation is for purposes of clarity when an ordinary or prevalent meaning is vague. Often the stipulation is only temporary and for a special purpose. For example, if the term "health" were defined as "the state of successful adaptation to the pressures of city life," such a definition would be stipulative. There are reasons of convenience and clarity for using stipulative definitions such as this one (imagine a study of the pressures of city life being presented to a convention of psychologists). It is not wrong to use such definitions as long as they are explicitly presented as stipulative and do not masquerade as descriptive. Unlike descriptive definitions, stipulative ones are neither true nor false, because they are announcements of a policy of usage. They might turn out to be good or bad for the purpose, but they cannot be mistaken.

3. *Reforming definitions* provide new meanings for old terms by suggesting new outlooks not incorporated in previous usage. They are not simply stipulative, because they try to illuminate and advance proper usage by giving a deeper insight into the meaning of a term. They may also attempt to reform ordinary usage, whereas stipulative definitions do not aim at reform, because they either introduce new meanings or are temporary and only for a special purpose.

In the readings in this chapter, Daniel Callahan mentions an example of a reforming definition. He notes that the task of defining "health" is often not merely descriptive but (as in the case of the WHO definition) "is nothing less than a way of deciding what should be valued, how life should be understood, and what principles should guide individual and social conduct." If Callahan is correct, reforming definitions may underlie programmatic attempts to change our health policies. Such definitions are usually the products of a theory—perhaps a social theory or a scientific theory. Assessment of the adequacy of the definition would thus probably require an assessment of the adequacy of the theory that generated it.

4. *Real definitions* are attempts to state what the real properties of something are. Such definitions are of special importance when (as in the case of reforming definitions) it is believed that ordinary usage is mistaken and therefore that descriptive definitions are inadequate. It might be, for example, that ordinary usage reflects Aristotle's belief that the term "man" means "rational animal." But perhaps it is not essential that man be rational; human infants do not appear to be rational, nor do humans in irreversible coma have rational processes. (These topics are discussed in Chapters 5 and 6.) If so, we may want to know what "man" really is, not just what the term might mean. Similarly, in the case of "mental illness," we want to know what such illness really is (if it is illness at all) and not simply what is commonly meant by the term. Such definitions are usually reforming definitions, but not all reforming definitions are real definitions. Many persons are now skeptical that real definitions can be given at all, because they doubt that language and theory are capable of grasping the real properties of things without recourse to an evaluative or theoretical perspective. Nonetheless, attempts to provide real definitions are frequent.

In assessing the definitions of "health," "disease," and "illness" in this chapter, it is important to analyze what type or mixture of types of definition is being offered, because only then can one be prepared to judge the definition's acceptability. This evaluation is especially critical if an author claims to be providing a descriptive or a real definition but is in fact providing a stipulative or a reforming definition.

T.L.B.

NOTES

1. See Raanan Gillon, "On Sickness and On Health," *British Medical Journal* 292 (February 1, 1986), p. 319.

2. Peter Sedgwick, "Illness—Mental and Otherwise," *Hastings Center Studies*, vol. 1, no. 3 (1973), pp. 19–40.

The Concept of Health

WORLD HEALTH ORGANIZATION

A Definition of Health

The States Parties to this Constitution declare, in conformity with the Charter of the United Nations, that the following principles are basic to the happiness, harmonious relations and security of all peoples:

Health is a state of complete physical, mental and social well-being and not merely the absence of disease or infirmity.

The enjoyment of the highest attainable standard of health is one of the fundamental rights of every human being without distinction of race, religion, political belief, economic or social condition.

The health of all peoples is fundamental to the attainment of peace and security and is dependent upon the fullest co-operation of individuals and States.

The achievement of any State in the promotion and protection of health is of value to all.

Unequal development in different countries in the promotion of health and control of disease, especially communicable disease, is a common danger.

Healthy development of the child is of basic importance; the ability to live harmoniously in a changing total environment is essential to such development.

The extension to all peoples of the benefits of medical, psychological and related knowledge is essential to the fullest attainment of health.

Informed opinion and active co-operation on the part of the public are of the utmost importance in the improvement of the health of the people.

Governments have a responsibility for the health of their peoples which can be fulfilled only by the provision of adequate health and social measures.

Accepting these principles, and for the purpose of co-operation among themselves and with others to promote and protect the health of all peoples, the Contracting Parties agree to the present Constitution and hereby establish the World Health Organization as a specialized agency within the terms of Article 57 of the Charter of the United Nations.

From the Preamble to the Constitution of the World Health Organization. Adopted by the International Health Conference held in New York from 19 June to 22 July 1946, and signed on 22 July 1946 by the representatives of sixty-one States (*Off. Rec. Wld Hlth Org.* 2, 100). Reprinted with permission of the publisher from *The First Ten Years of the World Health Organization*, WHO, 1958.

DANIEL CALLAHAN

The WHO Definition of "Health"

There is not much that can be called fun and games in medicine, perhaps because unlike other sports it is the only one in which everyone, participant and spectator, eventually gets killed playing. In the meantime, one of the grandest games is that version of king-of-the-hill where the aim of all players is to upset the World Health Organization (WHO) definition of "health." That definition, in case anyone could possibly forget it, is, "Health is a state of complete physical, mental, and social well-being and not merely the absence of disease or infirmity." Fair game, indeed. Yet somehow, defying all comers, the WHO definition endures; though literally every other aspirant to the crown has managed to knock it off the hill at least once. One possible reason for its presence is that it provides such an irresistible straw man; few there are who can resist attacking it in the opening paragraphs of papers designed to move on to more profound reflections.

But there is another possible reason which deserves some exploration, however unsettling the implications. It may just be that the WHO definition has more than a grain of truth in it, of a kind which is as profoundly frustrating as it is enticingly attractive. At the very least it is a definition which implies that there is some intrinsic relationship between the good of the body and the good of the self. The attractiveness of this relationship is obvious: it thwarts any movement toward a dualism of self and body, a dualism which in any event immediately breaks down when one drops a brick on one's toe; and it impels the analyst to work toward a conception of health which in the end is resistant to clear and distinct categories, closer to the felt experience. All that, naturally, is very frustrating.

Reprinted with permission of the author and the Institute of Society, Ethics and the Life Sciences from *The Hastings Center Studies*, Vol. 1, No. 3 (1973).

It seems simply impossible to devise a concept of health which is rich enough to be nutritious and yet not so rich as to be indigestible.

One common objection to the WHO definition is, in effect, an assault upon any and all attempts to specify the meaning of very general concepts. Who can possibly define words as vague as "health," a venture as foolish as trying to define "peace," "justice," "happiness," and other systematically ambiguous notions? To this objection the "pragmatic" clinicians (as they often call themselves) add that, anyway, it is utterly unnecessary to know what "health" means in order to treat a patient running a high temperature. Not only that, it is also a harmful distraction to clutter medical judgment with philosophical puzzles.

Unfortunately for this line of argument, it is impossible to talk or think at all without employing general concepts: without them, cognition and language are impossible. More damagingly, it is rarely difficult to discover, with a bit of probing, that even the most "pragmatic" judgment (whatever *that* is) presupposes some general values and orientations, all of which can be translated into definitions of terms as general as "health" and "happiness." A failure to discern the operative underlying values, the conceptions of reality upon which they are based, and the definitions they entail, sets the stage for unexamined conduct and, beyond that, positive harm both to patients and to medicine in general.

But if these objections to any and all attempts to specify the meaning of "health" are common enough, the most specific complaint about the WHO definition is that its very generality, and particularly its association of health and general well-being as a positive ideal, has given rise to a variety of evils. Among them are the cultural tendency to define all social problems, from war to crime in the streets, as "health" problems;

the blurring of lines of responsibility between and among the professions, and between the medical profession and the political order; the implicit denial of human freedom which results when failures to achieve social well-being are defined as forms of "sickness," somehow to be treated by medical means; and the general debasement of language which ensues upon the casual habit of labeling everyone from Adolf Hitler to student radicals to the brat next door as "sick." In short, the problem with the WHO definition is not that it represents an attempt to propose a general definition, but it is simply a bad one.

That is a valid line of objection, provided one can spell out in some detail just how the definition can or does entail some harmful consequences. Two lines of attack are possible against putatively hazardous social definitions of significant general concepts. One is by pointing out that the definition does not encompass all that a concept has commonly been taken to mean, either historically or at present, that it is a partial definition only. The task then is to come up with a fuller definition, one less subject to misuse. But there is still another way of objecting to socially significant definitions, and that is by pointing out some baneful effects of definitions generally accepted as adequate. Many of the objections to the WHO definition fall in the latter category, building upon the important insight that definitions of crucially important terms with a wide public use have ethical, social, and political implications; defining general terms is not an abstract exercise but a way of shaping the world metaphysically and structuring the world politically.

Wittgenstein's aphorism, "don't look for the meaning, look for the use," is pertinent here. The ethical problem in defining the concept of "health" is to determine what the implications are of the various uses to which a concept of "health" can be put. We might well agree that there are some uses of "health" which will produce socially harmful results. To carry Wittgenstein a step further, "don't look for the uses, look for the abuses." We might, then, examine some of the real or possible abuses to which the WHO definition leads, recognizing all the while that what we may term an "abuse" will itself rest upon some perceived *positive* good or value.

HEALTH AND HAPPINESS

Let us examine some of the principal objections to the WHO definition in more detail. One of them is that, by including the notion of "social well-being" under its rubric, it turns the enduring problem of human happiness into one more medical problem, to be dealt with by scientific means. That is surely an objectionable feature, if only because there exists no evidence whatever that medicine has anything more than a partial grasp of the sources of human misery. Despite [the optimism of Dr. Brock Chisholm, the first Director of WHO], medicine has not even found ways of dealing with more than a fraction of the whole range of physical diseases; campaigns, after all, are still being mounted against cancer and heart disease. Nor is there any special reason to think that future forays against those and other common diseases will bear rapid fruits. People will continue to die of disease for a long time to come, probably forever.

But perhaps, then, in the psychological and psychiatric sciences some progress has been made against what Dr. Chisholm called the "psychological ills," which lead to wars, hostility, and aggression. To be sure, there are many interesting psychological theories to be found about these "ills," and a few techniques which can, with some individuals, reduce or eliminate anti-social behavior. But so far as I can see, despite the mental health movement and the rise of the psychological sciences, war and human hostility are as much with us as ever. Quite apart from philosophical objections to the WHO definition, there was no empirical basis for the unbounded optimism which lay behind it at the time of its inception, and little has happened since to lend its limitless aspiration any firm support.

Common sense alone makes evident the fact that the absence of "disease or infirmity" by no means guarantees "social well-being." In one sense, those who drafted the WHO definition seem well aware of that. Isn't the whole point of their definition to show the inadequacy of negative definitions? But in another sense, it may be doubted that they really did grasp that point. For the third principle enunciated in the WHO Constitution says that "the health of all peoples is fundamental to the attainment of peace and security. . . ." Why is it fundamental, at least to peace? The worst wars of the twentieth century have been waged by countries with very high standards of health, by nations with superior life expectancies for individuals and with comparatively low infant mortality rates. The greatest present threats to world peace come in great part (though not entirely) from developed countries, those which have combated disease and illness most effectively. There seems to be no historical correlation whatever between health and peace, and that is true even if one includes "mental health."

How are human beings to achieve happiness? That is the final and fundamental question. Obviously illness, whether mental or physical, makes happiness less possible in most cases. But that is only because they are only one symptom of a more basic restriction, that of human finitude, which sees infinite human desires constantly thwarted by the limitations of reality. "Complete" well-being might, conceivably, be attainable, but under one condition only: that people ceased expecting much from life. That does not seem about to happen. On the contrary, medical and psychological progress have been more than outstripped by rising demands and expectations. What is so odd about that, if it is indeed true that human desires are infinite? Whatever the answer to the question of human happiness, there is no particular reason to believe that medicine can do anything more than make a modest, finite contribution.

Another objection to the WHO definition is that, by implication, it makes the medical profession the gate-keeper for happiness and social well-being. Or if not exactly the gate-keeper (since political and economic support will be needed from sources other than medical), then the final magic-healer of human misery. Pushed far enough, the whole idea is absurd, and it is not necessary to believe that the organizers of the WHO would, if pressed, have been willing to go quite that far. But even if one pushes the pretension a little way, considerable fantasy results. The mental health movement is the best example, casting the psychological professional in the role of high priest.

At its humble best, that movement can do considerable good; people do suffer from psychological disabilities and there are some effective ways of helping them. But it would be sheer folly to believe that all, or even the most important, social evils stem from bad mental health: political injustice, economic scarcity, food shortages, unfavorable physical environments have a far greater historical claim as sources of a failure to achieve "social well-being." To retort that all or most of these troubles can, nonetheless, be seen finally as symptoms of bad mental health is, at best, self-serving and, at worst, just plain foolish.

A significant part of the objection that the WHO definition places, at least by implication, too much power and authority in the hands of the medical profes-

sion need not be based on a fear of that power as such. There is no reason to think that the world would be any worse off if health professionals made all decisions than if any other group did; and no reason to think it would be any better off. That is not a very important point. More significant is that cultural development which, in its skepticism about "traditional" ways of solving social problems, would seek a technological and specifically a medical solution for human ills of all kinds. There is at least a hint in early WHO discussions that, since politicians and diplomats have failed in maintaining world peace, a more expert group should take over, armed with the scientific skills necessary to set things right; it is science which is best able to vanquish that old Enlightenment bogey-man, "superstition." More concretely, such an ideology has the practical effect of blurring the lines of appropriate authority and responsibility. If all problems—political, economic, and social—reduce to matters of "health," then there cease to be any ways to determine who should be responsible for what.

THE TYRANNY OF HEALTH

The problem of responsibility has at least two faces. One is that of a tendency to turn all problems of "social well-being" over to the medical professional, most pronounced in the instance of the incarceration of a large group of criminals in mental institutions rather than prisons. The abuses, both medical and legal, of that practice are, fortunately, now beginning to receive the attention they deserve, even if little corrective action has yet been taken. (Counterbalancing that development, however, are others, where some are seeking more "effective" ways of bringing science to bear on criminal behavior.)

The other face of the problem of responsibility is that of the way in which those who are sick, or purportedly sick, are to be evaluated in terms of their freedom and responsibility. Siegler and Osmond . . . discuss the "sick role," a leading feature of which is the ascription of blamelessness, of non-responsibility, to those who contract illness. There is no reason to object to this kind of ascription in many instances—one can hardly blame someone for contracting kidney disease—but, obviously enough, matters get out of hand when all physical, mental, and communal disorders are put under the heading of "sickness," and all sufferers (all of us, in the end) placed in the blameless "sick role." Not only are the concepts of "sickness" and "illness" drained of all content, it also becomes impossible to ascribe any freedom or responsibility to those caught up in the throes of sickness. The whole world is sick, and no one is responsible any longer for anything. That is determinism gone mad, a rather odd outcome of a development which began with attempts to bring unbenighted "reason" and free self-determination to bear for the release of the helpless captives of superstition and ignorance.

The final and most telling objection to the WHO definition has less to do with the definition itself than with one of its natural historical consequences. Thomas Szasz has been the most eloquent (and most single-minded) critic of that sleight-of-hand which has seen the concept of health moved from the medical to the moral arena. What can no longer be done in the name of "morality" can now be done in the name of "health": human beings labeled, incarcerated, and dismissed for their failure to toe the line of "normalcy" and "sanity."

At first glance, this analysis of the present situation might seem to be totally at odds with the tendency to put everyone in the blame-free "sick role." Actually, there is a fine, probably indistinguishable, line separating these two positions. For as soon as one treats all human disorders—war, crime, social unrest—as forms of illness, then one turns health into a normative concept, that which human beings must and ought to have if they are to live in peace with themselves and others. Health is no longer an optional matter, but the golden key to the relief of human misery. We *must* be well or we will all perish. "Health" can and must be imposed; there can be no room for the luxury of freedom when so much is at stake. Of course, the matter is rarely put so bluntly, but it is to Szasz's great credit that he has discerned what actually happens when "health" is allowed to gain the cultural clout which morality once had. (That he carries the whole business too far in his embracing of the most extreme moral individualism is another story, which cannot be dealt with here.) Something is seriously amiss when the "right" to have healthy children is turned into a further right for children not to be born defective, and from there into an obligation not to bring unhealthy children into the world as a way of respecting the right of those children to health! Nor is everything altogether lucid when abortion decisions are made a matter of "medical judgment" (see *Roe vs. Wade*); when decisions to provide psychoactive drugs for the relief of the ordinary stress of living are defined as no less

"medical judgment"; when patients are not allowed to die with dignity because of medical indications that they can, come what may, be kept alive; when prisoners, without their consent, are subjected to aversive conditioning to improve their mental health.

ABUSES OF LANGUAGE

In running through the litany of criticisms which have been directed at the WHO definition of "health," and what seem to have been some of its long-term implications and consequences, I might well be accused of beating a dead horse. My only defense is to assert, first, that the spirit of the WHO definition is by no means dead either in medicine or society. In fact, because of the usual cultural lag which requires many years for new ideas to gain wide social currency, it is only now coming into its own on a broad scale. (Everyone now talks about everybody and everything, from Watergate to Billy Graham to trash in the streets, as "sick.") Second, I believe that we are now in the midst of a nascent (if not actual) crisis about how "health" ought properly to be understood, with much dependent upon what conception of health emerges in the near future.

If the ideology which underlies the WHO definition has proved to contain many muddled and hazardous ingredients, it is not at all evident what should take its place. The virtue of the WHO definition is that it tried to place health in the broadest human context. Yet the assumptions behind the main criticisms of the WHO definition seem perfectly valid. Those assumptions can be characterized as follows: (1) health is only a part of life, and the achievement of health only a part of the achievement of happiness; (2) medicine's role, however important, is limited; it can neither solve nor even cope with the great majority of social, political, and cultural problems; (3) human freedom and responsibility must be recognized, and any tendency to place all deviant, devilish, or displeasing human beings into the blameless sick-role must be resisted; (4) while it is good for human beings to be healthy, medicine is not morality; except in very limited contexts (plagues and epidemics) "medical judgment" should not be allowed to become moral judgment; to be healthy is not to be righteous; (5) it is important to keep clear and distinct the different roles of different professions, with a clearly circumscribed role for medicine limited to those domains of life where the contribution of medicine is appropriate. Medicine can save some lives; it cannot save the life of society.

These assumptions, and the criticisms of the WHO definition which spring from them, have some important implications for the use of the words "health," "illness," "sick," and the like. It will be counted an abuse of language if the word "sick" is applied to all individual and communal problems, if all unacceptable conduct is spoken of in the language of medical pathologies, if moral issues and moral judgments are translated into the language of "health," if the lines of authority, responsibility, and expertise are so blurred that the health profession is allowed to pre-empt the rights and responsibilities of others by redefining them in its own professional language.

Abuses of that kind have no possibility of being curbed in the absence of a definition of health which does not contain some intrinsic elements of limitation—that is, unless there is a definition which, when abused, is self-evidently *seen* as abused by those who know what health means. Unfortunately, it is in the nature of general definitions that they do not circumscribe their own meaning (or even explain it) and contain no built-in safeguards against misuse, e.g., our "peace with honor" in Southeast Asia—"peace," "honor"? Moreover, for a certain class of concepts—peace, honor, happiness, for example—it is difficult to keep them free in ordinary usage from a normative content. In our own usage, it would make no sense to talk of them in a way which implied they are not desirable or are merely neutral: by well-ingrained social custom (resting no doubt on some basic features of human nature) health, peace, and happiness are both desired and desirable—good. For those and other reasons, it is perfectly plausible to say the cultural task of defining terms, and settling on appropriate and inappropriate usages, is far more than a matter of getting our dictionary entries right. It is nothing less than a way of deciding what should be valued, how life should be understood, and what principles should guide individual and social conduct.

Health is not just a term to be defined. Intuitively, if we have lived at all, it is something we seek and value. We may not set the highest value on health—other goods may be valued as well—but it would strike me as incomprehensible should someone say that health was a matter of utter indifference to him; we would

well doubt either his sanity or his maturity. The cultural problem, then, may be put this way. The acceptable range of uses of the term "health" should, at the minimum, capture the normative element in the concept as traditionally understood while, at the maximum, incorporating the insight (stemming from criticisms of the WHO definition) that the term "health" is abused if it becomes synonymous with virtue, social tranquility, and ultimate happiness. Since there are no instruction manuals available on how one would go about reaching a goal of that sort, I will offer no advice on the subject. I have the horrible suspicion, as a matter of fact, that people either have a decent intuitive sense on such matters (reflected in the way they use language) or they do not; and if they do not, little can be done to instruct them. One is left with the pious hope that, somehow, over a long period of time, things will change.

• • •

MODEST CONCLUSIONS

Two conclusions may be drawn. The first is that some minimal level of health is necessary if there is to be any possibility of human happiness. Only in exceptional circumstances can the good of self be long maintained in the absence of the good of the body. The second conclusion, however, is that one can be healthy without being in a state of "complete physical, mental, and social well-being." That conclusion can be justified in two ways: (a) because some degree of disease and infirmity is perfectly compatible with mental and social well-being; and (b) because it is doubtful that there ever was, or ever could be, more than a transient state of "complete physical, mental, and social well-being," for individuals or societies; that's just not the way life is or could be. Its attractiveness as an ideal is vitiated by its practical impossibility of realization. Worse than that, it positively misleads, for health becomes a goal of such all-consuming importance that it simply begs to be thwarted in its realization. The demands which the word "complete" entail set the stage for the worst false consciousness of all: the demand that life deliver perfection. Practically speaking, this demand has led, in the field of health, to a constant escalation of expectation and requirement, never ending, never satisfied.

What, then, would be a good definition of "health"? I was afraid someone was going to ask me that question. I suggest we settle on the following: "health is a state of physical well-being." That state need not be "complete," but it must be at least adequate, i.e., without significant impairment of function. It also need not encompass "mental" well-being; one can be healthy yet anxious, well yet depressed. And it surely ought not to encompass "social well-being," except insofar as that well-being will be impaired by the presence of large-scale, serious physical infirmities. Of course my definition is vague, but it would take some very fancy semantic footwork for it to be socially

misused; that brat next door could not be called "sick" except when he is running a fever. This definition would not, though, preclude all social use of the language of "pathology" for other than physical disease. The image of a physically well body is a powerful one and, used carefully, it can be suggestive of the kind of wholeness and adequacy of function one might hope to see in other areas of life.

The Concept of Disease

H. TRISTRAM ENGELHARDT, JR.

The Disease of Masturbation: Values and the Concept of Disease

Masturbation in the eighteenth and especially in the nineteenth century was widely believed to produce a spectrum of serious signs and symptoms, and was held to be a dangerous disease entity. Explanation of this phenomenon entails a basic reexamination of the concept of disease. It presupposes that one think of disease neither as an objective entity in the world nor as a concept that admits of a single universal definition: there is not, nor need there be, one concept of disease.[1] Rather, one chooses concepts for certain purposes, depending on values and hopes concerning the world.[2] The disease of masturbation is an eloquent example of the value-laden nature of science in general and of medicine in particular. In explaining the world, one judges what is to be significant or insignificant. For example, mathematical formulae are chosen in terms of elegance and simplicity, though elegance and simplicity are not attributes to be found in the world as such. The problem is even more involved in the case of medicine, which judges what the human organism should be (i.e., what counts as "health") and is thus involved in the entire range of human values. This paper will sketch the nature of the model of the disease of masturbation in the nineteenth century, particularly in America, and indicate the scope of this "disease entity" and the therapies it evoked. The goal will be to outline some of the interrelations between evaluation and explanation.

The moral offense of masturbation was transformed into disease with somatic not just psychological dimensions. Though sexual overindulgence generally was considered debilitating since at least the time of Hippocrates,[3] masturbation was not widely accepted as a disease until a book by the title *Onania* appeared anonymously in Holland in 1700 and met with great success.[4] This success was reinforced by the appearance of S. A. Tissot's book on onanism.[5] Tissot held that all sexual activity was potentially debilitating and

Reprinted with permission of the author and the publisher from *Bulletin of the History of Medicine*, Vol. 48, No. 2 (Summer, 1974), pp. 234–248. © 1974 by The Johns Hopkins University Press.

that the debilitation was merely more exaggerated in the case of masturbation. The primary basis for the debilitation was, according to Tissot, loss of seminal fluid, one ounce being equivalent to the loss of forty ounces of blood.[6] When this loss of fluid took place in an other than recumbent position (which Tissot held often to be the case with masturbation), this exaggerated the ill effects.[7] In attempting to document his contention, Tissot provided a comprehensive monograph on masturbation, synthesizing and appropriating the views of classical authors who had been suspicious of the effects of sexual overindulgence. He focused these suspicions clearly on masturbation. In this he was very successful, for Tissot's book appears to have widely established the medical opinion that masturbation was associated with serious physical and mental maladies.[8]

There appears to have been some disagreement whether the effect of frequent intercourse was in any respect different from that of masturbation. The presupposition that masturbation was not in accordance with the dictates of nature suggested that it would tend to be more subversive of the constitution than excessive sexual intercourse. Accounts of this difference in terms of the differential effect of the excitation involved are for the most part obscure. It was, though, advanced that "during sexual intercourse the expenditure of nerve force is compensated by the magnetism of the partner."[9] Tissot suggested that a beautiful sexual partner was of particular benefit or was at least less exhausting.[10] In any event, masturbation was held to be potentially more deleterious since it was unnatural, and, therefore, less satisfying and more likely to lead to a disturbance or disordering of nerve tone.

At first, the wide range of illnesses attributed to masturbation is striking. Masturbation was held to be the cause of dyspepsia,[11] constrictions of the urethra,[12] epilepsy,[13] blindness,[14] vertigo, loss of hearing,[15] headache, impotency, loss of memory, "irregular action of the heart," general loss of health and strength,[16] rickets,[17] leucorrhea in women,[18] and chronic catarrhal conjunctivitis.[19] Nymphomania was found to arise from masturbation, occurring more commonly in blonds than in brunettes.[20] Further, changes in the external genitalia were attributed to masturbation: elongation of the clitoris, reddening and congestion of the labia majora, elongation of the labia minora,[21] and a thinning and decrease in size of the penis.[22] Chronic

masturbation was held to lead to the development of a particular type, including enlargement of the superficial veins of the hands and feet, moist and clammy hands, stooped shoulders, pale sallow face with heavy dark circles around the eyes, a "draggy" gait, and acne.[23] Careful case studies were published establishing masturbation as a cause of insanity,[24] and evidence indicated that it was a cause of hereditary insanity as well.[25] Masturbation was held also to cause an hereditary predisposition to consumption.[26] Finally, masturbation was believed to lead to general debility. "From health and vigor, and intelligence and loveliness of character, they became thin and pale and cadaverous; their amiability and loveliness departed, and in their stead irritability, moroseness and anger were prominent characteristics. . . . The child loses its flesh and becomes pale and weak."[27] The natural history was one of progressive loss of vigor, both physical and mental.

In short, a broad and heterogeneous class of signs and symptoms were recognized in the nineteenth century as a part of what was tantamount to a syndrome, if not a disease: masturbation. If one thinks of a syndrome as the concurrence or running together of signs and symptoms into a recognizable pattern, surely masturbation was such a pattern. It was more, though, in that a cause was attributed to the syndrome, providing an etiological framework for a disease entity. That is, if one views the development of disease concepts as the progression from the mere collection of signs and symptoms to their interrelation in terms of a recognized causal mechanism, the disease of masturbation was fairly well evolved.

• • •

As mentioned, the concept of the disease of masturbation developed on the basis of a general suspicion that sexual activity was debilitating.[28] This development is not totally unexpected: if one examines the world with a tacit presupposition of a parallelism between what is good for one's soul and what is good for one's health, then one would expect to find disease correlates for immoral sexual behavior.[29] Also, this was influenced by a concurrent inclination to translate a moral issue into medical terms and relieve it of the associated moral opprobrium in a fashion similar to the translation of alcoholism from a moral into a medical problem.[30] Further, disease as a departure from a state of stability due to excess or under excitation offered the skeleton of a psychosomatic theory of the somatic alterations attributed to the excitation associated with masturbation.

. . .

Those who held the disease of masturbation to be more than a culturally dependent phenomenon often employed somewhat drastic therapies. Restraining devices were devised,[31] infibulation or placing a ring in the prepuce was used to make masturbation painful,[32] and no one less than Jonathan Hutchinson held that circumcision acted as a preventive.[33] Acid burns or thermoelectrocautery[34] were utilized to make masturbation painful and, therefore, to discourage it. The alleged seriousness of this disease in females led, as Professor John Duffy has shown, to the employment of the rather radical treatment of clitoridectomy.[35] The classic monograph recommending clitoridectomy, written by the British surgeon Baker Brown, advocated the procedure to terminate the "long continued peripheral excitement, causing frequent and increasing losses of nerve force. . . ."[36] Brown recommended that "the patient having been placed completely under the influence of chloroform, the clitoris [be] freely excised either by scissors or knife—I always prefer the scissors."[37] The supposed sequelae of female masturbation, such as sterility, paresis, hysteria, dysmenorrhea, idiocy, and insanity, were also held to be remedied by the operation.

Male masturbation was likewise treated by means of surgical procedures. Some recommended vasectomy[38] while others found this procedure ineffective and employed castration.[39] One illustrative case involved the castration of a physician who had been confined as insane for seven years and who subsequently was able to return to practice.[40]

. . .

There were, though, more tolerant approaches, ranging from hard work and simple diet[41] to suggestions that "If the masturbator is totally continent, sexual intercourse is advisable."[42] This latter approach to therapy led some physicians to recommend that masturbators cure their disease by frequenting houses of prostitution,[43] or acquiring a mistress.[44] Though these treatments would appear ad hoc, more theoretically sound proposals were made by many physicians in terms of the model of excitability. They suggested that the disease and its sequelae could be adequately controlled by treating the excitation and debility consequent upon masturbation. Towards this end, "active tonics" and the use of cold baths at night just before bedtime were suggested.[45] Much more in a "Brownian" mode was the proposal that treatment with opium would be effective. An initial treatment with $1/12$ of a grain of morphine sulfate daily by injection was followed after ten days by a dose of $1/16$ of a grain. This dose was continued for three weeks and gradually diminished to $1/30$ of a grain a day. At the end of the month the patient was dismissed from treatment "the picture of health, having fattened very much, and lost every trace of anaemia and mental imbecility."[46] The author, after his researches with opium and masturbation, concluded, "*We may find in opium a new and important aid in the treatment of the victims of the habit of masturbation by means of which their moral and physical forces may be so increased that they may be enabled to enter the true physiological path.*"[47] This last example eloquently collects the elements of the concept of the disease of masturbation as a pathophysiological entity: excitation leads to physical debilitation requiring a physical remedy. Masturbation as a pathophysiological entity was thus incorporated within an acceptable medical model of diagnosis and therapy.

In summary, in the nineteenth century, biomedical scientists attempted to correlate a vast number of signs and symptoms with a disapproved activity found in many patients afflicted with various maladies. Given an inviting theoretical framework, it was very conducive to think of this range of signs and symptoms as having one cause. The theoretical framework, though, as has been indicated, was not value free but structured by the values and expectations of the times. In the nineteenth century, one was pleased to think that not "one bride in a hundred, of delicate, educated, sensitive women, accepts matrimony from any desire of sexual gratification: when she thinks of this at all, it is with shrinking, or even with horror, rather than with desire."[48] In contrast, in the twentieth century, articles are published for the instruction of women in the use of masturbation to overcome the disease of frigidity or orgasmic dysfunction.[49] In both cases, expectations concerning what should be significant structure the appreciation of reality by medicine. The variations are not due to mere fallacies of scientific method[50] but involve a basic dependence of the logic of scientific discovery and explanation upon prior evaluations of reality.[51] A sought-for coincidence of morality and nature gives goals to explanation and therapy.[52] Values influence the purpose and direction of investigations and treatment. Moreover, the disease of masturbation has other analogues. In the nineteenth century, there were such diseases in the South as "Drapetomania, the disease causing slaves to run away," and the disease "Dysaesthesia Aethiopis or hebetude of mind and obtuse sensibility of body—a disease peculiar to Negroes—called by overseers 'rascality'."[53] In Europe, there was the disease of *morbus democritus*.[54] Some would hold that current analogues exist in diseases such as alcoholism and drug abuse.[55] In short, the disease of masturbation indicates that evaluations play a role in the development of explanatory models and that this may not be an isolated phenomenon.

This analysis, then, suggests the following conclusion: although vice and virtue are not equivalent to disease and health, they bear a direct relation to these concepts. Insofar as a vice is taken to be a deviation from an ideal of human perfection, or "well-being," it can be translated into disease language. In shifting to disease language, one no longer speaks in moralistic terms (e.g., "You are evil"), but one speaks in terms of a deviation from a norm which implies a degree of imperfection (e.g., "You are a deviant"). The shift is from an explicitly ethical language to a language of natural teleology. To be ill is to fail to realize the perfection of an ideal type; to be sick is to be defective rather than to be evil. The concern is no longer with what is naturally, morally good, but what is naturally beautiful. Medicine turns to what has been judged to be naturally ugly or deviant, and then develops etiological accounts in order to explain and treat in a coherent fashion a manifold of displeasing signs and symptoms. The notion of the "deviant" structures the concept of disease, providing a purpose and direction for explanation and for action, that is, for diagnosis and prognosis, and for therapy. A "disease entity" operates as a conceptual form organizing phenomena in a fashion deemed useful for certain goals. The goals, though, involve choice by man and are not objective facts, data "given" by nature. They are ideals imputed to nature. The disease of masturbation is an eloquent example of the role of evaluation in explanation and the structure values give to our picture of reality.

NOTES

1. Alvan R. Feinstein, "Taxonomy and logic in clinical data," *Ann. N.Y. Acad. Sci.*, 1969, *161*: 450–459.

2. Horacio Fabrega, Jr., "Concepts of disease: logical features and social implications," *Perspect. Biol. Med.*, 1972, *15*: 583–616.

3. For example, Hippocrates correlated gout with sexual intercourse, *Aphorisms*, VI, 30. Numerous passages in the *Corpus* recommend the avoidance of overindulgence especially during certain illnesses.

4. René A. Spitz, "Authority and masturbation. Some remarks on a bibliographical investigation," *Yb. Psychoanal.*, 1953, *9*: 116. Also, Robert H. MacDonald, "The frightful consequences of onanism: notes on the history of a delusion," *J. Hist. Ideas*, 1967, *28*: 423–431.

5. Simon-André Tissot, *Tentamen de Morbis ex Manustrupatione* (Lausannae: M. M. Bousquet, 1758). An anonymous American translation appeared in the early 19th century: *Onanism* (New York: Collins & Hannay, 1832).

6. Simon-André Tissot, *Onanism* (New York: Collins & Hannay, 1832), p. 5.

7. *Ibid.*, p. 50.

8. E. H. Hare, "Masturbatory insanity: the history of an idea," *J. Mental Sco.*, 1962, *108*: 2–3.

9. Joseph W. Howe, *Excessive Venery, Masturbation and Continence* (New York: Bermingham, 1884), pp. 76–77.

10. Tissot, *op. cit.* (n. 6 above), p. 51.

11. J. A. Mayes, "Spermatorrhoea, treated by the lately invented rings," *Charleston Med. J. & Rev.*, 1854, *9*: 352.

12. Allen W. Hagenbach, "Masturbation as a cause of insanity," *J. Ner. Ment. Dis.*, 1879, *6*: 609.

13. Baker Brown, *On the Curability of Certain Forms of Insanity, Epilepsy, Catalepsy, and Hysteria in Females* (London: Hardwicke, 1866). Brown phrased the cause discreetly in terms of "peripheral irritation, arising originally in some branches of the pudic nerve, more particularly the incident nerve supplying the clitoris. . . ." (p. 7).

14. F. A. Burdem, "Self pollution in children," *Mass. Med. J.*, 1896, *16*: 340.

15. Weber Liel, "The influence of sexual irritation upon the diseases of the ear," *New Orleans Med. & Surg. J.*, 1884, *11*: 786–788.

16. Joseph Jones, "Diseases of the nervous system," *Trans. La. Med. Soc.* (New Orleans: L. Graham & Son, 1889), p. 170.

17. Howe, *op. cit.* (n. 9 above), p. 93.

18. J. Castellanos, "Influence of sewing machines upon the health and morality of the females using them," *South. J. Med. Sci.*, 1866–1867, *I*: 495–496.

19. Comment, "Masturbation and ophthalmia," *New Orleans Med. & Surg. J.*, 1881–1882, *9*: 67.

20. Howe, *op. cit.* (n. 9 above), pp. 108–111.

21. *Ibid.*, pp. 41, 72.

22. *Ibid.*, p. 68.

23. *Ibid.*, p. 73.

24. Hagenbach, *op. cit.* (n. 12 above), pp. 603–612.

25. Jones, *op. cit.* (n. 16 above), p. 170.

26. Howe, *op. cit.* (n. 9 above), p. 95.

27. Burdem, *op. cit.* (n. 14 above), pp. 339, 341.

28. Even Boerhaave remarked that "an excessive discharge of semen causes fatigue, weakness, decrease in activity, convulsions, emaciation, dehydration, heat and pains in the membranes of the

brain, a loss in the acuity of the senses, particularly of vision, *tabes dorsalis*, simplemindedness, and various similar disorders." My translation of Hermanno Boerhaave's *Institutiones Medicae* (Viennae: J. T. Trattner, 1775), p. 315, paragraph 776.

29. "We have seen that masturbation is more pernicious than excessive intercourse with females. Those who believe in a special providence, account for it by a special ordinance of the Deity to punish this crime." Tissot, *op. cit.* (n. 6 above), p. 45.

30. ". . . the best remedy was not to tell the poor children that they were damning their souls, but to tell them that they might seriously hurt their bodies, and to explain to them the nature and purport of the functions they were abusing." Lawson Tait, "Masturbation. A clinical lecture," *Med. News*, 1888, *53*: 2.

31. C. D. W. Colby, "Mechanical restraint of masturbation in a young girl," *Med. Record in N.Y.*, 1897, *52*: 206.

32. Louis Bauer, "Infibulation as a remedy for epilepsy and seminal losses," *St. Louis Clin. Record*, 1879, 6: 163–165. See also Gerhart S. Schwarz, "Infibulation, population control, and the medical profession," *Bull. N.Y. Acad. Med.*, 1970, *46*: 979, 990.

33. Jonathan Hutchinson, "On circumcision as preventive of masturbation," *Arch. Surg.*, 1890–1891, 2: 267–269.

34. William J. Robinson, "Masturbation and its treatment," *Am. J. Clin. Med.*, 1907, *14*: 349.

35. John Duffy, "Masturbation and clitoridectomy. A nineteenth-century view," *J.A.M.A.*, 1963, *186*: 246–248.

36. Brown, *op. cit.* (n. 13 above), p. 11.

37. *Ibid.*, p. 17.

38. Timothy Haynes, "Surgical treatment of hopeless cases of masturbation and nocturnal emissions," *Boston Med. & Surg. J.*, 1883, *109*: 130.

39. J. H. Marshall, "Insanity cured by castration," *Med. & Surg. Reptr.*, 1865, *13*: 363–364.

40. "The patient soon evinced marked evidences of being a changed man, becoming quiet, kind, and docile." *Ibid.*, p. 363.

41. Editorial, "Review of European legislation for the control of prostitution," *New Orleans Med. & Surg. J.*, 1854–1855, *11*: 704.

42. Robinson, *op. cit.* (n. 34 above), p. 350.

43. Theophilus Parvin, "The hygiene of the sexual functions," *New Orleans Med. & Surg. J.*, 1884, *11*: 606.

44. Mayes, *op. cit.* (n. 11 above), p. 352.

45. Haynes, *op. cit.* (n. 38 above), p. 130.

46. B. A. Pope, "Opium as a tonic and alternative; with remarks upon the hypodermic use of the sulfate of morphia, and its use in the debility and amorosis consequent upon onanism," *New Orleans Med. & Surg. J.*, 1879, 6: 725.

47. *Ibid.*, p. 727.

48. Parvin, *op. cit.* (n. 43 above), p. 607.

49. Joseph LoPiccolo and W. Charles Lobitz, "The role of masturbation in the treatment of orgasmic dysfunction," *Arch. Sexual Behavior*, 1972, 2: 163–171.

50. E. Hare, *op. cit.* (n. 8 above), pp. 15–19.

51. Norwood Hanson, *Patterns of Discovery* (London: Cambridge University Press, 1965).

52. Tissot, *op. cit.* (n. 6 above), p. 45. As Immanuel Kant, a contemporary of S. A. Tissot remarked, "Also, in all probability, it was through this moral interest [in the moral law governing the world] that attentiveness to beauty and the ends of nature was first aroused." (*Kants Werke*, Vol. 5, *Kritik der Urtheilskraft* [Berlin: Walter de Gruyter & Co., 1968], p. 459, A 439. My translation.) That is, moral values influence the search for goals in nature, and direct attention to what will be considered natural, normal, and nondeviant. This would also imply a relationship between the aesthetic, especially what was judged to be naturally beautiful, and what was held to be the goals of nature.

53. Samuel A. Cartwright, "Report on the diseases and physical peculiarities of the Negro race," *New Orleans Med. & Surg. J.*, 1850–1851, 7: 707–709. An interesting examination of these diseases is given by Thomas S. Szasz, "The sane slave," *Am. J. Psychoth.*, 1971, *25*: 228–239.

54. Heinz Hartmann, "Towards a concept of mental health," *Brit. J. Med. Psychol.*, 1960, *33*: 248.

55. Thomas S. Szasz, "Bad habits are not diseases: a refutation of the claim that alcoholism is a disease," *Lancet*, 1972, 2: 83–84; and Szasz, "The ethics of addiction," *Am. J. Psychiatry*, 1971, *128*: 541–546.

CHRISTOPHER BOORSE

On the Distinction Between Disease and Illness

. . . With few exceptions, clinicians and philosophers are agreed that health is an essentially evaluative notion. According to this consensus view, a value-free science of health is impossible. This thesis I believe to be entirely mistaken. I shall argue in this essay that it rests on a confusion between the theoretical and the practical senses of "health," or in other words, between disease and illness.

Two presuppositions of my whole discussion should be noted at the outset. The first is substantive: with Szasz and Flew, I shall assume that the idea of health ought to be analyzed by reference to physiological medicine alone.[1] It is a mistake to view physical and mental health as equally well-entrenched species of a single conceptual genus. In most respects, our institutions of mental health are recent offshoots from physiological medicine, and their nature and future are under continual controversy. In advance of a clear analysis of health in physiological medicine, it seems an open question whether current applications of the health vocabulary to mental conditions have any justification at all. Such applications will therefore be put on probation in the first two sections below. The other presupposition of my discussion is terminological. For convenience in distinguishing theoretical from practical uses of "health," I shall adhere to the technical usage of "disease" found in textbooks of medical theory. In such textbooks "disease" is simply synonymous with "unhealthy condition." Readers who wish to preserve the much narrower ordinary usage of "disease" should therefore substitute "theoretically unhealthy condition" throughout.

Reprinted with permission of the publisher from *Philosophy and Public Affairs*, Vol. 5, No. 1 (Fall 1975), pp. 49–68. Copyright © 1975 by Princeton University Press.

NORMATIVISM ABOUT HEALTH

It is safe to begin any discussion of health by saying that health is normality, since the terms are interchangeable in clinical contexts. But this remark provides no analysis of health until one specifies the norms involved. The most obvious proposal, that they are pure statistical means, is widely recognized to be erroneous. On the one hand, many deviations from the average—e.g., unusual strength or vital capacity or eye color—are not unhealthy. On the other hand, practically everyone has some disease or other, and there are also particular diseases such as tooth decay and minor lung irritation that are nearly universal. Since statistical normality is therefore neither necessary nor sufficient for clinical normality, most writers take the following view about the norms of health: that they must be determined, in whole or in part, by acts of evaluation. More precisely, the orthodox view is that all judgments of health include value judgments as part of their meaning. To call a condition unhealthy is at least in part to condemn it; hence it is impossible to define health in nonevaluative terms. I shall refer to this orthodox view as *normativism*.

Normativism has many varieties, which are often not clearly distinguished from one another by the clinicians who espouse them. The common feature of healthy conditions may, for example, be held to be either their desirability for the individual or their desirability for society. The gap between these two values is a persistent source of controversy in the mental-health domain. One especially common variety of normativism combines the thesis that health judgments are value judgments with ethical relativism. The resulting view that society is the final authority on what counts as disease is typical of psychiatric texts, as illustrated by the following quotation:

While professionals have a major voice in influencing the judgment of society, it is the collective judgment of the larger social group that determines whether its members are to be viewed as sick or criminal, eccentric or immoral.[2]

For the most part my arguments against normativism will apply to all versions indiscriminately. It will, however, be useful to make a minimal division of normativist positions into strong and weak. Strong normativism will be the view that health judgments are pure evaluations without descriptive meaning; weak normativism allows such judgments a descriptive as well as a normative component.[3]

As an example of a virtually explicit statement of strong normativism by a clinician, consider Dr. Judd Marmor's remark in a recent psychiatric symposium on homosexuality:

. . . to call homosexuality the result of disturbed sexual development really says nothing other than that you disapprove of the outcome of the development.[4]

If we may substitute "unhealthy" for "disturbed," Marmor is claiming that to call a condition unhealthy is *only* to express disapproval of it. In other words—to collapse a few ethical distinctions—for a condition to be unhealthy it is necessary and sufficient that it be bad. Now at least half of this view, the sufficiency claim, is demonstrably false of physiological medicine. It is undesirable to be moderately ugly or, for that matter, to lack the manual dexterity of Liszt, but neither of these conditions is a disease. In fact, there are undesirable conditions regularly corrected by physicians which are not diseases: Jewish nose, sagging breasts, adolescent fertility, and unwanted pregnancies are only a few of many examples. Thus strong normativism is an erroneous account of health judgments in their paradigm area of application, and its influence upon mental-health theorists is regrettable.

Unlike Marmor, however, many clinical writers take positions that can be construed as committing them merely to weak normativism. A good example is Dr. Marie Jahoda, who concludes her survey of current criteria of psychological health with these words:

Actually, the discussion of the psychological meaning of various criteria could proceed without concern for value premises. Only as one calls these psychological phenomena "mental health" does the problem of values arise in full force. By this label, one asserts that these psychological attributes are "good." And, inevitably, the question is raised:

Good for what? Good in terms of middle class ethics? Good for democracy? For the continuation of the social *status quo*? For the individual's happiness? For mankind? . . . For the encouragement of genius or of mediocrity and conformity? The list could be continued.[5]

Jahoda may here mean to claim only that calling a condition healthy *involves* calling it good. Her remarks are at least consistent with the weak normativist thesis that healthy conditions are good conditions which satisfy some further descriptive property as well. On this view, "healthy" is a mixed normative-descriptive term of the same sort as "honest" and "courageous." The following passage by Dr. F. C. Redlich is likewise consistent with the weak view:

Most propositions about normal behavior refer implicitly or explicitly to ideal behavior. Deviations from the ideal obviously are fraught with value judgments; actually, all propositions on normality contain certain statements in various degrees.[6]

Redlich's term "contain" suggests that he too sees the goodness of something as merely one necessary condition of its healthiness, and similarly for badness and unhealthiness.

Yet even weak normativism runs into counterexamples within physiological medicine. It is obvious that a disease may be on balance desirable, as with the flat feet of a draftee or the mild infection produced by inoculation. It might be suggested in response that diseases must at any rate be prima facie undesirable. The trouble with this suggestion is that it is obscure. Consider the case of a disease that has infertility as its sole important effect. In what sense is infertility prima facie undesirable? Considered in abstraction from the actual effects of reproduction on human beings, it is hard to see how infertility is either desirable or undesirable. Possibly those who see it as "prima facie" undesirable assume that most people want to be able to have more children. But the corollary of this position will be that writers of medical texts must do an empirical survey of human preferences to be sure that a condition is a disease. No such considerations seem to enter into human physiological research, any more than they do into standard biological studies of the diseases of plants and animals. Here indeed is another difficulty for any normativist, weak or strong. It seems clear that one may speak of diseases in plants and animals without judging the conditions in question undesirable. Biologists who study the diseases of fruit flies or sharks need not assume that their health is a good thing for us. On the other hand, there is not much sense in talking about the best interests of, say, a begonia. So it seems that normativists must interpret health judgments about plants and lower animals as analogical, in the same way as would be statements about the courage or considerateness of wolves and rats.

If normativism about health is at once so influential and so objectionable, one must ask what persuasive arguments there are in its support. I know of only three arguments, of which one will be treated in the next section. A germ of an argument appears in the passage by Redlich just quoted. Health judgments involve a comparison to an ideal; hence, Redlich concludes, they are "fraught with value judgments." It seems evident, however, that Redlich is thinking of ideals such as beauty and holiness rather than the chemist's ideal gas or Weber's ideal bureaucrat. The fact that a gas or a bureaucrat deviates from the ideal type is nothing against the gas or the bureaucrat. There are normative and nonnormative ideals, as there are in fact normative and nonnormative norms. The question is which sort health is, and Redlich has here provided no grounds for an answer.

A second and equally incomplete argument for normativism is suggested by the first two chapters of Margolis' *Psychotherapy and Morality*.[7] Margolis argues in his first chapter that psychoanalysts have been mistaken in holding that their therapeutic activities can "escape moral scrutiny" (p. 13). From this he concludes that "it is reasonable to view therapeutic values as forming part of a larger system of moral values" (p. 37), and explicitly endorses normativism. But this inference is a non sequitur. From the fact that the promotion of health is open to moral review, it in no way follows that health judgments are value judgments. Wealth and power are also "values" in the sense that people pursue them in a morally criticizable fashion; neither is a normative concept. The pursuit of any descriptively definable condition, if it has effects on persons, will be open to moral review.

These two arguments, like the health literature generally, do next to nothing to rule out the alternative view that health is a descriptively definable property which is usually valuable. Why, after all, may not health be a concept of the same sort as intelligence, or deductive validity? Though the idea of intelligence is certainly vague, it does not seem to be normative. Intelligence is the ability to perform certain intellectual tasks, and one would expect that these intellectual tasks could be characterized without presupposing their value.[8] Similarly, a valid argument may, for theoretical purposes, be descriptively defined[9] roughly as one that has a form no instance of which could have true premises and a false conclusion. Intelligence in people and validity in arguments being generally valued, the statement that a person is intelligent or an argument valid does tend to have the force of a recommendation. But this fact is wholly irrelevant to the employment of the terms in theories of intelligence or validity. To insist that evaluation is still part of the very meaning of the terms would be to make an implausible claim to which there are obvious counterexamples. Exactly the same may be true of the concept of health. At any rate, we have already seen some of the counterexamples. . . .

The difference . . . emerges most clearly in the distinction between disease and illness. It is disease, the theoretical concept, that applies indifferently to organisms of all species. That is because, as we shall see, it is to be analyzed in biological rather than ethical terms. The point is that illnesses are merely a subclass of diseases, namely, those diseases that have certain normative features reflected in the institutions of medical practice. An illness must be, first, a reasonably *serious* disease with incapacitating effects that make it undesirable. A shaving cut or mild athlete's foot cannot be called an illness, nor could one call in sick on the basis of a single dental cavity, though all these conditions are diseases. Secondly, to call a disease an illness is to view its owner as deserving special treatment and diminished moral accountability. These requirements of "illness" will be discussed in some detail shortly, with particular attention to "mental illness." But they explain at once why the notion of illness does not apply to plants and animals. Where we do not make the appropriate normative judgments or activate the social institutions, no amount of disease will lead us to use the term "ill." Even if the laboratory fruit flies fly in listless circles and expire at our feet, we do not say they succumbed to an illness, and for roughly the same reasons as we decline to give them a proper funeral.

There are, then, two senses of "health." In one sense it is a theoretical notion, the opposite of "disease." In another sense it is a practical or mixed ethical notion, the opposite of "illness."[10] Let us now examine the relation between these two concepts more closely.

DISEASE AND ILLNESS

What is the theoretical notion of a disease? An admirable explanation of clinical normality was given thirty years ago by C. Daly King.

The normal . . . is objectively, and properly, to be defined as that which functions in accordance with its design.[11]

The root idea of this account is that the normal is the natural. The state of an organism is theoretically healthy, i.e., free of disease, insofar as its mode of functioning conforms to the natural design of that kind of organism. Philosophers have, of course, grown repugnant to the idea of natural design since its co-optation by natural-purpose ethics and the so-called argument from design. It is undeniable that the term "natural" is often given an evaluative force. Shakespeare as well as Roman Catholicism is full of such usages, and they survive as well in the strictures of state legislatures against "unnatural acts." But it is no part of biological theory to assume that what is natural is desirable, still less the product of divine artifice. Contemporary biology employs a version of the idea of natural design that seems ideal for the analysis of health.

The crucial element in the idea of a biological design is the notion of a natural function. I have argued elsewhere that a function in the biologist's sense is nothing but a standard causal contribution to a goal actually pursued by the organism.[12] Organisms are vast assemblages of systems and subsystems which, in most members of a species, work together harmoniously in such a way as to achieve a hierarchy of goals. . . . Whatever the correct analysis of function statements, there is no doubt that biological theory is deeply committed to attributing functions to processes in plants and animals. And the single unifying property of all recognized diseases of plants and animals appears to be this: that they interfere with one or more functions typically performed within members of the species. . . .

If what makes a condition a disease is its deviation from the natural functional organization of the species, then in calling tooth decay a disease we are saying that it is not simply in the nature of the species—and we say this because we think of it as mainly due to environmental causes. In general, deficiencies in the functional efficiency of the body are diseases when they are unnatural, and they may be unnatural either by being atypical or by being attributable mainly to the action of a hostile environment. If this explanation is accepted, then the functional account simultaneously avoids the pitfalls of statistical normality and also frees the idea of theoretical health of all normative content.

Theoretical health now turns out to be strictly analogous to the mechanical condition of an artifact. Despite appearances, "perfect mechanical condition" in, say, a 1965 Volkswagen is a descriptive notion. Such an artifact is in perfect mechanical condition when it conforms in all respects to the designer's detailed specifications. Normative interests play a crucial role, of course, in the initial choice of the design. But what the Volkswagen design actually *is* is an empirical matter by the time production begins. Thenceforward a car may be in perfect condition regardless of whether the design is good or bad. If one replaces its stock carburetor with a high-performance part, one may well produce a better car, but one does not produce a Volkswagen in better mechanical condition. Similarly, an automatic camera may function perfectly and take wretched pictures; guided missiles and instruments of torture in perfect mechanical condition may serve execrable ends. Perfect working order is a matter not of the worth of the product but of the conformity of the process to a fixed design. In the case of organisms, of course, the ideal of health must be determined by empirical analysis of the species rather than by the intentions of a designer. But otherwise the parallel seems exact. A person who by mutation acquires a sixth sense, or the ability to regenerate severed limbs, is not thereby healthier than we are. Sixth senses and limb regeneration are not part of the human design, which at any given time, for better or worse, just is what it is.

We have been arguing that health is descriptively definable within medical theory, as intelligence is in psychological theory or validity in logical theory. Nevertheless medical theory is the basis of medical practice, and medical practice unquestioningly presupposes the value of health. We must therefore ask how the functional view explains this presumption that health is desirable.

In the case of physiological health, there are at least two general reasons why the functional normality that defines it is usually worth having. In the first place, most people do want to pursue the goals with respect to which physiological functions are isolated. Not only do we want to survive and reproduce, but we also want to engage in those particular activities, such as eating and sex, by which these goals are typically achieved. In the second place—and this is surely the main reason the value of physical health seems indisputable—physiological functions tend to contribute to all manner of activities neutrally. Whether it is desirable for one's heart to pump, one's stomach to digest, or one's kidneys to eliminate hardly depends at all on what one wants to do. It follows that essentially all serious physiological diseases will satisfy the first requirement of an illness, namely, undesirability for its bearer.

This explanation of the fit between medical theory and medical practice has the virtue of reminding us that health, though an important value, is conceptually a very limited one. Health is not unconditionally worth promoting, nor is what is worth promoting necessarily health. Although mental-health writers are especially prone to ignore these points, even the constitution of the World Health Organization seems to embody a similar confusion:

Health is a state of complete physical, mental, and social well-being, and not merely the absence of disease or infirmity.

Unless one is to abandon the physiological paradigm altogether, this definition is far too wide. Health is functional normality, and as such is desirable exactly insofar as it promotes goals one can justify on independent grounds. But there is presumably no intrinsic value in having the functional organization typical of a species if the same goals can be better achieved by other means. A sixth sense, for example, would increase our goal-efficiency without increasing our health; so might the amputation of our legs at the knee and their replacement by a nuclear-powered air-cushion vehicle. Conversely, as we have seen, there is no a priori reason why ordinary diseases cannot contribute to well-being under appropriate circumstances.

In such cases, however, we will be reluctant to describe the person involved as ill, and that is because the term "ill" *does* have a negative evaluation built into it. Here again a comparison between health and other properties will be helpful. Disease and illness are related somewhat as are low intelligence and stupidity, or failure to tell the truth and speaking dishonestly. . . .

If we supplement this condition of undesirability with two further normative conditions, I believe we have the beginning of a plausible analysis of "illness."

A disease is an *illness* only if it is serious enough to be incapacitating, and therefore is

(i) undesirable for its bearer;
(ii) a title to special treatment; and
(iii) a valid excuse for normally criticizable behavior. . . .

I shall now argue . . . that conditions (i), (ii), and (iii) all present difficulties in the domain of mental health.

MENTAL ILLNESS

For the sake of discussion, let us simply assume that the mental conditions usually called pathological are in fact unhealthy by the theoretical standard sketched in the last section. That is, we shall assume both that there are natural mental functions and also that recognized types of psychopathology are unnatural interferences with these functions.[13] Is it reasonable to make a parallel extension of the vocabulary of medical practice by calling these mental diseases mental illnesses? Let us consider each condition on "illness."

Condition (i) was the undesirability of an illness for its bearer. Now there are obstacles to transferring our general arguments that physiological health is desirable to the psychological domain. Mental states are not nearly so neutral to the choice of actions as physiological states are. In particular, to evaluate the desirability of mental health we can hardly avoid consulting our desires; but in the mental-health context it could be those very desires that are judged unhealthy. From a theoretical standpoint desires must be assigned a motivational function in producing action. Thus our wants may or may not conform to the species design. But if our wants do not conform to the species design, it is not immediately obvious why we should want them to. If there is no good reason to want them to, then we have a disease which is not an illness. It is conceivable that this divergence between the two notions is illustrated by homosexuality. It can hardly be denied that one normal function of sexual desire is to promote reproduction. If one does not have a desire for heterosexual sex, however, the only good reason for wanting to have such a desire seems to be that one would be happier if one did. But this judgment needs to be supported by evidence. The desirability of having species-typical desires is not nearly so obvious on inspection as the desirability of having species-typical physiological functions. . . .

Since clinicians often assume that mental health involves social adjustment, it may be well to point out that the functional account of health shows this too to be a debatable assumption requiring empirical support. Certainly nothing in the mere statement that a person has a mental disease entails that he or she is contributing less to the social order than an arbitrary normal individual. There is no contradiction in calling van Gogh or Blake or Dostoyevsky mentally disturbed while admiring their work, even if they would have been less creative had they been healthier. Conversely, there is no a priori reason to assume that the healthy human personality will be morally worthy or socially acceptable. . . .

It must be conceded that *Homo sapiens* is a social species. Other organisms of this class, such as ants and bees, display elaborate fixed systems of social adaptations, and it would be remarkable if the human design included no standard functions at all promoting socialization. On the basis of the physiological paradigm, however, it is not at all clear that contributions to society can be viewed as requirements of health except when they also contribute to individual survival and reproduction. No matter how this issue is decided, the crucial point remains: the nature and extent of social functions in the human species can be discovered only empirically. Despite the contrary convictions of many clinicians, the concept of mental health itself provides no guarantee that healthy individuals will meet the standards or serve the interests of society at large. If it did, that would be one more reason to question the desirability of health for the individual.

Let us now go on to condition (ii) on a disease which is an illness: that it justify "special treatment" of its owner. It is this condition together with (iii) that gives some plausibility to the many recent attempts to explain mental illness as a "social status" or "role."[14] The idea that the "sick role" is a special one is consistent with the statistical normality of having some disease or other. Since illnesses are serious diseases that incapacitate at the level of gross behavior, everyone can be minimally diseased without being ill. In the realm of mental health, however, many psychiatrists suggest the stronger thesis that it is statistically normal to be significantly incapacitated by neurosis.[15] A similar problem may arise on Benedict's famous view that the characteristic personality type of some whole societies is clinically paranoid.[16] A statistically normal condition, according to our analysis, can be a disease

only if it can be blamed on the environment. But one might plausibly claim that most or all existing *cultural* environments do injure children, filling their minds with excessive anxiety about sexual pleasure, grotesque role models, absurd prejudices about reality, etc. It is at least possible that some degree of neurosis or psychosis is a nearly universal environmental injury in our species. Only an empirical inquiry into the incidence and etiology of neurosis can show whether this possibility is a reality. If it is, however, one can maintain the idea that serious diseases are illnesses only by abandoning one of the presuppositions of the illness concept: that not everyone can be ill.

The last and clearest difficulty with "mental illness" concerns condition (iii), the role of illness in excusing conduct. We said that the idea that serious diseases excuse conduct derives from the model of the relation of agents to their own physiology. Unfortunately the relation of agents to their own psychology is of a much more intimate kind. The puzzle about mental illness is that it seems to be an activity of the very seat of responsibility—the mind and character—and therefore to be beyond all hope of excuse.

This inference is hardly inescapable; there is room for considerable controversy to which I cannot do justice here. Strictly speaking, mental disorders are disturbances of the personality. It is persons, not personalities, who are held responsible for actions, and one central element in the idea of a person is certainly consciousness. This means that there may be some sense in contrasting responsible persons with their mental diseases insofar as these diseases lie outside their conscious personalities. Perhaps from a psychoanalytic standpoint this condition is often met in psychosis and neurosis. The unconscious processes that surface in these disorders seem at first sight more like things that happen within us, e.g., peristalsis, than like things we do. But several points make this classification look oversimplified. Unconscious ideas and wishes are still *our* ideas and wishes in a more compelling sense than movements of the gut are our movements. They may have been conscious at an earlier time or be made conscious in therapy, whereupon it becomes increasingly difficult to disclaim responsibility for them. It seems quite unclear that we are more responsible for many conscious desires and beliefs than for these unconscious ones. Finally, the hope for contrasting responsible people with their mental diseases grows vanishingly dim in the case of a character disorder, where the unhealthy condition seems to be integrated into the conscious personality.

In view of these points and the rest of the discussion, I think we must accept the following conclusion. While conditions (i), (ii), and (iii) apply fairly automatically to serious physical diseases, not one of them should be assumed to apply automatically to serious mental diseases. If the term "mental illness" is to be applied at all, it should probably be restricted to psychoses and disabling neuroses. But even this decision needs more analysis than I have provided in this essay. It seems doubtful that on any construal mental illness will ever be, in the mental-health movement's famous phrase, "just like any other illness." . . .

NOTES

1. Thomas S. Szasz, *The Myth of Mental Illness* (New York, 1961); Antony Flew, *Crime or Disease?* (New York, 1973), pp. 40, 42.

2. Ian Gregory, *Fundamentals of Psychiatry* (Philadelphia, 1968), p. 32.

3. R. M. Hare, in *Freedom and Reason* (New York, 1963), Chap. 2, argues that no terms have prescriptive meaning alone. If this view is accepted, the difference between strong and weak normativism concerns the question of whether "healthy" is "primarily" or "secondarily" evaluative.

4. Judd Marmor, "Homosexuality and Cultural Value Systems," *American Journal of Psychiatry* 130 (1973): 1208.

5. Marie Jahoda, *Current Concepts of Positive Mental Health* (New York, 1958), pp. 76–77. See also her remark in *Interrelations Between the Social Environment and Psychiatric Disorders* (New York, 1953), p. 142: ". . . inevitably at some place there is a value judgement involved. I think that mental health or mental sickness cannot be conceived of without reference to some basic value."

6. F. C. Redlich, "The Concept of Normality," *American Journal of Psychotherapy* 6 (1952): 553.

7. Joseph Margolis, *Psychotherapy and Morality* (New York, 1966).

8. Exactly what intellectual abilities are included in intelligence is, of course, unclear and may vary from culture to culture. (See N. J. Block and Gerald Dworkin, "IQ. Heritability and Inequality, Part I," *Philosophy and Public Affairs* 3, no. 4 [Summer, 1974]: 333.) But this does not show that for any particular group of speakers "intelligent" is a normative term, i.e., has positive evaluation as part of its meaning.

9. The contrary view, which might be called normativism about validity, is defended by J. O. Urmson in "Some Questions Concerning Validity," *Revue Internationale de Philosophie* 25 (1953): 217–229.

10. Thomas Nagel has suggested that the adjective "ill" may have its own special opposite "well." Our thinking about health might be greatly clarified if "wellness" had some currency.

11. C. Daly King, "The Meaning of Normal," *Yale Journal of Biology and Medicine* 17 (1945): 493–494. Most definitions of health in medical dictionaries include some reference to functions. Almost exactly King's formulation also appears in Fredrick C. Redlich and Daniel X. Freedman, *The Theory and Practice of Psychiatry* (New York, 1966), p. 113.

12. Christopher Boorse, "Wright on Functions," *The Philosophical Review* 85 (1976): 70–86.

13. The plausibility of these two claims is discussed at length in my essay, "What a Theory of Mental Health Should Be," *Journal for the Theory of Social Behavior* 6 (1976): 61–84.

14. An example of this approach is Robert B. Edgerton, "On The 'Recognition' of Mental Illness," in Stanley C. Plog and Robert B. Edgerton, *Changing Perspectives in Mental Illness* (New York, 1969), pp. 49–72.

15. Only one example of this suggestion is Dr. Reuben Fine's statement that neurosis afflicts 99 percent of the population. See Fine's "The Goals of Psychoanalysis," in *The Goals of Psychotherapy*, ed. Alvin R. Mahrer (New York, 1967), p. 95. I consider the issue of whether all neurosis can be called unhealthy in the essay cited in note 13.

16. See the descriptions of the Kwakiutl and the Dobu in Ruth Benedict, *Patterns of Culture* (Boston: Houghton Mifflin, 1934).

MICHAEL RUSE

Are Homosexuals Sick?

There is much controversy today about whether a homosexual orientation is in itself a disease or sickness. If one is attracted sexually to members of one's own sex rather than to members of the opposite sex, then is this a sign that one is ill—standing in need of a cure? Or is it the case that having a homosexual orientation is simply a matter of having an attribute different from heterosexuals—something on a par with having blue eyes rather than brown?

Not surprisingly, militant homosexuals tend to see homosexuality as nothing more than a variant form of sexual orientation. "I have come to an unshakable conclusion: the illness theory of homosexuality is a pack of lies, concocted out of the myths of a patriarchal society for a political purpose. Psychiatry dedicated to making sick people well has been the corner-stone of a system of oppression that makes gay people sick." (Gold, 1973, p. 1211) But there are medical people who argue in much the same way. The influential psychiatrist Judd Marmor states: "Surely the time has come for psychiatry to give up the archaic practice of classifying the millions of men and women who accept or prefer homosexual object choices as being, by virtue of that fact alone, mentally ill. The fact that their alternative lifestyle happens to be out of favor with current cultural conventions must not be a basis in itself for a diagnosis of psychopathology. It is our task as psychiatrists to be healers of the distressed, not watchdogs of our social mores." (Marmor, 1973, p. 1209)

Conversely, however, Irving Bieber states that "homosexuality is not an adaptation of choice: it is brought about by fears that inhibit satisfactory heterosexual functioning." (Bieber, 1973, p. 1210) Similarly, Charles Socarides states that "homosexuality repre-

Reprinted by permission of the author.

sents a disorder of sexual development and does not fall within the range of normal sexual behaviour." (Socarides, 1973, p. 1212) And in line with the views of these two psychiatrists, the endocrinologist Gunther Dörner speaks of homosexuality as involving "inborn disturbances of gonadal functions and sexual behaviour in man," and he thinks it is a "sexual deviation" in need of cure (Dörner, 1976).

Obviously whether or not homosexuality is to be judged a sickness or a disease or an illness depends in part on the facts, both at what one might call the "empirical" or "phenomenal" level and at the causal level. One wants to know something about homosexuality, how it affects people, and what putative causes have been proposed for it. But there is more than this. One must also learn how terms like "disease" and "illness" are used. Only when one has done a philosophical analysis at this level can one then examine the empirical and causal claims and properly judge how to assess the status of people's sexual orientations, and in particular to judge the healthiness or sickness of homosexuality.

This then is my task in this paper. I shall begin with brief exposition of two recently proposed philosophical models of health, disease, and illness. I shall not be critical of these models, although I do think that in the course of the discussion certain strains will appear in at least one of the models. Then I shall run quickly both through some recent findings about homosexuals at the empirical level and through the three main categories of putative explanatory causes for homosexuality: psychoanalytic, endocrinal, and sociobiological. Again, my main intent will be expository rather than critical. At each point I shall see what light is thrown on the "homosexuality as sickness" question by comparison of the scientific claims with the philosophical models. What I shall argue is that, given different scientific claims and different philosophical models, we get different answers to our main question. This, I shall suggest, is the reason why we get such a controversy over the medical status of homosexuality.

I. TWO MODELS OF HEALTH AND SICKNESS

There are I believe currently two main models of health and sickness. The first is due primarily to Christopher Boorse (1975, 1976, 1977) and for obvious reasons I shall label it the *naturalist* model. Boorse sees health and disease as being opposite sides of the same coin. Health is the absence of disease. Disease is what one has when one is not healthy. The key to Boorse's position is that one makes no judgments about good or bad, desirable or undesirable, when one judges something a disease. "On our view disease judgements are value-neutral . . . their recognition is a matter of natural science, not evaluative decision." (Boorse, 1977, p. 543) What then is disease (and health)? . . .

Against Boorse, we have the *normativist* position, endorsed in recent years particularly by Joseph Margolis and H. Tristram Engelhardt Jr. . . . Although both Margolis and Engelhardt agree with Boorse that disease involves functioning, or rather malfunctioning, of the body or person, they disagree in how they feel it should be regarded. For them, a disease is a bad thing. Consequently, obviously they do not tie functioning directly to the biological ends of survival and reproduction (although of course it could involve these). They see functioning as more "cultural": "working in a satisfactory manner," or the like.

We have now before us our two positions, the naturalist and the normativist models. We must now turn to what is known, or at least claimed, about homosexuality. . . .

II. THE EMPIRICAL FACTS
ABOUT HOMOSEXUALITY

For my empirical information I rely heavily on the recent Kinsey Institute-endorsed study of homosexuals (and heterosexuals) drawn from the San Francisco area. (Bell and Weinberg, 1978) This study will hardly be the last word on homosexuals, their perceptions of themselves, their lifestyles, and so forth. But it does seem to be the most comprehensive and best evidence that we have so far. The authors of the study, Alan Bell and Martin Weinberg, gave extensive questionnaires to 972 homosexuals and 477 heterosexuals. Since we are already in a situation where people are making judgments about health and illness with respect to homosexuality, it is not as if I am being that premature in thus turning to the Bell-Weinberg report. . . .

But what conclusions might we want to draw from [the] facts and figures [in the study]? Fairly obviously I think we would want to say that most homosexuals are pretty content with their lot. Some indeed . . . are very positive about their homosexuality, apparently being at least as satisfied if not happier than comparable heterosexuals. There really seems no reason to pretend otherwise. On the other hand, there are homosexuals who have trouble accepting their sexual orientation, and there are homosexuals (I would imagine much the same group) who are not very happy. Moreover, many homosexuals have gone through crises of one kind or another which have driven them to serious thoughts of, or even attempts at, suicide. One simply cannot deny this fact, or that we are looking at a minority of the order of 10 to 20 percent (admittedly, this might in part be a transitory phase of development, say pre-25, which is then followed by a happier maturity).

So, how do these empirical findings fit in with our models of health, disease, and illness? Taking first the naturalist position promulgated by Boorse, and concentrating on the negative notions (i.e., disease and illness), we have seen nothing directly about how homosexuality affects survival prospects. Only if we link attempted suicide with successful suicide (which seems a major assumption) can we suggest that homosexuality may in some respects reduce survival chances. However, we have got reasonably strong evidence that being a homosexual reduces reproduction, and this clearly seems to be a function of homosexuality itself, rather than something else. Hence, on one prong of Boorse's criterion, homosexuality must be judged a disease.

However, illness is another matter. Some homosexuals, indeed most homosexuals, cannot be judged ill by Boorse's criterion. They are at least as satisfied with their lot, specifically with their sexual orientation, as are heterosexuals. Nevertheless, I do think we have to allow that by the naturalist criterion, a small minority of homosexuals are ill, and that this illness must be laid at the feet of their homosexuality. There are, for instance, some who would really like to be heterosexual, to marry, and to have children, and because of their orientation they cannot and this makes them unhappy. These people are ill, as perhaps are others who at various times in their lives are driven to the brink because of their sexual orientation.

The normativist conclusion overlaps in part with the naturalist conclusion, but not entirely. Those homosexuals that the naturalist would judge to be *both* diseased and ill (because of their homosexuality) would seem to be judged both diseased and ill (because of their homosexuality) by the normativist. Certainly, these are people who are not much enjoying life because of their sexual orientation, and this all seems to fit the normativists' criteria for disease and illness. However, the normativist parts company with the naturalist's claim that, judgments of illness apart, homosexuality generally is a disease. For Boorse, homosexuality is a disease because it reduces biological fitness. For the normativist, whether loss of biological fitness is a disease is a contingent matter, dependent on whether such loss makes the loser in any way regretful or unhappy. And apparently, since many homosexuals are happy in their homosexuality, the normativist would have no reason to judge them diseased (or ill). One can put matters this way. Boorse would say of the integrated happy homosexual that he/she had a disease but was not thereby ill. (See Boorse, 1975) The normativist would deny both disease and illness.

In concluding this section, a number of points of clarification and qualification seem appropriate. First, even if one does judge (some) homosexuals diseased/ill on the basis of the empirical data, this does not imply that they are diseased/ill all of their lives. If anything, the data seem to imply that homosexuality-as-disease/illness is more of a young person's problem—perhaps giving the lie to the popular notion about the tragedy of the aging homosexual, a sentiment that Bell and Weinberg (1978) endorse. Whether spontaneously or through human intervention, the possibility that homosexuality-as-disease/illness will vanish is certainly not barred.

Second, if one talks in terms of "cure" at this point (and the argument does seem to imply that such talk is appropriate for some), note that such cure does not necessarily entail changing a person's sexual orientation (even if this be at all possible). The way to dissolve homosexuality-as-disease/illness may be to come to accept one's sexual orientation, and to appreciate and cherish it for its own values and virtues. Third, related to this point, total cure might well (undoubtedly will?) involve the heterosexual majority as well. If the majority stop thinking of homosexuality as a handicap and as something unpleasant, and if they stop hating homosexuals, then if nothing else we shall get a rise in the self-image of presently troubled homosexuals. (However, the evidence does seem to be that there is more to the problem than societal attitudes. For instance, some homosexuals dislike their homosexuality because they want to be heterosexual, get married, and have children. Admittedly society endorses the having of children, but the happiness of child-rearing transcends societal approval.)

The final point is directed against those who might be inclined to say that homosexual happiness cannot in any way be compared to heterosexual happiness—it is obviously lower and therefore even your integrated homosexual is sick as compared to your average heterosexual. All one can say in reply to an objection like this is that there is not the slightest bit of evidence for such an ad hoc assumption. . . .

However, . . . a look at causal claims might throw a different light on some of the answers to the empirical questions (although I hasten to add, not necessarily a *truer* light). One might for instance plausibly suggest that people tend to claim to be more happy than they really are (although this is not to deny my defense just above of the claim that a happy homosexual is apparently just as happy as a happy heterosexual). For these and like reasons, let us turn to causes.

III. PSYCHOANALYTIC CAUSAL EXPLANATIONS

I find two main explanations of homosexuality in the psychoanalytic literature. One I shall term the "classical Freudian" explanation; the other explanation stems from Freud's ideas but was developed in part in reaction to Freud, and is for fairly obvious reasons called the "adaptationist" or "phobic" theory.

Freud (1905) argues that we are all essentially, physiologically and psychologically, bisexual—with elements of male and female mingled in our nature. In the case of biological males (which was Freud's paradigm), psychologically speaking we start out with the male side predominant, as we are attracted to mother. Then the female side comes to the fore, as we turn narcissistically towards our own bodies. And then comes the swing back to the male side, first to mother again, and then hopefully with a successful resolution of the Oedipus complex, to other females at adolescence. Females take a comparable path, although as every critic has been happy and eager to point out, Freud gives female psychosexual development little study in its own right, and that shows a desperately sexist bias. Fortunately, Freud's problems are not our problems here.

For Freud, therefore, a person is not really turned into a homosexual—rather, it is more a question of the homosexual side of our nature coming to the front and pushing back or out our heterosexual side. . . .

Consequently, for Freud homosexuality was not so much "abnormal," but more a question of arrested development or regression to an earlier stage. This means that, in his language, it is a "perversion" rather than a "neurosis," which latter involves repression (of memories, ideas, and so forth, from full consciousness). Hence, the method of analysis is inappropriate, since this is designed to bring unconscious elements to the front. Freud was therefore not very sanguine about curing homosexuality (in the sense of changing one predominantly homosexual into one predominantly heterosexual). Indeed, as he explained in his famous "Letter to an American Mother," he did not even think that homosexuality is an illness.

The question we want to ask is whether, if one accepts Freud's position as true (please note the hypothetical), we would want to modify or in any way alter the conclusions arrived at in the last section. Freud himself seems to imply that if one regards homosexuality as a case of arrested development (which he does), then this means it cannot be an illness. However, this seems not to follow. In girls, if a piece of one of their sex chromosomes is missing, there is a failure to develop sexually at puberty. We would (and do) certainly want to classify this phenomenon, Turner's Syndrome, as a disease/illness. (Levitan and Montagu, 1977) Therefore, analogously, such judgments seem not to be ruled out in the case of homosexuality. But of course this is not to say conversely that even if homosexuality is arrested development, that it is thereby either a disease or an illness.

And in fact it would seem that accepting this classical Freudian position would not really much affect judgments made on the empirical evidence alone. The Freudian position implies nothing new about survival or reproduction, nor about the happiness or unhappiness of homosexuals. Perhaps indeed it does imply (as certainly Freud's letter assumes) that there is no reason why a homosexual cannot be perfectly happy and content with his/her lot—that such happiness is genuine. Some people are content to stay in or go back to a phase of childhood development. This being so, both naturalist and normativist can agree with Freud that many homosexuals are not ill at all. . . .

A number of analysts [have] developed [an] adaptationist or phobic theory. . . . Breaking from Freud, they see our natural state as heterosexual—we are not constitutionally bisexual. Normally a boy (they are good Freudians in that they continue to take males as the paradigm!) will grow up to be attracted to females, but certain things—fears—may deflect him into homosexuality. Homosexuality is therefore an adaptive move in the face of perceived threats. . . .

But whatever the cause, the homosexual male is deflected from his "true" heterosexual nature through fear. And unlike Freud, the phobic theorists think that cure (that is, change to heterosexuality) is theoretically and in many cases practically possible. . . .

The phobic theorists argue that these are not genuine homosexual phenomena—they are "pseudo." In fact, in an important sense they are not really sexual phenomena at all. Rather, they are defense, adaptive reactions to personal problems, like losing out on a professorship to a younger rival. (Ovesey, 1955a, 1955b, 1965)

The reaction can go one of two ways. Either one fantasizes about getting on top of things. In a case like that of the rival, one might dream about buggering him, thus acting out one's need to dominate, perhaps even kill, him. Or one retreats to safe ground. A typical pattern would be to identify the penis with that organ which is the symbol of security, the maternal breast. In this case, one wants to suck on the penis as on the breast, and subconsciously one draws up the simple equations: "penis = breast," and "semen = milk."

I take it that by definition a key aspect of this "pseudo-homosexuality" is that it is a fleeting aspect of a heterosexual's life, although one may need therapy to get over it entirely. I take it also that it is a rather unpleasant frightening phenomenon. Life is tense enough as it is, without losing grip on one's sense of sexual identity. I rather suspect however that at this point (if we accept the theorizing) we get an interesting reversal in our analyses. To now, it has been the naturalist who has been more ready than the normativist with his ascription of a disease. Clearly here the normativist could and would talk of disease and illness—certainly there is the drop in the quality of life that the normativist would seek in applying such labels. But could the naturalist even talk of disease here? I doubt it, because by definition we are dealing with people fundamentally and continuously heterosexual. I see no real loss of biological fitness. Hence, unless one commits suicide there is no loss of life or survival prospects: there is no disease. And hence there can be no illness either. At most, the naturalist seems locked in to regarding pseudo-homosexuality as one of those unpleasant things which happens to us in the course of life, like grief or fear. One is not sick when one grieves a loss or fears a bull, even though one is not happy. Perhaps this is how the naturalist must categorize pseudo-homosexuality.

IV. ENDOCRINOLOGICAL CAUSAL EXPLANATIONS OF HOMOSEXUALITY

There have been two main sets of attempts at pinning the causes of homosexual orientation on hormonal levels (specifically sex hormonal levels). One set argues that the crucial causal period is during development; the other that it is during adulthood. . . . For brevity in this section I shall concentrate exclusively on . . . developmental hypotheses, although I suspect that much (if not all) of what I have to say would apply to all endocrinological explanations.

Fundamentally, what is argued is about as simple as the psychoanalytic theories are complex. According to the chief spokesman of this position, Gunther Dörner in East Germany, the key organ in sexual orientation is the hypothalamus, and the key time is during its formation which is (approximately) from the third to sixth months of fetal development. Dörner argues straightforwardly that, for males, if at this time the androgen/estrogen level ratio surrounding (or in) the fetus is lower than normal, the adult will grow up sexually directed towards other males. Conversely, for females, if the androgen/estrogen level ratio is higher than normal, the adult will grow up sexually directed towards other females. And that is that. No change or cure is possible after the hypothalamus is fixed, beyond a vague as-yet-unrealized hope of psycho-surgery to alter sexual orientation. . . .

The question we want answered is to what extent (if at all), in the light of Dörner's scientific hypotheses, we must modify conclusions about homosexuality qua disease/illness drawn just on the empirical evidence.

First, there is the question of biological functioning. It will be remembered that Boorse explicated this both in terms of reproduction and of survival. In fact, biologists are concerned only with reproduction, but really Boorse cannot avoid mention of survival, because otherwise he would have to say that cancer in an old person is no disease. Now, as far as reproduction is

concerned, Dörner has nothing new to say. However, most interestingly, he does think his theory has implications about survival. In particular, Dörner suggests that life-expectancy is a direct function of sex-hormone levels as they have affected the developing hypothalamus. The owners of "male type" hypothalami live shorter lives than the owners of "female type" hypothalami. This is why, on average, females live ten years longer than males. The implication is therefore that male homosexuals will (on average) live longer lives than male heterosexuals, and female homosexuals will live shorter lives than female heterosexuals.

If this claim is true, what happens to an analysis of disease, considered from a Boorsian viewpoint? As far as lesbians are concerned, both reproduction and survival prospects are lowered, and so we have a disease either way. But as far as males are concerned, the model comes apart somewhat. From a reproductive viewpoint male homosexuals are diseased, but from a survival viewpoint male homosexuals are anything but! They are perfectly healthy.

Going on to illness, I think a major reason why Dörner thinks homosexuality must be an illness (and a disease too for that matter) is that he believes anything that comes about by accident, for instance atypical sex hormonal level ratios, must be bad for the organism. However, irrespective of whether homosexuality is really a disease, this argument seems not to hold. In the first place, if there is any truth in some of the sociobiological speculations (to be discussed shortly), it is a moot point whether the ratios are all that accidental. But this apart, even though accidents normally cause trouble, judgments of illness must be made solely on the effects. If by accident a child got more growth hormone, taking him from the expected 5′ 6″ to 6′, we would certainly not speak of illness. So similarly we must judge homosexuality.

Staying with Boorse's model, with illness as in the case of disease we get a certain amount of confusion. Dörner's ideas do not really seem to have any direct implications about how people feel about their homosexuality. Hence, if (concentrating on reproduction) one thinks of it as a disease, probably some will have it as an illness also. But not all. However, if by concentrating on survival, one thinks there is no disease, then there can be no illness (although no doubt some homosexuals are unhappy with their condition). Lesbians are easier to handle. By either criterion they have a disease. Some will be ill also (although this latter is not a judgment based directly on Dörner's work).

I suppose one might speculate about how homosexuals would feel about finding out about life expectancies! Presumably if anything this would tend to make lesbians more miserable (and hence more would be ill), whereas male homosexuals would be cheered (and hence fewer would be ill). But I wonder if at this point we are not entering the world of fantasy. My experience is that males (including myself) do not go around in a state of permanent gloom because our life expectancy is less than that of women. So I am not sure how relevant all of this is to the emotional states of homosexuals. . . .

V. SOCIOBIOLOGICAL CAUSAL EXPLANATIONS

We come now to the most recent set of explanations of human homosexual orientation. These are the explanations proposed primarily by biologists who want to explain human social behavior as a function of the genes, which have in turn been molded by the forces of evolution, primarily natural selection. (See Wilson, 1978; Caplan, 1978; Ruse, 1979) Since selection puts a premium on reproductive efficiency, indeed success in evolution is seen as a success in reproduction, and since prima facie homosexual orientation leads to a drop in reproductive efficiency, human homosexuality has attracted much attention from these thinkers, the "sociobiologists." At least four putative causal explanations have been proposed from this quarter, and I shall run quickly through [two of] them. . . .

The first explanation invokes the so-called phenomenon of "balanced heterozygote fitness." . . . The naturalist sees disease as a failure in proper or adequate functioning. But what is proper or adequate functioning? Not the absolute best in a species; but that which fits into the "species design." In other words, that which has been brought about and maintained by natural selection. (Hence, it is no disease that we cannot synthesize our own vitamin C, because that ability is not something selection has left us with.) But the whole point of the balanced heterozygote fitness explanation is that the homosexual homozygote is just as much a product of and just as much maintained by selection as its heterosexual siblings! In other words, the homosexual is part of the species design, and homosexuality cannot therefore be considered a disease. By definition consequently no homosexual can be made ill by his or her homosexuality, however unhappy it may make him or her feel.

The normativist seems unaffected by this line of reasoning. That the homosexuality might have been caused by homozygous possession of two alleles seems to make no difference at all to how one feels (except in the indirect and somewhat unpredictable way that knowledge that one's homosexuality is genetic may have on one). Hence, in this case there seems no reason to modify conclusions based on the empirical data.

The second sociobiological model takes us right to the heart of the new biological work on social behavior, for it rests on the most exciting mechanism yet proposed by the sociobiologists: kin selection. When one reproduces, one passes on one's genes—only not really, because what one is doing is passing on *copies* of one's genes. However, one shares genes with close relatives, and so there is really no reason why one should not reproduce by proxy, as it were. Inasmuch as relatives reproduce, one reproduces oneself (or rather, one reproduces a portion of oneself—relatives are not genetically identical, just genetically overlapping). Hence, a viable biological strategy (kin selection) is to aid relatives to reproduce, even though it may mean reduction of one's own direct reproductive effort. . . . If for some reason one's own reproduction is liable to be low, or one's skill at aiding relatives high, then kin selection and vicarious reproduction can come into play.

Some sociobiologists have seen in kin selection a mechanism for the production of homosexuals. (Weinrich, 1976; Wilson, 1978) If, for some reason people would be likely themselves to be low reproducers, or good at aiding relatives (or both), then there might be good biological sense in a condition which would turn one entirely or primarily from attempts at direct personal reproduction: such a condition being a homosexual orientation.

This kin selection explanation has rather interesting implications for the naturalist model of disease/illness. If nothing else, one suspects that Boorse had not thought too hard about kin selection when he set up his criteria. On the surface, the explanation seems to imply that homosexuals will themselves be rather poor reproducers. Furthermore, it rather seems to imply that homosexuals would be the kind of people who (homosexuality apart) would not be very good at reproducing anyway! One proponent of this model has suggested that the reasons for this might be a childhood illness (with possible long-term effects) like tuberculosis, or just general physical slightness or weakness. (Weinrich, 1976) Hence, even though one might not know much about the survival and reproductive chances of homosexuals, in Boorse's sense they seem diseased, and many if not all seem either to be or have been quite ill.

But there are two major points of qualification. First, the proponents suggest that kin selection might have been at work at fullest force amongst our ancestors, when we were all primitive people living close to nature. In such a state, it might have paid to switch sexual orientation, given a childhood disease. But in our modern society, biology might not have caught up to today's medicine. A childhood illness may still trigger homosexuality, even though today the child might recover completely (or alternatively, in today's society the fragility which would count against one in a hunter-gatherer society may be no handicap). Hence, we cannot immediately presume that all homosexuals today are either ill or show the effects of such illness.

Second, the explanation does not make homosexuality an illness, or even a disease for that matter. First there is the fact that the sexual orientation of the homosexual is supposed to have come about in part through selection and this in itself means that the naturalist has trouble talking in terms of "disease" at this point. But secondly, and more importantly, the whole point of the kin selection explanation is that one has reduced reproductive potential and one is perhaps also ill, in the first place. Homosexuality is a biologically adaptive move to *increase* one's reproduction in the face of this. In other words, from Boorse's viewpoint, homosexuality is no disease—it is a cure! What one is doing is exchanging the reasonably certain prospects of vicarious reproduction for the uncertain prospects of direct reproduction. On this model, therefore, we may be facing people with diseases and illnesses in Boorse's sense (although this is questionable)—but homosexuality itself seems no disease in Boorse's sense.

Turning to the normativists' analysis of disease and illness, little more needs to be added to what has just been said in the context of our discussion about Boorse's analysis. There is certainly no especial implication that homosexuality itself is a (normativist) disease or illness, although this is not to deny that it might be an adaptive move in the face of other disease and illness. The one thing about the normativist position different from the naturalist position that we can say is that, even supposing homosexuality is increasing someone's biological fitness, if the homosexuality makes the bearer unhappy, then we can start to think in

terms of disease and illness. I rather think that Boorse has cut off this option. However unhappy homosexuality makes someone, if it does not reduce reproductive (or survival) potential, then it is neither disease nor illness. . . .

VI. CONCLUSION

With this brief survey of the sociobiological explanations of homosexual orientation, we reach the end of our attempt to compare the two major models of disease and illness against the known and speculated facts about homosexuality, empirical and causal. Have we answered our initial question: "Are homosexuals sick?" In fact, we have done so rather too well, because we have come up with a whole set of answers—answers which are far from uniform. However, while in a sense having too many answers is almost as bad as having too few answers, all is far from lost. We now know at least three things we did not know when we set out. First, one of our models of illness and disease, the naturalist model, needs a certain amount of revision if it is to remain a plausible approach to analyzing ill-health. The model has led to counterintuitive results and shown internal strains. If one likes the general approach, it can probably be revised—but revision is necessary. Second, the reason why people differ on the homosexuality and health question is most probably because they bring different assumptions about disease, illness, and homosexuality to their arguments. Now, at least we are in a much better position than previously to sort out what information (or misinformation) is leading to what result. We are closer to finding out why particular people differ. And third, towards an adequate ultimate answer of our own, we do now know what the options are—philosophical and scientific. We have discovered what assumptions to check and evaluate. But this checking and evaluation is, I am afraid, going to need another paper.

REFERENCES

Alexander, R. D. 1974. The evolution of social behavior. *Ann. Rev. Ecology and Systematics* 5:325–84.

Bell, A. P., and Weinberg, M.S. 1978. *Homosexualities: A Study of Diversity Among Men and Women.* New York: Simon and Schuster.

Bieber, I. et al. 1962. *Homosexuality.* New York: Basic Books.

Bieber, I. 1965. Clinical aspects of male homosexuality. In *Sexual Inversion: The Multiple Roots of Homosexuality*, ed. J. Marmor, pp. 248–67. New York: Basic Books.

———. 1973. Homosexuality—An adaptive consequence of disorder in psychosexual development. A symposium: Should homosexuality be in the APA nomenclature? *Am. J. Psychiatry* 130:1209–11.

Boorse, C. 1975. On the distinction between disease and illness. *Philosophy and Public Affairs* 5:49–68. [Reprinted above.]

———. 1976. What a theory of mental health should be. *Journal for the Theory of Social Behaviour* 6:61–84.

———. 1977. Health as a theoretical concept. *Phil. Sci.* 44: 542–73.

Brown, R. 1977. Physical illness and mental health. *Philosophy and Public Affairs* 7:17–38.

Caplan, A., ed. 1978. *The Sociobiology Debate.* New York: Harper and Row.

Dörner, G. 1976. *Hormones and Brain Differentiation.* Amsterdam: Elsevier.

Engelhardt, H. T., Jr. 1975. The concepts of health and disease. In *Evaluation and Explanation in the Biomedical Sciences*, ed. H. T. Engelhardt, Jr., and S. Spicker. Dordrecht: Reidel.

Engelhardt, H. T. 1976. Ideology and etiology. *J. Med. and Phil.* 1:256–68.

Fisher, S., and Greenberg, R.P. 1977. *The Scientific Credibility of Freud's Theories and Therapy.* New York: Basic Books.

Flew, A. 1973. *Crime or Disease?* London: Macmillan and Co.

Freud, S. 1905. *Three Essays on the Theory of Sexuality.* In *Collected Works of Freud*, vol. 7, ed. J. Strachey. London: Hogarth, 1953.

———. 1913. *Totem and Taboo.* In *Collected Works of Freud*, vol. 13, ed. J. Strachey. London: Hogarth, 1953.

Gold, R. 1973. Stop it, you're making me sick! A symposium: Should homosexuality be in the APA nomenclature? *Am. J. Psychiatry* 130:1211–12.

Green, R. 1973. Should heterosexuality be in the APA nomenclature? A symposium: Should homosexuality be in the APA nomenclature? *Am. J. Psychiatry* 130:1213–14.

Hutchinson, G. E. 1959. A speculative consideration of certain possible forms of sexual selection in man. *Am. Nat.* 93:81–91.

Jones, E. 1958. *Sigmund Freud: Life and Work.* London: Hogarth Press.

Kardiner, A., Karush, A., and Ovesey, L. 1959a. A methodological study of Freudian theory: I. Basic Concepts. *Journal of Nervous and Mental Disease* 129:11–19.

———. 1959b. A methodological study of Freudian theory: II. The Libido Theory. *Journal of Nervous and Mental Disease* 129:133–143.

———. 1959c. A methodological study of Freudian theory: III. Narcissism, bisexuality and the dual instinct theory. *Journal of Nervous and Mental Disease* 129:207–221.

———. 1959d. A methodological study of Freudian theory: IV. The structural hypothesis, the problem of anxiety, and post-Freudian ego psychology. *J. Nerv. Ment. Dis.* 129:341–56.

Klerman, G. L. 1977. Mental illness, the medical model, and psychiatry. *J. Med. and Phil.* 2:220–43.

Levitan, M., and Montagu, A. 1977. *Textbook of Human Genetics*, 2d ed. New York: Oxford University Press.

Macklin, R. 1972. Mental health and mental illness: Some problems of definition and concept formation. *Phil. Sci.* 39 (1972): 341–65.

———. 1973. The medical model in psychotherapy and psychoanalysis. *Comprehensive Psychiatry* 14 (1973): 49–69.

Margolis, J. 1966. *Psychotherapy and Morality: A Study of Two Concepts.* New York: Random House.

———. 1976. The concept of disease. *J. Med. and Phil.* 1:238–55.

Marmor, J. 1973. Homosexuality and cultural value systems. A symposium: Should homosexuality be in the APA nomenclature? *Am. J. Psychiatry* 130 (1973): 1208–9.

Marston, King, and Marston. 1931. *Integrative Psychology.* New York: Harcourt, Brace, and World.

Meyer-Bahlburg, H. F. L. 1977. Sex hormones and male homosexuality in comparative perspective. *Arch. Sex. Beh.* 6:297–325.

Moore, M. 1975a. Some myths about mental illness. *Archives of General Psychiatry* 23:1483–97.

———. 1975b. Mental illness and responsibility. *Bulletin of the Menninger Clinic* 39:308–28.

Ovesey, L. 1954. The homosexual conflict: an adaptational analysis. *Psychiat.*, 17:243–50.

———. 1955a. The pseudohomosexual anxiety. *Psychiat.* 18: 17–25.

———. 1955b. Pseudohomosexuality, the paranoid mechanism, and paranoia: an adaptational revision of a classical Freudian theory. *Psychiat.* 18:163–73.

———. 1956. Masculine aspirations in women: an adaptational analysis. *Psychiat.* 19:341–51.

———. 1965. Pseudohomosexuality and homosexuality in men: Psychodynamics as a guide to treatment. In *Sexual Inversion: The Multiple Roots of Homosexuality*, ed. J. Marmor. New York: Basic Books, pp. 211–33.

Rado, S. 1940. A critical examination of the concept of bisexuality. *Psychosomatic Medicine* 2:459–67. Reprinted in *Sexual Inversion: The Multiple Roots of Homosexuality*, ed. J. Marmor. New York: Basic Books.

———. 1949. An adaptational view of sexual behaviour. In *Psychosexual development in Health and Disease*, ed. P. Hock and J. Zubin. New York: Grune and Stratton, pp. 186–213.

Ruse, M. 1973. *The Philosophy of Biology.* London: Hutchinson.

———. 1979. *Sociobiology: Sense or Nonsense.* Dordrecht: Reidel.

———. 1981. Are there gay genes? The sociobiology of homosexuality. *J. Homosexuality.*

———. (forthcoming). *Homosexuality: A Philosophical Perspective.* Calif.: University of California Press.

Salzman, L. 1965. "Latent" homosexuality. In *Sexual Inversion: The Multiple Roots of Homosexuality*, ed. J. Marmor. New York: Basic Books, pp. 234–47.

Socarides, C. W. 1973. Homosexuality: Findings derived from 15 years of clinical research. A symposium: Should homosexuality be in the APA nomenclature? *Am. J. Psychiatry* 130 (1973): 1212–13.

Spitzer, R. L. 1973. A proposal about homosexuality and the APA nomenclature. A symposium: Should homosexuality be in the APA nomenclature? *Am. J. Psychiatry* 130:1214–16.

Stoller, R. J. 1973. Criteria for psychiatric diagnosis. A symposium: Should homosexuality be in the APA nomenclature? *Am. J. Psychiatry* 130:1207–8.

Szasz, T. S. 1961. *The Myth of Mental Illness.* New York: Delta.

Trivers, R. L. 1974. Parent-offspring conflict. *Am. Zoo.* 14:249–64.

Wilson, E. O. 1975. *Sociobiology: The New Synthesis.* Cambridge, Mass.: Harvard University Press.

———. 1978. *On Human Nature.* Cambridge, Mass.: Harvard University Press.

Weinrich, J. D. 1976. *Human Reproductive Strategy.* Harvard Ph.D. thesis.

ARTHUR L. CAPLAN

The "Unnaturalness" of Aging— A Sickness unto Death?

NORMALITY, NATURALNESS, AND DISEASE

It may seem somewhat odd to question the "naturalness" of a process as familiar and as universal as aging. After all, if aging is not a natural process, what is? While the prospect of aging may be greeted with mixed feelings, there would seem to be little reason to doubt the fact that aging is understood to be a normal and inevitable feature of human existence.

The belief that aging is a normal and natural part of human existence is reflected in the practice of medicine. For example, no mention is made in most textbooks in the areas of medicine and pathology of aging as abnormal, unnatural, or indicative of disease. It is true that such texts often contain a chapter or two on the related subject of diseases commonly associated with aging or found in the elderly. But it is the diseases of the elderly, such as pneumonia, cancer, or atherosclerosis, rather than the aging process itself, that serve as the focus of description and analysis.

Why should this situation exist? What is so different about the physiological changes and deteriorations concurrent with the aging process that these events are considered to be unremarkable natural processes, while other debilitative changes are deemed to be diseases constituting health crises of the first order? Surely it cannot simply be the life-threatening aspects of diseases, such as cancer or atherosclerosis, that distinguish these processes from aging. For while it may be true that hardly anyone manages to avoid contracting a terminal disease at some point in life, aging itself produces the same ultimate consequence as these diseases. Nor can it be the familiarity and

universality of aging that inure medical science to its unnatural aspects. Malignant neoplasms, viral infections, and hypertension are all ubiquitous phenomena. Yet medicine maintains a radically different stance toward these physical processes from that which it holds toward the so-called "natural" changes that occur during aging.

It might be argued that the processes denoted by the term "aging" do not fit the standard conception of disease operative in clinical medicine. However, in medical dictionaries disease is almost always defined as any pathological change in the body. Pathological change is inevitably defined as constituting any morbid process in the body. Any morbid processes are usually defined in terms of disease states of the body. Regardless of the circularity surrounding this explication of the concept of somatic disease, aging would seem to have a prima facie claim to being counted as a disease. Pathological or morbid changes are often the sole criteria by which age is assessed in organic tissues.

What seems to differentiate aging from other processes or states traditionally classified as diseases is the fact that aging is perceived as a natural or normal process. Medicine has traditionally viewed its role as that of ameliorating or combating the abnormal, either through therapeutic interventions or preventive, prophylactic regimens. The natural and the normal, while not outside the sphere of medicine, are concepts that play key roles in licensing the intervention of the medical practitioner. For it is in response to or in anticipation of abnormality that physicians' activities are legitimated. And as E. A. Murphy, among others, has noted, "the clinician has tended to regard disease as that state in which the limits of the normal have been transgressed."[1] Naturalness and normality have, historically, been used as base lines to determine the presence of disease and the necessity of medical activity.

In light of the powerful belief that the abnormal and unnatural are indicative of medicine's range of interest, it is easy to see why many biological processes are not thought to be the proper subject of medical intervention of therapy. Puberty, growth, and maturation *as processes in themselves* all appear to stand outside the sphere of medical concern since they are normal and natural occurrences among human beings. Similarly, it seems odd to think of sexuality or fertilization as possible disease states precisely because these states are commonly thought to be natural and normal components of the human condition.

Nonetheless, it is true that certain biological processes, such as contraception, pregnancy, and fertility, have been the subject in recent years of heated debates as to their standing as possible disease states. The notions that it is natural and normal for only men and women to have sexual intercourse or for women to undergo menopause have been challenged in many quarters. The question arises as to whether the process of aging in and of itself can be classified as abnormal and unnatural in a way that will open the door for the reclassification of aging as a disease process and, thus, a proper subject of medical attention, concern, and control. . . .

WHAT IS AGING?

What are the grounds on which this label is applied? Why do we think of aging as a natural process? The reason that comes immediately to mind is that aging is a common and normal process. It occurs with a statistical frequency of one hundred percent. Inevitably and uniformly bones become brittle, vision dims, joints stiffen, and muscles lose their tone. The obvious question that arises is whether commonality, familiarity, and inevitability are sufficient conditions for referring to certain biological states as natural. To answer this question, it is necessary to first draw a distinction between aging and chronological age.

In a trivial sense, given the existence of a chronological device, all bodies that exist can be said to age relative to the measurements provided by that device. But since physicians have little practical interest in making philosophical statements about the time-bound nature of existence, or empirical claims about the relativity of space and time, it is evident that they do not have this chronological sense in mind in speaking about the familiarity and inevitability of aging. In speaking of aging, physicians are interested in a particular set of biological changes that occur with respect to time. In the aged individual, cells manifest a high frequency of visible chromosomal aberrations. The nuclei of nerve cells become distorted by clumps of chromatin and the surrounding cytoplasm contains fewer organelles, such as mitochondria. Collagen fibers become increasingly rigid and inflexible, as manifest in the familiar phenomenon of skin wrinkling. The aorta becomes wider and more tortuous. The immunological system weakens and the elderly person becomes more susceptible to infections. Melanin pigment formation decreases and, consequently, hair begins to whiten.[2] . . .

DOES AGING HAVE A FUNCTION?

Two purported explanations—one theological, one scientific—of the function or purpose of aging have been given. Both are flawed. While the theological explanation of aging may carry great weight for numerous individuals, it will simply not do as a scientific explanation of why aging occurs in humans. Medical professionals may have to cope with their patients' advocacy of this explanation and their own religious feelings on the subject. But, from a scientific perspective, it will hardly do to claim that aging, as a result of God's vindictiveness, is a natural biological process, and hence not a disease worthy of treatment.

More surprisingly, the scientific explanation of aging as serving an evolutionary role or purpose is also inadequate. It is simply not true that aging exists to serve any sort of evolutionary purpose or function. The claim that aging exists or occurs in individuals because it has a wider role or function in the evolutionary scheme of things rests on a faulty evolutionary analysis. The analysis incorrectly assumes that it is possible for biological processes to exist that directly benefit or advance the evolutionary success of a species or population. In other words, it supposes that processes such as aging exist because they serve a function or purpose in the life history of a species—in this case, that of removing the old to make way for the new. However, evolutionary selection rarely acts to advance the prospects of an entire species or population. Selection acts on individual organisms and their phenotypic traits and properties. Some traits or properties confer advantages in certain environments on the organisms that possess them and this fact increases the likelihood that the genes responsible for producing these traits will be passed on to future organisms.

Given that selective forces act on individuals and their genotypes and not species, it makes no sense to speak of aging as serving an evolutionary function or purpose to benefit the species. How then do evolutionary biologists explain the existence of aging? Briefly, the explanation is that features, traits, or properties in individual organisms will be selected for if they confer a relative reproductive advantage on the individual, or, his or her close kin. Any variation that increases inclusive reproductive fitness has a very high probability of being selected and maintained in the gene pool of a species. Selection, however, cannot look ahead to foresee the possible consequences of favoring certain traits at a given time; the environment selects for those traits and features that give an immediate return. An increased metabolic rate, for example, may prove advantageous early in life, in that it may provide more energy for seeking mates and avoiding predators; it may also result in early deterioration of the organism due to an increased accumulation of toxic wastes in the body of an individual thus endowed. Natural selection cannot foresee such delayed debilitating consequences.

Aging exists, then, as a consequence of lack of evolutionary foresight; it is simply a by-product of selective forces working to increase the chances of reproductive success in the life of an organism. Senescence has no function; it is simply the inadvertent subversion of organic function, later in life, in favor of maximizing reproductive advantage, early in life.

The common belief that aging serves a function or purpose, if this belief is based on a misapprehension of evolutionary theory, is mistaken. And, if this is so, it would seem that the common belief that aging is a natural process, as a consequence of the function or purpose it serves in the life of the species, is also mistaken. Consequently, unless it is possible to motivate the description on other grounds, it would seem that aging cannot be understood as a natural process. And if that is true, and if it is actually the case that what goes on during the aging process closely parallels the changes that occur during paradigmatic examples of disease,[3] then it would be unreasonable not to consider aging a disease.

THEORIES OF AGING AND
THE CONCEPT OF DISEASE

A consideration of the changes that constitute aging in human beings reinforces the similarities existing between aging and other clear-cut examples of somatic diseases. There is a set of external manifestations or symptoms: greying hair, increased susceptibility to infection, wrinkling skin, loss of muscular tone, and frequently, loss of mental ability. These manifestations seem to be causally linked to a series of internal cellular and subcellular changes. The presence of symptoms and an underlying etiology closely parallels the standard paradigmatic examples of disease. If the analogy is pushed a bit further, the cause for considering aging a disease appears to become even stronger.

There are many theories as to what causes changes at the cellular and subcellular level that produce the signs and symptoms associated with aging.[4] One view argues that aging is caused by an increase in the number of cross-linkages that exist in protein and nucleic acid molecules. Cross-linkages lower the biochemical efficiency and dependability of certain macromolecules involved in metabolism and other chemical reactions. Free radical by-products of metabolism are thought to accumulate in cells, thus allowing for an increase in available linkage sites for replicating nucleic acid strands and activating histone elements. This sort of cross-linkage is thought to be particularly important in the aging of collagen, the substance responsible for most of the overt symptoms we commonly associate with aging, such as wrinkled skin and loss of muscular flexibility.

Another view holds that aging results from an accumulation of genetic mutations in the chromosomes of cells in the body. The idea underlying this theory is that chromosomes are exposed over time to a steady stream of radiation and other mutagenic agents. The accumulation of mutational hits on the genes lying on the chromosomes results in the progressive inactivation of these genes. The evidence of a higher incidence of chromosomal breaks and aberrations in the aged is consistent with this mutational theory of aging.

Along with the cross-linkage and mutational theories, there is one other important hypothesis concerning the cause of aging. The autoimmune theory holds that, as time passes and the chromosomes of cells in the human body accumulate more mutations, certain key tissues begin to synthesize antibodies that can no longer distinguish between self and foreign material. Thus, a number of autoimmune reactions occur in the body as the immunological system begins to turn against the individual it was "designed" to protect. Arthritis and pernicious anemia are symptomatic of the sorts of debilities resulting from the malfunction of the immunological system. While this theory is closely allied to the mutation theory, the autoimmune view of aging holds that accumulated mutations do not simply result in deterioration of cellular activity, but, rather, produce lethal cellular end products that consume and destroy healthy tissue.

It would be rash to hold that any of the three hypotheses cited—the cross-linkage, mutational, or autoimmune hypotheses—will, in the end, turn out to be *the* correct explanation of aging. All three views are, in fact, closely related in that cross-linkages can result from periodic exposure to mutagenic agents and can, in turn, produce genetic aberrations that eventuate in cellular dysfunction or even autoimmunological reactions. What is important, however, is not whether *one* of these theories or *any* of them is in fact *the* correct theory of aging, but that all of them postulate mechanisms that are closely analogous to those mechanisms cited by clinicians in describing disease processes in the body.

The concept of disease is, without doubt, a slippery and evasive notion in medicine. Once one moves away from what can be termed "paradigmatic" examples of disease, such as tuberculosis or diphtheria, toward more nebulous examples, such as acne or jittery nerves, it becomes difficult to say exactly what are the criteria requisite for labeling a condition a somatic disease. However, even though it is notoriously difficult to concoct a set of necessary and sufficient conditions for employing the term "organic disease," it is possible to cite a list of general criteria that seem relevant in attempting to decide whether a bodily state or process is appropriately labeled a disease.

One criterion is that the state or process produces discomfort or suffering. A second is that the process or state can be traced back to a specific cause, event, or circumstance. A third is that there is a set of clear-cut structural changes, both macroscopic and microscopic, that follow in a uniform, sequential manner subsequent to the initial precipitating or causal event. A fourth is that there is a set of clinical symptoms or manifestations (headache, pain in the chest, rapid pulse, shortness of breath) commonly associated with the observed physiological alterations in structure. Finally,[5] there is usually some sort of functional impairment in the functions, behavior, or activity of a person thought to be diseased. Not all diseases will satisfy all or any of the criteria I have suggested. One need only consider the arguments surrounding the classification of astigmatism, alcoholism, drug-addiction, gambling,

and hyperactivity to realize the inadequacy of these criteria as necessary and sufficient conditions for the determination of disease. But that the suggested criteria are relevant to such determination is shown by the fact that advocates of all persuasions regarding controversial states and processes commonly resort to considerations of causation, clinical manifestations, etiology, functional impairment, and suffering in arguing the merits of their various views concerning the status of controversial cases.

With respect to the conceptual ambiguity surrounding the notion of disease, it is important to remember that medicine is by no means unique in being saddled with what might be termed "fuzzy-edged" concepts. One need only consider the status of terms such as "species," "adaptation," and "mutation" in biology, or "stimulus," "behavior," and "instinct" in psychology, to realize that medicine is not alone in the ambiguity of its key terms. It is also true that, just as the biologist is able to use biological theory to aid in the determination of relevant criteria for a concept, the physician is able to use his or her knowledge of the structure and function of the body to decide on relevant criteria for the determination of disease.

If one accepts the relevance of the five suggested criteria, aging, as a biological process, is seen to possess all the key properties of a disease. Unlike astigmatism or nervousness, aging possesses a definitive group of clinical manifestations or symptoms; a clear-cut etiology of structural changes at both the macroscopic and microscopic levels; a significant measure of impairment, discomfort, and suffering; and, if we are willing to grant the same tolerance to current theories of aging as we grant to theories in other domains of medicine, an explicit set of precipitating factors. Aging has all the relevant markings of a disease process. And if my earlier argument is sound, even if an additional criterion of unnaturalness were appended, aging would still meet all the requirements thought relevant to the classification of a process or state as indicative of disease.

SOME ETHICAL ARGUMENTS AGAINST TREATING AGING AS A DISEASE

What hinges on the decision to refer to a process or state such as aging by the word disease rather than by some other term? Obviously, a great deal. Medical attention, medical support, medical treatment, and medical research are devoted to the treatment, care, amelioration, and prevention of disease. While it is possible to view the activation of this vast professional machine either as a positive good or as a serious evil, an array of connotations and implications surrounds the medical profession's decision to consider a phenomenon worthy of its attention. Some groups have actively proselytized for the acceptance of certain conditions, such as alcoholism or gambling, as diseases. Other groups have worked to remove the label of disease from behavior such as homosexuality, masturbation, and schizophrenia. A number of motives and concerns underlie these arguments. The question is, what kinds of considerations should be considered relevant to the determination of whether a particular state, process, or condition is a disease?

I do not propose to try to answer the difficult question of what are the relevant nonorganic criteria affecting the choice of the disease label. Rather, I want to consider three specific arguments that might be raised against calling aging a disease—a classification that, of necessity, keeps the aged in touch with the medical profession.

The first counter-argument is that the decision to call aging a disease would be pointless, since doctors cannot at present intervene to treat or cure aging. This argument does not stand up to critical scrutiny. There are many diseases in existence today for which no cure is known, but no one proposes that these disorders are any less diseases as a consequence. Furthermore, the emphasis on treatment and cure implicit in this argument ignores the equally vital components of medical care involving understanding, education, and support. The profession's and the patient's interest in the healing function of medicine might make it difficult for physicians to accept aging as a disease, but the difficulty in achieving such acceptance does not provide a reason for rejecting the view.

The second argument is that to call aging a disease would involve the stigmatization of a large segment of the population; to view the aged as sick or diseased would only increase the burdens already borne by this much abused segment of society. The problem with this argument is that it tends to blend public perceptions of disease in general with the particular problem of whether seeing aging as a disease ought to carry negative and undesirable connotations. To deny that aging is a disease may be simply an easy way to avoid the more difficult problem of educating the medical profession and the lay public toward a better understanding of the threatening and nonthreatening aspects of disease. Contagiousness, death, disability, and ne-

glect may be the real objects of concern in speaking of disease, not disease in itself.

Finally, it might be claimed that there would be a tremendous social and economic cost to calling aging a disease. The claim is perhaps the most unconvincing of the three that I have offered. One factor especially relevant to the determination or diagnosis of disease would seem to be that the physician confine his or her concerns to the physical and mental state of the individual patient; social and economic considerations would appear to be quite out of place. Genetic and psychological diseases place a large burden on society: dialysis machines and tomography units are enormously expensive. But these facts do not in any way change the disease status of mongolism, schizophrenia, kidney failure or cancer. It may be the case that the government may decide not to spend one cent on research into aging or the treatment of aging. But such a decision should be consequent on, not prior to, a diagnosis of disease. This argument simply blurs the value questions relevant to a decision as to whether something is a disease, with value questions relevant to deciding what to do about something after it has been decided that it is a disease.

I have suggested a number of possible value issues and social problems that may enter into the decision of the medical profession to label a state or process a disease. I have also suggested that none of these issues and problems would seem to rule out a consideration of aging as a disease. The determination of disease status and the question of how physicians and society should react to disease are distinct issues. Considerations of the latter variety ought not to be allowed to color our decisions about what does and what does not constitute a disease.

Most persons in our society would be loath to see aging classified and treated as a disease. Much of the resistance to such a classification derives from the view that aging is a natural process and that, like other natural processes, it ought not, in itself, be the subject of medical intervention and therapeutic control. I have tried to show that much of the reasoning that tacitly underlies the categorization of aging as a natural or normal process rests on faulty biological analysis. Aging is not the goal or aim of the evolutionary process. Rather it is an accidental by-product of that process. Accordingly, it is incorrect to root a belief in the naturalness of aging in some sort of perceived biological design or purpose since aging serves no such end. It may be that good arguments can be adduced for excluding aging from the purview of medicine. However, if such arguments can be made, they must draw on considerations other than that of the naturalness of aging.

NOTES

1. E. A. Murphy, *The Logic of Medicine* (Baltimore: Johns Hopkins, 1976), p. 122. See also E. A. Murphy, "A Scientific Viewpoint on Normalcy," *Perspectives in Biology and Medicine*;

and G. B. Risse, "Health and Disease: History of the Concepts," in *Encyclopedia of Bioethics*, ed. W. T. Reich (New York: The Free Press, 1978), pp. 579–585.

2. Leonard Hayflick, "The Strategy of Senescence," *Gerontologist* 14 (1974):37–45.

3. For an interesting attempt to analyze the concepts of illness and disease, see C. Boorse, "On the Distinction Between Illness and Disease," *Philosophy and Public Affairs* 5, 1 (1975):49–68. [Reprinted above.]

4. A. Comfort, "Biological Theories of Aging," *Human Development* 13 (1970):127–39; L. Hayflick, "The Biology of Human Aging," *American Journal of Medical Sciences* 265, 6 (1973): 433–45; A. Comfort, *Aging: The Biology of Senescence* (New York: Holt, Rinehart and Winston, 1964).

5. See Boorse, "On the Distinction Between Illness and Disease."

The Concept of Mental Illness

THOMAS SZASZ

The Myth of Mental Illness

I

At the core of virtually all contemporary psychiatric theories and practices lies the concept of mental illness. A critical examination of this concept is therefore indispensable for understanding the ideas, institutions, and interventions of psychiatrists.

My aim in this essay is to ask if there is such a thing as mental illness, and to argue that there is not. Of course, mental illness is not a thing or physical object; hence it can exist only in the same sort of way as do other theoretical concepts. Yet, to those who believe in them, familiar theories are likely to appear, sooner or later, as "objective truths" or "facts." During certain historical periods, explanatory concepts such as deities, witches, and instincts appeared not only as theories but as *self-evident causes* of a vast number of

events. Today mental illness is widely regarded in a similar fashion, that is, as the cause of innumerable diverse happenings.

As an antidote to the complacent use of the notion of mental illness—as a self-evident phenomenon, theory, or cause—let us ask: What is meant when it is asserted that someone is mentally ill? In this essay I shall describe the main uses of the concept of mental illness, and I shall argue that this notion has outlived whatever cognitive usefulness it might have had and that it now functions as a myth.

II

The notion of mental illness derives its main support from such phenomena as syphilis of the brain or delirious conditions—intoxications, for instance—in which persons may manifest certain disorders of thinking and behavior. Correctly speaking, however, these are diseases of the brain, not of the mind. According to one school of thought, *all* so-called mental illness is of this type. The assumption is made that some neurological defect, perhaps a very subtle one, will ultimately be found to explain all the disorders of thinking and behavior. Many contemporary physicians, psychiatrists, and other scientists hold this view, which implies that people's troubles cannot be caused by conflicting personal needs, opinions, social aspirations, values, and so forth. These difficulties—which I think we may simply call *problems in living*—are thus attributed to physicochemical processes that in due time will be discovered (and no doubt corrected) by medical research.

Mental illnesses are thus regarded as basically similar to other diseases. The only difference, in this view, between mental and bodily disease is that the former, affecting the brain, manifests itself by means of mental symptoms; whereas the latter, affecting other organ systems—for example, the skin, liver, and so on—manifests itself by means of symptoms referable to those parts of the body.

In my opinion, this view is based on two fundamental errors. In the first place, a disease of the brain, analogous to a disease of the skin or bone, is a neurological defect, not a problem in living. For example, a *defect* in a person's visual field may be explained by correlating it with certain lesions in the nervous system. On the other hand, a person's *belief*—whether it be in Christianity, in Communism, or in the idea that his internal organs are rotting and that his body is already dead—cannot be explained by a defect or disease of the nervous system. Explanations of this sort of occurrence—assuming that one is interested in the belief itself and does not regard it simply as a symptom or expression of something else that is more interesting—must be sought along different lines.

The second error is epistemological. It consists of interpreting communications about ourselves and the world around us as symptoms of neurological functioning. This is an error not in observation or reasoning, but rather in the organization and expression of knowledge. In the present case, the error lies in making a dualism between mental and physical symptoms, a dualism that is a habit of speech and not the result of known observations. Let us see if this is so.

In medical practice, when we speak of physical disturbances we mean either signs (for example, fever) or symptoms (for example, pain). We speak of mental symptoms, on the other hand, when we refer to a patient's communications about himself, others, and the world about him. The patient might assert that he is Napoleon or that he is being persecuted by the Communists. These would be considered mental symptoms only if the observer believed that the patient was *not* Napoleon or that he was *not* being persecuted by the Communists. This makes it apparent that the statement "X is a mental symptom" involves rendering a judgment that entails a covert comparison between the patient's ideas, concepts, or beliefs and those of the observer and the society in which they live. The notion of mental symptom is therefore inextricably tied to the social, and particularly the ethical, context in which it is made, just as the notion of bodily symptom is tied to an anatomical and genetic context.

To sum up: For those who regard mental symptoms as signs of brain disease, the concept of mental illness is unnecessary and misleading. If they mean that people so labeled suffer from diseases of the brain, it would seem better, for the sake of clarity, to say that and not something else.

III

The term "mental illness" is also widely used to describe something quite different from a disease of the brain. Many people today take it for granted that living is an arduous affair. Its hardship for modern man derives, moreover, not so much from a struggle for biological survival as from the stresses and strains inherent in the social intercourse of complex human personalities. In this context, the notion of mental illness is used to identify or describe some feature of an individual's so-called personality. Mental illness—as a deformity of the personality, so to speak—is then regarded as the cause of human disharmony. It is implicit in this view that social intercourse between people is regarded as something inherently harmonious, its disturbance being due solely to the presence of "mental illness" in many people. Clearly, this is faulty reasoning, for it makes the abstraction "mental illness" into a cause of, even though this abstraction was originally created to serve only as a shorthand expression for, certain types of human behavior. It now becomes necessary to ask: What kinds of behavior are regarded as indicative of mental illness, and by whom?

The concept of illness, whether bodily or mental, implies deviation from some clearly defined norm. In the case of physical illness, the norm is the structural and functional integrity of the human body. Thus, although the desirability of physical health, as such, is an ethical value, what health is can be stated in anatomical and physiological terms. What is the norm, deviation from which is regarded as mental illness? This question cannot be easily answered. But whatever this norm may be, we can be certain of only one thing: namely, that it must be stated in terms of psychosocial, ethical, and legal concepts. For example, notions such as "excessive repression" and "acting out an unconscious impulse" illustrate the use of psychological concepts for judging so-called mental health and illness. The idea that chronic hostility, vengefulness, or divorce are indicative of mental illness is an illustration of the use of ethical norms (that is, the desirability of love, kindness, and a stable marriage relationship). Finally, the widespread psychiatric opinion that only a mentally ill person would commit homicide illustrates the use of a legal concept as a norm of mental health. In short, when one speaks of mental illness, the norm from which deviation is measured is a *psychosocial and ethical* standard. Yet, the remedy is sought in terms of *medical* measures that—it is hoped and assumed—are free from wide differences of ethical value. The definition of the disorder and the terms in which its remedy are sought are therefore at serious odds with one another. The practical significance of this covert conflict between the alleged nature of the defect and the actual remedy can hardly be exaggerated.

Having identified the norms used for measuring deviations in cases of mental illness, we shall now turn to the question, Who defines the norms and hence the deviation? Two basic answers may be offered: First, it may be the person himself—that is, the patient—who decides that he deviates from a norm; for example, an artist may believe that he suffers from a work inhibition; and he may implement this conclusion by seeking help *for himself* from a psychotherapist. Second, it may be someone other than the "patient" who decides that the latter is deviant—for example, relatives, physicians, legal authorities, society generally; a psychiatrist may then be hired by persons other than the "patient" to do something *to him* in order to correct the deviation.

These considerations underscore the importance of asking the question, Whose agent is the psychiatrist? and of giving a candid answer to it. The psychiatrist (or non-medical mental health worker) may be the agent of the patient, the relatives, the school, the military services, a business organization, a court of law, and so forth. In speaking of the psychiatrist as the agent of these persons or organizations, it is not implied that his moral values, or his ideas and aims concerning the proper nature of remedial action, must coincide exactly with those of his employer. For example, a patient in individual psychotherapy may believe that his salvation lies in a new marriage; his psychotherapist need not share this hypothesis. As the patient's agent, however, he must not resort to social or legal force to prevent the patient from putting his beliefs into action. If his *contract* is with the patient, the psychiatrist (psychotherapist) may disagree with him or stop his treatment, but he cannot engage others to obstruct the patient's aspirations. Similarly, if a psychiatrist is retained by a court to determine the sanity of an offender, he need not fully share the legal authorities' values and intentions in regard to the criminal, nor the means deemed appropriate for dealing with him; such a psychiatrist cannot testify, however, that the accused is not insane but that the legislators are—for passing the law that decrees the offender's actions illegal. This sort of opinion could be voiced, of course—but not in a courtroom, and not by a psychiatrist who is there to assist the court in performing its daily work.

To recapitulate: In contemporary social usage, the finding of mental illness is made by establishing a deviance in behavior from certain psychosocial, ethical, or legal norms. The judgment may be made, as in medicine, by the patient, the physician (psychiatrist), or others. Remedial action, finally, tends to be sought in a therapeutic—or covertly medical—framework. This creates a situation in which it is claimed that psychosocial, ethical, and legal deviations can be corrected by medical action. Since medical interventions are designed to remedy only medical problems, it is logically absurd to expect that they will help solve problems whose very existence has been defined and established on non-medical grounds.

• • •

IV

The position outlined above, according to which contemporary psychotherapists deal with problems in living, not with mental illnesses and their cures, stands in sharp opposition to the currently prevalent position, according to which psychiatrists treat mental diseases, which are just as "real" and "objective" as bodily diseases. I submit that the holders of the latter view have no evidence whatever to justify their claim, which is actually a kind of psychiatric propaganda: their aim is to create in the popular mind a confident belief that mental illness is some sort of disease entity, like an infection or a malignancy. If this were true, one could *catch* or *get* a mental illness, one might *have* or *harbor* it, one might *transmit* it to others, and finally one could *get rid* of it. Not only is there not a shred of evidence to support this idea, but, on the contrary, all the evidence is the other way and supports the view that what people now call mental illnesses are, for the most part, *communications* expressing unacceptable ideas, often framed in an unusual idiom.

This is not the place to consider in detail the similarities and differences between bodily and mental illnesses. It should suffice to emphasize that whereas the term "bodily illness" refers to physicochemical occurrences that are not affected by being made public, the term "mental illness" refers to sociopsychological events that are crucially affected by being made public. The psychiatrist thus cannot, and does not, stand apart from the person he observes, as the pathologist can and often does. The psychiatrist is committed to some picture of what he considers reality, and to what he thinks society considers reality, and he observes and judges the patient's behavior in the light of these beliefs. The very notion of "mental symptoms" or "mental illness" thus implies a covert comparison and often conflict, between observer and observed, psychiatrist and patient. Though obvious, this fact needs to be re-emphasized, if one wishes, as I do here, to counter the prevailing tendency to deny the moral aspects of psychiatry and to substitute for them allegedly value-free medical concepts and interventions.

Psychotherapy is thus widely practiced as though it entailed nothing other than restoring the patient from a state of mental sickness to one of mental health. While it is generally accepted that mental illness has something to do with man's social or interpersonal relations, it is paradoxically maintained that problems of values—that is, of ethics—do not arise in this process. Freud himself went so far as to assert: "I consider ethics to be taken for granted. Actually I have never done a mean thing."[1] This is an astounding thing to say, especially for someone who had studied man as a social being as deeply as Freud had. I mention it here to show how the notion of "illness"—in the case of

psychoanalysis, "psychopathology," or "mental illness"—was used by Freud, and by most of his followers, as a means of classifying certain types of human behavior as falling within the scope of medicine, and hence, by fiat, outside that of ethics. Nevertheless, the stubborn fact remains that, in a sense, much of psychotherapy revolves around nothing other than the elucidation and weighing of goals and values—many of which may be mutually contradictory—and the means whereby they might best be harmonized, realized, or relinquished.

Because the range of human values and of the methods by which they may be attained is so vast, and because many such ends and means are persistently unacknowledged, conflicts among values are the main source of conflicts in human relations. Indeed, to say that human relations at all levels—from mother to child, through husband and wife, to nation and nation—are fraught with stress, strain, and disharmony is, once again, to make the obvious explicit. Yet, what may be obvious may be also poorly understood. This, I think, is the case here. For it seems to me that in our scientific theories of behavior we have failed to accept the simple fact that human relations are inherently fraught with difficulties, and to make them even relatively harmonious requires much patience and hard work. I submit that the idea of mental illness is now being put to work to obscure certain difficulties that at present may be inherent—not that they need to be unmodifiable—in the social intercourse of persons. If this is true, the concept functions as a disguise: instead of calling attention to conflicting human needs, aspirations, and values, the concept of mental illness provides an amoral and impersonal "thing"—an "illness"—as an explanation for problems in living. We may recall in this connection that not so long ago it was devils and witches that were held responsible for man's problems in living. The belief in mental illness, as something other than man's trouble in getting along with his fellow man, is the proper heir to the belief in demonology and witchcraft. Mental illness thus exists or is "real" in exactly the same sense in which witches existed or were "real."

•   •   •

When I assert that mental illness is a myth, I am not saying that personal unhappiness and socially deviant behavior do not exist; what I am saying is that we categorize them as diseases at our own peril.

The expression "mental illness" is a metaphor that we have come to mistake for a fact. We call people physically ill when their body-functioning violates certain anatomical and physiological norms; similarly, we call people mentally ill when their personal conduct violates certain ethical, political, and social norms. This explains why many historical figures, from Jesus to Castro, and from Job to Hitler, have been diagnosed as suffering from this or that psychiatric malady.

NOTES

1. Quoted in E. Jones, *The Life and Work of Sigmund Freud* (New York: Basic Books, 1957), Vol. III, p. 247.

RUTH MACKLIN

Mental Health and Mental Illness: Some Problems of Definition and Concept Formation

INTRODUCTION

In recent years there has been considerable discussion and controversy concerning the concepts of mental health and mental illness. The controversy has centered around the problem of providing criteria for an adequate conception of mental health and illness, as well as difficulties in specifying a clear and workable system for the classification, understanding, and treatment of psychological and emotional disorders. In this paper I shall examine a cluster of these complex and important issues, focusing on attempts to define 'mental health' and 'mental illness'; diverse factors influencing the ascription of the predicates 'is mentally ill'; and 'is mentally healthy'; and some specific problems concerning these concepts as they appear in various theories of psychopathology. . . .

NORMALITY AND ABNORMALITY AS NORMATIVE AND AS STATISTICAL CONCEPTS

[One] set of problems emerges relating to the fact that normality is sometimes construed as a normative concept and sometimes as a statistical one. . . .

From *Philosophy of Science* 39(3) (1972). Reprinted by permission of the Philosophy of Science Association.

Noting that normality can be viewed either as a statistical frequency concept or as a normative idea of how people ought to function, Jahoda points out that a coincidence of statistical and normative correctness is, at best, fortuitous.

To believe that the two connotations always coincide leads to the assertion that whatever exists in the majority of cases is right by virtue of its existence. The failure to keep the two connotations of normality separate leads straight back into an extreme cultural relativism according to which the storm trooper, for example, must be considered as the prototype of integrative adjustment in Nazi culture. ([2], pp. 15–16)

The issue is now identified as the old problem in philosophical ethics: the is-ought gap. Although I am not concerned to argue here about whether there is or is not, or should or should not be such a gap, it seems that the significance of the distinction for the problem of defining 'mental health' in terms of some conception of normality is clear. As Jahoda correctly points out, "insofar as normality is used in the normative sense, it is a synonym for mental health, and the problems of concept definition are, of course, identical" ([2], p. 16).

Another difficulty with 'normality' as construed in

the normative sense is that the concept tends to function as an "ideal type," so that the actual behavior of persons is, at best, an approximation to some optimal conditions. The problem is, then, that according to some psychological theoretical frameworks it may be extraordinarily difficult or even impossible to draw the line between normality and abnormality (and, consequently, following Jahoda's insight, impossible to draw the line between mental illness and mental health). . . . This issue will be brought up again in connection with a problem to be discussed below: considerations *within* certain theories which preclude the possibility of a precise definition of mental health and illness. Let it suffice to note at this point that an attempt to define 'mental health' in terms of a normative conception of normality appears to lead either to circularity (as Jahoda claims), or else directly back to cultural relativism. We shall next examine the frequency concept of normality to see if it fares any better.

The most obvious difficulty with a statistical frequency concept of normality is that a majority of people may do many things we hesitate to call mentally healthy. Thus, "psychological health may, but need not be, the status of the majority of people" ([2], p. 16). That this is so might be illustrated by considering the case of physical illness and health. No one would be likely to urge a definition of 'physical health' based on statistical considerations, for it might turn out that a majority of the population is suffering from some form or other of physical ailment or disease (whether temporary or enduring). . . . It is true, of course, that there are much more systematic and comprehensive biological and physiological theories on the basis of which the concept of physical or bodily health may be constructed in medicine than now exist in the realm of psychological or psychiatric theory. But the inadequacy of a statistical conception of normality for physical health provides an instructive comparison for present purposes. It may be objected here that the example just given presupposes the applicability of the medical model and a conception of mental health based on the analogue of physical health. Although this is so, the reasons for questioning the adequacy of the frequency concept of normality for defining 'mental health' do not depend on the analogy with physical health.

An additional difficulty with the statistical approach is noted by Redlich and Freedman. This difficulty constitutes a methodological problem rather than an objection in principle, but presents obstacles nevertheless.

Few exact data . . . are available on the frequency and distribution of behavior traits. Such an approach presupposes that behavior is quantifiable and measurable, but obviously many forms of behavior are not . . . Few data . . . exist on the prevalence and the incidence of psychiatric symptoms, such as anxiety, hallucinations, phobias, and so forth. ([4], p. 113) . . .

THE CLINICAL APPROACH

. . . When construed in the normative sense, the concept of normality tends to function as an "ideal type" according to whatever theory is being employed. This is not the case, however, in the clinical approach, as Redlich and Freedman point out: "In general terms, clinical normality is not ideal performance but minimal performance, just above the level of pathological performance for a given individual" ([4], p. 113). But now the problem is to identify such "levels of performance," a task which is not only clinically difficult but also depends on some theoretical assumptions on the part of the clinician. Indeed, according to Redlich and Freedman:

The clinical approach defines as abnormal anything that does not function according to its design. This approach is useful in somatic illness, including brain disease, but it is less helpful in behavior disorders, because all too often we do not know what design or function a certain behavior pattern serves. ([4], p. 113)

Some criteria for normality which have been employed in the clinical approach are adaptation, maturity, "average expectable environment," and "predominance of conscious and preconscious motivations over unconscious motivation of behavioral acts" ([4], p. 113). But Redlich and Freedman find the concept of adaptation, "which is supposed to explain just about everything, only of very limited use in differentiating normal and abnormal behavior" ([4], p. 113); the conscious-unconscious criterion fails to apply to many forms of abnormal behavior determined by brain disease and ignores the fact that in many types of normal and socially desirable behavior, unconscious and preconscious motivations occur ([4], pp. 113–114). The criteria of "average expectable environment" and maturity are viewed more favorably, but the authors fail to note that 'maturity' and 'immaturity' are themselves value laden terms, depending for their application not only on the theoretical orientation of the clinician but also on a set of cultural and subcultural norms espoused by him. . . .

One large problem should be noted. . . . This is the absence of an overall scientific theory on which to base conceptions of mental health and illness, well-functioning and maladaptive behavior. It should be noted, however, that in this regard the concepts of health and disease face a number of similar problems in the domain of somatic medicine (i.e. the concepts are vague, there are multiple criteria for their application—criteria which may conflict occasionally, etc.). There is no general, well-integrated theory of the sort that exists in, say, physics, interconnecting the well-developed fields in medicine of physiology, anatomy, pathology, neurology, immunology, etc., with current developments in the biological sciences. The absence of bridging laws between these branches of medical and biological science, as well as the divergent theoretical and methodological approaches of experimental biologists, on the one hand, and medical scientists oriented towards pathology, on the other, all contribute to the present lack of systematization in the total field of biological science. So the absence of well-confirmed fundamental laws, from which other laws are derivable, and the absence of a systematic, general theory result in the situation that within medicine itself, there are no clear or precise formulations of the basic concepts of health and disease, and no set of necessary and sufficient conditions for their application. . . .

PROBLEMS WITH THE CONCEPTION OF PSYCHOLOGICAL DISORDERS AS "DISEASE" OR "ILLNESS"

A number of arguments have been put forth by some influential psychologists and psychiatrists who hold that the conceptualization of psychological disorders in terms of illness represents an adherence to a mistaken model—the medical model of health and disease. These criticisms of the continued use of the medical model rest partly on conceptual and theoretical grounds and partly on pragmatic considerations relating to the consequences for the individual and society of adhering to this model. There is, however, a good deal of confusion surrounding these issues—confusion which stems largely from a tendency to conflate epistemological, conceptual, and pragmatic

problems and attempts at solution to such problems. I shall concentrate on only a few of these issues here, specifically, those which relate most directly to the concerns of definition and concept formation.

The most outspoken opponent of the medical model is Dr. Thomas Szasz, a psychiatrist who holds the M.D. degree. Szasz claims that

. . . although the notion of mental illness made good *historical* sense—stemming as it does from the historical identity of medicine and psychiatry—it made no *rational* sense. Although mental illness might have been a useful concept in the nineteenth century, today it is scientifically worthless and socially harmful. ([5], p. ix)

Thus he argues that it is inappropriate or logically mistaken to construe emotional problems and psychological disorders as a species of illness, on an analogy with bodily disease. On Szasz's view, there exists a "*major logical and procedural error in the evolution of modern psychiatry*" ([5], p. 26). One "error" lay in decreeing that some malingerers be called "hysterics," which led to obscuring the similarities and differences between organic neurological diseases and phenomena that only looked like them ([5], p. 26). But it does not follow from the fact that hysteria (and other psychological disorders) are called "illness" that the similarities and differences between organic and nonorganic illness cannot be duly noted and treated accordingly. Indeed, the very introduction of the notion of *mental* illness to cover phenomena such as hysteria marks a decision to treat a class of seeming bodily disorders as different in relevant respects from organic neurological disease. The labelling itself need not involve a failure to attend to the relevant similarities and differences for the purpose of diagnosis, explanation, or treatment.

In general, the precise nature of Szasz's objection to construing psychological disorders as illnesses is not always clear. Sometimes he writes as though the reclassification and introduction of a set of "new rules of the medical game" consist in a sort of logical or conceptual error:

During [the past sixty or seventy years] a vast number of occurrences were reclassified as "illnesses." We have thus come to regard phobias, delinquencies, divorce, homicide, addiction, and so on almost without limit as psychiatric illnesses. This is a colossal and costly mistake. ([5], p. 43)

In answer to the question, "from what point of view is it a mistake to classify nonillnesses as illnesses?"

Szasz replies that "it is a mistake from the point of view of science and intellectual integrity." This would seem to imply that a proper scientific conception and a generally accepted classificatory schema preclude treating psychological disorders as illnesses. But there is no compelling evidence—either from Szasz's own account, or revealed in our inquiry in the preceding sections—to show that it is indeed the case that a clear "error" or "mistake" is involved in this type of classification. The consequence of the medical model approach and resulting reclassifications, according to Szasz, has been that although "some members of suffering humanity were promoted . . . to higher social rank, this was attained at the cost of obscuring the logical character of the observed phenomena" ([5], p. 295).

It is evident from the passages just cited that at least sometimes Szasz construes the reclassification of psychological disorders as illnesses to be a sort of error or mistake (logical or conceptual). At other times, however, he writes as though the change is "merely linguistic" and a matter of choice or preference of one classificatory schema rather than another. Thus he holds that it is "a matter of scientific and social choice whether we prefer to emphasize the similarities and, hence, place hysteria in the category of illness, or whether we prefer to emphasize the differences and place hysteria in a category of nonillness" ([5], p. 29). This view construes the issue as one of scientific and practical utility, rather than conceptual or logical error, and is borne out by Szasz's subsequent discussion. . . . It appears . . . that Szasz's position is at the very least, unclear, and at worst, inconsistent, with regard to the question of what is wrong with classifying behavioral disorders and disabling psychological difficulties as forms of "illness." We now turn to a brief discussion of Szasz's own view of what properly constitutes illness and some criticisms of his charge against those who have been engaged in reclassifying certain nonbodily disorders as forms of illness.

It is at least an implicit assumption of Szasz's—one which he sometimes makes explicit—that the only proper candidates for the notion of disease are those which refer to genuine *bodily* (organic or functional) ailments or involve a physical lesion. We need to examine this assumption in order to evaluate Szasz's contention that it is a mistake or error to construe nonbodily disorders as illness. The issue then becomes, on what grounds does Szasz reject mental "illnesses" as instances of some sort of disease, and are those grounds justifiable? He writes:

The adjectives "mental," "emotional," and "neurotic" are simply devices to codify—and at the same time obscure—the differences between two classes of disabilities or "problems" in meeting life. One category consists of bodily diseases—say, leprosy, tuberculosis, or cancer—which, by rendering imperfect the functioning of the human body as a machine, produce difficulties in social adaptation. In contrast to the first, the second category is characterized by difficulties in social adaptation not attributable to malfunctioning machinery but "caused" rather by the purposes the machine was made to serve . . . . ([5], pp. 41–42)

This view sets up two mutually exclusive categories of disability, such that an instance of the one category can never be construed as falling also under the second category. An antireductionist bias is evident in Szasz's remarks here and elsewhere, and it is legitimate to ask whether a clear distinction can be made between "the functioning of the human body as a machine" and "the purposes the machine was made to serve."

Moreover, it is certainly true, as Szasz contends ([5], pp. 79 ff.), that Freud continued to seek organic or physico-chemical *causes* of the psychological disorders and malfunctioning which he observed in his patients. But the question remains, *even if* Freud was mistaken in his continued search for neurological or some other physical bases for these behavioral disorders, does it follow that such disorders cannot properly be construed as forms of disease or illness nonetheless? Szasz's position seems to be that the absence of identifiable or probable physiological causes disqualifies a disorder or disability from the category of disease. Consequently, construing nonorganically based behavioral and personality disorders as diseases turns out to be *both* a logical and a scientific error. It is a logical error because the two categories of problems in facing life are mutually exclusive; and it is a scientific mistake because it erroneously presupposes an organic or neurological cause for every psychological, social, or ethical problem resulting from the malfunctioning of persons. Szasz wishes, therefore, to eliminate the entire notion of mental illness, claiming that "mental illness is a myth. Psychiatrists are not concerned with mental illnesses and their treatments. In actual practice they deal with personal, social, and ethical problems in living" ([5], p. 296).

Whereas Szasz chooses to *close* the concept of disease or illness, requiring as a necessary condition that there be a known or probable physiological basis, another view of the matter holds that the labors of

Freud and others resulted in a legitimate *extension* of the then existing concept of disease or illness. The strategy in replying to Szasz's position would thus consist in the following two-stage argument: (1) showing that Freud and his followers were not making a logical or conceptual *mistake* in treating psychological disorders as illnesses, but were rather engaged in the enterprise of extending or widening the concept of disease or illness; (2) showing that such extension in this case is *legitimate*, that is, can be justified by noting relevant and important similarities between cases of mental illness and cases of physical illness. I shall take the question, "Is it *ever* legitimate to extend or enlarge a concept?" as admitting of an uncontroversial affirmative answer. Accordingly, one reply to Szasz is given in the words of Joseph Margolis:

Szasz is absolutely right in holding that Freud reclassified types of suffering. But what he fails to see is that this is a perfectly legitimate (and even necessary) maneuver. In fact, this enlargement of the concept of illness does not obscure the differences between physical and mental illness—and the differences themselves are quite gradual, as psychosomatic disorder and hysterical conversion attest. On the contrary, these differences are preserved and respected in the very idea of an *enlargement* of the concept of illness. ([3], p. 73)

This passage serves not only to make the point about the legitimacy of enlarging the concept of illness to cover cases of mental or psychological illness, it also emphasizes that there is no clear and obvious line—as Szasz appears to think there is—between physical and mental illness, or between the "two categories" of problems in facing life. Indeed, it is apparent that Margolis has drawn this line in a different place from Szasz. While Szasz considers hysteria a nonbodily illness (hence, not an "illness" at all) on the grounds that it has no organic or neurological *causes*, Margolis construes hysterical conversion and other psychosomatic ailments at least as borderline cases, presumably on the grounds that such disorders are manifested in terms of observable and clear-cut bodily *symptoms* and *malfunctioning*. So it appears that there may be some genuine dispute as to the selection of criteria for an adequate or uncontroversial characterization of *physical* or *bodily* illness itself.

Once it is acknowledged that there are good reasons for construing Freud's maneuver as one of extending a concept rather than as a sort of logical or conceptual error, we may proceed to the second stage of the argument in reply to Szasz: the justification of the extension of the concept of illness to cover psychological problems and personality disorders. Margolis suggests the following, in answer to the question "Should mental 'disorders' be allowed, in a medical sense, to count as diseases or illnesses?"

If I were to describe a condition in which a patient suffers great pain in walking and is quickly overcome by fatigue, a condition which lasts for several years, and we were to find that there is an organic cause for this pattern, we should be strongly inclined to regard what we have before us as a *physical illness*. Now, if we have the same sort of pattern but are unable to find any organic cause, and begin to suspect that, in some inexplained way, the condition is due to the emotional or psychical life of the patient, we may have a reason for insisting that the pattern is still a *pattern of illness*. ([3], p. 74)

The reasonableness of this conclusion—Szasz's view notwithstanding—is shown by observing the affinities between the new cases and the standard ones. It should be noted, further, that the existence of unexplained phenomena and the absence at present of psychophysical laws (covering normal as well as abnormal behavior) do not in themselves compel theoretical conclusions and conceptual decisions of the sort that Szasz is prone to make.

There is a line of argument different from that employed by Margolis which can serve to show the relevant similarities between cases of physical disease and cases of putative mental illness. Whereas Margolis's method is a case by case approach, proceeding by comparison of new (mental) cases to old (physical) instances of disease and noting the affinities between them, the alternative method distinguishes general *categories* of behavioral symptoms and demonstrates that these categories are common both to bodily diseases and to disorders commonly construed as mental illness. David Ausubel uses this approach in arguing that "the plausibility of subsuming abnormal behavioral reactions to stress under the general rubric of disease is further enhanced by the fact that these reactions include the same three principal categories of symptoms found in physical illness" ([1], p. 262). Ausubel characterizes these categories as manifestations of impaired functioning, adaptive compensation, and defensive overreaction, and cites examples of both physical and mental diseases falling under each category, noting the relevant similarities between them. He concludes that there is no inherent contradiction in regarding mental symptoms *both* as expressions of "problems in living" (Szasz's preferred locution) *and* as manifestations of illness. "The latter situation results when individuals are for various reasons unable to cope with such problems, and react with seriously distorted or maladaptive behavior" ([1], p. 265). So according to some opponents of Szasz, the position is taken that in order to qualify as a genuine manifestation of disease, a symptom need not reflect a physical lesion.

We may conclude from the inquiry in this section that there appears to be no compelling reason to adopt Szasz's view that mental illness is a "myth" and that personality disorders and psychological problems are inappropriately viewed as illness and properly to be construed as "problems in living." In sum, there appear to be no logical or conceptual reasons why such difficulties cannot or should not be subsumed under the category of "illness." Moreover, whatever is gained in terms of social utility by viewing these problems as "problems in living" is not precluded by viewing them *also* as manifestations of disease, as Ausubel suggests. So whatever merits Szasz's position may have in terms of pragmatic consequences, these same results can be achieved if we retain the concept of mental *illness* along with the present classificatory schema.

By way of summary and conclusion, it would be well to note where the rejection of Szasz's antimedical model position leads us. Most of the problems discussed in this paper can be seen to re-emerge upon consideration of a brief quotation from Ausubel's paper. Arguing specifically against Szasz's contention that to qualify as a genuine manifestation of disease a given symptom must be caused by a physical lesion, Ausubel writes:

Adoption of such a criterion would be arbitrary and inconsistent both with medical and lay connotations of the term "disease," which in current usage is generally regarded as including any marked deviation, physical, mental, or behavioral, from normally desirable standards of structural and functional integrity. ([1], p. 259)

While this statement may appear sufficiently general to escape controversy, upon closer analysis a range of familiar problems can be identified in connection with the phrase 'normally desirable standards'. The immediate difficulty concerns whether the phrase is to be construed descriptively or normatively, but even if this question is decided, further problems remain. . . .

It may be, however, that we need to emphasize the further phrase: ". . . of structural and functional integrity" in analyzing Ausubel's statement. On this view, the appeal to "normally desirable standards of structural and functional integrity" presupposes some general theory which provides an account of an integrated, well-functioning system. Such an account is given, for the most part, in biological (anatomical and physiological) theories so that the notion of physical disease, although not without a number of problems, can be specified without engendering a great deal of controversy. With regard to mental health and illness, however, not only is there no generally accepted psychological or personality theory that can be presupposed, but the search for criteria of application for the basic concepts is itself an attempt to fill out such a theory and provide the very parameters which enable us to judge that a personality system possesses "structural and functional integrity."

In the words of Redlich and Freedman, "a completely acceptable supertheory on which psychiatry can generally rest its work does not exist" ([4], p. 79). But these authors would be quick to note that progress in the behavioral and biological sciences has been rapid and steadily advancing in recent years. So whatever pessimism may accrue to the observations made in this study about the concepts of mental health and mental illness as currently understood and employed by professionals and laymen alike, a measure of optimism exists in the belief that fruitful and systematic developments will continue to be forthcoming in the experimental, theoretical, and clinical areas of psychology and psychiatry.

REFERENCES

[1] Ausubel, D. P. "Personality Disorder *Is* Disease." *Mental Illness and Social Processes*. Edited by Thomas J. Scheff. New York: Harper and Row, 1967.

[2] Jahoda, M. *Current Concepts of Positive Mental Health*. New York: Basic Books, 1958.

[3] Margolis, J. *Psychotherapy and Morality*. New York: Random House, 1966.

[4] Redlich, F. C., and Freedman, D. X. *The Theory and Practice of Psychiatry*. New York: Basic Books, 1966.

[5] Szasz, T. S. *The Myth of Mental Illness*. New York: Harper and Row, 1961.

SUGGESTED READINGS FOR CHAPTER 3

Boorse, Christopher. "What a Theory of Mental Health Should Be." *Journal for the Theory of Social Behaviour* 6 (April 1976), 61–84.

———. "Health as a Theoretical Concept." *Philosophy of Science* 44 (December 1977), 542–573.

Breslow, Lester. "A Quantitative Approach to the World Health Organization Definition of Health: Physical, Mental, and Social Well-Being." *International Journal of Epidemiology* 1 (Winter 1972), 347–355.

Brown, W. Miller. "On Defining 'Disease.'" *Journal of Medicine and Philosophy* 10 (November 1985), 311–328.

Caplan, Arthur L., Engelhardt, H. Tristram, Jr., and McCartney, James J., eds. *Concepts of Health and Disease*. Reading, Mass.: Addison-Wesley, 1981.

Clouser, K. Danner, Culver, Charles M., and Gert, Bernard. "Malady: A New Treatment of Disease." *Hastings Center Report* 11 (June 1981), 29–37.

Eisenberg, Leon. "What Makes Persons 'Patients' and Patients 'Well'?" *American Journal of Medicine* 69 (August 1980), 277–286.

Engelhardt, H. Tristram, Jr. "The Concepts of Health and Disease." In Engelhardt, H. Tristram, Jr. and Spicker, Stuart F. eds. *Evaluation and Explanation in the Biomedical Sciences*. Boston: D. Reidel, 1975, pp. 125–141.

———. "Health and Disease: Philosophical Perspectives." In Reich, Warren T., ed. *Encyclopedia of Bioethics*. New York: Free Press, 1978. Vol. 2, pp. 599–606.

———. "Doctoring the Disease, Treating the Complaint, Helping the Patient." In Engelhardt, H. Tristram, Jr. and Callahan, Daniel, eds. *Knowing and Valuing*. Hastings-on-Hudson, N.Y.: The Hastings Center, 1980, pp. 225–249.

———. "Clinical Complaints and the *Ens Morbi*." *Journal of Medicine and Philosophy* 11 (August 1986), 207–214.

Fingarette, Herbert. *The Meaning of Criminal Insanity*. Berkeley, Calif.: University of California Press, 1972. Chap. 1.

Gert, Bernard, and Culver, Charles. *Philosophy in Medicine*. New York: Oxford University Press, 1982. Chap. 4.

———, Clouser, K. Danner, and Culver, Charles M. "Language and Social Goals." *Journal of Medicine and Philosophy* 11 (August 1986), 257–264.

Hoffman, Martin. "Philosophical Aspects of 'Mental Disease.'" *Australian and New Zealand Journal of Psychiatry* 12 (March 1978), 29–33.

Journal of Medicine and Philosophy. Vol. 1 (September 1976). Special issue on "Concepts of Health and Disease"; Vol. 2 (September 1977). Special issue on "Mental Health"; Vol. 5 (June 1980). Special issue on "Social and Cultural Perspectives on Disease."

Kass, Leon. "Regarding the End of Medicine and the Pursuit of Health." *Public Interest* 40 (Summer 1975), 11–42.

Kendell, R. E. "The Concept of Disease and Its Implications for Psychiatry." *British Journal of Psychiatry* 127 (1975), 305–315.

Kopelman, Loretta. "On Disease . . ." In Engelhardt, H. Tristram, Jr. and Spicker, Stuart F., eds. *Evaluation and Explanation in the Biomedical Sciences*. Boston: D. Reidel, 1975, pp. 143–150.

———, and Moskop, John. "The Holistic Health Movement: A Survey and Critique." *Journal of Medicine and Philosophy* 6 (May 1981), 209–235.

Macklin, Ruth. "Mental Health and Mental Illness: Some Problems of Definition and Concept Formation." *Philosophy of Science* 39 (September 1972), 341–365.

———. "The Medical Model in Psychoanalysis and Psychotherapy." *Comprehensive Psychiatry* 14 (January/February 1973), 49–69.

Margolis, Joseph. *Negativities: The Limits of Life*. Columbus, Ohio: Merrill, 1975. Chaps. 7 and 8.

———. "The Concept of Disease." *Journal of Medicine and Philosophy* 1 (September 1976), 238–255.

———. "Thoughts on Definitions of Disease." *Journal of Medicine and Philosophy* 11 (August 1986), 233–236.

Martin, Michael. "Malady and Menopause." *Journal of Medicine and Philosophy* 10 (November 1985), 329–337.

Mechanic, David. "The Concept of Illness Behavior." *Journal of Chronic Diseases* 15 (1962), 189–194.

Merskey, Harold. "Variable Meanings for the Definition of Disease." *Journal of Medicine and Philosophy* 11 (August 1986), 215–232.

Moore, Michael S. "Some Myths about 'Mental Illness.'" *Inquiry* 18 (Autumn 1975), 233–265.

———. *Law and Psychiatry: Rethinking the Relationship*. New York: Cambridge University Press, 1984.

Moreno, Jonathan. "The Continuity of Madness: Pragmatic Naturalism and Mental Health Care in America." In Caplan, Arthur L., et al., eds. *Concepts of Health and Disease*. Reading, Mass.: Addison-Wesley, 1981, pp. 645–664.

Murphy, Timothy F. "A Cure for Aging?" *Journal of Medicine and Philosophy* 11 (August 1986), 237–255.

Osmond, Humphrey. "The Medical Model in Psychiatry: Love It or Leave It." *Medical Annals of the District of Columbia* 41 (March 1972), 171–175.

Parsons, Talcott. "Health and Disease: A Sociological and Action Perspective." In Reich, Warren T., ed. *Encyclopedia of Bioethics*. New York: Free Press, 1978. Vol. 2, pp. 590–599.

Pflanz, Manfred, and Keupp, Heinrich. "A Sociological Perspective on Concepts of Disease." *International Social Science Journal* 29 (1977), 386–396.

Polgar, Stephen. "Health." In Sills, David L., ed., *International Encyclopedia of the Social Sciences*. New York: Free Press, 1968. Vol. 5, pp. 330–336.

Redlich, F. C. "The Concept of Health in Psychiatry." In Leighton, Alexander H., Claussen, John A., and Wilson, Robert N., eds. *Explorations in Social Psychiatry*. New York: Basic Books, 1957, pp. 138–158.

Risse, Guenter B. "Health and Disease: History of the Concepts." In Reich, Warren T., ed. *Encyclopedia of Bioethics*. New York: Free Press, 1978. Vol. 2, pp. 579–585.

Siegler, Mark. "The Doctor-Patient Encounter and Its Relationship to Theories of Health and Disease." In Caplan, Arthur L. et al., eds. *Concepts of Health and Disease*. Reading, Mass.: Addison-Wesley, 1981, pp. 627–644.

Szasz, Thomas. *The Manufacture of Madness*. New York: Harper & Row, 1970.

———. "Bad Habits Are Not Diseases." *Lancet* (July 8, 1972), 83–84.

———. *The Theology of Medicine: The Political-Philosophical Foundations of Medical Ethics*. New York: Harper & Row, 1977.

Whitbeck, Caroline. "A Theory of Health." In Caplan, Arthur L. et al., eds. *Concepts of Health and Disease*. Reading, Mass.: Addison-Wesley, 1981, pp. 611–626.

Wollheim, Richard. *The Thread of Life*. Cambridge, Mass.: Harvard University Press, 1984.

Goldstein, Doris Mueller. *Bioethics: A Guide to Information Sources*. Detroit: Gale Research Company, 1982. See under "Philosophy of Medicine" and "Psychotherapy and Psychopharmacology."

Lineback, Richard H., ed. *Philosopher's Index*. Vols. 1– . Bowling Green, Ohio: Philosophy Documentation Center, Bowling Green State University. Issued quarterly. See under "Health," "Illness," "Mental Health," "Mental Illness," and "Physicians."

Walters, LeRoy, and Kahn, Tamar Joy, eds. *Bibliography of Bioethics*. Vols. 1– . Washington, D.C.: Kennedy Institute of Ethics, Georgetown University. Issued annually. See under "Genetic Defects," "Health," and "Mental Health." (The information contained in the annual *Bibliography of Bioethics* can also be retrieved from BIOETHICSLINE, an online database of the National Library of Medicine.)

4.
Life, Death, and Personhood

This chapter explores two questions. The first is "When does (human) life begin and end?" This question includes both conceptual and empirical dimensions. We need to know exactly what we mean by the notion of "life"—and perhaps of its opposite, "death." Then, with that knowledge in hand, we can proceed to look for concrete evidence, tangible signs or indications, that life is present or absent. The second question addressed in the chapter is "Who are persons, and what difference does being a person make?" All conceptions of personhood, or at least all *philosophical* conceptions, presuppose that being alive is a necessary condition for being a person. However, in the literature of philosophy one encounters two distinct notions of personhood, which are not always clearly related to each other. The first is an ontological notion, in which descriptive characteristics of persons are listed and analyzed. The second is a moral notion, in which the capacity of a living individual to have moral rights and/or obligations is assessed.

THE BEGINNING AND END OF LIFE

The essays in this chapter by Michael Lockwood and Robert Veatch seek to elucidate the conceptual questions surrounding life and death. Lockwood distinguishes among living human organisms, (living) human beings, and (living) persons. He argues that a living human organism comes into being at the moment of conception and ceases to exist when the organism dies, decays, and turns to dust. In contrast, a human being comes into existence at some point after the human organism is already present and may cease to exist even though the human organism survives. What constitutes the life of a human being, on this view? According to Lockwood, it is a "continuity of physical organization within some part or parts of the brain persisting through time." When does the life of a human being, as Lockwood defines such beings, begin? Lockwood is not sure, but he argues that the beginning of life occurs between conception and birth, "certainly not *at* conception, and certainly not before my brain came into being."

Veatch finds it difficult to discuss definitions of life and death without at the same time treating the moral and legal standing of the living beings. Nonetheless, he examines four attributes of living beings that are often proposed as essential to their being alive: (1) the presence of a fixed genetic code; (2) the presence of the flowing of fluids; (3) the presence of the integrated functioning of the nervous system; and (4) the presence of the capacity for consciousness. Veatch argues that the first of these attributes can safely be ignored in the life-and-death discussion but that one's choice of attribute (2), (3), or (4) should be consistently applied at both the beginning and the end of life.

The question of life and death also has important empirical dimensions. These dimensions are featured in the essays by André Hellegers and Michael Flower and in a chapter from a presidential commission report entitled *Defining Death*. Hellegers and Flower present what might be called contrasting accounts of the facts about human embryonic and fetal development. Hellegers, founder and first director of the Kennedy Institute of Ethics and an articulate conservative on the abortion issue, presents the developing capacities of the fetus in their most favorable light. Flower, in a more technical mode, focuses primary attention on the anatomy and physiology of the fetal brain. He concludes that the key connections that would allow the neocortex to communicate with other parts of the brain are not made until the twentieth or twenty-first post-fertilization week. The President's Commission report recounts the evolution of standards for making decisions at the other end of the life spectrum. It notes that the brainstem can support respiration (and therefore heartbeat, as well) in some patients even when the cerebral neocortex, the anatomical locus of consciousness, has been irreversibly destroyed. Thus, a brainstem-oriented definition of death (and life) would classify as alive some patients who would be classified as dead by a cerebrally or neocortically oriented definition of death.

CONCEPTS OF PERSONHOOD

Discussions of personhood frequently adopt a purely descriptive approach. They ask the question: "What sorts of beings are persons, and how are persons to be distinguished from other entities present in the universe, for example, dogs, trees, or rocks?" These discussions belong to the branch of philosophy called metaphysics, and more particularly to the part of metaphysics called ontology, or the study of that which exists.

As philosophers have reflected on the problem of personhood, they have usually found it quite easy to categorize nonliving objects (for example, rocks) and many types of living things (for example, bacteria, plants, and invertebrate animals) as nonpersons. However, beyond this point the search for the criterion of personhood becomes much more complicated. Among the questions that have long puzzled philosophers are the following: Are some nonhuman beings—for example, chimpanzees—capable of becoming persons? And can there be other types of beings—for example, residents of unknown planets, angels, or robots—who should also be designated persons?

The standard philosophical approach to solving these puzzles has been to devise a list of necessary, and possibly sufficient, conditions for being a person. These conditions are often expressed in terms of properties that must be possessed by the being in question if it is to qualify as a person. Two properties, or characteristics, have been featured most prominently in ontological discussions of personhood—self-awareness and rationality. Other commentators have required the presence of a third characteristic, as well, namely, the capacity to be a moral agent. The German philosopher Immanuel Kant especially accented these moral characteristics of personhood. In a similar vein, contemporary philosopher Roland Puccetti distinguishes between C-predicates, which apply to all conscious beings, and P-predicates, which apply only to persons. Among the predicates applied by Puccetti to the two groups of subjects are the following:

C is in pain	P wants to secure justice
C feels hungry	P summarized the point nicely
C is excited	P is an astute judge of character
C is afraid of you	P is a smug hypocrite[1]

According to Puccetti, the C-predicates in the left-hand column can be applied to conscious nonpersons like dogs, whereas the P-predicates in the right-hand column presuppose the possession of a conceptual scheme and the capacity to act as a moral agent. This latter capacity is for Puccetti the primary distinguishing feature of personhood, for persons are the only conscious entities who can adopt moral attitudes toward moral objects.

It might seem that the preceding discussion has already crossed the line between ontological and moral notions of personhood. However, the authors cited to this point have only been involved in describing what sorts of beings persons are, not in prescribing how particular beings ought to be treated. Moral notions of personhood perform precisely this task. Ascribing moral personhood to an individual is tantamount to saying "I have moral obligations to this individual" or "This individual has moral rights." In the history of philosophy, Immanuel Kant was perhaps the most influential proponent of the moral personhood notion. Kant considered persons as beings whose rational nature "points them out as ends in themselves." Accordingly, Kant contended that the only appropriate attitude toward such beings is one of respect. (See the discussion of autonomy in Chapter 1. The difficulty inherent in specifying precisely what moral obligations are included in respect for persons is itself a complex philosophical problem. However, it need not detain us here. It is sufficient to observe the existence of at least minimal moral duties to all beings belonging to the category of persons.)

Given the moral obligations that are thought to be owed to persons, it is then an obvious strategy for anyone seeking to protect particular categories of beings to argue that those beings rightly belong to the category of (moral) persons. Conversely, it is sometimes thought that nonpersons do not deserve the same kind of respect, or even that any nonperson may be treated, in Kant's terms, merely as a means.

Whether and how one can move logically from ontology to ethics, or from "is" to "ought," is one of the most vigorously contested questions in philosophy. The problem of the relationship between ontological and moral notions of personhood is, from one perspective, simply an instance of this more generic question.

Some philosophers, among them R. M. Hare, have argued that there is no necessary logical connection between ontological personhood and moral personhood. According to Hare, one cannot infer from the assertion "X is a person" that "I ought to be kind to X."[2] In contrast, many other philosophers see an intimate connection between ontological and moral personhood.

There is an obverse side to the is-ought problem. The mere fact that a being is not ontologically a person does not logically entail the conclusion that we have no obligations to it or, correlatively, that it has no rights. Thus, there may be powerful arguments against infanticide, even if infants are not persons in the ontological sense. A similar question is explored in Chapter 9: "What moral obligations, if any, do we persons have toward animals that are not persons?"

In the latter part of this chapter, Joel Feinberg, Raanan Gillon, and Tristram Engelhardt explore the problem of moral personhood and the appropriate size and shape of the moral universe. Feinberg argues that nonhuman animals can have rights because they have, or can have, interests. Gillon's essay analyzes the strengths and weaknesses of four leading answers to the question "To what do we have moral obligations and why?" In contrast, Engelhardt argues that persons are by far the most important subjects and objects in the moral universe and that the moral status of nonpersons depends, and should depend, solely on the decisions made by persons.

L. W.

NOTES

1. Roland Puccetti, *Persons: A Study of Possible Moral Agents in the Universe* (New York: Herder and Herder, 1970), pp. 7–8. Puccetti's entire discussion of predicates builds upon P. F. Strawson's earlier work, *Individuals.* Whereas Strawson had distinguished only M-predicates (for material bodies) and P-predicates, Puccetti added the intermediate category of C-predicates.

2. R. M. Hare, *Freedom and Reason* (Oxford: Clarendon Press, 1963), pp. 212–213.

ANDRÉ E. HELLEGERS

Fetal Development

. . . Since society has imagery and definitions of its own, which it has inherited from the past, it may be well in the description which follows to highlight those stages of development to which, for one reason or another, [people] have attached importance in the past.[1]

I

First, let us ask in what way the ovum, or female egg, and the sperm, or male eggs, differ from the fertilized ovum. The essential difference is that an ovum or a sperm will inevitably die unless they are combined together in the process of fertilization, while the fertilized egg will automatically develop unless untoward events occur. The first definition of life, then, could be the ability to reproduce oneself, and this the fertilized egg has while the individual ovum and sperm do not.

How is this process of fertilization brought about? At intercourse, about 300,000,000 sperm are deposited in the vagina and will begin their journey upwards through the uterus, or womb, and up into the tube leading from the uterus towards the ovary. If an ovum has been released from the woman's ovary, it in turn will pass from the ovary down the same tube towards the uterus. The survival time of this ovum will be about twenty-four hours. If fertilization has not occurred in that time, both the ovum and the sperm will die. From a variety of mammalian species it has been learned that the sperm, as ejaculated, are not capable of immediately fertilizing an ovum. They must undergo a chemical change called "capacitation," without which they cannot fertilize the ovum.[2] The process is as yet little understood, but it is thought that a substance in the female uterus or tube changes the

sperm in such a way that they gain the ability to fertilize. In most species this process occurs in a matter of hours, say six or eight. Although the process has not yet been proven in the human, it is commonly assumed to exist, since it occurs in other mammalian species studied. Following intercourse, there would therefore be a period of several hours in which interference with reproduction would fall under the generally recognized heading of contraception rather than abortion, since no ovum would yet have been fertilized. Several hours after intercourse, then, fertilization may occur. The significance of this event lies in the fact that a totally new genetic package is now produced. The fertilized ovum contains genetic information brought from the father through the sperm, and from the mother through the ovum, so that a new combination of genetic information is created. This newly fertilized egg, sometimes called a zygote, has within it the hereditary characteristics of both the father and the mother, one half from each. The characteristics are derived from the genetic thread of life called DNA, contained in each.

This single fertilized cell will then proceed to divide into two cells, then four, then eight, etc., and this it will do at a rate of almost one division per day.[3]

It is well known that in this early stage of development the sphere of cells may split into identical parts to form identical twins. Twinning in the human may occur until the fourteenth day, when conjoined twins can still be produced. Less well known is the fact that it is also in these first few days that twins or triplets may be recombined into one single individual.

Experiments carried out in mice by Mintz showed that it was possible to recombine the early dividing cell stages from black parents and from white parents into a single black-and-white-striped mouse.[4] The significance of this phenomenon would seem to be that up

Reprinted with permission of the author and the publisher from *Theological Studies* 31 (1):3–9, March 1970.

until this stage the new individual mammal is not as yet irreversibly an individual, since it still may be recombined with others into one new, final being.

In the last few years this phenomenon has also been found in man. From the genetic make-up of these human individuals and from the make-up of their red blood cells it is clear that these human so-called chimeras, whose genetic type is XX-XY, are in fact recombinations into one human being of the products of more than one fertilization. The subject has recently been extensively reviewed by Benirschke,[5] and a prototype case can be found in the report of Myhre *et al*.[6] It is not as yet clear up to precisely what stage of development this can occur in the human, but in mice the recombination can still be performed at the 32-cell stage. The diagnostic criteria for such cases are that their genetic karyotype is XX-XY, that they are gonadally disturbed consisting as they do of a genetic mixture of male and female, that they can contain two different populations of red blood cells, and that they may have heterochromia of the eyes. Six human cases meeting these requirements have been reported up to the present time.

The initial stages of cell division of the fertilized egg do not seem to be dependent on any paternal genetic material brought to the fertilized egg by the sperm. It would seem as if genetic material brought to the fertilized egg in the mother's ovum suffices to take the fertilized egg through the earliest stages of cell division.

All these matters are brought forth to point out that, although at fertilization a new genetic package is brought into being within the confines of one cell, this anatomical fact does not necessarily mean that all of the genetic material in it becomes crucially activated at that point, or that final irreversible individuality has been achieved.

Modern genetic studies therefore suggest that, in old standard Catholic language, one could say: "If by means of two fertilizations two souls are infused, and if a single body only contains one soul, then we are beginning to see cases in which one of the two souls must have disappeared without any fertilized egg having died."

It is also important to realize that in these first few days of life it is quite impossible for the woman to know that she is pregnant, or for the doctor to diagnose the condition by a pregnancy test.

The fact that the first seven days of the reproductive process take place entirely in the tube, and not in the uterus itself, has several major implications for the subject of abortion. These should be fully understood. If within seven days of intercourse, as for instance following rape, the lining of the uterus is removed by curettage, abortion, in its legal sense, has not taken place. It would be impossible to prove that an abortion had been performed when all pregnancy tests were shown to be negative and the lining of the uterus was shown, under the microscope, to have contained no pregnancy. Indeed the operation of curettage is a common gynecological one, which is frequently carried out in the second half of the menstrual cycle, when a fertilized ovum may well be present in the tube. There has never been a medical tradition to perform the curettage only immediately following menstruation, in order to assure that no fertilized egg could be present in the tube (since ovulation would not as yet have occurred). By the same token, women scheduled to undergo a curettage are not instructed to forgo intercourse lest there be present in the tube a fertilized ovum which would be unable to implant into the uterus due to the removal of its lining. Moreover, there is some evidence that modern "contraceptive" techniques such as the intrauterine loop, and even some of the steroid pills, may well exert their effect in pregnancy prevention by acting after fertilization of the ovum has occurred, but before implantation in the uterus.[7] Although the action of these agents is not yet fully understood, there has never been a suggestion that they would be considered abortifacient under the civil law, since no evidence of pregnancy could possibly be obtained.

II

After approximately six or seven days of this cell-division process (all of which occurs in the tube), the next critical stage of development starts. The sphere of cells will now enter the uterus and implant itself into the uterine lining. This process of implantation is highly critical, for it is during these days that one pole of the sphere of cells, the trophoblast (later to become the placenta), burrows its way into the lining of the uterus. The opposite pole of this sphere will become the fetus. The part which becomes the placenta produces hormones. These enter the maternal blood stream and serve a critical function in preventing the mother from menstruating. Since the time interval between ovulation and menstruation is approximately fourteen days, and since the first seven days of the new life have been passed in the tube, it is obvious that the implanting trophoblast only has about seven days to produce enough hormone to stop the mother from menstruating and thus sloughing off the fetal life. These same hormones, circulating in the mother, form the basis for the chemical tests which enable us to diagnose pregnancy. After this second week of pregnancy the zygote rapidly becomes more complex and is now called the embryo. Somewhere between the third and fourth week the differentiation of the embryo will have been sufficient for heart pumping to occur,[8]

although the heart will by no means yet have reached its final configuration. At the end of six weeks all of the internal organs of the fetus will be present, but as yet in a rudimentary stage. The blood vessels leading from the heart will have been fully deployed, although they too will continue to grow in size with growth of the fetus. By the end of seven weeks tickling of the mouth and nose of the developing embryo with a hair will cause it to flex its neck, while at the end of eight weeks there will be readable electrical activity coming

Some Major Normal Stages in Fetal Development

Time	Cardiovascular system	Nervous system	Other criterion
Some Hours	—	—	Intercourse followed by "capacitation"
0 Hours	—	—	Fertilization; 1 cell, often called zygote
About 22 hours	—	—	2 cell ⎫ Possible recombi-
About 44 hours	—	—	4 cell ⎪ nation until day ?
About 66 hours	—	—	8 cell ⎬ Possible twinning
About 4 days	—	—	16 cell ⎭ until day 14 "Morula" stage
About 6–7 days	—	—	Implantation—often called "blastocyst" stage
2 weeks	—	—	Name changed from zygote to embryo
3–4 weeks	Heart pumping	—	—
6 weeks	—	—	All organs present
7–8 weeks	—	Mouth or nose tickling = neck flexing	—
8 weeks	—	Readable brain electric activity	Name change from embryo to fetus. Length 3 cm.
9–10 weeks	—	Swallowing, squinting, local reflexes	—
10 weeks	—	Spontaneous movement	—
11 weeks	—	—	Thumb sucking
12 weeks	Fetal EKG via mother	—	Brain structure complete Length 10 cm.
13 weeks*	—	—	D & C contraindicated hereafter
12–16 weeks*	—	—	"Quickening." Length 18 cm. at 16 weeks
16–20 weeks*	Fetal heart heard	—	Length 25 cm. at 20 weeks
20 weeks*	—	—	Name change from abortus to premature infant
20–28 weeks*	—	—	10% survive
28 weeks*	—	—	Fetus said to be "viable" in some definitions
40 weeks*	—	—	Birth

*Calculated from the first day of the last menstrual period.

from the brain.[9] The meaning of the activity cannot be interpreted. By now also the fingers and toes will be fully recognizable. Sometime between the ninth and the tenth week local reflexes appear such as swallowing, squinting, and tongue retraction. By the tenth week spontaneous movement is seen, independent of stimulation. By the eleventh week thumb-sucking has been observed and X rays of the fetus at this time show clear details of the skeleton. After twelve weeks the fetus, now 3½ inches in size, will have completed its brain structure, although growth of course will continue. By this time also it has become possible to pick up the fetal heart by modern electrocardiographic techniques, via the mother.

The twelve-week stage is also important for an entirely different reason. It is after this stage that the performance of an abortion by the relatively simple D&C (scraping of the womb) becomes dangerous. Thereafter abortion must be performed either by abdominal operation or by the more recently developed technique of the injection of a concentrated fluid into the amniotic cavity.

Sometime between the twelfth and sixteenth week "quickening" will occur. This event, long considered important in law, denotes the fact that fetal movements are first felt by the mother. Quickening, therefore, is a phenomenon of maternal perception rather than a fetal achievement. It is subjective and varies with the degree of experience and obesity of the mother.

Sometime between the sixteenth and twentieth week it will also become possible to hear the fetal heart, not just by the refined EKG, but also by the simple stethoscope.

The twentieth-week stage again has definite importance. Before this date delivery of the product of conception is called an abortion in medical terminology. After this date we no longer speak of abortion but of premature delivery. The fetus at this stage will weigh about one pound. Between the twentieth and twenty-eighth week fetuses born have an approximately 10% chance of survival. At twenty-eight weeks the fetus will weigh slightly over two pounds. In former days the medical profession defined fetuses of less than twenty-eight weeks of age as abortions, but this was impossible to maintain when 10% of such infants might survive. As a consequence, a discrepancy may now exist between possible definitions of viability in legal and in medical circles; at least the ability to

ensure survival of fetuses has progressively occurred at earlier stages.

After the twenty-eighth week little change in outward appearance of the fetus occurs, although growth obviously continues, and with this growth the chances of survival also increase.

These, then, are the major stages of fetal development in the order of their occurrence. Grouped systematically, and therefore rather arbitrarily, by genetic factors, by cardiovascular or nervous system development, and by chances of survival, they can be summarized as in the accompanying Table.

Throughout the analysis of the beginning of life it is important to bear several factors in mind. First, the understanding of the processes described is the understanding of today. The eliciting of fetal responses depends on the methods available today. Second, it is not a function of science to prove, or disprove, where in this process *human* life begins, in the sense that those discussing the abortion issue so frequently use the word "life," i.e., human dignity, human personhood, or human inviolability. Such entities do not pertain to the science or art of medicine, but are rather a societal judgment. Science cannot prove them; it can only describe the biological development and predict what will occur to it with an accuracy that depends on the stage of development of the particular science. In the ultimate analysis the question is not just to forecast when life begins, but rather: How should one behave when one does not know whether dignity is or is not present in the fetus?

NOTES

1. I shall stress heavily the new biology on the developmental processes in the first seven days, while the "fetus" is in the tube. This is crucial, I believe, (1) by reason of its own biological interest; (2) because of the action of the pill and intrauterine devices, which may act during these seven days; (3) because this stage precedes the period when a diagnosis of pregnancy can be made, i.e., it is the stage commonly described as "the normal second half of the normal menstrual cycle"; (4) because it is the stage when the "morning-after pill" may act; (5) because it is not presently covered under abortion laws, inasmuch as it precedes the stage when the woman knows she is pregnant (for she has not yet missed a period) and precedes the stage when a diagnosis can be made; (6) because it is a stage upon which the Catholic Hospital Association has not yet reflected, since we frequently do operations after ovulation but before a period is missed, i.e., during these seven days.

2. Cf. C. E. Adams, "The Influence of Maternal Environment on Preimplantation Stages of Pregnancy in the Rabbit," in *Preimplantation Stages of Pregnancy*, ed. G. E. W. Wolstenholme and M. O'Connor (Boston, 1965) p. 345; K. A. Rafferty, "The Beginning of Development," in *Intrauterine Development*, ed. A. C. Barnes (Philadelphia, 1968).

3. Cf. Rafferty, *op. cit.*

4. Cf. B. Mintz, "Experimental Genetic Mosaicism in the Mouse," in *Preimplantation Stages of Pregnancy* (n. 1 above) p. 194.

5. Cf. K. Benirschke, *Current Topics in Pathology* 1 (1969) 1.

6. Cf. A. Myhre, T. Meyer, J. N. Opitz, R. R. Race, R. Sanger, and T. J. Greenwalt, "Two Populations of Erythrocytes Associated with XX-XY Mosaicism," *Transfusion* 5 (1965) 501.

7. Cf. P. A. Corfman and S. J. Segal, "Biologic Effects of Intrauterine Devices," *American Journal of Obstetrics and Gynecol-* ogy 100 (1968) 448; also "Hormonal Steroids in Contraception," *WHO Technical Report Series, 1968* (Geneva, 1968) p. 386.

8. Cf. J. W. C. Johnson, "Cardio-Respiratory Systems," in *Intrauterine Development* (n. 1 above).

9. Cf. D. Goldblatt, "Nervous System and Sensory Organs," in *Intrauterine Development* (n. 1 above).

M I C H A E L   J .   F L O W E R

Neuromaturation of the Human Fetus*

If once the fetus was a stranger to us, such is not the case today. The fetal human no longer develops unseen but is photographed *in utero*, with images of its changing form being circulated to millions in news magazines. With the aid of ultrasonography, a woman can view the fetus within her body, seeing it move about long before she will be able to feel its stirrings. Fetuses are also the subjects of medical scrutiny and intervention. They can be examined for genetic defects, as well as become patients for corrective surgery. At the same time, the fetus is the subject of agonizing decisions about whether to terminate pregnancy and of political battles to circumscribe such decisions. Quite simply, our relations with the fetal human have multiplied, heightening the need for surer foundations to guide those relations.

What we know or might learn of fetal neural function has become part of that search. No longer is an interest in prenatal neuromaturation linked only to the general goal of understanding the ontogenetic underpinnings of mature brain function or neural disorder. Now it is also important to know when the fetus is likely to become sentient, feel pain, and register intrauterine experience. Further, some (Goldenring, 1982; Veatch, 1983) have argued that if we can agree that the loss of integral brain function, coordination of bodily functions and the sponsorship of consciousness constitutes *death* (President's Commission, 1981, p. 34) then—assuming we can delineate the emergence of the same integral function in the fetus—we ought to be able to locate the *coming into being* of a human subject with significant moral claims upon us.

It is the purpose of this essay to examine what we know about the development of the central nervous system of the fetal human. Four processes will be featured: appearance of fetal motor activity, development of the neocortex,[a] establishment of the crucial connection between the neocortex and its major input channel (the thalamus), and maturation of the electrical activity of the brain. Some of the evidence in hand is fragmentary. Opportunities to study the human fetus are rare, and ethically permissible methods are often not very informative. As a result, we know less about the fetus than we would like. Still, there are numerous observations, some old and some recent, which taken together yield a useful picture of fetal neuromaturation.

FETAL MOTOR ACTIVITY AND ITS NEURAL BASIS

It has been known for at least a century that the fetus is capable of sustained motor activity well before quickening. Systematic study of this activity is much more recent, the earliest carefully planned and recorded

From *Journal of Medicine and Philosophy* Vol. 10, No. 3 (August 1985), pp. 237–251. Copyright © 1985 by D. Reidel Publishing Company. Reprinted by permission of Kluwer Academic Publishers.

a. Ed. note: The part of the brain involved in thinking and remembering.

work being that which began in the 1930s, by Hooker and his colleagues (reviewed by Humphrey, 1978). As we shall see, their observations of the reflex patterns of previable fetuses can be used to advantage in light of more recent findings.

The elicitation of a reflex response from a 7.5 week fetus[1] *ex utero* is the earliest reported in a study maintaining cinematic records (Fitzgerald and Windle, 1942). Humphrey (1978, p. 655) describes this first reflex as a contralateral flexion of the head, a movement *away* from a gentle stroking stimulus applied to regions around the mouth. Through the eighth week, in fact, nearly 95% of responses were contralateral. The responses were also stereotypic and involved the whole body; they were predictable 'total pattern' reflexes. In the middle of the ninth week, a transition began. Ipsilateral responses (*toward* a stimulus) began to appear with much greater frequency. Also, the first local reflexes were elicited—only parts of the fetal body moved. By 12–13 weeks, local reflexes had almost completely replaced the total pattern response, combining in variable and unpredictable motor behaviors.

One might reasonably ask whether the motor activities demonstrated in these early studies were representative of normal fetal behavior. After all, the fetuses were observed following therapeutic termination of pregnancy. They lived but a short time and rapidly became anoxic.[b] Fortunately, several recent studies have utilized real-time ultrasonography to follow motor activity *in utero*, and all confirm a transition from simple whole body movements to complex motor repertoires. The simplest movements are detected in a few embryos as early as the sixth week (Van Dongen and Goudie, 1980, p. 192), whereas most embryos begin moving during the seventh week and exhibit more complex motor activity a week later. One longitudinal study (de Vries *et al.*; 1982, p. 311) followed eleven individual pregnancies from 5 to 18 weeks of development with the finding that the *sequence* of embryonic and fetal motor behaviors and their *time of first appearance* . . . did not differ significantly from the situation *ex utero*. Thus, our continued use of earlier accounts is warranted.

What [can we] say about the neural basis of these motor patterns and the transition in quality of response near the end of the first trimester? First, the conditions

necessary for a reflex arc can be demonstrated prior to the first observed embryonic and fetal movements. Okado (1981, pp. 212, 215) has shown that synapses[c] between interneurons and motoneurons (an output connection) first appear in the embryonic lateral motor column of the cervical spinal cord during the fifth week (at 30–32 days), while the first synapses in the dorsal marginal layer—representing (input) connections between sensory fibers and interneurons—appear about four days later (Figure 1). Thus, the very first reflexes at 7.5 weeks (as well as the earliest movements detected *in utero*) can be accounted for by simple, three-neuron circuits.

Within a few days, however, the situation becomes more complex. By the end of the eighth week, the trunk and pelvis are incorporated into the whole body response to a stimulus about the mouth. However, the nerve stimulated in this way (the trigeminal) does not carry fibers that extend to the trunk region. Additional circuitry is required. Probably involved are intersegmental neurons (they 'bridge' sections of the spinal cord) and a phylogenetically-old[d] region of the brainstem known as the reticular[e] formation (Humphrey, 1978, p. 661). The latter is a richly interconnected neuronal network which, in the adult, has the ability to self-generate an ongoing neural activity, i.e., it can function as an impulse generator. As it does in the adult, this region very likely receives and 'processes' signals whenever sensory information is imparted from the surface (or interior) of the fetus. The reticular formation, in turn, can impart electrical impulses along (reticulospinal) fibers that project from it down the spinal cord, branching and synapsing with motoneurons along the way.

With such circuitry in place, a fetus would no longer be restricted to simplex reflex arcs. It would possess a rudimentary information processor, the brainstem reticular formation. It could produce a repeated output that was a modulated version of its intrinsic neural activity *and* sensory inputs received. This sort of system might then account for motor activity *in utero*. As de Vries and her co-workers (1982, p. 317) point out, early activity is not merely reflexive but is spontaneously generated. Also, components of the behavior exhibit patterns of expression that change in frequency and duration as development proceeds.

---

b. Ed. note: Severely depleted in its oxygen supply.

c. Ed. note: Sites where nervous impulses are transmitted from one nerve cell to another.

d. Ed. note: Old in terms of evolutionary history.

e. Ed. note: Network-like.

Thus, as in other mammals (such as the guinea pig (Bergström, 1969, p. 25)), it may be that fetal motor activity is subject to brainstem[f] influence (one hesitates to say control) within days of its first appearance.

But what of the transition from whole body to local reflex response? It is likely to be the composite result of several developmental changes. First, the electrical activity pattern of the brainstem changes as development proceeds, becoming increasingly regular after ten weeks of gestation (Bergström, 1969, p. 20). Interestingly, it is near this time that general movement of the fetus begins to occur as a series of relatively discrete bursts of repeated activity in place of an earlier intermittent pattern (de Vries *et al.*, 1982, p. 312). Second, local reflexes can occur only if other neuro-muscular systems come under inhibitory influence from higher centers. If such is the case, we should be able to identify inhibitory circuitry in the spinal cord. In fact, the number of synapses within the cord increases sevenfold during the eighth week, with a second increase (more than four-fold) from week 11 to week 13 (Okado, 1980, p. 508). An increasing number of these are axosomatic, a synapse type that is generally inhibitory.

f. Ed. note: The part of the brain that controls noncognitive functions like respiration.

A third change is an increase in the fetal somatosensorium, the fetus's capacity to respond to external (exteroceptive) and internal (proprioceptive) stimulation. At 7.5 weeks only the mouth region is sensitive to an external stimulus, whereas by nine to ten weeks reflex activity can be initiated by stimulating the palm of the hands, the genital area, the soles of the feet, the arm, back, and shoulder (Humphrey, 1964, p. 96). In addition, receptors specialized for the detection of muscle stretch (the muscle spindles) first appear at nine weeks and are present in most muscles by the fourteenth week (Humphrey, 1964, p. 121). Thus, the sensation of fetal movement is an increasing part of the sensory input to the brainstem. If the reticular formation is indeed a rudimentary signal processor, it receives an increasingly more complex array of information as the fetus moves about.

DEVELOPMENT OF THE NEOCORTEX

The neocortex begins its long period of development during the eighth week (52–54 days; Molliver *et al.*, 1973, p. 406; Marin-Padilla, 1983, p. 34). The first of the prospective neocortical neurons migrate from a

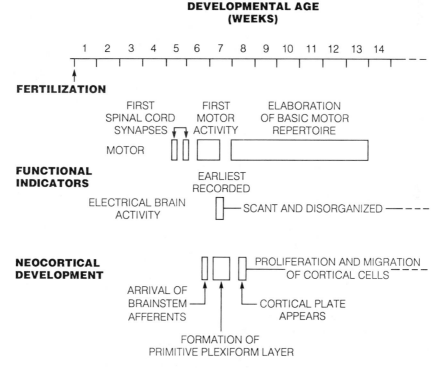

Figure 1. Neuromaturational Processes During Early Fetal Human Life.

proliferative zone near the ventricular border of the cerebrum, halt before reaching the pial margin, and form a cortical plate of cells—the neocortical anlage.[2] The plate forms in the middle of another band of cells formed about a week earlier (Figure 1), the primitive plexiform layer. This latter band of cells is phylogenetically old and may represent what Marin-Padilla (1978) considers a premammalian cerebral structure. Coursing through the plexiform layer and forming occasional synapses as early as the seventh week (Larroche, 1981, p. 309) are axonal fibers[g] thought to originate in the brainstem.

As a result of this mode of corticogenesis, the rudimentary neocortex comes to lie between two early-differentiating neuronal populations that are in synaptic contact with the brainstem (Molliver *et al.*, 1973, p. 404; Larroche *et al.*, 1981, p. 354). Furthermore, these sandwiching layers are considered to be functionally active, perhaps influencing the subsequent enlargement and organization of the cortical plate (Poliakov, 1961; Schlumpf *et al.*, 1980, p. 375; Marin-Padilla, 1983, p. 37). The mode of possible developmental influence is not clear. It may be that electrical activity originating in the brainstem is important; alternatively, the influences may be due to the release of trophic[h] factors, a possibility made more likely by the knowledge that cortically-projecting brainstem systems . . . can modulate later neuronal activity through the direct, non-synaptic release of neurotransmitters and peptides (Vale and Brown, 1979). Added to its earlier discussed role as a rudimentary modulator of fetal sensory and motor activity, the demonstration of a brainstem influence on the development of the neocortex would certainly raise its stock as a pivotal link in early neuromaturation.

Regardless of whether the brainstem plays a significant developmental role, the process of proliferation and cell migration is certainly a precise one (Rakic, 1981). It continues for more than three months, producing a succession of layers within which specialized cortical neurons of differing function (Peters and Jones, 1984) develop and begin forming synapses. Synaptogenesis within the cortical plate does not begin until migration of neocortical cells is nearly complete.

The first synapses appear some time between 19 and 22 weeks (Figure 2), having been found at 23 but not 18 weeks (Molliver *et al.*, 1973, p. 404). The period of greatest synaptic connection begins several weeks later when the predominant neuronal classes . . . differentiate by producing prodigiously branched dendritic[i] arbors along which hundreds or thousands of small protuberances or spines appear. These spines are the synaptic targets of incoming as well as intracortical neural pathways; therefore, their appearance marks neocortical readiness to establish functional circuitry.

THE THALAMOCORTICAL CONNECTION

With only a few exceptions, all pathways to the neocortex pass through the thalamus, a multi-component structure which modulates sensory input just before relaying it to the cerebrum. The time of thalamocortical connection is therefore of crucial importance. In the absence of this linkage, the developing neocortex is relatively isolated. When are the connections made? Our best answer is a relatively imprecise one—a bit past mid-gestation.

Studying non-human primates, Rakic (1981) has shown that cells of the lateral geniculate[j] (a portion of the thalamus responsible for the passage of visual information) produce axons that exit the thalamus during the first third of gestation, and arrive in the cerebrum prior to mid-gestation. There they 'wait' just below the neocortex proper until the neocortical cells have completed their migration and the cortex is in place. The thalamic fibers then penetrate the cortex and begin establishing precise synaptic connections.

While it is likely that events in the fetal human progress along an analogous time course (with connection at about 21 weeks), one would like a direct demonstration if possible. However, information of this exact sort cannot be gotten for the human being using Rakic's informative methods. To trace the development of this connection, Rakic had to gain access to a series of monkey fetuses by caesarian section, inject circuit-tracing molecules into the eye, return the fetuses to the uterus, and then repeat the caesarian and sacrifice the fetuses at a later time. Quite obviously, no such human experiment would be ethically acceptable.

Recently, however, two studies (Kostovic and Goldman-Rakic, 1983; Kostovic and Rakic, 1984) have

---

g. Ed. note: The wire-like structures that conduct electrical impulses in the nervous system.

h. Ed. note: Regulatory.

i. Ed. note: Pertaining to a dendrite, a branch-like structure that conducts electrical impulses.

j. Ed. note: A structure that is bent like a knee.

appeared which take advantage of the fact that two regions of the thalamus (the pulvinar[k] and mediodorsal[l]) possess a "natural marker" by which the thalamocortical connection could be traced. They were able to reconstruct the developmental process by use of sequentially staged human fetuses. They confirmed the events found in the monkey and showed that pulvinar and mediodorsal thalamic fibers pass into the human neocortex at about 22–23 weeks' gestation (Figure 2).

There are other regions of the thalamus about whose time course of connection with the neocortex we know nothing. Their fibers might conceivably arrive earlier. But even if they do, there is no evidence of neocortical synapse formation before 19–22 weeks as already noted. Even the simplest involvement of the neocortex in fetal human life must await the second half of gestation.

k. Ed. note: Relating to the posterior extremity of the thalamus.
l. Ed. note: In the middle, toward the back.

ELECTRICAL ACTIVITY OF THE FETAL BRAIN

It is probably reasonable to assume that nearly all of the electrical brain activity present during the first half of gestation originates in the brainstem. Certainly in the earliest reported case at 6.5 weeks this is so (Borkowski and Bernstine, 1955, p. 363). The two synapse-containing layers of the original primitive plexiform layer might conceivably form active local circuits; it is more likely, however, that the activity they exhibit follows from the fact of their brainstem innervation.

The first patterned electroencephalograms (EEGs)[m] are obtained from premature fetal-infants near midgestation—about the time cortical synaptogenesis begins (Figure 2). Occasional time-patterned EEGs are

m. Ed. note: Recordings of electrical activity in the cerebrum of the brain.

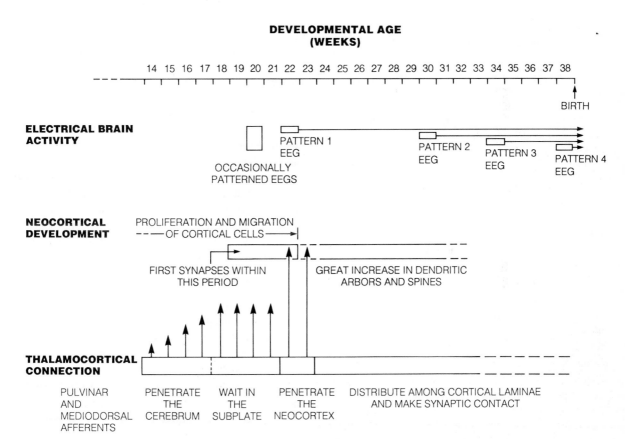

Figure 2. Neuromaturational Processes during Mid-to-Late Gestation Fetal Human Life.

seen at 20 weeks; the first sustained EEGs, at 22 weeks (Spehlmann, 1981, p. 159). This latter activity, the so-called pattern 1 EEG, is discontinuous, occurring in bursts in both cerebral hemispheres simultaneously (with individual waves within the bursts becoming bilaterally synchronous at 26–27 weeks).

Later EEG patterns (Figure 2; Spehlmann, 1981, pp. 163–165) appear only after considerable synaptogenesis has taken place. The emergence of pattern 2 EEGs (continuous electrical activity) at about 30 weeks marks the distinction of wakefulness and sleep. Pattern 2 EEGs are observed during waking and active sleep, while slightly modified pattern 1 EEGs occur during quiet sleep. To what degree waking/sleep states are a matter of neocortical maturation or a consequence of changing brainstem control (Vertes, 1984) is not known. Finally, as the normal time of birth nears, alternative waking/active sleep (pattern 3) and quiet sleep (pattern 4) EEGs make their appearance.

IMPLICATIONS OF THE FINDINGS

Our examination of neuromaturational events has emphasized two transitional periods: a possible consolidation of brainstem influence over motor activity and sensory input near the end of the first trimester, and establishment of the sensory input channel to the neocortex via the thalamocortical connection around mid-gestation. Beyond the scientific interest of such findings is the matter of their implications for debates about fetal experience and fetal personhood (see, for example, the essay by Tauer (1985) . . .).

FETAL SENTIENCE

When talking about the nature of fetal experience, we can easily locate the limits within which it must lie— somewhere between simple sensation and intentional awareness. An eighth week fetus is certainly capable of a limited response to stimulation, while a growing infant gradually begins to pay attention to its surroundings. We have left, however, a large gap about which we know little. Because of their accessibility as a result of premature birth, we may be able to gain a fuller understanding of the experiential capacity of late-stage human fetuses than we now possess. These direct observations may be complemented by laboratory studies of adult non-human mammals, where considerable progress has been made in locating the specific brainstem regions controlling the events

of active sleep and return to consciousness (Vertes, 1984). Also, recent evidence suggests that selective awareness involves a thin sheet of neurons . . . interposed between the thalamus and the neocortex (Scheibel, 1980; Crick, 1984; Steriade and Deschenes, 1984). As more is learned about these structures, there may be lessons applicable to the waking fetus *in utero*.

But what of the early fetus? In what way might it be sentient? Grobstein (1981, pp. 83–85) has provided an opening move. Between simple sensation and clear awareness, he suggests that a rudimentary individualized self could be characterized as "a bounded sentient locus". Might it not be possible to consider the fetus with a system-modulating brainstem (at 12–14 weeks' gestation) as an approximation of what Grobstein has in mind? Perhaps the key defining property would be a proprioceptive[n] sense, the integrated link between brainstem-generated fetal motility and brainstem modulation of proprioceptive feedback resulting from that motility. That the rudimentary proprioceptive function bounds the fetus as a sensate locus seems an idea worth pursuing.

FETAL PAIN

When the fetal human might begin to experience discomfort and pain, to know hurt, is a question whose answer is tied to our understanding of adult pain. The answer would seem to turn on whether there can be anything like the affective dimension of pain ('it hurts') without cortical participation. Ralston (1984) has reviewed what is known about the pathways linking peripheral pain receptors with the central nervous system. He finds evidence (in monkeys and other species) that somatosensory neurons of the neocortex respond to noxious stimuli and he concludes that "it does not appear necessary to postulate a subcortical mechanism for appreciation of pain" (p. 189). For Ralston, 'it hurts' is a neocortical state. If his assessment of the scientific findings is correct, the fetal human cannot experience hurt before the thalamocortical connection is made (at mid-gestation), since the noxious stimulus pathways pass through the thalamus.

SEEKING CONSISTENCY BETWEEN BEGINNINGS AND ENDINGS

The most widely accepted definition of brain death is the irreversible loss of all functions of the entire brain (President's Commission, 1981, p. 1). To possess

---

n. Ed. note: Having to do with the capacity to perceive stimuli originating within the body.

lower brain function, even though the capacity for consciousness is destroyed, is to be alive. If we look to the emergence of such functions rather than to their loss, are the consequences obvious? Goldenring (1982) is certain that they are. He claims that physicians "know how to define a human being" and "should have the scientific courage and consistency to say so". For Goldenring the eight-week fetus is *fully* human—the "coordinating and individuating" functions of the brain demonstrated by the presence of recordable electrical activity. While we might agree that the brainstem plays an initial coordinating role as early as this, it is more likely that substantial integrative function emerges several weeks later. Also, it is difficult to know what would count as individuation in the absence of the neocortex.

Veatch (1983) also looks for consistency, but he is willing to settle for "the first presence of integrated brain activity" until a time when we can better judge the capacity for consciousness. The difficulty, of course, is deciding what counts as integrated brain activity. For Veatch there is enough of it at "perhaps the tenth week". Unfortunately, he provides no reasons for his choice. We could offer him evidence of the transition in fetal motor behavior (from the ninth to the thirteenth weeks) as an indicator of growing brainstem influence. Until we know more about early brainstem function, however, we cannot be certain whether or how to draw lines.

CONCLUSION

We can say a few things about fetal neuromaturation with some assurance: central nervous system activity begins early in development; fetal motor activity is spontaneous; and the neocortex completes its inclusion into the neuraxis[o] after mid-gestation. On the other hand, these findings fall far short of serving the tasks we would like to ask of them. They permit us to make very little headway on the question of fetal sentience, for example. In other cases, findings have been stretched thin—how significant is the motor activity transition which appears to signal greater brainstem modulatory function? Perhaps we shall see greater attention paid to the role of brainstem systems in fetuses as a complement to the attention they are receiving in mature organisms. In light of the crucial issues of which the fetus is a part, it will be important to follow a variety of approaches to brain function for any clues they may provide us.

o. Ed. note: The brainstem and spinal cord.

NOTES

* Supported by grant PRA-8020679 from the National Science Foundation.

1. Unless otherwise indicated, fetal ages are expressed in terms of developmental age (in weeks). The more frequently used designation, menstrual age, is measured from the first day of a woman's last menstrual period and is approximately two weeks greater than the developmental ages referred to in the text.

2. Rakic (1981) provides an excellent account of the details of cortex formation as they are illustrated in non-human primates.

REFERENCES

Bergström, R. M.: 1969, 'Electrical parameters of the brain during ontogeny,' in R. J. Robinson (ed.), *Brain and Early Behavior: Development in the Fetus and Infant*, Academic Press, New York, pp. 15–37.

Borkowski, W. J., and Bernstine, R. L.: 1955, 'Electroencephalography of the fetus,' *Neurology* 5, 362–365.

Crick, F.: 1984, 'Function of the thalamic reticular complex: the searchlight hypothesis,' *Proceedings of the National Academy of Sciences, U.S.A.* 81, 4586–4590.

de Vries, J. I. P., Visser, G. H. A., and Prechtl, H. F. R.: 1982, 'The emergence of fetal behaviour. I. Qualitative aspects,' *Early Human Development* 7, 301–322.

Fitzgerald, J. E., and Windle, W. F.: 1942, 'Some observations on early human fetal movements,' *Journal of Comparative Neurology* 76, 159–167.

Goldenring, J. M.: 1982, 'Development of the fetal brain,' *New England Journal of Medicine* 307, 564.

Grobstein, C.: 1981, *From Chance to Purpose: An Appraisal of External Human Fertilization*, Addison-Wesley, Reading, Massachusetts.

Humphrey, T.: 1964, 'Some correlations between the appearance of human fetal reflexes and the development of the nervous system,' *Progress in Brain Research* 4, 93–135.

Humphrey, T.: 1978, 'Function of the nervous system during prenatal life,' in U. Stave (ed.), *Perinatal Physiology*, Plenum, New York, pp. 651–683.

Kostovic, I., and Goldman-Rakic, P. S.: 1983, 'Transient cholinesterase staining in the mediodorsal nucleus of the thalamus and its connections in the developing human and monkey brain,' *Journal of Comparative Neurology* 219, 413–447.

Kostovic, I., and Rakic, P.: 1984, 'Development of prestriate visual projections in the monkey and human fetal cerebrum revealed by transient cholinesterase staining,' *Journal of Neuroscience* 4, 25–42.

Larroche, J.-C.: 1981, 'The marginal layer in the neocortex of a 7 week-old human embryo. A light and electron microscopic study,' *Anatomy and Embryology* 162, 301–312.

Larroche, J.-C., Privat, A., and Jardin, L.: 1981, 'Some fine structures of the human fetal brain,' in A. Minkowski (ed.), *Physiological and Biochemical Basis for Perinatal Medicine*, Karger, Basel, pp. 350–358.

Marin-Padilla, M.: 1978, 'Dual origin of the mammalian neocortex and evolution of the cortical plate,' *Anatomy and Embryology* 152, 109–126.

Marin-Padilla, M.: 1983, 'Structural organization of the human cerebral cortex prior to the appearance of the cortical plate,' *Anatomy and Embryology* 168, 21–40.

Molliver, M. E., Kostovic, I., and Van Der Loos, H.: 1973, 'The development of synapses in cerebral cortex of the human fetus,' *Brain Research* 50, 403–407.

Okado, N.: 1980, 'Development of the human cervical spinal cord with reference to synapse formation in the motor nucleus,' *Journal of Comparative Neurology* 191, 495–513.

Okado, N.: 1981, 'Onset of synapse formation in the human spinal cord,' *Journal of Comparative Neurology* 201, 211–219.

O'Rahilly, R.: 1979, 'Early human development and the chief sources of information on staged human embryos,' *European Journal of Obstetrics and Gynecology and Reproductive Biology* 9, 273–280.

Peters, A., and Jones, E. G.: 1984, *Cerebral Cortex, Volume 1: Cellular Components of the Cerebral Cortex*, Plenum, New York.

Poliakov, G. I.: 1961, 'Some results of research into the development of the neuronal structure of the cortical ends of the analyzers in man,' *Journal of Comparative Neurology* 117, 197–212.

President's Commission for the Study of Ethical Problems in Medicine and Biomedical and Behavioral Research: 1981, *Defining Death: Medical, Legal and Ethical Issues in the Determination of Death*, U.S. Government Printing Office, Washington, D.C.

Rakic, P.: 1981, 'Developmental events leading to laminar and areal organization of the neocortex,' in F. O. Schmitt, F. G. Worden, and G. Adelman (eds.), *The Organization of the Cerebral Cortex*, MIT Press, Cambridge, pp. 7–28.

Ralson, H. J.: 1984, 'Synaptic organization of spinothalamic tract projections to the thalamus, with special reference to pain,' in L.

Kruger and J. C. Liebeskind (eds.), *Advances in Pain Research and Therapy*, Vol. 6, Raven Press, New York, pp. 183–195.

Robinson, H. P., and Fleming, J. E. E.: 1975, 'A critical evaluation of sonar "crown-rump length" measurements,' *British Journal of Obstetrics and Gynaecology* 82, 702–710.

Scheibel, A. B.: 1980, 'Anatomical and physiological substrates of arousal: a view from the bridge,' in J. A. Hobson and M. A. B. Brazier (eds.), *The Reticular Formation Revisited*, Raven Press, New York, pp. 55–56.

Schlumpf, M., Shoemaker, W. J., and Bloom, F. E.: 1980, 'Innervation of embryonic rat cerebral cortex by catecholamine-containing fibers,' *Journal of Comparative Neurology* 192, 361–376.

Steriade, M., and Deschenes, M.: 1984, 'The thalamus as a neuronal oscillator,' *Brain Research Reviews* 8, 1–63.

Spehlmann, R.: 1981, *EEG Primer*, Elsevier-Holland, New York.

Tauer, C. A.: 1985, 'Personhood and human embryos and fetuses,' *Journal of Medicine and Philosophy* 10, 253–266.

Vale, W., and Brown, M.: 1979, 'Neurobiology of peptides,' in F. O. Schmitt and F. G. Worden (eds.), *The Neurosciences Fourth Study Program*, MIT Press, Cambridge, pp. 1027–1041.

Van Dongen, L. G. R., and Goudie, E. G.: 1980, 'Fetal movement patterns in the first trimester of pregnancy,' *British Journal of Obstetrics and Gynaecology* 87, 191–193.

Veatch, R. M.: 1983, 'Definitions of life and death: should there be consistency?' in M. W. Shaw and A. E. Doudera (eds.), *Defining Human Life: Medical, Legal, and Ethical Implications*, AUPHA Press, Ann Arbor, pp. 99–113.

Vertes, R. P.: 1984, 'Brainstem control of the events of REM sleep,' *Progress in Neurobiology* 22, 241–288.

MICHAEL LOCKWOOD

When Does a Life Begin?

. . . I shall argue that there is a right answer to the question of when a human life begins, and that philosophical reflection can make a substantial contribution to revealing what that right answer is. This, I shall argue, is an area where philosophy can be of considerable practical value, even if that is not the main reason for doing philosophy.

One source of confusion in this debate is the rather careless bandying about of three notions which ought

Reprinted with permission of the publisher from *Moral Dilemmas in Modern Medicine* (Oxford: Oxford University Press, 1985), pp. 10–14, 16–19, 20–23.

to be kept distinct from each other. These are the concepts of (a) a *living human organism* (in the rest of this paper I shall omit 'living' but it should be understood), (b) a *human being*, and (c) a *person*. For the purposes of this paper, 'human organism' is to be understood in a biological sense: a human organism is simply a (complete) living organism of the species *Homo sapiens*. 'Person', on the other hand, is not a biological concept at all. A person is a being that is conscious, in the sense of having the capacity for conscious thought and experiences, but not only that: it must have the capacity for reflective consciousness and self-consciousness. It must have, or at any rate have the ability to acquire, a concept of itself, as a being with a past and a future. Mere sentience is not enough to qualify a being as a person. But a person, in this sense, need not be human. Perhaps some non-human higher primates—chimpanzees for example—are persons in this sense; perhaps dolphins are. Probably there are persons, though not of course human persons, on planets of distant stars. Perhaps we shall one day be able to create persons artificially out of non-organic material (though it is not clear how we should know when we had done so; it is not behaviour that makes something a person, but rather the possession of an 'inner life' of the appropriate degree of richness and depth[1]).

I shall explain in a moment just how I intend to use the term 'human being'. First, however, I want to consider two fallacious, and indeed rather crude, arguments designed to show, respectively, that you and I came into existence at the moment of conception, and, on the contrary, that we came into existence much later than that, probably subsequent to birth. I have no idea whether either of these arguments has ever been put forward in the literature, at least in such a bald form; but that doesn't matter for my purposes. The first argument runs: You and I are human organisms; a human organism comes into existence at the moment of conception; therefore, we came into existence at the moment of conception. The second argument runs: You and I are persons; but a fetus is not a person; indeed, it seems likely that several months have to elapse before the new-born baby acquires any capacity for reflective consciousness or self-consciousness; therefore, it seems likely that we did not come into existence until some time after birth.

Both arguments are unsound. The first is valid, but its premiss is false. You and I are not human organisms. Consider the human organism corresponding to some given human being. If that human being were the very same thing as that organism, he would not only come into existence at the same time as the organism; he would also cease to exist at the same time as the organism ceased to exist. But hardly any reflective person believes this to be the case, at any rate invariably. Those who believe in the existence of an immortal soul do not believe this, because they believe that we continue to exist, even when the corresponding human organisms die, decay, and turn to dust. But those who do not believe in an immortal soul mostly do not believe either that the time at which a human being ceases to exist is necessarily the same as the time at

which the corresponding organism dies. (I am assuming that a living human organism ceases to exist when it dies, so that a corpse is merely the remains of such an organism.) This is because most people are prepared to accept the concept of brain death. That is to say, most people accept that certain sorts of brain damage would constitute the end of our (mortal) existence, even if they did not prevent the continuation of such lower brain functions as are necessary to maintain respiration, circulation, and so forth. Suitable destruction of higher brain centres, coupled with the maintenance of such lower functions, would in most people's eyes mean that the living human organism remained, even though we were no more. That view now enjoys the status of scientifically educated common sense. I shall nevertheless attempt shortly to give a philosophical justification for it.

The second argument fails for quite different reasons. Its premiss is true, but not in such a sense as to support the conclusion drawn. Or at least, it has not been shown that it is true in the required sense. Consider the following parody of the argument: I am a philosopher; but the individual bearing my name in 1954 was not a philosopher; therefore, I did not exist in 1954. The point is that 'philosopher' is what is known as a 'phase sortal':[2] one and the same individual can be a philosopher at one time yet not be a philosopher at another earlier or later time. There are, on the other hand, some things which an object is, if at all, for the entire period of its existence, things which it cannot become or cease to be: we may call these *temporally essential* attributes. The property of being a building is in this sense temporally essential. You can reduce a building to a pile of rubble; but then the building no longer exists. Likewise, the building did not itself exist when the bricks of which it was composed had not yet been assembled. To cease to be a building is, for a building, to cease to be. Is personhood a temporally essential attribute of you or me? Personhood, that is to say, as I stipulatively defined it above. If it were, the second of our two arguments would be valid. Could I cease to be a person without ceasing to be? It seems pretty clear to me that I could. I want you to engage in the following thought experiment.[3] Suppose that you knew that you were going to suffer from a terrible disease, which would slowly extinguish your mental capacity for reflective consciousness or self-consciousness—those attributes that mark us off from at any rate most lower animals. But imagine that this disease still left the organism capable of sentience: it would still be aware, still be capable of experiencing sounds, colours, pleasure and pain, and so forth. Only higher cognitive functions would have gone. Now suppose this being were to be subjected to the most excruciating pain imaginable for some extended period. If you knew that it was going to be you that suffered the disease, and that it would be the brain you now possess, albeit pathetically reduced in cognitive capacity, whose pain centres were going to be stimulated, what would your attitude be towards the pain? Would you consider that it was going to happen to you? Would you deem it rational to fear this pain in a self-interested way? Or would you think of it as something that was going to happen to someone or something that was not, after all, you? So that, at most, you would view the prospect of this pain as you would view the prospect of it happening to a dog, say, of whom you were fond. If you think, as I do, that it would be rational to fear this pain in a self-interested way, then you will be forced to conclude that being a person is not a temporally essential attribute but merely a phase sortal. I could cease to be a person and yet still exist; and if so, then by the same token, it makes perfectly good sense to say that I did exist before I became a person, just as I existed before I became an adult, and existed before I became a philosopher. Some may disagree with this view. Some of you may think that it is not rational to fear the pain, in the example just given, as something that would be happening to you. All well and good: my point at the moment is just that it would not be absurd for someone to take the opposite view. If being a person is indeed a temporally essential attribute, that needs to be argued for; it is not obviously so, if indeed it is so at all. . . .

The above discussion reveals that we need a term for whatever it is that you and I are essentially, what we can neither become nor cease to be, without ceasing to exist. I use the term *human being* to fill this slot. Some might think *conscious being* a better term: on the grounds that one could perhaps turn into a frog without ceasing to exist, but would then hardly be a *human* being, or on the grounds that the souls of the departed, if such there be, have ceased to be *human* beings without ceasing to be, or that Pinocchio existed, as a conscious being, before he became human. On this view, 'human being' means a conscious being with a human body: and since in principle one could acquire or cease to possess a human body without ceasing to

be, 'human being' is really just a phase sortal. Perhaps. But I shall ignore these niceties: there is a point beyond which pedantry ceases to be profitable.

We have thus refined our question: it is the question 'When does a human being come into existence?' And we have seen this to be a different question from that of when a human organism comes into existence or when personhood is attained. How are we to set about answering this question? Well there is one thing that seems to me now quite obvious, something that should be obvious to anyone with a philosophical training, though I have never heard any philosopher say it; and indeed, it only occurred to me relatively recently. It is this: The question of when a human being comes into existence is really the same question as that of what constitutes the identity of a human being over time: the so-called problem of personal identity. . . .

Consider the following two imaginary cases. Case 1. You are in hospital suffering from an inoperable brain tumour. The prognosis is exceedingly bleak; the doctors are clearly very worried. Then one day, the consultant comes to your bedside surprisingly cheerful. 'I think', he says, 'we might be able to do something for you, after all.' Hope surges within your breast. 'Yes', the consultant continues, 'we've made a lot of progress lately in microsurgical techniques enabling us to suture ruptured nerve fibres. Indeed, we can do this, in suitable cases, even with fibres coming from different individuals. We've been experimenting with animals; and we're now ready to try the technique on a human being. In another ward, we have a very sad case of a woman involved in a car accident. Her body is hopelessly smashed up; but we've been able to maintain a supply of blood to her brain. We now intend, with your consent, to give you a new brain—by transplanting her brain into your skull.' How do you react? Do you think: 'Gosh, I'm going to live after all'? No. The doctor is surely wrong. What he is proposing is not so much giving you a new brain as giving the accident victim a new body. Transplanting the woman's brain into your skull is fine for her (though if you're a man, it might create problems of adjustment), but it will do nothing for *you* at all. You are still going to die—even sooner, in fact, assuming that your brain is to be discarded after the operation.

Now consider another case, only more fantastic. Case 2. Freddy Laker, trying to make a come-back after the collapse of his Skytrain operation, announces a splendid new way of crossing the Atlantic. It's much simpler than anything yet devised. He has set up a series of booths on Victoria Station. What you do is step into a booth, insert your credit card, which is promptly returned to you, and dial your intended destination—say, New York, Chicago, Dallas, or San Francisco. Assume you choose New York. You press a button and . . . whoosh! You find yourself standing in a somewhat similar booth in Grand Central Station on Park Avenue. This, at any rate, is the claim. And several people who have already tried it attest that it really works. It is relatively cheap and involves none of the hassle that surrounds conventional air travel. It rapidly becomes *the* way to travel. You, who haven't yet travelled this way, are invited to attend a conference in San Francisco, and are tempted to use the new Laker service. But you are curious about just how it works. You make enquiries and learn that the principle is as follows. When the button is pressed, the body in the booth is scanned by an intense beam of high-energy radiation that maps the position and chemical constitution of every molecule in your body. This information is digitally recorded and beamed as a radio message via satellite, to the corresponding booth in San Francisco, where a new body is almost instantaneously assembled, drawing on material from a molecule bank. Meanwhile, the intensity of the scanning beam has had the effect of vaporizing the original body. It is hardly surprising that the person finding himself in the booth in San Francisco should possess all the memories of the person who stepped into the booth on Victoria Station, and indeed, have the impression that he was, a moment ago, in London, given that the two bodies are, as near as makes no difference, qualitatively identical down to the last molecule. But is the person who steps out of the booth in San Francisco right in thinking that *he* was, a moment ago, in London? Is it really the same person? Is this, in fact, a neat way of crossing the Atlantic, or just a rather bizarre way of committing suicide? Now you will doubtless be able to find some philosophers who at an impressionable age have been made to read Locke and his successors, who will insist that it is the same human being who both steps into the booth in London and subsequently steps out of the booth in San Francisco. But what do *you* think? What do you think intuitively? It seems to me quite clear that if I were to step into the booth in London, what would step out of the booth in San Francisco would not be me, but a newly created individual possessed of the illusion of being me. (Of course, if it was me that stepped into the original booth, then, given that I knew the facts about how the system worked, the individual stepping out of the other booth wouldn't actually *think* that he was me,

since he would be bound to share my philosophical convictions.) If this seems unclear to you, imagine now that Freddy Laker were to develop a Mark 2 model, that could work the same trick with a less intense beam of radiation, that left the original body intact. Then almost everybody would come to see that even the original device was not, as it purported to be, a 'tele*transporter*', but merely a human being duplicator. Nobody, I take it, would think that the identity of what comes out the other end can depend on whether or not the original body remains. (To say, as some philosophers might, that this latter was a case of one human being *splitting* into two seems to me desperately implausible.) In short, I put it to you that what emerges at the other end is merely a copy, not the original article. If I am right about that, then it would show that continuity of memory, indeed psychological continuity generally, is not only not a necessary condition of continuing identity, as is shown by the amnesia example, but that it is not a sufficient condition of continuing identity either. For clearly the person who emerges from the booth in San Francisco does stand in Locke's relation to the person who enters the booth in London.

What both these examples seem to me to suggest is that a human being cannot be me unless he has my brain, or at any rate some crucial part of my brain. That is why *I* want to insist that the individual emerging from the booth in San Francisco is not me: he doesn't have *my* brain. Of course, he has a brain that is qualitatively indistinguishable from mine, but that isn't good enough. A fake Rembrandt is still a fake, even if it is a perfect copy of a genuine Rembrandt; a copy is still a copy, even if it is a perfect copy. No power on Earth would induce *me* to use Freddy Laker's machine.

Assuming that all this is correct, it has immediate implications for the kinds of medical ethical dilemma that I cited at the beginning of this paper. Take, for example, the recent controversies surrounding the 'morning after' pill and Robert Edwards's supposed mistreatment of human embryos a few days old.[4] The worry, in each case, stems from the fear that what is being destroyed or damaged is an innocent human being. That, on the present view, cannot be true. For newly fertilized human ova and week-old human embryos *do not yet have brains*. If the brain is what is crucial here, then we must conclude that, before the brain comes into being, there is no human being there to worry about. Of course, there is a potential for a human being. But then that is equally true of a sperm and an ovum before conception. Suppose we have sperm and an ovum in a Petri dish. We're observing through a microscope and find one sperm that is clearly just about to fertilize the ovum. We then, just in the nick of time, drop a glass partition between them to prevent fertilization taking place. Is there anything intrinsically wrong with that? Surely not; no more than there is with ordinary contraception. Yet there is a potential, here, for the coming into existence of a specific human being, which is thereby being prevented from being realized. But if the brain is what is important, then if it is not wrong to thwart this potential at that point, then no more is it wrong to thwart this potential at any later point before brain development. That, at least, seems to be the logical conclusion to draw. . . .

Philosophers have traditionally seen the problem of personal (or perhaps we should really say 'human') identity as one of coming up with an acceptable definition or conceptual analysis. Now it is generally agreed that reference to the brain simply does not belong in any analysis of what is *meant* when one speaks of a given later human being as being identical with a given earlier one. It does not belong to the *concept* of personal identity. Aristotle, after all, presumably had the same concept of personal identity as we do, and meant the same by whatever Greek words would express that notion as we mean by the corresponding English words. Yet he, as is well known, considered that the brain was merely an instrument for cooling the blood. And there is another consideration. Many people believe that the self, the human being (or, at least, the conscious being) survives the death of the body and *a fortiori* that of the brain. There is, surely, nothing in that that runs contrary to what we *mean* by the continuing identity of a human being. (To be sure, there are some philosophers who think that materialism is somehow true by definition, a conceptual truth; but they've never succeeded in making out a plausible case.) Also, we have no difficulty in understanding science fiction stories in which people switch bodies, including their brains. For this reason, even materialistically minded philosophers have, for the most part, resisted accounts of personal identity that make essential appeal to what is really just a matter of scientific theory.

What I want to suggest here is that the question

'What do we mean when we speak of the identity through time of a human being?' and the question 'What does that identity actually consist in?' are two distinct questions, and that an answer to the first, supposing it could be given, would still leave the second unresolved. Consider the analogy (inspired by Saul Kripke[5]) of gold. (I was rather proud of having thought of this analogy, until I discovered that John Mackie uses precisely the same analogy in his *Problems from Locke* to make essentially the same point.[6]) The question 'What do we mean by "gold"?' clearly is not the same question as the question 'What does gold actually consist in? What is it about what we call "gold" that makes it gold?' The way the concept of gold functions is roughly as follows. We find a certain kind of stuff lying around—a stuff distinguished by certain readily discernible attributes. These would include yellowish hue, metallic, heavy, resists most acids but not aqua regia, excellent conductor of electricity, and so on. But these attributes do not make gold gold. The concept allows for the possibility that some quite distinct substance might possess all of these attributes and yet not really be gold: a kind of super fool's gold. No, the assumption is, and has always been, that what makes gold gold, what being gold actually consists in, is the possession by a stuff of the appropriate underlying nature, whatever that might be. (This point has been urged by a number of philosophers in the last decade or so, most notably Hilary Putnam[7] and Saul Kripke.) This underlying nature, when properly understood, would be expected to explain why, under normal conditions, gold displays the discernible attributes that it does. But at the same time, it is possible that something might have the right underlying nature to be genuine gold, and yet for other reasons, not display the attributes by which we normally recognize gold as gold. Perhaps there could be a state of gold in which it appears, for example, as a blue liquid. The same goes for any substance term. (That is why it was not absurd for Thales, the earliest philosopher of whose thought we have any record, to suggest that everything might be water.) In the light of recent scientific developments, we now think we know what underlying nature constitutes a given stuff as gold: it is the possession of the right atomic structure. Specifically, something is gold, it is now believed, in virtue of being made up of atoms with the atomic number 79. That, we now think, is what being gold actually consists in. That is what gold is as a matter of fact, not definition. (The scientists just conceivably could have got it wrong.)

Exactly the same, I believe, goes for personal identity. There is a variety of discernible continuities within the biography of a given human being. Memory is one: the capacity to remember, at later times, experiences had and actions performed at earlier times. But there are others: knowledge of facts and of skills, continuity of attitudes, of behavioural dispositions, and of character traits. These can change, of course. But they usually change gradually, and they certainly do not, as a rule, change suddenly all together. Further, there is a causal continuity. Later actions flow from earlier intentions. Later attitudes are explainable in terms of earlier occurrences and so forth. Also, we have an introspective awareness of continuity within ourselves, of which memory, long and short term, is perhaps the principal ingredient. What philosophers have tried to do is *define* personal identity (or some kindred notion such as survival) in terms of these discernible continuities—mostly in terms of memory, though some writers, most notably Parfit,[8] have appreciated the importance of the other continuities as well. But this I believe to be a mistake. It is mistaken for exactly the same reason that it would be a mistake to try to *define* 'gold' in terms of yellowness, malleability, and so forth. For our ordinary concept of identity through time of a human being is not of something that is *constituted* by these discernible continuities, but as something that *underlies* these continuities and accounts for them—something of which these discernible continuities are merely a manifestation. Just what this underlying continuity might consist in is left open in our concept of personal identity; it is left open as far as the *meaning* of the relevant words goes. Thus, it is open to someone to hold, as do most Christians, that what underlies the discernible continuities of human personality is ultimately an immaterial soul—a soul that survives the death of the body. That is a logical possibility; though I must admit that I see not the slightest reason for believing it to be true. The view that I favour, and that I think is favoured by the available scientific evidence, is that what underlies the discernible continuities of memory and personality is a continuity of physical organization within some part or parts of a living human brain persisting through time.[9]

If this is right, then our earlier, tentative conclusion is sustained. Just as I shall live only as long as the relevant part of my brain remains essentially intact, so I came into existence only when the appropriate part or parts of my brain came into existence, or more precisely, reached the appropriate stage of development to sustain my identity as a human being, with the capacity for consciousness. When I came into existence is a matter of how far back the relevant neurophysiological continuity can be traced. Presumably, then, my life began somewhere between conception and birth. Certainly not *at* conception, and certainly not before my brain came into being. A more precise determination would require more scientific knowledge than I possess and probably more than anyone possesses at present. And ultimately, of course, the attempt to fix a precise point would founder, even against a background of scientific omniscience, on the imprecision of the concepts I've been invoking. 'Human being' is not itself a completely precise concept, and *a fortiori* nor is that of a human life. But nor is it so vague that absolutely any view on the question of when, between conception and early infancy, a life begins is philosophically sustainable. . . .

NOTES

1. This point is made very clearly in an excellent article by D. M. MacKay: 'The Use of Behavioural Language to Refer to Mechanical Processes,' *British Journal for the Philosophy of Science*, XIII, 50 (1962), pp. 89–103.

2. This term is originally due to David Wiggins. See his *Identity and Spatio-Temporal Continuity* (Oxford: Basil Blackwell, 1967), pp. 7, 29.

3. The idea, also exploited in one of my later examples, of using imagined future pain as a way of testing our intuitions about identity, is one I have borrowed from Bernard Williams. See his 'The Self and the Future,' *Philosophical Review*, 79, No. 2 (April, 1970), pp. 161–80, reprinted in John Perry (ed.), *Personal Identity* (Berkeley: University of California Press, 1975), pp. 179–98.

4. Reports that Edwards had been experimenting on live human embryos first appeared in September 1982, in the *Daily Express* and the *Daily Star*, based on a Press Association report. . . .

5. S. Kripke, *Naming and Necessity* (Oxford: Basil Blackwell, 1980), pp. 116–44 (original version published 1972).

6. J. L. Mackie, *Problems from Locke* (Oxford: Oxford University Press, 1976), pp. 199–203.

7. H. Putnam, 'Meaning and Reference,' *Journal of Philosophy* (1973), reprinted in S. P. Schwartz (ed.), *Naming, Necessity and Natural Kinds* (Ithaca, NY: Cornell University Press, 1977), and H. Putnam, *Philosophical Papers*, Vol. 2 (Cambridge: Cambridge University Press, 1975).

8. See Derek Parfit, *Reasons and Persons* (Oxford: Oxford University Press, 1984), pp. 205–8.

9. The emphasis here on neural organization, as opposed to function, means that the beginning of human life may be antecedent to the onset of awareness: the fetus may start life in a state of dreamless sleep or even coma. The brain structures whose continuity over time are, in my view, constitutive of a human being's continuing identity have in some sense to be structures that are capable of sustaining awareness.

ROBERT M. VEATCH

Definitions of Life and Death: Should There Be Consistency?

On the surface, it is puzzling to consider whether the definitions of two different words in the English language ought to be consistent. In fact, I am not sure how definitions of two unlinked terms could be consistent—or inconsistent. But let me tip my hand: if I understand what the question really means, if I am allowed to reformulate the question in terms I can understand, then the answer must be "yes." Not only that, but by clarifying what is often called the definition of death we may learn a great deal about the problem of when fetuses acquire moral or legal standing.

REFORMULATING THE QUESTION

THE DEFINITION OF DEATH

Let me start reformulating the question by looking at the definition-of-death debate. Dictionaries define death as the permanent cessation of vital or life-giving functions, the end of life. Since death is the negation of life, the definition of death contains the definition of life, and in this sense they must be consistent. Death is nothing more than the loss of that which is essential to being alive.

However, the point of the debate is not a linguistic or conceptual analysis of the term "death." We are not even interested in a theological account of the meaning of death, or a scientific account of the biological events that take place in the brain or the heart when an individual dies. Then what is the point of controversy, and why might it be of some interest to those con-

cerned about abortion, genetic engineering, fetal experimentation, and the rights of postnatal humans?

The definition-of-death debate is really a front for a crucial question in public policy and ethics over when it is appropriate to stop treating certain individuals as if we had a particular set of ethical and legal duties toward them. It is a debate over when we should begin treating them the way we treat the newly dead. It is a debate over what I would call the "social system of death behavior."

Traditionally, certain behaviors are viewed as appropriate only at the point at which we agree to call an individual dead. Important social and cultural changes such as the following are then signalled.

1) We stop treatments that would otherwise continue.
2) We begin mourning.
3) We refer to the person in the past tense.
4) We start processes leading to the reading of the will.
5) We start processes leading to the burial, the assumption of the role of widowhood, or the procurement of organs under the Uniform Anatomical Gift Act.
6) If the individual labelled dead is President of the United States, the Vice President is automatically elevated to the presidency.

There is a radical shift in moral, social, and political standing for someone who is labelled dead.[1] But the public policy question raised by the so-called definition-of-death debate is whether we can continue to identify a single point in time when all of these behavioral shifts ought to take place. As we become more sophisticated in stretching out the dying process, we

Reprinted with permission of the author and publisher from Margery W. Shaw and Edward A. Doudera, eds., *Defining Human Life: Medical, Legal and Ethical Implications* (Ann Arbor: AUPHA Press, 1983), pp. 104–113.

can stand face-to-face with an individual whose heart beats but whose brain is dead. We are forced to become much more precise in identifying the moment of death—that is, the moment when these behaviors become appropriate. We now face patients whose higher brain centers have decayed to the point of putrefaction, but who continue to breathe either on a respirator, or occasionally, spontaneously because of intact lower brain centers. What we really want to know is precisely when an individual loses the legal and moral standing that we attribute to human beings so that this cluster of behaviors I have called "death behaviors" is appropriate.

It may, of course, turn out that there is no single point where all these behaviors become appropriate. We may decide to remove organs for transplantation when the brain is irreversibly destroyed, read the will when and only when the heart stops, and begin mourning at some point not precisely aligned with either of these. If that turns out to be the case, then the definition-of-death debate will cease to be of interest for public policy purposes. It will no longer be meaningful to say someone has died. Different behavioral events will be triggered at different points in the dying trajectory, and death really will become a process rather than an event.[2]

As a society, however, we are continuing to behave as if all (or at least many) of these death behaviors should be triggered at a single point. We want to continue to call that point the point of death. If we can agree morally, legally, and politically on that point, we shall have recovered for our society a definition of death. We also may have learned something about what it means morally, legally, and politically to be alive and what the rights of fetuses are.

It is interesting to note that some people, as they attempt to define life, have been tempted to conclude that different definitions should be used for different purposes. They are saying, in effect, that different behaviors we associate with those given full standing should be initiated at different points in human development, and that in the various contexts we can call each of those points "the beginning of life." What is striking is that if there is any one point over which there is consensus in the definition-of-death debate, it is that there must be one definition for all purposes. Some early definitions implied that a brain-oriented definition of death should be used in cases where organ donation was planned, while older, heart-lung-oriented definitions should be used for other purposes.

This raised practical problems, such as what should happen if a person were pronounced dead because he or she was scheduled to donate an organ, only to have the potential recipient die before the donor's organ could be removed. In order to avoid the terrible confusion that different definitions for different purposes might create, a substantial consensus has emerged that one definition should be used for all purposes. (Of course according to this view, some behaviors, such as turning off a respirator, might still be considered appropriate even if someone is not dead.)

It should now be clear that insofar as medicine is a body of knowledge about the human body and a set of procedures that can be applied to a human body, there are absolutely no medical implications of defining life or death. Whatever we can say about a human body—its anatomy, its physiology, our capacities to intervene to affect its functioning—we can say it regardless of whether we decide to call that body dead or alive. Deciding to call a body dead is essentially making a moral, legal, or political decision about how a body ought to be treated. There are moral, legal, or political implications for defining death or life. Such definitions will tell us what we ought to do, including what medical professionals ought to do, but they have no bearing on what can be done medically.

The definition-of-death debate, then, is a debate over when we ought to stop treating an individual as a full member of the human community with moral and/or legal standing, as a citizen with all the accompanying rights.

THE DEFINITION OF LIFE

The question of the definition of life presents a problem precisely parallel to that of the definition of death. We can develop an analytical definition probably beginning with some minimal constellation of features, such as cells containing a fixed genetic material carrying out certain processes essential to life (respiration and motility, for example). Identifying features of this sort, however, has no bearing upon the central focus of this paper—that is, clarifying the point at which moral and/or legal standing should be attributed to this living tissue. The interesting moral, legal, and political question concerns what features of human life imply standing so that the claims of an individual are comparable, at least for most purposes, to those of other living human beings.

There is systematic ambiguity in the project of defining life and death. Sometimes the moral or legal baggage is attached to the definition of life analytically, in that we simply define life to *mean* the point at which full moral or legal standing accrues. Likewise, we define death to *mean* the point at which that standing ceases. In that mode, the terms life and death must have moral or legal policy implications. We know that moral shifts take place when life begins or ends, but it is in principle impossible to determine biologically when those points are. If death means the end of legal standing it cannot simultaneously mean the death of the brain or the stopping of the heart. If it is linked to one of those physiological events, it is linked synthetically. It is linked by argument, intuition, or conviction that legal standing ought to cease when the heart or the brain irreversibly ceases to function.

Alternatively, life and death can be defined without reference to moral or legal evaluations. Life could simply mean the beating of the heart or the capacity of the body to integrate its functions, leaving open the moral or legal question of whether not-yet-living bodies and dead bodies still have the same standing as living ones.

The definition-of-death debate has taken our society far down the road of linking the concept of death to this radical shift in standing *by definition*, that is, analytically. If that is the case, then the argument reduces to a debate over what features of a human are so essential that their loss causes this shift in standing and that, therefore, the body can be called dead.

Unfortunately there is no such clear pattern in the use of language regarding the definition of life. Many people are saying that whatever point we determine to be the commencement of standing comparable to that of other human beings shall be called the beginning point of life.[3] The more dominant notion is that we shall define life independent of the judgment about standing. Life will be said to begin when the genetic code is fixed, or when critical cellular activities begin, or when essential organ system functioning begins.[4]

This suggests an initial inconsistency in the use of the terms life and death. While we may be beginning to use "death" so that it has policy content by definition, "life" continues to be used ambiguously, sometimes having policy content and sometimes not. We could avoid all of this linguistic and policy confusion if we dropped all of the talk about the definition of life

and the definition of death and simply talked about the beginning and the ending points of that special moral or legal standing that we attribute to human beings.

THE RELATION TO PERSONHOOD

Our problem is made more complex with the introduction of the term personhood. Some people want to say that the beginning and ending of life can be identified without moral or legal judgment, but that personhood is necessarily linked to questions of standing.[5] This is the move that gives rise to the slogan, "Embryos don't have rights; only persons have rights." Of course, if personhood is defined as all those who possess full standing in the human community, then only persons have full standing. It does not follow from that, however, that embryos do not have standing unless we can establish that independently.

To make matters even more complicated, some define person quite apart from the attribution of rights or standing. Persons are self-conscious entities,[6] those capable of communicating or manipulating symbol systems,[7] or those possessing personal identity.[8] Such nonmoral usage leaves open the question of whether those who are persons (because they are self-conscious entities, etc.) have full moral or legal standing. It also leaves open the question of whether those who are not yet persons or never again will be persons have such standing. One could sensibly say that someone has ceased to be a person, but still has the full standing of a citizen of the human community.

In effect, this means that individuals can be classified in three independent ways: whether they are living, whether they are persons, and whether they have standing. Only the last label is necessarily evaluative. Only that one by definition says anything about whether the individual is a bearer of moral or legal claims of a particular type that we attribute to human beings.

SHOULD THERE BE CONSISTENCY?

According to the preceding reasoning, the question of whether or not definitions of life and death should be consistent may be restated in the following way: if there are some features, the initial presence of which signals the beginning of full moral or legal standing, should the loss of those features correspondingly signal the loss of that standing?

If we can identify some feature about human life—the presence of a fixed genetic code, a beating heart, a functioning nervous system, or the presence of consciousness—which we can agree is the essential feature for treating that individual as a full member of the human community, does it make sense to say that the irreversible loss of that same feature would imply the loss of that standing to be treated as a full member of the same community?

Put that way it is difficult to answer anything but "yes." Some feature is a necessary and sufficient condition for an entity to be included in the category of members in full standing in the human community, although it is conceivable that the feature that brings one into the community would not be the same as that which ushers one out. This would be the case, for instance, if there were two or more features, each of which was sufficient for standing but no one of which was necessary, and these features came and departed in a different time sequence. It is hard to imagine, however, that these conditions would ever be met. It seems that the obvious, most straightforward position is the one favoring consistency: if there is some essential feature that gives individuals moral or legal claims comparable to other members of the human community, loss of that feature implies that one no longer relates to the community in the same way. We can safely begin an examination of the definition-of-death debate with a strong presumption in favor of consistency.

IMPLICATIONS FOR THE DEFINITION OF DEATH AND THE DEFINITION OF LIFE

On the presumption, then, that we may learn something about the point where full human standing begins by examining when it ends and vice versa, let us examine four possible answers to the question of what that essential feature may be.

THE PRESENCE OF A FIXED GENETIC CODE

The first, most striking observation is that one major candidate for this feature is never mentioned in the definition-of-death debate. It is widely held that the critical feature that gives a fetus standing is the development of a fixed genetic code. At some point following the fertilization of the egg, a genetically unique individual is created. In a simpler era this could safely be taken to occur at the "moment" of conception. Now, thanks to the pioneering work of geneticists such as Jerome Lejeune[9] and the application of that work to the question of abortion by people like André Hellegers,[10] many argue that a truly unique genetic code is not fixed until the time when twinning can no longer take place—perhaps two weeks after fertilization. This move alone opens the possibility that abortifa-

cient-like procedures (such as the morning-after pill) might be more acceptable morally than abortions after the second week of pregnancy. For our purposes, the interesting point is that people following this line of reasoning—whether they take the genetic code to be fixed at conception or some weeks later—consider the fixation of the genetic material to be critical for full standing. Of course, even prior to that time humans may bear some obligation toward the treatment of human material—eggs, sperm, or zygotes. Full human standing, however, is seen as coming when the genetic code first becomes unique. Individuation, as signalled by fixing of the genetic code, is said to be critical.

What is striking is that nobody is claiming that moral standing ends—that is, an individual is "dead"—when the fixed genetic code is destroyed. It is obvious that many people are pronounced dead (by any definition of death) when their genetic patterns are still intact. In fact living cells survive for minutes, hours, perhaps even days after the point when it is appropriate to treat someone as dead even based on the most traditional definitions related to heart function. The full complement of genetic information about an individual is contained in each of those living cells. It is potentially possible to clone those remaining cells so that a new individual with the identical genetic composition would continue living for years after what we would all agree is the death of the individual. If there is to be consistency in establishing the beginning and end points of human standing, either we must radically change the end point or we must reformulate the beginning point. The mere presence of a fixed genetic code will not do the job consistently.

THE PRESENCE OF THE FLOWING OF FLUIDS

We have traditionally pronounced death based on conditions related to the heart and lungs, which suggests that the critical feature we are seeking might be related to heart or lung activity. At first, one might think that the mere beating of the heart was this feature, and the policy claim could then be, "When and only when a beating heart is present, moral and/or legal standing is present."

Consider, however, the possibility that the heart of a terminally ill patient might be removed and attached to a machine so that it continued to beat, perhaps for weeks or months if we were technologically clever enough. The human heart would be reminiscent of the beating frog's heart that we learned to prepare for study in college physiology labs. Yet even in those labs we knew the difference between a living frog and a beating frog heart.

Those who look to heart and lung activity as definitive probably are not really interested in the beating heart per se, but rather in what that beating normally implies: the flowing of so-called vital bodily fluids—blood and breath. What would be the implication of this focus for the abortion debate?

If cardiac function is critical for standing, significant life could not begin before the appearance of the first cardiac tissues, at approximately the fourth week of gestation. But with only a few specialized cells in existence, full cardiac function does not begin at that point. If we are really interested in the more integrated functioning of the circulatory system, we are identifying a point that comes much later in fetal development—probably no earlier than the twelfth week.

This suggests a problem that those involved in the definition-of-death debate have had to face recently. Whatever function is identified as critical, cellular level function may remain intact long after supercellular, organ system functioning ceases. When we shift our attention to brain-oriented conceptions of when we ought to treat people as dead, we shall see that isolated, perfused brain cells may continue intracellular activity long after organ level brain function stops. Thus electrical activity will remain, even when we say a brain is "dead," meaning that the brain has irreversibly lost its capacity to carry out its traditional organ-level functions.

In principle, there is no scientific way to choose whether the cellular level functions or the supercellular level functions are critical. We simply must make a choice based on philosophical, theological, and other evaluative views of what is important in being a human. Most have reached the conclusion that isolated cellular level function is insignificant—that it is the supercellular level that is critical.[11] If isolated heart or brain cells remain living after the organ level functions of these cells have been irreversibly lost, then the continuing presence of the living cells here and there means nothing.

If that is the answer given in the definition-of-death debate and if we seek consistency, then we have an answer to the question of whether cellular activity per se is critical in deciding when a human first gains human standing. In the case of those who focus on cardiac activity, the mere presence of the first differentiated cardiac cells is no more important than the presence of a few living cardiac cells would be in a patient whose heart has stoppped providing its traditional supercellular functions. The crucial process is the flowing of the vital fluids in the circulatory and respiratory system. Those who choose to treat a person as dead when these functions cease would, if they are to be consistent, vest a human with full standing when those more integrated, supercellular functions begin. If my reading of embryology is correct, supercellular cardiac function commences at a point no earlier than the twelfth week. If capacity for lung function is included, this point may be established as late as the twenty-fourth week. If it is the actual flowing of the air in the lungs and exchange of respiratory gases that are critical, then one might consistently adopt the position that "life is breath"—that full standing as a member of the human community begins only at birth when the first breath is taken. This leads to identifying a point essentially identical to that sometimes considered significant in traditional Judaism: when the head has emerged from the womb.[12]

Adopting the view that the critical function has to do with circulation and respiration leaves one in a strange position, because [the] abortion policy implied by this view is somewhat liberal in the context of current debate[s]. One would accept or at least tolerate abortion through the first trimester and maybe up until the beginning of the third trimester. Some lesser moral standing might be assigned to fetuses prior to that time, just as special moral obligations exist in many societies for the care and treatment of a new corpse after the critical moment of death. Compromises with the welfare of the fetus prior to the development of circulation would be tolerated, however, at least if good reasons are offered for what is sometimes viewed as a tragic moral compromise. If breath rather than circulation is critical, then similar compromises up to the moment of birth might be acceptable.

At the other end of the spectrum, those focusing on circulatory or respiratory function represent the conservative rear guard. What we might crudely call the "heart-lung people" are thus simultaneously pushing toward liberal abortion policy and conservative death definition policy.

But they face an even more serious problem. They have adopted a view that the essence of being a human has to do with something as crass, as animalistic, as biological as whether liquids are being pumped through the plumbing and gases are properly maintaining the ventilation system. There is nothing unscientific about such a view; it is fundamentally not a scientific judgment. It represents, however, a very limited view of human nature. It rejects the mainstream of the Western Judeo-Christian tradition that says the human is far more than a mere body. It is even more decisively at odds with the Greek emphasis on the soul as man's essence, temporarily entrapped in the flesh.

THE PRESENCE OF THE INTEGRATED FUNCTIONING OF THE NERVOUS SYSTEM

Two developments have forced us to rethink what it really means to die—that is, when we want to initiate the range of behaviors I have called death behaviors. These are, first, our new capacity to maintain people with dead brains and beating hearts and, second, our philosophical dissatisfaction with that animalistic view of human nature. This discomfort began in 1968 within months after the first heart transplant made the question of when we can treat someone as dead a crucial and emotionally exciting question. It soon gave rise to the idea that we really should start treating people as dead when their brain function ceases, even if the heart and lungs continue to function.[13]

Supporters of this notion (let's call them the "brain people") say that the essence of human existence is not related to mere fluid flow, but to something far more complicated and subtle having to do with the integration of bodily functions by the nervous system. When that is present, we have a "person as a whole" and not merely a collection of cells, tissues, and organs carrying on independent functions. The President's Commission for the Study of Ethical Problems in Medicine and Biomedical and Behavioral Research adopted this position in July of [1981] when it adopted its report endorsing a brain-oriented definition of death.[14] It has also been officially adopted by 27 states.

The implications for the abortion debate are less striking than they might at first appear. If one adopts a position that central nervous system functioning is critical for moral standing, a determination must be made about when this activity begins in a fetus. Once again, it will depend upon whether we are interested in cellular activity or supercellular activity. The first signs of nervous tissue cells appear at about the third week, while more complex integrated nervous system functioning does not appear until perhaps the tenth week and becomes substantial at about the twenty-fourth week when integration is sufficiently complete

so that the fetus can survive independently of its mother. Assuming that we follow the answer being given by those in the definition-of-death debate, we will identify the later time as the critical point to give full moral standing to fetuses—an answer somewhat later than, but still close to, that which would be given by one who applied a heart-oriented definition of death consistently to the abortion question.

In this case, however, there is more consistency in where one ends up on the public policy spectrum for the two issues. One who adopts the more liberal view on the definition of death, perhaps being willing to run the risk of being philosophically wrong when he treats the irreversibly comatose patient as dead, will also adopt a relatively liberal view on abortion, being willing to run the risk of being morally wrong in treating a midterm fetus as having, at most, only limited moral claims. Thus, one who is willing to apply the brain-oriented formulation consistently to matters of life and death has to reject the "safer course arguments" reminiscent of the probabiliorism of moral theologians.[15] It seems reasonable that if one has seen the way clear to reject the safer course arguments at one end of the spectrum, he or she would be willing to reject them at the other end for similar reasons.

PRESENCE OF THE CAPACITY FOR CONSCIOUSNESS

While the abortion debate seems almost stagnant in the murky confusion of policy debate, the definition-of-death debate has continued to evolve. The "brain people" have recently split into two major camps. What is now the old school continues to insist that integrating capacities are critical and that the entire brain—as the primary organ of integration—must be dead for death behavior to be appropriate. A newer school of brain-oriented advocates of a new definition of death says that the "whole brain people" have not gone far enough.[16] Those who focus on the whole brain and its integrating capacities still see the human as essentially a biological creature.

The test case is the patient who retains substantial capacity to integrate respiration, heart rate, cranial reflexes, and the like, but who has irreversibly lost the capacity for consciousness because all higher brain tissues have been destroyed. To use Henry Beecher's language (which now seems inappropriate for defending the whole brain view),[17] advocates of the newer "higher-brain-oriented" definition of death say that a person should be considered dead when the capacity for consciousness, for thinking, feeling, reasoning, and remembering is irreversibly lost. The real argument today is no longer between heart- and brain-oriented formulations, but between whole-brain and higher-brain or cerebral formulations.

What would a higher-brain-oriented definition of death mean in relation to the beginning of full standing? If one opted for this view, presumably such standing would begin when and only when an individual had some capacity for consciousness. However, determining precisely when this capacity for consciousness begins may turn out to be as difficult as determining when it ends. We have had considerable uncertainty over measuring the irreversible loss of the capacity for consciousness. Stories of patients with "locked [in] syndrome," the condition in which someone is conscious but lacks all motor capacity and therefore the capacity to communicate, abound. As a result, many who in principle favor a concept of death related to loss of consciousness fall back in practice to using the destruction of the entire brain as the clinical point at which we are first really sure consciousness is no longer possible.

A similar practical, clinical, and legal implication may be in store for the abortion debate for those who identify consciousness as critical. There is good reason to think that the capacity for consciousness may be present in some crude way well before birth, but since we may not be able to determine its starting point, we may have to fall back on the first presence of integrated brain activity as the decisive point in establishing full standing. If at some later time, however, we could more accurately measure the capacity for consciousness, the higher-brain and whole-brain people would part company at the practical level as well as the theoretical.

POTENTIAL VS. CAPACITY

The search for consistency between the definition of life and the definition of death leaves us with some insights as well as some confusion. Fixation of the genetic code has no defenders in the definition-of-death debate. All three of the plausible definitions of death (heart-, whole-brain-, and higher-brain-oriented) identify supercellular capacities as necessary for full standing in the human community. Only one of them, the higher-brain formulation, insists on a necessary combination of mental and bodily functions. For that reason, many are beginning to argue that it alone is

consistent with our Judeo-Christian and Greek heritage. Regardless of whether that conclusion is accepted, all three of the plausible definitions of death imply a somewhat late point in fetal development as the starting point for full human standing. Circulatory function, nervous system integrating functions, and consciousness are all rather late arrivals in fetal development. The heart-oriented formulation has the unpleasant feature of requiring both a late point for the beginning of standing and an early point for the end of it, while the brain-oriented formulations are at least consistently liberal at both ends of the spectrum.

Why is it, then, that the definition-of-death debate, which seems to have rich practical implications, is relatively uncontroversial while the abortion debate lingers, frustratingly unresolvable? I suggest that it is because the definition-of-death debate is able to finesse a critical question that is both decisive and unresolvable in the abortion debate. When one irreversibly loses the critical capacity—circulatory, integrative, or mental—one simultaneously loses any *potential* for that capacity. It will never return again. However, at the beginning of life the potential for a capacity far precedes the presence of the capacity itself. In fact, as the genetic code becomes fixed many characteristics of those capacities are predetermined. To be sure, they are not completely determined and anyone who follows the sociobiology fight wants to hold on to the idea that social and other factors may be decisive in determining capacities as well as actual performance. Still, at the beginning of life potential predates capacity. In order to know when one should be treated as a member in full standing of the human community, one must know whether the elusive critical feature we have been searching for is a capacity or a potential. Since capacity and potential depart at the same time, we need not have tackled this issue in the definition-of-death debate.

In the debate over when standing begins, however, some choice between the options must be made. As we have witnessed throughout this debate, there is no scientific way to choose. Whether potential counts or only the actual capacities is a fundamental question of choice, just the way we are forced to choose on faith whether there is an external world, or to decide whether rights really are inalienable.

It now appears that there are several plausible positions in the definition-of-death debate that reasonable people may take. I am increasingly convinced that there will never be agreement on any one of these. Some tolerable compromise will have to result, possibly including limited freedom of choice.

In the abortion debate, things are a little different. If capacities are critical, all of the capacities we have identified occur late enough so that substantial policy agreement can be achieved. Supporters of the circulation, integrating capacity, and consciousness theories do not have to fight among themselves. What cannot be agreed upon, however, is whether capacity or potential is critical. On that question the definition of death can tell us nothing, just as medical facts can tell us nothing. We almost certainly will be forced to live with the frustrating and perpetual uncertainty this creates, just as we live with uncertainty over when we should treat people as dead.

NOTES

1. Here, and throughout this paper, I am using the concept of "standing" to refer to a status typically assigned to typical members of a society. It is approximately the same notion as "prime moral status" developed by Daniel Wikler elsewhere in [the original] volume. The concept is built on the idea that full standing or prime moral status is attributed to members of society when rights and claims of a moral or legal sort are justifiably exercised by such an individual in exactly the same way as they are by others given similar status. In practice this means in law that the rights and responsibilities of the Constitution, statutory law, and common law attach to such individuals. In ethics, moral claims and moral responsibilities attach to them. I am using the term "standing" in this paper in a way that can be interpreted as either moral or legal standing. As long as one is consistent throughout, one could thus apply this analysis to either law or ethics.

2. *See* Morison, R., *Death—Process or Event?* SCIENCE 173(3998):694–98 (1971); Kass, L., *Death as an Event: A Commentary on Robert Morison*, SCIENCE 173(3998):698–702 (1971).

3. *See* S. 158, 97th Cong., 1st Sess., 127 Cong. Rec. 570 (1981); Fletcher, J., *Medicine and the Nature of Man*, in THE TEACHING OF MEDICAL ETHICS (R. M. Veatch, W. Gaylin, C. Morgan, eds.) (Hastings Center, Hastings-on-Hudson, N.Y.) (1973) at 47–58.

4. R. McCormick, *How Brave a New World?* (Doubleday & Co., Garden City, N.Y.) (1981) at 194–95; Engelhardt, Jr., H. T., *On the Bounds of Freedom: From the Treatment of Fetuses to Euthanasia*, Connecticut Medicine 40(1):51 (January 1976).

5. Tooley, M., *Abortion and Infanticide*, PHILOSOPHY AND PUBLIC AFFAIRS 2(1):37, 42 (Fall 1972); Becker, L. C., *Human Being: The Boundaries of the Concept*, PHILOSOPHY AND PUBLIC AFFAIRS 4(4):334, 348 (Spring 1975).

6. Warren, M., *On the Moral and Legal Status of Abortion*, MONIST 57(1):43, 55 (January 1973); Tooley, *supra* note 5, at 44.

7. Warren, *supra* note 6, at 55.

8. Green, M. B., and Wikler, D., *Brain Death and Personal Identity*, PHILOSOPHY AND PUBLIC AFFAIRS 9(2):105–33 (Winter 1980).

9. Lejeune, J., *Wann Beginnt das Leben des Menschen?* PÄDIATRIE UND PÄDOLOGIE 16:11–18 (1981).

10. *See* Hellegers, A., *Fetal Development*, THEOLOGICAL STUDIES 31(1):4 (March 1970).

11. Veatch, R. M., *The Definition of Death: Ethical, Philosophical and Policy Confusion*, in BRAIN DEATH: INTERRELATED MEDICAL AND SOCIAL ISSUES (J. Korein, ed.) (New York Academy of Sciences, New York City) (1978) at 310–13, 315.

12. I. Jakobovits, *Jewish Medical Ethics* (Block Publishing Co., New York City) (1967) at 184, 190, 191; *see also* F. Rosner, *Studies in Torah Judaism: Modern Medicine and Jewish Law* (Yeshiva University, Department of Special Publications, New York City) (1972) at 65, 83.

13. *See* Ad Hoc Committee of the Harvard Medical School to Examine the Definition of Brain Death, *A Definition of Irreversible Coma*, JOURNAL OF THE AMERICAN MEDICAL ASSOCIATION 205(6): 337–40 (1968); Institute of Society, Ethics and the Life Sciences, Task Force on Death and Dying, *Refinements in Criteria for the Determination of Death*, JOURNAL OF THE AMERICAN MEDICAL ASSOCIATION 221(1):48–53 (1972); Capron, A. M., and Kass., L. R., *A Statutory Definition of the Standards for Determining Human Death: An Appraisal and a Proposal*, UNIVERSITY OF PENNSYLVANIA LAW REVIEW 121(1):87–118 (November 1972).

14. President's Commission for the Study of Ethical Problems in Medicine and Biomedical and Behavioral Research, *Defining Death: A Report on the Medical, Legal and Ethical Issues in the Determination of Death* (U.S. Gov't Printing Office, Washington, D.C.) (1981).

15. C. J. McFadden, *Medical Ethics* (F. A. Davis Co., Philadelphia, Pa.) (1967) at 19–20.

16. Veatch, R. M., *The Whole-Brain-Oriented Concept of Death: An Outmoded Philosophical Formulation*, JOURNAL OF THANATOLOGY 3(1):13–30 (1975); Green, Wikler, *supra* note 8, at 105–33; Engelhardt, Jr., H. T., *Defining Death: A Philosophical Problem for Medicine and Law*, AMERICAN REVIEW OF RESPIRATORY DISEASE 112(5):587 (1975); Brierley, J. B., *et al.*, *Neocortical Death after Cardiac Arrest*, LANCET 2(7724):560–65 (September 11, 1971); Institute of Society, Ethics and the Life Sciences, Task Force on Death and Dying, *supra* note 13, at 53.

17. Beecher, H. K., "The New Definition of Death: Some Opposing Views" (paper presented at the meeting of the American Association for the Advancement of Science) (December 1970).

PRESIDENT'S COMMISSION FOR THE STUDY OF ETHICAL PROBLEMS IN MEDICINE AND BIOMEDICAL AND BEHAVIORAL RESEARCH

Why "Update" Death?

For most of the past several centuries, the medical determination of death was very close to the popular one. If a person fell unconscious or was found so, someone (often but not always a physician) would feel for the pulse, listen for breathing, hold a mirror before the nose to test for condensation, and look to see if the pupils were fixed. Although these criteria have been used to determine death since antiquity, they have not always been universally accepted.

DEVELOPING CONFIDENCE IN THE HEART-LUNG CRITERIA

In the eighteenth century, macabre tales of "corpses" reviving during funerals and exhumed skeletons found to have clawed at coffin lids led to widespread fear of premature burial. Coffins were developed with elaborate escape mechanisms and speaking tubes to the world above (Figure 1), mortuaries employed guards to monitor the newly dead for signs of life, and legislatures passed laws requiring a delay before burial.[1]

The medical press also paid a great deal of attention to the matter. In *The Uncertainty of the Signs of Death and the Danger of Precipitate Interments* in 1740, Jean-Jacques Winslow advanced the thesis that putrefaction was the only sure sign of death. In the years following, many physicians published articles agreeing with him. This position had, however, notable logistic and public health disadvantages. It also disparaged, sometimes with unfair vigor, the skills of physicians as diagnosticians of death. In reply, the French surgeon Louis published in 1752 his influential *Letters on the Certainty of the Signs of Death*. The debate dissipated in the nineteenth century because of the gradual improvement in the competence of physicians and a concomitant increase in the public's confidence in them.

Physicians actively sought to develop this competence. They even held contests encouraging the search for a cluster of signs—rather than a single infallible sign—for the diagnosis of death.[2] One sign did, however, achieve prominence. The invention of the stethoscope in the mid-nineteenth century enabled physicians to detect heartbeat with heightened sensitivity. The use of this instrument by a well-trained physician, together with other clinical measures, laid to rest public fears of premature burial. The twentieth century brought even more sophisticated technological means to determine death, particularly the electrocardiograph (EKG), which is more sensitive than the stethoscope in detecting cardiac functioning.

THE INTERRELATIONSHIPS OF BRAIN, HEART, AND LUNG FUNCTIONS

The brain has three general anatomic divisions: the cerebrum, with its outer shell called the cortex; the cerebellum; and the brainstem, composed of the midbrain, the pons, and the medulla oblongata. Tradi-

Reprinted from President's Commission for the Study of Ethical Problems in Medicine and Biomedical and Behavioral Research, *Defining Death: Medical, Legal and Ethical Issues in the Determination of Death* (Washington, D.C.: U.S. Government Printing Office, 1981), pp. 13–20.

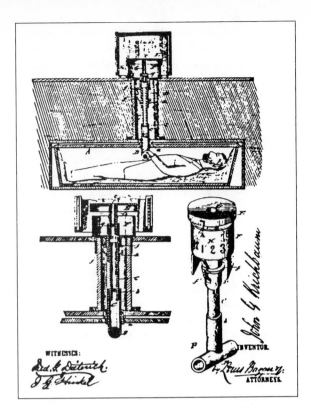

Figure 1. Kirchbaum's device for indicating life in buried persons, Patent sketch, 1882.

tionally, the cerebrum has been referred to as the "higher brain" because it has primary control of consciousness, thought, memory and feeling. The brainstem has been called the "lower brain," since it controls spontaneous, vegetative functions such as swallowing, yawning and sleep-wake cycles. It is important to note that these generalizations are not entirely accurate. Neuroscientists generally agree that such "higher brain" functions as cognition or consciousness probably are not mediated strictly by the cerebral cortex; rather, they probably result from complex interrelations between brainstem and cortex.

Respiration is controlled in the brainstem, particularly the medulla. Neural impulses originating in the respiratory centers of the medulla stimulate the diaphragm and intercostal[a] muscles, which cause the lungs to fill with air. Ordinarily, these respiratory centers adjust the rate of breathing to maintain the correct levels of carbon dioxide and oxygen. In certain circumstances, such as heavy exercise, sighing,

a. Ed. note: Between the ribs.

coughing or sneezing, other areas of the brain modulate the activities of the respiratory centers or even briefly take direct control of respiration.

Destruction of the brain's respiratory center stops respiration, which in turn deprives the heart of needed oxygen, causing it too to cease functioning. The traditional signs of life—respiration and heartbeat—disappear: the person is dead. The "vital signs" traditionally used in diagnosing death thus reflect the direct interdependence of respiration, circulation and the brain.

The artificial respirator and concomitant life-support systems have changed this simple picture. Normally, respiration ceases when the functions of the diaphragm and intercostal muscles are impaired. This results from direct injury to the muscles or (more commonly) because the neural impulses between the brain and these muscles are interrupted. However, an artificial respirator (also called a ventilator) can be used to compensate for the inability of the thoracic muscles to fill the lungs with air. Some of these machines use negative pressure to expand the chest wall (in which case they are called "iron lungs"); others use positive pressure to push air into the lungs. The respirators are equipped with devices to regulate the rate and depth of "breathing," which are normally controlled by the respiratory centers in the medulla. The machines cannot compensate entirely for the defective neural connections since they cannot regulate blood gas levels precisely. But, provided that the lungs themselves have not been extensively damaged, gas exchange can continue and appropriate levels of oxygen and carbon dioxide can be maintained in the circulating blood.

Unlike the respiratory system, which depends on the neural impulses from the brain, the heart can pump blood without external control. Impulses from brain centers modulate the inherent rate and force of the heartbeat but are not required for the heart to contract at a level of function that is ordinarily adequate. Thus, when artificial respiration provides adequate oxygenation and associated medical treatments regulate essential plasma components and blood pressure, an intact heart will continue to beat, despite loss of brain functions. At present, however, no machine can take over the functions of the heart except for a very limited time and in limited circumstances (e.g., a heart-lung machine used during surgery). Therefore, when a severe injury to the heart or major blood vessels prevents the circulation of the crucial blood supply to the brain, the loss of brain functioning is inevitable because no oxygen reaches the brain.

LOSS OF VARIOUS BRAIN FUNCTIONS

The most frequent causes of irreversible loss of functions of the whole brain are: (1) direct trauma to the head, such as from a motor vehicle accident or a gunshot wound, (2) massive spontaneous hemorrhage into the brain as a result of ruptured aneurysm or complications of high blood pressure, and (3) anoxic[b] damage from cardiac or respiratory arrest or severely reduced blood pressure.[3]

Many of these severe injuries to the brain cause an accumulation of fluid and swelling in the brain tissue, a condition called cerebral edema. In severe cases of edema, the pressure within the closed cavity increases until it exceeds the systolic blood pressure, resulting in a total loss of blood flow to both the upper and lower portions of the brain. If deprived of blood flow for at least 10–15 minutes, the brain, including the brainstem, will completely cease functioning.[4] Other pathophysiologic mechanisms also result in a progressive and, ultimately, complete cessation of intracranial circulation.

Once deprived of adequate supplies of oxygen and glucose, brain neurons will irreversibly lose all activity and ability to function. In adults, oxygen and/or glucose deprivation for more than a few minutes causes some neuron loss.[5] Thus, even in the absence of direct trauma and edema, brain functions can be lost if circulation to the brain is impaired. If blood flow is cut off, brain tissues completely self-digest (autolyze) over the ensuing days.

When the brain lacks all functions, consciousness is, of course, lost. While some spinal reflexes often persist in such bodies (since circulation to the spine is separate from that of the brain), all reflexes controlled by the brainstem as well as cognitive, affective and integrating functions are absent. Respiration and circulation in these bodies may be generated by a ventilator together with intensive medical management. In adults who have experienced irreversible cessation of the functions of the entire brain, this mechanically generated functioning can continue only a limited time because the heart usually stops beating within two to ten days. (An infant or small child who has lost all brain functions will typically suffer cardiac arrest within several weeks, although respiration and heartbeat can sometimes be maintained even longer.[6])

Less severe injury to the brain can cause mild to profound damage to the cortex, lower cerebral structures, cerebellum, brainstem, or some combination thereof. The cerebrum, especially the cerebral cortex, is more easily injured by loss of blood flow or oxygen than is the brainstem. A 4–6 minute loss of blood flow—caused by, for example, cardiac arrest—typically damages the cerebral cortex permanently, while the relatively more resistant brainstem may continue to function.[7]

When brainstem functions remain, but the major components of the cerebrum are irreversibly destroyed, the patient is in what is usually called a "persistent vegetative state" or "persistent noncognitive state."[8] Such persons may exhibit spontaneous, involuntary movements such as yawns or facial grimaces, their eyes may be open and they may be capable of breathing without assistance. Without higher brain functions, however, any apparent wakefulness does not represent awareness of self or environment (thus, the condition is often described as "awake but unaware"). The case of Karen Ann Quinlan has made this condition familiar to the general public. With necessary medical and nursing care—including feeding through intravenous or nasogastric tubes, and antibiotics for recurrent pulmonary infections—such patients can survive months or years, often without a respirator. (The longest survival exceeded 37 years.[9])

CONCLUSION: THE NEED FOR RELIABLE POLICY

Medical interventions can often provide great benefit in avoiding *irreversible* harm to a patient's injured heart, lungs, or brain by carrying a patient through a period of acute need. These techniques have, however, thrown new light on the interrelationship of these crucial organ systems. This has created complex issues for public policy as well.

For medical and legal purposes, partial brain impairment must be distinguished from complete and irreversible loss of brain functions or "whole brain death." The President's Commission . . . regards the cessation of the vital functions of the entire brain—and not merely portions thereof, such as those responsible for cognitive functions—as the only proper neurologic basis for declaring death. This conclusion

---

b. Ed. note: Severely depleted in its oxygen supply.

accords with the overwhelming consensus of medical and legal experts and the public.

Present attention to the "definition" of death is part of a process of development in social attitudes and legal rules stimulated by the unfolding of biomedical knowledge. In the nineteenth century increasing knowledge and practical skill made the public confident that death could be diagnosed reliably using cardiopulmonary criteria. The question now is whether, when medical intervention may be responsible for a patient's respiration and circulation, there are other equally reliable ways to diagnose death.

The Commission recognizes that it is often difficult to determine the severity of a patient's injuries, especially in the first few days of intensive care following a cardiac arrest, head trauma, or other similar event. Responsible public policy in this area requires that physicians be able to distinguish reliably those patients who have died from those whose injuries are less severe or are reversible. . . .

NOTES

1. Marc Alexander, "The Rigid Embrace of the Narrow House: Premature Burial and the Signs of Death," 10 *Hastings Ctr. Rpt.* 25 (1980); John D. Arnold, Thomas F. Zimmerman and Daniel C. Martin, "Public Attitudes and the Diagnosis of Death," 206 *J.A.M.A.* 1949 (1968).

2. Alexander, *op. cit.* at 30, citing, Orifila, *A Popular Treatise on the Remedies to be Employed in Case of Poisoning and Apparent Death; Including Means of Detecting Poisons, of Distinguishing Real From Apparent Death, and of Ascertaining the Adulteration of Wines*, trans. from French, Philadelphia (1818) at 154; G. Tourdes, "Mort (Medicine legate)," *Dictionnaire Encyclopedique des Sciences Medicales*, Ser. II, X (1875) at 579–708, 603.

3. Ronald E. Cranford and Harmon L. Smith, "Some Critical Distinctions Between Brain Death and Persistent Vegetative State" 6 *Ethics in Sci. and Med.* 199, 201 (1979).

4. H. A. H. van Till-d'Aulnis de Bourouill, "Diagnosis of Death in Comatose Patients under Resuscitation Treatment: A Critical Review of the Harvard Report," 2 *Am. J. L. & Med.* 1, 21–22 (1976).

5. One exception to this general picture requires brief mention. Certain drugs or low body temperature (hypothermia) can place the neurons in "suspended animation." Under these conditions, the neurons may receive virtually no oxygen or glucose for a significant period of time without sustaining irreversible damage. This effect is being used to try to limit brain injury in patients by giving them barbiturates or reducing temperature; the use of such techniques will, of course, make neurological diagnoses slower or more complicated.

6. Julius Korein, "Brain Death," in J. Cottrell and H. Turndorf (eds.), *Anesthesia and Neurosurgery*, C. V. Mosby & Co., St. Louis (1980) at 282, 284, 292–293.

7. Cranford and Smith, *op. cit.* at 203.

8. Bryan Jennett and Fred Plum, "The Persistent Vegetative State: A Syndrome in Search of a Name," 1 *Lancet* 734 (1972); Fred Plum and Jerome B. Posner, *The Diagnosis of Stupor and Coma*, F. A. David Co., Philadelphia (1980 3rd ed.) at 6–7.

9. See Norris McWhirter (ed.), *The Guinness Book of World Records*, Bantam Books, New York (1981) at 42, citing the case of Elaine Esposito who lapsed into coma following surgery on August 6, 1941, and died on November 25, 1978, 37 years and 111 days later.

JOEL FEINBERG

The Rights of Animals
and Unborn Generations

Every philosophical paper must begin with an un-proved assumption. Mine is the assumption that there will still be a world five hundred years from now, and that it will contain human beings who are very much like us. We have it within our power now, clearly, to affect the lives of these creatures for better or worse by contributing to the conservation or corruption of the environment in which they must live. I shall assume furthermore that it is psychologically possible for us to care about our remote descendants, that many of us in fact do care, and indeed that we ought to care. My main concern then will be to show that it makes sense to speak of the rights of unborn generations against us, and that given the moral judgment that we ought to conserve our environmental inheritance for them, and its grounds, we might well say that future generations *do* have rights correlative to our present duties toward them. Protecting our environment now is also a matter of elementary prudence, and insofar as we do it for the next generation already here in the persons of our children, it is a matter of love. But from the perspective of our remote descendants it is basically a matter of justice, of respect for their rights. My main concern here will be to examine the concept of a right to better understand how that can be.

THE PROBLEM

To have a right is to have a claim[1] *to* something and *against* someone, the recognition of which is called for by legal rules or, in the case of moral rights, by the principles of an enlightened conscience. In the famil-

Reprinted from *Philosophy and Environmental Ethics*, pp. 43–60. Edited by William T. Blackstone. © 1974 by permission of the University of Georgia Press.

iar cases of rights, the claimant is a competent adult human being, and the claimee is an officeholder in an institution or else a private individual, in either case, another competent adult human being. Normal adult human beings, then, are obviously the sorts of beings of whom rights can meaningfully be predicated. Everyone would agree to that, even extreme misanthropes who deny that anyone in fact has rights. On the other hand, it is absurd to say that rocks can have rights, not because rocks are morally inferior things unworthy of rights (that statement makes no sense either), but because rocks belong to a category of entities of whom rights cannot be meaningfully predicated. That is not to say that there are no circumstances in which we ought to treat rocks carefully, but only that the rocks themselves cannot validly claim good treatment from us. In between the clear cases of rocks and normal human beings, however, is a spectrum of less obvious cases, including some bewildering borderline ones. Is it meaningful or conceptually possible to ascribe rights to our dead ancestors? to individual animals? to whole species of animals? to plants? to idiots and madmen? to fetuses? to generations yet unborn? Until we know how to settle these puzzling cases, we cannot claim fully to grasp the concept of a right, or to know the shape of its logical boundaries.

One way to approach these riddles is to turn one's attention first to the most familiar and unproblematic instances of rights, note their most salient characteristics, and then compare the borderline cases with them, measuring as closely as possible the points of similarity and difference. In the end, the way we classify the borderline cases may depend on whether we are more impressed with the similarities or the differences between them and the cases in which we have the most confidence.

It will be useful to consider the problem of individual animals first because their case is the one that has already been debated with the most thoroughness by philosophers so that the dialectic of claim and rejoinder has now unfolded to the point where disputants can get to the end game quickly and isolate the crucial point at issue. When we understand precisely what *is* at issue in the debate over animal rights, I think we will have the key to the solution of all the other riddles about rights.

INDIVIDUAL ANIMALS

Almost all modern writers agree that we ought to be kind to animals, but that is quite another thing from holding that animals can claim kind treatment from us as their due. Statutes making cruelty to animals a crime are now very common, and these, of course, impose legal duties on people not to mistreat animals; but that still leaves open the question whether the animals, as beneficiaries of those duties, possess rights correlative to them. We may very well have duties *regarding* animals that are not at the same time duties *to* animals, just as we may have duties regarding rocks, or buildings, or lawns, that are not duties *to* the rocks, buildings, or lawns. Some legal writers have taken the still more extreme position that animals themselves are not even the directly intended beneficiaries of statutes prohibiting cruelty to animals. During the nineteenth century, for example, it was commonly said that such statutes were designed to protect human beings by preventing the growth of cruel habits that could later threaten human beings with harm too. Prof. Louis B. Schwartz finds the rationale of the cruelty-to-animals prohibition in its protection of animal lovers from affronts to their sensibilities. "It is not the mistreated dog who is the ultimate object of concern," he writes. "Our concern is for the feelings of other human beings, a large proportion of whom, although accustomed to the slaughter of animals for food, readily identify themselves with a tortured dog or horse and respond with great sensitivity to its sufferings."[2] This seems to me to be factitious. How much more natural it is to say with John Chipman Gray that the true purpose of cruelty-to-animals statutes is "to preserve the dumb brutes from suffering."[3] The very people whose sensibilities are invoked in the alternative explanation, a group that no doubt now includes most of us, are precisely those who would insist that the protection belongs primarily to the animals themselves, not merely to their own tender feelings. Indeed, it would be difficult even to account for the existence of such feelings in the absence of a belief that the animals deserve the protection in their own right and for their own sakes.

Even if we allow, as I think we must, that animals are the intended direct beneficiaries of legislation forbidding cruelty to animals, it does not follow directly that animals have legal rights, and Gray himself, for one,[4] refused to draw this further inference. Animals cannot have rights, he thought, for the same reason they cannot have duties, namely, that they are not genuine "moral agents." Now, it is relatively easy to see why animals cannot have duties, and this matter is largely beyond controversy. Animals cannot be "reasoned with" or instructed in their responsibilities; they are inflexible and unadaptable to future contingencies; they are subject to fits of instinctive passion which they are incapable of repressing or controlling, postponing or sublimating. Hence, they cannot enter into contractual agreements, or make promises; they cannot be trusted; and they cannot (except within very narrow limits and for purposes of conditioning) be blamed for what would be called "moral failures" in a human being. They are therefore incapable of being moral subjects, of acting rightly or wrongly in the moral sense, of having, discharging, or breeching duties and obligations.

But what is there about the intellectual incompetence of animals (which admittedly disqualifies them for duties) that makes them logically unsuitable for rights? The most common reply to this question is that animals are incapable of *claiming* rights on their own. They cannot make motion, on their own, to courts to have their claims recognized or enforced; they cannot initiate, on their own, any kind of legal proceedings; nor are they capable of even understanding when their rights are being violated, of distinguishing harm from wrongful injury, and responding with indignation and an outraged sense of justice instead of mere anger or fear.

No one can deny any of these allegations, but to the claim that they are the grounds for disqualification of rights of animals, philosophers on the other side of this controversy have made convincing rejoinders. It is simply not true, says W. D. Lamont,[5] that the ability to understand what a right is and the ability to set legal machinery in motion by one's own initiative are necessary for the possession of rights. If that were the case, then neither human idiots nor wee babies would have any legal rights at all. Yet it is manifest that both of these classes of intellectual incompetents have legal rights recognized and easily enforced by the courts. Children and idiots start legal proceedings, not on their own direct initiative, but rather through the actions of proxies or attorneys who are empowered to speak in their names. If there is no conceptual absurdity in this situation, why should there be in the case where a proxy makes a claim on behalf of an animal? People commonly enough make wills leaving money to trustees for the care of animals. Is it not natural to speak of the animal's right to his inheritance in cases of this kind? If a trustee embezzles money from the animal's account,[6] and a proxy speaking in the dumb brute's behalf presses the animal's claim, can he not be described as asserting the animal's *rights*? More exactly, the animal itself claims its rights through the vicarious actions of a human proxy speaking in its name and in its behalf. There appears to be no reason why we should require the animal to understand what is going on (so the argument concludes) as a condition for regarding it as a possessor of rights.

Some writers protest at this point that the legal relation between a principal and an agent cannot hold between animals and human beings. Between humans, the relation of agency can take two very different forms, depending upon the degree of discretion granted to the agent, and there is a continuum of combinations between the extremes. On the one hand, there is the agent who is the mere "mouthpiece" of his principal. He is a "tool" in much the same sense as is a typewriter or telephone; he simply transmits the instructions of his principal. Human beings could hardly be the agents or representatives of animals in this sense, since the dumb brutes could no more use human "tools" than mechanical ones. On the other hand, an agent may be some sort of expert hired to exercise his professional judgment on behalf of, and in the name of, the principal. He may be given, within some limited area of expertise, complete independence to act as he deems best, binding his principal to all the beneficial or detrimental consequences. This is the role played by trustees, lawyers, and ghost-writers. This type of representation requires that the agent have great skill, but makes little or no demand upon the principal, who may leave everything to the judgment of his agent. Hence, there appears, at first, to be no

reason why an animal cannot be a totally passive principal in this second kind of agency relationship.

There are still some important dissimilarities, however. In the typical instance of representation by an agent, even of the second, highly discretionary kind, the agent is hired by a principal who enters into an agreement or contract with him; the principal tells his agent that within certain carefully specified boundaries "You may speak for me," subject always to the principal's approval, his right to give new directions, or to cancel the whole arrangement. No dog or cat could possibly do any of those things. Moreover, if it is the assigned task of the agent to defend the principal's rights, the principal may often decide to release his claimee, or to waive his own rights, and instruct his agent accordingly. Again, no mute cow or horse can do that. But although the possibility of hiring, agreeing, contracting, approving, directing, canceling, releasing, waiving, and instructing is present in the typical (all-human) case of agency representation, there appears to be no reason of a logical or conceptual kind why that *must* be so, and indeed there are some special examples involving human principals where it is not in fact so. I have in mind legal rules, for example, that require that a defendant be represented at his trial by an attorney, and impose a state-appointed attorney upon reluctant defendants, or upon those tried *in absentia*, whether they like it or not. Moreover, small children and mentally deficient and deranged adults are commonly represented by trustees and attorneys, even though they are incapable of granting their own consent to the representation, or of entering into contracts, of giving directions, or waiving their rights. It may be that it is unwise to permit agents to represent principals without the latters' knowledge or consent. If so, then no one should ever be permitted to speak for an animal, at least in a legally binding way. But that is quite another thing than saying that such representation is logically incoherent or conceptually incongruous—the contention that is at issue.

H. J. McCloskey,[7] I believe, accepts the argument up to this point, but he presents a new and different reason for denying that animals can have legal rights. The ability to make claims, whether directly or through a representative, he implies, is essential to the possession of rights. Animals obviously cannot press their claims on their own, and so if they have rights, these rights must be assertable by agents. Animals, however, cannot be represented, McCloskey contends, and not for any of the reasons already discussed, but rather because representation, in the requisite sense, is always of interests, and animals (he says) are incapable of having interests.

Now, there is a very important insight expressed in the requirement that a being have interests if he is to be a logically proper subject of rights. This can be appreciated if we consider just why it is that mere things cannot have rights. Consider a very precious "mere thing"—a beautiful natural wilderness, or a complex and ornamental artifact, like the Taj Mahal. Such things ought to be cared for, because they would sink into decay if neglected, depriving some human beings, or perhaps even all human beings, of something of great value. Certain persons may even have as their own special job the care and protection of these valuable objects. But we are not tempted in these cases to speak of "thing-rights" correlative to custodial duties, because, try as we might, we cannot think of mere things as possessing interests of their own. Some people may have a duty to preserve, maintain, or improve the Taj Mahal, but they can hardly have a duty to help or hurt it, benefit or aid it, succor or relieve it. Custodians may protect it for the sake of a nation's pride and art lovers' fancy; but they don't keep it in good repair for "its own sake," or for "its own true welfare," or "well-being." A mere thing, however valuable to others, has no good of its own. The explanation of that fact, I suspect, consists in the fact that mere things have no conative life: no conscious wishes, desires, and hopes; or urges and impulses; or unconscious drives, aims, and goals; or latent tendencies, direction of growth, and natural fulfillments. Interests must be compounded somehow out of conations; hence mere things have no interests. *A fortiori*, they have no interests to be protected by legal or moral rules. Without interests a creature can have no "good" of its own, the achievement of which can be its due. Mere things are not loci of value in their own right, but rather their value consists entirely in their being objects of other beings' interests.

So far McCloskey is on solid ground, but one can quarrel with his denial that any animals but humans have interests. I should think that the trustee of funds willed to a dog or cat is more than a mere custodian of the animal he protects. Rather his job is to look out for the interests of the animal and make sure no one denies it its due. The animal itself is the beneficiary of his dutiful services. Many of the higher animals at least have appetites, conative urges, and rudimentary purposes, the integrated satisfaction of which constitutes

their welfare or good. We can, of course, with consistency treat animals as mere pests and deny that they have any rights; for most animals, especially those of the lower orders, we have no choice but to do so. But it seems to me, nevertheless, that in general, animals *are* among the sorts of beings of whom rights can meaningfully be predicated and denied.

Now, if a person agrees with the conclusion of the argument thus far, that animals are the sorts of beings that *can* have rights, and further, if he accepts the moral judgment that we ought to be kind to animals, only one further premise is needed to yield the conclusion that some animals do in fact have rights. We must now ask ourselves for whose sake ought we to treat (some) animals with consideration and humaneness? If we conceive our duty to be one of obedience to authority, or to one's own conscience merely, or one of consideration for tender human sensibilities only, then we might still deny that animals have rights, even though we admit that they are the kinds of beings that *can* have rights. But if we hold not only that we ought to treat animals humanely but also that we should do so for the animals' own sake, that such treatment is something we owe animals as their due, something that can be claimed for them, something the withholding of which would be an injustice and a wrong, and not merely a harm, then it follows that we do ascribe rights to animals. I suspect that the moral judgments most of us make about animals do pass these phenomenological tests, so that most of us do believe that animals have rights, but are reluctant to say so because of the conceptual confusions about the notion of a right that I have attempted to dispel above.

Now we can extract from our discussion of animal rights a crucial principle for tentative use in the resolution of the other riddles about the applicability of the concept of a right, namely, that the sorts of beings who *can* have rights are precisely those who have (or can have) interests. I have come to this tentative conclusion for two reasons: (1) because a right holder must be capable of being represented and it is impossible to represent a being that has no interests, and (2) because a right holder must be capable of being a beneficiary in his own person, and a being without interests is a being that is incapable of being harmed or benefited, having no good or "sake" of its own. Thus, a being without interests has no "behalf" to act in, and no "sake" to act for. . . .

HUMAN VEGETABLES

Mentally deficient and deranged human beings are hardly ever so handicapped intellectually that they do not compare favorably with even the highest of the lower animals, though they are commonly so incompetent that they cannot be assigned duties or be held responsible for what they do. Since animals can have rights, then, it follows that human idiots and madmen can too. It would make good sense, for example, to ascribe to them a right to be cured whenever effective therapy is available at reasonable cost, and even those incurables who have been consigned to a sanatorium for permanent "warehousing" can claim (through a proxy) their right to decent treatment.

Human beings suffering extreme cases of mental illness, however, may be so utterly disoriented or insensitive as to compare quite unfavorably with the brightest cats and dogs. Those suffering from catatonic schizophrenia may be barely distinguishable in respect to those traits presupposed by the possession of interests from the lowliest vegetables. So long as we regard these patients as potentially curable, we may think of them as human beings with interests in their own restoration and treat them as possessors of rights. We may think of the patient as a genuine human person inside the vegetable casing struggling to get out, just as in the old fairy tales a pumpkin could be thought of as a beautiful maiden under a magic spell waiting only the proper words to be restored to her true self. Perhaps it is reasonable never to lose hope that a patient can be cured, and therefore to regard him always as a person "under a spell" with a permanent interest in his own recovery that is entitled to recognition and protection.

What if, nevertheless, we think of the catatonic schizophrenic and the vegetating patient with irreversible brain damage as absolutely incurable? Can we think of them at the same time as possessed of interests and rights too, or is this combination of traits a conceptual impossibility? Shocking as it may at first seem, I am driven unavoidably to the latter view. If redwood trees and rosebushes cannot have rights, neither can incorrigible human vegetables.[8] The trustees who are designated to administer funds for the care of these unfortunates are better understood as mere custodians than as representatives of their interests since these patients no longer have interests. It does not follow that they should not be kept alive as long as possible: that is an open moral question not foreclosed by conceptual analysis. Even if we have duties to keep human vegetables alive, however, they cannot be duties *to* them. We may be obliged to keep them alive to protect the sensibilities of others, or to foster humanitarian tendencies in ourselves, but we cannot keep them alive for their own good, for they are no longer capable of having a "good" of their own. Without awareness, expectation, belief, desire, aim, and purpose, a being can have no interests; without interests, he cannot be benefited; without the capacity to be a beneficiary, he can have no rights. But there may nevertheless be a dozen other reasons to treat him as if he did.

FETUSES

If the interest principle is to permit us to ascribe rights to infants, fetuses, and generations yet unborn, it can only be on the grounds that interests can exert a claim upon us even before their possessors actually come into being, just the reverse of the situation respecting dead men where interests are respected even after their possessors have ceased to be. Newly born infants are surely noisier than mere vegetables, but they are just barely brighter. They come into existence, as Aristotle said, with the capacity to acquire concepts and dispositions, but in the beginning we suppose that their consciousness of the world is a "blooming, buzzing confusion." They do have a capacity, no doubt from the very beginning, to feel pain, and this alone may be sufficient ground for ascribing both an interest and a right to them. Apart from that, however, during the first few hours of their lives, at least, they may well lack even the rudimentary intellectual equipment necessary to the possession of interests. Of course, this induces no moral reservations whatever in adults. Children grow and mature almost visibly in the first few months so that those future interests that are so rapidly emerging from the unformed chaos of their earliest days seem unquestionably to be the basis of their present rights. Thus, we say of a newborn infant that he has a right now to live and grow into his adulthood, even though he lacks the conceptual equipment at this very moment to have this or any other desire. A new infant, in short, lacks the traits necessary for the possession of interests, but he has the capacity to acquire those traits, and his inherited potentialities are moving quickly toward actualization even as we watch him. Those proxies who make claims in behalf of infants, then, are more than mere custodians: they are (or can be) genuine representatives of the child's emerging interests, which may need protection even now if they are to be allowed to come into existence at all.

The same principle may be extended to "unborn persons." After all, the situation of fetuses one day before birth is not strikingly different from that a few hours after birth. The rights our law confers on the unborn child, both proprietary and personal, are for the most part, placeholders or reservations for the rights he shall inherit when he becomes a full-fledged interested being. The law protects a potential interest in these cases before it has even grown into actuality, as a garden fence protects newly seeded flower beds long before blooming flowers have emerged from them. The unborn child's present right to property, for example, is a legal protection offered now to his future interest, contingent upon his birth, and instantly voidable if he dies before birth. As Coke put it: "The law in many cases hath consideration of him in respect of the apparent expectation of his birth";[9] but this is quite another thing than recognizing a right actually to be born. Assuming that the child will be born, the law seems to say, various interests that he will come to have after birth must be protected from damage that they can incur even before birth. Thus prenatal injuries of a negligently inflicted kind can give the newly born child a right to sue for damages which he can exercise through a proxy-attorney and in his own name any time *after* he is born.

There are numerous other places, however, where our law seems to imply an unconditional right to be born, and surprisingly no one seems ever to have found that idea conceptually absurd. One interesting example comes from an article given the following headline by the *New York Times*: "Unborn Child's Right Upheld Over Religion."[10] A hospital patient in her eighth month of pregnancy refused to take a blood transfusion even though warned by her physician that "she might die at any minute and take the life of her child as well." The ground of her refusal was that blood transfusions are repugnant to the principles of her religion (Jehovah's Witnesses). The Supreme Court of New Jersey expressed uncertainty over the constitutional question of whether a nonpregnant adult might refuse on religious grounds a blood transfusion pronounced necessary to her own survival, but the court nevertheless ordered the patient in the present case to receive the transfusion on the grounds that "the unborn child is entitled to the law's protection."

It is important to reemphasize here that the questions of whether fetuses do or ought to have rights are substantive questions of law and morals open to argument and decision. The prior question of whether fetuses are the kind of beings that can have rights, however, is a conceptual, not a moral, question, amenable only to what is called "logical analysis," and irrelevant to moral judgment. The correct answer to the conceptual question, I believe, is that unborn children are among the sorts of beings of whom possession of rights can meaningfully be predicated, even though they are (temporarily) incapable of having interests, because their future interests can be protected now, and it does make sense to protect a potential interest even before it has grown into actuality. The interest principle, however, makes perplexing, at best, talk of a noncontingent fetal right to be born; for fetuses, lacking actual wants and beliefs, have no actual interest in being born, and it is difficult to think of any other reason for ascribing any rights to them other than on the assumption that they will in fact be born.[11]

FUTURE GENERATIONS

We have it in our power now to make the world a much less pleasant place for our descendants than the world we inherited from our ancestors. We can continue to proliferate in ever greater numbers, using up fertile soil at an even greater rate, dumping our wastes into rivers, lakes, and oceans, cutting down our forests, and polluting the atmosphere with noxious gases. All thoughtful people agree that we ought not to do these things. Most would say that we have a duty not to do these things, meaning not merely that conservation is morally required (as opposed to merely desirable) but also that it is something due our descendants, something to be done for their sakes. Surely we owe it to future generations to pass on a world that is not a used up garbage heap. Our remote descendants are not yet present to claim a livable world as their right, but there are plenty of proxies to speak now in their behalf. These spokesmen, far from being mere custodians, are genuine representatives of future interests.

Why then deny that the human beings of the future have rights which can be claimed against us now in their behalf? Some are inclined to deny them present rights out of a fear of falling into obscure metaphysics, by granting rights to remote and unidentifiable beings who are not yet even in existence. Our unborn great-great-grandchildren are in some sense "potential" persons, but they are far more remotely potential, it may seem, than fetuses. This, however, is not the real difficulty. Unborn generations are more remotely potential than fetuses in one sense, but not in another. A much greater period of time with a far greater number of causally necessary and important events must pass before their potentiality can be actualized, it is true; but our collective posterity is just as certain to come into existence "in the normal course of events" as is any given fetus now in its mother's womb. In that sense the existence of the distant human future is no more remotely potential than that of a particular child already on its way.

The real difficulty is not that we doubt whether our descendants will ever be actual, but rather that we don't know who they will be. It is not their temporal remoteness that troubles us so much as their indeterminacy—their present facelessness and namelessness. Five centuries from now men and women will be living where we live now. Any given one of them will have an interest in living space, fertile soil, fresh air, and the like, but that arbitrarily selected one has no other qualities we can presently envision very clearly. We don't even know who his parents, grandparents, or great-grandparents are, or even whether he is related to us. Still, whoever these human beings may turn out to be, and whatever they might reasonably be expected to be like, they will have interests that we can affect, for better or worse, right now. That much we can and do know about them. The identity of the owners of these interests is now necessarily obscure, but the fact of their interest-ownership is crystal clear, and that is all that is necessary to certify the coherence of present talk about their rights. We can tell, sometimes, that shadowy forms in the spatial distance belong to human beings, though we know not who or how many they are; and this imposes a duty on us not to throw bombs, for example, in their direction. In like manner, the vagueness of the human future does not weaken its claim on us in light of the nearly certain knowledge that it will, after all, be human.

Doubts about the existence of a right to be born transfer neatly to the question of a similar right to come into existence ascribed to future generations. The rights that future generations certainly have against us are contingent rights: the interests they are sure to have when they come into being (assuming of course that they will come into being) cry out for protection from invasions that can take place now. Yet there are no actual interests, presently existent, that future generations, presently nonexistent, have now. Hence, there is no actual interest that they have in simply coming into being, and I am at a loss to think of any other reason for claiming that they have a right to come into existence (though there may well be such a reason). Suppose then that all human beings at a given time voluntarily form a compact never again to produce children, thus leading within a few decades to the end of our species. This of course is a wildly improbable hypothetical example but a rather crucial one for the position I have been tentatively considering. And we can imagine, say, that the whole world is converted to a strange ascetic religion which absolutely requires sexual abstinence for everyone. Would this arrangement violate the rights of anyone? No one can complain on behalf of presently nonexistent future generations that their future interests which give them a contingent right of protection have been violated since they will never come into existence to be wronged. My inclination then is to conclude that the suicide of our species would be deplorable, lamentable, and a deeply moving tragedy, but that it would violate no one's rights. Indeed if, contrary to fact, all human beings could ever agree to such a thing, that very agreement would be a symptom of our species' biological unsuitability for survival anyway.

CONCLUSION

For several centuries now human beings have run roughshod over the lands of our planet, just as if the animals who do live there and the generations of humans who will live there had no claims on them whatever. Philosophers have not helped matters by arguing that animals and future generations are not the kinds of beings who can have rights now, that they don't presently qualify for membership, even "auxiliary membership," in our moral community. I have tried in this essay to dispel the conceptual confusions that make such conclusions possible. To acknowledge their rights is the very least we can do for members of endangered species (including our own). But that is something.

NOTES

1. I shall leave the concept of a claim unanalyzed here, but for a detailed discussion, see my "The Nature and Value of Rights," *Journal of Value Inquiry* 4 (Winter 1971): 263–277.

2. Louis B. Schwartz, "Morals, Offenses and the Model Penal Code," *Columbia Law Review* 63 (1963): 673.

3. John Chipman Gray, *The Nature and Sources of the Law*, 2d ed. (Boston: Beacon Press, 1963), p. 43.

4. And W. D. Ross for another. See *The Right and the Good* (Oxford: Clarendon Press, 1930), app. I, pp. 48–56.

5. W. D. Lamont, *Principles of Moral Judgment* (Oxford: Clarendon Press, 1946), pp. 83–85.

6. Cf. H. J. McCloskey, "Rights," *Philosophical Quarterly* 15 (1965): 121, 124.

7. Ibid.

8. Unless, of course, the person in question, before he became a "vegetable," left testamentary directions about what was to be done with his body just in case he should ever become an incurable vegetable. He may have directed either that he be preserved alive as long as possible, or else that he be destroyed, whichever he preferred. There may, of course, be sound reasons of public policy why we should not honor such directions, but if we did promise to give legal effect to such wishes, we would have an example of a man's earlier interest in what is to happen to his body surviving his very competence as a person, in quite the same manner as that in which the express interest of a man now dead may continue to exert a claim on us.

9. As quoted by Salmond, *Jurisprudence*, p. 303. Simply as a matter of policy the potentiality of some future interests may be so remote as to make them seem unworthy of present support. A testator may leave property to his unborn child, for example, but not to his unborn grandchildren. To say of the potential person presently in his mother's womb that he owns property now is to say that certain property must be held for him until he is "real" or "mature" enough to possess it. "Yet the law is careful lest property should be too long withdrawn in this way from the uses of living men in favor of generations yet to come; and various restrictive rules have been established to this end. No testator could now direct his fortune to be accumulated for a hundred years and then distributed among his descendants"—Salmond, ibid.

10. *New York Times*, 17 June 1966, p. 1.

11. In an essay entitled "Is There a Right to be Born?" I defend a negative answer to the question posed, but I allow that under certain very special conditions, there can be a "right *not* to be born." See *Abortion*, ed. J. Feinberg (Belmont, Calif.: Wadsworth, 1973).

RAANAN GILLON

To What Do We Have Moral Obligations and Why?

The moral prosecution of Dr Arthur* began by claiming that innocent human beings have a fundamental right to life and that this entailed that it was both wrong to kill them and wrong to deny them reasonably straightforward protection against life threatening conditions. . . . I shall look at rights subsequently. Here I wish to look at another profound moral question raised by these claims: to what do we have moral obligations and why? For example, and in John Harris's memorable phraseology,[1] by what criteria might we decide, on meeting a creature from outer space, to have him for dinner in one sense rather than the other?

If it is wrong to shoot peasants but OK to shoot pheasants this might be a matter that has nothing to do with the nature of pheasants and peasants; it might be an arbitrary (that is, discretionary) matter arising from some decision taken by people to allow pheasant shooting and forbid peasant shooting. Some moral obligations certainly do arise in this way. If I arbitrarily and knowingly promise to give Oxfam or the National Front £50 I am then morally obliged to honour my promise and this—assuming certain obvious stage setting—has nothing to do with the nature of Oxfam or the National Front but arises from what I have arbitrarily decided and undertaken to do. On the other hand, some of our moral obligations are, it seems fairly clear, not arbitrary and stem directly from the nature of the entities to which we owe those obligations.

WHICH ENTITIES ARE OWED A MORAL OBLIGATION?

It is widely agreed (though it was not always so) that our moral obligation not to shoot peasants is precisely not the sort of moral obligation that we are free to accept or reject but that it resides in the nature of

*Ed. note: A British physician charged with causing the death of a newborn infant.

Reprinted by permission from *British Medical Journal* Vol. 290 (June 1 and 8, 1985), pp. 1646–1647, 1734–1736.

peasants, in particular in their human nature. Conversely, there is wide disagreement about our obligation to pheasants. Supporters of "animal rights" claim that the nature of pheasants is such that it does impose a moral obligation on us not to shoot them (or at least not to shoot them for fun: the claims vary), while those who accept the moral legitimacy of shooting pheasants argue that the nature of pheasants, unlike the nature of peasants, is such that shooting them (and again the permitted circumstances are disputed) is morally permissible.

The claim of the moral prosecution of Dr Arthur was that all innocent human beings have a moral right not to be killed and that this includes a right to some straightforward help in the face of life threatening conditions. Infants with Down's syndrome are undeniably innocent human beings and therefore have this moral right. Similarly, most antiabortionists argue that human fetuses and indeed all human embryos from fertilisation onwards are innocent human beings and have this right. Some supporters of animal rights argue that all animals have this right, and some people, who really do believe in the "sanctity of life," believe that all living things have this right. Indeed, this is an implied premise in some strands of Buddhism[2] and was central to the philosophy of Albert Schweitzer.[3] In all cases it is something about the nature of the entities that is supposed to ground the moral obligation we are claimed to have towards them.

FOUR MORAL POSITIONS

In this . . . article I shall consider four moral positions offered as justifications for differentiating morally between different sorts of beings because of differences in their nature. That is, I shall consider ways of deciding the scope of certain moral obligations, and especially the obligation not to kill, on the basis of the characteristics possessed by potential candidates for our moral concern. Obviously there are many more moral positions than the four I have chosen but these seem particularly relevant in the context of medical ethics. I shall also indicate some awkward implications of each of these positions, for I have yet to encounter a moral stance on this issue that is free from awkward implications.

Of the four positions I shall consider, the first is the Benthamite claim that all sentient beings (beings that can experience pleasure and pain) are morally equivalent and that whether or not to kill them depends entirely on calculations of pleasure and pain of all potentially affected. The second is that membership of the species *Homo sapiens* confers a unique moral importance and that all (living and innocent) human beings have the moral right not to be killed and the moral right not to be denied reasonably straightforward help in life threatening conditions (for brevity I propose to call all this "the right to life," though such abbreviation presents problems that I shall consider in later articles on rights and on acts and omissions).

The third position is that all "viable" innocent human beings have this right to life and is commonly held by doctors who accept abortion but who also believe in the right to life of fetuses late on in pregnancy. The fourth, while usually accepting that sentience confers some moral importance, holds that within the class of sentient beings there is a morally more important subclass that possesses the special attributes grounding the unique moral importance due to people, including their right to life.

SENTIENCE

Jeremy Bentham, a founder of modern utilitarianism, argued that sentience was the fundamental moral criterion and that all others were ultimately reducible to it. He believed that animals were morally equivalent to humans and that the utilitarian calculus, the basis of all morality, applied to them as much as to humans: "The question is not whether they can reason but whether they can suffer." He reflected that "the day may come when the rest of the animal creation may acquire those rights which never could have been withholden from them but by the hand of tyranny."[4] (Like many modern utilitarians Bentham actually thought that the concept of rights was nonsense . . .; but this does not seem to stop many such critics from using the term, usually, to be fair, in actual or implied inverted commas).

. . . [T]his simple claim that all sentient beings are morally equivalent is highly counterintuitive. Although most people would grant some moral importance to the need to avoid suffering and to promote pleasure, few are prepared to accept this as of equal importance in animals and humans, and few are prepared to accept it as the only or overriding moral obligation. Most people would argue that people are simply more important morally speaking than (other) animals and that this is so for reasons that are independent of considerations of pain and pleasure. How, however, are such intuitions to be justified?

One standard response, typified by Roman Catholic theology, is to claim that all innocent, living human beings from the beginning to the end of their lives are morally equivalent in having equal natural rights including an equal right to life. It would be a mistake to see this as grounded merely in membership of the species *Homo sapiens*; rather the claim is that all human beings who possess the morally crucial gift of a soul are in this special moral category and that their lives as human beings start at the time of this "ensoulment" or "hominisation."

When precisely it occurs is still today, as it has been throughout the history of the Roman Catholic Church, a matter of disagreement and debate. Current orthodoxy, though explicitly uncertain about this according to Father John Mahoney (the Second Vatican Council "deliberately leaves aside at what moment in time the spiritual soul is infused" and the Roman Congregation for the Doctrine of Faith acknowledges disagreement about this point and "does not proceed to adjudicate"), none the less requires Roman Catholics to behave as though it occurred at fertilisation and thus proscribes all abortion however early, including any destruction of the fertilised ovum before implantation by contraceptive methods having this effect.[5]

Mahoney himself, a Jesuit philosopher and theologian and a past principal of London University's Jesuit Heythrop College, argues that hominisation or ensoulment at fertilisation is highly improbable—rather it is more coherently understood as a process that must occur at or after the time at which (*a*) the developing embryo is no longer able to divide into twins, (*b*) coalescence of embryos is no longer possible, and (*c*) cell differentiation rather than mere cell division has started.[6]

Other contemporary Roman Catholic theorists, deploying classical Thomist arguments, argue that hominisation could not occur until even later, perhaps after the development of neural tissue.[7] On the other hand, Iglesias[8] and also Grisez and Boyle in their powerful modern defence of the Roman Catholic "pro-life" position argue inter alia that any such theory whereby moral personality "joins" the developing human after its beginning at conception must entail a version of mind body dualism against which there are powerful philosophical arguments.[9] Roman Catholic counterarguments, however, to this claim by Iglesias, Grisez, and Boyle can either deny the need for dualism, using the Aristotelian theory of hylomorphism adopted by Aquinas whereby the human soul is seen as the "form"

of a sufficiently complex human body (a form which a less complex human body simply could not have), or they can argue the case for dualism, as Mahoney at least implicitly does.[10]

Such disagreements are not new in Roman Catholicism, for long ago that church's greatest philosopher, Thomas Aquinas, accepted the Aristotelian claims that ensoulment does not occur until 40 days for boys and 90 days for girls.[11] None the less, there is no doubt that so far as practical issues are concerned it is widely accepted within that faith that all living human beings from fertilisation onwards are to be treated as morally equal and as possessing the full human rights possessed by all people, including the right to life.

A WIDESPREAD MORAL INTUITION

Such a view is not limited to Roman Catholicism; certain protestants also accept it.[12] [13] Such positions are not, however, generally shared by all protestant strands of Christianity,[14] [15] by Judaism,[16] or by Islam.[17] In general, it would be fair to say that the stance of no killing from conception runs counter to a widespread intuition that newly fertilised ovums and developing embryos and fetuses are not in the same moral category as people and that unlike people they may legitimately be killed for the sake of (sufficient) benefits to others. Moreover, when the position that all human life has a right to life from conception onwards is combined with the view that man properly has "dominion" over (including the right to kill) other animals the combination also runs counter to an increasingly strongly held view that such a straightforward moral division between members of our species and members of other animal species is not morally defensible. How, however, are such moral intuitions to be justified? . . .

"SPECIESISM"

Professor Peter Singer, a contemporary utilitarian, argues against both the simple Benthamite moral equating of humans and other sentient animals and what he dubs the prejudice of "speciesism" (a neologism attributed to Richard Ryder and intended to be a pejorative term analogous to racism and sexism—"specism" would have been better). Thus, so far as pain and suffering go, Singer argues that "pains of the same intensity and duration are equally bad whether felt by humans or animals."[18] To be prepared to inflict such pain on animals but not on humans, other circumstances being the same, is irredeemably speciesist. On the other hand, argues Singer, human beings tend to have many interests that most other sorts of animals do not and cannot have. It is possession of such differing interests that can ground different moral rights and moral evaluation of human beings who possess these interests. Thus human lives that have a capacity for self awareness, ability to plan for the future, ability to have relationships with others and close family and personal ties, importance to other affected human beings, and other attributes such as the capacity for abstract thought and complex communication may, claims Singer, be legitimately valued more than lives that do not have these qualities.

This, he argues (somewhat contentiously), in no way undermines the principle that in making any moral decision the interests of all sentient beings affected by that decision must be taken equally into account; it is just that those interests are often vastly different. Such differences, however, are not determined simply by membership of a species. For instance, so far as a right to life is concerned "mere membership of our own biological species cannot be a morally relevant criterion. . . . A chimpanzee, dog, or pig, for instance, will have a higher degree of self awareness and a greater capacity for meaningful relations with others than a severely retarded infant or someone in a state of advanced senility. So if we base the right to life on these characteristics we must grant these animals a right to life as good as, or better than, such retarded or senile humans."[19]

Dame Mary Warnock doubtless speaks for many when she summarily rejects arguments against speciesism as "absurd." Such speciesism, she claims, far from being arbitrary prejudice "is a supremely important moral principle. . . . To live in a universe in which we were genuinely species-indifferent would be impossible, or if not impossible, then in the highest degree undesirable."[20] She does not, however, give much argument for her position and, like many doctors, she none the less wishes to differentiate morally between those very young human beings whom, or which, doctors are prepared to kill or let die in various circumstances and those to whom they wish to attribute a right to life that would prevent them doing so. Her answer is not quite clear but seems to require distinctions based on whether the embryo or fetus is (1) "plainly human" (in this context she offers as two exemplifying criteria the ability "to experience pain [and] to perceive their environment"); and (2) "a full human being" (alas, she does not say what she means by this). Over and above distinctions based on the nature of the developing human embryo or fetus she also puts great emphasis on respecting other people's moral outrage at any proposed action.

The trouble with all this is that in so far as it is clear it does not hold together. As Dame Mary writes, "human is a biological term"; but as such it cannot (in the absence of some additional moral criterion) give us a basis for the "supremely important" moral principle she desires. In any case, if her pro-human principle is to be understood biologically it will claim that all human beings are of equal moral importance, and this she clearly rejects. Furthermore, her criteria of experiencing pain and perceiving the environment cannot in themselves make the embryo or fetus "plainly human," either biologically construed (for many non-human biological species have these attributes) or morally construed, for there is nothing morally speaking specifically human about feeling pain and perceiving the environment. She may even be implicitly accepting such criticisms when she adds that it should be "absolutely prohibited" to anaesthetise the sentient human embryo for the purpose of experimenting on it. If, however, capacity for sentience and perception are to be her moral cut off points in the developing human embryo (1) she is no longer relying on specifically human attributes as she claims and (2) she offers no moral justification for rejection of the same moral cut off points in relation to other animal species.

TECHNICAL DIFFERENTIA

Dame Mary's dividing lines (if such they be) are among an enormous variety of such lines that have been proposed to distinguish morally between embryos and fetuses at different stages of development,[21] including the simple and widely accepted distinction between being unborn and born. Few, however, who think critically about the problem can justify this simple distinction (essentially based on the position of the infant relative to the mother's vulva) as being of moral importance.

A common medical fallback position is to claim that it is viability of the fetus that makes the moral difference. Before a fetus is viable it is seen as a morally acceptable candidate for abortion; after viability abortion becomes morally indefensible. (A less extreme version of this position has found its way into American law[22] via the Supreme Court's ruling in Roe v Wade.)

There are numerous problems with this position, among them the ambiguity, perhaps even incoherence, of the concept of viability. If, however, viability is taken to denote the stage of fetal development at which it becomes possible to maintain the fetus alive after it has left the uterus the alleged moral criterion turns out to be a (merely) technological criterion and a constantly changing one as medical technology makes it ever more possible to preserve the lives of premature infants. In theory any human embryo at any stage is viable with appropriate technology. Given the evidence of man's existing technological wizardry there seems to be no reason why Aldous Huxley's prediction of such complete mechanical incubation of human embryos should not become possible in reality, in which case the criterion of viability would collapse into the orthodox Roman Catholic criterion of fertilisation.

Viability, like so many other technical differentia, offers no (direct) moral rationale to justify treating previable human fetuses differently from viable fetuses. In any case, even without technology, are not most fetuses viable in the ordinary sense provided they are left alone to develop in the uterus?[23]

PERSONHOOD

So far I have suggested that a simple reliance on sentience, or on membership of the human species, or on technical differentia such as viability are highly implausible candidates on which to ground the scope of our moral obligations, including our recognition of a right to life.

In an earlier article about deontological theories of ethics I wrote about the radically different theoretical approach to problems about the scope of morality offered by Kant, for whom it was rational willing agency that afforded the moral criterion for distinguishing entities that had and were owed moral obligations from entities that were not. Such rational willing agents he called persons. John Locke, that most illustrious physician philosopher, also differentiated the "forensic" category of persons, to which praise and blame and other forensic attitudes were appropriate from other entities. Like Kant, and unlike many contemporary philosophers, Locke distinguished between the moral or forensic strand in the concept of a person and what might be called the ontological strand (ontology being the study of what is or what exists). While Kant saw rational willing agency as the essential characteristic of persons, Locke saw the ability to think combined with self awareness over time as the essence of personhood. Thus for Locke a person was "a thinking intelligent being that has reason and reflection and can consider itself as itself, the same thinking being in different times and place; which it does only by that consciousness which is inseparable from thinking and as it seems to me essential to it."[24]

One of the consequences of adopting either the Lockean or the Kantian criteria for personhood is that not all living human beings are persons. Embryos, fetuses, very young infants, and humans with severely damaged or severely defective brains may be able neither to think nor to be self-aware, and if the Kantian requirement of rational agency is to be met many older children and some adults will fail to fall into the net of personhood. Yet the idea that a single living human being starts its existence not being a person, develops into a person, and then at some stage may stop being a person while remaining a living human being seems to be intuitively plausible both as an account of what happens and also as a basis for at least some sorts of important moral distinction. Indeed, it may be some such assumptions that prompted the World Medical Association in its Declaration of Sydney (about death) to assert, "clinical interest lies not in the state of preservation of isolated cells but in the fate of a person."[25]

Quite apart, however, from producing conflicting moral intuitions of this sort, the idea that living human beings can be persons at some stages of their lives and not at others produces many other sorts of philosophical difficulty, especially problems clustering around the concept of identity. Attempts to overcome such difficulties are legion in philosophical works and include three broad categories.

The first resorts to dualism, whereby physical bodies are understood to be composed of substances ontologically distinct from spiritual substances, minds or souls, with personhood being understood necessarily to require some non-material substance. (Descartes offers the classic dualist position in his sixth meditation, and Popper and Eccles argue for dualism,[26] though it is generally speaking out of philosophical favour.)

The second uses some variant of the identity theory whereby persons are identified with their bodies or some part or parts of their bodies, notably their brains.[27]

The third approach is to deny that personhood is an intrinsic property of any human being and instead to postulate it as a "social construct"—that is, an attribute socially conferred on some but not all human beings by other human beings.[28]

Problems with all these approaches are shown in the vast amount of philosophical writing discussing personal identity,[29] often by means of imaginary problem cases. These range from Locke's own example of the prince and the cobbler who swap souls and Shoemaker's modern analogue in which Brown's brain is successfully transplanted into Robinson's head (who is the result?) to real cases of the so called "multipersonality syndrome" and brain bisection at the corpus callosum with one half of the brain implicitly answering the same question differently from the other half.

Some philosophers have argued that the moral and philosophical problems of personhood are resoluble on the basis of the Lockean intuition that persons are essentially self conscious. Professor Michael Tooley, for example, has argued that self awareness is at least a necessary feature for being a person in the morally important sense of having a right to life.[30] As fetuses are not self aware they do not have a right to life. He confronts the obvious intuitive objection to this stance head on: newborn infants are not self aware either and therefore they too by parity of reasoning do not have a right to life and thus infanticide may be morally permissible. Tooley argues that, far from being a disadvantage of his position, this is a positive advantage in that it corresponds to a further widespread moral intuition; "most people would prefer to raise children who do not suffer from gross deformities or from severe physical emotional or intellectual handicaps. If it could be shown that there is no moral objection to infanticide the happiness of society could be significantly and justifiably increased."[31] He has recently changed his mind,[32] but the change is based on philosophically rather technical distinctions, and even under his new formulation persons necessarily possess, either now or in the past, a sense of time, a concept of a continuing subject of mental states, and a capacity for episodes of thought.[33]

Professor Tristram Engelhardt, an American physician philosopher, also argues that self consciousness is a necessary (though not sufficient) condition of being a person,[34] as does Professor David Wiggins (but in a very different way and for very different reasons).[35]

Among the many problems faced by this sort of position are the widespread and deeply felt intuitions (a) that newborn infants are of the same moral importance as the rest of us and have the same right to life; and (b) the slippery slope intuition that once handicapped infants are deprived of a right to life other infants and other handicapped people are at risk, as, ultimately are all human beings. Indeed, there are undoubtedly grave problems associated with any of these theories about what properties ground a right to life, and the problems are manifested particularly clearly in consideration of the moral standing of very young human beings, of live but brain dead and live but permanently unconscious human beings, and of animals of varying attributes. Although such issues have received considerable philosophical attention fairly recently, the subject still represents a lacuna in ethics as a whole and medical ethics in particular.

REFERENCES

1. Harris J. *The value of life: an introduction to medical ethics.* London: Routledge and Kegan Paul (in press).

2. Edwards E., ed. *The encyclopedia of philosophy.* London: Collier Macmillan, 1967:1,417.

3. Schweitzer A. *Philosophy of civilisation.* Part 2. *Civilisation and ethics.* Chapters 19–22. London: A and C Black, 1929.

4. Bentham J. Introduction to the principles of morals and legislation. In: Harrison W, ed. *Jeremy Bentham's fragment on government and introduction to the principles of morals and legislation.* Oxford: Blackwell, 1948.

5. Mahoney J. *Bioethics and belief.* London: Sheed and Ward, 1984:52–86.

6. Mahoney J. *Bioethics and belief.* London: Sheed and Ward, 1984:67,69,85.

7. Donceel FJ. Immediate animation and delayed hominisation. *Theological studies* 1970;31:76–105.

8. Iglesias T. In vitro fertilisation: the major issues. *J Med Ethics* 1984;10:32–7.

9. Grisez G, Boyle JM. *Life and death with liberty and justice.* Notre Dame, Indiana: University of Notre Dame Press, 1979: 375–80.

10. Mahoney J. *Bioethics and belief.* London: Sheed and Ward, 1984:57.

11. Mahoney J. *Bioethics and belief.* London: Sheed and Ward, 1984:58–9,71.

12. Stirrat G. From your letters. *Journal of the Christian Medical Fellowship* 1984;30:23.

13. Vere DW. Working out salvation: is there a Christian Ethic? *Journal of the Christian Medical Fellowship* 1984;30:14.

14. Dunstan GR. The moral status of the human embryo: a tradition recalled. *J Med Ethics* 1984;10:38–44.

15. Church of England Board for Social Responsibility. *Abortion: an ethical discussion.* London: Church Information Office, 1965.

16. Jakobovits I. *Jewish medical ethics.* New York: Bloch Publishing Company, 1975:273–5.

17. Musallam BF. Population ethics: Islamic perspectives. In: Reich WT, ed. *Encyclopedia of bioethics.* Vol. 3. London: Collier Macmillan, 1978:1267.

18. Singer P. *Animal liberation.* Wellingborough: Thorsons, 1976:19.

19. Singer P. *Animal liberation.* Wellingborough: Thorsons, 1976:22.

20. Warnock M. In vitro fertilisation: the ethical issues. II. *The Philosophical Quarterly* 1983;33:238–49.

21. Veatch RM. Case studies in medical ethics. London: Harvard University Press, 1977:170.

22. Finnis JM. Abortion: legal aspects. In: Reich WT, ed. *Encyclopedia of bioethics*. Vol 1. London: Collier Macmillan, 1978:30.

23. Engelhardt TH. Viability and the use of the fetus. In: Bondeson WB, Engelhardt HT, Spicker SF, Winship DH. *Abortion and the status of the fetus*. Dordrecht: Reidel, 1983:183–208. This gives a slightly more sympathetic approach to viability as a moral criterion.

24. Locke J. *Essay concerning human understanding*. (Yolton JW, ed.) London: Dent, 1972:280.

25. World Medical Association. Declaration of Sydney—a statement on death. In: Duncan AS, Dunstan GR, Welbourn RB, eds. *Dictionary of medical ethics*. London: Darton Longman and Todd, 1981:135–6.

26. Popper K, Eccles J. *The self and its brain*. New York: Springer International, 1977.

27. Borst CV, ed. *The mind brain identity theory*. London: Macmillan, 1970.

28. Shorter JM. Personal identity, personal relationships and criteria. *Proceedings of the Aristotelian Society* 1970/71;1:165–86.

29. Rorty AD, ed. *The identities of persons*. London: University of California Press, 1976.

30. Tooley M. Abortion and infanticide. *Philosophy and Public Affairs* 1972;2:37–65, especially at 44.

31. Tooley M. Abortion and infanticide. *Philosophy and Public Affairs* 1972;2:39.

32. Tooley M. *Abortion and infanticide*. Oxford: Clarendon Press, 1983:142–6.

33. Tooley M. *Abortion and infanticide*. Oxford: Clarendon Press, 1983:419–20.

34. Engelhardt HT. Some persons are humans, some humans are persons, and the world is what we persons make of it. In: Spicker SF, Engelhardt HT, eds. *Philosophical medical ethics: its nature and significance*. Dordrecht: Reidel, 1977:183–98, especially 190–3.

35. Wiggins D. *Sameness and substance*. Oxford: Blackwell, 1980:148–89.

H. TRISTRAM ENGELHARDT, JR.

The Context of Health Care: Persons, Possessions, and States

Not all humans are equal. Health care confronts individuals of apparently widely divergent capacities: competent adults, mentally retarded adults, children, infants, and fetuses. These differences are the bases of morally relevant inequalities. Competent adults have a moral position not held by fetuses or infants. In addition, there are social inequalities among competent adults as a consequence of disparities in wealth. The wealthy may buy goods and services not available to the less fortunate. These inequalities reach into the central fabric of health care decisions. Finally, special questions of equality and inequality among persons are raised by the existence of states. States frequently claim special moral prerogatives to regulate health care and to distribute health care resources. To come to

terms with bioethical issues as they arise for patients and health care professionals within the embrace of states, one will need to know how seriously one ought to take the various moral and financial inequalities among humans and the supposed moral prerogatives of states.

THE SPECIAL PLACE OF PERSONS

Persons, not humans, are special. Adult competent humans have much higher intrinsic moral standing than human fetuses or adult frogs. It is important to understand the nature of these inequalities in some detail, for physicians and medical scientists intervene in numerous ways in the lives of adult humans, children, infants, fetuses, and laboratory mice. There is a need to understand in some detail why obligations of respect or of beneficence vary according to the moral status of the entities involved.

Reprinted from *The Foundations of Bioethics* (New York: Oxford University Press, 1986), pp. 104–109, 110–117, 121–123, 145–153.

Only persons write or read books on philosophy. As my arguments have already shown, it is persons who are the constituents of the moral community. Only persons are concerned about moral arguments and can be convinced by them. The very notion of a moral community presumes a community of entities that are self-conscious, rational, free to choose, and in possession of a sense of moral concern. It is only when these entities are interested in understanding when they or others are acting in a blameworthy or praiseworthy fashion that there comes into existence a sphere of moral discourse I have termed the peaceable community. The peaceable community exists both actually and potentially. It exists potentially as a moral standpoint in terms of which self-conscious rational entities can speak of blame and praise. It is an intellectual standpoint in the sense that once one understands what it means justly to blame or praise, one realizes that such activities presuppose entities worthy of blame and praise, beings that could have abided by the conditions for the possibility of a peaceable community. In terms of this possible moral standpoint, persons can at any time in any place conceive of themselves as belonging to, and being bound by the rules of the peaceable community. An examination of moral language reveals a very important intellectual standpoint: the *mundus intelligibilis* of Kant.[1] Competent physicians and patients of any rational species anywhere in the cosmos can participate in this moral standpoint, which embraces not only the staff and patients of terrestrial hospitals, but also ships' doctors and their patients on flying saucers, should such exist. It is in terms of this intellectual possibility or standpoint[2] that persons can think of themselves as free; as Kant put it, ". . . we think of ourselves as free, we transport ourselves into the intelligible world as members of it and know the autonomy of the will together with its consequence, morality . . ."[3] When persons actually deport themselves in accord with the notion of the peaceable community, they can come to live in a general moral community with real boundaries, so that those persons that act against the peaceable community are by their own choices moral outlaws of all and any particular moral community. In summary, all persons can envisage (1) the *notion of the peaceable (moral) community*. (2) Insofar as they act in accord with this notion they participate with others in *the peaceable (moral) community* (i.e., defined by general secular pluralist morality), and (3) have the opportunity to fashion with consenting others a *particular* moral community (defined in addition by its particular view of the good life).

By examining the foundations of morals, Kant offered what could be termed the grammar of a major dimension of human thought. It is impossible for rational, self-reflective entities coherently to construe themselves except as moral, responsible entities. To protest that they ought to have been treated differently, to blame themselves or others for their actions, is to enter the domain of moral discourse, and at once to place all entities that engage in that discourse in a special light. The self-reflective character of our thought commits us to certain ways of regarding ourselves and similar entities. We cannot coherently regard ourselves solely as caused to do the things we do. An entity that asserted that all of its assertions were simply caused, not rationally affirmed, would at that point abandon any truth claim to that assertion regarding determinism. It would be holding, instead, that it had been caused to make that statement (i.e., "I am determined") independently of considered reflections or rational bases for assent. The domain of morality in which we think of ourselves as free and responsible is inescapable. On the other hand, there is, as Kant also recognizes, the domain of scientific and empirical reflections where we do indeed treat the world as determined. This is for Kant a second standpoint, as equally unavoidable as the moral point of view.[4] For Kant, persons are put in the peculiar predicament of having to conceive of themselves as determined, caused to do the things they do, while on the other hand conceiving of themselves and other persons as moral entities, worthy of blame and praise and therefore free.[5] It is important to realize that Kant is not advancing a metaphysical proposition. He is rather indicating two major and inescapable domains of human reasoning and experience. Our very notion of ourselves as self-conscious, rational entities requires us to treat ourselves as moral agents, as persons, and as knowers.

As a consequence, persons stand out as possessing a special importance for moral discussions, for it is such entities who have rights to forbearance and who may not be used without their permission. This moral concern, it must be stressed, focuses *not on humans but on persons*. That an entity belongs to a particular species is not important unless that membership results in that entity's being in fact a moral agent. This should be fairly clear if one reflects on what it means to be a human, a member of a particular species. First one must note that there have in fact been a number of human species within the genus *Homo*. To identify an entity as a member of *Homo sapiens* is to place it in a particular taxonomic locus. The genus *Homo* shares with the genera *Ramapithecus* and *Australopithecus* membership in the family Hominidae of the suborder Anthropoidea of the order primates of the class Mammalia. In identifying an entity as human, one indicates that it possesses primate characteristics, such as long limbs and pentadactyl hands and feet, along with an increased specialization of the nervous system. With the family Hominidae one would want to note the development of tool-making capacities, language, and other symbol-related or -dependent behaviour. If one were in the future to possess a galactic study of rational species in the cosmos, one would likely find that numerous, somewhat different biological bases lead to the ability to use tools, language, and abstract symbols. Humans would be distinguished primarily through their biological peculiarities as primates. But insofar as one characterizes the peculiar anatomical structures and physiological capacities of humans as primates, one advances a set of biological characteristics that take on moral significance only insofar as they support the special characteristics of persons, namely, their capacity to play a role in the moral community. It is because members of *Homo sapiens* are usually self-conscious, rational, and possess a moral sense that being a human is so significant.

As talk of angels and of gods and goddesses, not to mention current science-fictional speculation regarding rational, selfconscious entities on other planets, indicates, not all persons need be humans. The archangel Gabriel appearing to Mohammed in the desert, and E.T. going through a modern twentieth-century American town, provide examples of entities that are persons, though they are clearly not human. What distinguishes persons is their capacity to be self-conscious, rational, and concerned with worthiness of blame and praise. The possibility of such entities grounds the possibility of the moral community. It offers us a way of reflecting on the rightness and wrongness of actions and the worthiness or unworthiness of actors.

On the other hand, not all humans are persons. Not all humans are self-conscious, rational, and able to conceive of the possibility of blaming and praising. Fetuses, infants, the profoundly mentally retarded, and the hopelessly comatose provide examples of human nonpersons. Such entities are members of the human species. They do not in and of themselves have

standing in the moral community. They cannot blame or praise or be worthy of blame or praise. They are not prime participants in the moral endeavor. Only persons have that status.

It is because of interest in morality that talk about persons as moral agents occurs. One speaks of persons in order to identify entities one can with warrant blame and praise, which can themselves blame and praise, and which can as a result play a role in the core of the moral life. In order to engage in moral discourse, such entities will need to reflect on themselves; they must therefore be *self-conscious*. They will need in addition to be able to conceive of rules of action for themselves and others in order to envisage the possibility of the moral community. They will need to be *rational* beings. That rationality must include an understanding of the notion of worthiness of blame and praise: *a minimal moral sense*. Sociopaths would cease to be moral agents (persons in the moral sense), only if they lost even the capacity to understand blameworthiness to the point that they could not blame those who might injure them. These three characteristics of self-consciousness, rationality, and moral sense identify those entities capable of moral discourse. These characteristics give to those entities the rights and obligations of the morality of self-respect. The principle of autonomy and its elaboration in the morality of mutual respect applies only to autonomous beings. It concerns only persons. The morality of autonomy is the morality of persons.

For this reason it is nonsensical to speak of respecting the autonomy of fetuses, infants, or profoundly retarded adults, who have never been rational. There is no autonomy to affront.[6] Treating such entities without regard for that which they do not possess, and never have possessed, despoils them of nothing. They fall outside the inner sanctum of morality. Just as this concern with respecting moral agents excludes some humans, it may in fact include nonhuman persons, should such exist. Though failing to treat a fetus or an infant as a person in the strict sense shows no disrespect to that fetus or infant, to fail to treat E.T. or a peaceable extraterrestrial at a *Star Wars* bar scene without such respect would be to act immorally in a fundamental fashion. It would mean that one had acted against the very possibility of *the* peaceable community.

What is important about us as humans is not our membership in the species *Homo sapiens* as such, but the fact that we are persons. This distinction between persons and humans will have important consequences for the ways in which one treats human personal life versus merely human biological life. Once these distinctions are clearly drawn, one can disclose some of the conceptual confusions that have plagued the moral debates regarding abortion. One will not be interested in when human life begins, unless one is attempting to determine when the human species evolved. Life, it would appear, is an unbroken continuum some four billion years old, and human life a phenomenon some two million years or more old. One is, or should be, concerned with determining when in human ontogeny humans become persons.

In summary to this point: not all persons need be human, and not all humans are persons. In order to understand the geography of obligations in health care regarding fetuses, infants, the profoundly mentally retarded, and the severely brain damaged, one will need to determine the moral status of persons and of mere human biological life, and then develop criteria to distinguish between these classes of entities. Further, even if infants are not persons in the strict sense that E.T. would be, there still may be important reasons for according special rights to infants. In order to sort out and distinguish the obligations one holds to competent adults, infants, fetuses, and the severely brain damaged, one will need to assess the moral significance of different categories of human life.

Such categorizations require no metaphysical commitments or doctrines. Nor do reflections about the status of persons commit one either to affirming or to denying traditional religious or metaphysical views regarding the existence of the soul or its entrance into the human body at some particular point in human ontogeny. One must, rather, ignore such for the purposes of these considerations. In general secular reflections, one must presume that beings are rational beings whenever they show evidence of being rational. One will not assume that fetuses in some occult or hidden fashion are in fact rational beings. One will not assume that there is a rational soul in some fashion lying hidden and undisclosed. Persons are persons when they have the characteristics of persons, when they are self-conscious, rational, and in possession of a minimal moral sense. . . . [S]uch entities are *persons in the strict sense*.

Though this approach simplifies matters by freeing discussions of metaphysical quandaries, it begets some special problems and puzzles of its own. First, one might object that this way of construing things creates an unduly person-centered or person-oriented construal of the moral universe. This difficulty is inescapable. Since it is only persons who reflect on the world and fashion accounts of its meaning, all accounts will perforce be developed in the rational language of persons, such that rational beings and their concerns will recurringly be central to moral accounts. One cannot give a rational account of the nature of things except from the point of view of rational beings: persons. It is for this reason that respect of persons is so central to moral discourse.

This orientation marks the morality of welfare and social sympathies. It is persons who can define for themselves their own best interests. They can place themselves and their concerns in their own terms for any calculations made under the principle of beneficence. But for nonpersonal organisms, others must choose on their behalf. Others must determine for those entities what their best interests are. A competent adult patient can define in his own terms his own best interests. It is surely the case that rational individuals can make mistakes in such calculations. But their judgments about themselves have a cardinal significance in that persons can decide for themselves the ordering of costs and benefits that they wish to take seriously for their lives, including the risk they are willing to run. Persons are in this very important sense self-legislating. This is not the case in the instance of infants, the profoundly mentally retarded, and other individuals who cannot determine for themselves their own hierarchy of costs and benefits. Persons must choose for them. Since such choices will depend on the moral sense of the chooser, and since there is not one univocal moral sense to deliver a single authoritative hierarchy of costs and benefits, nonpersons will have imposed on their destiny the particular choices of particular persons or communities of persons. Both the morality of mutual respect and the morality of welfare and mutual sympathies are inextricably person-centered.

When persons must calculate the weight that should be given to the interests of persons versus nonpersons, it is quite likely that the position of persons will remain central. Persons can appreciate harm and good, pleasure and pain, in intricate, reflective fashions. It would appear likely that rational beings after careful reflection will hold that it is better first to test pain-killing substances on animals, even when such experiments will mean suffering for the animals, rather than to move directly to trials on persons. The greater good of persons will likely be seen as having a higher position in the hierarchy of goods than the good of experimental animals who will need to be sacrificed in the course of medical experimentation and research. The hunter will decide that the delectation of the hunt, and the refined recall of the kill in sharing stories with other hunters, is a good that outweighs the value of the life of the animal to be hunted and killed. The same will be the case for those individuals who plan to raise animals for food. There will be none but persons to adjudicate which goods are to be given greater weight. Moreover, when such arguments come to a complete standstill and fail to deliver a view as to which side ought to be given precedence, when the problem is TEYKU, then it is not unreasonable for persons to choose on the side of their intuitions. This is not a consequence of mere prejudice or idiosyncratic bias. It reflects what it means to give rational moral arguments in these circumstances and what as a consequence will appear as rational, defensible choices. Even animals who are not persons, and will never be persons, are thus placed inescapably within the bounds of a person-centered morality, dominated by person-centered interests.

One should note that prejudice in favor of persons is not like prejudice in favor of humans versus other possible rational species. If, for instance, we ever needed to compare the competing claims of humans and extraterrestrial persons, we could never morally use them merely as means, as one may use animals.

POTENTIALITY AND PROBABILITY

What is one to make of those entities such as embryos, fetuses, and infants who will with great likelihood develop into moral agents? It might appear that one could in such circumstances appeal to a notion of potentiality in order to argue that since fetuses and children are potential persons, they must *eo ipso* be accorded the rights and standing of persons. This argument cannot succeed. This was already clear to the theologians of the Middle Ages who approached the issue of abortion within the compass of an Aristotelian world view and its commitment to a doctrine of potentiality. St. Thomas Aquinas argued that taking the life of an early fetus did not involve the evil of murder, even though the early fetus or embryo was potentially a

person.[7] This view was reflected in Roman Catholic theology and in canon law from the time of St. Thomas until 1869, except for a brief period between 1588 and 1591.[8] During that time, taking the life of an early fetus or embryo was held usually to be a mortal sin, somewhat analogous to the mortal sin of contraception.[9] However, it did not involve the sin of murder. The Catholic church correctly perceived that human life developed only over time into the life of a person. It recognized that a sort of human life preceded the human life of persons. This issue surfaced in an interesting fashion in speculations regarding the doctrine of the Immaculate Conception of the Blessed Virgin Mary. If Mary's body only later developed into being a body for a rational soul, then the immaculate conception of her *soul* could only take place sometime after the physical conception of her *body*. "Before the creation of Mary's soul, that which was to become her body shared the common lot; but before the creation of her soul *Mary* did not yet exist."[10]

If X is a potential Y, it follows that X is not a Y. If fetuses are potential persons, it follows clearly that fetuses are not persons. As a consequence, X does not have the actual rights of Y, but only potentially has the rights of Y. If fetuses are only potential persons, they do not have the rights of persons. To take an example from S. I. Benn, if X is a potential president, it follows from that fact alone that X does not yet have the rights and prerogatives of actual presidents.[11]

Undoubtedly, the language of potentiality is itself misleading, for it is often taken to suggest that an X that is a potential Y in some mysterious fashion already possesses the being and significance of Y. It is therefore perhaps better to speak not of X's being a potential Y but rather of its having a certain probability of developing into Y. One can then assign a probability value to that outcome. Recent research concerning zygotes suggests that there is a great amount of zygote wastage. Since only 40–50 percent of zygotes survive to be persons (i.e., adult, competent human beings), it might be best to speak of human zygotes as 0.4 probable persons. In this fashion one can indicate that they are the kinds of entities likely with that probability to develop into full-fledged moral agents, without suggesting that they are in some mysterious fashion already persons.

It follows from these considerations that one harms *no person* either by not conceiving that entity or by aborting the body from which it would develop. Though one is bound morally to respect persons in the sense of forbearing from unconsented-to harms against them and acting to aid them in achieving their good, it does not follow that one is bound to increase the number of such entities to which one has obligations. One might very well come to the reasonable conclusion that there are sufficient persons already to whom one has obligations. Reflections on the consequences of overpopulation may lead to the rational conclusion that it would be best if there were not more persons to feed, care, and respect. In addition, one might conclude that persons of a particular sort, such as those with severe physical or mental impairments, would create particularly severe moral obligations, which would be best avoided. In such circumstances, one might decide to prevent such obligations from coming into existence by using abortion. That zygotes, embryos, or fetuses are human rather than simian or canine would be of significance primarily in terms of one's interest in having more humans rather than more individuals of a different species. One might indeed imagine circumstances in which one would be very pleased regarding the high likelihood that a whooping crane embryo would go to term, but disvalue the likelihood that a human embryo (e.g., one likely to lead to the birth of a severely deformed infant) would go to term.

The value of animal life, which is not the life of a person, must be determined by other persons. Since in the case of such animals there is no person to respect, the issue is the value that must be imputed to the entity and the regard one must give to the pains and pleasures of that animal. The more an organism's life is characterized not just by sensations but by consciousness of objects and goals, the more one can plausibly hold that the organism's life has value for it. The more an organism can direct itself with appreciation and subtlety to certain objects and away from others, the more plausible it is that it has an inner life with some prereflective anticipations of values as values are understood by self-conscious free agents. Adult higher mammals enjoy their lives, pursue their pleasures, and avoid sufferings in elaborate and complex ways. Their lives in this very straightforward sense can have both value and disvalue for them. But since they are not persons, they cannot require that they be respected. They cannot as persons set moral limits to the extent to which they can be used by others. They cannot refuse

with moral authority to participate in the results of comparisons of the value of being beneficent to them versus being beneficent to other entities. They are not members of the moral community but are rather objects of its beneficence. The value of an animal's quality of life is thus set by persons in two senses. First, if the animal has no developed conscious life, persons may find little intrinsic value in such life and the predominant value may be the value that the life has as an object for persons. Second, even if the animal has an inward life that in a prereflective sense has a value for that organism, persons must still compare that value with other competing values.

It is for these reasons that the value of zygotes, embryos, and fetuses is to be primarily understood in terms of the values they have for actual persons. Zygotes, fetuses, and embryos do not have the rich inward life of adult mammals. Thus, if the zygote promises to be the long-awaited child of a couple that has been struggling for years to have another child, it is very likely to be highly valued by the couple and by all who are sympathetic with the would-be parents' hopes. On the other hand, if the zygote is in an unwed graduate student for whom the pregnancy would mean a major disruption of study plans, the zygote will likely be highly disvalued by her and by all who are sympathetic with her plans. Or if the zygote has a trisomy of chromosome 21, not only will the parents and those close to the parents likely disvalue the zygote, but so will society, which will need to participate in the costs of raising a defective child, should the pregnancy be uninterrupted. Some value is likely to be assigned to the zygote simply because it is human. However, one must remember that the sentience of a zygote, embryo, or fetus is much less than that of an adult mammal. One might even develop a suggestion of the natural theologian Charles Hartshorne so as to argue that from the perspective of the Deity the intrinsic value of a human fetus will be less than that of an adult normal member of some other mammalian species.[12] One might still be concerned that the processes of abortion might cause pain to the fetus. But one must remember that the level of obligations one has to a fetus in this regard is the same as one would have to an animal with a similar level of sensorimotor integration and perception.

To put this into perspective, one must realize that circumcisions are routinely performed for ritual and so-called medical reasons on male infants without the benefit of anesthesia. The basis for this practice is the incapacity of the newborn infant to integrate experiences sufficiently so as to actually suffer. For suffering to occur, there must be some fairly well-developed frontal lobe connections to allow the entity not only to experience the pain, but to recognize the pain over time as a noxious quale that must be avoided.[13] The capacities of fetuses give no indication that they approach the capacities for suffering of adult mammals. As a result, one's moral obligations will simply be to make sure that the good pursued, such as avoiding the birth of a Down's syndrome child, outweighs the evil of the pain to the animal organism to be killed.

AN EXCURSUS REGARDING ANIMALS

Some have found this assessment of the comparative standing of persons and animals to be improper. Robert Nozick speaks critically of the maxim "Utilitarianism for animals, Kantianism for people."[14] He speaks against the notion that "human beings may not be used or sacrificed for the benefit of others; animals may be used or sacrificed for the benefit of other people or animals, *only if* those benefits are greater than the loss inflicted."[15] This position derives from the Kantian moral contrast between persons and things. This moral position, in fact, is presupposed by the industry of medical research and investigation that first studies drugs through animal models. Persons are then used only after animal research has indicated that such a course is relatively safe. Such an approach is Kantian. Persons for Kant are subjects whose actions can be imputed.[16] There may be grounds for suspecting that certain nonhuman mammals are indeed not only animals but also persons as we are. If they are persons, then we owe them respect. However, the behavior of all but perhaps the higher apes shows no evidence of a rational appreciation of the moral life. Persons are moral agents, entities that can with justification be blamed and praised. They are entities that can be a part of the community of ends. In contrast, nonpersons are not worthy of blame or praise. As a consequence, "Every object of free choice that itself lacks freedom is therefore called a thing (*res corporalis*)."[17] For Kant one has duties to persons, and duties to persons regarding things, including animals.[18] This duty to other persons regarding animals is constituted in part out of an obligation to act in ways that will enhance and protect moral sensibilities. Thus, Kant argues that "tender feelings towards dumb animals develop humane feelings toward mankind."[19] Certain rules or practices of kindness and consideration toward animals work to the advantage of moral practices established to secure respect for persons.[20]

One must go beyond the Kantian perspective. One ought, in addition to recognizing duties to other persons regarding animals, recognize as well a duty directly to regard the pain and suffering of animals. One has duties of beneficence to animals, even if the strongest of such duties are usually simply negative ones of beneficence, that is, duties of nonmaleficence. Though one does not have duties of respect to animals because they fall outside the bounds of the morality of mutual respect, one has duties to them in terms of the morality of welfare and mutual sympathies. Here it might be useful to distinguish between persons, who ought to be objects of respect, and animals, which ought to be objects of beneficent regard. We owe to persons both respect and beneficent regard. To animals we owe only beneficent regard.

One can in part take account of Nozick's concerns and bring them within a reformed Kantian viewpoint in which one recognizes that it is only persons who are the judges of the relative significance of harms and benefits and the objects of our respect and beneficent regard, while animals are the objects of our beneficent regard. When persons are dealing with entities that are not persons, it is persons who will make the judgment regarding the significance of any exchanges of harms and benefits. It is persons who fashion actual moral communities with their particular moral senses, histories, and practices. Nonpersonal animals do not constitute moral communities, nor do they have a history. Moreover, there is no border of respect protecting organisms that are not persons. Animals are protected rather through a web of moral concerns regarding welfare and sympathies, which also protects persons. Respect of persons springs from the concern to act in ways in which persons can be justified as praiseworthy or blameworthy. In contrast, caring for animals springs from the concern to have a world that maximizes welfare and sustains a web of sympathies.

This web of sympathy binds us most tightly to those animals with which we can actually share sympathies—usually mammals and perhaps some birds. These bonds of sympathy are most fully drawn between humans and mature primates; they can also reach between human persons and human zygotes or fetuses. This web of sympathies justifies a wide range of beneficent action, not only to laboratory animals, but to human fetuses as well. Such concerns may influence the kind of abortifacient one might choose, all else being equal. They will as well have implications for the ways in which animals are treated generally. They strongly support policies of kindness and sympathy toward animals. However, they do not foreclose the raising of animals for meat or hunting, much less for use in research, whether it be medical research in the strict sense or even the testing of the safety of new cosmetics.

INFANTS, THE PROFOUNDLY RETARDED, AND SOCIAL SENSES OF "PERSON"

These conclusions raise a third and very vexatious difficulty. What is one to make of the status of infants, the profoundly mentally retarded, and those who are suffering from very advanced stages of Alzheimer's disease? Such entities are not persons in any strict sense. Yet we are concerned usually to accord such entities many of the rights normally possessed by adult persons. In the case of rules against maiming and injuring but not killing fetuses and infants, one can advance a justification of our moral concerns in terms of respect for the future person that such a fetus or infant will likely become. Even if one does not accord special moral rights to merely possible persons (e.g., the persons who could be conceived were the readers of this volume engaged in fruitful sexual congress rather than philosophical study) or probable persons (e.g., zygotes that would develop into competent persons, were the women carrying them not to seek an abortion in order to complete their graduate studies in theology), one can still understand the status of fetuses in the light of the standing of future actual persons. Future persons can have the standing of actual persons who we know will in the future exist. If one plants a bomb in the foundations of a grammar school with a timing device so that it will explode in fifteen years, one is intending to murder actual persons who will in the future exist. So, too, if one injures a fetus or infant, but does not kill it, one then sets in train a series of events that will in fact injure a future actual person.[21] In these terms one can secure certain moral protections (and moral grounds for the legal protection) of infants.

Considerations of beneficence protect animals, which are not persons, against being tortured uselessly, whether or not they are human. Considerations of the contingent rights of future persons protect entities that will become persons from being maimed. They do not protect infants, the profoundly mentally retarded, or those suffering from advanced Alzheimer's disease

from being killed painlessly at whim. What one must seek are the grounds that may justify the practices through which infants, the profoundly mentally retarded, and the very senile are customarily assigned a proportion of the rights possessed by entities who are persons strictly, including being protected from being killed at whim. Here, perhaps, one can take a suggestion from Kant regarding the need to support practices that will, in general, lead to the protection of persons. To find grounds for protecting such entities, one will need to look at the justification for certain social practices in terms of their importance for persons so as to justify a social role one might term "being a person for social considerations." Since this sense of person cannot be justified in terms of the basic grammar of mortality (i.e., because such entities do not have intrinsic moral standing through being moral agents), one will need rather to justify a social sense of person in terms of the usefulness of the practice of treating certain entities as if they were persons. If such a practice can be justified, one will have, in addition to a strict sense of persons as moral agents, a social sense of persons justified in terms of various utilitarian and other consequentialist considerations.

Most societies in fact have such a social sense of person, which is usually assigned to human beings at birth, or at some time soon after birth. In ancient Greek law an infant could be exposed with impunity up to the time it would be admitted into the family through a special ceremony, the *amphidromia*. After that the infant had standing and received some of the major rights of persons.[22] In other societies the line has been less clearly drawn. To take one example, a strain of Jewish interpretation holds that the death of an infant during the first thirty days of life should be considered a miscarriage. Such an infant had not yet been given the full standing of children that have survived beyond this point.[23] Even in contemporary American society one can note a greater acceptance of the cessation of treatment for severely defective newborns than would be the case with young children fully socialized within the role of child. It is as if the full conveying of social personhood does not occur immediately for many neonates.[24] . . . [T]his informal distinction between the treatment accorded to neonates versus other children has come under critical attack from some quarters. In many societies, and to some extent in ours, there remain informal distinctions between the standing accorded to neonates and that given to infants who have been brought fully within the role of the child and accorded robust rights similar to those possessed by persons in the strict sense.

A social role of person can be justified for infants and others in terms of (1) the role's supporting important virtues such as sympathy and care for human life, especially when that life is fragile and defenseless, and (2) the role's offering a protection against the uncertainties as to when exactly humans become persons strictly, as well as protecting persons during various vicissitudes of competence and incompetence, while (3) in addition securing the important practice of child-rearing through which humans develop as persons in the strict sense.

Since the assigning of the status of person in the social sense on the basis of such concerns must be justified in terms of utilitarian and consequentialist considerations, the justifications will be somewhat different, depending on whether the practice concerns (1) humans who in the past were persons in the strict sense (e.g, individuals now suffering from severe Alzheimer's disease); (2) humans who are likely to become persons and have been brought within a social role giving them special social standing (e.g., infants); (3) neonates who could become persons, but who have not yet been brought within a social role giving them special social standing (e.g., neonates in an intensive care unit who have not yet been fully accepted by the parents); (4) neonates who, because of their serious handicaps, will not be accorded strong social rights; and (5) those humans who have not, and never will, become persons in the strict sense (e.g., the profoundly mentally retarded). There are likely to be somewhat different justifications for the protection afforded in each instance. In each case, one will find a special social role justified in terms of a set of important moral considerations sustained by a major social practice, such as child rearing. . . .

SLEEPING PERSONS AND THE PROBLEM OF EMBODIMENT

There is yet another major puzzle to face. What are we to make of the status of sleeping individuals? If being a person depends on being a moral agent, and if one does not have a metaphysical doctrine of the soul to explain where persons go when they are asleep, what is the moral standing of a sleeping person?[25] Do personhood and its rights go away while one sleeps? This puzzle can be answered without metaphysical assumptions concerning souls of similar substances, through

an analysis of what it means to be a person, and to possess moral claims on the peaceable community of persons generally. This analysis depends on at least two major factors, the satisfactory resolution of either of which should dispel the puzzle sufficiently to give sleeping persons a standing tantamount to those who are persons strictly.

The first point turns on what it means to be an embodied person. Persons do not disappear to themselves as discontinuous. They sew together their various episodes of wakefulness and presence within a single identity. Alfred Schutz has explored this in his phenomenological account of going to sleep and awakening. The very sense of a person includes its unifying various temporally discontinuous episodes into one life.[26] Of course these attempts can fail. John Hughlings Jackson was one of the first clearly to recognize that our integration as one continuous person is a precarious and difficult undertaking.[27] To be a finite, spatiotemporal, sensibly intuiting person is to have the task of constantly constituting temporally diverse experiences as one's own. This point is appreciated by Kant in his characterizations of person or subjects in terms of the transcendental unity of apperception, the capacity to unite experiences under an "I think," to make a diverse manifold of experiences one's own. Those experiences that one can unite within one's unity of apperception under one's "I think," one's "I experience," become one's own. Persons, if they are not free of spatiotemporal extension (e.g., angels or gods), will be subject to the difficulty of integrating various experiences as their own. Sleep constitutes simply one example of such a problem for integration.

This can be better appreciated in terms of an understanding of the mind–brain relationship. To talk of minds that are finite, spatio–temporal, and sensibly perceiving presumes that they will span spatial and temporal extension as a part of their very being.[28] Their embodiment is their spatially and temporally extended place in this world. The integrative function of the brain must span brief pulsations of attention that are experienced in a single act of self-consciousness. As a result, what one can minimally mean by a person in such circumstances cannot be an unbroken godlike continuity of self-consciousness. Rather it is a self-consciousness, as a recurring integration of experience spanning discontinuities. This analysis does not require metaphysical presuppositions or a doctrine of potentiality, such as that required for those who hold that since fetuses are potential persons, they should count as persons. The question is not whether to regard an entity that has never shown the capacities of a person, as if it were a person. The question is rather how to regard an entity that intermittently shows the full capacities of a moral agent. How should one regard that entity during a period of time when it is not showing those capacities, but when one believes it will again in the future demonstrate those capacities?

To begin with, there is a difference in kind between a body that *is* someone's body, and a body that *may become* someone's body. With respect to a zygote, fetus, or even young infant, one does not yet know the person who will come to be "in" (or perhaps better, in, through, and with) that body. With respect to a sleeping person, one knows whose body it is. One knows who is there. The person will again awaken, make judgments, and answer questions. The body with the full capacities of sensorimotor integration that are the physical expression of a person's life is that person in the world. The body's capacities are the capacities of a person. One will need to distinguish between the potentiality *to become* a person and the potentialities *of* a person. There is a difference in kind between knowing who is sleeping, in the case of an adult competent human, and knowing who a fetus will be.

The point is that the very meaning of a spatiotemporally extended, sensibly intuiting person involves the spanning of, and the integration of, temporal extension. The existence of such persons will therefore not be set aside by temporal discontinuities across which their identity can reasonably be presumed to span. Talking about persons as spatiotemporally extended entities will therefore mean regarding their intact embodiment as them, as long as that embodiment maintains the full capacities that are the physical substrata of moral agents.

This point can be put a second way. The very language of blame and praise presumes that moral agents span discontinuities of experience. If interruptions in attention or self-consciousness shattered the identity of persons, the minimum moral fabric of the peaceable moral community would be set aside. Given the discontinuous nature of finite, spatiotemporal moral agents, discontinuity would make the moral community impossible, if strict continuity were required. If one allowed moral agents who are fully self-conscious to exterminate without the permission of those innocent moral agents whose attention had temporarily waned, had become temporarily obtunded, or had fallen asleep, one would be allowing them to act against the peaceable moral community insofar as it exists. Since spatiotemporal persons fashion moral actions over time and across moments of attention and of sleep, they are the sort of entity, should they come into existence, that would need to be treated with respect even when they were inattentive or sleeping.

These considerations do not lead one to the position that one is morally obliged to bring moral agents into existence so as to continue the moral community as an actual community through history. Such an argument would turn the moral community into a goal to be pursued. Rather, what has been advanced is a sketch of the minimal conceptual conditions for the notion of a moral community of spatiotemporal persons. Insofar as we think of ourselves as moral agents, we must think of ourselves as acting across these discontinuities in self-consciousness that occur, though our brains, our embodiments, remain intact. It is a condition of understanding ourselves within the practice of morality. One cannot respect other moral agents, while willing to destroy their unique place in the world, their embodiment. To will to destroy the embodiment of actual persons is to will to act against the very morality of mutual respect. The very notion of mutual respect and of moral authority would have to be rejected. This situation contrasts with the killing of fetuses or infants. In the case of competent adults not only does one know whose embodiment is at stake (unlike fetuses and infants, whose bodies are not yet anyone's embodiment), but taking a view that would allow the killing of sleeping persons would make a coherent portrayal of a moral community of spatiotemporally extended persons impossible. Killing fetuses only prevents possible persons from becoming persons and therefore members of the moral community. Finally, if the embodiment of a person is so compromised as to preclude any future states of consciousness, the person has ceased to exist. The person has died. But beforehand the person perdures.

The reader may suspect that such reflections are the contemporary equivalent of the supposed medieval theological pursuit of a census of the number of angels dancing on the pins of Christendom. However, since moral questions are intellectual questions, they commit us to tracing out the implications of moral theories. The controversies regarding the moral significance of killing fetuses force us to explore the differences between actual moral agents (e.g., competent, adult patients) and fetuses, while paying attention to those borderline cases that might constrain us to reaccept a doctrine of potentiality, or even to speak of souls within the context of general secular ethics. . . .

HUMAN BIOLOGICAL VERSUS HUMAN PERSONAL LIFE: SOME SUMMARIES

Given these reflections on the character of persons and animals, . . . some general classifications can be offered regarding the moral standing of such entities.

PERSONS STRICTLY

Such entities are moral agents, rational, able to choose freely according to a rational plan of life, and are possessed of a notion of blameworthiness and praiseworthiness. Persons strictly are protected by the moralities of mutual respect and of beneficence. They may not be treated or experimented on without their consent (unless they have ceded that right).

Free Persons. This group encompasses those who are not substantially restricted in their liberty to accept or refuse medical treatment for themselves due to agreements made explicitly or implicitly with other persons, e.g., most adult competent humans other than those serving in the armed forces.

Persons in the Possession of Others. Here one would have to include not only nonemancipated minors, but also indentured servants and members of the military. Such individuals are characterized by their having given to others the right to make important choices on their behalf. The rights of parents to choose medical treatment for their adolescent children must be understood in this light.

HUMAN BIOLOGICAL LIFE

Human biological life is protected by the morality of beneficence insofar as such life is capable of suffering, and insofar as such life is of significance to other persons. To the extent that such life is owned by other persons, the morality of mutual respect is also involved. One should note that concerns of beneficence toward such life will vary widely. One can have substantial concerns with beneficence toward severely mentally retarded humans. However, the opportunities to be beneficent toward a brain-dead but otherwise alive human organism vanish to the point of nonexistence.

Social Persons. Some instances of human life, because of their capacity to interact in social roles, are accorded some of the rights of persons strictly. Here one finds infants, very young children, the profoundly and many of the severely mentally retarded, the severely demented, including those suffering from advanced stages of senile dementia. Distinctions will need to be made among different classes of social persons: (a) infants and young children, (b) neonates prior to a commitment to full treatment, (c) the very senile who once were moral agents, and (d) the very severely and profoundly mentally retarded and demented who never were and never will be persons in the strict sense.

Human Life Accorded Special Levels of Protection. Out of considerations of utility, one may accord a special protection to viable fetuses. Though they are not given the rights of persons, one may wish to encourage respectful treatment. . . . [S]uch treatment of fetuses ought not to include actions on the behalf of fetuses against the wishes of the women bearing them except in very specific circumstances in order to protect the future person whom that fetus is likely to become.

Other Instances of Human Biological Life. These need not be accorded special protection, unless there are clear utilitarian arguments to support such protection, and then only when such protection does not violate the rights of persons strictly. Examples of such instances of human life would include human gametes and cells in culture. They need not be accorded any special respect. Consider, for instance, what it might mean to treat human sperm with respect.

ANIMAL LIFE

Animals are protected by the morality of beneficence. Since the range of the capacity for animals to suffer or achieve pleasure and fulfillment spans from that of the higher primates to that of one-cell animals, the strength of claims to beneficence will vary dramatically. The more animals can feel, suffer, and have affection for others, the more the concerns of beneficence toward them may plausibly have weight. On the other hand, concerns of beneficence with respect to roaches and amoebas are much less substantial. Still, capriciously to torment a paramecium for sport, if one were of the opinion that paramecia can be the subjects of torment, would be an act against the morality of beneficence (unless one held that a proportionate good was to be realized in or through that sport). One would need also to classify animals in terms of whether they are (1) owned by individuals or groups, or (2) unowned, in order to be clear with respect to one's duties regarding them. These considerations would place few restrictions on the use of animals in bona fide medical research. . . .

NOTES

1. Kant, *Grundlegung zur Metaphysik der Sitten*, Akademie Textausgabe, vol. 4 (Berlin: Walter de Gruyter, 1968), p. 438.

2. Ibid., p. 452.

3. Ibid., p. 453; *Foundations of the Metaphysics of Morals*, trans. Lewis White Beck (Indianapolis: Bobbs-Merrill, 1959), p. 72.

4. *Grundlegung zur Metaphysik der Sitten*, p. 452.

5. This point is explored at great length by Kant in his treatment of the third antinomy in the *Critique of Pure Reason*.

6. Ramsey has been reluctant to allow experimentation on fetuses and children because they cannot consent. Such a line of argument presumes that fetuses can sensibly be the object of such respect. Ramsey also objects to the use of children in research not aimed at their benefit, because such would entail using that individual "without his will." However, there is no will to respect in the case of infants. Paul Ramsey, *The Patient as Person* (New Haven, Conn.: Yale University Press, 1970), p. 35.

7. St. Thomas Aquinas distinguishes between the status of the early and late fetus in *Summa Theologica* I, 118, art. 2.

8. A good overview of the history of abortion in canon law is provided by John T. Noonan, Jr., "An Almost Absolute Value in History," in John T. Noonan, Jr. (ed.), *The Morality of Abortion* (Cambridge, Mass.: Harvard University Press, 1971). . . .

9. For an excellent study of the significance of the sin of contraception and its relation to the sin of abortion, see John T. Noonan, Jr., *Contraception* (Cambridge, Mass.: Harvard University Press, 1965). See also, for a helpful treatment of current Catholic viewpoints in this matter, James J. McCartney, "Some Roman Catholic Concepts of Person and Their Implications for the Ontological Status of the Unborn," in W. B. Bondeson et al. (eds.), *Abortion and the Status of the Fetus* (Dordrecht: Reidel, 1983), pp. 313–23.

10. Marie-Joseph Nicolas, "The Meaning of the Immaculate Conception in the Perspectives of St. Thomas," in E. D. O'Connor (ed.), *The Dogma of the Immaculate Conception* (Notre Dame, Ind.: University of Notre Dame Press, 1958), p. 333.

11. S. I. Benn, "Abortion, Infanticide, and Respect for Persons," in Joel Feinberg (ed.), *The Problem of Abortion* (Belmont, Calif.: Wadsworth, 1973), pp. 92–104.

12. As Charles Hartshorne suggests, whales may have a higher intrinsic significance than human fetuses, since whales may be able intellectually to recognize their significance for the Deity, though human fetuses and infants cannot. This greater complexity of adult whales would then itself have a significance for the Deity in contributing more richly to the Deity's life. See, for example, Charles Hartshorne, "Scientific and Religious Aspects of Bioethics," in Earl E. Shelp (ed.), *Theology and Bioethics* (Dordrecht: Reidel, 1985), p. 42.

13. The distinction between pain and suffering is explored by George Pitcher, "Pain and Unpleasantness," pp. 181–96; David Bakan, "Pain—The Existential Symptom," pp. 197–207; Bernard Tursky, "The Evaluation of Pain Responses: A Need for Improved Measures," pp. 209–19; and Jerome A. Shaffer, "Pain and Suffering," pp. 221–33, in *Philosophical Dimensions of the Neuro-Medical Sciences*, ed. S. F. Spicker and H. T. Engelhardt, Jr. (Dordrecht: Reidel, 1976).

14. Robert Nozick, *Anarchy, State, and Utopia* (New York: Basic Books, 1974), p. 39.

15. Ibid.

16. One must in fact acknowledge the wide range of ways in which Kant treats persons, the ego, or the subject. Kant employs at least six different senses.

17. *Metaphysik der Sitten*, in *Kants Werke* (Berlin: Walter de Gruyter, 1968), vol. 6, p. 223; *Metaphysical Principles of Virtue*, trans. J. Ellington (Indianapolis: Bobbs-Merrill, 1964), p. 23.

18. Immanuel Kant, *Lectures on Ethics*, trans. Louis Infield (Indianapolis: Hackett, 1979), p. 240.

19. Ibid. Kant argues that one should keep an old dog until it dies, for "such action helps to support us in our duties towards human beings, where they are bounden duties." Ibid. However, if the man shoots his dog, according to Kant, he does not fail in his duty to the dog, "but his act is inhuman and damages in himself that humanity which it is his duty to show towards mankind." The dog owner has no duty to the dog, but a duty to humanity regarding the dog. In my arguments I have indicated that the dog owner in addition has a duty of beneficence to the dog. I agree with Kant that the purposes of humans can outweigh the considerations of beneficence to animals. "Vivisectionists, who use living animals for their experiments, certainly act cruelly, although their aim is praiseworthy, and they can justify their cruelty, since animals must be regarded as man's instruments, but any such cruelty for sport cannot be justified." Ibid., pp. 240–1. The arguments in this book do not preclude the use of animals for purposes of sport. As an example, consider the report of a gun club using live pigeons for target practice. Olive Talley, "Gun Club Again Using Live Pigeons," *Houston Chronicle* (February 16, 1985), sec. 1, p. 32.

20. For a recent discussion of the use of animals for medical and other research, see R. G. Frey, "Vivisection, Morals and Medicine," *Journal of Medical Ethics* 9 (June 1983): 94–7.

21. For an overview of the issues raised by tort-for-wrongful-life cases, see Angela Holder, "Is Existence Ever an Injury?: The Wrongful Life Cases," in S. F. Spicker et al. (eds.), *The Law-Medicine Relation: A Philosophical Exploration* (Dordrecht: Reidel, 1981), pp. 225–39.

22. Richard H. Feen, "Abortion and Exposure in Ancient Greece: Assessing the Status of the Fetus and 'Newborn' from Classical Sources," in Bondeson et al. (eds.), *Abortion and the Status of the Fetus*, pp. 283–300.

23. This point is noted in *Kitzur Shulhan Arukh*, by Rabbi Solomon Ganzfried (the standard condensed version of the code of Jewish religious law, entitled *Shulhan Arukh*, compiled by Joseph Karo [1488–1575], sec. 203, par. 3): ". . . if an infant dies within the first 30 days of its life, or even on the 30th day of its life, and even if there has been growth of its hair and nails, you do not follow any of the observances of mourning, because it is as if there had been a miscarriage" (adapted and translated by Professor Isaac Franck).

24. Stopping treatment on defective newborns seems to have been fairly well accepted. One might think here of the suggestions by Raymond S. Duff and A. G. M. Campbell regarding the ways in which parents may be assisted in making responsible choices regard-

ing when to refuse treatment for their severely defective newborn. "Moral and Ethical Dilemmas in the Special Care Nursery," *New England Journal of Medicine* 289 (Oct. 25, 1973): 890–4. See also Anthony Shaw, "Dilemmas of Informed Consent in Children," *New England Journal of Medicine* 289 (Oct. 25, 1973): 885–90.

25. Gary E. Jones, "Engelhardt on the Abortion and Euthanasia of Defective Infants," *Linacre Quarterly* 50 (May 1983): 172–81.

26. Alfred Schutz and Thomas Luckmann, *The Structures of the Life-World*, trans. R. M. Zaner and H. T. Engelhardt, Jr. (Evanston, Ill.: Northwestern University Press, 1973), p. 47.

27. John Hughlings Jackson (1835–1902), the father of modern neurology, examined this issue in a number of his writings. See, in particular, "Evolution and Dissolution of Nervous System," in *John Hughlings Jackson: Selected Writings*, ed. James Taylor (London: Staples Press, 1958), vol. 2, pp. 45–75.

28. H. T. Engelhardt, Jr., *Mind-Body: A Categorical Relation* (The Hague: Martinus Nijhoff, 1973).

SUGGESTED READINGS FOR CHAPTER 4

CONCEPTS OF PERSONHOOD

Atkinson, Gary M. "Persons in the Whole Sense." *American Journal of Jurisprudence* 22 (1977), 86–117.

Ayer, A. J. *The Concept of a Person*. London: Macmillan, 1963. Chap. 4.

Becker, Lawrence C. "Human Being: The Boundaries of the Concept." *Philosophy and Public Affairs* 4 (Summer 1975), 334–358.

Bok, Sissela. "Who Shall Count as a Human Being? A Treacherous Question in the Abortion Discussion." In Perkins, Robert L., ed., *Abortion: Pro and Con*. Cambridge, Mass.: Schenkman, 1974, pp. 91–105.

Danto, Arthur C. "Persons." In Taylor, Paul, ed., *Encyclopedia of Philosophy*. New York: Free Press, 1967. Vol. 4, pp. 110–114.

Dennett, Daniel C. *Brainstorms: Philosophical Essays on Mind and Psychology*. Montgomery, Vt.: Bradford Books, 1978. Chap. 14.

Engelhardt, H. Tristram, Jr. "The Ontology of Abortion." *Ethics* 84 (April 1974), 217–234.

Fletcher, Joseph. "Four Indicators of Humanhood—The Enquiry Matures." *Hastings Center Report* 4 (December 1974), 4–7.

Frankfurt, Harry G. "Freedom of the Will and the Concept of a Person." *Journal of Philosophy* 68 (January 14, 1971), 5–20.

Gaylin, Willard. "In Defense of Being Human." *Hastings Center Report* (August 1984), 18–22.

Macklin, Ruth. "Personhood in the Bioethics Literature." *Milbank Memorial Fund Quarterly/Health and Society* 61 (Winter 1983), 35–57.

Margolis, Joseph. *Persons and Minds: The Prospects of Nonreductive Materialism*. Boston: D. Reidel, 1978.

Newton, Lisa. "Humans and Persons: A Reply to Tristram Engelhardt." *Ethics* 85 (July 1975), 332–336.

Puccetti, Roland. *Persons: A Study of Possible Moral Agents in the Universe*. London: Macmillan, 1968. New York: Herder and Herder, 1969.

Rorty, Amélie O. "Persons, Policies, and Bodies." *International Philosophical Quarterly* 13 (March 1973), 63–80.

Sellars, Wilfrid. "Metaphysics and the Concept of Person." In Lambert, K., ed., *The Logical Way of Doing Things*. New Haven, Conn.: Yale University Press, 1969.

Shaffer, Jerome A. *Philosophy of Mind*. Englewood Cliffs, N.J.: Prentice-Hall, 1968.

Strawson, P. F. *Individuals: An Essay in Descriptive Metaphysics*. London: Methuen, 1959.

Weiss, Roslyn. "The Perils of Personhood." *Ethics* 89 (October 1978), 66–75.

THE BEGINNING OF LIFE

Fleming, Lorette. "The Moral Status of the Fetus: A Reappraisal." *Bioethics* 1 (January 1987), 15–34.

Gertler, Gary B. "Brain Birth: A Proposal for Defining When a Fetus Is Entitled to Human Life Status." *Southern California Law Review*, Vol. 59, No. 5 (July 1986), pp. 1061–1078.

Goldenring, John. "The Brain-Life Theory: Towards a Consistent Biological Definition of Humaneness." *Journal of Medical Ethics* 11 (December 1985), 194–204.

Grobstein, Clifford. "The Early Development of Human Embryos." *Journal of Medicine and Philosophy* 10 (August 1985), 213–236.

Iglesias, Teresa. "In Vitro Fertilization: The Major Issues." *Journal of Medical Ethics* 10 (March 1987), 32–37.

Kushner, Thomasine. "Having a Life Versus Being Alive." *Journal of Medical Ethics* 10 (March 1984), 5–8.

Mahoney, John. "The Beginning of Life." In his *Bioethics and Beliefs: Religion and Medicine in Dialogue*. London: Sheed and Ward, 1984, 52–86.

Shea, M. C. "Embryonic Life and Human Life." *Journal of Medical Ethics* 11 (June 1984), 79–81.

Tauer, Carol. "Personhood and Human Embryos and Fetuses." *Journal of Medicine and Philosophy* 10 (August 1985), 253–266.

United Kingdom, Department of Health and Social Security. *Report of the Committee of Inquiry into Human Fertilisation and Embryology* [The Warnock Committee Report]. London: Her Majesty's Stationery Office (July 1984), pp. 58–60.

THE END OF LIFE

Beauchamp, Tom L., and Perlin, Seymour, eds. *Ethical Issues in Death and Dying*. Englewood Cliffs, N.J.: Prentice-Hall, 1978. Chap. 1.

Beecher, Henry K. "Ethical Problems Created by the Hopelessly Unconscious Patient." *New England Journal of Medicine* 278 (June 27, 1968), 1425–1430.

———. "After the 'Definition of Irreversible Coma.'" *New England Journal of Medicine* 281 (November 6, 1969), 1070–1071.

Bernat, James L., et al. "On the Definition and Criterion of Death." *Annals of Internal Medicine* 94 (March 1981), 389–394.

Black, Peter M. "Three Definitions of Death." *Monist* 60 (January 1977), 136–146.

———. "Brain Death." *New England Journal of Medicine* 299 (August 17 and 24, 1978), 338–344, 393–401.

Brierley, J. B., et al. "Neocortical Death After Cardiac Arrest." *Lancet* 2 (September 11, 1971), 560–565.

Browne, Alister. "Whole-Brain Death Reconsidered." *Journal of Medical Ethics* 9 (March 1983), 28–31, 44.

Byrne, Paul A., et al. "Brain Death—An Opposing Viewpoint." *Journal of the American Medical Association* 242 (November 2, 1979), 1985–1990.

Canada, Law Reform Commission. *Criteria for the Determination of Death*. Ottawa: Law Reform Commission of Canada, 1979.

Capron, Alexander M. "Death, Definition and Determination of: Legal Aspects of Pronouncing Death." In Reich, Warren T., ed., *Encyclopedia of Bioethics*. New York: Free Press, 1978. Vol. 1, pp. 296–301.

Conference of Medical Royal Colleges and Faculties of the United Kingdom. "Diagnosis of Brain Death." *Lancet* 2 (November 13, 1976), 1069–1070.

Engelhardt, H. Tristram, Jr. "Definition of Death: Where to Draw the Lines and Why." In McMullin, Ernan, ed., *Death and Decision*. Boulder, Colo.: Westview Press, 1978, pp. 15–34.

Gaylin, Willard. "Harvesting the Dead." *Harper's* 249 (September 1974), 23–28 +.

Green, Michael, and Wikler, Daniel. "Brain Death and Personal Identity." *Philosophy and Public Affairs* 9 (Winter 1980), 105–133.

Green, Ronald M. "Toward a Copernican Revolution in Our Thinking About Life's Beginning and Life's End." *Soundings* 66 (Summer 1983), 152–173.

High, Dallas M. "Death, Definition and Determination of: Philosophical and Legal Foundations." In Reich, Warren T., ed., *Encyclopedia of Bioethics*. New York: Free Press, 1978. Vol. 1, pp. 301–307.

Institute of Society, Ethics and the Life Sciences, Task Force on Death and Dying. "Refinements in Criteria for the Determination of Death." *Journal of the American Medical Association* 221 (July 3, 1972), 48–53.

Jennett, Bryan, et al. "Brain Death in Three Neurosurgical Units." *British Medical Journal* 282 (February 14, 1981), 553–559.

Korein, Julius, ed. "Brain Death: Interrelated Medical and Social Issues." *Annals of the New York Academy of Sciences* 315 (1978), 1–454.

Margolis, Joseph. *Negativities*. Columbus, Ohio: Merrill, 1975. Chap. 1.

Molinari, Gaetano F. "Death, Definition and Determination of: Criteria for Death." In Reich, Warren T., ed., *Encyclopedia of Bioethics*. New York: Free Press, 1978. Vol. 1, pp. 292–296.

Pallis, Christopher. "Whole Brain Death Reconsidered—Physiological Facts and Philosophy." *Journal of Medical Ethics* 9 (March 1983), 32–37.

———. "Defining Death." *British Medical Journal* 291 (September 1985), 666–667.

Ramsey, Paul. "On Updating Procedures for Stating That a Man Has Died." In his *Patient as Person*. New Haven, Conn.: Yale University Press, 1970, 59–112.

Shrader, Douglas. "On Dying More Than One Death." *Hastings Center Report* 16 (February 1986), 12–17.

United States, President's Commission for the Study of Ethical Problems in Medicine and Biomedical and Behavioral Research. *"Defining Death": A Report on the Medical, Legal, and Ethical Issues in the Determination of Death*. Washington, D.C.: President's Commission, 1981.

Van Till, H. A. H. "Diagnosis of Death in Comatose Patients Under Resuscitation Treatment: A Critical Review of the Harvard Report." *American Journal of Law and Medicine* 2 (Summer 1976), 1–40.

Veatch, Robert M. *Death, Dying and the Biological Revolution: Our Last Quest for Responsibility*. New Haven, Conn.: Yale University Press, 1976. Chap. 2.

Veith, Frank, et al. "Brain Death." *Journal of the American Medical Association* 238 (October 10 and 17, 1977), 1651–1655, 1744–1748.

BIBLIOGRAPHIES

Goldstein, Doris Mueller. *Bioethics: A Guide to Information Sources*. Detroit: Gale Research Company, 1982. See under "Philosophy of Medicine" and "Definition and Determination of Death."

Lineback, Richard H., ed. *Philosopher's Index*. Vols. 1– . Bowling Green, Ohio: Philosophy Documentation Center, Bowling Green State University. Issued quarterly. See under "Brain Death," "Death," "Humans," "Individuals," "Life," and "Person(s)."

Walters, LeRoy, and Kahn, Tamar Joy, eds. *Bibliography of Bioethics*. Vols. 1– . Washington, D.C.: Kennedy Institute of Ethics, Georgetown University. Issued annually. See under "Brain Death," "Determination of Death," and "Personhood." (The information contained in the annual *Bibliography of Bioethics* can also be retrieved from BIOETHICSLINE, an online database of the National Library of Medicine.)

5.
Abortion

In recent legal developments, laws that restrict abortion have either been sharply modified or struck down by courts in several Western nations, including the United States. Despite the legal permissibility of abortion in these nations, questions of its ethical acceptability continue to be widely debated, and some high government officials stand morally opposed to the law of their land. At the same time, the adequacy of court decisions that have determined antiabortion laws to be unconstitutional is also debated. In this chapter these and other contemporary ethical and legal issues about abortion will be examined.

THE PROBLEM OF MORAL JUSTIFICATION

An abortion might be desired for many reasons: cardiac complications; a suicidal condition of mind; psychological trauma; pregnancy caused by rape; the inadvertent use of fetus-deforming drugs; genetic predisposition to disease; prenatally diagnosed birth defects; and many personal and family reasons, such as the financial burden or intrusiveness of a child. These reasons explain why an abortion is often viewed as a desirable way to extricate a woman or a family from an undesired circumstance. But explanations of this sort do not answer the problem of *justification*: What reasons, if any, are sufficient to justify the act of aborting a human fetus?

One who is concerned to defend abortion through ethical theory seeks a principled justification where ethical reasons are given in support of one's conclusions. It might be decided that in only some of the above-mentioned circumstances would an abortion be morally allowable, whereas in others it would not be justified, but any decision presupposes some set of general criteria that enables one to discriminate justified abortions from unjustified ones.

The central moral problem of abortion is how to specify the conditions, if any, under which abortion is ethically permissible. Some contend that abortion is never acceptable, or at most is permissible only under the condition that it is required to save the pregnant woman's life or for some other similarly serious reason. This view is commonly called the conservative theory of abortion because of its emphasis on conserving life. Roman Catholics have traditionally been exponents of the conservative approach, but they are by no means its only advocates. John Noonan presents the case for this point of view in this chapter.

Others hold that abortion is always permissible, whatever the state of fetal development. This view is commonly termed the liberal theory of abortion because of the emphasis on freedom of choice. The theory has frequently been advocated by those adherents of women's rights who emphasize the right of a woman to make decisions that affect her body, but the position is advocated by others as well. Mary Anne Warren defends this approach in this chapter.

Finally, many defend intermediate or moderate theories, according to which abortion is ethically permissible up to a specified stage of fetal development or for some limited set of moral reasons believed to be sufficient to warrant abortions under special circumstances. Baruch Brody discusses possible intermediate theories leaning toward conservatism, while Judith Thomson's essay suggests an intermediate theory that leans toward liberalism. However, it is worth noting that the traditional terminology of "liberal" and "conservative" can be both distracting and inaccurate. The issues before us are not directly linked to *political* liberalism and conservatism.

THE ONTOLOGICAL STATUS OF THE FETUS

Recent controversies about abortion focus on ethical problems of our obligations to fetuses and on what rights, if any, fetuses possess. A more basic issue, some say, concerns the *kind of entities* fetuses are. Following current usage, we can refer to this as the problem of *ontological status*. An account of what kind of entities fetuses are will have important implications for the issues of our obligations to fetuses and their rights, but the two issues are distinct.

Several layers of questions may be distinguished about ontological status: (1) Is the fetus *an individual organism*? (2) Is the fetus *biologically a human being*? (3) Is the fetus *psychologically a human being*? (4) Is the fetus *a person*? Some who write on problems of ontological status attempt to develop a theory that specifies the conditions under which the fetus can be said to be independent and alive, while others focus on the conditions, if any, under which the fetus is human, and still others are concerned with explaining the conditions, if any, under which the fetus is a person. It would be generally agreed that one attributes a more significant status to the fetus by granting that it is fully a human being (biologically and psychologically), rather than by saying merely that it is an individual organism, and that one enhances its status still further by attributing personhood to the fetus.

Many would be willing to concede that an individual life begins at fertilization without conceding that there is a human being or a person at fertilization. Others claim that the fetus is human at fertilization but not a person. Still others grant full personhood at fertilization. Those who espouse these views sometimes differ because they define one or the other of these terms differently, but many differences also derive from theoretical disagreements about what constitutes life or humanity or personhood.

THE CONCEPT OF HUMANITY

The concept of human life has long been at the center of the abortion discussion, but it is a confusing term, because "human life" can take two very different meanings. On the one hand, it can mean *biological human life*, that set of biological characteristics (for example, genetic ones) that set the human species apart from nonhuman species. On the other hand, "human life" can also be used to mean *life that is distinctively human*—that is, a life characterized by those properties that define the essence of humanity through distinctive psychological rather than biological properties. It is often said, for example, that the ability to use symbols, to imagine, to love, and to perform higher intellectual skills are among the most distinctive human properties. To have these properties, we sometimes imply, is to be a "human being."

A simple example will illustrate the differences between these two senses. Some seriously handicapped infants die shortly after birth. They are born of human parents, and biologically they are human. However, they never exhibit any distinctively human psychological traits, and (in many cases) have no potential to do so. For these individuals it is not possible to make human life in the "biological" sense human in the "distinctively human" or "psychological" sense. We do not differentiate these two aspects of life in discourse about any other animal species. We do not, for example, speak of making feline life more distinctively feline. But we do meaningfully speak of making human life human, and this usage makes sense precisely because there exists in the language the dual meaning just discussed. In discussions of abortion, it is important to be clear about which meaning is being employed when using the expression "the taking of human life." Many proponents of abortion, and some opponents as well, would agree that while biological human life is taken by abortions, human life in the second or psychological sense is not taken.

THE CONCEPT OF PERSONHOOD

The concept of personhood was discussed in Chapter 4. Here it need only be observed that personhood may or may not be different from either the biological sense or the psychological sense of "human life." That is, one might claim that what it means to be a person is simply to have some properties that make an organism human in one or both of these senses. But other writers have suggested a list of more demanding criteria for being a person. A list of conditions for being a person, similar to the following, is advanced by Warren and has been put forward by several recent writers:

(1) Consciousness
(2) Self-consciousness
(3) Freedom to act on one's own reasons
(4) Capacity to communicate with other persons
(5) Capacity to make moral judgments
(6) Rationality

Sometimes it is said by those who propose such a list that in order to be a person an entity need only satisfy some one criterion on the list—for example, it must be conscious (1) but need not also satisfy the other conditions (2)–(6). Others say that all of these conditions must be satisfied in order to be a person. It again can make a major difference which of these two views one accepts. But the dominant and prior question is whether any list approximating (1)–(6) is acceptable. Noonan, Brody, and Thomson tend not to view the core problems of abortion as turning on the acceptance or rejection of such a list.

Two issues have emerged in the abortion controversy concerning the proper analysis of the concept of person. First, the *factual characteristics* an entity must possess in order to be a person are disputed. One might analyze personhood in terms of a rather abbreviated list of factual though not necessarily biological characteristics—for example, in terms of physical characteristics such as genetic structure, characteristics of consciousness such as rationality and free choice, and perhaps characteristics that can at present be applied only to human developmental histories, such as having learned a language. If personhood can be explicated through elementary properties such as genetic structure, then fetuses might well qualify as persons. But one might also analyze personhood in terms of a more demanding list of presumably factual properties, such as conditions (2)–(6) above. Clearly the burden of argument is heavy to show that a fetus is a person if these criteria must be satisfied.

A second dispute has emerged in connection with the first. Several writers have suggested that the concept of personhood must be analyzed in terms of properties *bestowed by human evaluation*. For example, it has been argued that in order to be a person in any meaningful sense one must be the bearer of legal rights and social responsibilities and must be capable of being judged by others as morally praiseworthy or blameworthy. The central question is whether it is appropriate to value fetuses in this way. This issue is closely related to what we shall discuss momentarily as the moral status of the fetus.

The problem of ontological status is complicated by a further factor related to the biological development of the fetus. It is important to many writers on the subject of abortion to state *at what point of development* an entity achieves significant status as a human or a person. This involves specifying criteria that nonarbitrarily delineate a developmental stage at which significant (perhaps full) ontological status is gained—for fetuses or for anyone. In Brody's essay and also in the opinion in *Roe* v. *Wade* by the U.S. Supreme Court, locating the crucial point of development is taken to be the central task.

The problem of drawing the line between that which has full status and that which has not has long been a major hurdle in advancing the controversy over abortion. One polar position (said to be the extreme liberal position) is that the fetus never satisfies any of the criteria mentioned above and therefore has *no ontological status* of any importance. Warren defends this view. The polar opposite position (often said to be the extreme conservative position) is that the fetus always has *full ontological status* in regard to all of the significant measures of status. John Noonan supports this view. Those who defend it typically claim that the line is properly drawn at conception, so that the fetus is always an individual human person. Obviously there can be many intermediate positions, which are generally defended by drawing the line somewhere between the extremes of conception and birth. For example, the line may be drawn at quickening or viability—or perhaps at the time when brain waves are first present (as Brody argues).

Whichever point is chosen, it is essential that any theory be clear on two crucial matters: (1) It should be specified whether the ontological status of persons or human beings or some other category is under discussion; and (2) whatever the point at which the line is drawn (viability, conception, birth, and so on), it should be argued that the line can be justifiably drawn at that point so that the theory is therefore not an arbitrarily chosen line.

THE MORAL STATUS OF THE FETUS

The notion of "moral status" has been explicated in several ways but probably is best analyzed in terms of *rights*:[1] To say that a being possesses moral status is to attribute rights to the being. If, for example, the unborn have *full moral status*, then they possess all the same rights as those who are born. Brody holds this thesis for at least some periods of fetal development, and Noonan holds it for all periods. By contrast, at least some moderates hold that fetuses have only a *partial moral status* and therefore only a partial set of rights. Many liberals maintain that fetuses possess *no moral status* and therefore no rights, as Warren maintains. If this liberal account is accepted, then the unborn and animals have no more right to life than a bodily cell or a tumor, and an abortion is no more morally objectionable than surgery to remove the tumor. But if the conservative view is accepted, the unborn possess all the rights possessed by human beings and an abortion is as objectionable as any common killing of the innocent.

Theories of moral status are often directly connected with prior theories of ontological status. A typical conservative thesis is that because the line between the human and the nonhuman is properly drawn at conception, the fetus has full ontological status and *therefore* full moral status. A typical liberal claim is that the line between the human and the nonhuman must be drawn at birth; the fetus has no significant ontological status and *therefore* no moral status. Some liberals argue that even though the fetus is biologically human, it nonetheless is not human in a morally significant sense and hence has no significant moral status. This claim is usually accompanied by the thesis that only persons constitute the moral community, and because fetuses are not persons they do not have a moral status (see Warren).

Moderates use a diverse mixture of arguments, which sometimes do and sometimes do not combine an ontological account with a moral one. Typical of moderate views is the claim that the line between the human and the nonhuman or the line between persons and nonpersons should be drawn at some point between conception and birth. Therefore, the fetus has no significant moral status during some stages of growth but does have significant moral status beginning at some later stage. In many recent theories, viability has been an especially popular point at which to draw the line, with the result that the fetus is given either full moral status or partial moral status at viability. This is a major premise in the majority opinion in *Roe* v. *Wade*, as delivered by Justice Blackmun. It is also a major premise attacked in the minority opinion in *City of Akron*, as written by Justice Sandra Day O'Connor.

THE PROBLEM OF CONFLICTING RIGHTS

If either the liberal or the conservative view of the moral status of the fetus is adopted, the problem of morally justifying abortion may at first seem uncomplicated. If one endorses the theory that a fetus does not enjoy an ethically significant claim to treatment as a human being, it can then be argued that abortions are not morally reprehensible and are prudentially justified just as other surgical procedures are. On the other hand, if one endorses the theory that a fetus at any stage of development is a human life with full moral status, and is possibly a person, then the equation "abortion is murder" seems in order. By this reasoning abortion is never justified under any conditions, or at least it can be permitted only if it is an instance of "justified homicide."

However, finding a position on abortion is not quite so straightforward. Even on a conservative theory there may be cases of justified homicide involving the unborn. For example, it might be argued that a pregnant woman may legitimately "kill" the fetus in "self-defense" if only one of the two can survive or if both will die unless the life of the fetus is terminated. In order to claim that abortion is *always* wrong, one must justify maintaining the position that the fetus's "right to life" *always* overrides (or at least is equal to) all the pregnant woman's rights, including her rights to life and liberty.

Even if the conservative theory is construed so that it entails that human fetuses have equal rights because of their moral status, nothing in the theory requires that these moral rights *always override* all other moral rights. Here a proponent of this theory bluntly confronts the problem of conflicting rights: The unborn possess some rights (including a right to life) and pregnant women also possess rights (including a right to life). Those who possess the rights have a (*prima facie*) moral claim to be treated in accordance with their rights. But what is to be done when these rights conflict?

This problem is no less formidable for those who hold a moderate theory of the moral status of the fetus. These theories provide moral grounds against arbitrary termination of fetal life (the fetus has some claim to protection against the actions of others), yet do not grant to the unborn (at least in some stages) the same rights to life possessed by those already born. Accordingly, advocates of these theories are faced with the problem of specifying which rights or claims are sufficiently weighty to take precedence over which other rights or claims. Is the woman's right to decide what happens to her body sufficient to justify abortion? Is pregnancy as a result of rape sufficient? Is the likely death of the mother sufficient? Is psychological damage (sometimes used to justify "therapeutic abortion") sufficient? Is knowledge of a grossly deformed fetus, which produces severe mental suffering in the pregnant woman, sufficient? And further, does the fetus have a right to a "minimum quality of life," that is, to protection against wrongful life? Some of these issues of conflicting rights are raised in a striking manner by Thomson, who in turn is criticized by both Brody and Warren.

LAW, TECHNOLOGY, AND EVOLVING SOCIAL POLICY

The problem of conflicting rights has always been at the forefront of the discussions in the U.S. Supreme Court's decisions on abortion. In the 1973 case of *Roe* v. *Wade*, the Court addressed the social problem of how abortion legislation may and may not be formulated in the attempt to protect the fetus against abortion. In the majority opinion in this case, the right to privacy implicit in the Fourteenth Amendment is held to be broad enough to encompass a woman's decision to have an abortion. This right is regarded as a right that overrides all other concerns until the fetus reaches the point of viability. After that point, the Court finds that state statutes may be constructed to protect the life of the fetus. The Court reasons that the fact of viability provides sufficient interest on the state's part to provide the fetus protection, even if offering that protection directly competes with the woman's interest in liberty (but not if the protection interferes with maternal health).

In addition to the viability criterion, the Court correspondingly divides pregnancy into three periods, called trimesters. Because the fetus becomes viable in roughly the third trimester, it is in this period that the Court determines it may be protected by laws. (These laws may take the form of prohibiting third-trimester abortions unless there is a question of protecting *maternal* health.) The Court's conception of a solution to the social problem of abortion has increasingly come under attack, both from external critics and internally from a minority of Supreme Court justices who have filed dissenting opinions. O'Connor represents these justices in the aforementioned *Akron* case. The nature of the Court's reasoning in its string of cases on abortion and the ongoing dispute surrounding those opinions are outlined in this chapter by Leonard Glantz, who presents an analysis of what the Court did in *Roe*, what it did after *Roe*, and where the substantive controversies have emerged over the Court's arguments.

An argument of particular importance against the Court's stand is that advances in biomedical technology are undermining the use of the criteria of viability and trimesters as a means of defending a woman's freedom of choice in seeking abortion. Both Ken Martyn and Justice O'Connor present variants of this argument in their selections in this chapter. Martyn focuses on how the biotechnology of sustaining premature infants has important implications for abortion. He argues that these developments will force changes in the way we conceive and attempt to resolve the abortion problem. His own solution is to use a criterion of when human life *ends* in order to determine when life begins in the unborn. Using this solution he tries to show that the abortion issue can be understood in terms of a unified legal theory of what constitutes a human being.

Justice O'Connor offers a particularly blistering attack on her colleagues in the Court majority. She maintains that the Court's reasoning is not sufficient to justify its fundamental analytical framework of "stages" of pregnancy. She accuses the Court of inconsistency both in handling abortion cases and in processing cases involving fundamental rights in other areas. Like Martyn, she lands on the issue of how the state's compelling interests in maternal and fetal health must change as medical technology changes.

The problem they envision is the following: If the woman's right to privacy overrides the state's interest in protecting fetal health only up to the point of viability, then as the point of viability is pushed back by technological advancement the point at which abortion is legally allowed must also be pushed back. O'Connor argues that as medical practices improve, the need to protect maternal health will also be reduced. These two considerations taken together lead her to argue that *Roe* necessitates continuous, ongoing medical review by the Court, an obvious impossibility. She concludes that the *Roe* framework is unworkable and "on a collision course with itself." She leaves us with the question of whether new abortion criteria must be established in the law that will give more protection to the fetus throughout pregnancy. Her opinion indicates that the legal issues surrounding abortion are no more resolved than the moral issues.

T. L. B.

NOTES

1. The notion of moral status could be explicated in ways other than by reference to rights. To say that a fetus possesses some form of moral status might be simply to say that it is *wrong* to do certain things to it. This observation is important because some who deny that fetuses have rights still believe that certain ways of treating fetuses are wrong, just as some who believe that animals do not have rights nonetheless believe that it is wrong to do certain things to them.

Moral Analyses

JOHN T. NOONAN, JR.

An Almost Absolute Value in History

The most fundamental question involved in the long history of thought on abortion is: How do you determine the humanity of a being? To phrase the question that way is to put in comprehensive humanistic terms what the theologians either dealt with as an explicitly theological question under the heading of "ensoulment" or dealt with implicitly in their treatment of abortion. The Christian position as it originated did not depend on a narrow theological or philosophical concept. It had no relation to theories of infant baptism.[1] It appealed to no special theory of instantaneous ensoulment. It took the world's view on ensoulment as that view changed from Aristotle to Zacchia. There was, indeed, theological influence affecting the theory of ensoulment finally adopted, and, of course, ensoulment itself was a theological concept, so that the

position was always explained in theological terms. But the theological notion of ensoulment could easily be translated into humanistic language by substituting "human" for "rational soul"; the problem of knowing when a man is a man is common to theology and humanism.

If one steps outside the specific categories used by the theologians, the answer they gave can be analyzed as a refusal to discriminate among human beings on the basis of their varying potentialities. Once conceived, the being was recognized as man because he had man's potential. The criterion for humanity, thus, was simple and all-embracing: if you are conceived by human parents, you are human.

The strength of this position may be tested by a review of some of the other distinctions offered in the contemporary controversy over legalizing abortion. Perhaps the most popular distinction is in terms of viability. Before an age of so many months, the fetus is not viable, that is, it cannot be removed from the mother's womb and live apart from her. To that extent, the life of the fetus is absolutely dependent on the life of the mother. This dependence is made the basis of denying recognition to its humanity.

There are difficulties with this distinction. One is that the perfection of artificial incubation may make the fetus viable at any time: it may be removed and artificially sustained. Experiments with animals already show that such a procedure is possible. This hypothetical extreme case relates to an actual difficulty: there is considerable elasticity to the idea of viability. Mere length of life is not an exact measure. The viability of the fetus depends on the extent of its anatomical and functional development. The weight and length of the fetus are better guides to the state of its development than age, but weight and length vary. Moreover, different racial groups have different ages at which their fetuses are viable. Some evidence, for example, suggests that Negro fetuses mature more quickly than white fetuses. If viability is the norm, the standard would vary with race and with many individual circumstances.

The most important objection to this approach is that dependence is not ended by viability. The fetus is still absolutely dependent on someone's care in order to continue existence; indeed a child of one or three or even five years of age is absolutely dependent on another's care for existence; uncared for, the older fetus or the younger child will die as surely as the early fetus detached from the mother. The unsubstantial lessening in dependence at viability does not seem to signify any special acquisition of humanity.

A second distinction has been attempted in terms of experience. A being who has had experience, has lived and suffered, who possesses memories, is more human than one who has not. Humanity depends on formation by experience. The fetus is thus "unformed" in the most basic human sense.

This distinction is not serviceable for the embryo which is already experiencing and reacting. The embryo is responsive to touch after eight weeks and at least at that point is experiencing. At an earlier stage the zygote is certainly alive and responding to its environment. The distinction may also be challenged by the rare case where aphasia has erased adult memory: has it erased humanity? More fundamentally, this distinction leaves even the older fetus or the younger child to be treated as an unformed inhuman thing. Finally, it is not clear why experience as such confers humanity. It could be argued that certain central experiences such as loving or learning are necessary to make a man human. But then human beings who have failed to love or to learn might be excluded from the class called man.

A third distinction is made by appeal to the sentiments of adults. If a fetus dies, the grief of the parents is not the grief they would have for a living child. The fetus is an unnamed "it" till birth, and is not perceived as personality until at least the fourth month of existence when movements in the womb manifest a vigorous presence demanding joyful recognition by the parents.

Yet feeling is notoriously an unsure guide to the humanity of others. Many groups of humans have had difficulty in feeling that persons of another tongue, color, religion, sex, are as human as they. Apart from reactions to alien groups, we mourn the loss of a ten-year-old boy more than the loss of his one-day-old brother or his 90-year-old grandfather. The difference felt and the grief expressed vary with the potentialities extinguished, or the experience wiped out; they do not seem to point to any substantial difference in the humanity of baby, boy, or grandfather.

Distinctions are also made in terms of sensation by the parents. The embryo is felt within the womb only after about the fourth month. The embryo is seen only at birth. What can be neither seen nor felt is different from what is tangible. If the fetus cannot be seen or touched at all, it cannot be perceived as man.

Yet experience shows that sight is even more untrustworthy than feeling in determining humanity. By sight, color became an appropriate index for saying who was a man, and the evil of racial discrimination was given foundation. Nor can touch provide the test; a being confined by sickness, "out of touch" with others, does not thereby seem to lose his humanity. To the extent that touch still has appeal as a criterion, it appears to be a survival of the old English idea of "quickening"—a possible mistranslation of the Latin *animatus* used in the canon law. To that extent touch as a criterion seems to be dependent on the Aristotelian notion of ensoulment, and to fall when this notion is discarded.

Finally, a distinction is sought in social visibility. The fetus is not socially perceived as human. It cannot communicate with others. Thus, both subjectively and objectively, it is not a member of society. As moral rules are rules for the behavior of members of society to each other, they cannot be made for behavior toward what is not yet a member. Excluded from the society of men, the fetus is excluded from the humanity of men.[2]

By force of the argument from the consequences, this distinction is to be rejected. It is more subtle than that founded on an appeal to physical sensation, but it is equally dangerous in its implications. If humanity depends on social recognition, individuals or whole groups may be dehumanized by being denied any status in their society. Such a fate is fictionally portrayed in *1984* and has actually been the lot of many men in many societies. In the Roman empire, for example, condemnation to slavery meant the practical denial of most human rights; in the Chinese Communist world, landlords have been classified as enemies of the people and so treated as nonpersons by the state. Humanity does not depend on social recognition, though often the failure of society to recognize the prisoner, the alien, the heterodox as human has led to the destruction of human beings. Anyone conceived by a man and a woman is human. Recognition of this condition by society follows a real event in the objective order, however imperfect and halting the recognition. Any attempt to limit humanity to exclude some group runs the risk of furnishing authority and precedent for excluding other groups in the name of the consciousness or perception of the controlling group in the society.

A philosopher may reject the appeal to the humanity of the fetus because he views "humanity" as a secular view of the soul and because he doubts the existence of anything real and objective which can be identified as humanity. One answer to such a philosopher is to ask how he reasons about moral questions without supposing that there is a sense in which he and the others of whom he speaks are human. Whatever group is taken as the society which determines who may be killed is thereby taken as human. A second answer is to ask if he does not believe that there is a right and wrong way of deciding moral questions. If there is such a difference, experience may be appealed to: to decide who is human on the basis of the sentiment of a given society has led to consequences which rational men would characterize as monstrous.

The rejection of the attempted distinctions based on viability and visibility, experience and feeling, may be buttressed by the following considerations: Moral judgments often rest on distinctions, but if the distinctions are not to appear arbitrary *fiat*, they should relate to some real difference in probabilities. There is a kind of continuity in all life, but the earlier stages of the elements of human life possess tiny probabilities of development. Consider, for example, the spermatozoa in any normal ejaculate: There are about 200,000,000

in any single ejaculate, of which one has a chance of developing into a zygote. Consider the oocytes which may become ova: there are 100,000 to 1,000,000 oocytes in a female infant, of which a maximum of 390 are ovulated. But once spermatozoon and ovum meet and the conceptus is formed, such studies as have been made show that roughly in only 20 percent of the cases will spontaneous abortion occur. In other words, the chances are about 4 out of 5 that this new being will develop. At this stage in the life of the being there is a sharp shift in probabilities, an immense jump in potentialities. To make a distinction between the rights of spermatozoa and the rights of the fertilized ovum is to respond to an enormous shift in possibilities. For about twenty days after conception the egg may split to form twins or combine with another egg to form a chimera, but the probability of either event happening is very small.

It may be asked, What does a change in biological probabilities have to do with establishing humanity? The argument from probabilities is not aimed at establishing humanity but at establishing an objective discontinuity which may be taken into account in moral discourse. As life itself is a matter of probabilities, as most moral reasoning is an estimate of probabilities, so it seems in accord with the structure of reality and the nature of moral thought to found a moral judgment on the change in probabilities at conception. The appeal to probabilities is the most commonsensical of arguments; to a greater or smaller degree all of us base our actions on probabilities, and in morals, as in law, prudence and negligence are often measured by the account one has taken of the probabilities. If the chance is 200,000,000 to 1 that the movement in the bushes into which you shoot is a man's, I doubt if many persons would hold you careless in shooting; but if the chances are 4 out of 5 that the movement is a human being's, few would acquit you of blame. Would the argument be different if only one out of ten children conceived came to term? Of course this argument would be different. This argument is an appeal to probabilities that actually exist, not to any and all states of affairs which may be imagined.

The probabilities as they do exist do not show the humanity of the embryo in the sense of a demonstration in logic any more than the probabilities of the movement in the bush being a man demonstrate beyond all doubt that the being is a man. The appeal is a "buttressing" consideration, showing the plausibility of the standard adopted. The argument focuses on the decisional factor in any moral judgment and assumes that part of the business of a moralist is drawing lines. One evidence of the nonarbitrary character of the line drawn is the difference of probabilities on either side of it. If a spermatozoon is destroyed, one destroys a being which had a chance of far less than 1 in 200 million of developing into a reasoning being, possessed of the genetic code, a heart and other organs, and capable of pain. If a fetus is destroyed, one destroys a being already possessed of the genetic code, organs, and sensitivity to pain, and one which had an 80 percent chance of developing further into a baby outside the womb who, in time, would reason.

The positive argument for conception as the decisive moment of humanization is that at conception the new being receives the genetic code. It is this genetic information which determines his characteristics, which is the biological carrier of the possibility of human wisdom, which makes him a self-evolving being. A being with a human genetic code is man.

This review of current controversy over the humanity of the fetus emphasizes what a fundamental question the theologians resolved in asserting the inviolability of the fetus. To regard the fetus as possessed of equal rights with other humans was not, however, to decide every case where abortion might be employed. It did decide the case where the argument was that the fetus should be aborted for its own good. To say a being was human was to say it had a destiny to decide for itself which could not be taken from it by another man's decision. But human beings with equal rights often come in conflict with each other, and some decision must be made as to whose claims are to prevail. Cases of conflict involving the fetus are different only in two respects: the total inability of the fetus to speak for itself and the fact that the right of the fetus regularly at stake is the right to life itself.

The approach taken by the theologians to these conflicts was articulated in terms of "direct" and "indirect." Again, to look at what they were doing from outside their categories, they may be said to have been drawing lines or "balancing values." "Direct" and "indirect" are spatial metaphors; "line-drawing" is another. "To weigh" or "to balance" values is a metaphor of a more complicated mathematical sort hinting at the process which goes on in moral judgments. All the metaphors suggest that, in the moral judgments made, comparisons were necessary that no value completely controlled. The principle of double effect was no doctrine fallen from heaven, but a method of analysis appropriate where two relative values were being compared. In Catholic moral theology, as it developed, life even of the innocent was not taken as an absolute. Judgments on acts affecting life issued from a process of weighing. In the weighing, the fetus was always given a value greater than zero, always a value separate and independent from its parents. The valuation was crucial and fundamental in all Christian thought on the subject and marked it off from any approach which considered that only the parents' interests needed to be considered.

Even with the fetus weighed as human, one interest could be weighed as equal or superior: that of the mother in her own life. The casuists between 1450 and 1895 were willing to weigh this interest as superior. Since 1895, that interest was given decisive weight only in the two special cases of the cancerous uterus and the ectopic pregnancy. In both of these cases the fetus itself had little chance of survival even if the abortion were not performed. As the balance was once struck in favor of the mother whenever her life was endangered, it could be so struck again. The balance reached between 1895 and 1930 attempted prudentially and pastorally to forestall a multitude of exceptions for interests less than life.

The perception of the humanity of the fetus and the weighing of fetal rights against other human rights constituted the work of the moral analysts. But what spirit animated their abstract judgments? For the Christian community it was the injunction of Scripture to love your neighbor as yourself. The fetus as human was a neighbor; his life had parity with one's own. The commandment gave life to what otherwise would have been only rational calculation.

The commandment could be put in humanistic as well as theological terms: Do not injure your fellow man without reason. In these terms, once the humanity of the fetus is perceived, abortion is never right except in self-defense. When life must be taken to save life, reason alone cannot say that a mother must prefer a child's life to her own. With this exception, now of great rarity, abortion violates the rational humanist tenet of the equality of human lives.

For Christians the commandment to love had received a special imprint in that the exemplar proposed of love was the love of the Lord for his disciples. In the light given by this example, self-sacrifice carried to the point of death seemed in the extreme situations not without meaning. In the less extreme cases, preference for one's own interests to the life of another seemed to express cruelty or selfishness irreconcilable with the demands of love.

NOTES

1. According to Glanville Williams (*The Sanctity of Human Life supra* n. 169, at 193), "The historical reason for the Catholic objection to abortion is the same as for the Christian Church's historical opposition to infanticide: the horror of bringing about the death of an unbaptized child." This statement is made without any citation of evidence. As has been seen, desire to administer baptism could, in the Middle Ages, even be urged as a reason for procuring an abortion. It is highly regrettable that the American Law Institute was apparently misled by Williams' account and repeated after him the same baseless statement. See American Law Institute, *Model Penal Code: Tentative Draft No. 9* (1959), p. 148, n. 12.

2. . . . Thomas Aquinas gave an analogous reason against baptizing a fetus in the womb: "As long as it exists in the womb of the mother, it cannot be subject to the operation of the ministers of the Church as it is not known to men" (*In sententias Petri Lombardi* 4.6 1.1.2).

JUDITH JARVIS THOMSON

A Defense of Abortion[1]

Most opposition to abortion relies on the premise that the fetus is a human being, a person, from the moment of conception. The premise is argued for, but, as I think, not well. Take, for example, the most common argument. We are asked to notice that the development of a human being from conception through birth into childhood is continuous; then it is said that to draw a line, to choose a point in this development and say "before this point the thing is not a person, after this point it is a person" is to make an arbitrary choice, a choice for which in the nature of things no good reason can be given. It is concluded that the fetus is, or anyway that we had better say it is, a person from the moment of conception. But this conclusion does not follow. Similar things might be said about the development of an acorn into an oak tree, and it does not follow that acorns are oak trees, or that we had better say they are. Arguments of this form are sometimes called "slippery slope arguments"—the phrase is perhaps self-explanatory—and it is dismaying that opponents of abortion rely on them so heavily and uncritically.

I am inclined to agree, however, that the prospects for "drawing a line" in the development of the fetus look dim. I am inclined to think also that we shall probably have to agree that the fetus has already become a human person well before birth. Indeed, it comes as a surprise when one first learns how early in its life it begins to acquire human characteristics. By the tenth week, for example, it already has a face, arms and legs, fingers and toes; it has internal organs, and brain activity is detectable.[2] On the other hand, I think that the premise is false, that the fetus is not a person from the moment of conception. A newly fertilized ovum, a newly implanted clump of cells, is no more a person than an acorn is an oak tree. But I shall not discuss any of this. For it seems to me to be of great interest to ask what happens if, for the sake of argument, we allow the premise. How, precisely, are we supposed to get from there to the conclusion that abortion is morally impermissible? Opponents of abortion commonly spend most of their time establishing that the fetus is a person, and hardly any time explaining the step from there to the impermissibility of abortion. Perhaps they think the step too simple and obvious to require much comment. Or perhaps instead they are simply being economical in argument. Many of those who defend abortion rely on the premise that

Reprinted with permission of the publisher from *Philosophy and Public Affairs*, Vol. 1, No. 1 (1971), pp. 47–66. Copyright © 1971 by Princeton University Press.

the fetus is not a person, but only a bit of tissue that will become a person at birth; and why pay out more arguments than you have to? Whatever the explanation, I suggest that the step they take is neither easy nor obvious, that it calls for closer examination than it is commonly given, and that when we do give it this closer examination we shall feel inclined to reject it.

I propose, then, that we grant that the fetus is a person from the moment of conception. How does the argument go from here? Something like this, I take it. Every person has a right to life. So the fetus has a right to life. No doubt the mother has a right to decide what shall happen in and to her body; everyone would grant that. But surely a person's right to life is stronger and more stringent than the mother's right to decide what happens in and to her body, and so outweighs it. So the fetus may not be killed; an abortion may not be performed.

It sounds plausible. But now let me ask you to imagine this. You wake up in the morning and find yourself back to back in bed with an unconscious violinist. A famous unconscious violinist. He has been found to have a fatal kidney ailment, and the Society of Music Lovers has canvassed all the available medical records and found that you alone have the right blood type to help. They have therefore kidnapped you, and last night the violinist's circulatory system was plugged into yours, so that your kidneys can be used to extract poisons from his blood as well as your own. The director of the hospital now tells you, "Look, we're sorry the Society of Music Lovers did this to you—we would never have permitted it if we had known. But still, they did it, and the violinist now is plugged into you. To unplug you would be to kill him. But never mind, it's only for nine months. By then he will have recovered from his ailment, and can safely be unplugged from you." Is it morally incumbent on you to accede to this situation? No doubt it would be very nice of you if you did, a great kindness. But do you *have* to accede to it? What if it were not nine months, but nine years? Or longer still? What if the director of the hospital says, "Tough luck, I agree, but you've now got to stay in bed, with the violinist plugged into you, for the rest of your life. Because remember this. All persons have a right to life, and violinists are persons. Granted you have a right to decide what happens in and to your body, but a person's right to life outweighs your right to decide what happens in and to your body. So you cannot ever be

unplugged from him." I imagine you would regard this as outrageous, which suggests that something really is wrong with that plausible-sounding argument I mentioned a moment ago.

In this case, of course, you were kidnapped; you didn't volunteer for the operation that plugged the violinist into your kidneys. Can those who oppose abortion on the ground I mentioned make an exception for a pregnancy due to rape? Certainly. They can say that persons have a right to life only if they didn't come into existence because of rape; or they can say that all persons have a right to life, but that some have less of a right to life than others, in particular, that those who came into existence because of rape have less. But these statements have a rather unpleasant sound. Surely the question of whether you have a right to life at all, or how much of it you have, shouldn't turn on the question of whether or not you are the product of a rape. And in fact the people who oppose abortion on the ground I mentioned do not make this distinction, and hence do not make an exception in case of rape.

Nor do they make an exception for a case in which the mother has to spend the nine months of her pregnancy in bed. They would agree that would be a great pity, and hard on the mother; but all the same, all persons have a right to life, the fetus is a person, and so on. I suspect, in fact, that they would not make an exception for a case in which, miraculously enough, the pregnancy went on for nine years, or even the rest of the mother's life.

Some won't even make an exception for a case in which continuation of the pregnancy is likely to shorten the mother's life; they regard abortion as impermissible even to save the mother's life. Such cases are nowadays very rare, and many opponents of abortion do not accept this extreme view. All the same, it is a good place to begin: a number of points of interest come out in respect to it.

1. Let us call the view that abortion is impermissible even to save the mother's life "the extreme view." I want to suggest first that it does not issue from the argument I mentioned earlier without the addition of some fairly powerful premises. Suppose a woman has become pregnant, and now learns that she has a cardiac condition such that she will die if she carries the baby to term. What may be done for her? The fetus, being a person, has a right to life, but as the mother is a person too, so has she a right to life. Presumably they have an equal right to life. How is it supposed to come out that an abortion may not be performed? If mother and child have an equal right to life, shouldn't we

perhaps flip a coin? Or should we add to the mother's right to life her right to decide what happens in and to her body, which everybody seems to be ready to grant—the sum of her rights now outweighing the fetus's right to life?

The most familiar argument here is the following. We are told that performing the abortion would be directly killing[3] the child, whereas doing nothing would not be killing the mother, but only letting her die. Moreover, in killing the child, one would be killing an innocent person, for the child has committed no crime, and is not aiming at his mother's death. And then there are a variety of ways in which this might be continued. (a) But as directly killing an innocent person is always and absolutely impermissible, an abortion may not be performed. Or, (b) as directly killing an innocent person is murder, and murder is always and absolutely impermissible, an abortion may not be performed.[4] Or, (c) as one's duty to refrain from directly killing an innocent person is more stringent than one's duty to keep a person from dying, an abortion may not be performed. Or, (d) if one's only options are directly killing an innocent person or letting a person die, one must prefer letting the person die, and thus an abortion may not be performed.[5]

Some people seem to have thought that these are not further premises which must be added if the conclusion is to be reached, but that they follow from the very fact that an innocent person has a right to life.[6] But this seems to me to be a mistake, and perhaps the simplest way to show this is to bring out that while we must certainly grant that innocent persons have a right to life, the theses in (a) through (d) are all false. Take (b), for example. If directly killing an innocent person is murder, and thus is impermissible, then the mother's directly killing the innocent person inside her is murder, and thus is impermissible. But it cannot seriously be thought to be murder if the mother performs an abortion on herself to save her life. It cannot seriously be said that she *must* refrain, that she *must* sit passively by and wait for her death. Let us look again at the case of you and the violinist. There you are, in bed with the violinist, and the director of the hospital says to you, "It's all most distressing, and I deeply sympathize, but you see this is putting an additional strain on your kidneys, and you'll be dead within the month. But you *have* to stay where you are all the same. Because unplugging you would be directly killing an innocent violinist, and that's murder, and that's impermissible." If anything in the world is true, it is that you do not commit murder, you do not do what is impermissible,

if you reach around to your back and unplug yourself from that violinist to save your life.

The main focus of attention in writings on abortion has been on what a third party may or may not do in answer to a request from a woman for an abortion. This is in a way understandable. Things being as they are, there isn't much a woman can safely do to abort herself. So the question asked is what a third party may do, and what the mother may do, if it is mentioned at all, is deduced, almost as an afterthought, from what it is concluded that third parties may do. But it seems to me that to treat the matter in this way is to refuse to grant to the mother that very status of person which is so firmly insisted on for the fetus. For we cannot simply read off what a person may do from what a third party may do. Suppose you find yourself trapped in a tiny house with a growing child. I mean a very tiny house, and a rapidly growing child—you are already up against the wall of the house and in a few minutes you'll be crushed to death. The child on the other hand won't be crushed to death; if nothing is done to stop him from growing he'll be hurt, but in the end he'll simply burst open the house and walk out a free man. Now I could well understand it if a bystander were to say, "There's nothing we can do for you. We cannot choose between your life and his, we cannot be the ones to decide who is to live, we cannot intervene." But it cannot be concluded that you too can do nothing, that you cannot attack it to save your life. However innocent the child may be, you do not have to wait passively while it crushes you to death. Perhaps a pregnant woman is vaguely felt to have the status of house, to which we don't allow the right of self-defense. But if the woman houses the child, it should be remembered that she is a person who houses it.

I should perhaps stop to say explicitly that I am not claiming that people have a right to do anything whatever to save their lives. I think, rather, that there are drastic limits to the right of self-defense. If someone threatens you with death unless you torture someone else to death, I think you have not the right, even to save your life, to do so. But the case under consideration here is very different. In our case there are only two people involved, one whose life is threatened, and one who threatens it. Both are innocent: the one who is threatened is not threatened because of any fault, the one who threatens does not threaten because of any fault. For this reason we may feel that we bystanders cannot intervene. But the person threatened can.

In sum, a woman surely can defend her life against the threat to it posed by the unborn child, even if doing so involves its death. And this shows not merely that the theses in (a) through (d) are false; it shows also that the extreme view of abortion is false, and so we need not canvass any other possible ways of arriving at it from the argument I mentioned at the outset.

2. The extreme view could of course be weakened to say that while abortion is permissible to save the mother's life, it may not be performed by a third party, but only by the mother herself. But this cannot be right either. For what we have to keep in mind is that the mother and the unborn child are not like two tenants in a small house which has, by an unfortunate mistake, been rented to both: the mother *owns* the house. The fact that she does adds to the offensiveness of deducing that the mother can do nothing from the supposition that third parties can do nothing. But it does more than this: it casts a bright light on the supposition that third parties can do nothing. Certainly it lets us see that a third party who says "I cannot choose between you" is fooling himself if he thinks this is impartiality. If Jones has found and fastened on a certain coat, which he needs to keep him from freezing, but which Smith also needs to keep him from freezing, then it is not impartiality that says "I cannot choose between you" when Smith owns the coat. Women have said again and again "This body is *my* body!" and they have reason to feel angry, reason to feel that it has been like shouting into the wind. Smith, after all, is hardly likely to bless us if we say to him, "Of course it's your coat, anybody would grant that it is. But no one may choose between you and Jones who is to have it."

We should really ask what it is that says "no one may choose" in the face of the fact that the body that houses the child is the mother's body. It may be simply a failure to appreciate this fact. But it may be something more interesting, namely, the sense that one has a right to refuse to lay hands on people, even where it would be just and fair to do so, even where justice seems to require that somebody do so. Thus justice might call for somebody to get Smith's coat back from Jones, and yet you have a right to refuse to be the one to lay hands on Jones, a right to refuse to do physical violence to him. This, I think, must be granted. But then what should be said is not "no one may choose," but only "*I* cannot choose," and indeed not even this, but "*I* will not *act*," leaving it open that somebody else can or should, and in particular that anyone in a posi-

tion of authority, with the job of securing people's rights, both can and should. So this is no difficulty. I have not been arguing that any given third party must accede to the mother's request that he perform an abortion to save her life, but only that he may.

I suppose that in some views of human life the mother's body is only on loan to her, the loan not being one which gives her any prior claim to it. One who held this view might well think it impartiality to say "I cannot choose." But I shall simply ignore this possibility. My own view is that if a human being has any just, prior claim to anything at all, he has a just, prior claim to his own body. And perhaps this needn't be argued for here anyway, since, as I mentioned, the arguments against abortion we are looking at do grant that the woman has a right to decide what happens in and to her body.

But although they do grant it, I have tried to show that they do not take seriously what is done in granting it. I suggest the same thing will reappear even more clearly when we turn away from cases in which the mother's life is at stake, and attend, as I propose we now do, to the vastly more common cases in which a woman wants an abortion for some less weighty reason than preserving her own life.

3. Where the mother's life is not at stake, the argument I mentioned at the outset seems to have a much stronger pull. "Everyone has a right to life, so the unborn person has a right to life." And isn't the child's right to life weightier than anything other than the mother's own right to life, which she might put forward as ground for an abortion?

This argument treats the right to life as if it were unproblematic. It is not, and this seems to me to be precisely the source of the mistake.

For we should now, at long last, ask what it comes to, to have a right to life. In some views having a right to life includes having a right to be given at least the bare minimum one needs for continued life. But suppose that what in fact *is* the bare minimum a man needs for continued life is something he has no right at all to be given. If I am sick unto death, and the only thing that will save my life is the touch of Henry Fonda's cool hand on my fevered brow, then all the same, I have no right to be given the touch of Henry Fonda's cool hand on my fevered brow. It would be frightfully nice of him to fly in from the West Coast to provide it. It would be less nice, though no doubt well meant, if my friends flew out to the West Coast and carried Henry Fonda back with them. But I have no right at all against anybody that he should do this for me. Or again, to return to the story I told earlier, the fact that for continued life that violinist needs the continued use of your kidneys does not establish that he has a right to be given the continued use of your kidneys. He certainly has no right against you that *you* should give him continued use of your kidneys. For nobody has any right to use your kidneys unless you give him such a right; and nobody has the right against you that you shall give him this right—if you do allow him to go on using your kidneys, this is a kindness on your part, and not something he can claim from you as his due. Nor has he any right against anybody else that *they* should give him continued use of your kidneys. Certainly he had no right against the Society of Music Lovers that they should plug him into you in the first place. And if you now start to unplug yourself, having learned that you will otherwise have to spend nine years in bed with him, there is nobody in the world who must try to prevent you, in order to see to it that he is given something he has a right to be given.

Some people are rather stricter about the right to life. In their view, it does not include the right to be given anything, but amounts to, and only to, the right not to be killed by anybody. But here a related difficulty arises. If everybody is to refrain from killing that violinist, then everybody must refrain from doing a great many different sorts of things. Everybody must refrain from slitting his throat, everybody must refrain from shooting him—and everybody must refrain from unplugging you from him. But does he have a right against everybody that they shall refrain from unplugging you from him? To refrain from doing this is to allow him to continue to use your kidneys. It could be argued that he has a right against us that *we* should allow him to continue to use your kidneys. That is, while he had no right against us that we should give him the use of your kidneys, it might be argued that he anyway has a right against us that we shall not now intervene and deprive him of the use of your kidneys. I shall come back to third-party interventions later. But certainly the violinist has no right against you that *you* shall allow him to continue to use your kidneys. As I said, if you do allow him to use them, it is a kindness on your part, and not something you owe him.

The difficulty I point to here is not peculiar to the right to life. It reappears in connection with all the other natural rights; and it is something which an adequate account of rights must deal with. For present purposes it is enough just to draw attention to it. But I would stress that I am not arguing that people do not have a right to life—quite to the contrary, it seems to

me that the primary control we must place on the acceptability of an account of rights is that it should turn out in that account to be a truth that all persons have a right to life. I am arguing only that having a right to life does not guarantee having either a right to be given the use of or a right to be allowed continued use of another person's body—even if one needs it for life itself. So the right to life will not serve the opponents of abortion in the very simple and clear way in which they seem to have thought it would.

4. There is another way to bring out the difficulty. In the most ordinary sort of case, to deprive someone of what he has a right to is to treat him unjustly. Suppose a boy and his small brother are jointly given a box of chocolates for Christmas. If the older boy takes the box and refuses to give his brother any of the chocolates, he is unjust to him, for the brother has been given a right to half of them. But suppose that, having learned that otherwise it means nine years in bed with that violinist, you unplug yourself from him. You surely are not being unjust to him for you gave him no right to use your kidneys, and no one else can have given him any such right. But we have to notice that in unplugging yourself, you are killing him; and violinists, like everybody else, have a right to life, and thus in the view we were considering just now, the right not to be killed. So here you do what he supposedly has a right you shall not do, but you do not act unjustly to him in doing it.

The emendation which may be made at this point is this: the right to life consists not in the right not to be killed, but rather in the right not to be killed unjustly. This runs a risk of circularity, but never mind: it would enable us to square the fact that the violinist has a right to life with the fact that you do not act unjustly toward him in unplugging yourself, thereby killing him. For if you do not kill him unjustly, you do not violate his right to life, and so it is no wonder you do him no injustice.

But if this emendation is accepted, the gap in the argument against abortion stares us plainly in the face: It is by no means enough to show that the fetus is a person, and to remind us that all persons have a right to life—we need to be shown also that killing the fetus violates its right to life, i.e., that abortion is unjust killing. And is it?

I suppose we may take it as a datum that in a case of pregnancy due to rape the mother has not given the unborn person a right to the use of her body for food and shelter. Indeed, in what pregnancy could it be supposed that the mother has given the unborn person such a right? It is not as if there were unborn persons drifting about the world, to whom a woman who wants a child says "I invite you in."

But it might be argued that there are other ways one can have acquired a right to the use of another person's body than by having been invited to use it by that person. Suppose a woman voluntarily indulges in intercourse, knowing of the chance it will issue in pregnancy, and then she does become pregnant; is she not in part responsible for the presence, in fact the very existence, of the unborn person inside her? No doubt she did not invite it in. But doesn't her partial responsibility for its being there itself give it a right to the use of her body?[7] If so, then her aborting it would be more like the boy's taking away the chocolates, and less like your unplugging yourself from the violinist—doing so would be depriving it of what it does have a right to, and thus would be doing it an injustice.

And then, too, it might be asked whether or not she can kill it even to save her own life: If she voluntarily called it into existence, how can she now kill it, even in self-defense?

The first thing to be said about this is that it is something new. Opponents of abortion have been so concerned to make out the independence of the fetus, in order to establish that it has a right to life, just as its mother does, that they have tended to overlook the possible support they might gain from making out that the fetus is *dependent* on the mother, in order to establish that she has a special kind of responsibility for it, a responsibility that gives it rights against her which are not possessed by any independent person—such as an ailing violinist who is a stranger to her.

On the other hand, this argument would give the unborn person a right to its mother's body only if her pregnancy resulted from a voluntary act, undertaken in full knowledge of the chance a pregnancy might result from it. It would leave out entirely the unborn person whose existence is due to rape. Pending the availability of some further argument, then, we would be left with the conclusion that unborn persons whose existence is due to rape have no right to the use of their mothers' bodies, and thus that aborting them is not depriving them of anything they have a right to and hence is not unjust killing.

And we should also notice that it is not at all plain that this argument really does go even as far as it purports to. For there are cases and cases, and the details make a difference. If the room is stuffy, and I therefore open a window to air it, and a burglar climbs in, it would be absurd to say, "Ah, now he can stay, she's given him a right to the use of her house—for she is partially responsible for his presence there, having voluntarily done what enabled him to get in, in full knowledge that there are such things as burglars, and that burglars burgle." It would be still more absurd to say this if I had had bars installed outside my windows, precisely to prevent burglars from getting in, and a burglar got in only because of a defect in the bars. It remains equally absurd if we imagine it is not a burglar who climbs in, but an innocent person who blunders or falls in. Again, suppose it were like this: people-seeds drift about in the air like pollen, and if you open your windows, one may drift in and take root in your carpets or upholstery. You don't want children, so you fix up your windows with fine mesh screens, the very best you can buy. As can happen, however, and on very, very rare occasions does happen, one of the screens is defective; and a seed drifts in and takes root. Does the person-plant who now develops have a right to the use of your house? Surely not—despite the fact that you voluntarily opened your windows, you knowingly kept carpets and upholstered furniture, and you knew that screens were sometimes defective. Someone may argue that you are responsible for its rooting, that it does have a right to your house, because after all you *could* have lived out your life with bare floors and furniture, or with sealed windows and doors. But this won't do—for by the same token anyone can avoid a pregnancy due to rape by having a hysterectomy, or anyway by never leaving home without a (reliable!) army.

It seems to me that the argument we are looking at can establish at most that there are *some* cases in which the unborn person has a right to the use of its mother's body, and therefore *some* cases in which abortion is unjust killing. There is room for much discussion and argument as to precisely which, if any. But I think we should sidestep this issue and leave it open, for at any rate the argument certainly does not establish that all abortion is unjust killing.

5. There is room for yet another argument here, however. We surely must all grant that there may be cases in which it would be morally indecent to detach a person from your body at the cost of his life. Suppose you learn that what the violinist needs is not nine years of your life, but only one hour: All you need do to save his life is to spend one hour in that bed with him.

Suppose also that letting him use your kidneys for that one hour would not affect your health in the slightest. Admittedly you were kidnapped. Admittedly you did not give anyone permission to plug him into you. Nevertheless it seems to me plain you *ought* to allow him to use your kidneys for that hour—it would be indecent to refuse.

Again, suppose pregnancy lasted only an hour, and constituted no threat to life or health. And suppose that a woman becomes pregnant as a result of rape. Admittedly she did not voluntarily do anything to bring about the existence of a child. Admittedly she did nothing at all which would give the unborn person a right to the use of her body. All the same it might well be said, as in the newly emended violinist story, that she *ought* to allow it to remain for that hour—that it would be indecent in her to refuse.

Now some people are inclined to use the term "right" in such a way that it follows from the fact that you ought to allow a person to use your body for the hour he needs, that he has a right to use your body for the hour he needs, even though he has not been given that right by any person or act. They may say that it follows also that if you refuse, you act unjustly toward him. This use of the term is perhaps so common that it cannot be called wrong; nevertheless it seems to me to be an unfortunate loosening of what we would do better to keep a tight rein on. Suppose that box of chocolates I mentioned earlier had not been given to both boys jointly, but was given only to the older boy. There he sits, stolidly eating his way through the box, his small brother watching enviously. Here we are likely to say "You ought not to be so mean. You ought to give your brother some of those chocolates." My own view is that it just does not follow from the truth of this that the brother has any right to any of the chocolates. If the boy refuses to give his brother any, he is greedy, stingy, callous—but not unjust. I suppose that the people I have in mind will say it does follow that the brother has a right to some of the chocolates, and thus that the boy does act unjustly if he refuses to give his brother any. But the effect of saying this is to obscure what we should keep distinct, namely the difference between the boy's refusal in this case and the boy's refusal in the earlier case, in which the box was given to both boys jointly, and in which the small brother thus had what was from any point of view clear title to half.

A further objection to so using the term "right" that from the fact that A ought to do a thing for B, it follows that B has a right against A that A do it for him, is that it is going to make the question of whether or not a man has a right to a thing turn on how easy it is to provide him with it; and this seems not merely unfortunate, but morally unacceptable. Take the case of Henry Fonda again. I said earlier that I had no right to the touch of his cool hand on my fevered brow, even though I needed it to save my life. I said it would be frightfully nice of him to fly in from the West Coast to provide me with it, but that I had no right against him that he should do so. But suppose he isn't on the West Coast. Suppose he has only to walk across the room, place a hand briefly on my brow—and lo, my life is saved. Then surely he ought to do it, it would be indecent to refuse. Is it to be said "Ah well, it follows that in this case she has a right to the touch of his hand on her brow, and so it would be an injustice in him to refuse"? So that I have a right to it when it is easy for him to provide it, though no right when it's hard? It's rather a shocking idea that anyone's rights should fade away and disappear as it gets harder and harder to accord them to him.

So my own view is that even though you ought to let the violinist use your kidneys for the one hour he needs, we should not conclude that he has a right to do so—we would say that if you refuse, you are, like the boy who owns all the chocolates and will give none away, self-centered and callous, indecent in fact, but not unjust. And similarly, that even supposing a case in which a woman pregnant due to rape ought to allow the unborn person to use her body for the hour he needs, we should not conclude that he has a right to do so; we should conclude that she is self-centered, callous, indecent, but not unjust, if she refuses. The complaints are no less grave; they are just different. However, there is no need to insist on this point. If anyone does wish to deduce "he has a right" from "you ought," then all the same he must surely grant that there are cases in which it is not morally required of you that you allow that violinist to use your kidneys, and in which he does not have a right to use them, and in which you do not do him an injustice if you refuse. And so also for mother and unborn child. Except in such cases as the unborn person has a right to demand it—and we were leaving open the possibility that there may be such cases—nobody is morally *required* to make large sacrifices, of health, of all other interests and concerns, of all other duties and commitments, for nine years, or even for nine months, in order to keep another person alive.

6. We have in fact to distinguish between two kinds of Samaritan: the Good Samaritan and what we might call the Minimally Decent Samaritan. The story of the Good Samaritan, you will remember, goes like this:

A certain man went down from Jerusalem to Jericho, and fell among thieves, which stripped him of his raiment, and wounded him, and departed, leaving him half dead.

And by chance there came down a certain priest that way; and when he saw him, he passed by on the other side.

And likewise a Levite, when he was at the place, came and looked on him, and passed by on the other side.

But a certain Samaritan, as he journeyed, came where he was; and when he saw him he had compassion on him.

And went to him, and bound up his wounds, pouring in oil and wine, and set him on his own beast, and brought him to an inn, and took care of him.

And on the morrow, when he departed, he took out two pence, and gave them to the host, and said unto him, "Take care of him; and whatsoever thou spendest more, when I come again, I will repay thee."

(Luke 10:30–35)

The Good Samaritan went out of his way, at some cost to himself, to help one in need of it. We are not told what the options were, that is, whether or not the priest and the Levite could have helped by doing less than the Good Samaritan did, but assuming they could have, then the fact they did nothing at all shows they were not even Minimally Decent Samaritans, not because they were not Samaritans, but because they were not even minimally decent.

These things are a matter of degree, of course, but there is a difference, and it comes out perhaps most clearly in the story of Kitty Genovese, who, as you will remember, was murdered while thirty-eight people watched or listened, and did nothing at all to help her. A Good Samaritan would have rushed out to give direct assistance against the murderer. Or perhaps we had better allow that it would have been a Splendid Samaritan who did this, on the ground that it would have involved a risk of death for himself. But the thirty-eight not only did not do this, they did not even trouble to pick up a phone to call the police. Minimally Decent Samaritanism would call for doing at least that, and their not having done it was monstrous.

After telling the story of the Good Samaritan, Jesus said, "Go, and do thou likewise." Perhaps he meant that we are morally required to act as the Good Samaritan did. Perhaps he was urging people to do more than is morally required of them. At all events it seems plain that it was not morally required of any of the thirty-eight that he rush out to give direct assistance at the risk of his own life, and that it is not morally required of anyone that he give long stretches of his life—nine years or nine months—to sustaining the life of a person who has no special right (we were leaving open the possibility of this) to demand it.

Indeed, with one rather striking class of exceptions, no one in any country in the world is *legally* required to do anywhere near as much as this for anyone else. The class of exceptions is obvious. My main concern here is not the state of the law in respect to abortion, but it is worth drawing attention to the fact that in no state in this country is any man compelled by law to be even a Minimally Decent Samaritan to any person; there is no law under which charges could be brought against the thirty-eight who stood by while Kitty Genovese died. By contrast, in most states in this country women are compelled by law to be not merely Minimally Decent Samaritans, but Good Samaritans to unborn persons inside them. This doesn't by itself settle anything one way or the other, because it may well be argued that there should be laws in this country—as there are in many European countries—compelling at least Minimally Decent Samaritanism.[8] But it does show that there is a gross injustice in the existing state of the law. And it shows also that the groups currently working against liberalization of abortion laws, in fact working toward having it declared unconstitutional for a state to permit abortion, had better start working for the adoption of Good Samaritan laws generally, or earn the charge that they are acting in bad faith.

I should think, myself, that Minimally Decent Samaritan laws would be one thing, Good Samaritan laws quite another, and in fact highly improper. But we are not here concerned with the law. What we should ask is not whether anybody should be compelled by law to be a Good Samaritan, but whether we must accede to a situation in which somebody is being compelled—by nature, perhaps—to be a Good Samaritan. We have, in other words, to look now at third-party interventions. I have been arguing that no person is morally required to make large sacrifices to sustain the life of another who has no right to demand them, and this even where the sacrifices do not include life itself; we are not morally required to be Good Samaritans or anyway Very Good Samaritans to one another. But what if a man cannot extricate himself from such a situation? What if he appeals to us to extricate him? It seems to me plain that there are cases in which we can, cases in which a Good Samaritan would extricate him. There you are, you were kidnapped, and nine years in bed with that violinist lie ahead of you. You have your own life to lead. You are sorry, but you simply cannot see giving up so much of your life to the sustaining of his. You cannot extricate yourself, and ask us to do so. I should have thought that—in light of his having no right to the use of your body—it was obvious that we do not have to accede to your being forced to give up so much. We can do what you ask. There is no injustice to the violinist in our doing so.

7. Following the lead of the opponents of abortion, I have throughout been speaking of the fetus merely as a person, and what I have been asking is whether or not the argument we began with, which proceeds only from the fetus's being a person, really does establish its conclusion. I have argued that it does not.

But of course there are arguments and arguments, and it may be said that I have simply fastened on the wrong one. It may be said that what is important is not merely the fact that the fetus is a person, but that it is a person for whom the woman has a special kind of responsibility issuing from the fact that she is its mother. And it might be argued that all my analogies are therefore irrelevant—for you do not have that special kind of responsibility for that violinist, Henry Fonda does not have that special kind of responsibility for me. And our attention might be drawn to the fact that men and women both *are* compelled by law to provide support for their children.

I have in effect dealt (briefly) with this argument in section 4 above; but a (still briefer) recapitulation now may be in order. Surely we do not have any such "special responsibility" for a person unless we have assumed it, explicitly or implicitly. If a set of parents do not try to prevent pregnancy, do not obtain an abortion, and then at the time of birth of the child do not put it out for adoption, but rather take it home with them, then they have assumed responsibility for it, they have given it rights, and they cannot *now* withdraw support from it at the cost of its life because they now find it difficult to go on providing for it. But if they have taken all reasonable precautions against having a child, they do not simply by virtue of their biological relationship to the child who comes into existence have a special responsibility for it. They may wish to assume responsibility for it, or they may not wish to. And I am suggesting that if assuming responsibility for it would require large sacrifices, then they may refuse. A Good Samaritan would not refuse—or anyway, a Splendid Samaritan, if the sacrifices that

had to be made were enormous. But then so would a Good Samaritan assume responsibility for that violinist; so would Henry Fonda, if he is a Good Samaritan, fly in from the West Coast and assume responsibility for me.

8. My argument will be found unsatisfactory on two counts by many of those who want to regard abortion as morally permissible. First, while I do argue that abortion is not impermissible, I do not argue that it is always permissible. There may well be cases in which carrying the child to term requires only Minimally Decent Samaritanism of the mother, and this is a standard we must not fall below. I am inclined to think it a merit of my account precisely that it does *not* give a general yes or a general no. It allows for and supports our sense that, for example, a sick and desperately frightened fourteen-year-old schoolgirl, pregnant due to rape, may *of course* choose abortion, and that any law which rules this out is an insane law. And it also allows for and supports our sense that in other cases resort to abortion is even positively indecent. It would be indecent in the woman to request an abortion, and indecent in a doctor to perform it, if she is in her seventh month and wants the abortion just to avoid the nuisance of postponing a trip abroad. The very fact that the arguments I have been drawing attention to treat all cases of abortion, or even all cases of abortion in which the mother's life is not at stake, as morally on a par ought to have made them suspect at the outset.

Secondly, while I am arguing for the permissibility of abortion in some cases, I am not arguing for the right to secure the death of the unborn child. It is easy to confuse these two things in that up to a certain point in the life of the fetus it is not able to survive outside the mother's body; hence removing it from her body guarantees its death. But they are importantly different. I have argued that you are not morally required to spend nine months in bed, sustaining the life of that violinist; but to say this is by no means to say that if, when you unplug yourself, there is a miracle and he survives, you then have a right to turn round and slit his throat. You may detach yourself even if this costs him his life; you have no right to be guaranteed his death, by some other means, if unplugging yourself does not kill him. There are some people who will feel dissatisfied by this feature of my argument. A woman may be utterly devastated by the thought of a child, a bit of herself, put out for adoption and never seen or heard of again. She may therefore want not merely that the child be detached from her, but more, that it die. Some opponents of abortion are inclined to regard this as beneath contempt—thereby showing insensitivity to what is surely a powerful source of despair. All the same, I agree that the desire for the child's death is not one which anybody may gratify, should it turn out to be possible to detach the child alive.

At this place, however, it should be remembered that we have only been pretending throughout that the fetus is a human being from the moment of conception. A very early abortion is surely not the killing of a person, and so is not dealt with by anything I have said here.

NOTES

1. I am very much indebted to James Thomson for discussion, criticism, and many helpful suggestions.

2. Daniel Callahan, *Abortion: Law, Choice and Morality* (New York, 1970), p. 373. This book gives a fascinating survey of the available information on abortion. The Jewish tradition is surveyed in David M. Feldman, *Birth Control in Jewish Law* (New York, 1968), Part 5; the Catholic tradition in John T. Noonan, Jr., "An Almost Absolute Value in History," in *The Morality of Abortion*, ed. John T. Noonan, Jr. (Cambridge, Mass., 1970).

3. The term "direct" in the arguments I refer to is a technical one. Roughly, what is meant by "direct killing" is either killing as an end in itself, or killing as a means to some end, for example, the end of saving someone else's life. See note 6, below, for an example of its use.

4. Cf. *Encyclical Letter of Pope Pius XI on Christian Marriage*, St. Paul Editions (Boston, n.d.), p. 32: "however much we may pity the mother whose health and even life is gravely imperiled in the performance of the duty allotted to her by nature, nevertheless what could ever be a sufficient reason for excusing in any way the direct murder of the innocent? This is precisely what we are dealing with here." Noonan (*The Morality of Abortion*, p. 43) reads this as follows: "What cause can ever avail to excuse in any way the direct killing of the innocent? For it is a question of that."

5. The thesis in (d) is in an interesting way weaker than those in (a), (b), and they rule out abortion even in cases in which both mother *and* child will die if the abortion is not performed. By contrast, one who held the view expressed in (d) could consistently say that one needn't prefer letting two persons die to killing one.

6. Cf. the following passage from Pius XII, *Address to the Italian Catholic Society of Midwives*: "The baby in the maternal breast has the right to life immediately from God.—Hence there is no man, no human authority, no science, no medical eugenic, social, economic or moral 'indication' which can establish or grant a valid juridical ground for a direct deliberate disposition of an innocent human life, that is a disposition which looks to its destruction either as an end or as a means to another end perhaps in itself not illicit.—The baby, still not born, is a man in the same degree and for the same reason as the mother" (quoted in Noonan, *The Morality of Abortion*, p. 45).

7. The need for a discussion of this argument was brought home to me by members of the Society for Ethical and Legal Philosophy, to whom this paper was originally presented.

8. For a discussion of the difficulties involved, and a survey of the European experience with such laws, see *The Good Samaritan and the Law*, ed. James M. Ratcliffe (New York, 1966).

BARUCH BRODY

The Morality of Abortion*

THE WOMAN'S RIGHT TO HER BODY

It is a common claim that a woman ought to be in control of what happens to her body to the greatest extent possible, that she ought to be able to use her body in ways that she wants to and refrain from using it in ways that she does not want to. This right is particularly pressed where certain uses of her body have deep and lasting effects upon the character of her life, personal, social, and economic. Therefore, it is argued, a woman should be free either to carry her fetus to term, thereby using her body to support it, or to abort the fetus, thereby not using her body for that purpose.

In some contexts in which this argument is advanced, it is clear that it is not addressed to the issue of the morality of abortion at all. Rather, it is made in opposition to laws against abortion on the ground that the choice to abort or not is a moral decision that should belong only to the mother. But that specific direction of the argument is irrelevant to our present purposes; I will consider it [later] when I deal with the

From *Abortion and the Sanctity of Human Life: A Philosophical View* (Cambridge, Mass.: MIT Press, 1975), pp. 26–32, 37–39, 44–47, 123–129, 131, and "Fetal Humanity and the Theory of Essentialism," in *Philosophy and Sex*, Robert Baker and Frederick Elliston, eds. (Buffalo, N.Y.: Prometheus Books, 1975), pp. 348–352. (Some parts of these essays were later revised by Professor Brody.) Reprinted by permission.

Ed. note: This selection from the writings of Professor Brody is divided into five sections. Section 1 discusses whether abortions can be justified on the grounds that the woman owns her own body if the fetus is a human being. Section 2 discusses whether abortions can be justified by a wide variety of special circumstances if the fetus is a human being. Both sections conclude that on this assumption abortions cannot be justified. Section 3 justifies the claim that, from an early stage after conception, the fetus is a human being. The last two sections discuss the implications of this position for the law, focusing on a criticism of the Supreme Court's opinion.

issues raised by laws prohibiting abortions. For the moment, I am concerned solely with the use of this principle as a putative ground tending to show the permissibility of abortion, with the claim that because it is the woman's body that carries the fetus and upon which the fetus depends, she has certain rights to abort the fetus that no one else may have.

We may begin by remarking that it is obviously correct that, as carrier of the fetus, the mother has it within her power to choose whether or not to abort the fetus. And, as an autonomous and responsible agent, she must make this choice. But let us notice that this in no way entails either that whatever choice she makes is morally right or that no one else has the right to evaluate the decision that she makes.

• • •

At first glance, it would seem that this argument cannot be used by anyone who supposes, as we do for the moment, that there is a point in fetal development from which time on the fetus is a human being. After all, people do not have the right to do anything whatsoever that may be necessary for them to retain control over the uses of their bodies. In particular, it would seem wrong for them to kill another human being in order to do so.

In a recent article,[1] Professor Judith Thomson has, in effect, argued that this simple view is mistaken. How does Professor Thomson defend her claim that the mother has a right to abort the fetus, even if it is a human being, whether or not her life is threatened and whether or not she has consented to the act of intercourse in which the fetus is conceived? At one point,[2] discussing just the case in which the mother's life is threatened, she makes the following suggestion:

In [abortion], there are only two people involved, one whose life is threatened and one who threatens it. Both are innocent: the one who is threatened is not threatened because of any fault, the one who threatens does not threaten because of any fault. For this reason, we may feel that we bystanders cannot intervene. But the person threatened can.

But surely this description is equally applicable to the following case: *A* and *B* are adrift on a lifeboat, *B* has a disease that he can survive, but *A*, if he contracts it, will die, and the only way that *A* can avoid that is by killing *B* and pushing him overboard. Surely, *A* has no right to do this. So there must be some special reason why the mother has, if she does, the right to abort the fetus.

There is, to be sure, an important difference between our lifeboat case and abortion, one that leads us to the heart of Professor Thomson's argument. In the case that we envisaged, both *A* and *B* have equal rights to be in the lifeboat, but the mother's body is hers and not the fetus's and she has first rights to its use. The primacy of these rights allow an abortion whether or not her life is threatened. Professor Thomson summarizes this argument in the following way:[3]

I am arguing only that having a right to life does not guarantee having either a right to be given the use of, or a right to be allowed continued use of, another person's body—even if one needs it for life itself.

One part of this claim is clearly correct. I have no duty to *X* to save *X*'s life by giving him the use of my body (or my life savings, or the only home I have, and so on), and *X* has no right, even to save his life, to any of those things. Thus, the fetus conceived in the laboratory that will perish unless it is implanted into a woman's body has in fact no right to any woman's body. But this portion of the claim is irrelevant to the abortion issue, for in abortion of the fetus that is a human being the mother must kill *X* to get back the sole use of her body, and that is an entirely different matter.

This point can also be put as follows: . . . we must distinguish the taking of *X*'s life from the saving of *X*'s life, even if we assume that one has a duty not to do the former and to do the latter. Now that latter duty, if it exists at all, is much weaker than the first duty; many circumstances may relieve us from the latter duty that will not relieve us from the former one. Thus, I am

certainly relieved from my duty to save *X*'s life by the fact that fulfilling it means the loss of my life savings. It may be noble for me to save *X*'s life at the cost of everything I have, but I certainly have no duty to do that. And the same observation may be made about cases in which I can save *X*'s life by giving him the use of my body for an extended period of time. However, I am not relieved of my duty not to take *X*'s life by the fact that fulfilling it means the loss of everything I have and not even by the fact that fulfilling it means the loss of my life. . . .

At one point in her paper, Professor Thomson does consider this objection. She has previously imagined the following case: a famous violinist, who is dying from a kidney ailment, has been, without your consent, plugged into you for a period of time so that his body can use your kidneys:

Some people are rather stricter about the right to life. In their view, it does not include the right to be given anything, but amounts to, and only to, the right not to be killed by anybody. But here a related difficulty arises. If everybody is to refrain from killing that violinist, then everybody must refrain from doing a great many different sorts of things . . . everybody must refrain from unplugging you from him. But does he have a right against everybody that they shall refrain from unplugging you from him? To refrain from doing this is to allow him to continue to use your kidneys . . . certainly the violinist has no right against you that you shall allow him to continue to use your kidneys.

Applying this argument to the case of abortion, we can see that Professor Thomson's argument would run as follows:

    a. Assume that the fetus's right to life includes the right not to be killed by the woman carrying him.
    b. But to refrain from killing the fetus is to allow him the continued use of the woman's body.
    c. So our first assumption entails that the fetus's right to life includes the right to the continued use of the woman's body.
    d. But we all grant that the fetus does not have the right to the continued use of the woman's body.
    e. Therefore, the fetus's right to life cannot include the right not to be killed by the woman in question.

And it is also now clear what is wrong with this argument. When we granted that the fetus has no right to the continued use of the woman's body, all that we meant was that he does not have this right merely because the continued use saves his life. But, of course, there may be other reasons why he has this right. One would be that the only way to take the use of the woman's body away from the fetus is by killing him, and that is something that neither she nor we have the right to do. So, I submit, the way in which Assumption d is true is irrelevant, and cannot be used by Professor Thomson, for Assumption d is true only in cases where the saving of the life of the fetus is at stake and not in cases where the taking of his life is at stake.

I conclude therefore that Professor Thomson has not established the truth of her claims about abortion, primarily because she has not sufficiently attended to the distinction between our duty to save X's life and our duty not to take it. Once one attends to that distinction, it would seem that the mother, in order to regain control over her body, has no right to abort the fetus from the point at which it becomes a human being.

It may also be useful to say a few words about the larger and less rigorous context of the argument that the woman has a right to her own body. It is surely true that one way in which women have been oppressed is by their being denied authority over their own bodies. But it seems to me that, as the struggle is carried on for meaningful amelioration of such oppression, it ought not to be carried so far that it violates the steady responsibilities all people have to one another. Parents may not desert their children, one class may not oppress another, one race or nation may not exploit another. For parents, powerful groups in society, races or nations in ascendancy, there are penalties for refraining from these wrong actions, but those penalties can in no way be taken as the justification for such wrong actions. Similarly, if the fetus is a human being, the penalty of carrying it cannot, I believe, be used as the justification for destroying it.

• • •

THE MODEL PENAL CODE CASES

All of the arguments that we have looked at so far are attempts to show that there is something special about abortion that justifies its being treated differently from other cases of the taking of human life. We shall now consider claims that are confined to certain special cases of abortion: the case in which the mother has been raped, the case in which bearing the child would be harmful to her health, and the case in which having the child may cause a problem for the rest of her family (the latter case is a particular case of the societal

argument). In addressing these issues, we shall see whether there is any point to the permissibility of abortions in some of the cases covered by the Model Penal Code[4] proposals.

When the expectant mother has conceived after being raped, there are two different sorts of considerations that might support the claim that she has the right to take the life of the fetus. They are the following: (A) the woman in question has already suffered immensely from the act of rape and the physical and/or psychological aftereffects of that act. It would be particularly unjust, the argument runs, for her to have to live through an unwanted pregnancy owing to that act of rape. Therefore, even if we are at a stage at which the fetus is a human being, the mother has the right to abort it; (B) the fetus in question has no right to be in that woman. It was put there as a result of an act of aggression upon her by the rapist, and its continued presence is an act of aggression against the mother. She has a right to repel that aggression by aborting the fetus.

The first argument is very compelling. We can all agree that a terrible injustice has been committed on the woman who is raped. The question that we have to consider, however, is whether it follows that it is morally permissible for her to abort the fetus. We must make that consideration reflecting that, however unjust the act of rape, it was not the fetus who committed or commissioned it. The injustice of the act, then, should in no way impinge upon the rights of the fetus, for it is innocent. What remains is the initial misfortune of the mother (and the injustice of her having to pass through the pregnancy, and, further, to assume responsibility of at least giving the child over for adoption or assuming the burden of its care). However unfortunate that circumstance, however unjust, the misfortune and the injustice are not sufficient cause to justify the taking of the life of an innocent human being as a means of mitigation.

It is at this point that Argument B comes in, for its whole point is that the fetus, by its mere presence in the mother, is committing an act of aggression against her, one over and above the one committed by the rapist, and one that the mother has a right to repel by abortion. But . . . (1) the fetus is certainly innocent (in the sense of not responsible) for any act of aggression against the mother and . . . (2) the mere presence of the fetus in the mother, no matter how unfortunate for her, does not constitute an act of aggression by the fetus against the mother. Argument B fails then at just that point at which Argument A needs its support, and we can therefore conclude that the fact that pregnancy is the result of rape does not give the mother the right to abort the fetus.

We turn next to the case in which the continued existence of the fetus would threaten the mental and/or physical health but not necessarily the life of the mother. Again, . . . the fact that the fetus's continued existence poses a threat to the life of the mother does not justify her aborting it.* It would seem to be true, a fortiori, that the fact that the fetus's continued existence poses a threat to the mental and/or physical health of the mother does not justify her aborting it either.

We come finally to those cases in which the continuation of the pregnancy would cause serious problems for the rest of the family. There are a variety of cases that we have to consider here together. Perhaps the health of the mother will be affected in such a way that she cannot function effectively as a wife and mother during, or even after, the pregnancy. Or perhaps the expenses incurred as a result of the pregnancy would be utterly beyond the financial resources of the family. The important point is that the continuation of the pregnancy raises a serious problem for other innocent people involved besides the mother and the fetus, and it may be argued that the mother has the right to abort the fetus to avoid that problem.

By now, the difficulties with this argument should be apparent. We have seen earlier that the mere fact that the continued existence of the fetus threatens to harm the mother does not, by itself, justify the aborting of the fetus. Why should anything be changed by the fact that the threatened harm will accrue to the other members of the family and not to the mother? Of course, it would be different if the fetus were committing an act of aggression against the other members of the family. But, once more, this is certainly not the case.

We conclude, therefore, that none of these special circumstances justifies an abortion from that point at which the fetus is a human being.

• • •

FETAL HUMANITY AND BRAIN FUNCTION

The question which we must now consider is the question of fetal humanity. Some have argued that the fetus is a human being with a right to life (or, for convenience, just a human being) from the moment of conception. Others have argued that the fetus only becomes a human being at the moment of birth. Many positions in between these two extremes have also been suggested. How are we to decide which is correct?

The analysis which we will propose here rests upon certain metaphysical assumptions which I have defended elsewhere. These assumptions are: (a) the question is when has the fetus acquired all the properties essential (necessary) for being a human being, for when it has, it is a human being; (b) these properties are such that the loss of any one of them means that the human being in question has gone out of existence and not merely stopped being a human being; (c) human beings go out of existence when they die. It follows from these assumptions that the fetus becomes a human being when it acquires all those characteristics which are such that the loss of any one of them would result in the fetus's being dead. We must, therefore, turn to the analysis of death.

• • •

We will first consider the question of what properties are essential to being human if we suppose that death and the passing out of existence occur only if there has been an irreparable cessation of brain function (keeping in mind that that condition itself, as we have noted, is a matter of medical judgment). We shall then consider the same question on the supposition that [Paul] Ramsey's more complicated theory of death (the modified traditional view) is correct.

*Ed. note: Professor Brody provided a lengthy argument to this effect in a chapter not here excerpted. His summary of that argument is as follows: "Is it permissible, as an act of killing a pursuer, to abort the fetus in order to save the mother? The first thing that we should note is that Pope Pius's objection to aborting the fetus as a permissible act of killing a pursuer is mistaken. His objection is that the fetus shows no knowledge or intention in his attempt to take the life of the mother, that the fetus is, in a word, innocent. But that only means that the condition of guilt is not satisfied, and we have seen that its satisfaction is not necessary.

"Is, then, the aborting of the fetus, when necessary to save the life of the mother, a permissible act of killing a pursuer? It is true that in such cases the fetus is a danger to the mother. But it is also clear that the condition of attempt is not satisfied. The fetus has neither the beliefs nor the intention to which we have referred. Furthermore, there is on the part of the fetus no action that threatens the life of the mother. So not even the condition of action is satisfied. It seems to follow, therefore, that aborting the fetus could not be a permissible act of killing a pursuer."

According to what is called the brain-death theory, as long as there has not been an irreparable cessation of brain function the person in question continues to exist, no matter what else has happened to him. If so, it seems to follow that there is only one property—leaving aside those entailed by this one property—that is essential to humanity, namely, the possession of a brain that has not suffered an irreparable cessation of function.

Several consequences follow immediately from this conclusion. We can see that a variety of often advanced claims about the essence of humanity are false. For example, the claim that movement, or perhaps just the ability to move, is essential for being human is false. A human being who has stopped moving, and even one who has lost the ability to move, has not therefore stopped existing. Being able to move, and a fortiori moving, are not essential properties of human beings and therefore are not essential to being human. Similarly, the claim that being perceivable by other human beings is essential for being human is also false. A human being who has stopped being perceivable by other humans (for example, someone isolated on the other side of the moon, out of reach even of radio communication) has not stopped existing. Being perceivable by other human beings is not an essential property of human beings and is not essential to being human. And the same point can be made about the claims that viability is essential for being human, that independent existence is essential for being human, and that actual interaction with other human beings is essential for being human. The loss of any of these properties would not mean that the human being in question had gone out of existence, so none of them can be essential to that human being and none of them can be essential for being human.

Let us now look at the following argument: (1) A functioning brain (or at least, a brain that, if not functioning, is susceptible of function) is a property that every human being must have because it is essential for being human. (2) By the time an entity acquires that property, it has all the other properties that are essential for being human. Therefore, when the fetus acquires that property it becomes a human being. It is clear that the property in question is, according to the brain-death theory, one that is had essentially by all human beings. The question that we have to consider is whether the second premise is true. It might appear that its truth does follow from the brain-death theory. After all, we did see that the theory entails that only one property (together with those entailed by it) is

essential for being human. Nevertheless, rather than relying solely on my earlier argument, I shall adopt an alternative approach to strengthen the conviction that this second premise is true: I shall note the important ways in which the fetus resembles and differs from an ordinary human being by the time it definitely has a functioning brain (about the end of the sixth week of development). It shall then be evident, in light of our theory of essentialism, that none of these differences involves the lack of some property in the fetus that is essential for its being human.

Structurally, there are few features of the human being that are not fully present by the end of the sixth week. Not only are the familiar external features and all the internal organs present, but the contours of the body are nicely rounded. More important, the body is functioning. Not only is the brain functioning, but the heart is beating sturdily (the fetus by this time has its own completely developed vascular system), the stomach is producing digestive juices, the liver is manufacturing blood cells, the kidney is extracting uric acid from the blood, and the nerves and muscles are operating in concert, so that reflex reactions can begin.

What are the properties that a fetus acquires after the sixth week of its development? Certain structures do appear later. These include the fingernails (which appear in the third month), the completed vocal chords (which also appear then), taste buds and salivary glands (again, in the third month), and hair and eyelashes (in the fifth month). In addition, certain functions begin later than the sixth week. The fetus begins to urinate (in the third month), to move spontaneously (in the third month), to respond to external stimuli (at least in the fifth month), and to breathe (in the sixth month). Moreover, there is a constant growth in size. And finally, at the time of birth the fetus ceases to receive its oxygen and food through the placenta and starts receiving them through the mouth and nose.

I will not examine each of these properties (structures and functions) to show that they are not essential for being human. The procedure would be essentially the one used previously to show that various essentialist claims are in error. We might, therefore, conclude, on the supposition that the brain-death theory is correct, that the fetus becomes a human being about the end of the sixth week after its development.

There is, however, one complication that should be noted here. There are, after all, progressive stages in the physical development and in the functioning of the brain. For example, the fetal brain (and nervous system) does not develop sufficiently to support spontaneous motion until some time in the third month after conception. There is, of course, no doubt that that stage of development is sufficient for the fetus to be human. No one would be likely to maintain that a spontaneously moving human being has died; and similarly, a spontaneously moving fetus would seem to have become human. One might, however, want to claim that the fetus does not become a human being until the point of spontaneous movement. So then, on the supposition that the brain-death theory of death is correct, one ought to conclude that the fetus becomes a human being at some time between the sixth and twelfth week after its conception.

But what if we reject the brain-death theory, and replace it with its equally plausible contender, Ramsey's theory of death? According to that theory—which we can call the brain, heart, and lung theory of death—the human being does not die, does not go out of existence, until such time as the brain, heart and lungs have irreparably ceased functioning naturally. What are the essential features of being human according to this theory?

Actually, the adoption of Ramsey's theory requires no major modifications. According to that theory, what is essential to being human, what each human being must retain if he is to continue to exist, is the possession of a functioning (actually or potentially) heart, lung, or brain. It is only when a human being possesses none of these that he dies and goes out of existence; and the fetus comes into humanity, so to speak, when he acquires one of these.

On Ramsey's theory, the argument would now run as follows: (1) The property of having a functioning brain, heart, or lungs (or at least organs of the kind that, if not functioning, are susceptible of function) is one that every human being must have because it is essential for being human. (2) By the time that an entity acquires that property it has all the other properties that are essential for being human. Therefore, when the fetus acquires that property it becomes a human being. There remains, once more, the problem of the second premise. Since the fetal heart starts operating rather early, it is not clear that the second premise is correct. Many systems are not yet operating, and many structures are not yet present. Still, following our theory of essentialism, we should conclude that the fetus becomes a human being when it acquires a functioning heart (the first of the organs to function in the fetus).

There is, however, a further complication here, and it is analogous to the one encountered if we adopt the brain-death theory: When may we properly say that the fetal heart begins to function? At two weeks, when occasional contractions of the primitive fetal heart are present? In the fourth to fifth week, when the heart, although incomplete, is beating regularly and pumping blood cells through a closed vascular system, and when the tracings obtained by an ECG exhibit the classical elements of an adult tracing? Or after the end of the seventh week, when the fetal heart is functionally complete and "normal"?

We have not reached a precise conclusion in our study of the question of when the fetus becomes a human being. We do know that it does so some time between the end of the second week and the end of the third month. But it surely is not a human being at the moment of conception and it surely is one by the end of the third month. Though we have not come to a final answer to our question, we have narrowed the range of acceptable answers considerably.

[In summary] we have argued that the fetus becomes a human being with a right to life some time between the second and twelfth week after conception. We have also argued that abortions are morally impermissible after that point except in rather unusual circumstances. What is crucial to note is that neither of these arguments appeal to any theological considerations. We conclude, therefore, that there is a human-rights basis for moral opposition to abortions.

• • •

LAW AND SOCIETY IN A DEMOCRACY

Before turning to such considerations, however, we must first examine several important assertions about law and society that, if true, would justify the joint assertion of the principles that abortion is murder but nevertheless should be or remain legal. The first is the assertion that citizens of a pluralistic society must forgo the use of the law as a method of enforcing what are their private moralities. It might well be argued that in our pluralistic society, in which there are serious disagreements about the status of the fetus and about the rightness and wrongness of abortion in consequence, it would be wrong (or inappropriate) to legislate against abortion.

Such assertions about a pluralistic society are difficult to evaluate because of their imprecision. So let us first try to formulate some version of them more carefully. Consider the following general principle: Principle [1]. When the citizens of a society strongly disagree about the rightness and wrongness of a given action, and a considerable number think that such an action is right (or, at least, permissible), then it is wrong (or inappropriate) for that society to prohibit that action by law, even if the majority of citizens believe such an action to be wrong.

There are a variety of arguments that can be offered in support of the principle. One appeals to the right of the minority to follow its own conscience rather than being compelled to follow the conscience of the majority. That right has a theoretical political justification, but it also is practically implicit in the inappropriateness in the members of the majority imposing this kind of enforcement upon the minority that would be opposed were they the minority and were the enforcement being imposed upon them. Another argument appeals to the detrimental consequences to a society of the sense on the part of a significant minority that the law is being used by the majority to coerce. Such considerations make it seem that a principle like [1] is true.

If Principle [1] is true, it is easy to offer a defense of the joint assertion of the principles that abortion is murder but nevertheless should be or remain legal. All we need are the additional obvious assumptions that the citizens of our society strongly disagree about the morality of abortion and that at least a significant minority of individuals believe that there are many cases in which abortion is permissible. From these assumptions and Principle [1] it follows that abortions should be or remain legal even if they are murders.

The trouble with this argument is that it depends upon Principle [1]. I agree that, because of the considerations mentioned already, something like Principle [1] must be true. But Principle [1] as formulated is much too broad to be defensible. Consider, after all, a society in which a significant number of citizens think that it is morally permissible, and perhaps even obligatory, to kill Blacks or Jews, for example, because they are seen as being something less than fully human. It would seem to follow from Principle [1] that the law should not prohibit such actions. Surely this consequence of Principle [1] is wrong. Even if a pluralistic society should forgo passing many laws out of deference to the views of those who think that the actions

that would thereby be prevented are not wrong, there remain some cases in which the force of the law should be applied because of the evil of the actions it is intended to prevent. If such actions produce very harmful results and infringe upon the rights of a sufficiently large number of individuals, then the possible benefits that may be derived from passing and enforcing a law preventing those actions may well override the rights of the minority (or even of the majority) to follow its conscience.

Principle [1] must therefore be modified as follows: Principle [2]. When the citizens of a society strongly disagree about the rightness and wrongness of a given action, and a considerable number think that such an action is right (or, at least, permissible), then it is wrong (or inappropriate) for that society to prohibit that action by law, even if the majority of citizens believe such an action to be wrong, unless the action in question is so evil that the desirability of legal prohibition outweighs the desirability of granting to the minority the right to follow its own conscience.

Principle [2] is, of course, rather vague. In particular, its last clause needs further clarification. But Principle [2] is clear enough for us to see that it cannot be used to justify the joint assertibility of the principles that abortion is murder but should nevertheless be or remain legal. Principle [2], conjoined with the obvious truths that the citizens of our society strongly disagree about the rightness and wrongness of abortion and that a significant number of citizens believe that, in certain circumstances, the right (or, at least, a permissible) thing to do is to have an abortion, does not yield the conclusion that abortion should be or remain legal if abortion is murder. After all, if abortion is murder, then the action in question is the unjustifiable taking of a human life and may well fall under the last clause of Principle [2]. The destruction of a fetus may not be unlike the killing of a Black or Jew. They may all be cases of the unjust taking of a human life.

• • •

THE DECISION IN *ROE V. WADE*

Two decisions were announced by the [United States Supreme] Court on January 22 [1973]. The first (*Roe v. Wade*) involved a challenge to a Texas law prohibiting all abortions not necessary to save the life of the mother. The second (*Doe v. Bolton*) tested a Georgia law incorporating many of the recommendations of the Model Penal Code as to the circumstances under which abortion should be allowed (in the case of rape and of a defective fetus, as well as when the pregnancy threatens the life or health of the mother), together with provisions regulating the place where abortions can be performed, the number of doctors that must concur, and other factors.

Of these two decisions, the more fundamental was *Roe v. Wade*. It was in this case that the Court came to grips with the central legal issue, namely, the extent to which it is legitimate for the state to prohibit or regulate abortion. In *Doe v. Bolton*, the Court was more concerned with subsidiary issues involving the legitimacy of particular types of regulations.

The Court summarized its decision in *Roe v. Wade* as follows:[5]

(a) For the stage prior to approximately the end of the first trimester/three months the abortion decision and its effectuation must be left to the medical judgment of the pregnant woman's attending physician.

(b) For the stage subsequent to approximately the end of the first trimester, the state, in promoting its interest in the health of the mother, may, if it chooses, regulate the abortion procedure in ways that are reasonably related to maternal health.

(c) For the stage subsequent to viability, the state, in promoting its interest in the potentiality of human life, may, if it chooses, regulate, and even proscribe, abortion except where it is necessary, in appropriate medical judgment, for the preservation of the life or health of the mother.

In short, the Court ruled that abortion can be prohibited only after viability and then only if the life or health of the mother is not threatened. Before viability, abortions cannot be prohibited, but they can be regulated after the first trimester if the regulations are reasonably related to maternal health. This last clause is taken very seriously by the Court. In *Doe v. Bolton*, instances of regulation in the Georgia code were found unconstitutional on the ground that they were not reasonably related to maternal health.

How did the Court arrive at this decision? In Sections V and VII of the decision, it set out the claims on both sides. Jane Roe's argument was summarized in these words:[6]

The principal thrust of appellant's attack on the Texas statutes is that they improperly invade a right, said to be possessed by the pregnant woman, to choose to terminate her pregnancy.

On the other hand, the Court saw as possible legitimate interests of the state the regulation of abortion, like other medical procedures, so as to ensure maximum safety for the patient and the protection of prenatal life. At this point in the decision, the Court added the following very significant remark:[7]

Logically, of course, a legitimate state interest in this area need not stand or fall on acceptance of the belief that life begins at conception or at some other point prior to live birth. In assessing the state's interest, recognition may be given to the less rigid claim that as long as at least potential life is involved, the state may assert interests beyond the protection of the pregnant woman alone.

In Sections VIII to X, the Court stated its conclusion. It viewed this case as one presenting a conflict of interests, and it saw itself as weighing these interests. It began by agreeing that the woman's right to privacy did encompass her right to decide whether or not to terminate her pregnancy. But it argued that this right is not absolute, since the state's interests must also be considered:[8]

We therefore conclude that the right of personal privacy includes the abortion decision, but that this right is not unqualified and must be considered against important state interests in regulation.

The Court had no hesitation in ruling that the woman's right can be limited after the first trimester because of the state's interest in preserving and protecting maternal health. But the Court was less prepared to agree that the woman's right can be limited because of the state's interest in protecting prenatal life. Indeed, the Court rejected Texas's strong claim that life begins at conception, and that the state therefore has a right to protect such life by prohibiting abortion. The first reason advanced for rejecting that claim was phrased in this way:[9]

We need not resolve the difficult question of when life begins. When those trained in the respective disciplines of medicine, philosophy, and theology are unable to arrive at any consensus, the judiciary, at this point in the development of man's knowledge, is not in a position to speculate as to the answer.

Its second reason was that[10]

In areas other than criminal abortion, the law has been reluctant to endorse any theory that life, as we recognize it, begins before live birth or to accord legal rights to the unborn except in narrowly defined situations and except when the rights are contingent upon live birth.

The Court accepted the weaker claim that the state has an interest in protecting the potential of life. But when does that interest become compelling enough to enable the state to prohibit abortion? The Court said:[11]

. . . the compelling point is at viability. This is so because the fetus then has the capacity of meaningful life outside the mother's womb. State regulation protective of fetal life after viability thus has both logical and biological justifications. If the state is interested in protecting fetal life after viability, it may go so far as to proscribe abortion during that period except where it is necessary to preserve the life or health of the mother.

THE COURT ON POTENTIAL LIFE

I want to begin by considering that part of the Court's decision that allows Texas to proscribe abortions after viability so as to protect its interest in potential life. I note that it is difficult to evaluate that important part of the decision because the Court had little to say in defense of it other than the paragraph just quoted.

There are three very dubious elements of this ruling:

1. Why is the state prohibited from proscribing abortions when the life or health of the mother is threatened? Perhaps the following argument may be offered in the case of threat to maternal life: the mother is actually alive but the fetus is only potentially alive, and the protection of actual life takes precedence over the protection of potential life. Even if we grant this argument, why is the state prevented from prohibiting abortion when only maternal health is threatened? What is the argument against the claim that protecting potential life takes precedence in that case?

2. Why does the interest in potential life become compelling only when the stage of viability is reached? The Court's whole argument for this claim is[12]

This is so because the fetus then presumably has the capacity of meaningful life outside the mother's womb.

There is, no doubt, an important type of potential for life, the capacity of meaningful life outside the mother's womb, that the fetus acquires only at the time of viability. But there are other types of potential for life that it acquires earlier. At conception, for example, the fertilized cell has the potential for life in the sense that it will, in the normal course of events, develop into a human being. A six-week-old fetus has the potential for life in the stronger sense that all of the major organs it needs for life are already functioning. Why then does the state's interest in protecting potential life become compelling only at the point of viability? The Court failed to answer that question.

3. It can fairly be said that those trained in the respective disciplines of medicine, philosophy, and theology are unlikely to be able to arrive at any consensus on the question of when the fetus becomes potentially alive and when the state's interest in protecting this potential life becomes compelling enough to outweigh the rights of the mother. Why then did not the Court conclude, as it did when it considered the question of fetal humanity, that the judiciary cannot rule on such a question?

In pursuit of this last point, we approach the Court's more fundamental arguments against prohibiting abortion before viability.

THE COURT ON ACTUAL LIFE

The crucial claim in the Court's decision is that laws prohibiting abortion cannot be justified on the ground that the state has an interest in protecting the life of the fetus who is a human being. The Court offered two reasons for this claim: that the law has never yet accorded the fetus this status, and that the matter of fetal humanity is not one about which it is appropriate for the courts to speculate.

The first of the Court's reasons is not particularly strong. Whatever force we want to ascribe to precedent in the law, the Court has in the past modified its previous decisions in light of newer information and insights. In a matter as important as the conflict between the fetus's right to life and the rights of the mother, it would have seemed particularly necessary to deal with the issues rather than relying upon precedent.

In its second argument, the Court did deal with those issues by adopting the following principle:

1. It is inappropriate for the Court to speculate about the answer to questions about which relevant

professional specialists cannot arrive at a consensus. This principle seems irrelevant. The issue before the Court was whether the Texas legislature could make a determination in light of the best available evidence and legislate on the basis of it. Justice White, in his dissent, raised this point:[13]

The upshot is that the people and legislatures of the fifty states are constitutionally disentitled to weigh the relative importance of the continued existence and development of the fetus on the one hand against the spectrum of possible impacts on the mother on the other hand.

This objection could be met, however, if we modified the Court's principle in the following way:

2. It is inappropriate for a legislature to write law upon the basis of its best belief when the relevant professional specialists cannot agree that that belief is correct.

On the basis of such a principle, the Court could argue that Texas had no right to protect by law the right of the fetus to life, thereby acknowledging it to be a human being with such a right, because the relevant specialists do not agree that the fetus has that right. As it stands, however, Principle 2 is questionable. In a large number of areas, legislatures regularly do (and must) act upon issues upon which there is a wide diversity of opinion among professional specialists. So Principle 2 has to be modified to deal with only certain cases, and the obvious suggestion is:

3. It is inappropriate for the legislature, on the ground of belief, to write law in such a way as to violate the basic rights of some individuals, when professional specialists do not agree that that belief is correct.

This principle could be used to defend the Court's decision. But is there any reason to accept it as true? Two arguments for this principle immediately suggest themselves: (a) If the relevant professional specialists do not agree, then there cannot be any proof that the answer in question is the correct one. But a legislature should not infringe the rights of people on the basis of unproved belief. (b) When the professional specialists do not agree, there must be legitimate and reasonable alternatives of belief, and we ought to respect the rights of believers in each of these alternatives to act on their own judgments.

• • •

We have already discussed . . . the principles that lie behind these arguments. We saw . . . that neither of these arguments, as applied to abortion, is acceptable if the fetus is a human being. To employ these arguments correctly, the Court must presuppose that the fetus is not a human being. And that, of course, it cannot do, since the aim of its logic is the view that courts and legislatures, at least at this juncture, should remain neutral on the issue of fetal humanity.

There is a second point that should be noted about Principles 1 to 3. There are cases in which, by failing to deal with an issue, an implicit, inevitable decision is in fact reached. We have before us such a case. The Court was considering Texas's claim that it had the right to prohibit abortion in order to protect the fetus. The Court conceded that if the fetus had a protectable right to life, Texas could prohibit abortions. But when the Court concluded that it (and, by implication, Texas) could not decide whether the fetus is a human being with the right to life, Texas was compelled to act as if the fetus had no such right that Texas could protect. Why should Principles like 1 to 3 be accepted if the result is the effective endorsement of one disputed claim over another?[14]

There is an alternative to the Court's approach. It is that each of the legislatures should consider the vexing problems surrounding abortions, weigh all of the relevant fractors, and write law on the basis of its conclusions. The legislature would, undoubtedly, have to consider the question of fetal humanity, but, I submit, the Court is wrong in supposing that there is a way in which that question can be avoided.

• • •

CONCLUSION

The Supreme Court has ruled, and the principal legal issues in this country are, at least for now, resolved. I have tried to show, however, that the Court's ruling was in error, that it failed to grapple with the crucial issues surrounding the laws prohibiting abortion. The serious public debate about abortion must, and certainly will, continue.

NOTES

1. J. Thomson, "A Defense of Abortion," *Philosophy and Public Affairs*, Vol. 1 (1971), pp. 47–66.

2. *Ibid.*, p. 53.

3. *Ibid.*, p. 56.

4. On the Model Penal Code provisions, see American Law Institute, *Model Penal Code*: Tentative Draft No. 9 (1959).

5. *Roe v. Wade*, 41 *LW* 4229.

6. *Roe*, 41 *LW* 4218.

7. *Roe*, 41 *LW* 4224.

8. *Roe*, 41 *LW* 4226.

9. *Roe*, 41 *LW* 4227.

10. *Roe*, 41 *LW* 4228.

11. *Roe*, 41 *LW* 4228–4229.

12. *Ibid.*

13. *Roe*, 41 *LW* 4246.

14. This argument is derived from one used (for very different purposes) by William James in *The Will to Believe*, reprinted in William James, *The Will to Believe and Other Essays on Popular Philosophy* (New York: Dover, 1956), pp. 1–31.

MARY ANNE WARREN

On the Moral and Legal Status of Abortion

We will be concerned with both the moral status of abortion, which for our purposes we may define as the act which a woman performs in voluntarily terminating, or allowing another person to terminate, her pregnancy, and the legal status which is appropriate for this act. I will argue that, while it is not possible to produce a satisfactory defense of a woman's right to obtain an abortion without showing that a fetus is not a human being, in the morally relevant sense of that term, we ought not to conclude that the difficulties involved in determining whether or not a fetus is human make it impossible to produce any satisfactory solution to the problem of the moral status of abortion. For it is possible to show that, on the basis of intuitions which we may expect even the opponents of abortion to share, a fetus is not a person, and hence not the sort of entity to which it is proper to ascribe full moral rights.

Of course, while some philosophers would deny the possibility of any such proof,[1] others will deny that there is any need for it, since the moral permissibility of abortion appears to them to be too obvious to require proof. But the inadequacy of this attitude should be evident from the fact that both the friends and the foes of abortion consider their position to be morally self-evident. Because proabortionists have never adequately come to grips with the conceptual issues surrounding abortion, most, if not all, of the arguments which they advance in opposition to laws restricting access to abortion fail to refute or even weaken the traditional antiabortion argument, i.e., that a fetus is a human being, and therefore abortion is murder.

These arguments are typically of one of two sorts. Either they point to the terrible side effects of the restrictive laws, e.g., the deaths due to illegal abortions, and the fact that it is poor women who suffer the most as a result of these laws, or else they state that to deny a woman access to abortion is to deprive her of her right to control her own body. Unfortunately, however, the fact that restricting access to abortion has tragic side effects does not, in itself, show that the restrictions are unjustified, since murder is wrong regardless of the consequences of prohibiting it; and the appeal to the right to control one's body, which is generally construed as a property right, is at best a rather feeble argument for the permissibility of abortion. Mere ownership does not give me the right to kill innocent people whom I find on my property, and indeed I am apt to be held responsible if such people injure themselves while on my property. It is equally unclear that I have any moral right to expel an innocent person from my property when I know that doing so will result in his death.

Furthermore, it is probably inappropriate to describe a woman's body as her property, since it seems natural to hold that a person is something distinct from her property, but not from her body. Even those who

Reprinted from *The Monist*, Vol. 57, No. 1 (January 1973) with the permission of the publisher. Copyright © 1973, *The Monist*.

would object to the identification of a person with his body, or with the conjunction of his body and his mind, must admit that it would be very odd to describe, say, breaking a leg, as damaging one's property, and much more appropriate to describe it as injuring one*self*. Thus it is probably a mistake to argue that the right to obtain an abortion is in any way derived from the right to own and regulate property.

But however we wish to construe the right to abortion, we cannot hope to convince those who consider abortion a form of murder of the existence of any such right unless we are able to produce a clear and convincing refutation of the traditional antiabortion argument, and this has not, to my knowledge, been done. With respect to the two most vital issues which that argument involves, i.e., the humanity of the fetus and its implication for the moral status of abortion, confusion has prevailed on both sides of the dispute.

Thus, both proabortionists and antiabortionists have tended to abstract the question of whether abortion is wrong to that of whether it is wrong to destroy a fetus, just as though the rights of another person were not necessarily involved. This mistaken abstraction has led to the almost universal assumption that if a fetus is a human being, with a right to life, then it follows immediately that abortion is wrong (except perhaps when necessary to save the woman's life), and that it ought to be prohibited. It has also been generally assumed that unless the question about the status of the fetus is answered, the moral status of abortion cannot possibly be determined.

Two recent papers, one by B. A. Brody,[2] and one by Judith Thomson,[3] have attempted to settle the question of whether abortion ought to be prohibited apart from the question of whether or not the fetus is human. Brody examines the possibility that the following two statements are compatible: (1) that abortion is the taking of innocent human life, and therefore wrong; and (2) that nevertheless it ought not to be prohibited by law, at least under the present circumstances.[4] Not surprisingly, Brody finds it impossible to reconcile these two statements since, as he rightly argues, none of the unfortunate side effects of the prohibition of abortion is bad enough to justify legalizing the *wrongful* taking of human life. He is mistaken, however, in concluding that the incompatibility of (1) and (2), in itself, shows that "the legal problem about abortion cannot be resolved independently of the status of the fetus problem" (p. 369).

What Brody fails to realize is that (1) embodies the questionable assumption that if a fetus is a human being, then of course abortion is morally wrong, and that an attack on *this* assumption is more promising, as a way of reconciling the humanity of the fetus with the claim that laws prohibiting abortion are unjustified, than is an attack on the assumption that if abortion is the wrongful killing of innocent human beings then it ought to be prohibited. He thus overlooks the possibility that a fetus may have a right to life and abortion still be morally permissible, in that the right of a woman to terminate an unwanted pregnancy might override the right of the fetus to be kept alive. The immorality of abortion is no more demonstrated by the humanity of the fetus, in itself, than the immorality of killing in self-defense is demonstrated by the fact that the assailant is a human being. Neither is it demonstrated by the *innocence* of the fetus, since there may be situations in which the killing of innocent human beings is justified.

It is perhaps not surprising that Brody fails to spot this assumption, since it has been accepted with little or no argument by nearly everyone who has written on the morality of abortion. John Noonan is correct in saying that "the fundamental question in the long history of abortion is, How do you determine the humanity of a being?"[5] He summarizes his own antiabortion argument, which is a version of the official position of the Catholic Church, as follows:

. . . it is wrong to kill humans, however poor, weak, defenseless, and lacking in opportunity to develop their potential they may be. It is therefore morally wrong to kill Biafrans. Similarly, it is morally wrong to kill embryos.[6]

Noonan bases his claim that fetuses are human upon what he calls the theologians' criterion of humanity: that whoever is conceived of human beings is human. But although he argues at length for the appropriateness of this criterion, he never questions the assumption that if a fetus is human then abortion is wrong for exactly the same reason that murder is wrong.

Judith Thomson is, in fact, the only writer I am aware of who has seriously questioned this assumption; she has argued that, even if we grant the antiabortionist his claim that a fetus is a human being, with the same right to life as any other human being, we can still demonstrate that, in at least some and perhaps most cases, a woman is under no moral obligation to complete an unwanted pregnancy.[7] Her argument is worth examining, since if it holds up it may enable us to establish the moral permissibility of abortion without becoming involved in problems about what entitles an entity to be considered human, and accorded full moral rights. To be able to do this would be a great gain in the power and simplicity of the pro-abortion position, since, although I will argue that these problems can be solved at least as decisively as can any other moral problem, we should certainly be pleased to be able to avoid having to solve them as part of the justification of abortion.

On the other hand, even if Thomson's argument does not hold up, her insight, i.e., that it requires *argument* to show that if fetuses are human then abortion is properly classified as murder, is an extremely valuable one. The assumption she attacks is particularly invidious, for it amounts to the decision that it is appropriate, in deciding the moral status of abortion, to leave the rights of the pregnant woman out of consideration entirely, except possibly when her life is threatened. Obviously, this will not do; determining what moral rights, if any, a fetus possesses is only the first step in determining the moral status of abortion. Step two, which is at least equally essential, is finding a just solution to the conflict between whatever rights the fetus may have, and the rights of the woman who is unwillingly pregnant. While the historical error has been to pay far too little attention to the second step, Ms. Thomson's suggestion is that if we look at the second step first we may find that a woman has a right to obtain an abortion *regardless* of what rights the fetus has.

Our own inquiry will also have two stages. In Section I, we will consider whether or not it is possible to establish that abortion is morally permissible even on the assumption that a fetus is an entity with a full-fledged right to life. I will argue that in fact this cannot be established, at least not with the conclusiveness which is essential to our hopes of convincing those who are skeptical about the morality of abortion, and that we therefore cannot avoid dealing with the question of whether or not a fetus really does have the same right to life as a (more fully developed) human being.

In Section II, I will propose an answer to this question, namely, that a fetus cannot be considered a member of the moral community, the set of beings with full and equal moral rights, for the simple reason that it is not a person, and that it is personhood, and not genetic humanity, i.e., humanity as defined by Noonan, which is the basis for membership in this community. I will argue that a fetus, whatever its stage of development, satisfies none of the basic criteria of personhood, and is not even enough *like* a person to be accorded even some of the same rights on the basis of this resemblance. Nor, as we will see, is a fetus's *potential* personhood a threat to the morality of abortion, since, whatever the rights of potential people may be, they are invariably overridden in any conflict with the moral rights of actual people.

I

We turn now to Professor Thomson's case for the claim that even if a fetus has full moral rights, abortion is still morally permissible, at least sometimes, and for some reasons other than to save the woman's life. Her argument is based upon a clever, but I think faulty, analogy. She asks us to picture ourselves waking up one day, in bed with a famous violinist. Imagine that you have been kidnapped, and your bloodstream hooked up to that of the violinist, who happens to have an ailment which will certainly kill him unless he is permitted to share your kidneys for a period of nine months. No one else can save him, since you alone have the right type of blood. He will be unconscious all that time, and you will have to stay in bed with him, but after the nine months are over he may be unplugged, completely cured, that is, provided that you have cooperated.

Now then, she continues, what are your obligations in this situation? The antiabortionist, if he is consistent, will have to say that you are obligated to stay in bed with the violinist: for all people have a right to life, and violinists are people, and therefore it would be murder for you to disconnect yourself from him and let him die (p. 49). But this is outrageous, and so there must be something wrong with the same argument when it is applied to abortion. It would certainly be commendable of you to agree to save the violinist, but it is absurd to suggest that your refusal to do so would be murder. His right to life does not obligate you to do whatever is required to keep him alive; nor does it justify anyone else in forcing you to do so. A law which required you to stay in bed with the violinist would clearly be an unjust law, since it is no proper function of the law to force unwilling people to make huge sacrifices for the sake of other people toward whom they have no such prior obligation.

Thomson concludes that, if this analogy is an apt one, then we can grant the antiabortionist his claim that a fetus is a human being, and still hold that it is at least sometimes the case that a pregnant woman has the right to refuse to be a Good Samaritan towards the fetus, i.e., to obtain an abortion. For there is a great gap between the claim that x has a right to life, and the claim that y is obligated to do whatever is necessary to keep x alive, let alone that he ought to be forced to do so. It is y's duty to keep x alive only if he has somehow contracted a *special* obligation to do so; and a woman who is unwillingly pregnant, e.g., who was raped, has done nothing which obligates her to make the enormous sacrifice which is necessary to preserve the conceptus.

This argument is initially quite plausible, and in the extreme case of pregnancy due to rape it is probably conclusive. Difficulties arise, however, when we try to specify more exactly the range of cases in which abortion is clearly justifiable even on the assumption that the fetus is human. Professor Thomson considers it a virtue of her argument that it does not enable us to conclude that abortion is *always* permissible. It would, she says, be "indecent" for a woman in her seventh month to obtain an abortion just to avoid having to postpone a trip to Europe. On the other hand, her argument enables us to see that "a sick and desperately frightened schoolgirl pregnant due to rape may *of course* choose abortion, and that any law which rules this out is an insane law" (p. 65). So far, so good; but what are we to say about the woman who becomes pregnant not through rape but as a result of her own carelessness, or because of contraceptive failure, or who gets pregnant intentionally and then changes her mind about wanting a child? With respect to such cases, the violinist analogy is of much less use to the defender of the woman's right to obtain an abortion.

Indeed, the choice of a pregnancy due to rape, as an example of a case in which abortion is permissible even if a fetus is considered a human being, is extremely significant; for it is only in the case of pregnancy due to rape that the woman's situation is adequately analogous to the violinist case for our intuitions about the latter to transfer convincingly. The crucial difference between a pregnancy due to rape and the *normal* case of an unwanted pregnancy is that in the normal case we cannot claim that the woman is in no way responsible for her predicament; she could have remained chaste, or taken her pills more faithfully, or abstained on dangerous days, and so on. If on the other hand, you are kidnapped by strangers, and hooked up to a strange violinist, then you are

free of any shred of responsibility for the situation, on the basis of which it would be argued that you are obligated to keep the violinist alive. Only when her pregnancy is due to rape is a woman clearly just as nonresponsible.[8]

Consequently, there is room for the antiabortionist to argue that in the normal case of unwanted pregnancy a woman has, by her own actions, assumed responsibility for the fetus. For if x behaves in a way which he could have avoided, and which he knows involves, let us say, a 1 percent chance of bringing into existence a human being, with a right to life, and does so knowing that if this should happen then that human being will perish unless x does certain things to keep him alive, then it is by no means clear that when it does happen x is free of any obligation to what he knew in advance would be required to keep that human being alive.

The plausibility of such an argument is enough to show that the Thomson analogy can provide a clear and persuasive defense of a woman's right to obtain an abortion only with respect to those cases in which the woman is in no way responsible for her pregnancy, e.g., where it is due to rape. In all other cases, we would almost certainly conclude that it was necessary to look carefully at the particular circumstances in order to determine the extent of the woman's responsibility, and hence the extent of her obligation. This is an extremely unsatisfactory outcome, from the viewpoint of the opponents of restrictive abortion laws, most of whom are convinced that a woman has a right to obtain an abortion regardless of how and why she got pregnant.

Of course a supporter of the violinist analogy might point out that it is absurd to suggest that forgetting her pill one day might be sufficient to obligate a woman to complete an unwanted pregnancy. And indeed it *is* absurd to suggest this. As we shall see, the moral right to obtain an abortion is not in the least dependent upon the extent to which the woman is responsible for her pregnancy. But unfortunately, once we allow the assumption that a fetus has full moral rights, we cannot avoid taking this absurd suggestion seriously. Perhaps we can make this point more clear by altering the violinist story just enough to make it more analogous to a normal unwanted pregnancy and less to a pregnancy due to rape, and then seeing whether it is still obvious that you are not obligated to stay in bed with the fellow.

Suppose, then, that violinists are peculiarly prone to the sort of illness the only cure for which is the use of someone else's bloodstream for nine months, and that because of this there has been formed a society of music lovers who agree that whenever a violinist is stricken they will draw lots and the loser will, by some means, be made the one and only person capable of saving him. Now then, would you be obligated to cooperate in curing the violinist if you had voluntarily joined this society, knowing the possible consequences, and then your name had been drawn and you had been kidnapped? Admittedly, you did not promise ahead of time that you would, but you did deliberately place yourself in a position in which it might happen that a human life would be lost if you did not. Surely this is at least a prima facie reason for supposing that you have an obligation to stay in bed with the violinist. Suppose that you had gotten your name drawn deliberately; surely *that* would be quite a strong reason for thinking that you had such an obligation.

It might be suggested that there is one important disanalogy between the modified violinist case and the case of an unwanted pregnancy, which makes the woman's responsibility significantly less, namely, the fact that the fetus *comes into existence* as the result of the woman's actions. This fact might give her a right to refuse to keep it alive, whereas she would not have had this right had it existed previously, independently, and then as a result of her actions become dependent upon her for its survival.

My own intuition, however, is that x has no more right to bring into existence, either deliberately or as a foreseeable result of actions he could have avoided, a being with full moral rights (y), and then refuse to do what he knew beforehand would be required to keep that being alive, than he has to enter into an agreement with an existing person, whereby he may be called upon to save that person's life, and then refuse to do so when so called upon. Thus, x's responsibility for y's existence does not seem to lessen his obligation to keep y alive, if he is also responsible for y's being in a situation in which only he can save him.

Whether or not this intuition is entirely correct, it brings us back once again to the conclusion that once we allow the assumption that a fetus has full moral rights it becomes an extremely complex and difficult question whether and when abortion is justifiable. Thus the Thomson analogy cannot help us produce a clear and persuasive proof of the moral permissibility of abortion. Nor will the opponents of the restrictive laws thank us for anything less; for their conviction (for the most part) is that abortion is obviously *not*

a morally serious and extremely unfortunate, even though sometimes justified act, comparable to killing in self-defense or to letting the violinist die, but rather is closer to being a morally neutral act, like cutting one's hair.

The basis of this conviction, I believe, is the realization that a fetus is not a person, and thus does not have a full-fledged right to life. Perhaps the reason why this claim has been so inadequately defended is that it seems self-evident to those who accept it. And so it is, insofar as it follows from what I take to be perfectly obvious claims about the nature of personhood, and about the proper grounds for ascribing moral rights, claims which ought, indeed, to be obvious to both the friends and foes of abortion. Nevertheless, it is worth examining these claims, and showing how they demonstrate the moral innocuousness of abortion, since this apparently has not been adequately done before.

II

The question which we must answer in order to produce a satisfactory solution to the problem of the moral status of abortion is this: How are we to define the moral community, the set of beings with full and equal moral rights, such that we can decide whether a human fetus is a member of this community or not? What sort of entity, exactly, has the inalienable rights to life, liberty, and the pursuit of happiness? Jefferson attributed these rights to all *men*, and it may or may not be fair to suggest that he intended to attribute them *only* to men. Perhaps he ought to have attributed them to all human beings. If so, then we arrive, first, at Noonan's problem of defining what makes a being human, and second, at the equally vital question which Noonan does not consider, namely, What reason is there for identifying the moral community with the set of all human beings, in whatever way we have chosen to define that term?

ON THE DEFINITION OF "HUMAN"

One reason why this vital second question is so frequently overlooked in the debate over the moral status of abortion is that the term "human" has two distinct, but not often distinguished, senses. This fact results in a slide of meaning, which serves to conceal the fallaciousness of the traditional argument that since (1) it is wrong to kill innocent human beings, and (2) fetuses are innocent human beings, then (3) it is wrong to kill fetuses. For if "human" is used in the same sense in both (1) and (2) then, whichever of the two senses is meant, one of these premises is question-begging. And if it is used in two different senses, then of course the conclusion doesn't follow.

Thus, (1) is a self-evident moral truth,[9] and avoids begging the question about abortion, only if "human being" is used to mean something like "a full-fledged member of the moral community." (It may or may not also be meant to refer exclusively to members of the species *Homo sapiens*.) We may call this the *moral* sense of "human." It is not to be confused with what we will call the *genetic* sense, i.e., the sense in which *any* member of the species is a human being, and no member of any other species could be. If (1) is acceptable only if the moral sense is intended, (2) is non-question-begging only if what is intended is the genetic sense.

In "Deciding Who Is Human," Noonan argues for the classification of fetuses with human beings by pointing to the presence of the full genetic code, and the potential capacity for rational thought (p. 135). It is clear that what he needs to show, for his version of the traditional argument to be valid, is that fetuses are human in the moral sense, the sense in which it is analytically true that all human beings have full moral rights. But, in the absence of any argument showing that whatever is genetically human is also morally human, and he gives none, nothing more than genetic humanity can be demonstrated by the presence of the human genetic code. And, as we will see, the *potential* capacity for rational thought can at most show that an entity has the potential for *becoming* human in the moral sense.

DEFINING THE MORAL COMMUNITY

Can it be established that genetic humanity is sufficient for moral humanity? I think that there are very good reasons for not defining the moral community in this way. I would like to suggest an alternative way of defining the moral community, which I will argue for only to the extent of explaining why it is, or should be, self-evident. The suggestion is simply that the moral community consists of all and only *people*, rather than all and only human beings;[10] and probably the best way of demonstrating its self-evidence is by considering the concept of personhood, to see what sorts of entity are and are not persons, and what the decision that a being is or is not a person implies about its moral rights.

What moral characteristics entitle an entity to be considered a person? This is obviously not the place to attempt a complete analysis of the concept of personhood, but we do not need such a fully adequate analysis just to determine whether and why a fetus is or isn't a person. All we need is a rough and approximate list of the most basic criteria of personhood, and some idea of which, or how many, of these an entity must satisfy in order to properly be considered a person.

In searching for such criteria, it is useful to look beyond the set of people with whom we are acquainted, and ask how we would decide whether a totally alien being was a person or not. (For we have no right to assume that genetic humanity is necessary for personhood.) Imagine a space traveler who lands on an unknown planet and encounters a race of beings utterly unlike any he has ever seen or heard of. If he wants to be sure of behaving morally toward these beings, he has to somehow decide whether they are people, and hence have full moral rights, or whether they are the sort of thing which he need not feel guilty about treating as, for example, a source of food.

How should he go about making this decision? If he has some anthropological background he might look for such things as religion, art, and the manufacturing of tools, weapons, or shelters, since these factors have been used to distinguish our human from our pre-human ancestors, in what seems to be closer to the moral than the genetic sense of "human." And no doubt he would be right to consider the presence of such factors as good evidence that the alien beings were people, and morally human. It would, however, be overly anthropocentric of him to take the absence of these things as adequate evidence that they were not, since we can imagine people who have progressed beyond, or evolved without ever developing, these cultural characteristics.

I suggest that the traits which are most central to the concept of personhood, or humanity in the moral sense, are, very roughly, the following:

1. Consciousness (of objects and events external and/or internal to the being), and in particular the capacity to feel pain;
2. Reasoning (the *developed* capacity to solve new and relatively complex problems);
3. Self-motivated activity (activity which is relatively independent of either genetic or direct external control);

4. The capacity to communicate, by whatever means, messages of an indefinite variety of types, that is, not just with an indefinite number of possible contents, but on indefinitely many possible topics;

5. The presence of self-concepts, and self-awareness, either individual or racial, or both.

Admittedly, there are apt to be a great many problems involved in formulating precise definitions of these criteria, let alone in developing universally valid behavioral criteria for deciding when they apply. But I will assume that both we and our explorer know approximately what (1)–(5) mean, and that he is also able to determine whether or not they apply. How, then, should he use his findings to decide whether or not the alien beings are people? We needn't suppose that an entity must have *all* of these attributes to be properly considered a person; (1) and (2) alone may well be sufficient for personhood, and quite probably (1)–(3) are sufficient. Neither do we need to insist that any one of these criteria is *necessary* for personhood, although once again (1) and (2) look like fairly good candidates for necessary conditions, as does (3), if "activity" is construed so as to include the activity of reasoning.

All we need to claim, to demonstrate that a fetus is not a person, is that any being which satisfies *none* of (1)–(5) is certainly not a person. I consider this claim to be so obvious that I think anyone who denied it, and claimed that a being which satisfied none of (1)–(5) was a person all the same, would thereby demonstrate that he had no notion at all of what a person is— perhaps because he had confused the concept of a person with that of genetic humanity. If the opponents of abortion were to deny the appropriateness of these five criteria, I do not know what further arguments would convince them. We would probably have to admit that our conceptual schemes were indeed irreconcilably different, and that our dispute could not be settled objectively.

I do not expect this to happen, however, since I think that the concept of a person is one which is very nearly universal (to people), and that it is common to both proabortionists and antiabortionists, even though neither group has fully realized the relevance of this concept to the resolution of their dispute. Furthermore, I think that on reflection even the antiabortionists ought to agree not only that (1)–(5) are central to the concept of personhood, but also that it is a part of this concept that all and only people have full moral rights. The concept of a person is in part a moral concept; once we have admitted that x is a person we have recognized, even if we have not agreed to respect, x's right to be treated as a member of the moral community. It is true that the claim that x is a *human being* is more commonly voiced as part of an appeal to treat x decently than is the claim that x is a person, but this is either because "human being" is here used in the sense which implies personhood, or because the genetic and moral senses of "human" have been confused.

Now if (1)–(5) are indeed the primary criteria of personhood, then it is clear that genetic humanity is neither necessary nor sufficient for establishing that an entity is a person. Some human beings are not people, and there may well be people who are not human beings. A man or woman whose consciousness has been permanently obliterated but who remains alive is a human being which is no longer a person; defective human beings, with no appreciable mental capacity, are not and presumably never will be people; and a fetus is a human being which is not yet a person, and which therefore cannot coherently be said to have full moral rights. Citizens of the next century should be prepared to recognize highly advanced, self-aware robots or computers, should such be developed, and intelligent inhabitants of other worlds, should such be found, as people in the fullest sense, and to respect their moral rights. But to ascribe full moral rights to an entity which is not a person is as absurd as to ascribe moral obligations and responsibilities to such an entity.

FETAL DEVELOPMENT AND THE RIGHT TO LIFE

Two problems arise in the application of these suggestions for the definition of the moral community to the determination of the precise moral status of a human fetus. Given that the paradigm example of a person is a normal adult being, then (1) How like this paradigm, in particular how far advanced since conception, does a human being need to be before it begins to have a right to life by virtue, not of being fully a person as of yet, but of being *like* a person? and (2) To what extent, if any, does the fact that a fetus has the *potential* for becoming a person endow it with some of the same rights? Each of these questions requires some comment.

In answering the first question, we need not attempt a detailed consideration of the moral rights of organisms which are not developed enough, aware enough, intelligent enough, etc., to be considered people, but which resemble people in some respects. It does seem reasonable to suggest that the more like a person, in the relevant respects, a being is, the stronger is the case for regarding it as having a right to life, and indeed the stronger its right to life is. Thus we ought to take seriously the suggestion that, insofar as "the human individual develops biologically in a continuous fashion . . . the rights of a human person might develop in the same way."[11] But we must keep in mind that the attributes which are relevant in determining whether or not an entity is enough like a person to be regarded as having some of the same moral rights are no different from those which are relevant to determining whether or not it is fully a person—i.e., are no different from (1)–(5)—and that being genetically human, or having recognizably human facial and other physical features, or detectable brain activity, or the capacity to survive outside the uterus, are simply not among these relevant attributes.

Thus it is clear that even though a seven- or eight-month fetus has features which make it apt to arouse in us almost the same powerful protective instinct as is commonly aroused by a small infant, nevertheless it is not significantly more personlike than is a very small embryo. It is *somewhat* more personlike; it can apparently feel and respond to pain, and it may even have a rudimentary form of consciousness, insofar as its brain is quite active. Nevertheless, it seems safe to say that it is not fully conscious, in the way that an infant of a few months is, and that it cannot reason, or communicate messages of indefinitely many sorts, does not engage in self-motivated activity, and has no self-awareness. Thus, in the *relevant* respects, a fetus, even a fully developed one, is considerably less personlike than is the average mature mammal, indeed the average fish. And I think that a rational person must conclude that if the right to life of a fetus is to be based upon its resemblance to a person, then it cannot be said to have any more right to life than, let us say, a newborn guppy (which also seems to be capable of feeling pain), and that a right of that magnitude could never override a woman's right to obtain an abortion, at any stage of her pregnancy.

There may, of course, be other arguments in favor of placing legal limits upon the stage of pregnancy in which an abortion may be performed. Given the relative safety of the new techniques of artificially inducing labor during the third trimester, the danger to the woman's life or health is no longer such an argument.

Neither is the fact that people tend to respond to the thought of abortion in the later stages of pregnancy with emotional repulsion, since mere emotional responses cannot take the place of moral reasoning in determining what ought to be permitted. Nor, finally, is the frequently heard argument that legalizing abortion, especially late in the pregnancy, may erode the level of respect for human life, leading, perhaps to an increase in unjustified euthanasia and other crimes. For this threat, if it is a threat, can be better met by educating people to the kinds of moral distinctions which we are making here than by limiting access to abortion (which limitation may, in its disregard for the rights of women, be just as damaging to the level of respect for human rights).

Thus, since the fact that even a fully developed fetus is not personlike enough to have any significant right to life on the basis of its person-likeness shows that no legal restrictions upon the stage of pregnancy in which an abortion may be performed can be justified on the grounds that we should protect the rights of the older fetus; and since there is no other apparent justification for such restrictions, we may conclude that they are entirely unjustified. Whether or not it would be *indecent* (whatever that means) for a woman in her seventh month to obtain an abortion just to avoid having to postpone a trip to Europe, it would not, in itself, be *immoral*, and therefore it ought to be permitted.

POTENTIAL PERSONHOOD AND THE RIGHT TO LIFE

We have seen that a fetus does not resemble a person in any way which can support the claim that it has even some of the same rights. But what about its *potential*, the fact that if nurtured and allowed to develop naturally it will very probably become a person? Doesn't that alone give it at least some right to life? It is hard to deny that the fact that an entity is a potential person is a strong prima facie reason for not destroying it; but we need not conclude from this that a potential person has a right to life, by virtue of that potential. It may be that our feeling that it is better, other things being equal, not to destroy a potential person is better explained by the fact that potential people are still (felt to be) an invaluable resource, not to be lightly squandered. Surely, if every speck of dust were a potential person, we would be much less apt to conclude that every potential person has a right to become actual.

Still, we do not need to insist that a potential person has no right to life whatever. There may well be something immoral, and not just imprudent, about wantonly destroying potential people, when doing so isn't necessary to protect anyone's rights. But even if a potential person does have some prima facie right to life, such a right could not possibly outweigh the right of a woman to obtain an abortion, since the rights of any actual person invariably outweigh those of any potential person, whenever the two conflict. Since this may not be immediately obvious in the case of a human fetus, let us look at another case.

Suppose that our space explorer falls into the hands of an alien culture, whose scientists decide to create a few hundred thousand or more human beings, by breaking his body into its component cells, and using these to create fully developed human beings, with, of course, his genetic code. We may imagine that each of these newly created men will have all of the original man's abilities, skills, knowledge, and so on, and also have an individual self-concept, in short that each of them will be a bona fide (though hardly unique) person. Imagine that the whole project will take only seconds, and that its chances of success are extremely high, and that our explorer knows all of this, and also knows that these people will be treated fairly. I maintain that in such a situation he would have every right to escape if he could, and thus to deprive all of these potential people of their potential lives; for his right to life outweighs all of theirs together, in spite of the fact that they are all genetically human, all innocent, and all have a very high probability of becoming people very soon, if only he refrains from action.

Indeed, I think he would have a right to escape even if it were not his life which the alien scientists planned to take, but only a year of his freedom, or, indeed, only a day. Nor would he be obligated to stay if he had gotten captured (thus bringing all these people-potentials into existence) because of his own carelessness, or even if he had done so deliberately, knowing the consequences. Regardless of how he got captured, he is not morally obligated to remain in captivity for *any* period of time for the sake of permitting any number of potential people to come into actuality, so great is the margin by which one actual person's right to liberty outweighs whatever right to life even a hundred thousand potential people have. And it seems reasonable to conclude that the rights of a woman will outweigh by a similar margin whatever right to life a fetus may have by virtue of its potential personhood.

Thus, neither a fetus's resemblance to a person, nor its potential for becoming a person provides any basis whatever for the claim that it has any significant right to life. Consequently, a woman's right to protect her health, happiness, freedom, and even her life,[12] by terminating an unwanted pregnancy will always override whatever right to life it may be appropriate to ascribe to a fetus, even a fully developed one. And thus, in the absence of any overwhelming social need for every possible child, the laws which restrict the right to obtain an abortion, or limit the period of pregnancy during which an abortion may be performed, are a wholly unjustified violation of a woman's most basic moral and constitutional rights.[13]

POSTSCRIPT ON INFANTICIDE

Since the publication of this [essay], many people have written to point out that my argument appears to justify not only abortion, but infanticide as well. For a new-born infant is not significantly more person-like than an advanced fetus, and consequently it would seem that if the destruction of the latter is permissible so too must be that of the former. Inasmuch as most people, regardless of how they feel about the morality of abortion, consider infanticide a form of murder, this might appear to represent a serious flaw in my argument.

Now, if I am right in holding that it is only people who have a full-fledged right to life, and who can be murdered, and if the criteria of personhood are as I have described them, then it obviously follows that killing a new-born infant isn't murder. It does *not* follow, however, that infanticide is permissible, for two reasons. In the first place, it would be wrong, at least in this country and in this period of history, and other things being equal, to kill a new-born infant, because even if its parents do not want it and would not suffer from its destruction, there are other people who would like to have it, and would, in all probability, be deprived of a great deal of pleasure by its destruction. Thus, infanticide is wrong for reasons analogous to those which make it wrong to wantonly destroy natural resources, or great works of art.

Secondly, most people, at least in this country, value infants and would much prefer that they be preserved, even if foster parents are not immediately available. Most of us would rather be taxed to support orphanages than allow unwanted infants to be destroyed. So long as there are people who want an infant preserved, and who are willing and able to provide the means of caring for it, under reasonably humane conditions, it is, *certeris paribus*, wrong to destroy it.

But, it might be replied, if this argument shows that infanticide is wrong, at least at this time and in this country, doesn't it also show that abortion is wrong?

After all, many people value fetuses, are disturbed by their destruction, and would much prefer that they be preserved, even at some cost to themselves. Furthermore, as a potential source of pleasure to some foster family, a fetus is just as valuable as an infant. There is, however, a crucial difference between the two cases: so long as the fetus is unborn, its preservation, contrary to the wishes of the pregnant woman, violates her rights to freedom, happiness, and self-determination. Her rights override the rights of those who would like the fetus preserved, just as if someone's life or limb is threatened by a wild animal, his right to protect himself by destroying the animal overrides the rights of those who would prefer that the animal not be harmed.

The minute the infant is born, however, its preservation no longer violates any of its mother's rights, even if she wants it destroyed, because she is free to put it up for adoption. Consequently, while the moment of birth does not mark any sharp discontinuity in the degree to which an infant possesses the right to life, it does mark the end of its mother's right to determine its fate. Indeed, if abortion could be performed without killing the fetus, she would never possess the right to have the fetus destroyed, for the same reasons that she has no right to have an infant destroyed.

On the other hand, it follows from my argument that when an unwanted or defective infant is born into a society which cannot afford and/or is not willing to care for it, then its destruction is permissible. This conclusion will, no doubt, strike many people as heartless and immoral; but remember that the very existence of people who feel this way, and who are willing and able to provide care for unwanted infants, is reason enough to conclude that they should be preserved.

NOTES

1. For example, Roger Wertheimer, who in "Understanding the Abortion Argument" (*Philosophy and Public Affairs*, 1, No. 1 [Fall, 1971], 67–95), argues that the problem of the moral status of abortion is insoluble, in that the dispute over the status of the fetus is not a question of fact at all, but only a question of how one responds to the facts.

2. B. A. Brody, "Abortion and the Law," *The Journal of Philosophy*, 68, No. 12 (June 17, 1971), 357–69.

3. Judith Thomson, "A Defense of Abortion," *Philosophy and Public Affairs*, 1, No. 1 (Fall, 1971), 47–66.

4. I have abbreviated these statements somewhat, but not in a way which affects the argument.

5. John Noonan, "Abortion and the Catholic Church: A Summary History," *Natural Law Forum*, 12 (1967), 125.

6. John Noonan, "Deciding Who Is Human," *Natural Law Forum*, 13 (1968), 134.

7. "A Defense of Abortion."

8. We may safely ignore the fact that she might have avoided getting raped, e.g., by carrying a gun, since by similar means you might likewise have avoided getting kidnapped, and in neither case does the victim's failure to take all possible precautions against a highly unlikely event (as opposed to reasonable precautions against a rather likely event) mean that he is morally responsible for what happens.

9. Of course, the principle that it is (always) wrong to kill innocent human beings is in need of many other modifications, e.g., that it may be permissible to do so to save a greater number of other innocent human beings, but we may safely ignore these complications here.

10. From here on, we will use "human" to mean genetically human, since the moral sense seems closely connected to, and perhaps derived from, the assumption that genetic humanity is sufficient for membership in the moral community.

11. Thomas L. Hayes, "A Biological View," *Commonweal*, 85 (March 17, 1967), 677–78; quoted by Daniel Callahan, in *Abortion, Law, Choice, and Morality* (London: Macmillan & Co., 1970).

12. That is, insofar as the death rate, for the woman, is higher for childbirth than for early abortion.

13. My thanks to the following people, who were kind enough to read and criticize an earlier version of this paper: Herbert Gold, Gene Glass, Anne Lauterbach, Judith Thomson, Mary Mothersill, and Timothy Binkley.

UNITED STATES SUPREME COURT

Roe v. Wade: Majority Opinion and Dissent

[Mr. Justice Blackmun delivered the opinion of the Court.]

It is . . . apparent that at common law, at the time of the adoption of our Constitution, and throughout the major portion of the nineteenth century, abortion was viewed with less disfavor than under most American statutes currently in effect. Phrasing it another way, a woman enjoyed a substantially broader right to terminate a pregnancy than she does in most states today. At least with respect to the early stage of pregnancy, and very possibly without such a limitation, the opportunity to make this choice was present in this country well into the nineteenth century. Even later, the law continued for some time to treat less punitively an abortion procured in early pregnancy. . . .

Three reasons have been advanced to explain historically the enactment of criminal abortion laws in the nineteenth century and to justify their continued existence.

It has been argued occasionally that these laws were the product of a Victorian social concern to discourage illicit sexual conduct. Texas, however, does not advance this justification in the present case, and it appears that no court or commentator has taken the argument seriously. . . .

A second reason is concerned with abortion as a medical procedure. When most criminal abortion laws were first enacted, the procedure was a hazardous one for the woman. This was particularly true prior to the development of antisepsis. Antiseptic techniques, of course, were based on discoveries by Lister, Pasteur, and others first announced in 1867, but were not generally accepted and employed until about the turn of the century. Abortion mortality was high. Even after 1900, and perhaps until as late as the development of antibiotics in the 1940s, standard modern techniques such as dilation and curettage were not nearly so safe as they are today. Thus it has been argued that a state's real concern in enacting a criminal abortion law was to protect the pregnant woman, that is, to restrain her from submitting to a procedure that placed her life in serious jeopardy.

Modern medical techniques have altered this situation. Appellants and various *amici* refer to medical data indicating that abortion in early pregnancy, that is, prior to the end of first trimester, although not without its risk, is now relatively safe. Mortality rates for women undergoing early abortions, where the procedure is legal, appear to be as low as or lower than the rates for normal childbirth. Consequently, any interest of the state in protecting the woman from an inherently hazardous procedure, except when it would be equally dangerous for her to forgo it, has largely disappeared. Of course, important state interests in the area of health and medical standards do remain. The state has a legitimate interest in seeing to it that abortion like any other medical procedure, is performed under circumstances that insure maximum safety for the patient. This interest obviously extends at least to the performing physician and his staff, to the facilities involved, to the availability of after-care, and to adequate provision for any complication or emergency that might arise. The prevalence of high mortality rates at illegal "abortion mills" strengthens, rather than weakens, the state's interest in regulating the conditions under which abortions are performed. Moreover,

Reprinted from 410 *United States Reports* 113; decided January 22, 1973.

the risk to the woman increases as her pregnancy continues. Thus the state retains a definite interest in protecting the woman's own health and safety when an abortion is performed at a late stage of pregnancy.

The third reason is the state's interest—some phrase it in terms of duty—in protecting prenatal life. Some of the argument for this justification rests on the theory that a new human life is present from the moment of conception. The state's interest and general obligation to protect life then extends, it is argued, to prenatal life. Only when the life of the pregnant mother herself is at stake, balanced against the life she carries within her, should the interest of the embryo or fetus not prevail. Logically, of course, a legitimate state interest in this area need not stand or fall on acceptance of the belief that life begins at conception or at some other point prior to live birth. In assessing the state's interest, recognition may be given to the less rigid claim that as long as at least *potential* life is involved, the state may assert interests beyond the protection of the pregnant woman alone.

Parties challenging state abortion laws have sharply disputed in some courts the contention that a purpose of these laws, when enacted, was to protect prenatal life. Pointing to the absence of legislative history to support the contention, they claim that most state laws were designed solely to protect the woman. Because medical advances have lessened this concern, at least with respect to abortion in early pregnancy, they argue that with respect to such abortions the laws can no longer be justified by any state interest. There is some scholarly support for this view of original purpose. The few states courts called upon to interpret their laws in the late nineteenth and early twentieth centuries did focus on the state's interest in protecting the woman's health rather than in preserving the embryo and fetus. . . .

The Constitution does not explicitly mention any right of privacy. In a line of decisions, however, going back perhaps as far as *Union Pacific R. Co. v. Botsford* (1891), the Court has recognized that a right of personal privacy, or a guarantee of certain areas or zones of privacy, does exist under the Constitution. In varying contexts the Court or individual Justices have indeed found at least the roots of that right in the First Amendment, . . . in the Fourth and Fifth Amendments, . . . in the penumbras of the Bill of Rights, . . . in the Ninth Amendment, . . . or in the concept of liberty guaranteed by the first section of the Fourteenth Amendment. . . . These decisions make it clear that only personal rights that can be deemed "fundamental" or "implicit in the concept of ordered liberty" . . . are included in this guarantee of personal privacy. They also make it clear that the right has some extension to activities relating to marriage, . . . procreation, . . . contraception, . . . family relationships, . . . and child rearing and education. . . .

This right of privacy, whether it be founded in the Fourteenth Amendment's concept of personal liberty and restrictions upon state action, as we feel it is, or, as the District Court determined, in the Ninth Amendment's reservation of rights to the people, is broad enough to encompass a woman's decision whether or not to terminate her pregnancy. . . .

Appellants and some *amici* argue that the woman's right is absolute and that she is entitled to terminate her pregnancy at whatever time, in whatever way, and for whatever reason she alone chooses. With this we do not agree. Appellants' arguments that Texas either has no valid interest at all in regulating the abortion decision, or no interest strong enough to support any limitation upon the woman's sole determination, is unpersuasive. The Court's decisions recognizing a right of privacy also acknowledge that some state regulation in areas protected by that right is appropriate. As noted above, a state may properly assert important interests in safeguarding health, in maintaining medical standards, and in protecting potential life. At some point in pregnancy, these respective interests become sufficiently compelling to sustain regulation of the factors that govern the abortion decision. The privacy right involved, therefore, cannot be said to be absolute. . . .

We therefore conclude that the right of personal privacy includes the abortion decision, but that this right is not unqualified and must be considered against important state interests in regulation.

We note that those federal and state courts that have recently considered abortion law challenges have reached the same conclusion. . . .

Although the results are divided, most of these courts have agreed that the right of privacy, however based, is broad enough to cover the abortion decision; that the right, nonetheless, is not absolute and is subject to some limitations; and that at some point the state interests as to protection of health, medical standards, and prenatal life, become dominant. We agree with this approach. . . .

The appellee and certain *amici* argue that the fetus is a "person" within the language and meaning of the

Fourteenth Amendment. In support of this they outline at length and in detail the well-known facts of fetal development. If this suggestion of personhood is established, the appellant's case, of course, collapses, for the fetus's right to life is then guaranteed specifically by the Amendment. The appellant conceded as much on reargument. On the other hand, the appellee conceded on reargument that no case could be cited that holds that a fetus is a person within the meaning of the Fourteenth Amendment. . . .

All this, together with our observation, *supra*, that throughout the major portion of the nineteenth century prevailing legal abortion practices were far freer than they are today, persuades us that the word "person," as used in the Fourteenth Amendment, does not include the unborn. . . . Indeed, our decision in *United States v. Vuitch* (1971), inferentially is to the same effect, for we there would not have indulged in statutory interpretation favorable to abortion in specified circumstances if the necessary consequence was the termination of life entitled to Fourteenth Amendment protection.

. . . As we have intimated above, it is reasonable and appropriate for a state to decide that at some point in time another interest, that of health of the mother or that of potential human life, becomes significantly involved. The woman's privacy is no longer sole and any right of privacy she possesses must be measured accordingly.

Texas urges that, apart from the Fourteenth Amendment, life begins at conception and is present throughout pregnancy, and that, therefore, the state has a compelling interest in protecting that life from and after conception. We need not resolve the difficult question of when life begins. When those trained in the respective disciplines of medicine, philosophy, and theology are unable to arrive at any consensus, the judiciary, at this point in the development of man's knowledge, is not in a position to speculate as to the answer.

It should be sufficient to note briefly the wide divergence of thinking on this most sensitive and difficult question. There has always been strong support for the view that life does not begin until live birth. This was the belief of the Stoics. It appears to be the predominant, though not the unanimous, attitude of the Jewish faith. It may be taken to represent also the position of a large segment of the Protestant community, insofar as that can be ascertained; organized groups that have taken a formal position on the abortion issue have generally regarded abortion as a matter for the conscience of the individual and her family. As we have noted, the common law found greater significance in quickening. Physicians and their scientific colleagues have regarded that event with less interest and have tended to focus either upon conception or upon live birth or upon the interim point at which the fetus becomes "viable," that is, potentially able to live outside the mother's womb, albeit with artificial aid. Viability is usually placed at about seven months (28 weeks) but may occur earlier, even at 24 weeks. . . .

In areas other than criminal abortion the law has been reluctant to endorse any theory that life, as we recognize it, begins before live birth or to accord legal rights to the unborn except in narrowly defined situations and except when the rights are contingent upon live birth. . . . In short, the unborn have never been recognized in the law as persons in the whole sense.

In view of all this, we do not agree that, by adopting one theory of life, Texas may override the rights of the pregnant woman that are at stake. We repeat, however, that the state does have an important and legitimate interest in preserving and protecting the health of the pregnant woman, whether she be a resident of the state or a nonresident who seeks medical consultation and treatment there, and that it has still *another* important and legitimate interest in protecting the potentiality of human life. These interests are separate and distinct. Each grows in substantiality as the woman approaches term and, at a point during pregnancy, each becomes "compelling."

With respect to the state's important and legitimate interest in the health of the mother, the "compelling" point, in the light of present medical knowledge, is at approximately the end of the first trimester. This is so because of the now established medical fact . . . that until the end of the first trimester mortality in abortion is less than mortality in normal childbirth. It follows that, from and after this point, a state may regulate the abortion procedure to the extent that the regulation reasonably relates to the preservation and protection of maternal health. Examples of permissible state regulation in this area are requirements as to the qualifications of the person who is to perform the abortion; as to the licensure of that person; as to the facility in which the procedure is to be performed, that is, whether it must be a hospital or may be a clinic or some other place of less-than-hospital status; as to the licensing of the facility; and the like.

This means, on the other hand, that, for the period of pregnancy prior to this "compelling" point, the attending physician, in consultation with his patient, is free to determine, without regulation by the state, that in his medical judgment the patient's pregnancy should be terminated. If that decision is reached, the judgment may be effectuated by an abortion free of interference by the state.

With respect to the state's important and legitimate interest in potential life, the "compelling" point is at viability. This is so because the fetus then presumably has the capability of meaningful life outside the mother's womb. State regulation protective of fetal life after viability thus has both logical and biological justifications. If the state is interested in protecting fetal life after viability, it may go so far as to proscribe abortion during that period except when it is necessary to preserve the life or health of the mother. . . .

To summarize and repeat:

1. A state criminal abortion statute of the current Texas type, that excepts from criminality only a *life-saving* procedure on behalf of the mother, without regard to pregnancy stage and without recognition of the other interests involved, is violative of the Due Process Clause of the Fourteenth Amendment.

(a) For the stage prior to approximately the end of the first trimester, the abortion decision and its effectuation must be left to the medical judgment of the pregnant woman's attending physician.

(b) For the stage subsequent to approximately the end of the first trimester, the state, in promoting its interest in the health of the mother, may, if it chooses, regulate the abortion procedure in ways that are reasonably related to maternal health.

(c) For the stage subsequent to viability the state, in promoting its interest in the potentiality of human life, may, if it chooses, regulate, and even proscribe, abortion except where it is necessary, in appropriate medical judgment, for the preservation of the life or health of the mother.

2. The state may define the term "physician" . . . to mean only a physician currently licensed by the state, and may proscribe any abortion by a person who is not a physician as so defined.

. . . The decision leaves the state free to place increasing restrictions on abortion as the period of pregnancy lengthens, so long as those restrictions are tailored to the recognized state interests. The decision vindicates the right of the physician to administer medical treatment according to his professional judg-ment up to the points where important state interests provide compelling justifications for intervention. Up to those points the abortion decision in all its aspects is inherently, and primarily, a medical decision, and basic responsibility for it must rest with the physician. If an individual practitioner abuses the privilege of exercising proper medical judgment, the usual reme-dies, judicial and intraprofessional, are available. . . .

[Mr. Justice White, with whom Mr. Justice Rehn-quist joins, dissenting.]

At the heart of the controversy in these cases are those recurring pregnancies that pose no danger what-soever to the life or health of the mother but are, nevertheless, unwanted for any one or more of a vari-ety of reasons—convenience, family planning, eco-nomics, dislike of children, the embarrassment of illegitimacy, etc. The common claim before us is that for any one of such reasons, or for no reason at all, and without asserting or claiming any threat to life or health, any woman is entitled to an abortion at her request if she is able to find a medical advisor willing to undertake the procedure.

The Court for the most part sustains this position: During the period prior to the time the fetus becomes viable, the Constitution of the United States values the convenience, whim, or caprice of the putative mother more than the life or potential life of the fetus; the Constitution, therefore, guarantees the right to an abortion as against any state law or policy seeking to protect the fetus from an abortion not prompted by more compelling reasons of the mother.

With all due respect, I dissent. I find nothing in the language or history of the Constitution to support the Court's judgment. The Court simply fashions and an-nounces a new constitutional right for pregnant mothers and, with scarcely any reason or authority for its ac-tion, invests that right with sufficient substance to override most existing state abortion statutes. The upshot is that the people and the legislatures of the 50 states are constitutionally disentitled to weigh the relative importance of the continued existence and development of the fetus, on the one hand, against a spectrum of possible impacts on the mother, on the other hand. As an exercise of raw judicial power, the Court perhaps has authority to do what it does today; but in my view its judgment is an improvident and extravagant exercise of the power of judicial review that the Constitution extends to this Court.

The Court apparently values the convenience of the pregnant mother more than the continued existence and development of the life or potential life that she carries. Whether or not I might agree with that marshaling of values, I can in no event join the Court's judgment because I find no constitutional warrant for imposing such an order of priorities on the people and legislatures of the states. In a sensitive area such as this, involving as it does issues over which reasonable men may easily and heatedly differ, I cannot accept the Court's exercise of its clear power of choice by interposing a constitutional barrier to state efforts to protect human life and by investing mothers and doctors with the constitutionally protected right to exterminate it. This issue, for the most part, should be left with the

people and to the political processes the people have devised to govern their affairs.

It is my view, therefore, that the Texas statute is not constitutionally infirm because it denies abortions to those who seek to serve only their convenience rather than to protect their life or health. Nor is this plaintiff, who claims no threat to her mental or physical health, entitled to assert the possible rights of those women whose pregnancy assertedly implicated their health. This, together with *United States v. Vuitch*, 402 U.S. 62 (1971), dictates reversal of the judgment of the District Court.

UNITED STATES SUPREME COURT

City of Akron v. Akron Center for Reproductive Health

[Justice O'Connor delivered this dissenting opinion.]

I

The trimester or "three-stage" approach adopted by the Court in *Roe*, and, in a modified form, employed by the Court to analyze the state regulations in these cases, cannot be supported as a legitimate or useful framework for accommodating the woman's right and the State's interests. The decision of the Court today graphically illustrates why the trimester approach is a completely unworkable method of accommodating the conflicting personal rights and compelling state interests that are involved in the abortion context.

As the Court indicates today, the State's compelling interest in maternal health changes as medical technology changes, and any health regulation must not "depart from accepted medical practice." . . . In applying

Reprinted from 462 *United States Reports* 416; decided June 15, 1983.

this standard, the Court holds that "the safety of second-trimester abortions has increased dramatically" since 1973, when *Roe* was decided. . . .

It is not difficult to see that despite the Court's purported adherence to the trimester approach adopted in *Roe*, the lines drawn in that decision have now been "blurred" because of what the Court accepts as technological advancement in the safety of abortion procedure. The State may no longer rely on a "bright line" that separates permissible from impermissible regulation, and it is no longer free to consider the second trimester as a unit and weigh the risks posed by all abortion procedures throughout that trimester. Rather, the State must continuously and conscientiously study contemporary medical and scientific literature in order to determine whether the effect of a particular regulation is to "depart from accepted medical practice" insofar as particular procedures and particular periods within the trimester are concerned. Assuming that legislative bodies are able to engage in this exacting task, it is difficult to believe that our Constitution *requires* that they do it as a prelude to protecting the health of their citizens. . . . As today's decision indicates, medical technology is changing, and this change will necessitate our continued functioning as the nation's "*ex officio* medical board with powers to approve or disapprove medical and operative practices and standards throughout the United States." [*Planned Parenthood* v. *Danforth*, 428 U. S. 52, 99 (1976) (White, J., concurring in part and dissenting in part).]

Just as improvements in medical technology inevitably will move *forward* the point at which the State may regulate for reasons of maternal health, different technological improvements will move *backward* the point of viability at which the State may proscribe abortions except when necessary to preserve the life and health of the mother.

In 1973, viability before 28 weeks was considered unusual. The fourteenth edition of L. Hellman & J. Pritchard, Williams Obstetrics, on which the Court relied in *Roe* for its understanding of viability, stated that "[a]ttainment of a [fetal] weight of 1,000 g [or a fetal age of approximately 28 weeks gestation] is . . . widely used as the criterion of viability." *Id.*, at 493. However, recent studies have demonstrated increasingly earlier fetal viability. It is certainly reasonable to believe that fetal viability in the first trimester of pregnancy may be possible in the not too distant future. Indeed, the Court has explicitly acknowledged that *Roe* left the point of viability "flexible for anticipated advancements in medical skill." *Colautti* v. *Franklin*, 439 U. S. 379, 387 (1979). "[W]e recognized in *Roe* that viability was a matter of medical judgment, skill, and technical ability, and we preserved the flexibility of the term." *Danforth, supra*, 428 U. S. at 64.

The *Roe* framework, then, is clearly on a collision course with itself. As the medical risks of various abortion procedures decrease, the point at which the State may regulate for reasons of maternal health is moved further forward to actual childbirth. As medical science becomes better able to provide for the separate existence of the fetus, the point of viability is moved further back toward conception. . . . The *Roe* framework is inherently tied to the state of medical technology that exists whenever particular litigation ensues.

Although legislatures are better suited to make the necessary factual judgments in this area, the Court's framework forces legislatures, as a matter of constitutional law, to speculate about what constitutes "accepted medical practice" at any given time. Without the necessary expertise or ability, courts must then pretend to act as science review boards and examine those lesiglative judgments. . . .

II

The Court in *Roe* correctly realized that the State has important interests "in the areas of health and medical standards" and that "[t]he State has a legitimate interest in seeing to it that abortion, like any other medical procedure, is performed under circumstances that insure maximum safety for the patient." . . . The Court also recognized that the State has "*another* important and legitimate interest in protecting the potentiality of human life." I agree completely that the State has these interests, but in my view, the point at which these interests become compelling does not depend on the trimester of pregnancy. Rather, these interests are present *throughout* pregnancy. . . .

The fallacy inherent in the *Roe* framework is apparent: just because the State has a compelling interest in ensuring maternal safety once an abortion may be more dangerous in childbirth, it simply does not follow that the State has *no* interest before that point that justifies state regulation to ensure that first-trimester abortions are performed as safely as possible.

The state interest in potential human life is likewise extant throughout pregnancy. In *Roe*, the Court held that although the State had an important and legitimate interest in protecting potential life, that interest could not become compelling until the point at which the fetus was viable. The difficulty with this analysis is clear: *potential* life is no less potential in the first weeks of pregnancy than it is at viability or afterward. At any stage in pregnancy, there is the *potential* for human life. Although the Court refused to "resolve the difficult question of when life begins," *id.*, at 159, the Court chose the point of viability—when the fetus is *capable* of life independent of its mother—to permit the complete proscription of abortion. The choice of viability as the point at which the state interest in *potential* life becomes compelling is no less arbitrary than choosing any point before viability or any point afterward. Accordingly, I believe that the State's interest in protecting potential human life exists throughout the pregnancy.

. . . The Court's reliance on increased abortion costs and decreased availability is misplaced. As the City of Akron points out, there is no evidence in this case to show that the two Akron hospitals that performed second-trimester abortions denied an abortion to any woman, or that they would not permit abortion by the D&E procedure. In addition, there was no evidence presented that other hospitals in nearby areas did not provide second-trimester abortions. Further, almost *any* state regulation, including the licensing requirements that the Court *would* allow, inevitably and necessarily entails increased costs for *any* abortion. In *Simopoulos* v. *Virginia*, the Court upholds the State's stringent licensing requirements that will clearly involve greater cost because the State's licensing scheme "is not an unreasonable means of furthering the State's compelling interest in" preserving maternal health. Although the Court acknowledges this indisputably correct notion in *Simopoulos*, it inexplicably refuses to apply it in this case. A health regulation, such as the hospitalization requirement, simply does not rise to the level of "official interference" with the abortion decision. . . .

Section 1870.05(B) of the Akron ordinance provides that no physician shall perform an abortion on a minor under 15 years of age unless the minor gives written consent, and the physician first obtains the informed written consent of a parent or guardian, or unless the minor first obtains "an order from a court having jurisdiction over her that the abortion be performed or induced." Despite the fact that this regulation has yet to be construed in the state courts, the Court holds that the regulation is unconstitutional because it is not "reasonably susceptible of being construed to create an 'opportunity for case-by-case evaluations of the maturity of pregnant minors.'" [*Ante*, at 23 (quoting *Bellotti II, supra*, 443 U. S., at 643–644, n. 23 (plurality opinion)).] I believe that the Court should have abstained from declaring the ordinance unconstitutional.

In *Bellotti I, supra*, the Court abstained from deciding whether a state parental consent provision was unconstitutional as applied to mature minors. The Court recognized and respected the well-settled rule that abstention is proper "where an unconstrued state statute is susceptible of a construction by the state judiciary 'which might avoid in whole or in part the necessity for federal constitutional adjudication, or at least materially change the nature of the problem.'" [428 U. S., at 147 (quoting *Harrison* v. *NAACP*, 360

U. S. 167, 177, (1959)).] While acknowledging the force of the abstention doctrine, see *ante*, at 22, the Court nevertheless declines to apply it. Instead, it speculates that a state juvenile court *might* inquire into a minor's maturity and ability to decide to have an abortion in deciding whether the minor is being provided "'surgical care . . . necessary for his health, morals, or well being,'" *ante* at 23, n. 31 (quoting Ohio Rev. Code Ann. § 2151.03). The Court ultimately rejects this possible interpretation of state law, however, because filing a petition in juvenile court requires parental notification, an unconstitutional condition insofar as mature minors are concerned.

Assuming *arguendo* that the Court is correct in holding that a parental notification requirement would be unconstitutional as applied to mature minors, I see no reason to assume that the Akron ordinance and the state juvenile court statute compel state judges to notify the parents of a mature minor if such notification was contrary to the minor's best interests. Further, there is no reason to believe that the state courts would construe the consent requirement to impose any type of parental or judicial veto on the abortion decisions of mature minors. . . .

The Court invalidates the informed consent provisions of § 1870.06(B) and § 1870.06(C) of the Akron ordinance.[1] . . .

We have approved informed consent provisions in the past even though the physician was required to deliver certain information to the patient. In *Danforth, supra*, the Court upheld a state informed consent requirement because "[t]he decision to abort, indeed, is an important, and often a stressful one, and it is desirable and imperative that it be made with full knowledge of its nature and consequences." 428 U. S., at 67.[2] In *H.L.* v. *Matheson, supra*, the Court noted that the state statute in the case required that the patient "be advised at a minimum about available adoption services, about fetal development, and about forseeable complications and risks of an abortion. . . .

The remainder of § 1870.06(B), and § 1870.06(C), impose no undue burden or drastic limitation on the abortion decision. The City of Akron is merely attempting to ensure that the decision to abort is made in light of that knowledge that the City deems relevant to informed choice. As such, these regulations do not impermissibly affect any privacy right under the Fourteenth Amendment.

Section 1870.07 of the Akron ordinance requires a 24-hour waiting period between the signing of a consent form and the actual performance of the abortion, except in cases of emergency. See § 1870.12. The court below invalidated this requirement because it affected abortion decisions during the first trimester of pregnancy. The Court affirms the decision below, not on the ground that it affects early abortions, but because "Akron has failed to demonstrate that any legitimate state interest is furthered by an arbitrary and inflexible waiting period." . . .

The State's compelling interests in maternal physical and mental health and protection of fetal life clearly justify the waiting period. As we acknowledged in *Danforth, supra*, 428 U. S., at 67, the decision to abort is "a stressful one," and the waiting period reasonably relates to the State's interest in ensuring that a woman does not make this serious decision in undue haste. The decision also has grave consequences for the fetus, whose life the State has a compelling interest to protect and preserve. "No other [medical] procedure involves the purposeful termination of a potential life." [*Harris, supra*, 448 U. S., at 325.] The waiting period is surely a small cost to impose to ensure that

the woman's decision is well-considered in light of its certain and irreparable consequences on fetal life, and the possible effects on her own. . . .

IV

For the reasons set forth above, I dissent from the judgment of the Court in these cases.

NOTES

1. Section 1870.06(B) requires that the attending physician orally inform the pregnant woman: (1) that she is pregnant; (2) the probable number of weeks since conception; (3) that the unborn child is a human being from the moment of conception, and has certain anatomical and physiological characteristics; (4) that the unborn child may be viable and if so, the physician has a legal responsibility to try to save the child; (5) that abortion is a major surgical procedure that can result in serious physical and psychological complications; (6) that various agencies exist that will provide the pregnant woman with information about birth control; and (7) that various agencies exist that will assist the woman through pregnancy should she decide not to undergo the abortion. Section 1870.06(C) requires the attending physician to inform the woman of risks associated with her particular pregnancy and proposed abortion technique, as well as information that the physician deems relevant "in his own medical judgment."

2. The Court in *Danforth* did not even view the informed consent requirement as having a "legally significant impact" on first-trimester abortions that would trigger the *Roe* and *Doe* proscriptions against state interference in the decision to seek a first-trimester abortion. See 428 U. S., at 81 (recordkeeping requirements).

LEONARD H. GLANTZ

Abortion: A Decade of Legal Decisions

In 1973, the Supreme Court of the United States struck down all restrictive state abortion statutes in *Roe v. Wade*.[1] In doing so, it set forth a scheme by which the constitutionality of future statutes could be measured. In essence, the court ruled that, during the first trimester of pregnancy, the state could have essentially no role in the regulation of abortion; that in the second trimester, the state could regulate abortions in ways

designed to further maternal health; and that after fetal viability (*not* the third trimester), in furtherance of the state's interest in protecting fetal life, the state could prohibit abortions except those that were necessary to protect the life or health of the pregnant woman. On the face of it, these are simple rules. However, over the last decade, many states have tried to pass the most restrictive abortion statutes possible under these rules, and indeed, some states have passed clearly unconstitutional abortion legislation. As a result of these state efforts, innumerable lawsuits have been brought in state and federal courts, and the U.S. Supreme

From *Genetics and the Law III*, ed. George J. Annas and Aubrey Milunsky (Plenum Press, 1985), pp. 295–307. Reprinted by permission of the author and publisher.

Court has decided at least 14 abortion cases since *Roe v. Wade*. This activity indicates at least two things. First, the deceptively simple rules set forth in *Roe* are much more difficult to apply than they initially appeared to be. Second, those who are opposed to legalized abortion will work very diligently to have their voices heard and respected by state legislatures. It would also seem to indicate that the legal battles fought over abortion will not soon be settled.

This chapter will explore how the U.S. Supreme Court has dealt with various abortion issues presented to it since the last Genetics and the Law Conference in 1979, with the goal of ascertaining the constitutional boundaries regarding the regulation of abortion as the court sees them.

An important tactic that the "prolife" forces have adopted is withholding state or federal funding of abortions for poor women. The goal has been to reduce the total number of abortions performed. In 1977, the U.S. Supreme Court decided two cases that involved the public funding of "unnecessary" or "nontherapeutic" abortions. In the first case, *Beal v. Doe*,[2] the court decided that the Medicaid statute did not require states to pay for these abortions. In the second case, *Maher v. Roe*,[3] the court decided that a state policy that offered payment for the costs incident to childbirth, but not to abortion, did not violate the Equal Protection Clause of the U.S. Constitution.

At the time of the last Genetics and the Law Conference, I pointed out that these cases had been rather narrowly decided.[4] First, they dealt with "unnecessary" procedures that are usually not covered by Medicaid in any event. Second, the availability of funds was dependent on a determination of "medical necessity," which is left to the discretion of the women's physician. Finally, these cases allowed the withholding of funds in situations where the woman would not suffer any physical or mental harm from the continuation of the pregnancy. As it turns out, however, these factors were apparently not important to a majority of the court.

Harris v. McCrae[5] involved the constitutionality of the "Hyde amendment." The *Hyde amendment*, named after its congressional sponsor, is a term used to describe a [number] of federal restrictions on abortion funding. In 1980, the Hyde amendment forbade the use of federal funds to perform abortions except where the life of the mother would be endangered if the fetus were carried to term; or except for such medical procedures necessary for the victims of rape or incest when such rape or incest has been reported promptly to a law enforcement agency or public health service.[6]

However, there have been a variety of Hyde amendments over the years. In 1977, there was no rape or incest exception, and in 1979, there was an additional exception for instances where two physicians determined that a woman would suffer "severe and long-lasting physical health damage" if the pregnancy were carried to term. The court stated in footnote 4 that its opinion referred to all the versions of the Hyde amendment. This means that the court was rendering an opinion about the constitutionality of withholding funds for abortions except in life-threatening situations. Put another way, the issue was: Could the federal government deny funds to women who would suffer severe and long-lasting physical harm unless they had abortions, while providing funds for women who would undergo normal labor and deliver? The court, in a 5–4 decision, decided that the Hyde amendment was constitutional.

In rendering its decision, the court relied extensively on *Maher*, which involved nontherapeutic abortions, whereas this case involved therapeutic abortions. The court concluded that this distinction is without constitutional significance. In *Maher*, the court held that denying funding for nontherapeutic abortions did not impinge on a woman's right to privacy as described in *Roe*. Under *Roe*, the court explained, a woman must be free to decide whether or not to terminate her pregnancy, and the state must not place obstacles of its own making in front of a woman who wishes to act on her decision. However, by refusing to pay for abortions, the *state* has not placed any obstacles in front of her. As the court stated in *Maher*,

The indigency that may make it difficult—and in some cases, perhaps, impossible—for some women to have abortions is neither created nor in any way affected by the [lack of state funding].[7]

In essence, the court was saying that one can have a right to make a choice, but, if poor, is not entitled to have the state pay for the exercise of that choice. The court adopted this reasoning in *McCrae* and held that the state need not pay for therapeutic abortions.

There were vigorous, and even bitter dissents, in this case. Justice Stevens, who was a member of the majority in the nontherapeutic abortion cases, was a dissenter here. He felt that, once the government decided to alleviate some of the hardships of poverty by providing "necessary medical care," the government must use neutral criteria in distributing benefits. He was particularly concerned about the fact that, if the government decided to cut off funds for abortions that a woman needed to save her life, it would be constitutional to do so after *McCrae*. Indeed, the Solicitor General agreed with this proposition at the oral argument.[8]

This case stands for several propositions. The clearest is that neither states nor the federal government must pay for abortions for poor women. However, it also stands for the proposition that no government is required by the Constitution to pay for any medical care for the indigent no matter how necessary it may be, as long as the refusal to pay for such service is "rationally related to a legitimate government interest." Advocates for the poor see this case as an ominous foreshadowing of things to come. For example, anyone who ever believed that there is a "right to health care" will find that a constitutional basis for such a right has been undercut by *McCrae*.

Needless to say, both "prolife" and "prochoice" advocates tried to determine what *McCrae* meant in terms of the direction the Supreme Court was taking on abortion. Regardless of the fact that the court stated in *Maher* and *McCrae* that these cases did not lessen the right to privacy set forth in *Roe*, both sides of the abortion issue wondered if this was really the case. The vitality of *Roe* after *McCrae* is discussed in a later section.

ABORTION AND MINORS

Perhaps the most controversial issue that the U.S. Supreme Court has had to contend with in the abortion area is the access of minor women to abortion services. In *Planned Parenthood of Missouri v. Danforth*,[9] the court struck down a Missouri statute that required the written consent of a parent of a woman who was under the age of 18 and who was unmarried. The court noted that "constitutional rights do not mature and come into being magically only when one attains the state-defined age of majority."[10] Furthermore, the court argued that the "State does not have the constitutional authority to give a third party an absolute, and possibly arbitrary veto over the decision of the physician and his patient to terminate the patient's pregnancy."[11] The minor's right to consent to abortion on her own does

not apply to every minor regardless of age or maturity; rather, it applies to a minor who is "sufficiently mature to understand the procedure and to make an intelligent assessment of her circumstances with the advice of her physician."[12] In effect, the court held that if the state could not veto a woman's decision to have an abortion, it could not give anyone else veto power over a woman who could maturely and intelligently decide whether or not to have an abortion, regardless of the woman's age. . . .

In *Akron v. Center for Reproductive Health*,[13] the court was asked to determine the constitutionality of a municipal ordinance that prohibited a minor from receiving an abortion without obtaining the "informed written consent" of one of her parents or "an order from a court having jurisdiction over her that the abortion be performed or induced." The court struck down this provision as unconstitutional. . . .

THE RESURRECTION
OF *ROE V. WADE*

As we discussed earlier, following the court's decisions in the Medicaid cases, which held that neither the state nor the federal government was obliged to pay for abortions for poor women, there was a question concerning whether that decision signaled a retreat from *Roe*. This question was answered in June 1983, 10 years after *Roe*, when the court issued its opinions in *City of Akron v. Akron Center for Reproductive Health*[14] and *Planned Parenthood Association of Kansas City, Missouri v. Ashcroft*.[15]

Akron concerned the constitutionality of a restrictive municipal ordinance that contained the following provisions:

1. All abortions performed after the first trimester of pregnancy had to be performed in a general hospital that was accredited by the Joint Commission on Accreditation of Hospitals (JCAH) or the American Osteopathic Association.

2. The woman's physician was required to inform her of the status of her pregnancy, the development of the fetus, the date of possible viability, the physical and emotional complications that might result from an abortion, and the availability of agencies that would provide her with assistance and information with respect to birth control, abortion, and childbirth. The physician was specifically required to state

That abortion is a major surgical procedure which can result in serious complications, including hemorrhage, perforated uterus, infection, menstrual disturbances, sterility and miscarriage and prematurity in subsequent pregnancies and that abortion may leave essentially unaffected or may worsen any existing psychological problems she may have, and can result in severe emotional disturbances.[16]

The physician was also required by the ordinance to state that "the unborn child is a human life from the moment of conception," and to describe the anatomical and physiological characteristics of the fetus in some detail.

3. The attending physician was required to inform the woman of "the particular risks associated with her own pregnancy and the abortion technique to be employed" and other information that, in his or her medical judgment, he or she believed would be relevant to the woman's decision regarding the abortion.

4. At least a 24-hour waiting period was required between the time the woman signed the consent form and the performance of the abortion.

5. Physicians performing abortions were required to dispose of the fetal remains in a "humane and sanitary manner."

At the beginning of its opinion, the U.S. Supreme Court repeated the doctrines that it had set forth in *Roe*. Perhaps more significantly the court stated,

arguments continue to be made . . . that we erred in interpreting the Constitution [in *Roe*]. Nonetheless, the doctrine of *stare decisis*, while perhaps never entirely persuasive on a constitutional question, is a doctrine that demands respect in a society governed by the rule of law. We respect it today, and reaffirm *Roe v. Wade*.[17]

Arguably, the court went even further than in *Roe*, as will be seen in the following analysis.

The court struck down the requirement that all abortions performed after the first trimester be performed in a general hospital. In *Roe*, the court had held that, subsequent to the first trimester, a state could regulate abortions to the extent that "the regulation reasonably relates to the preservation and protection of maternal health"[18] because the state's interest in maternal health becomes "compelling" at this point in the pregnancy. Needless to say, the city argued that the hospitalization requirement was designed to further its interest in maternal health.

In striking down this requirement, the court noted that a second-trimester abortion costs $850–$900 in a hospital, whereas it costs $350–$400 in a clinic. It also pointed out that hospitals in Akron only rarely performed second-trimester abortions, so that women who wished to obtain such an abortion were subjected

to the additional financial burdens and health risks associated with travel. It concluded from these facts that the hospitalization requirement "may significantly limit a woman's ability to obtain an abortion."[19]

At the same time, the court noted that both the American Public Health Association (APHA) and the American College of Obstetrics and Gynecology (ACOG) had abandoned their recommendations that all second-trimester abortions be performed in hospitals, a standard that existed at the time of *Roe*. Instead, both organizations agreed that second-trimester abortions could be performed safely in adequately equipped clinics until 18 weeks of pregnancy. As a result, the court concluded that requiring *all* second-trimester abortions to be performed in a general hospital could not now be justified on the grounds of protecting maternal health, especially when the requirement placed a "heavy, and unnecessary, burden on women's access to a relatively inexpensive, otherwise accessible, and safe abortion procedure."

There are a number of important lessons in this part of the decision. First, a regulation that significantly increases the expense of an abortion, or that has the effect of requiring women to travel to obtain an abortion, can be seen as placing an "undue burden" on the women's abortion decision. Second, the court ruled that regulations designed to protect maternal health may not "depart from accepted medical practice."[20] Not only does this statement show tremendous deference to the medical profession, but it also indicates that, as medical standards evolve, the constitutionality of laws that restrict abortion practices may be affected. In this instance, a city ordinance that may have been constitutional in 1973 was unconstitutional in 1983 because the APHA and the ACOG had changed their standards as to the acceptability of performing abortions on an outpatient basis. This means that legislative bodies must pay close attention to standard medical practice when trying to restrict post-first-trimester abortions. It also means that those who wish to challenge such restrictive laws may be unsuccessful at one time but may succeed at a later date if accepted practice changes.

The court also struck down the detailed informed-consent requirement described in Point 2 above. The court's first opportunity to deal with the issue of informed consent occurred in *Danforth*.[21] In that case, the court upheld a Missouri statute that required a pregnant woman to verify in writing that her consent was "informed and freely given." In upholding this requirement, the court noted that the "right" set forth in *Roe* is to allow the woman to make a decision about whether or not to have an abortion. Therefore, by requiring a woman to give an informed consent, the state is enhancing her capacity to make an intelligent decision. As the court put it, "the decision to abort . . . is an important, and often a stressful one, and it is desirable and imperative that it be made with full knowledge of its nature and consequences."[22]

In *Danforth*, the challengers argued that the term *informed consent* was too vague. In a footnote, the court construed the term to mean

the giving of information to the patient as to just what would be done and as to its consequences. To ascribe more meaning than this might well confine the attending physician in an undesired and uncomfortable straitjacket in the practice of his profession.[23]

The issue was whether Akron's informed consent requirements met this standard. The court struck down this portion of the ordinance for a number of reasons. First, the court said the purpose of the information required was designed not to inform the woman but rather "to persuade her to withhold it altogether." Second, the court held that the requirement to inform the woman that "the unborn child is a human life from the moment of conception" was inconsistent with the court's holding in *Roe* that a state may not adopt one theory of when life begins to justify its abortion regulations. Third, the court stated that to require a detailed anatomical description would force a physician to speculate about the particular fetus. Fourth, the requirement that a woman be told that abortion is a major surgical procedure followed by numerous possible physical and psychological complications was described as a "parade of horribles" intended to make the woman believe that abortion is a particularly dangerous procedure. Fifth, the requirement was seen as an "intrusion upon the discretion of the pregnant woman's physician," forcing him or her to recite the same "litany" of "information" to every patient regardless of the physician's judgment about the relevance of the information to a particular patient.

Again, we see the court being very protective of physicians' prerogatives. Additionally, it is very clear that the court discerned Akron's motives for passing this ordinance and refused to allow the city to turn a physician into a "mouthpiece" for the expression of its unscientific and biased views to individual patients. . . .

The Court did indicate that a physician could be required to verify that adequate counseling had been provided and that the woman's consent was informed. The state may also establish "reasonable" qualifications for counselors.

The court spent little time striking down the 24-hour waiting period. The district court had found that the 24-hour waiting period might increase the cost of abortions by requiring two trips, and that scheduling difficulties might increase the wait to more than 24 hours. Also, Akron was unable to demonstrate that any legitimate state interest was furthered by an "arbitrary and inflexible" waiting period. The court once again noted that this requirement interfered with the physician's discretion in the exercise of his or her "medical judgment."

If we read between the lines, the court viewed this provision as designed to make it more difficult for a woman to obtain an abortion and essentially as a form of state harassment. The judges on the court know that limbs are amputated and risky neurosurgery and heart transplants are performed without waiting periods: How could they possibly view this waiting period as anything less than arbitrary?

The court also struck down the provision requiring the "humane and sanitary" disposal of the fetal remains. It was unclear what this requirement meant, and in a criminal statute, which is what this is, such vagueness is a fatal flaw.

The *Planned Parenthood*[24] case involved the constitutionality of a Missouri statute that required,

1. Abortions performed after 12 weeks of pregnancy be performed in a hospital.
2. A pathology report for each abortion performed.
3. The presence of a second physician during abortions performed after viability.[25]

The hospitalization requirement was struck down for the same reasons stated in *City of Akron*.

The court upheld the requirement that a second physician be present at postviability abortions. The court noted that, in *Roe*, it had recognized the state's compelling interest in the protection of potential human life after viability, and that a state could prohibit postviability abortions except where the abortion was necessary to preserve the life or health of the woman. Given this fact, and given the fact that in a postviability abortion the operating physician has to direct his or her attention and skills to the care of the woman, the court found that the presence of a second physician would serve to assure the state's interest in protecting the life of a live-born child.

The court also upheld the requirement of a pathologist's report. In Missouri, there is a statute requiring that most tissue surgically removed in a *hospital* be examined by a pathologist. The question in this case was: Can that requirement be constitutionally applied to tissue removed in a *clinic* during an abortion? The court found that the examination of tissue by a pathologist is a legitimate means of protecting maternal health, and that both medical testimony and the medical literature support the desirability of this practice. . . .

There was a strong dissent in these cases against the court's actions striking down the various provisions in these laws, written by Justice O'Connor, joined by Justices White and Rehnquist, both of whom had been strong opponents of the court's prior decisions striking down restrictive abortions laws. The position that Justice O'Connor took was of particular interest because she is the first female Supreme Court Justice and because "prolife" advocates opposed her nomination because of their perception that she was too "prochoice." Justice O'Connor's opinion was essentially a dissent from *Roe v. Wade*. She argued that the trimester scheme is "completely unworkable" and was especially unhappy with the court's use of changing medical standards to determine the constitutionality of state laws. She was concerned that "without the necessary expertise or ability, courts must . . . pretend to act as science review boards."[25]

Justice O'Connor's opinion raises a serious generic question about the role that the courts should play when they are confronted with scientific evidence and scientific disputes. But it also indicates a lack of general awareness of the increasing role of scientific evidence in courts. More and more courts deal with public health regulations, the validity (or invalidity) of which is based on scientific evidence, whether one is talking about compulsory vaccination, using x-ray machines to determine if shoes fit, cotton dust standards, or nuclear-power-plant regulations. . . .

In order to try to determine the direction that the court has taken on abortion generally, it is useful to see which regulations regarding abortion the court has upheld and which it has struck down over the last 10 years (see Table 1). We will put aside the cases regarding minors because that area is still unsettled, as discussed earlier.

What is striking about these lists is that, with one exception, the provisions that the court has struck down involve regulations that apply to the abortion procedure itself or to activities that occur prior to the abortion. On the list of provisions that are upheld, with one exception (C), they all apply to postabortion regulations. The general informed-consent regulation that was upheld does not single out abortion for special treatment, as informed consent is a requirement for all surgeries.

Based on this list and the recent and past U.S. Supreme Court cases, we can glean the following tests to determine the validity of state regulations of abortions.

Table 1. Abortion Regulations Struck Down and Upheld by the Court

Struck down	Upheld
1. Recital of a "parade of horribles"	A. Pathological examination of tissue
2. Hospitalization in second trimester	B. Record keeping and reporting if not burdensome and confidentiality is assured
3. "Humane and sanitary" disposal of fetal remains	C. General informed-consent provisions
4. Twenty-four-hour waiting period	D. Presence of second doctor at postviability abortions
5. Legislative determinations of viability	
6. Spousal consent	
7. Ban on use of saline amniocentesis	
8. Requiring a *physician* to obtain informed consent	

These are not necessarily independent tests; they can be used in various combinations:

1. Has a state placed an obstacle in front of the woman or otherwise significantly burdened the pregnant woman's ability to choose or obtain an abortion?
2. Is abortion being treated differently from other similar medical or surgical procedures? This is a critical point in the early stages of pregnancy and is much less important after the fetus is viable.
3. Does the regulation interfere with the treating physician's exercise of professional judgment?
4. Does the regulation conflict with, or is it stricter than, accepted medical and scientific norms?
5. Is the regulation designed to protect maternal health?
6. If it is designed to protect maternal health, is there a less intrusive or less expensive alternative? . . .

Over the past decade, it is quite remarkable how consistent the court has been in protecting a woman's right to obtain an abortion and a physician's right to perform one. As to the latter point, what is striking about the *City of Akron* decision is just how zealously the majority of the court acted to protect the right of the physician to exercise individual medical judgment—it is an extremely prophysician case and will be of as much use in protecting "physicians' rights" in areas other than abortion, as it will be to argue for a woman's right to obtain an abortion. The problem with the "parade of horribles" was not so much that a woman had to listen to it as that a physician had to recite it.

As it turns out, the Medicaid cases really meant what they said: they were restricted to the issue of the governmental obligation to pay for abortions. These cases have not been cited by the Court as a means of regulating abortion, although dissenters have used them in this manner.

City of Akron is not the last abortion case that will ever be heard. There are still many ambiguities and, questions, and the strong feelings and the political power that the members of the "right-to-life" movement have will continue to cause restrictive abortion legislation to be passed. What *City of Akron* does, however, is clarify the court's strong feelings about limiting the states' power to pass restrictive abortion laws, at least as the court is currently constituted.

NOTES

1. 410 U.S. 113 (1973).
2. 432 U.S. 438 (1977).
3. 432 U.S. 464 (1977).
4. Glantz, L. H. Recent developments in abortion law, in *Genetics and the Law II* (A. Milunsky and G. J. Annas, eds.), Plenum Press, Boston (1979), 217.
5. 448 U.S. 297 (1980).
6. P.L. No. 96–123 Sec. 109, 93 Stat. 926.
7. 432 U.S. at 474.
8. *Supra* note 5 at page 354, n. 6.
9. 428 U.S. 52 (1976).
10. *Id*. at 74.
11. *Id*.
12. *Id*. at 73–74, citing the Dissenting Judge in District Court, 392 F. Supp. 1362, 1376 (E.D. Mo. 1975).
13. 103 S.Ct. 2481 (1983).
14. *Id*.
15. 103 S. Ct. 2517 (1983)
16. Akron Codified Ordinances Ch. 1870.05 (5) as cited in 103 S.Ct. 2489 n.5.
17. 103 S.Ct. at 2487.
18. 410 U.S. at 163.
19. 103 S.Ct. at 2493.
20. *Id*.
21. 428 U.S. 52 (1976).
22. *Id*. at 67.
23. *Id*. at 67 n.8.
24. 103 S.Ct. 2517 (1983).
25. 103 S.Ct. at 2507 (O'Connor, dissenting).

KEN MARTYN

Technological Advances and *Roe v. Wade*: The Need to Rethink Abortion Law

In *Roe v. Wade*, the Supreme Court held that a state may prohibit the abortion of a viable fetus, provided that the abortion is not necessary to preserve the life or health of the mother. A fetus becomes viable when there is a reasonable likelihood of its sustained survival outside the womb, *with or without artificial support*. . . .

The Court reaffirmed its position that the Constitution protects an individual's right to privacy even though this right is not explicitly mentioned in the Constitution. The Court cited a long list of cases going back to 1886 in which it had found a right to privacy in some form. In previous cases, the Court had found evidence of the right to privacy in the first, third, fourth, and ninth amendments, and in the concept of personal liberty guaranteed by the first section of the fourteenth amendment. In *Roe*, the Court held that only personal rights can be included in this zone of privacy. Thus, the Constitution protects the privacy of certain matters relating to marriage, procreation, contraception, child rearing, and education.

The Court held that the concept of personal liberty contained in the fourteenth amendment protects a woman's decision whether or not to undergo an abortion. While the woman's right to decide whether to have an abortion is fundamental, it is not absolute. The woman's right must be balanced against important state interests. . . .

The *Roe* Court recognized that the state has two "important and legitimate" interests: protecting maternal health, and protecting the potential life of the fetus. These state interests grow in importance "as the

Originally published in *UCLA Law Review* 29 (5–6): 1194–1215, June–August 1982. © 1982 The Regents of the University of California. All rights reserved.

woman approaches term and, at a point during pregnancy, each becomes 'compelling.' . . ."[1]

Regardless of any subtle differences between the terms "viable" and "may be viable," viability is defined in terms of our technological ability to sustain a fetus' life. As a result, the point in time at which the fetus becomes viable is not fixed. Rather, it varies depending on the state of medical technology. As the technology of sustaining premature infants improves, the point of viability for fetuses will move back toward an earlier stage of the pregnancy.

IMPLICATIONS OF ADVANCES IN THE TECHNOLOGY OF SUSTAINING PREMATURE INFANTS

VIABILITY AND TECHNOLOGY

Once the decision is made to select viability as the determinative point in balancing the interests of the woman and the state, there is almost no choice but to include, as the Court in *Roe* did, room for technological change. There could not be any constitutionally defensible reason for tying a fundamental right to the state of medical technology at some arbitrary date. Nor can the problem be solved by claiming that a fetus is viable when it has a reasonable likelihood of survival outside the womb *without* technological support. Where would we draw the line? Is an incubator a form of technological support? Is an artificially controlled ambient room temperature a form of technological support? Does a germ-free environment qualify? It seems clear that once we adopt the medical concept of viability as the standard we are compelled to accept it lock, stock, and barrel. That includes taking account of changes in technology.

The net result of what the Court has done by choosing viability as its standard is to place the focus of the abortion inquiry on the existing state of medical technology, rather than on the state of fetal development. The determining factor is now whether and to what degree the medical profession has the technological capacity to sustain the fetus outside the womb. If, in the opinion of the attending physician, there is a reasonable likelihood that the fetus can be sustained outside the womb, then the state can prohibit the abortion regardless of the extent of fetal development. As the technology for keeping premature infants alive improves, the point of viability will move closer to the beginning of the term of pregnancy. Thus, if current law remains static as the technology of sustaining premature infants improves, a woman's right to an abortion will diminish.

RECENT DEVELOPMENTS IN THE TECHNOLOGY OF SUSTAINING PREMATURE INFANTS

A generation ago the major threat to premature infants' survival was their susceptibility to infection. The advent of antibiotics has made infection a minor problem. Advances are still being made in techniques for combating various diseases and syndromes which frequently affect premature infants. "There is absolutely no question that in the current era there has been a sustained and progressive improvement in the outlook for survival of small premature infants."[2] . . .

THE LEGAL IMPLICATIONS OF FUTURE ADVANCES IN THE TECHNOLOGY OF SUSTAINING PREMATURE INFANTS

Under *Roe*, the states have two independent interests that are considered to be important and legitimate: protecting maternal health and protecting the potential life of the fetus. The states cannot regulate abortion during the first stage of pregnancy because neither interest is compelling at that time. If technological improvements move the point of viability to a time within the first twelve weeks of pregnancy, the states' compelling interest in protecting a viable fetus will correspondingly attach during the first twelve weeks of pregnancy. In other words, if the legal system adheres to the reasoning of *Roe*, there is no limit to the extent to which advances in technology may diminish a woman's right to an abortion.

CHANGING THE FOCUS OF THE ABORTION QUESTION

If the focus is placed on viability, then advances in technology will eventually destroy a woman's right to an abortion. If, however, the focus is placed upon the degree of fetal development, the courts can avoid the problems resulting from technological advances.

The ultimate question should be at what point does the fetus become a human being. If the fetus is a human being, then the states clearly have the right to protect it. In other words, the state's interest in protecting the fetus would be compelling, so it could override the woman's right of privacy with respect to procreation. On the other hand, if the fetus is not a human being the decision whether to bear it to full term would rest with the pregnant woman.

Some commentators have argued that this last proposition is wrong because a state may constitutionally protect things that are not human beings, for example, draft cards and post offices. What this argument overlooks is that if the fetus is not a separate human being, then it is a part of the woman's body. This is not true of draft cards and post offices. The right of privacy that attaches to a person's own body clearly does not attach to draft cards and post offices. More importantly, a law that forbids the destruction of draft cards or post offices does not impinge upon the right of privacy with respect to procreation.

If the standard for deciding when the states may outlaw abortion is when the fetus becomes a human being, then we will need some kind of criterion by which we can decide when human life begins. On the one extreme are those who argue that the fetus becomes a human being at the moment of conception. On the other extreme are those who argue that the fetus is not a human being until the end of the term of pregnancy.[3] Although significant support exists for each of these positions, the Supreme Court would probably not adopt either. The latter position would give the woman an absolute right to an abortion, while the former would give her no right at all to an abortion. The Court in *Roe*, however, was apparently seeking some sort of compromise.

In addition to the pragmatic concern for reaching a compromise, the definition of what constitutes the beginning of human life should comport with our notions of what it is about a human life that makes it sacred. While some would argue that it is because humans have souls that human life is sacred, a standard for determining when life begins which was based upon the existence of a soul would be unworkable. There is no way to prove that humans have souls, let alone to determine when a soul comes into existence. In addition, such a standard would probably be unconstitutional: the soul is clearly a religious notion. Under the first amendment, laws that restrict a person's liberty may not be based on purely religious notions. By focusing on the human capacity for thought, these problems can be avoided.

One unique characteristic of humans is our status as thinking, conscious beings. The fetus' capacity for thought can be evaluated, at least indirectly, by measuring the degree of its brain development. An appropriate standard for determining the beginning of human life is when the fetal brain is developed to the point where the fetus is a thinking, conscious being.

INDICATORS OF FETAL CONSCIOUSNESS

A survey of existing scientific research indicates that a fetus becomes a thinking, conscious being sometime between twelve and thirty-two weeks after conception. A reasonable estimate is that the development of fetal consciousness takes place primarily between nineteen and thirty weeks after conception.

The development of the brain can be assessed in terms of its weight and structure. . . . The development of the brain can also be measured by the complexity of its electrical activity. Electrical activity can be measured with an electroencephalogram ("E.E.G."). . . .

The fetus is clearly not a conscious being twelve weeks after conception. It has a brain mass of only about ten grams, there are no fissures in the cerebral cortex, and electrical activity is scant and unorganized. In contrast, at thirty-two weeks the fetal brain weighs about 280 grams, has a well developed cerebral cortex (complete with complex fissures and cell layering comparable to adult brains), and displays electrical activity which is very similar to that of a full-term infant, including E.E.G. patterns characteristic of sleeping and being awake.

There is, of course, no way to be absolutely sure of the extent of the correlation between thought processes and the brain's physical and electrical development, though a strong correlation probably exists between them. The most rapid physical and electrical development of the brain appears to occur between nineteen and thirty weeks after conception. If the beginning of human life is defined in terms of consciousness and

thought, then human life probably begins during this period.

ADVANTAGES OF DEFINING THE BEGINNING OF LIFE IN TERMS OF BRAIN FUNCTION

Avoiding the Problems Associated with Viability. The problems outlined in Section II can be avoided by focusing the abortion inquiry on the point at which the fetus becomes a human being rather than on viability. . . . It is entirely appropriate for the Court to decide when the fetus becomes a human being and thus acquires a fourteenth amendment right to life.

In determining what sort of criteria to apply in deciding when the fetus becomes a human being entitled to fourteenth amendment protection, the Court would have wide latitude, but it would not be wholly without constitutional constraint. For example, although it is perfectly legitimate to base one's personal belief as to when human life begins on religious concepts, it would not be appropriate for our legal system to do so. A standard for determining when human life begins based on brain function would, however, provide a workable and religiously neutral resolution of the competing interests of the woman and the fetus.

Creation of a Unified Legal Theory of What Constitutes a Human Being. After many years, American law has finally begun to define death as a lack of brain function. By determining the beginning of life by brain capacity, a symmetry would be created between the definitions for the beginning and end of life. . . .

Life would be said to begin when the fetal brain develops to the point that the fetus is a conscious entity. This would be determined on the basis of the physical and electrical development of the fetal brain. Correspondingly, life would be said to end when the brain permanently ceases to function electrically. There would thus be a single legal theory of what constitutes a human being.

A Final Consideration. There is a fundamental difference between the beginning of life and the termination of life. Death is an event. Although some people may be terminally ill for a long period of time, death is usually a fairly discrete occurrence. In contrast, the beginning of life is a process. The change from embryo to fetus and the development of the fetus are gradual. Scientific evidence indicates that the development of consciousness is also a gradual process. This gradual progression raises an additional issue: should the states be allowed to prohibit abortions when the development of consciousness begins, or should government prohibition be allowed only when the development of consciousness is largely complete?

The states should be allowed to prohibit those abortions at the beginning of the development of consciousness that are not necessary to protect the life or health of the mother. State intervention at this stage would allow a full vindication of the rights of the fetus while imposing only a minor restriction on the woman's right to decide whether to have an abortion. The period during which consciousness develops probably does not begin until about nineteen weeks after conception. Adoption of this standard would allow the woman well over four months in which to discover the pregnancy and to obtain an abortion if that is her choice. . . .

A standard for deciding when human life begins based on the degree of fetal brain development would provide a workable solution to the abortion issue. It would avoid the problems associated with the concept of viability, it is constitutionally justifiable, and it would not require a major change with respect to the time at which the states are currently allowed to prohibit abortions. . . .

NOTES

1. *Roe*, 410 U.S. at 162.

2. Stern, *Intensive Care of the Pre-term Infant*, 26 DANISH MED. BULL. 144 (1979). *See generally* Kopelman, *The Smallest Preterm Infants—Reasons for Optimism and New Dilemmas*, 132 AM. J. DISEASES CHILDREN 278 (1979).

3. Both positions seem extremely arbitrary. To say that a fetus just before the onset of labor is not a human being seems ridiculous, since there are no significant physical differences between it and a newborn baby. It has a functioning heart and brain. *See* K. MOORE, THE DEVELOPING HUMAN 1–5, 239–64 (2d ed. 1977). The only arguably significant difference is that it does not yet breathe air and it is still physically attached to the mother. But would it not be murder if someone shot it before the doctor was able to cut the umbilical cord? Yet, during this period, it does not breathe air and is still physically attached to the mother.

The only possible justification for claiming that an embryo several days after conception *is* a human being would be the claim that it has a soul. In a pluralistic society such as ours, everyone is entitled to his or her religious beliefs, and entitled to act (or not act) accordingly. Thus, if someone's religious beliefs convince her that a small clump of four cells (the number of cells present three days after conception) has a soul, and that every thing which has a soul is a human being, she is entitled to act in accordance with her beliefs if she becomes pregnant. But one wishing to use the legal system to restrict the actions of other adults who are clearly human beings (i.e., the women seeking a legal abortion) must come up with something stronger than merely postulating the existence of an incorporeal entity (the soul), ascribing it to the embryo, and claiming that all things which possess such an entity are human beings.

The argument that an embryo is entitled to protection from the moment of conception because it has human genes is also unpersuasive. Although having human genes is certainly a necessary condition to being human, it is far from sufficient. For example, people who have recently died have human genes, yet we have no qualms about allowing them to be cremated or otherwise destroyed. At best, the argument proves that the embryo has the potential to *become* a human being.

SUGGESTED READINGS FOR CHAPTER 5

Annas, George J. "The Supreme Court and Abortion: The Irrelevance of Medical Judgment." *Hastings Center Report* 10 (October 1980), 23–24.

Brandt, Richard B. "The Morality of Abortion." *The Monist* 36 (October 1972), 503–526.

Brock, Dan W. "Taking Human Life." *Ethics* 95 (July 1985), 851–865.

Brody, Baruch A. "Abortion and the Sanctity of Human Life." *American Philosophical Quarterly* 10 (April 1973), 133–140.

Callahan, Daniel. *Abortion: Law, Choice and Morality*. New York: Macmillan, 1970.

———. "How Technology Is Reframing the Abortion Debate." *Hastings Center Report* 16 (February 1986), 33–42.

———, and Callahan, Sidney, eds. *Abortion: Understanding Differences*. New York: Plenum Press, 1984.

Chervenak, Frank, et al. "When Is Termination of Pregnancy During the Third Trimester Morally Justifiable?" *New England Journal of Medicine* 310 (February 23, 1984), 501–504.

Connery, John R. *Abortion: The Development of the Roman Catholic Perspective*. Chicago: Loyola University Press, 1977.

Daniels, Charles B. "Abortion and Potential." *Dialogue* 18 (June 1979), 220–223.

Davis, Michael. "Fetuses, Famous Violinists, and the Right to Continued Aid." *Philosophical Quarterly* 33 (July 1983), 259–278.

Davis, Nancy. "Abortion and Self-Defense." *Philosophy and Public Affairs* 13 (Summer 1984), 175–207.

Devine, Philip E. *The Ethics of Homicide*. Ithaca, N.Y.: Cornell University Press, 1978.

Dworkin, Gerald. "Morality, Legality, and Abortion." *Society* 19 (May/June 1982), 51–53.

Ely, John Hart. "The Wages of Crying Wolf: A Comment on *Roe* v. *Wade*." *Yale Law Journal* 82 (April 1973), 920–949.

Engelhardt, H. Tristram, Jr. "The Ontology of Abortion." *Ethics* 84 (April 1974), 217–234.

———. *The Foundations of Bioethics*. New York: Oxford University Press, 1986. Chap. 6.

English, Jane. "Abortion and the Concept of a Person." *Canadian Journal of Philosophy* 5 (October 1975), 233–243.

Feinberg, Joel, ed. *The Problem of Abortion*. 2nd edition. Belmont, Calif.: Wadsworth Publishing Company, 1984.

———. "Abortion." In Regan, Tom, ed. *Matters of Life and Death*. New York: Random House, 1980, pp. 183–217.

Finnis, John. "The Rights and Wrongs of Abortion: A Reply to Judith Thomson." *Philosophy and Public Affairs* 2 (Winter 1973), 117–145.

———. "Abortion: Legal Aspects." In Reich, Warren T., ed. *Encyclopedia of Bioethics*. New York: Free Press, 1978. Vol. 1, pp. 26–32.

Fleming, Lorette. "The Moral Status of the Fetus: A Reappraisal." *Bioethics* 1 (January 1987), 15–34.

Foot, Philippa. "The Problem of Abortion and the Doctrine of Double Effect." *The Oxford Review* 5 (1967), 59–70.

Glantz, Leonard H. "Abortion and the Supreme Court: Why Legislative Motive Matters." *American Journal of Public Health* 76 (December 1986), 1452–1455.

Glover, Jonathan. *Causing Death and Saving Lives.* Harmondsworth, England: Penguin Books, 1977.

Goldman, Alan H. "Abortion and the Right to Life." *Personalist* 60 (October 1979), 402–406.

Hare, R. M. "Abortion and the Golden Rule." *Philosophy and Public Affairs* 4 (Spring 1975), 201–222.

Kapp, Marshall B. "Abortion and Informed Consent Requirements." *American Journal of Obstetrics and Gynecology* 144 (September 1, 1982), 1–4.

King, Patricia A. "The Juridical Status of the Fetus: A Proposal for Legal Protection of the Unborn." *Michigan Law Review* 77 (August 1979), 1647–1687.

Kushner, Thomasine. "Having a Life Versus Being Alive." *Journal of Medical Ethics* 10 (March 1984), 5–8.

Mechanic, David. "The Supreme Court and Abortion: Sidestepping Social Realities." *Hastings Center Report* 10 (December 1980), 17–19.

Nicholson, Susan Teft. *Abortion and the Roman Catholic Church.* Knoxville, Tenn.: *Journal of Religious Ethics* Monographs (1978).

Noonan, John T., Jr., ed. *The Morality of Abortion: Legal and Historical Perspectives.* Cambridge, Mass.: Harvard University Press, 1970.

———. *A Private Choice: Abortion in America in the Seventies.* New York: Free Press, 1979.

———. "The Supreme Court and Abortion: Upholding Constitutional Principles." *Hastings Center Report* 10 (December 1980), 14–16.

Quinn, Warren. "Abortion: Identity and Loss." *Philosophy and Public Affairs* 13 (Winter 1984), 24–54.

Ramsey, Paul. "The Morality of Abortion." In Labby, Daniel H., ed. *Life or Death: Ethics and Options.* Seattle, Wash.: University of Washington Press, 1968, pp. 60–93.

Singer, Peter. *Practical Ethics.* New York: Cambridge University Press, 1979. Chap. 6.

Sterba, James P. "Abortion, Distant Peoples and Future Generations." *Journal of Philosophy* 77 (July 1980), 424–440.

Sumner, L. W. *Abortion and Moral Theory.* Princeton, N.J.: Princeton University Press, 1981.

Thomson, Judith Jarvis. "Rights and Deaths." *Philosophy and Public Affairs* 2 (Winter 1973), 146–155.

Tooley, Michael. "Abortion and Infanticide." *Philosophy and Public Affairs* 2 (Fall 1972), 37–65.

———. "In Defense of Abortion and Infanticide." In Feinberg, Joel, ed. *The Problem of Abortion.* 2nd edition. Belmont, Calif.: Wadsworth Publishing Company, 1984, pp. 120–134.

Tribe, Laurence H. "Toward a Model of Roles in the Due Process of Life and Law." *Harvard Law Review* 87 (November 1973), 1–53.

Tushnet, Mark, and Seidman, Louis Michael. "A Comment on Tooley's *Abortion and Infanticide.*" *Ethics* 96 (January 1986), 350–355.

U.S. Supreme Court. *Thornburgh v. American College of Obstetricians. Supreme Court Reporter* 106 (June 11, 1986), 2169–2216.

VanDeVeer, Donald. "Justifying 'Wholesale Slaughter.'" *Canadian Journal of Philosophy* 5 (October 1975), 245–258.

Veatch, Robert M. *Case Studies in Medical Ethics.* Cambridge, Mass.: Harvard University Press, 1977. Chap. 7.

Werner, Richard. "Abortion: The Ontological and Moral Status of the Unborn." In Wasserstrom, Richard A., ed. *Today's Moral Problems.* 2nd edition. New York: Macmillan, 1979, pp. 51–74.

Wertheimer, Roger. "Understanding the Abortion Argument." *Philosophy and Public Affairs* 1 (Fall 1971), 67–95.

Winkler, Earl R. "Abortion and Victimisability." *Journal of Applied Philosophy* 1 (October 1984), 305–318.

Winston, M. E. "Abortion and Parental Responsibility." *Journal of Medical Humanities and Bioethics* 7 (Spring/Summer 1986), 33–56.

Zaitchik, Alan. "Viability and the Morality of Abortion." *Philosophy and Public Affairs* 10 (Winter 1981), 18–26.

BIBLIOGRAPHIES

Goldstein, Doris Mueller. *Bioethics: A Guide to Information Sources.* Detroit, Mich.: Gale Research Company, 1982. See under "Abortion" and "Treatment for Defective Newborns and Infanticide."

Lineback, Richard H., ed. *Philosopher's Index.* Vols. 1– . Bowling Green, Ohio: Philosophy Documentation Center, Bowling Green State University. Issued quarterly. See under "Abortion," "Dignity," "Fetus(es)," "Infanticide," "Life," "Mentally Retarded," "Persons," "Right to Life," "Sanctity of Life," and "Therapeutic Abortion."

Walters, LeRoy, and Kahn, Tamar Joy, eds. *Bibliography of Bioethics.* Vols. 1– . Washington, D.C.: Kennedy Institute of Ethics, Georgetown University. Issued annually. See under "Abortion," "Selective Abortion," and "Therapeutic Abortion." (The information contained in the annual *Bibliography of Bioethics* can also be retrieved from BIOETHICSLINE, an on-line database of the National Library of Medicine.)

6.
Euthanasia and the Prolongation of Life

Chapter 4 examined concepts of death and the standards for recognizing when death has occurred. The present chapter considers ethical issues in the treatment of living human beings who are seriously or terminally ill. In the discussion of these issues a variety of words and phrases have been employed, including "death with dignity," "euthanasia," "the prolongation of life," "allowing to die," and even "mercy killing." As we shall see, alternative ways of conceptualizing the topic of this chapter are sometimes correlated with divergent ethical perspectives.

GENERAL CONCEPTUAL AND ETHICAL QUESTIONS

Three major conceptual issues frequently arise in discussions of euthanasia and the prolongation of life: (1) the distinction between killing and allowing to die; (2) the distinction between "voluntary" and "involuntary" decisions concerning death; and (3) the proper usage of the term "euthanasia."

The killing/allowing to die debate includes two distinct subquestions: Is it possible to draw a clear, logical distinction between actions and omissions? And, if such a distinction can be drawn, is it morally relevant? Several commentators assert that a meaningful logical distinction can be drawn between killing and allowing to die. Two major arguments are commonly adduced in support of this distinction:

1. Ordinary language: Speakers of English regularly distinguish without difficulty between "causing harm or death" and "permitting harm or death to occur." Most English speakers would classify "allowing to die" as an instance of the latter category, "killing," of the former.
2. Causation: In cases where a terminally ill or seriously injured patient dies following nontreatment, the proximate cause of death is the patient's disease or injury, not nontreatment, a principle traditionally recognized in the law.

James Rachels, on the other hand, argues that the cessation of treatment in terminal cases is "the intentional termination of the life of one human being by another" and, more generally, that letting a patient die is an action, not merely an omission. He therefore questions whether any clear conceptual distinction between killing and allowing to die can be sustained.

On the second subquestion, the moral relevance of the killing/allowing-to-die distinction, Rachels holds that if it is morally permissible to intend that a patient die, then acting directly to terminate a patient's life is justified if it causes less suffering to the patient than simply allowing him or her to die. By contrast, Tom Beauchamp argues that active or direct killing may not be justified in a *particular* case even if it causes less suffering for the patient, on grounds that seriously harmful consequences might occur if the active/passive distinction were generally viewed as morally irrelevant.

On this subquestion, however, there is some measure of agreement between Rachels and his opponents. Neither side accepts a simple correlation between the killing/letting-die distinction and the wrong/right distinction. For example, Rachels and Beauchamp agree that certain omissions that allow another to die are morally or legally blameworthy. Even the American Medical Association (AMA) statement (cited by Rachels) implicitly recognizes the moral accountability of physicians for some types of omissions by carefully circumscribing the conditions in which the cessation of treatment is considered to be justified: Only "extraordinary" means may be withheld and then only in cases in which there is "irrefutable evidence" that biological death is imminent. On the other hand, the AMA statement seems to regard the killing of a patient, even for humane reasons, as morally wrong; thus in its view there is a close connection between killing (a patient) and morally wrong action. Rachels obviously disagrees. Beauchamp adopts an intermediate position, arguing that there are rule-utilitarian reasons for preserving the killing/letting-die distinction; however, he does not regard killing for humane reasons as necessarily correlated with morally wrong action.

The conceptual distinction between "voluntary" and "involuntary" decisions about death is less controversial; however, the term "involuntary" is ambiguous. Voluntary decisions about death are those in which a competent patient requests or gives informed consent to a particular course of treatment or nontreatment. The term "involuntary," however, is not generally applied to situations in which the expressed will of a competent patient is overridden but rather to cases in which the patient—because of age, mental impairment, or unconsciousness—is not competent to give informed consent to life-death decisions. In such cases, where decisions must be made by others on the patient's behalf, the term "nonvoluntary" might be more appropriate, since it lacks the coercive overtones of "involuntary." However, the term "involuntary" is well established in the discussion of life-and-death questions and will therefore be employed in its noncoercive sense in the remainder of this introduction.

The third issue identified above is perhaps the most difficult: What is the proper usage of the term "euthanasia"? The answer to this question is complicated by the fact that the *descriptive definition* (see Chapter 3) of the term may be in transition. Originally, euthanasia was derived from two Greek roots meaning simply "good death." In *Webster's Third New International Dictionary (Unabridged)*, first published in 1961, the definition of euthanasia was further specified as (1) "an easy death or means of inducing one" and (2) "the act or practice of painlessly putting to death persons suffering from incurable conditions or diseases." Two features of these definitions may be noted: Both seem to employ the language of acting rather than omitting to act, or killing rather than allowing to die; and the second definition suggests that the action is performed by a party other than the patient. By contrast, a 1975 reference work, the *New Columbia Encyclopedia*, defines euthanasia as "either painlessly putting to death or failing to prevent death from natural causes in cases of terminal illness." The euthanasia entry continues:

The term formerly referred only to the act of painlessly putting incurably ill patients to death. However, technological advances in medicine, which have made it possible to prolong the lives of patients who have no hope of recovery, have led to the use of the term *negative euthanasia*, i.e., the withdrawing of extraordinary means used to preserve life.[1]

If Webster's definition is accepted, then the paradigm case of euthanasia is the (active) termination of a suffering patient's life by a second party. If the termination is requested or consented to by the patient, then the action is called "voluntary euthanasia." In cases where the patient is not mentally competent to give consent, the action is called "involuntary euthanasia." If, however, one accepts the definition proposed by the *New Columbia Encyclopedia*, two discrete subtypes of euthanasia are distinguishable, active (or positive) euthanasia and passive (or negative) euthanasia. On this view, the paradigm case of euthanasia just described is an instance of active euthanasia. The combination of the voluntary/involuntary distinction with the *New Columbia Encyclopedia* definition of euthanasia would thus yield four subtypes of euthanasia, which can be represented schematically as follows:

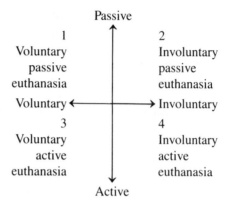

Adherents of Webster's definition, however, would insist on a sharp conceptual distinction between euthanasia and allowing to die and would probably deny that both concepts can be included on a single graph.

As we shall see, the first and third of these conceptual issues have been complicated in the 1980s by a new debate, namely, the debate about withholding or withdrawing "artificial" nutrition and hydration from patients. Whereas the earlier discussion about killing and allowing to die adopted decisions about the use of respirators as the standard paradigm, more recent commentators have focused considerable attention on the use of intravenous lines, stomach tubes, or total parenteral nutrition (the introduction of nutrients into major blood vessels of the upper chest) to provide food and water to patients. An important element of the earlier debate was the uncertainty about what would happen to a patient if a respirator were removed. Think, for example, of Karen Ann Quinlan, who, contrary to expectations, survived for ten years after she was taken off the respirator. However, much less uncertainty attends the withholding or withdrawal of nutrition and hydration from patients who cannot take food and fluids by mouth. Within a few days virtually all of them will be dead.

ISSUES INVOLVING ADULTS

Adult patients can be divided into two groups—individuals who have the mental capacity to make decisions about their treatment and those who do not. In some cases a court of law makes a formal determination that particular individuals either have or lack such a capacity, and the individuals are declared to be either "competent" or "incompetent" to make decisions in certain matters. In the following paragraphs these technical legal terms will be employed in an extended, nontechnical sense to characterize individuals who seem to have or to lack decision-making capacity.

While the most fundamental distinction among adult patients is the competent-incompetent distinction, there is a further important distinction between two kinds of incompetent patients. Some were competent at an earlier point in their lives but have since become incompetent; others are incompetent now and never were competent at any point in their lives. These two kinds of incompetent patients can be called "once-competent" and "never-competent." This distinction is important because once-competent individuals have at least had an *opportunity* to declare their wishes about life-sustaining treatment.

Two court decisions in cases involving adults are reprinted in this chapter. The first involved Mr. Abe Perlmutter, a formerly competent, terminally ill patient, and a decision about the removal of a mechanical ventilator. In the second case the central figure was Ms. Elizabeth Bouvia, a competent but physically disabled woman who requested court assistance in her attempt to secure the removal of a nasogastric tube through which she was being fed.

The remaining three essays in this section illustrate important aspects of the current death-and-dying debate, both in the United States and abroad. Joanne Lynn and James Childress discuss the generic issues raised by cases like that involving Elizabeth Bouvia. They conclude that the provision of artificial nutrition and hydration is not always a moral obligation. The summary of a Dutch commission report indicates that the active killing of patients by physicians at the patients' request, as well as physicians' assistance in the provision of lethal medications to patients, is an established practice in the Netherlands. One procedural approach to death-and-dying decisions is typified by the California durable power of attorney form. This advance directive, or "living will" as such documents are sometimes called, allows competent individuals to specify what intensity of life-sustaining care they wish to receive. In addition, the form encourages the appointment of a proxy, or agent, to make decisions on behalf of the patient, if the patient becomes incompetent.

ISSUES INVOLVING INFANTS

Infants are by definition never-competent individuals. Thus, decisions about their care must of necessity be made by others. Two questions immediately arise: Who should make such decisions? and, On the basis of what substantive criteria should such decisions be made?

Three general answers to the second question can be identified. The first is that every infant with a life-threatening condition should receive whatever treatments are required to save the infant's life, if such salvage seems medically possible. On this view, both killing and allowing to die are excluded as morally acceptable options. The primary justifications for this position are, negatively, that no one should be authorized to make life-and-death decisions on behalf of (at least) never-competent individuals and, positively, that every patient, regardless of his or her physical or mental condition, has an overriding right to life. A second general answer is that life-and-death decisions should be made on the basis of the patient's best interests alone. This answer would generally be implemented with the aid of a proxy's judgment about the quality of life that the patient is likely to experience as balanced against the suffering that the patient is likely to endure.

A third answer would allow decisions concerning the treatment of infants to be determined, or at least strongly influenced, by familial and broader social considerations. According to this view, if the patient's continued existence would be likely to undermine a marriage, adversely affect other family members, or claim an undue share of society's resources, then a decision to allow the patient to die (or possibly to kill the patient) would be morally justifiable. A benefit-harm calculus is involved in the implementation of this answer, as it was in the case of the second. However, factors other than patient benefit are also included in the calculus.

Who should select among these answers and apply them in specific cases? The parent or parents of an infant are generally regarded as the principal protectors of the infant's interests, unless they disqualify themselves through neglectful or abusive behavior. Health professionals—including physicians, nurses, and perhaps other groups, as well—possess kinds of information that are clearly relevant to such decisions and often devote enormous effort to preserving the lives and promoting the health of infants. Other possible participants in decisions about life-sustaining treatment for infants include hospital administrators, hospital ethics committees (see below), attorneys, and public officials acting to protect what they perceive to be the interests of society.

The "Johns Hopkins case" in the excerpt from James Gustafson's essay and the case history of Andrew Stinson narrated by his parents graphically illustrate the moral dilemmas raised by newborn care. During the Reagan administration, one response to more recent cases like the Hopkins case has been to involve the federal government in the setting of standards for legally acceptable newborn care; an excerpt from the April 1985 government regulations is reprinted in this chapter. John Moskop and Rita Saldanha object to what they regard as unwarranted governmental intrusion into decision making that is both medically and morally complex.

THE ROLE OF HOSPITAL ETHICS COMMITTEES

A recently developed procedural approach to death-and-dying decisions, especially in cases involving incompetent patients, has been the establishment of hospital (or institutional) ethics committees. Such committees may have been modeled on similar bodies that now provide prior review to most research involving human subjects (see Chapter 9). One major goal of hospital committees has been to keep difficult or controversial decisions about life support out of the courts, where considerable expense, long delays, and unwanted publicity are often involved. Norman Fost and Ronald Cranford survey the multiple possible roles of hospital ethics committees and welcome their creation as a useful adjunct to traditional decision-making mechanisms. In contrast, Robert Veatch sees serious ambiguities, if not fundamental contradictions, in both the goals of and the ethical standards governing hospital ethics committees.

L. W.

NOTES

1. William H. Harris and Judith S. Levey, eds., *The New Columbia Encyclopedia* (New York: Columbia University Press, 1975), p. 904.

JAMES RACHELS

Active and Passive Euthanasia

The distinction between active and passive euthanasia is thought to be crucial for medical ethics. The idea is that it is permissible, at least in some cases, to withhold treatment and allow a patient to die, but it is never permissible to take any direct action designed to kill the patient. This doctrine seems to be accepted by most doctors, and it was endorsed in a statement adopted by the House of Delegates of the American Medical Association on December 4, 1973:

The intentional termination of the life of one human being by another—mercy killing—is contrary to that for which the medical profession stands and is contrary to the policy of the American Medical Association.

The cessation of the employment of extraordinary means to prolong the life of the body when there is irrefutable evidence that biological death is imminent is the decision of the patient and/or his immediate family. The advice and judgment of the physician should be freely available to the patient and/or his immediate family.

However, a strong case can be made against this doctrine. In what follows I will set out some of the relevant arguments, and urge doctors to reconsider their views on this matter.

To begin with a familiar type of situation, a patient who is dying of incurable cancer of the throat is in terrible pain, which can no longer be satisfactorily alleviated. He is certain to die within a few days, even if present treatment is continued, but he does not want to go on living for those days since the pain is unbearable. So he asks the doctor for an end to it, and his family joins in the request.

Reprinted with permission from *The New England Journal of Medicine*, Vol. 292, No. 2 (January 9, 1975), pp. 78–80.

Suppose the doctor agrees to withhold treatment, as the conventional doctrine says he may. The justification for his doing so is that the patient is in terrible agony, and since he is going to die anyway, it would be wrong to prolong his suffering needlessly. But now notice this. If one simply withholds treatment, it may take the patient longer to die, and so he may suffer more than he would if more direct action were taken and a lethal injection given. This fact provides strong reason for thinking that, once the initial decision not to prolong his agony has been made, active euthanasia is actually preferable to passive euthanasia, rather than the reverse. To say otherwise is to endorse the option that leads to more suffering rather than less, and is contrary to the humanitarian impulse that prompts the decision not to prolong his life in the first place.

Part of my point is that the process of being "allowed to die" can be relatively slow and painful, whereas being given a lethal injection is relatively quick and painless. Let me give a different sort of example. In the United States about one in 600 babies is born with Down's syndrome. Most of these babies are otherwise healthy—that is, with only the usual pediatric care, they will proceed to an otherwise normal infancy. Some, however, are born with congenital defects such as intestinal obstructions that require operations if they are to live. Sometimes, the parents and the doctor will decide not to operate, and let the infant die. Anthony Shaw describes what happens then.

When surgery is denied [the doctor] must try to keep the infant from suffering while natural forces sap the baby's life away. As a surgeon whose natural inclination is to use the scalpel to fight off death, standing by and watching a salvageable baby die is the most emotionally exhausting experience I know. It is easy at a conference, in a theoretical discussion, to decide that such infants should be allowed to die. It is altogether different to stand by in the nursery and watch as dehydration and infection wither a tiny being over hours and days. This is a terrible ordeal for me and the hospital staff—much more so than for the parents who never set foot in the nursery.[1]

I can understand why some people are opposed to all euthanasia, and insist that such infants must be allowed to live. I think I can also understand why other people favor destroying these babies quickly and painlessly. But why should anyone favor letting "dehydration and infection wither a tiny being over hours and days"? The doctrine that says that a baby may be allowed to dehydrate and wither, but may not be given an injection that would end its life without suffering, seems so patently cruel as to require no further refutation. The strong language is not intended to offend, but only to put the point in the clearest possible way.

My second argument is that the conventional doctrine leads to decisions concerning life and death made on irrelevant grounds.

Consider again the case of the infants with Down's syndrome who need operations for congenital defects unrelated to the syndrome to live. Sometimes there is no operation, and the baby dies, but when there is no such defect, the baby lives on. Now, an operation such as that to remove an intestinal obstruction is not prohibitively difficult. The reason why such operations are not performed in these cases is, clearly, that the child has Down's syndrome and the parents and doctor judge that because of that fact it is better for the child to die.

But notice that this situation is absurd, no matter what view one takes of the lives and potentials of such babies. If the life of such an infant is worth preserving, what does it matter if it needs a simple operation? Or, if one thinks it better that such a baby should not live on, what difference does it make that it happens to have an unobstructed intestinal tract? In either case, the matter of life and death is being decided on irrelevant grounds. It is the Down's syndrome, and not the intestines, that is the issue. The matter should be decided, if at all, on that basis, and not be allowed to depend on the essentially irrelevant question of whether the intestinal tract is blocked.

What makes this situation possible, of course, is the idea that when there is an intestinal blockage, one can "let the baby die," but when there is no such defect there is nothing that can be done, for one must not "kill" it. The fact that this idea leads to such results as deciding life or death on irrelevant grounds is another good reason why the doctrine should be rejected.

One reason why so many people think that there is an important moral difference between active and passive euthanasia is that they think killing someone is morally worse than letting someone die. But is it? Is killing, in itself, worse than letting die? To investigate this issue, two cases may be considered that are exactly alike except that one involves killing whereas the other involves letting someone die. Then, it can be asked whether this difference makes any difference to the moral assessments. It is important that the cases be exactly alike, except for this one difference, since otherwise one cannot be confident that it is this difference and not some other that accounts for any variation in the assessments of the two cases. So, let us consider this pair of cases:

In the first, Smith stands to gain a large inheritance if anything should happen to his six-year-old cousin. One evening while the child is taking his bath, Smith sneaks into the bathroom and drowns the child, and then arranges things so that it will look like an accident.

In the second, Jones also stands to gain if anything should happen to his six-year-old cousin. Like Smith, Jones sneaks in planning to drown the child in his bath. However, just as he enters the bathroom Jones sees the child slip and hit his head, and fall face down in the water. Jones is delighted; he stands by, ready to push the child's head back under if it is necessary, but it is not necessary. With only a little thrashing about, the child drowns all by himself, "accidentally," as Jones watches and does nothing.

Now Smith killed the child, whereas Jones "merely" let the child die. That is the only difference between them. Did either man behave better, from a moral point of view? If the difference between killing and letting die were in itself a morally important matter, one should say that Jones's behavior was less reprehensible than Smith's. But does one really want to say that? I think not. In the first place, both men acted from the same motive, personal gain, and both had exactly the same end in view when they acted. It may be inferred from Smith's conduct that he is a bad man, although that judgment may be withdrawn or modified if certain further facts are learned about him—for example, that he is mentally deranged. But would not the very same thing be inferred about Jones from his conduct? And would not the same further considerations also be relevant to any modification of this judgment? Moreover, suppose Jones pleaded, in his own defense, "After all, I didn't do anything except just stand there and watch the child drown. I didn't kill him; I only let him die." Again, if letting die were in itself less bad than killing, this defense should have at least some weight. But it does not. Such a "defense" can only be regarded as a grotesque perversion of moral reasoning. Morally speaking, it is no defense at all.

Now it may be pointed out, quite properly, that the cases of euthanasia with which doctors are concerned are not like this at all. They do not involve personal gain or the destruction of normal healthy children. Doctors are concerned only with cases in which the patient's life is of no further use to him, or in which the patient's life has become or will soon become a terrible burden. However, the point is the same in these cases: the bare difference between killing and letting die does not, in itself, make a moral difference. If a doctor lets a patient die, for humane reasons, he is in the same moral position as if he had given the patient a lethal injection for humane reasons. If his decision was wrong—if, for example, the patient's illness was in fact curable—the decision would be equally regrettable no matter which method was used to carry it out. And if the doctor's decision was the right one, the method used is not in itself important.

The AMA policy statement isolates the crucial issue very well; the crucial issue is "the intentional termination of the life of one human being by another." But after identifying this issue, and forbidding "mercy killing," the statement goes on to deny that the cessation of treatment is the intentional termination of a life. This is where the mistake comes in, for what is the cessation of treatment, in these circumstances, if it is not "the intentional termination of the life of one human being by another?" Of course it is exactly that, and if it were not, there would be no point to it.

Many people will find this judgment hard to accept. One reason, I think, is that it is very easy to conflate the question of whether killing is, in itself, worse than letting die, with the very different question of whether most actual cases of killing are more reprehensible than most actual cases of letting die. Most actual cases of killing are clearly terrible (think, for example, of all the murders reported in the newspapers), and one hears of such cases every day. On the other hand, one hardly ever hears of a case of letting die, except for the actions of doctors who are motivated by humanitarian reasons. So one learns to think of killing in a much worse light than of letting die. But this does not

mean that there is something about killing that makes it in itself worse than letting die, for it is not the bare difference between killing and letting die that makes the difference in these cases. Rather, the other factors—the murderer's motive of personal gain, for example, contrasted with the doctor's humanitarian motivation—account for different reactions to the different cases.

I have argued that killing is not in itself any worse than letting die; if my contention is right, it follows that active euthanasia is not any worse than passive euthanasia. What arguments can be given on the other side? The most common, I believe, is the following:

"The important difference between active and passive euthanasia is that, in passive euthanasia, the doctor does not do anything to bring about the patient's death. The doctor does nothing, and the patient dies of whatever ills already afflict him. In active euthanasia, however, the doctor does something to bring about the patient's death: he kills him. The doctor who gives the patient with cancer a lethal injection has himself caused his patient's death; whereas if he merely ceases treatment, the cancer is the cause of the death."

A number of points need to be made here. The first is that it is not exactly correct to say that in passive euthanasia the doctor does nothing, for he does do one thing that is very important: he lets the patient die. "Letting someone die" is certainly different, in some respects, from other types of action—mainly in that it is a kind of action that one may perform by way of not performing certain other actions. For example, one may let a patient die by way of not giving medication, just as one may insult someone by way of not shaking his hand. But for any purpose of moral assessment, it is a type of action nonetheless. The decision to let a patient die is subject to moral appraisal in the same way that a decision to kill him would be subject to moral appraisal: it may be assessed as wise or unwise, compassionate or sadistic, right or wrong. If a doctor deliberately let a patient die who was suffering from a routinely curable illness, the doctor would certainly be to blame for what he had done, just as he would be to blame if he had needlessly killed the patient. Charges against him would then be appropriate. If so, it would be no defense at all for him to insist that he didn't "do anything." He would have done something very serious indeed, for he let his patient die.

Fixing the cause of death may be very important from a legal point of view, for it may determine whether criminal charges are brought against the doctor. But I do not think that this notion can be used to show a moral difference between active and passive euthanasia. The reason why it is considered bad to be the cause of someone's death is that death is regarded as a great evil—and so it is. However, if it has been decided that euthanasia—even passive euthanasia—is desirable in a given case, it has also been decided that in this instance death is no greater an evil than the patient's continued existence. And if this is true, the usual reason for not wanting to be the cause of someone's death simply does not apply.

Finally, doctors may think that all of this is only of academic interest—the sort of thing that philosophers may worry about but that has no practical bearing on their own work. After all, doctors must be concerned about the legal consequences of what they do, and active euthanasia is clearly forbidden by the law. But even so, doctors should also be concerned with the fact that the law is forcing upon them a moral doctrine that may well be indefensible, and has a considerable effect on their practices. Of course, most doctors are not now in the position of being coerced in this matter, for they do not regard themselves as merely going along with what the law requires. Rather, in statements such as the AMA policy statement that I have quoted, they are endorsing this doctrine as a central point of medical ethics. In that statement, active euthanasia is condemned not merely as illegal but as "contrary to that for which the medical profession stands," whereas passive euthanasia is approved. However, the preceding considerations suggest that there is really no moral difference between the two, considered in themselves (there may be important moral differences in some cases in their *consequences*, but, as I pointed out, these differences may make active euthanasia, and not passive euthanasia, the morally preferable option). So, whereas doctors may have to discriminate between active and passive euthanasia to satisfy the law, they should not do any more than that. In particular, they should not give the distinction any added authority and weight by writing it into official statements of medical ethics.

NOTES

1. A. Shaw, "Doctor, Do We Have a Choice?" *The New York Times Magazine*, January 30, 1972, p. 54.

TOM L. BEAUCHAMP

A Reply to Rachels on Active and Passive Euthanasia

James Rachels has recently argued that the distinction between active and passive euthanasia is neither appropriately used by the American Medical Association nor generally used for the resolution of moral problems of euthanasia.[1] Indeed he believes this distinction—which he equates with the killing/letting die distinction—does not in itself have any moral importance. The chief object of his attack is the following statement adopted by the House of Delegates of the American Medical Association in 1973:

> The intentional termination of the life of one human being by another—mercy killing—is contrary to that for which the medical profession stands and is contrary to the policy of the American Medical Association.

The cessation of the employment of extraordinary means to prolong the life of the body when there is irrefutable evidence that biological death is imminent is the decision of the patient and/or his immediate family. The advice and judgment of the physician should be freely available to the patient and/or his immediate family (p. 313).

From Tom L. Beauchamp and Seymour Perlin, eds., *Ethical Issues in Death and Dying* (Englewood Cliffs, N.J.: Prentice-Hall, 1978), pp. 246–258. This is a heavily revised version of an article by the same title first published in Thomas Mappes and Jane Zembaty, eds., *Social Ethics* (New York: McGraw-Hill, 1976). Reprinted by permission.

Rachels constructs a powerful and interesting set of arguments against this statement. In this paper I attempt the following: (1) to challenge his views on the grounds that he does not appreciate the moral reasons which give weight to the active/passive distinction; (2) to provide a constructive account of the moral relevance of the active/passive distinction; and (3) to offer reasons showing that Rachels may nonetheless be correct in urging that we *ought* to abandon the active/passive distinction for purposes of moral reasoning.

I

I would concede that the active/passive distinction is *sometimes* morally irrelevant. Of this Rachels convinces me. But it does not follow that it is *always* morally irrelevant. What we need, then, is a case where the distinction is a morally relevant one and an explanation why it is so. Rachels himself uses the method of examining two cases which are exactly alike except that "one involves killing whereas the other involves letting die" (p. 314). We may profitably begin by comparing the kinds of cases governed by the AMA's doctrine with the kinds of cases adduced by Rachels in order to assess the adequacy and fairness of his cases.

The second paragraph of the AMA statement is confined to a narrowly restricted range of passive euthanasia cases, viz., those (a) where the patients are on extraordinary means, (b) where irrefutable evidence of imminent death is available, and (c) where patient or family consent is available. Rachels' two cases involve conditions notably different from these:

In the first, Smith stands to gain a large inheritance if anything should happen to his six-year-old cousin. One evening while the child is taking his bath, Smith sneaks into the bathroom and drowns the child, and then arranges things so that it will look like an accident.

In the second, Jones also stands to gain if anything should happen to his six-year-old cousin. Like Smith, Jones sneaks in planning to drown the child in his bath. However, just as he enters the bathroom Jones sees the child slip and hit his head, and fall face down in the water. Jones is delighted; he stands by, ready to push the child's head back under if it is necessary, but it is not necessary. With only a little thrashing about, the child drowns all by himself, "accidentally," as Jones watches and does nothing.

Now Smith killed the child, whereas Jones "merely" let the child die. That is the only difference between them (p. 314).

Rachels says there is no moral difference between the cases in terms of our moral assessments of Smith and Jones' behavior. This assessment seems fair enough, but what can Rachels' cases be said to prove, as they are so markedly disanalogous to the sorts of cases envisioned by the AMA proposal? Rachels concedes important disanalogies, but thinks them irrelevant:

The point is the same in these cases: the bare difference between killing and letting die does not, in itself, make a moral difference. If a doctor lets a patient die, for humane reasons, he is in the same moral position as if he had given the patient a lethal injection for humane reasons (p. 315).

Three observations are immediately in order. First, Rachels seems to infer that from such cases we can conclude that the distinction between killing and letting die is *always* morally irrelevant. This conclusion is fallaciously derived. What the argument in fact shows, being an analogical argument, is only that in all *relevantly similar* cases the distinction does not in itself make a moral difference. Since Rachels concedes that other cases are disanalogous, he seems thereby to concede that his argument is as weak as the analogy itself. Second, Rachels' cases involve two *unjustified* actions, one of killing and the other of letting die. The AMA statement distinguishes one set of cases of unjustified killing and another of *justified* cases of allowing to die. Nowhere is it claimed by the AMA that what makes the difference in these cases is the active/passive distinction itself. It is only implied that one set of cases, the justified set, *involves* (passive) letting die while the unjustified set *involves* (active) killing. While it is said that justified euthanasia cases are passive ones and unjustified ones active, it is not said either that what makes some acts justified is the fact of their being passive or that what makes others unjustified is the fact of their being active. This fact will prove to be of vital importance.

The third point is that in both of Rachels' cases the respective moral agents—Smith and Jones—are morally responsible for the death of the child and are morally blameworthy—even though Jones is presumably not causally responsible. In the first case death is caused by the agent, while in the second it is not; yet the second agent is no less morally responsible. While the law might find only the first homicidal, morality condemns the motives in each case as equally wrong, and it holds that the duty to save life in such cases is as compelling as the duty not to take life. I suggest that it is largely because of this equal degree of moral responsibility that there is no morally relevant difference in Rachels' cases. In the cases envisioned by the AMA, however, an agent is held to be responsible for taking life by actively killing but is not held to be morally required to preserve life, and so not responsible for death, when removing the patient from extraordinary means (under conditions a–c above). I shall elaborate this latter point momentarily. My only conclusion thus far is the negative one that Rachels' arguments rest on weak foundations. His cases are not relevantly similar to euthanasia cases and do not support his apparent conclusion that the active/passive distinction is *always* morally irrelevant.

II

I wish first to consider an argument that I believe has powerful intuitive appeal and probably is widely accepted as stating the main reason for rejecting Rachels' views. I will maintain that this argument fails, and so leaves Rachels' contentions untouched.

I begin with an actual case, the celebrated Quinlan case.[2] Karen Quinlan was in a coma, and was on a mechanical respirator which artificially sustained her vital processes and which her parents wished to cease. At least some physicians believed there was irrefutable evidence that biological death was imminent and the coma irreversible. This case, under this description, closely conforms to the passive cases envisioned by the AMA. During an interview the father, Mr. Quinlan, asserted that he did not wish to kill his daughter, but only to remove her from the machines in order to see whether she would live or would die a natural death.[3] Suppose he had said—to envision now a second and hypothetical, but parallel case—that he wished only to see her die painlessly and therefore wished that the doctor could induce death by an overdose of morphine. Most of us would think the second act, which involves active killing, morally unjustified in these circumstances, while many of us would think the first act morally justified. (This is not the place to consider whether in fact it is justified, and if so under what conditions.) What accounts for the apparent morally relevant difference?

I have considered these two cases together in order to follow Rachels' method of entertaining parallel cases where the only difference is that the one case involves killing and the other letting die. However, there is a further difference, which crops up in the euthanasia context. The difference rests in our judg-

ments of medical fallibility and moral responsibility. Mr. Quinlan seems to think that, after all, the doctors might be wrong. There is a remote possibility that she might live without the aid of a machine. But whether or not the medical prediction of death turns out to be accurate, if she dies then no one is morally responsible for directly bringing about or causing her death, as they would be if they caused her death by killing her. Rachels finds explanations which appeal to causal conditions unsatisfactory; but perhaps this is only because he fails to see the nature of the causal link. To bring about her death is by that act to preempt the possibility of life. To "allow her to die" by removing artificial equipment is to allow for the possibility of wrong diagnosis or incorrect prediction and hence to absolve oneself of moral responsibility for the taking of life under false assumptions. There may, of course, be utterly no empirical possibility of recovery in some cases since recovery would violate a law of nature. However, judgments of empirical impossibility in medicine are notoriously problematic—the reason for emphasizing medical fallibility. And in all the hard cases we do not *know* that recovery is empirically impossible, even if good *evidence* is available.

The above reason for invoking the active/passive distinction can now be generalized: Active termination of life removes all possibility of life for the patient, while passively ceasing extraordinary means may not. This is not trivial since patients have survived in several celebrated cases where, in knowledgeable physicians' judgments, there was "irrefutable" evidence that death was imminent.[4]

One may, of course, be entirely responsible and culpable for another's death either by killing him or by letting him die. In such cases, of which Rachels' are examples, there is no morally significant difference between killing and letting die precisely because whatever one does, omits, or refrains from doing does not absolve one of responsibility. Either active or passive involvement renders one responsible for the death of another, and both involvements are equally wrong for the same principled moral reason: it is (prima facie) morally wrong to bring about the death of an innocent person capable of living whenever the causal intervention or negligence is intentional. (I use causal terms here because causal involvement need not be active, as when by one's negligence one is nonetheless causally responsible.) But not all cases of killing and letting die fall under this same moral principle. One is sometimes culpable for killing, because morally responsible as the agent for death, as when one pulls the plug on a respirator sustaining a recovering patient (a murder). But one is sometimes not culpable for letting die because one is not morally responsible as agent, as when one pulls the plug on a respirator sustaining an irreversibly comatose and unrecoverable patient (a routine procedure, where one is *merely* causally responsible).[5] Different degrees and means of involvement assess different degrees of responsibility, and our assessments of culpability can become intricately complex. The only point which now concerns us, however, is that because different moral principles may govern very similar circumstances, we are sometimes morally culpable for killing but not for letting die. And to many people it will seem that in passive cases we are not morally responsible for causing death, though we are responsible in active cases.

This argument is powerfully attractive. Although I was once inclined to accept it in virtually the identical form just developed,[6] I now think that, despite its intuitive appeal, it cannot be correct. It is true that different degrees and means of involvement entail different degrees of responsibility, but it does not follow that we are *not* responsible and therefore are absolved of possible culpability in *any* case of intentionally allowing to die. We are responsible and *perhaps* culpable in either active or passive cases. Here Rachels' argument is entirely to the point: It is not primarily a question of greater or lesser responsibility by an active or a passive means that should determine culpability. Rather, the question of culpability is decided by the moral *justification* for choosing either a passive or an active means. What the argument in the previous paragraph overlooks is that one might be unjustified in using an active means or unjustified in using a passive means, and hence be culpable in the use of either; yet one might be justified in using an active means or justified in using a passive means, and hence not be culpable in using either. Fallibility might just as well be present in a judgment to use one means as in a judgment to use another. (A judgment to allow to die is just as subject to being based on *knowledge which is fallible* as a judgment to kill.) Moreover, in either case, it is a matter of what one knows and believes, and not a matter of a particular kind of causal connection or causal chain. If we kill the patient, then we are certainly causally responsible for his death. But, similarly, if we cease treatment, and the patient dies, the patient might have recovered if treatment had been continued. The patient might have been saved in either case, and hence there is no morally relevant difference between the two cases. It is, therefore,

simply beside the point that "one is sometimes culpable for killing . . . but one is sometimes not culpable for letting die"—as the above argument concludes.

Accordingly, despite its great intuitive appeal and frequent mention, this argument from responsibility fails.

III

There may, however, be more compelling arguments against Rachels, and I wish now to provide what I believe is the most significant argument that can be adduced in defense of the active/passive distinction. I shall develop this argument by combining (1) so-called wedge or slippery slope arguments with (2) recent arguments in defense of rule utilitarianism. I shall explain each in turn and show how in combination they may be used to defend the active-passive distinction.

(1) *Wedge arguments* proceed as follows: if killing were allowed, even under the guise of a merciful extinction of life, a dangerous wedge would be introduced which places all "undesirable" or "unworthy" human life in a precarious condition. Proponents of wedge arguments believe the initial wedge places us on a slippery slope for at least one of two reasons: (i) It is said that our justifying principles leave us with no principled way to avoid the slide into saying that all sorts of killings would be justified under similar conditions. Here it is thought that once killing is allowed, a firm line between justified and unjustified killings cannot be securely drawn. It is thought best not to redraw the line in the first place, for redrawing it will inevitably lead to a downhill slide. It is then often pointed out that as a matter of historical record this is precisely what has occurred in the darker regions of human history, including the Nazi era, where euthanasia began with the best intentions for horribly ill, non-Jewish Germans and gradually spread to anyone deemed an enemy of the people. (ii) Second, it is said that our basic principles against killing will be gradually eroded once some form of killing is legitimated. For example, it is said that permitting voluntary euthanasia will lead to permitting involuntary euthanasia, which will in turn lead to permitting euthanasia for those who are a nuisance to society (idiots, recidivist criminals, defective newborns, and the insane, e.g.). Gradually other principles which instill respect for human life will be eroded or abandoned in the process.

I am not inclined to accept the first reason (i).[7] If our justifying principles are themselves justified, then any action they warrant would be justified.

Accordingly, I shall only be concerned with the second approach (ii).

(2) *Rule utilitarianism* is the position that a society ought to adopt a rule if its acceptance would have better consequences for the common good (greater social utility) than any comparable rule could have in that society. Any action is right if it conforms to a valid rule and wrong if it violates the rule. Sometimes it is said that alternative rules should be measured against one another, while it has also been suggested that whole moral *codes* (complete sets of rules) rather than individual rules should be compared. While I prefer the latter formulation (Brandt's), this internal dispute need not detain us here. The important point is that a particular rule or a particular code of rules is morally justified if and only if there is no other competing rule or moral code whose acceptance would have a higher utility value for society, and where a rule's acceptability is contingent upon the consequences which would result if the rule were made current.

Wedge arguments, when conjoined with rule utilitarian arguments, may be applied to euthanasia issues in the following way. We presently subscribe to a no-active-euthanasia rule (which the AMA suggests we retain). Imagine now that in our society we make current a restricted-active-euthanasia rule (as Rachels seems to urge). Which of these two moral rules would, if enacted, have the consequence of maximizing social utility? Clearly a restricted-active-euthanasia rule would have *some* utility value, as Rachels notes, since some intense and uncontrollable suffering would be eliminated. However, it may not have the highest utility value in the structure of our present code or in any imaginable code which could be made current, and therefore may not be a component in the ideal code for our society. If wedge arguments raise any serious questions at all, as I think they do, they rest in this area of whether a code would be weakened or strengthened by the addition of active euthanasia principles. For the disutility of introducing legitimate killing into one's moral code (in the form of active euthanasia rules) may, in the long run, outweigh the utility of doing so, as a result of the eroding effect such a relaxation would have on rules in the code which demand respect for human life. If, for example, rules permitting active killing were introduced, it is not implausible to suppose that destroying defective newborns (a form of involuntary euthanasia) would become an accepted and common practice, that as population

increases occur the aged will be even more neglectable and neglected than they now are, that capital punishment for a wide variety of crimes would be increasingly tempting, that some doctors would have appreciably reduced fears of actively injecting fatal doses whenever it seemed to them propitious to do so, and that laws of war against killing civilians would erode in efficacy even beyond their already abysmal level.

A hundred such possible consequences might easily be imagined. But these few are sufficient to make the larger point that such rules permitting killing could lead to a general reduction of respect for human life. Rules against killing in a moral code are not *isolated* moral principles; they are pieces of a web of rules against killing which forms the code. The more threads one removes, the weaker the fabric becomes. And if, as I believe, moral principles against active killing have the deep and continuously civilizing effect of promoting respect for life, and if principles which allow passively letting die (as envisioned in the AMA statement) do not themselves cut against this effect, then this seems an important reason for the maintenance of the active/passive distinction. (By the logic of the above argument, passively letting die would also have to be prohibited if a rule permitting it had the serious adverse consequence of eroding acceptance or rules protective of respect for life. While this prospect seems to me improbable, I can hardly claim to have refuted those conservatives who would claim that even rules that sanction letting die place us on a precarious slippery slope.)

A troublesome problem, however, confronts my use of utilitarian and wedge arguments. Most all of us would agree that both killing and letting die are justified under some conditions. Killings in self-defense and in "just" wars are widely accepted as justified because the conditions excuse the killing. If society can withstand these exceptions to moral rules prohibiting killing, then why is it not plausible to suppose society can accept another excusing exception in the form of justified active euthanasia? This is an important and worthy objection, but not a decisive one. The defenseless and the dying are significantly different classes of persons from aggressors who attack individuals and/or nations. In the case of aggressors, one does not confront the question whether their lives are no longer *worth living*. Rather, we reach the judgment that the aggressors' morally blameworthy actions justify counteractions. But in the case of the dying and the otherwise ill, there is no morally blameworthy action to justify our own. Here we are required to accept the judgment that their lives are no longer *worth living* in order to believe that the termination of their lives is justified. It is the latter sort of judgment which is feared by those who take the wedge argument seriously. We do not now permit and never have permitted the taking of morally blameless lives. I think this is the key to understanding why recent cases of intentionally allowing the death of defective newborns (as in the now famous case at the Johns Hopkins Hospital) have generated such protracted controversy. Even if such newborns could not have led meaningful lives (a matter of some controversy), it is the wedged foot in the door which creates the most intense worries. For if we once take a decision to allow a restricted infanticide justification or any justification at all on grounds that a life is not meaningful or not worth living, we have qualified our moral rules against killing. That this qualification is a matter of the utmost seriousness needs no argument. I mention it here only to show why the wedge argument may have moral force even though we *already* allow some very different conditions to justify intentional killing.

There is one final utilitarian reason favoring the preservation of the active/passive distinction.[8] Suppose we distinguish the following two types of cases of wrongly diagnosed patients:

1. Patients wrongly diagnosed as hopeless, and who will survive even if a treatment *is* ceased (in order to allow a natural death).
2. Patients wrongly diagnosed as hopeless, and who will survive only if the treatment is *not ceased* (in order to allow a natural death).

If a social rule permitting only passive euthanasia were in effect, then doctors and families who "allowed death" would lose only patients in class 2, not those in class 1; whereas if active euthanasia were permitted, at least some patients in class 1 would be needlessly lost. Thus, the consequence of a no-active-euthanasia rule would be to save some lives which could not be saved if both forms of euthanasia were allowed. This reason is not a *decisive* reason for favoring a policy of passive euthanasia, since these classes (1 and 2) are likely to be very small and since there might be counterbalancing reasons (extreme pain, autonomous expression of the patient, etc.) in favor of active euthanasia. But certainly it is *a* reason favoring only passive euthanasia and one which is morally relevant and ought to be considered along with other moral reasons.

IV

It may still be insisted that my case has not touched Rachels' leading claim, for I have not shown, as Rachels puts it, that it is "the bare difference between killing and letting die that makes the difference in these cases" (p. 315). True, I have not shown this and in my judgment it cannot be shown. But this concession does not require capitulation to Rachels' argument. I adduced a case which is at the center of our moral intuition that killing is morally different (in at least some cases) from letting die; and I then attempted to account for at least part of the grounds for this belief. The grounds turn out to be other than the *bare* difference, but nevertheless *make* the distinction morally relevant. The identical point can be made regarding the voluntary/involuntary distinction, as it is commonly applied to euthanasia. It is not the bare difference between voluntary euthanasia (i.e., euthanasia with patient consent) and involuntary euthanasia (i.e., without patient consent) that makes one justifiable and one not. Independent moral grounds based on, for example, respect for autonomy or beneficence, or perhaps justice will alone make the moral difference.

In order to illustrate this general claim, let us presume that it is sometimes justified to kill another person and sometimes justified to allow another to die. Suppose, for example, that one may kill in self-defense and may allow to die when a promise has been made to someone that he would be allowed to die. Here conditions of self-defense and promising justify actions. But suppose now that someone A promises in exactly similar circumstances to kill someone B at B's request, and also that someone C allows someone D to die in an act of self-defense. Surely A is obliged equally to kill or to let die if he promised; and surely C is permitted to let D die if it is a matter of defending C's life. If this analysis is correct, then it follows that killing is sometimes right, sometimes wrong, depending on the circumstances, and the same is true of letting die. It is the justifying reasons which make the difference whether an action is right, not merely the kind of action it is.

Now, *if* letting die led to disastrous conclusions but killing did not, then letting die but not killing would be wrong. Consider, for example, a possible world in which dying would be indefinitely prolongable even if all extraordinary therapy were removed and the patient were allowed to die. Suppose that it costs over one million dollars to let each patient die, that nurses consistently commit suicide from caring for those being "allowed to die," that physicians are constantly being successfully sued for malpractice for allowing death by cruel and wrongful means, and that hospitals are uncontrollably overcrowded and their wards filled with communicable diseases which afflict only the dying. Now suppose further that killing in this possible world is quick, painless, and easily monitored. I submit that in this world we would believe that *killing is morally acceptable but that allowing to die is morally unacceptable*. The point of this example is again that it is the circumstances that make the difference, not the bare difference between killing and letting die.

It is, however, worth noticing that there is nothing in the AMA statement which says that the bare difference between killing and letting die itself and alone makes the difference in our differing moral assessments of rightness and wrongness. Rachels forces this interpretation on the statement. Some philosophers may have thought bare difference makes the difference, but there is scant evidence that the AMA or any thoughtful ethicist *must* believe it in order to defend the relevance and importance of the active/passive distinction. When this conclusion is coupled with my earlier argument that from Rachels' paradigm cases it follows only that the active/passive distinction is sometimes, but not always, morally irrelevant, it would seem that his case against the AMA is rendered highly questionable.

V

There remains, however, the important question as to whether we *ought* to accept the distinction between active and passive euthanasia, now that we are clear about (at least one way of drawing) the moral grounds for its invocation. That is, should we employ the distinction in order to judge some acts of euthanasia justified and others not justified? Here, as the hesitant previous paragraph indicates, I am uncertain. This problem is a substantive moral issue—not merely a conceptual one—and would require at a minimum a lengthy assessment of wedge arguments and related utilitarian considerations. In important respects empirical questions are involved in this assessment. We should like to know, and yet have hardly any evidence to indicate, what the consequences would be for our society if we were to allow the use of active means to produce death. The best hope for making such an assessment has seemed to some to rest in analogies to suicide and capital punishment statutes. Here it may reasonably be asked whether recent liberalizations of laws limiting these forms of killing have served as the thin end of a wedge leading to a breakdown of principles protecting life or to widespread violations of moral principles. Nonetheless, such analogies do not seem to me promising, since they are still fairly remote from the pertinent issue of the consequences of allowing active humanitarian killing of one person by another.

It is interesting to notice the outcome of the Kamisar-Williams debate on euthanasia—which is almost exclusively cast by both writers in a consequential, utilitarian framework.[9] At one crucial point in the debate, where possible consequences of laws permitting euthanasia are under discussion, they exchange "perhaps" judgments:

I [Williams] will return Kamisar the compliment and say: "Perhaps." We are certainly in an area where no solution is going to make things quite easy and happy for everybody, and all sorts of embarrassments may be conjectured. But these embarrassments are not avoided by keeping to the present law: we suffer from them already.[10]

Because of the grave difficulties which stand in the way of making accurate predictions about the impact of liberalized euthanasia laws—especially those that would permit active killing—it is not surprising that those who debate the subject would reach a point of exchanging such "perhaps" judgments. And that is why, so it seems to me, we are uncertain whether to perpetuate or to abandon the active-passive distinction in our moral thinking about euthanasia. I think we *do* perpetuate it in medicine, law, and ethics because we are still somewhat uncertain about the conditions under which *passive* euthanasia should be permitted by law (which is one form of social *rule*). We are unsure about what the consequences will be of the California "Natural Death Act" and all those similar acts passed by other states which have followed in its path. If no untoward results occur, and the balance of the results seems favorable, then we will perhaps be less concerned about further liberalizations of euthanasia laws. If untoward results do occur (on a widespread scale), then we would be most reluctant to accept further liberalizations and might even abolish natural death acts.

In short, I have argued in this section that euthanasia in its active and its passive forms presents us with a dilemma which can be developed by using powerful consequentialist arguments on each side, yet there is little clarity concerning the proper resolution of the dilemma precisely because of our uncertainty regarding proclaimed consequences.

VI

I reach two conclusions at the end of these several arguments. First, I think Rachels is incorrect in arguing that the distinction between active and passive is (always) morally irrelevant. It may well be relevant, and for moral reasons—the reasons adduced in section III above. Second, I think nonetheless that Rachels may ultimately be shown correct in his contention that we ought to dispense with the active-passive distinction—for reasons adduced in sections IV–V. But if he is ultimately judged correct, it will be because we have come to see that some forms of active killing have generally acceptable social consequences, and not primarily because of the arguments he adduces in his paper—even though *something* may be said for each of these arguments. Of course, in one respect I have conceded a great deal to Rachels. The bare difference argument is vital to his position, and I have fully agreed to it. On the other hand, I do not see that the bare difference argument does play or need play a major role in our moral thinking—or in that of the AMA.

NOTES

1. "Active and Passive Euthanasia," *New England Journal of Medicine* 292 (January 9, 1975), 78–80. [All page references in parentheses refer to Rachels' article as reprinted in this chapter.]

2. As recorded in the Opinion of Judge Robert Muir, Jr., Docket No. C-201-75 of the Superior Court of New Jersey, Chancery Division, Morris County (November 10, 1975).

3. See Judge Muir's Opinion, p. 18—a slightly different statement but on the subject.

4. This problem of the strength of evidence also emerged in the Quinlan trial, as physicians disagreed whether the evidence was "irrefutable." Such disagreement, when added to the problems of medical fallibility and causal responsibility just outlined, provides in the eyes of some one important argument against the *legalization* of active euthanasia, as perhaps the AMA would agree. Cf. Kamisar's arguments in this chapter.

5. Among the moral reasons why one is held to be responsible in the first sort of case and not responsible in the second sort are, I believe, the moral grounds for the active/passive distinction under discussion in this section.

6. In *Social Ethics*, as cited in the permission note to this [essay].

7. An argument of this form, which I find unacceptable for reasons given below, is Arthur Dyck, "Beneficent Euthanasia and Benemortasia: Alternative Views of Mercy," in M. Kohl, ed., *Beneficent Euthanasia* (Buffalo: Prometheus Books, 1975), pp. 121f.

8. I owe most of this argument to James Rachels, whose comments on an earlier draft of this paper led to several significant alterations.

9. Williams bases his pro-euthanasia argument on the prevention of two consequences: (1) loss of liberty and (2) cruelty. Kamisar bases his anti-euthanasia position on three projected consequences of euthanasia laws: (1) mistaken diagnosis, (2) pressured decisions by seriously ill patients, and (3) the wedge of the laws will lead to legalized involuntary euthanasia. Kamisar admits that individual acts of euthanasia are sometimes justified. It is the rule that he opposes. He is thus clearly a rule-utilitarian, and I believe Williams is as well (cf. his views on children and the senile). Their assessments of wedge arguments are, however, radically different.

10. Glanville Williams, "Mercy-Killing Legislation—A Rejoinder," *Minnesota Law Review* 43, no. 1 (1958), 5.

FLORIDA DISTRICT COURT OF APPEAL, FOURTH DISTRICT

Satz v. Perlmutter

DECIDED SEPTEMBER 13, 1978

LETTS, JUDGE.

The State here appeals a trial court order permitting the removal of an artificial life sustaining device from a competent, but terminally ill adult. . . .

Seventy-three year old Abe Perlmutter lies mortally sick in a hospital, suffering from amyotrophic lateral sclerosis (Lou Gehrig's disease) diagnosed in January 1977. There is no cure and normal life expectancy, from time of diagnosis, is but two years. In Mr. Perlmutter, the affliction has progressed to the point of virtual incapability of movement, inability to breathe without a mechanical respirator and his very speech is an extreme effort. Even with the respirator, the prognosis is death within a short time. Notwithstanding, he remains in command of his mental faculties and legally competent. He seeks, with full approval of his adult family, to have the respirator removed from his trachea, which act, according to his physician, based upon medical probability, would result in "a reasonable life expectancy of less than one hour." Mr. Perlmutter is fully aware of the inevitable result of such removal, yet has attempted to remove it for himself (hospital personnel, activated by an alarm, reconnected it). He has repeatedly stated to his family, "I'm miserable, take it out" and at a bedside hearing, told the obviously concerned trial judge that whatever would be in store for him if the respirator were removed, "it can't be worse than what I'm going through now."

Pursuant to all of the foregoing, and upon the petition of Mr. Perlmutter himself, the trial judge entered a

Reprinted from the *Southern Reporter*, 362 So. 2d 160; affirmed 379 So. 2d 359.

detailed and thoughtful final judgment which included the following language:

ORDERED AND ADJUDGED that Abe Perlmutter, in the exercise of his right of privacy, may remain in defendant hospital or leave said hospital, free of the mechanical respirator now attached to his body and all defendants and their staffs are restrained from interfering with Plaintiff's decision.

We agree with the trial judge.

The State's position is that it (1) has an overriding duty to preserve life, and (2) that termination of supportive care, whether it be by the patient, his family or medical personnel, is an unlawful killing of a human being under the Florida Murder Statute Section 782.04, Florida Statutes (1977) or Manslaughter under Section 782.08. The hospital, and its doctors, while not insensitive to this tragedy, fear not only criminal prosecution if they aid in removal of the mechanical device, but also civil liability. In the absence of prior Florida law on the subject, their fears cannot be discounted.

The pros and cons involved in such tragedies which bedevil contemporary society, mainly because of incredible advancement in scientific medicine, are all exhaustively discussed in Superintendent of Belchertown v. Saikewicz, Mass., 370 N.E.2d 417 (1977). As *Saikewicz* points out, the right of an individual to refuse medical treatment is tempered by the State's:

1. Interest in the preservation of life.
2. Need to protect innocent third parties.
3. Duty to prevent suicide.
4. Requirement that it help maintain the ethical integrity of medical practice.

In the case at bar, none of these four considerations surmount the individual wishes of Abe Perlmutter.

Thus we adopt the view of the line of cases discussed in *Saikewicz* which would allow Abe Perlmutter the right to refuse or discontinue treatment based upon "the constitutional right to privacy . . . an expression of the sanctity of individual free choice and self-determination." (Id. 426.) We would stress that this adoption is limited to the specific facts now before us, involving a competent adult patient. The problem is less easy of solution when the patient is incapable of understanding and we, therefore, postpone a crossing of that more complex bridge until such time as we are required to do so.

PRESERVATION OF LIFE

There can be no doubt that the State *does* have an interest in preserving life, but we again agree with *Saikewicz* that "there is a substantial distinction in the State's insistence that human life be saved where the affliction is curable, as opposed to the State interest where, as here, the issue is not whether, but when, for how long and at what cost to the individual [his] life may be briefly extended." (Id. 425–426.) In the case at bar the condition is terminal, the patient's situation wretched and the continuation of his life temporary and totally artificial.

Accordingly, we see no compelling State interest to interfere with Mr. Perlmutter's expressed wishes.

PROTECTION OF THIRD PARTIES

Classically, this protection is exemplified in the case Application of the President and Directors of Georgetown College, Inc., 118 U.S.App.D.C. 80, 331 F.2d 1000, cert. denied, 377 U.S. 978 (1964), where the patient, by refusing treatment, is said to be abandoning his minor child, which abandonment the State as *parens patriae* sought to prevent. We point out that Abe Perlmutter is 73, his family adult and all in agreement with his wishes. The facts do not support abandonment.

As to suicide, the facts here unarguably reveal that Mr. Perlmutter would die, but for the respirator. The disconnecting of it, far from causing his unnatural death by means of a "death producing agent" in fact will merely result in his death, if at all, from natural causes, *Saikewicz*, Id., 426, fn. 11. The testimony of Mr. Perlmutter, like the victim in the *Georgetown College* case, supra, is that he really wants to live, but to do so, God and Mother Nature willing, under his own power. This basic wish to live, plus the fact that he did not self-induce his horrible affliction, precludes

his further refusal of treatment being classed as attempted suicide.

Moreover we find no requirement in the law that a competent, but otherwise mortally sick, patient undergo the surgery or treatment which constitutes the only hope for temporary prolongation of his life. This being so, we see little difference between a cancer ridden patient who declines surgery, or chemotherapy, necessary for his temporary survival and the hopeless predicament which tragically afflicts Abe Perlmutter. It is true that the latter appears more drastic because affirmatively, a mechanical device must be disconnected, as distinct from mere inaction. Notwithstanding, the principle is the same, for in both instances the hapless, but mentally competent, victim is choosing not to avail himself of one of the expensive marvels of modern medical science.

The State argues that a patient has *no right* to refuse treatment and cites several of the familiar blood transfusion cases. However, a reading of these reveal substantial distinctions between them and the case at bar. In the blood transfusion cases, the patient is either incompetent to make a medical decision, equivocal about making it ("he would not agree to be transfused but would not resist a court order permitting it because it would be the court's will and not his own.") or it is a family member making the decision for an inert or minor third party patient. By contrast, we find, and agree with, several cases upholding the right of a competent adult patient to refuse treatment for himself. From this agreement, we reach our conclusion that, because Abe Perlmutter has a right to refuse treatment in the first instance, he has a concomitant right to discontinue it.

ETHICS OF MEDICAL PRACTICE

Lastly, as to the ethical integrity of medical practice, we again adopt the language of *Saikewicz*:

Prevailing medical ethical practice does not, without exception, demand that all efforts toward life prolongation be made in all circumstances. Rather, as indicated in *Quinlan*, the prevailing ethical practice seems to be to recognize that the dying are more often in need of comfort than treatment. Recognition of the right to refuse necessary treatment in appropriate circumstances is consistent with existing medical mores; such a doctrine does not threaten either the integrity of the medical profession, the proper role of hospitals in caring for such patients or the State's interest in protecting the same. It is not necessary to deny a right of self-determination to a patient in order to recognize the interests of doctors, hospitals, and medical personnel in attendance on the patient. . . .

It is our conclusion, therefore, under the facts before us, that when these several public policy interests are weighed against the rights of Mr. Perlmutter, the latter must and should prevail. Abe Perlmutter should be allowed to make his choice to die with dignity, notwithstanding over a dozen legislative failures in this state to adopt suitable legislation in this field. It is all very convenient to insist on continuing Mr. Perlmutter's life so that there can be no question of foul play, no resulting civil liability and no possible trespass on medical ethics. However, it is quite another matter to do so at the patient's sole expense and against his competent will, thus inflicting never ending physical torture on his body until the inevitable, but artificially suspended, moment of death. Such a course of conduct invades the patient's constitutional right of privacy, removes his freedom of choice and invades his right to self-determine.

The judgment of the trial court is hereby affirmed. . . .

CALIFORNIA COURT OF APPEALS, SECOND DISTRICT

Bouvia v. Superior Court

DECIDED APRIL 16, 1986

Elizabeth BOUVIA, Petitioner.

v.

SUPERIOR COURT of the State of California For the County of Los Angeles, Respondent

(Glenchur)

OPINION AND ORDER FOR A PEREMPTORY WRIT OF MANDATE

BEACH, ASSOCIATE JUSTICE.

Petitioner, Elizabeth Bouvia, a patient in a public hospital seeks the removal from her body of a nasogastric tube inserted and maintained against her will and without her consent by physicians who so placed it for the purpose of keeping her alive through involuntary forced feeding. . . .

The trial court denied petitioner's request for the immediate relief she sought. It concluded that leaving the tube in place was necessary to prolong petitioner's life, and that it would, in fact, do so. With the tube in place petitioner probably will survive the time required to prepare for trial, a trial itself and an appeal, if one proved necessary. The real party physicians also assert, and the trial court agreed, that physically petitioner tolerates the tube reasonably well and thus is not in great physical discomfort. . . .

FACTUAL BACKGROUND

Petitioner is a 28-year-old woman. Since birth she has been afflicted with and suffered from severe cerebral palsy. She is quadriplegic. She is now a patient at a public hospital maintained by one of the real parties in interest, the County of Los Angeles. . . . Petitioner's physical handicaps of palsy and quadriplegia have progressed to the point where she is completely bedridden. Except for a few fingers of one hand and some slight head and facial movements, she is immobile. She is physically helpless and wholly unable to care for herself. She is totally dependent upon others for all of her needs. These include feeding, washing, cleaning, toileting, turning, and helping her with elimination and other bodily functions. She cannot stand or sit upright in bed or in a wheelchair. She lies flat in bed and must do so the rest of her life. She suffers also

Reprinted from the *California Reporter*, 225 Cal.Rptr. 297 (Cal.App. 2 Dist.).

from degenerative and severely crippling arthritis. She is in continual pain. Another tube permanently attached to her chest automatically injects her with periodic doses of morphine which relieves some, but not all of her physical pain and discomfort.

She is intelligent, very mentally competent. She earned a college degree. She was married but her husband has left her. She suffered a miscarriage. She lived with her parents until her father told her that they could no longer care for her. She has stayed intermittently with friends and at public facilities. A search for a permanent place to live where she might receive the constant care which she needs has been unsuccessful. She is without financial means to support herself and, therefore, must accept public assistance for medical and other care.

She has on several occasions expressed the desire to die. In 1983 she sought the right to be cared for in a public hospital in Riverside County while she intentionally "starved herself to death." A court in that county denied her judicial assistance to accomplish that goal. She later abandoned an appeal from that ruling. Thereafter, friends took her to several different facilities, both public and private, arriving finally at her present location. . . .

Petitioner must be spoon fed in order to eat. Her present medical and dietary staff have determined that she is not consuming a sufficient amount of nutrients. Petitioner stops eating when she feels she cannot orally swallow more, without nausea and vomiting. As she cannot now retain solids, she is fed soft liquid-like food. Because of her previously announced resolve to starve herself, the medical staff feared her weight loss might reach a life-threatening level. Her weight since admission to real parties' facility seems to hover between 65 and 70 pounds. Accordingly, they inserted the subject tube against her will and contrary to her express written instructions.[1] . . .

THE RIGHT TO REFUSE
MEDICAL TREATMENT

"[A] person of adult years and in sound mind has the right, in the exercise of control over his own body, to determine whether or not to submit to lawful medical treatment." (*Cobbs v. Grant* (1972) 8 Cal.3d 229, 242, 104 Cal.Rptr. 505, 502 P.2d 1.) It follows that such a patient has the right to refuse *any* medical treatment, even that which may save or prolong her life. (*Barber v. Superior Court* (1983) 147 Cal.App.3d 1006, 195 Cal.Rptr. 484; *Bartling v. Superior Court* (1984) 163

Cal.App.3d 186, 209 Cal.Rptr. 220.) In our view the foregoing authorities are dispositive of the case at bench. Nonetheless, the County and its medical staff contend that for reasons unique to this case, Elizabeth Bouvia may not exercise the right available to others. Accordingly, we again briefly discuss the rule in the light of real parties' contentions.

The right to refuse medical treatment is basic and fundamental. It is recognized as a part of the right of privacy protected by both the state and federal constitutions. (Calif.Const., art. I, § 1; *Griswold v. Connecticut* (1965) 381 U.S. 479, 484, 85 S.Ct. 1678, 1681, 14 L.Ed.2d 510; *Bartling v. Superior Court, supra*, 163 Cal.App.3d 186, 209 Cal.Rptr. 220.) Its exercise requires no one's approval. It is not merely one vote subject to being overridden by medical opinion.

In *Barber v. Superior Court, supra*, 147 Cal.App.3d 1006, 195 Cal.Rptr. 484, we considered this same issue although in a different context. Writing on behalf of this division, Justice Compton thoroughly analyzed and reviewed the issue of withdrawal of life-support systems beginning with the seminal case of the *Matter of Quinlan* (N.J. 1976) 355 A.2d 647, *cert. den.* 429 U.S. 922, 97 S.Ct. 319, 50 L.Ed.2d 289, and continuing on to the then recent enactment of the California Natural Death Act (Health & Saf. Code. §§ 7185–7195). His opinion clearly and repeatedly stresses the fundamental underpinning of its conclusion, i.e., the patient's right to decide: 147 Cal.App.3d at page 1015, 195 Cal.Rptr. 484, "In this state a clearly recognized legal right to control one's own medical treatment predated the Natural Death Act. A long line of cases, approved by the Supreme Court in *Cobbs v. Grant* (1972) 8 Cal.3d 229 [104 Cal.Rptr. 505, 502 P.2d 1] . . . have held that where a doctor performs treatment in the absence of an informed consent, there is an actionable battery. The obvious corollary to this principle is that *a competent adult patient has the legal right to refuse medical treatment*" (emphasis added); 147 Cal.App.3d at page 1019, 195 Cal.Rptr. 484, "[T]he *patient's interests and desires are the key* ingredients of the decision-making process" (emphasis added); at page 1020, 195 Cal.Rptr. 484, "Given the general standards for determining when there is a duty to provide medical treatment of debatable value, the question still remains as to who should make these vital decisions. Clearly, the medical diagnoses and prognoses must be determined by the treating and consulting physicians under the generally accepted standards of medical practice in the community and, *whenever possible, the patient himself should then be the ultimate decisionmaker*" (emphasis added); at page 1021, 195 Cal.Rptr. 484, "The authorities are in agreement that any surrogate, court appointed or otherwise, ought to be guided in his or her decisions first by his knowledge of *the patient's own desires* and feelings, to the extent that they were expressed before the patient became incompetent." (Emphasis added.)

Bartling v. Superior Court, supra, 163 Cal.App.3d 186, 209 Cal.Rptr. 220, was factually much like the case at bench. Although not totally identical in all respects, the issue there centered on the same question here present: i.e., "May the patient refuse even life continuing treatment?" Justice Hastings, writing for another division of this court, explained: "In this case we are called upon to decide whether a competent adult patient, with serious illnesses which are probably incurable but have not been diagnosed as terminal, has the right, over the objection of his physicians and the hospital, to have life-support equipment disconnected despite the fact that withdrawal of such devices will surely hasten his death." (At p. 189, 209 Cal.Rptr. 220.) . . .

The description of Mr. Bartling's condition fits that of Elizabeth Bouvia. The holding of that case applies here and compels real parties to respect her decision even though she is not "terminally" ill. The trilogy of *Cobbs v. Grant, supra*, 8 Cal.3d 229, 104 Cal.Rptr. 505, 502 P.2d 1, *Barber v. Superior Court, supra*, 147 Cal.App.3d 1006, 195 Cal.Rptr. 484, and *Bartling v. Superior Court, supra*, 163 Cal.App.3d 186, 209 Cal.Rptr. 220, with their thorough explanation and discussion, are authority enough and in reality provide a complete answer to the position and assertions of real parties' medical personnel.

But if additional persuasion be needed, there is ample. As indicated by the discussion in *Bartling* and *Barber*, substantial and respectable authority throughout the country recognize the right which petitioner seeks to exercise. Indeed, it is neither radical nor startlingly new. It is a basic and constitutionally predicated right. More than seventy years ago, Judge Benjamin Cardozo observed: "Every human being of adult years and sound mind has a right to determine what shall be done with his own body. . . ." (*Schloendorff v. Society of New York Hospital* (1914) 211 N.Y. 125, 105 N.E. 92, 93.) . . .

. . . At bench the trial court concluded that with sufficient feeding petitioner could live an additional 15 to 20 years; therefore, the preservation of petitioner's life for that period outweighed her right to decide. In so holding the trial court mistakenly attached undue importance to the *amount of time* possibly available to petitioner, and failed to give equal weight and consideration for the *quality* of that life; an equal, if not more significant, consideration.

All decisions permitting cessation of medical treatment or life-support procedures to some degree hastened the arrival of death. In part, at least, this was permitted because the quality of life during the time remaining in those cases had been terribly diminished. In Elizabeth Bouvia's view, the quality of her life has been diminished to the point of hopelessness, uselessness, unenjoyability and frustration. She, as the patient, lying helplessly in bed, unable to care for herself, may consider her existence meaningless. She cannot be faulted for so concluding. If her right to choose may not be exercised because there remains to her, in the opinion of a court, a physician or some committee, a certain arbitrary number of years, months, or days, her right will have lost its value and meaning.

Who shall say what the minimum amount of available life must be? Does it matter if it be 15 to 20 years, 15 to 20 months, or 15 to 20 days, if such life has been physically destroyed and its quality, dignity and purpose gone? As in all matters lines must be drawn at some point, somewhere, but that decision must ultimately belong to the one whose life is in issue.

Here Elizabeth Bouvia's decision to forego medical treatment or life-support through a mechanical means belongs to her. It is not a medical decision for her physicians to make. Neither is it a legal question whose soundness is to be resolved by lawyers or judges. It is not a conditional right subject to approval by ethics committees or courts of law. It is a moral and philosophical decision that, being a competent adult, is hers alone.

Adapting the language of *Satz v. Perlmutter* [(Fla. 1980) 379 So.2d, affd. 362 So.2d 160 (Fla.App. 1978)], "It is all very convenient to insist on continuing [Elizabeth Bouvia's] life so that there can be no question of foul play, no resulting civil liability and no possible trespass on medical ethics. However, it is quite another matter to do so at the patient's sole expense and against [her] competent will, thus inflicting never ending physical torture on [her] body until the inevitable, but artificially suspended, moment of death. Such a course of conduct invades the patient's constitutional right of privacy, removes [her] freedom of choice and invades [her] right to self-determination." (*Satz v. Perlmutter, supra*, at pp. 162–163.)

Here, if force fed, petitioner faces 15 to 20 years of a painful existence, endurable only by the constant administrations of morphine. Her condition is irreversible. There is no cure for her palsy or arthritis. Petitioner would have to be fed, cleaned, turned, bedded, toileted by others for 15 to 20 years! Although alert, bright, sensitive, perhaps even brave and feisty, she must lie immobile, unable to exist except through physical acts of others. Her mind and spirit may be free to take great flights but she herself is imprisoned and must lie physically helpless subject to the ignominy, embarrassment, humiliation and dehumanizing aspects created by her helplessness. We do not believe it is the policy of this State that all and every life must be preserved against the will of the sufferer. It is incongruous, if not monstrous, for medical practitioners to assert their right to preserve a life that someone else must live, or, more accurately, endure, for "15 to 20 years." We cannot conceive it to be the policy of this State to inflict such an ordeal upon anyone.

It is, therefore, immaterial that the removal of the nasogastric tube will hasten or cause Bouvia's eventual death. Being competent she has the right to live out the remainder of her natural life in dignity and peace. It is precisely the aim and purpose of the many decisions upholding the withdrawal of life-support systems to accord and provide as large a measure of dignity, respect and comfort as possible to every patient for the remainder of his days, whatever be their number. This goal is not to hasten death, though its earlier arrival may be an expected and understood likelihood. . . .

It is not necessary to here define or dwell at length upon what constitutes suicide. Our Supreme Court dealt with the matter in the case of *In re Joseph G.* (1983) 34 Cal.3d 429, 194 Cal.Rptr. 163, 667 P.2d 1176, wherein declaring that the State has an interest in preserving and recognizing the sanctity of life, it observed that it is a crime to aid in suicide. But it is significant that the instances and the means there discussed all involved affirmative, assertive, proximate, direct conduct such as furnishing a gun, poison, knife, or other instrumentality or usable means by which another could physically and immediately inflict some death producing injury upon himself. Such situations

are far different than the mere presence of a doctor during the exercise of his patient's constitutional rights.

This is the teaching of *Bartling* and *Barber*. No criminal or civil liability attaches to honoring a competent, informed patient's refusal of medical service.

We do not purport to establish what will constitute proper medical practice in all other cases or even other aspects of the care to be provided petitioner. We hold only that her right to refuse medical treatment even of the life-sustaining variety, entitles her to the immediate removal of the nasogastric tube that has been involuntarily inserted into her body. The hospital and medical staff are still free to perform a substantial, if not the greater part of their duty, i.e., that of trying to alleviate Bouvia's pain and suffering.

Petitioner is without means to go to a private hospital and, apparently, real parties' hospital as a public facility was required to accept her. Having done so it may not deny her relief from pain and suffering merely because she has chosen to exercise her fundamental right to protect what little privacy remains to her.

Personal dignity is a part of one's right of privacy. Such a right of bodily privacy led the United States Supreme Court to hold that it shocked its conscience to learn that a state, even temporarily, had put a tube into the stomach of a criminal defendant to recover swallowed narcotics. (*Rochin v. California* (1952) 342 U.S. 165, 72 S.Ct. 205, 96 L.Ed. 183.) Petitioner asks for no greater consideration.

IT IS ORDERED:

Let a peremptory writ of mandate issue commanding the Los Angeles Superior Court immediately upon receipt thereof, to make and enter a new and different order granting Elizabeth Bouvia's request for a preliminary injunction, and the relief prayed for therein; in particular to make an order (1) directing real parties in interest forthwith to remove the nasogastric tube from petitioner, Elizabeth Bouvia's, body, and (2) prohibiting any and all of the real parties in interest from replacing or aiding in replacing said tube or any other or similar device in or on petitioner without her consent. . . .

COMPTON, Associate Justice, concurring opinion.

I have no doubt that Elizabeth Bouvia wants to die; and if she had the full use of even one hand, could probably find a way to end her life—in a word—commit suicide. In order to seek the assistance which she needs in ending her life by the only means she sees available—starvation—she has had to stultify her position before this court by disavowing her desire to end her life in such a fashion and proclaiming that she will eat all that she can physically tolerate. Even the majority opinion here must necessarily "dance" around the issue.

Elizabeth apparently has made a conscious and informed choice that she prefers death to continued existence in her helpless and, to her, intolerable condition. I believe she has an absolute right to effectuate that decision. This state and the medical profession instead of frustrating her desire, should be attempting to relieve her suffering by permitting and in fact assisting her to die with ease and dignity. The fact that she is forced to suffer the ordeal of self-starvation to achieve her objective is in itself inhumane.

The right to die is an integral part of our right to control our own destinies so long as the rights of others are not affected. That right should, in my opinion, include the ability to enlist assistance from others, including the medical profession, in making death as painless and quick as possible. . . .

NOTE

1. Her instructions were dictated to her lawyers, written by them and signed by her by means of her making a feeble "x" on the paper with a pen which she held in her mouth.

J O A N N E   L Y N N   A N D
J A M E S   F .   C H I L D R E S S

Must Patients Always Be Given Food and Water?

Many people die from the lack of food or water. For some, this lack is the result of poverty or famine, but for others it is the result of disease or deliberate decision. In the past, malnutrition and dehydration must have accompanied nearly every death that followed an illness of more than a few days. Most dying patients do not eat much on their own, and nothing could be done for them until the first flexible tubing for instilling food or other liquid into the stomach was developed about a hundred years ago. Even then, the procedure was so scarce, so costly in physician and nursing time, and so poorly tolerated that it was used only for patients who clearly could benefit. With the advent of more reliable and efficient procedures in the past few decades, these conditions can be corrected or ameliorated in nearly every patient who would otherwise be malnourished or dehydrated. In fact, intravenous lines and nasogastric tubes have become common images of hospital care.

Providing adequate nutrition and fluids is a high priority for most patients, both because they suffer directly from inadequacies and because these deficiencies hinder their ability to overcome other diseases. But are there some patients who need not receive these treatments? This question has become a prominent public policy issue in a number of recent cases. In May 1981, in Danville, Illinois, the parents and the physician of newborn conjoined twins with shared abdominal organs decided not to feed these children. Feeding and other treatments were given after court intervention, though a grand jury refused to indict the parents.[1] Later that year, two physicians in Los Angeles discontinued intravenous nutrition to a patient who had severe brain damage after an episode involving loss of oxygen following routine surgery. Murder charges were brought, but the hearing judge dismissed the charges at a preliminary hearing. On appeal, the charges were reinstated and remanded for trial.[2]

In April 1982, a Bloomington, Indiana, infant who had tracheoesophageal fistula and Down Syndrome was not treated or fed, and he died after two courts

Reprinted by permission of the authors and reproduced by permission of The Hastings Center from *Hastings Center Report* 13 (October 1983), pp. 17–21.

ruled that the decision was proper but before all appeals could be heard.[3] When the federal government then moved to ensure that such infants would be fed in the future,[4] the Surgeon General, Dr. C. Everett Koop, initially stated that there is never adequate reason to deny nutrition and fluids to a newborn infant.

While these cases were before the public, the nephew of Claire Conroy, an elderly incompetent woman with several serious medical problems, petitioned a New Jersey court for authority to discontinue her nasogastric tube feedings. Although the intermediate appeals court has reversed the ruling,[5] the trial court held that he had this authority since the evidence indicated that the patient would not have wanted such treatment and that its value to her was doubtful.

In all these dramatic cases and in many more that go unnoticed, the decision is made to deliberately withhold food or fluid known to be necessary for the life of the patient. Such decisions are unsettling. There is now widespread consensus that sometimes a patient is best served by not undertaking or continuing certain treatments that would sustain life, especially if these entail substantial suffering.[6] But food and water are so central to an array of human emotions that it is almost impossible to consider them with the same emotional detachment that one might feel toward a respirator or a dialysis machine.

Nevertheless, the question remains: Should it ever be permissible to withhold or withdraw food and nutrition? The answer in any real case should acknowledge the psychological contiguity between feeding and loving and between nutritional satisfaction and emotional satisfaction. Yet this acknowledgment does not resolve the core question.

Some have held that it is intrinsically wrong not to feed another. The philosopher G. E. M. Anscombe contends: "For wilful starvation there can be no excuse. The same can't be said quite without qualification about failing to operate or to adopt some courses of treatment."[7] But the moral issues are more complex than Anscombe's comment suggests. Does correcting nutritional deficiencies always improve patients' wellbeing? What should be our reflective moral response to withholding or withdrawing nutrition? What moral principles are relevant to our reflections? What medical facts about ways of providing nutrition are relevant? And what policies should be adopted by the society, hospitals, and medical and other health care professionals?

In our effort to find answers to these questions, we will concentrate upon the care of patients who are incompetent to make choices for themselves. Patients who are competent to determine the course of their therapy may refuse any and all interventions proposed by others, as long as their refusals do not seriously harm or impose unfair burdens upon others.[8] A competent patient's decision regarding whether or not to accept the provision of food and water by medical means such as tube feeding or intravenous alimentation is unlikely to raise questions of harm or burden to others.

What then should guide those who must decide about nutrition for a patient who cannot decide? As a start, consider the standard by which other medical decisions are made: one should decide as the incompetent person would have if he or she were competent, when that is possible to determine, and advance that person's interests in a more generalized sense when individual preferences cannot be known.

THE MEDICAL PROCEDURES

There is no reason to apply a different standard to feeding and hydration. Surely, when one inserts a feeding tube, or creates a gastrostomy opening, or inserts a needle into a vein, one intends to benefit the patient. Ideally, one should provide what the patient believes to be of benefit, but at least the effect should be beneficial in the opinions of surrogates and caregivers.

Thus, the question becomes, is it ever in the patient's interest to become malnourished and dehydrated, rather than to receive treatment? Posing the question so starkly points to our need to know what is entailed in treating these conditions and what benefits the treatments offer.

The medical interventions that provide food and fluids are of two basic types. First, liquids can be delivered by a tube that is inserted into a functioning gastrointestinal tract, most commonly through the nose and esophagus into the stomach or through a surgical incision in the abdominal wall and directly into the stomach. The liquids used can be specially prepared solutions of nutrients or a blenderized version of an ordinary diet. The nasogastric tube is cheap; it may lead to pneumonia and often annoys the patient and family, sometimes even requiring that the patient be restrained to prevent its removal.

Creating a gastrostomy is usually a simple surgical procedure, and, once the wound is healed, care is very simple. Since it is out of sight, it is aesthetically more acceptable and restraints are needed less often. Also, the gastrostomy creates no additional risk of pneumonia. However, while elimination of a nasogastric tube requires only removing the tube, a gastrostomy is fairly permanent, and can be closed only by surgery.

The second type of medical intervention is intravenous feeding and hydration, which also has two major forms. The ordinary hospital or peripheral IV, in which fluid is delivered directly to the bloodstream through a small needle, is useful only for temporary efforts to improve hydration and electrolyte concentrations. One cannot provide a balanced diet through the veins in the limbs: to do that requires a central line, or a special catheter placed into one of the major veins in the chest. The latter procedure is much more risky and vulnerable to infections and technical errors, and it is much more costly than any of the other procedures. Both forms of intravenous nutrition and hydration commonly require restraining the patient, cause minor infections and other ill effects, and are costly, especially since they ordinarily require the patient to be in a hospital.

None of these procedures, then, is ideal; each entails some distress, some medical limitations, and some costs. When may a procedure be forgone that might improve nutrition and hydration for a given patient? Only when the procedure and the resulting improvement in nutrition and hydration do not offer the patient a net benefit over what he or she would otherwise have faced.

Are there such circumstances? We believe that there are; but they are few and limited to the following three kinds of situations: (1) the procedures that would be required are so unlikely to achieve improved nutritional and fluid levels that they could be correctly considered futile; (2) the improvement in nutritional and fluid balance, though achievable, could be of no benefit to the patient; (3) the burdens of receiving the treatment may outweigh the benefit.

WHEN FOOD AND WATER MAY BE WITHHELD

Futile Treatment. Sometimes even providing "food and water" to a patient becomes a monumental task. Consider a patient with a severe clotting deficiency and a nearly total body burn. Gaining access to the central veins is likely to cause hemorrhage or infection, nasogastric tube placement may be quite painful,

and there may be no skin to which to suture the stomach for a gastrostomy tube. Or consider a patient with severe congestive heart failure who develops cancer of the stomach with a fistula that delivers food from the stomach to the colon without passing through the intestine and being absorbed. Feeding the patient may be possible, but little is absorbed. Intravenous feeding cannot be tolerated because the fluid would be too much for the weakened heart. Or consider the infant with infarction of all but a short segment of bowel. Again, the infant can be fed, but little if anything is absorbed. Intravenous methods can be used, but only for a short time (weeks or months) until their complications, including thrombosis, hemorrhage, infections, and malnutrition, cause death.

In these circumstances, the patient is going to die soon, no matter what is done. The ineffective efforts to provide nutrition and hydration may directly cause suffering that offers no counterbalancing benefit for the patient. Although the procedures might be tried, especially if the competent patient wanted them or the incompetent patient's surrogate had reason to believe that this incompetent patient would have wanted them, they cannot be considered obligatory. To hold that a patient must be subjected to this predictably futile sort of intervention just because protein balance is negative or the blood serum is concentrated is to lose sight of the moral warrant for medical care and to reduce the patient to an array of measurable variables.

No Possibility of Benefit. Some patients can be reliably diagnosed to have permanently lost consciousness. This unusual group of patients includes those with anencephaly, persistent vegetative state, and some preterminal comas. In these cases, it is very difficult to discern how any medical intervention can benefit or harm the patient. These patients cannot and never will be able to experience any of the events occurring in the world or in their bodies. When the diagnosis is exceedingly clear, we sustain their lives vigorously mainly for their loved ones and the community at large.

While these considerations probably indicate that continued artificial feeding is best in most cases, there may be some cases in which the family and the caregivers are convinced that artificial feeding is offensive and unreasonable. In such cases, there seems to be no adequate reason to claim that withholding food and water violates any obligations that these parties or the general society have with regard to permanently unconscious patients. Thus, if the parents of an anencephalic infant or of a patient like Karen Quinlan in a persistent vegetative state feel strongly that no medical procedures should be applied to provide nutrition and hydration, and the caregivers are willing to comply, there should be no barrier in law or public policy to thwart the plan.[9]

Disproportionate Burden. The most difficult cases are those in which normal nutritional status or fluid balance could be restored, but only with a severe burden for the patient. In these cases, the treatment is futile in a broader sense—the patient will not actually benefit from the improved nutrition and hydration. A patient who is competent can decide the relative merits of the treatment being provided, knowing the probable consequences, and weighing the merits of life under various sets of constrained circumstances. But a surrogate decision maker for a patient who is incompetent to decide will have a difficult task. When the situation is irremediably ambiguous, erring on the side of continued life and improved nutrition and hydration seems the less grievous error. But are there situations that would warrant a determination that this patient, whose nutrition and hydration could surely be improved, is not thereby well served?

Though they are rare, we believe there are such cases. The treatments entailed are not benign. Their effects are far short of ideal. Furthermore, many of the patients most likely to have inadequate food and fluid intake are also likely to suffer the most serious side effects of these therapies.

Patients who are allowed to die without artificial hydration and nutrition may well die more comfortably than patients who receive conventional amounts of intravenous hydration.[10] Terminal pulmonary edema, nausea, and mental confusion are more likely when patients have been treated to maintain fluid and nutrition until close to the time of death.

Thus, those patients whose "need" for artificial nutrition and hydration arises only near the time of death may be harmed by its provision. It is not at all clear that they receive any benefit in having a slightly prolonged life, and it does seem reasonable to allow a surrogate to decide that, for this patient at this time, slight prolongation of life is not warranted if it involves measures that will probably increase the patient's suffering as he or she dies.

Even patients who might live much longer might not be well served by artificial means to provide fluid and food. Such patients might include those with fairly severe dementia for whom the restraints required could be a constant source of fear, discomfort, and struggle. For such a patient, sedation to tolerate the feeding mechanisms might preclude any of the pleasant experiences that might otherwise have been available. Thus, a decision not to intervene, except perhaps briefly to ascertain that there are no treatable causes, might allow such a patient to live out a shorter life with fair freedom of movement and freedom from fear, while a decision to maintain artificial nutrition and hydration might consign the patient to end his or her life in unremitting anguish. If this were the case a surrogate decision-maker would seem to be well justified in refusing the treatment.

INAPPROPRIATE MORAL CONSTRAINTS

Four considerations are frequently proposed as moral constraints on forgoing medical feeding and hydration. We find none of these to dictate that artificial nutrition and hydration must always be provided.

The Obligation to Provide "Ordinary" Care. Debates about appropriate medical treatment are often couched in terms of "ordinary" and "extraordinary" means of treatment. Historically, this distinction emerged in the Roman Catholic tradition to differentiate optional treatment from treatment that was obligatory for medical professionals to offer and for patients to accept.[11] These terms also appear in many secular contexts, such as court decisions and medical codes. The recent debates about ordinary and extraordinary means of treatment have been interminable and often unfruitful, in part because of a lack of clarity about what the terms mean. Do they represent the premises of an argument or the conclusion, and what features of a situation are relevant to the categorization as "ordinary" or "extraordinary"?[12]

Several criteria have been implicit in debates about ordinary and extraordinary means of treatment; some of them may be relevant to determining whether and which treatments are obligatory and which are optional. Treatments have been distinguished according to their simplicity (simple/complex), their naturalness (natural/artificial), their customariness (usual/unusual), their invasiveness (noninvasive/invasive), their chance of success (reasonable chance/futile), their balance of benefits and burdens (proportionate/disproportionate), and their expense (inexpensive/costly). Each set of paired terms or phrases in the parentheses suggests a continuum: as the treatment moves from the first of the paired terms to the second, it is said to become less obligatory and more optional.

However, when these various criteria, widely used in discussions about medical treatment, are carefully examined, most of them are not morally relevant in distinguishing optional from obligatory medical treatments. For example, if a rare, complex, artificial, and invasive treatment offers a patient a reasonable chance of nearly painless cure, then one would have to offer a substantial justification not to provide that treatment to an incompetent patient.

What matters, then, in determining whether to provide a treatment to an incompetent patient is not a prior determination that this treatment is "ordinary" per se, but rather a determination that this treatment is likely to provide this patient benefits that are sufficient to make it worthwhile to endure the burdens that accompany the treatment. To this end, some of the considerations listed above are relevant: whether a treatment is likely to succeed is an obvious example. But such considerations taken in isolation are not conclusive. Rather, the surrogate decision-maker is obliged to assess the desirability to this patient of each of the options presented, including nontreatment. For most people at most times, this assessment would lead to a clear obligation to provide food and fluids.

But sometimes, as we have indicated, providing food and fluids through medical interventions may fail to benefit and may even harm some patients. Then the treatment cannot be said to be obligatory, no matter how usual and simple its provision may be. If "ordinary" and "extraordinary" are used to convey the conclusion about the obligation to treat, providing nutrition and fluids would have become, in these cases, "extraordinary." Since this phrasing is misleading, it is probably better to use "proportionate" and "disproportionate," as the Vatican now suggests,[13] or "obligatory" and "optional."

Obviously, providing nutrition and hydration may sometimes be necessary to keep patients comfortable while they are dying even though it may temporarily prolong their dying. In such cases, food and fluids constitute warranted palliative care. But in other cases, such as a patient in a deep and irreversible coma, nutrition and hydration do not appear to be needed or helpful, except perhaps to comfort the staff and family.[14] And sometimes the interventions needed for nutrition and hydration are so burdensome that they are harmful and best not utilized.

The Obligation to Continue Treatments Once Started. Once having started a mode of treatment, many caregivers find it very difficult to discontinue it. While this strongly felt difference between the ease of withholding a treatment and the difficulty of withdrawing it provides a psychological explanation of certain actions, it does not justify them. It sometimes even leads to a thoroughly irrational decision process. For example, in caring for a dying, comatose patient, many physicians apparently find it harder to stop a functioning peripheral IV than not to restart one that has infiltrated (that is, has broken through the blood vessel and is leaking fluid into surrounding tissue), especially if the only way to reestablish an IV would be to insert a central line into the heart or to do a cutdown (make an incision to gain access to the deep large blood vessels).[15]

What factors might make withdrawing medical treatment morally worse than withholding it? Withdrawing a treatment seems to be an action, which, when it is likely to end in death, initially seems more serious than an omission that ends in death. However, this view is fraught with errors. Withdrawing is not always an act: failing to put the next infusion into a tube could be correctly described as an omission, for example. Even when withdrawing is an act, it may well be morally correct and even morally obligatory. Discontinuing intravenous lines in a patient now permanently unconscious in accord with that patient's well-informed advance directive would certainly be such a case. Furthermore, the caregiver's obligation to serve the patient's interests through both acts and omissions rules out the exculpation that accompanies omissions in the usual course of social life. An omission that is not warranted by the patient's interests is culpable.

Sometimes initiating a treatment creates expectations in the minds of caregivers, patients, and family that the treatment will be continued indefinitely or until the patient is cured. Such expectations may provide a reason to continue the treatment as a way to keep a promise. However, as with all promises, caregivers could be very careful when initiating a treatment to explain the indications for its discontinuation, and they could modify preconceptions with continuing reevaluation and education during treatment. Though all patients are entitled to expect the continuation of care in the patient's best interests, they are not and should not be entitled to the continuation of a particular mode of care.

Accepting the distinction between withholding and withdrawing medical treatment as morally significant also has a very unfortunate implication: caregivers may become unduly reluctant to begin some treatments precisely because they fear that they will be locked into continuing treatments that are no longer of value to the patient. For example, the physician who had been unwilling to stop the respirator while the infant Andrew Stinson died over several months is reportedly "less eager to attach babies to respirators now."[16] But if it were easier to ignore malnutrition and dehydration and to withhold treatments for these problems than to discontinue the same treatments when they have become especially burdensome and insufficiently beneficial for the patient, then the incentives would be perverse. Once a treatment has been tried, it is often much clearer whether it is of value to the patient, and the decision to stop it can be made more reliably.

The same considerations should apply to starting as to stopping a treatment, and whatever assessment warrants withholding should also warrant withdrawing.

The Obligation to Avoid Being the Unambiguous Cause of Death. Many physicians will agree with all that we have said and still refuse to allow a choice to forgo food and fluid because such a course seems to be a "death sentence." In this view death seems to be more certain from malnutrition and dehydration than from forgoing other forms of medical therapy. This implies that it is acceptable to act in ways that are likely to cause death, as in not operating on a gangrenous leg, only if there remains a chance that the patient will survive. This is a comforting formulation for caregivers, to be sure, since they can thereby avoid feeling the full weight of the responsibility for the time and manner of a patient's death. However, it is not a persuasive moral argument.

First, in appropriate cases discontinuing certain medical treatments is generally accepted despite the fact that death is as certain as with nonfeeding. Dialysis in a patient without kidney function or transfusions in a patient with severe aplastic anemia are obvious examples. The dying that awaits such patients often is not greatly different from dying of dehydration and malnutrition.

Second, the certainty of a generally undesirable outcome such as death is always relevant to a decision, but it does not foreclose the possibility that this course

is better than others available to this patient.[17] Ambiguity and uncertainty are so common in medical decision-making that caregivers are tempted to use them in distancing themselves from direct responsibility. However, caregivers are in fact responsible for the time and manner of death for many patients. Their distaste for this fact should not constrain otherwise morally justified decisions.

The Obligation to Provide Symbolically Significant Treatment. One of the most common arguments for always providing nutrition and hydration is that it symbolizes, expresses, or conveys the essence of care and compassion. Some actions not only aim at goals, they also express values. Such expressive actions should not simply be viewed as means to ends; they should also be viewed in light of what they communicate. From this perspective food and water are not only goods that preserve life and provide comfort; they are also symbols of care and compassion. To withhold or withdraw them—to "starve" a patient—can never express or convey care.

Why is providing food and water a central symbol of care and compassion? Feeding is the first response of the community to the needs of newborns and remains a central mode of nurture and comfort. Eating is associated with social interchange and community, and providing food for someone else is a way to create and maintain bonds of sharing and expressing concern. Furthermore, even the relatively low levels of hunger and thirst that most people have experienced are decidedly uncomfortable, and the common image of severe malnutrition or dehydration is one of unremitting agony. Thus, people are rightly eager to provide food and water. Such provision is essential to minimally tolerable existence and a powerful symbol of our concern for each other.

However, *medical* nutrition and hydration, we have argued, may not always provide net benefits to patients. Medical procedures to provide nutrition and hydration are more similar to other medical procedures than to typical human ways of providing nutrition and hydration, for example, a sip of water. It should be possible to evaluate their benefits and burdens, as we evaluate any other medical procedure. Of course, if family, friends, and caregivers feel that such procedures affirm important values even when they do not benefit the patient, their feelings should not be ignored. We do not contend that there is an obligation to withhold or to withdraw such procedures (unless consideration of the patient's advance directives or current best interest unambiguously dictates that conclusion); we only contend that nutrition and hydration may be forgone in some cases.

The symbolic connection between care and nutrition or hydration adds useful caution to decision making. If decision makers worry over withholding or withdrawing medical nutrition and hydration, they may inquire more seriously into the circumstances that putatively justify their decisions. This is generally salutary for health care decision making. The critical inquiry may well yield the sad but justified conclusion that the patient will be served best by not using medical procedures to provide food and fluids.

A LIMITED CONCLUSION

Our conclusion—that patients or their surrogates, in close collaboration with their physicians and other caregivers and with careful assessment of the relevant information, can correctly decide to forgo the provision of medical treatments intended to correct malnutrition and dehydration in some circumstances—is quite limited. Concentrating on incompetent patients, we have argued that in most cases such patients will be best served by providing nutrition and fluids. Thus, there should be a presumption in favor of providing nutrition and fluids as part of the broader presumption to provide means that prolong life. But this presumption may be rebutted in particular cases.

We do not have enough information to be able to determine with clarity and conviction whether withholding or withdrawing nutrition and hydration was justified in the cases that have occasioned public concern, though it seems likely that the Danville and Bloomington babies should have been fed and that Claire Conroy should not.

It is never sufficient to rule out "starvation" categorically. The question is whether the obligation to act in the patient's best interests was discharged by withholding or withdrawing particular medical treatments. All we have claimed is that nutrition and hydration by medical means need not always be provided. Sometimes they may not be in accord with the patient's wishes or interests. Medical nutrition and hydration do not appear to be distinguishable in any morally relevant way from other life-sustaining medical treatments that may on occasion be withheld or withdrawn.

NOTES

1. John A. Robertson, "Dilemma in Danville," *Hastings Cent. Rep.* 11: 5–8 (October 1981).

2. T. Rohrlich, "2 Doctors Face Murder Charges in Patient's Death," *L.A. Times*, August 19, 1982, A-1; Jonathan Kirsch, "A Death at Kaiser Hospital," *Calif. Mag.* (1982), 79ff; Magistrate's findings, California v. Barber and Nejdl, No. A 925586, Los Angeles Mun. Ct. Cal. (March 9, 1983); Superior Court of California, County of Los Angeles, California v. Barber and Nejdl, No. A0 25586k tentative decision May 5, 1983.

3. *In re* Infant Doe, No. GU 8204-00 (Cir. Ct. Monroe County, Ind., April 12, 1982), *writ of mandamus dismissed sub nom.* State ex rel. Infant Doe v. Baker, No. 482 S140 (Indiana Supreme Ct., May 27, 1982).

4. Office of the Secretary, Department of Health and Human Services, "Nondiscrimination on the Basis of Handicap," *Federal Register* 48 (1983), 9630–32. (Interim final rule modifying 45 C.F.R. #84.61.) See Judge Gerhard Gesell's decision, American Academy of Pediatrics v. Heckler, No. 83–0774, U.S. District Court, D.C., April 24, 1983; and also George J. Annas, "Disconnecting the Baby Doe Hotline," *Hastings Cent. Rep.* 13:14–16 (June 1983).

5. *In re* Conroy, 190 N.J. Super. 453, 464 A.2d 303 (App. Div. 1983).

6. President's Commission for the Study of Ethical Problems in Medicine and Biomedical and Behavioral Research, *Deciding to Forego Life-Sustaining Treatment*, Washington, D.C.: U.S. Government Printing Office (1982).

7. G. E. M. Anscombe, "Ethical Problems in the Management of Some Severely Handicapped Children: Commentary 2," *J. Med. Ethics* 7:117–124 (1981).

8. See, e.g., President's Commission for the Study of Ethical Problems in Medicine and Biomedical and Behavioral Research, *Making Health Care Decisions*, Washington, D.C.: U.S. Government Printing Office (1982).

9. President's Commission, *Deciding to Forego*, at 171–196.

10. Joyce V. Zerwekh, "The Dehydration Question," *Nursing83*, 47–51 (1983) with comments by Judith R. Brown and Marion B. Dolan. See also chapter 3.

11. James J. McCartney, "The Development of the Doctrine of Ordinary and Extraordinary Means of Preserving Life in Catholic Moral Theology before the Karen Quinlan Case," *Linacre Q.* 47:215 (1980).

12. President's Commission, *Deciding to Forego*, at 82–90. For an argument that fluids and electrolytes can be "extraordinary," see Carson Strong, "Can Fluids and Electrolytes be 'Extraordinary' Treatment?" *J. Med. Ethics* 7:83–85 (1981).

13. The Sacred Congregation for the Doctrine of the Faith, Declaration on Euthanasia, Vatican City, May 5, 1980.

14. Paul Ramsey, *The Patient as Person*, New Haven: Yale University Press (1970), 128–129; Paul Ramsey, *Ethics at the Edges of Life: Medical and Legal Intersections*, New Haven: Yale University Press (1978), 275; Bernard Towers, "Irreversible Coma and Withdrawal of Life Support: Is It Murder If the IV Line is Disconnected?" *J. Med. Ethics* 8:205 (1982).

15. See Kenneth C. Micetich, Patricia H. Steinecker, and David C. Thomasma, "Are Intravenous Fluids Morally Required for a Dying Patient?" *Arch. Intern. Med.* 143:975–978 (1983), also chapter 4.

16. Robert and Peggy Stinson, *The Long Dying of Baby Andrew*, Boston: Little, Brown and Co. (1983), 355.

17. See chapter 4 [in original volume].

THE NETHERLANDS STATE COMMISSION ON EUTHANASIA

Final Report: An English Summary

INTRODUCTION

The State Commission on Euthanasia was set up in the Netherlands in 1982 at the instigation of the then Minister of Health and Environmental Protection and Minister of Justice with a view to advising on future governmental policy on euthanasia and assistance with suicide, with particular reference to legislation and the application of the law.

RECOMMENDATIONS IN RELATION TO ARTICLES 293 AND 294 OF THE CRIMINAL CODE

The State Commission defines euthanasia as the intentional termination of life by another party at the request of the person concerned.

The majority of the Commission support the view that, in certain circumstances and subject to certain conditions, euthanasia should not be an offence. These members unanimously support the requirement that euthanasia be carried out solely by physicians and endorse the stipulations concerning careful medical procedure and safeguards with respect to supervision.

Unanimity could not be reached on one point. The majority proposed that euthanasia should enjoy immunity from prosecution provided 'that the patient be in an untenable situation with no prospect of improvement' to which four members would add 'and at the point where death will inevitably ensue.'

Two members did not share the rest of the Commission's viewpoint on the question of whether euthanasia should be exempt from punishment in certain circum-

stances and subject to certain conditions. These two members have set out their views in an extensive minority report, rejecting any change in or modification of the law leading to a justification of euthanasia. The main arguments for this view are based on their concept of human dignity, a strict interpretation of the European Convention of Human Rights and Fundamental Freedom and the conviction that, once such a step has been taken, further infringements of the protection of human life would appear to be unavoidable.

With respect to a request to terminate life, the State Commission takes the view that a written request to that end must be treated as an indication of the patient's wishes, subject to the proviso that such a declaration of intention only assumes relevance once the patient is no longer capable of expressing his or her will. As long as the patient does remain capable of doing so, only the verbal expression of intent is relevant and the written instructions can be revoked or amended at any time.

The State Commission deems it essential for Parliament to make plain its position on euthanasia. The Commission shares the fear that the issue could become politicized, and to this end would urge that a free vote be allowed on the question in which Members of Parliament could vote in accordance with their conscience. The Commission bases this judgement on the grounds that widespread uncertainty exists concerning the scope of Article 293 of the Criminal Code in relation to euthanasia.

In the Commission's view, the development of relevant case law will take so long that it will be many years before the exact definition emerges of what is and what is not an offence. Nor does the fact that prosecution policy has been under discussion by the

Reprinted with permission of the publisher from *Bioethics*, Vol. 1, No. 2 (1987), pp. 163–169, 172–174.

Conference of Procurator Generals since February 1982 provide the necessary clarity and legal certainty.

As regards the task of the legislature, the State Commission notes that the former will need to consider whether and to what extent the removal of legal sanctions against euthanasia would be consistent with Article 2 of the European Convention for the Protection of Human Rights and Fundamental Freedoms, the first sentence of clause one of which states: 'Everyone's right to life shall be protected by law'. In view of the formulation of this obligation under international law, the State Commission has worked on the assumption that under the Convention the member states have a large measure of freedom in deciding on the form in which life is to be protected under their legal system. Parliament does, however, need to proceed with great caution in removing the existing legal sanctions against euthanasia.

With respect to assistance with suicide given by a physician, the majority of the State Commission takes the view that this should cease to be an offence in the same circumstances and under the same conditions as those applying to the termination of life on request. The signatories to the minority report similarly reject this proposal. The Commission does not regard as warranted the removal of legal sanctions against other cases of assistance with suicide—including in particular 'rational' suicide—in view of the fact that social and professional opinion in these areas has not yet crystallised. Rational suicide is understood to mean the termination of a life regarded as unacceptable or meaningless by an individual who is not mentally disturbed and who may be deemed, on the basis of his or her mental state, to be capable of satisfactorily assessing his or her own psychological and social situation and the social consequences of the proposed suicide.

The Commission proposes that Article 293 of the Criminal Code be amended in such a way that the intentional termination of another person's life at the latter's express and earnest request would not be an offence, provided this is carried out by a doctor in the context of careful medical procedure in respect of a patient who is in an untenable situation with no prospect of improvement. The Commission did not elaborate on the meaning of this term since the situations of unbearable suffering in which consideration could be given to terminating life vary too widely to be incorporated into a statute. Such an untenable situation may be caused by both physical and mental suffering.

The State Commission set out its recommendation in the form of a proposal for the amendment of Title XIX of Book II of the Criminal Code. The Commission was of the opinion that a decision to terminate life should be implemented by a physician and cannot be delegated by the latter to a third party, for example a relative or nurse. The same applies mutatis mutandis to assistance with suicide. In its proposal to amend the legislation, the State Commission drew up a number of safeguards to be complied with in order to ensure proper medical procedure. One of these would be the requirement to consult another physician designated by the Minister of Welfare, Health and Cultural Affairs.

The State Commission made one exception to its basic premise that euthanasia presupposes a request on the part of the person concerned. It considers that the intentional termination of the life of a person unable to express his or her will should not be an offence provided this is performed by a physician in the context of careful medical procedure in respect of a patient who, according to the current state of medical knowledge, has irreversibly lost consciousness, and provided also that treatment has been suspended as pointless. In the event of an irreversible coma where objective medical criteria provide no grounds for hope of improvement, the State Commission takes the view that the termination of life by a physician is justified, but only after treatment has been suspended as pointless. Once again the Commission would deem it essential that another physician be consulted.

The State Commission believes it to be so important that another doctor be consulted that it proposes the introduction of a separate punitive sanction (Article 293 *bis*) to cover any case where the physician in charge omits to take this step. To help ensure compliance with the procedures proposed by the State Commission in relation to funeral arrangements, the Commission proposes that deliberate failure to fulfil the obligation to furnish particulars, or provision of incorrect particulars, in cases where life has been terminated, should be made a separate offence (Article 293 *ter*).

During the hearings the attention of the State Commission was drawn to the fact that in practice there is widespread uncertainty as to what actions may be said to constitute euthanasia. In the belief that potential uncertainty should be avoided, the Commission has summarized various types of action in its proposed Article 293 *quater* which in its view do not constitute the termination of deprivation of life as referred to in Title XIX of Book II of the Criminal Code. Examples include the withholding or suspension of treatment at the patient's request deemed pointless according to prevailing medical opinion. . . .

APPENDIX . . .

PROPOSED AMENDMENTS TO TITLE XIX OF BOOK 2
OF THE CRIMINAL CODE

Article 292 bis

1. Any person who intentionally terminates the life of another person on account of serious physical or mental illnesses or disorders suffered by that person, if the latter is incapable of expressing his will shall be liable to a term of imprisonment not exceeding six years or to a fourth category fine.
2. The action defined in paragraph 1 shall not be an offence if termination of life is carried out by a physician as part of careful medical procedure in respect of a patient who, according to prevailing medical opinion, has irreversibly lost consciousness, provided also that treatment has previously been suspended as pointless.
3. Careful medical procedure, as referred to in paragraph 2, shall in any event mean that the physician shall have consulted an expert designated by Our Minister of Welfare, Health, and Cultural Affairs.

Article 293

1. Any person who intentionally terminates the life of another person at the latter's express and earnest request shall be liable to a term of imprisonment not exceeding four years and six months or a fourth category fine.
2. The action defined in paragraph 1 shall not be an offence if termination of life is carried out by a physician as part of a careful medical procedure in respect of patient in an untenable situation with no prospect of improvement.
3. With respect to the application of paragraph 2 the termination of life shall be taken to include the provision as part of careful medical procedure of drugs to make it possible to commit suicide and to render assistance therewith.
4. Proper medical procedure as referred to in paragraphs 2 and 3 shall in any event mean that:
   a. the patient has been informed of his particular circumstances;

   b. the physician has satisfied himself that the patient has made his request for life to be terminated after careful consideration and voluntarily abides by that decision;
   c. the physician has decided that termination of life on the basis of his findings would be justified because he has reached the conclusion with the patient that there is no other solution to the patient's untenable situation;
   d. the physician has consulted an expert designated by Our Minister of Welfare, Health and Cultural Affairs.
5. With respect to a patient who has submitted a written request for his life to be terminated and who is incapable of expressing his will, proper medical procedure as referred to in paragraph 2 shall in any event mean that:
   a. the physician has satisfied himself that the patient made the request for his life to be terminated voluntarily and after careful consideration;
   b. the physician has decided that termination of life on the basis of his findings would be justified because he has reached the conclusion that there is no other solution to the patient's untenable situation;
   c. the physician has consulted an expert designated by Our Minister of Welfare, Health and Cultural Affairs.

Article 293 bis

A physician as referred to in paragraph 2 of Articles 292 bis and 293 who fails to consult an expert designated by Our Minister of Welfare, Health and Cultural Affairs prior to the termination of life shall be liable to a term of imprisonment not exceeding three years or a fourth category fine.

Article 293 ter

Without prejudice to the provisions of Article 228, a physician as referred to in paragraph 2 of Articles 292 bis and 293 who intentionally fails to fulfil the statutory requirements to furnish particulars, shall be liable to a term of imprisonment not exceeding three years or a fourth category fine.

Article 293 quater

For the purpose of the application of the provisions of

this Title, the deprivation or termination of life shall be understood to exclude:

a. the withholding or suspension of treatment at the express and earnest request of the patient;

b. the withholding or suspension of treatment in cases where such treatment is deemed pointless according to prevailing medical opinion;

c. failure to treat a secondary illness or disorder in the case of a patient who, according to prevailing medical opinion, has irreversibly lost consciousness;

d. acceleration of death as a secondary effect of treatment specifically designed to relieve severe suffering on the part of the patient and essential for that purpose.

Article 294

Any person who deliberately incites another to suicide or who assists suicide and provides drugs to that end shall, where suicide eventuates, be liable to a term of imprisonment not exceeding three years or a fourth category fine.

CALIFORNIA

Durable Power of Attorney for Health Care

1. CREATION OF DURABLE POWER OF ATTORNEY FOR HEALTH CARE

By this document I intend to create a durable power of attorney by appointing the person designated above to make health care decisions for me as allowed by Sections 2410 to 2443, inclusive, of the California Civil Code. This power of attorney shall not be affected by my subsequent incapacity.

2. DESIGNATION OF HEALTH CARE AGENT

(Insert the name and address of the person you wish to designate as your agent to make health care decisions for you. None of the following may be designated as your agent: (1) your treating health care provider, (2) a nonrelative *employee of your treating health care provider, (3) an operator of a community care facility, or (4) a* nonrelative *employee of an operator of a community care facility.)*

I, _____
(insert your name)

do hereby designate and appoint: Name: _____

Address: _____

Telephone Number: _____ as my attorney-in-fact (agent) to make health care decisions for me as authorized in this document.

3. GENERAL STATEMENT OF AUTHORITY GRANTED

If I become incapable of giving informed consent to health care decisions, I hereby grant to my agent full power and authority to make health care decisions for me including the right to consent, refuse consent, or withdraw consent to any care, treatment, service, or procedure to maintain, diagnose or treat a physical or mental condition, and to receive and to consent to the release of medical information, subject to the statement of desires, special provisions and limitations set out in paragraph 4.

4. STATEMENT OF DESIRES, SPECIAL PROVISIONS, AND LIMITATIONS

(Your agent must make health care decisions that are consistent with your known desires. You can, but are not required to, state your desires in the space provided below. You should consider whether you want to include a statement of your desires concerning decisions to withhold or remove life-sustaining treatment. For your convenience, some general statements concerning the withholding and removal of life-sustaining treatment are set out below. If you agree with one of these statements, you may INITIAL that statement. READ ALL OF THESE STATEMENTS CAREFULLY BEFORE YOU SELECT ONE TO INITIAL. You can also write your own statement concerning life-sustaining treatment and/or other matters relating to your health care. BY LAW, YOUR AGENT IS NOT PERMITTED TO CONSENT ON YOUR BEHALF TO ANY OF THE FOLLOWING: COMMITMENT TO OR PLACEMENT IN A MENTAL HEALTH TREATMENT FACILITY, CONVULSIVE TREATMENT, PSYCHOSURGERY, STERILIZATION OR ABORTION. In every other respect, your agent may make health care decisions for you to the same extent you could make them for yourself if you were capable of doing so. If you want to limit in any other way the authority given your agent by this document, you should state the limits in the space below. If you do not initial one of the printed statements or write your own statement, your agent will have the broad powers to make health care decisions on your behalf which are set forth in Paragraph 3, except to the extent that there are limits provided by law.)

I do **not** want my life to be prolonged and I do **not** want life-sustaining treatment to be provided or continued if the burdens of the treatment outweigh the expected benefits. I want my agent to consider the relief of suffering and the quality as well as the extent of the possible extension of my life in making decisions concerning life-sustaining treatment.

If this statement reflects your desires, initial here ⎯⎯⎯⎯⎯⎯⎯⎯⎯⎯⎯⎯⎯⎯⎯⎯.

I want my life to be prolonged and I want life-sustaining treatment to be provided **unless I am in a coma** which my doctors reasonably believe to be irreversible. Once my doctors have reasonably concluded I am in an irreversible coma, I do **not** want life-sustaining treatment to be provided or continued.

If this statement reflects your desires, initial here ⎯⎯⎯⎯⎯⎯⎯⎯⎯⎯⎯⎯⎯⎯⎯⎯.

I want my life to be prolonged to the greatest extent possible without regard to my condition, the chances I have for recovery or the cost of the procedures.

If this statement reflects your desires, initial here ⎯⎯⎯⎯⎯⎯⎯⎯⎯⎯⎯⎯⎯⎯⎯⎯.

Other or additional statements or desires, special provisions, or limitations.

⎯⎯

⎯⎯

⎯⎯

(You may attach additional pages if you need more space to complete your statement. If you attach additional pages, you must DATE and SIGN EACH PAGE.)

I sign my name to this Durable Power of Attorney for Health Care on

_____ at
(Date)

_____ , _____
(City)   *(State)*

_____
(Signature of Principal)

(THIS POWER OF ATTORNEY WILL NOT BE VALID FOR MAKING HEALTH CARE DECISIONS UNLESS IT IS EITHER: (1) SIGNED BY TWO QUALIFIED ADULT WITNESSES WHO ARE PERSONALLY KNOWN TO YOU AND WHO ARE PRESENT WHEN YOU SIGN OR ACKNOWLEDGE YOUR SIGNATURE OR (2) ACKNOWLEDGED BEFORE A NOTARY PUBLIC IN CALIFORNIA.)

Issues Involving Children

J A M E S   M .   G U S T A F S O N

The Johns Hopkins Case

THE PROBLEM

THE FAMILY SETTING

Mother, 34 years old, hospital nurse.
Father, 35 years old, lawyer.
Two normal children in the family.

In late fall of 1963, Mr. and Mrs. ——— gave birth to a premature baby boy. Soon after birth, the child was diagnosed as a "mongoloid" (Down's syndrome) with the added complication of an intestinal blockage (duodenal atresia). The latter could be corrected with

Reprinted by permission of the author and publisher The University of Chicago Press from "Mongolism, Parental Desires, and the Right to Life," *Perspectives in Biology and Medicine*, Vol. 16, No. 4 (Summer 1973), pp. 529–531.

an operation of quite nominal risk. Without the operation, the child could not be fed and would die.

At the time of birth Mrs. ——— overheard the doctor express his belief that the child was a mongol. She immediately indicated she did not want the child. The next day, in consultation with a physician, she maintained this position, refusing to give permission for the corrective operation on the intestinal block. Her husband supported her in this position, saying that his wife knew more about these things (i.e., mongoloid children) than he. The reason the mother gave for her position—"It would be unfair to the other children of the household to raise them with a mongoloid."

The physician explained to the parents that the degree of mental retardation cannot be predicted at birth—running from very low mentality to borderline subnormal. As he said: "Mongolism, it should be stressed, is one of the milder forms of mental retardation. That is, mongols' IQs are generally in the 50–80 range, and sometimes a little higher. That is, they're almost always trainable. They can hold simple jobs. And they're famous for being happy children. They're perennially happy and usually a great joy." Without other complications, they can anticipate a long life.

Given the parents' decision, the hospital staff did not seek a court order to override the decision (see "Legal Setting" below). The child was put in a side room and, over an 11-day period, allowed to starve to death.

Following this episode, the parents undertook genetic counseling (chromosome studies) with regard to future possible pregnancies.

THE LEGAL SETTING

Since the possibility of a court order reversing the parents' decision naturally arose, the physician's opinion in this matter—and his decision not to seek such an order—is central. As he said: "In the situation in which the child has a known, serious mental abnormality, and would be a burden both to the parents financially and emotionally and perhaps to society, I think it's unlikely that the court would sustain an order to operate on the child against the parents' wishes." He went on to say: "I think one of the great difficulties, and I hope [this] will be part of the discussion relative to this child, is what happens in a family where a court order is used as the means of correcting a congenital abnormality. Does that child ever really become an accepted member of the family? And what are all of the feelings, particularly guilt and coercion feelings that the parents must have following that type of extraordinary force that's brought to bear upon them for making them accept a child that they did not wish to have?"

Both doctors and nursing staff were firmly convinced that it was "clearly illegal" to hasten the child's death by the use of medication.

One of the doctors raised the further issue of consent, saying: "Who has the right to decide for a child anyway? . . . The whole way we handle life and death is the reflection of the long-standing belief in this country that children don't have any rights, that they're not citizens, that their parents can decide to kill them or to let them live, as they choose."

THE HOSPITAL SETTING

When posed the question of whether the case would have been taken to court had the child had a normal IQ, with the parents refusing permission for the intestinal operation, the near unanimous opinion of the doctors: "Yes, we would have tried to override their decision." Asked why, the doctors replied: "When a retarded child presents us with the same problem, a different value system comes in; and not only does the staff acquiesce in the parent's decision to let the child die, but it's probable that the courts would also. That is, there is a different standard. . . . There is this tendency to value life on the basis of intelligence. . . . [It's] a part of the American ethic."

The treatment of the child during the period of its dying was also interesting. One doctor commented on "putting the child in a side room." When asked about medication to hasten the death, he replied: "No one would ever do that. No one would ever think about it, because they feel uncomfortable about it. . . . A lot of the way we handle these things has to do with our own anxieties about death and our own desires to be separated from the decisions that we're making."

The nursing staff who had to tend to the child showed some resentment at this. One nurse said she had great difficulty just in entering the room and watching the child degenerate—she could "hardly bear to touch him." Another nurse, however, said: "I didn't mind coming to work. Because like I would rock him. And I think that kind of helped me some—to be able to sit there and hold him. And he was just a tiny little thing. He was really a very small baby. And he was cute. He had a cute little face to him, and it was easy to love him, you know?" And when the baby died, how did she feel?—"I was glad that it was over. It was an end for him."

ROBERT AND PEGGY STINSON

On the Death of a Baby

Andrew was a desperately premature baby, weighing under two pounds. He died after months of "heroic" efforts in an intensive care facility. The story of his short, cruel, institutionalized life is a case study in the limits and excesses of modern medicine.

The night he told us our son, Andrew, was about to die, the doctor who had taken charge of him six months before also told us we were "intellectually tight," that we had "no feelings, only thoughts and words and strategies." We were "bad parents." As the parents of a five-year-old daughter, we knew the love a mother and father feel for children. Yet, as Andrew's parents, we were used to condemnation and insult.

Andrew was a baby born 15½ weeks prematurely, weighing only 1 lb. 12 oz., and in a state of painful deterioration almost from the start. We wanted him to be allowed to die a natural death. Andrew's story is the story of what can happen when a baby becomes hopelessly entrapped in an intensive care unit where the machinery is more sophisticated than the codes of law and ethics governing its use.

The letter printed below was sent to the administrator and numerous personnel of the hospital that controlled the life and death of our son. The physician in chief of that hospital characterized it as a "carefully documented critique." The letter appears here somewhat edited and abridged; the names of people and institutions have been changed, all but our own. It is the personal record of what happened to our baby and to us.

August 29, 1977

Dear Mr. Clark:

This letter concerns the case of Andrew Stinson, who was a patient in the Infant Intensive Care Unit

(IICU) of Pediatric Hospital from December 24, 1976, to June 14, 1977.

Andrew was born at Community Hospital in our town on December 17, 1976, at a gestational age of 24½ weeks and a weight of 800 grams (1 lb. 12 oz.), at the extreme margin of human viability. He was admitted to the Pediatric Hospital Center (PHC) weighing 600 grams (1 lb. 5 oz.) on December 24, was placed on a respirator against our wishes and without our consent on January 13, and remained dependent on the respirator until he was finally permitted to die on the evening of June 14.

The sad list of Andrew's afflictions, almost all of which were iatrogenic, reveals how disastrous this hospitalization was. Andrew had a month-long, unresolved case of bronchopulmonary dysplasia, sometimes referred to as "respirator lung syndrome." He was "saved" by the respirator to endure countless episodes of bradycardia and cyanosis, countless suctionings and tube insertions and blood samplings and blood transfusions, "saved" to develop retrolental fibroplasia, numerous infections, demineralized and fractured bones, an iatrogenic cleft palate, and, finally, as his lungs became irreparably diseased, pulmonary artery hypertension and seizures of the brain. He was, in effect, "saved" by the respirator to die five long, painful and expensive months later of the respirator's side effects.

The IICU's attempt to nourish Andrew artificially was nearly as successful as its attempt to breathe for him. His bone problems, which included severe rickets secondary to hyperalimentation, testify to the large amount of research still required before the nutritional needs of extremely premature, crucially ill infants can be competently met. The notes in the medical record by those called in to consult about Andrew's problems show that research interest in our baby's problems was indeed high. "The incidence of rickets here and in

This article originally appeared in the *Atlantic Monthly* (July 1979). It is reprinted with permission of Robert and Peggy Stinson.

other IICU units is very interesting," one consultant began, "and points out the need for data. . . . The endocrine section, with your help, would be interested in exploring this area."

"Thank you," another note reads, "for interesting consult on this 'syndrome.' . . . The only time I have seen X-rays of more fractured bones was in an air force crash victim." One of the reasons a doctor once gave to explain Andrew's dependence on the respirator and lack of effort to breathe for himself was that, with all those broken ribs, it "hurts like hell everytime he takes a breath."

Andrew's fractures did heal, but he continued to suffer from "severe failure to thrive"—his height, weight, and head circumference were listed as "much less than third percentile," and by the final six weeks his head (i.e., brain) had stopped growing altogether. Clearly, no one really knew how to provide our baby with the nourishment he needed for normal growth and development. The extraordinary technology that was marshaled to keep Andrew from dying was sufficient only to the production of new, "interesting" problems which no one as yet understands.

Complicating Andrew's respiratory and nutritional difficulties was the fact that the IICU could not protect him from recurring rounds of infection. During his stay at Pediatric Hospital, Andrew suffered through a prolonged case of E. coli septicemia, related abscesses at the arterial line sites which necessitated surgical removal of gangrene and necrotic muscle down to the bone of his right leg (it was noted in the record in May that "right foot remains limited due to severed and removed muscle tissue"), several urinary tract infections, and "multiple courses of pneumonia."

And this was not yet the end of Andrew's problems. He also suffered from a heart defect and possible stress ulcers. He experienced a pulmonary hemorrhage in January. The question of whether there were also intracranial hemorrhages in December or January was never successfully settled, but as the months went by, the record noted cortical atrophy, enlarged ventricles, chronic encephalopathy, microcephaly, and "severe developmental delay."

We have begun with a chronicle of Andrew's afflictions because we think the magnitude of the medical failure involved is quite obviously staggering. It can be argued, of course, that this could all have turned out differently. But the only reality now is that it turned out disastrously for all of us. And the meager statistics available in this very new, still largely experimental effort to save babies at 800 grams and 25 weeks or less

of gestation who need extensive respiratory support indicate that the chances for survival, and certainly for intact neurological survival, were and are grim.

It was our position at the beginning of this case that medical knowledge was not sufficient to justify the no-holds-barred, heroic attempt to simulate the last 15½ weeks of pregnancy. It is hard to feel now that our pessimism was unreasonable. We can only hope that Andrew's case has been, for the doctors involved, an object lesson in humility—a reminder of how pathetically doctors can still fail and how much suffering that failure can inflict on other human beings, on tiny patients and on their families.

We think the question must be raised as to whose interests were really served by this six months of imposed hospitalization. Certainly not Andrew's. He had the misfortune of being declared "salvageable" (the IICU's word) by people who knew neither how to "salvage" him nor when or how to stop. Certainly not ours. Those six months were for us a nightmare of anguish, frustration, and despair. It seems clear to us that all the benefits in this case went to Pediatric Hospital and its staff. The medical residents got a chance to broaden their education by working with a baby with malfunctions of virtually every system of his body, the specialists took part in some "interesting consults" and gathered some data, and the hospital collected the mind-boggling sum of $102,303.20 from our insurance company.

Although we signed a general consent form when Andrew was admitted to the hospital, we did not know that we were signing away control over the events of the next months or, until later, that we could withdraw our consent. However, in our opinion, the hospital did not accord us, Andrew's parents and legal guardians, our rights of informed consent in decisions about his care. From the very first, we were treated as wholly external to the case. Our wishes, judgments, and thoughts were rarely of interest to the IICU's medical staff, who arrogated decisions to themselves as though we did not exist.

Thus, we often telephoned the hospital or arrived for a conference to discover that major decisions, literally involving life and death, had been taken with little effort to explain the problem, let alone to obtain our specific consent one way or the other. On our first visit to the hospital in December, for example, we met Dr. Carvalho, the IICU's attending physician, and explained that we opposed extraordinary efforts to keep Andrew alive. If his troubled breathing failed, we opposed placing him on a respirator. Dr. Carvalho told us that he and his colleagues had already decided that if the baby's severe episodes of apnea and bradycardia continued to worsen, Andrew would be ventilated (put on a respirator). When parents dissented from its decisions, he said, the hospital's policy was to obtain a court order.

A few days later we drove the many miles to Pediatric Hospital again, and this time a doctor we had not met before explained that Andrew had suffered an intracranial hemorrhage and that Dr. Craft, now the IICU's attending physician, had decided that the baby would *not* be attached to a respirator after all.

Again a few more days passed, and now we met Dr. Farrell. Dr. Craft, we discovered, had been attending physician only over the New Year's weekend; now it was January and Dr. Farrell's turn, and he had already made yet another decision. Andrew *would* be ventilated after all, Dr. Farrell said, for he was not so sure now that the baby had had an intracranial bleed. There was no effort made to win our consent to this reversal; we couldn't determine whether the reversal was due to a change in Andrew's prognosis or to the change in personnel. When we objected to the decision, Dr. Farrell accused us of wanting to "play God" and to "go back to the law of the jungle." Apparently not recognizing his responsibility to obtain our informed consent to Andrew's treatment, he reduced the issue to its most absurd level. "I would not presume," he told us, "to tell my auto mechanic how to fix my car."

Drs. Carvalho, Craft, and Farrell did not even discuss with us the long list of risks they knew were involved in ventilating infants as tiny as Andrew. Within a few more days, Andrew's breathing collapsed and he was attached to the mechanical respirator upon which he would be dependent for the rest of his life.

The EMI scan performed on April 19 is another example of serious blocking out of parental knowledge and consent. The baby's medical record shows that the staff was attempting to schedule a computer scan of Andrew's brain for nearly two weeks before it was done, but no one told us about it until it was over. The anesthetist cautioned in the record for April 18, "Plan & risk of anes. will be discussed w. parents." But *no one called*—not an attending physician, not a resident, not an anesthetist—to discuss the "plan and

risk" which were obviously present in their minds but were kept from us.

One curious deviation from this pattern of exclusion occurred in May. When we sought out Dr. Craft during a visit to the hospital on May 5, he told us of several new developments in Andrew's case and said he now regarded Andrew as terminally ill, though Andrew could remain on the respirator for a long time before his respirator-caused lung and heart disease progressed to the point where he would die. Meanwhile, his current case of pneumonia was being successfully treated with antibiotics, and Dr. Craft was close to ordering a tracheostomy because the tube connecting Andrew to the respirator kept coming out and it was becoming more difficult to get it back in.

Then Dr. Craft amazed us by doing something no one at PHC had ever done: he asked our consent. When we refused to give it, we were assured that the hospital had the power to go ahead and operate anyway. But we were by this time more cognizant of our rights—and of the hospital's penchant for not advising us fully and accurately of those rights—than we had been at the beginning of Andrew's case, and after Dr. Craft received a call from our lawyer, plans for the tracheostomy were dropped.

When, at the beginning of Andrew's hospitalization, we asked specific questions about the prognosis for a baby of Andrew's severe prematurity—what, in other words, was the theoretical basis justifying the decision to place Andrew on a respirator?—the medical staff's answers were vague and unrealistically optimistic. Dr. Farrell assured us that statistics show that, thanks to modern medical expertise, almost all premature babies survive and grow up to have no problems of any kind. When we pointed out that such "statistics" were skewed because they lumped together babies of 800 grams with babies of 2000 grams and everything in between, his answer was that we should not adopt this sort of adversary relationship with the medical staff.

Dr. Craft did cite evidence to support his optimism about Andrew: the "Vanderbilt study," which, he said, showed that of 22 babies born at under 1000 grams who survived, 18 turned out to be totally normal. This seemed encouraging until we went, two months later, to the medical school library and discovered that there was no "Vanderbilt study" showing anything of the kind. There had been a study of premature infants done at Vanderbilt, but it dealt with another question. We did discover the study (done in Seattle) dealing with 22 babies born at under 1000 grams (the study included 161 babies, but 87 percent died); it showed that *none* of the babies of Andrew's weight, gestational age, and respiratory status had been successfully "salvaged." (The results of other studies we found later were not quite so bleak, but the prognosis in January 1977 for a baby in Andrew's condition could hardly be seen as encouraging.)

Should a parent have to spend hours in the library of a medical school to obtain answers to his or her questions? We were told later that our questions were inappropriate because the effort to save babies like Andrew is still too new for reliable data to exist, but that was, of course, precisely our point. The attending physicians were not, as they had at first maintained, guided by data; they were creating it.

Nor were our questions about the specifics of Andrew's case answered fully and candidly. Andrew was making good progress, Dr. Farrell assured one of us in late January (though he had developed a major infection, couldn't breathe without the respirator, was off his regular feedings, and had problems with a distended abdomen); he might, said Dr. Farrell, be a "colicky baby" when he came home. Andrew was still "doing all right" on February 9 when we talked to Dr. Craft, though the baby was still dependent on the respirator, still hadn't been cured of the weeks-long bloodstream infection, still hadn't resumed his feedings, and hadn't been gaining weight. All this was, we were assured, "just a technical management problem." In March, Dr. Carvalho was "optimistic" about Andrew, though his bones were breaking because of then unresolved dietary deficiencies and he had developed more infection. Andrew, Dr. Carvalho said, should be off the respirator in "a couple of weeks."

The situation became particularly grotesque at the end of March. The resident then in charge discussed with us the high risk that Andrew had by that time suffered serious brain damage. But when we sought an assessment of Andrew's problems and how they would affect his future from Dr. Carvalho, he replied that premature babies tend to be shorter than their siblings, though we shouldn't worry that Andrew's shortness would be so pronounced as to affect him socially.

A severe crisis of confidence developed as we despaired of getting any believable information. And evidence confirms that our cynicism was not out of place. Even *we* were surprised when we obtained a copy of Andrew's medical record and compared the information there with the version we had been given. Andrew's bronchopulmonary dysplasia had first been noted nearly two months before we were informed of it. He had had more infections than had been reported to us, had been on more drugs of a seemingly experimental nature than we knew of, and had bone problems more severe and fractures more numerous than we had been told. We found out that Andrew had developed an iatrogenic cleft palate. We learned for the first time about the gangrene that had developed in his infected leg and of the tissue and muscle that had been cut away down to the bone; we had been told only that Andrew had an abscess which had been drained and which had "healed nicely."

Perhaps most serious was our discovery that pessimistic assessments of Andrew's condition and prognosis had been made by the Neurology Department, though they were never mentioned to us by anyone. How many other parents would discover such omissions and distortions in what they were told about their children's cases, we wonder, if they too were to request their children's medical records?

We recognize that there are very real legal and ethical problems in the area of consent for medical treatment when children are involved. We were told repeatedly that "someone must be the child's advocate." But how is it possible to be sure in a case like Andrew's just what that means? Who can determine whether or at what point the child's true advocate is the person proclaiming his right to life or the person proclaiming his right to death? We felt that we as the child's parents were more likely to have feelings of concern for his suffering than the necessarily detached medical staff busy with scores of other cases and "interesting" projects.

However, the "someone" who became our child's self-appointed advocate was the attending physician of the IICU. It was argued that we were not the baby's advocates but merely the parents' advocates. By that logic, why are Drs. Farrell, Craft, and Carvalho not recognized as the *doctors'* advocates? For it is useless to pretend that there was ever such a thing as an objective advocate of Andrew's rights. Is any neonatologist, who has, in addition to his ethical commitments as a human being, a professional interest in a baby's problems, a pride in his expertise and in the statistics of success in his unit, and concerns about protecting his reputation in the eyes of his associates, really the right person to be trusted as the baby's sole advocate?

Of course, we were self-interested too. As Andrew's parents, we had a heightened sense of his suffering. Also, we feared the prospect of having to care for the rest of our lives for a pathetically handicapped, retarded child. If this is considered less than noble, what then is the appropriate label for the willingness to apply the latest experimental technology to salvage such a high-risk child and then to hand him over to the life-long care of someone else?

We believe there is a moral and ethical problem of the most fundamental sort involved in a system which allows complicated decisions of this nature to be made unilaterally by people who do not have to live with the consequences of their decisions. A minister—to whom we went for counseling when our family life began to fall apart under the pressures of the hospital's handling of Andrew's case—was direct in his assessment: "This tragedy is not an act of God but an act of man. Don't let yourselves be its victims."

The tube connecting Andrew to the respirator came out of his throat on the night of June 9, and when he began breathing on his own, the decision was made that when his breathing proved inadequate, as it surely must in a baby with "irreversible lung disease," Andrew would not be reattached to the respirator even though that meant he would die. All of this happened without our knowing anything about it. Only the accident of our telephone call to the hospital on the afternoon of June 10 revealed that Andrew was off the respirator and that the attending physicians had conferred and made their decision. It should not have surprised us that none of them thought it useful to have explicit, current expressions of our opinion or to include us in their conference. Andrew was more their baby than ours.

One of the ironic "Catch-22's" of our relationship with PHC is that we were treated in a way practically guaranteed to produce profound psychological upset and then blamed and dismissed from further consideration because we were upset. We were categorized as "hostile," "emotionally fragile," "under psychiatric care."

When Andrew was transferred from our community hospital to PHC, he was already one week old. During that first week we visited him each day, brought him breast milk, talked with both doctor and nurses daily, and together worked out a plan for his care. We agreed that Andrew would be made comfortable and given a chance to thrive if he was able, but that there

would be no heroics. Community Hospital, his physician there advised us, had all the equipment and staff necessary to safeguard the baby if he should be strong enough to do well. But, unlike an intensive care center, they did not have so much equipment that he could be subjected to extraordinary measures which might keep alive a baby whose prognosis didn't warrant aggressive intervention.

After Andrew had done surprisingly well for a week, he developed what was described to us as a minor fluid adjustment and measurement problem. "The time for heroics is past," his doctor assured us, and we agreed to his transfer to PHC. Three obstetricians, a pediatrician, and numerous nurses at Community Hospital had taken our viewpoints and our anguish seriously and had treated us with competence and concern and simple human understanding. We signed the transfer paper in the naive belief that the same atmosphere would prevail at PHC.

Our initial visit to Andrew at Pediatric Hospital gave us the first shocking insight into the error we had made. When we tried to raise the same issues of extraordinary treatment and quality of life that we had all been discussing at Community Hospital, Dr. Carvalho responded coolly that "these children are precious to most parents."

The succession of six principal residents, and others on night or weekend and holiday assignment, created a major obstacle to effective parent-doctor communication. Having to depend for crucial information on people we hardly knew, and having to express our deepest frustrations and most vulnerable feelings to a new stranger every month, built a special and destructive tension through all the months of Andrew's crisis.

We were told that continuity was assured by the presence of the IICU's three attending physicians, but they rotated too, and it was common knowledge that the philosophy of neonatal care varied from one attending doctor to the next. The medical record ought to have been a guarantor of continuity for Andrew. But even the record contains surprising errors and discontinuities, while basic facts concerning the circumstances of Andrew's birth and our family life are creatively elaborated from one resident to the next like whispered stories in a parlor game.

The residents' written comments reflect the lack of understanding we felt from many of them as we were dealing with them. The doctor who wrote the "discharge summary" at the end of Andrew's life felt qualified to state definitively that we "clearly never wanted to have Andrew." That was not true. Another doctor concluded a discussion of Andrew's birth with: "Not to worry tho. The parents were assured by the obstetrician that the child would die and everyone could be happy."

What possible excuse can there be for this sort of callousness becoming a part of the official information that is reported from one doctor to another just coming on the case? How can anyone be so insensitive to the pain involved when the parents' hope for a new baby takes such a disastrous turn? We wondered frequently how many of the young doctors and nurses who felt so qualified to judge us and our feelings had ever experienced a problem pregnancy, had ever had a child at all, had ever been in a situation even remotely like the one that befell us after Andrew's birth and during his stay at Pediatric Hospital.

We do not entirely blame the residents for all of this. They too were in a real sense victims of the rotation system. It was hard for them to know us, though some tried. But in the end they all went on to other cases. We were the only ones who were not allowed to rotate. (The situation was made bearable only by the chance fact that the first resident with whom we dealt was an unusually understanding person who was willing to remain in contact with us and with Andrew's case for all the months which followed his official tour of duty in the IICU. We are grateful to Dr. Perlman for his attempt to reach out beyond the confines of an impersonal system.)

The medical record contains the following brief summary of Andrew's case, dated only June: "6 months bronchopulmonary dysplasia, pulmonary artery hypertension, cerebral atrophy now with seizures—? current status. Difficult parents as per chart."

We asked ourselves again and again what the staff at PHC could have expected people in our situation to do. Did they think we didn't really mean it when we said we believed it was morally wrong to keep Andrew alive? Did anyone consider the impossible psychological position we were put into when we were systematically and casually overruled?

The whole sad case of Andrew Stinson could have been avoided if we had been given complete, accurate information about the policies and ideologies of those in charge of the IICU of Pediatric Hospital *before* we signed the admission forms, for then we would certainly never have allowed Andrew's transfer.

We recognize, of course, that providing accurate, candid information about hospital policies is not so simple as it sounds. But after spending six months agonizing over what was right and what was wrong at every stage of Andrew's medical treatment, after ex-

tensive reading in the field of bioethics, after discussions with acquaintances and colleagues who are by profession philosophers, ministers, theologians, biologists, psychologists, lawyers, and doctors, we can perhaps be excused for saying quite frankly that we are fed up with simplistic discussions of this problem. We are fed up with having to listen to the self-righteous and self-protective rhetoric of "brain death" and "flat EEG's"—as if those concepts weren't irrelevant to the way deaths must really be "orchestrated" (as one more candid doctor put it) in intensive care units. We are fed up with being told that it is illegal and immoral to turn off a respirator at PHC when it is somehow both legal and moral to turn it off somewhere else. We are fed up with the assumption that people disagree on "right-to-life" issues because some of us are moral and some of us are not.

After the responses we got for daring to raise the question of when or in what circumstances Andrew's respirator could be turned off ("What do you want me to do?" asked Dr. Farrell on one memorable occasion. "Go in and put a pillow over his head?"), is it any wonder that we were surprised (and bitter about the hypocrisy of it all) when a variant of respirator withdrawal was in fact arranged—while most of the staff pretended officially that Andrew's death on June 14 was an inevitable occurrence and not arranged at all? Is waiting for a baby who is described as respirator-dependent to dislodge his own breathing tube, chance to breathe for a while for himself, and then, predictably, fail to survive, either moral or "dignified"?

The situation now exists in which it is very easy to turn on a respirator—no one's consent is even needed—and almost impossible to turn one off. Until our legal and moral codes become sophisticated enough to cope with our machinery, parents must have the right to decide whether or in what circumstances their tiny babies should be attached to respirators. Meanwhile, patients, families, hospitals, and society as a whole will continue to be plagued by new and agonizing problems created by the boom in life-support technology. As one attending physician remarked of Andrew's case after it was finally over: "We were all lucky to get out of this as easily as we did."

At the end came a notice from the PHC business office, announcing in passionless figures that the hospital costs alone for Andrew Stinson's treatment came to $104,403.20 (of which all but $2100 has been paid). The bill is more than an accounting of charges for daily treatment. It is a reminder that through the six months of hospital experiments, failures, and arrogance, the meter was ticking—but someone else would pay. The IICU could continue to operate in splendid isolation, not only from our protests, but also from any sense of the financial impact of their solitary decisions.

The bill also reminds us of other financial burdens, and of the many times we tried to give attending physicians, residents, nurses, and business office clerks a sense of how financially destructive this experience was. Our marriage and family life came under substantial pressure, and we began to run up uninsured bills with a family counselor. At the same time we were forced to incur the cost of enunciating and protecting our legal rights when we retained an attorney. Hanging over our heads throughout the spring was the thought that while our medical insurance would probably pay most of the bills that were strictly medical, it listed exclusions and deductions. No matter how expensive our daily lives had become, we knew there would be hundreds and hundreds more to pay at the end.

When this nightmare began, we had a small savings account, but this spring we saw it dwindle to nothing. An annual salary of $13,600 was enough in normal times to maintain a modest living for our family. Since December, when Andrew entered PHC, we have not been able to make ends meet and will do no better in the foreseeable future.

None of this seemed intelligible to the personnel of PHC. It was a problem, perhaps, but it was, again, someone else's problem. We tried, during an extraordinary meeting with him in February, to make Dr. Craft see how serious the situation was. Andrew's hospitalization seemed completely open-ended, we said, and we were afraid that the expenses would run over the limit of our insurance. "What will they do?" we asked. "Will they make us declare bankruptcy and lose everything?" His reply left us speechless: "I guess they will," was all he said. What we needed at that moment was assurance, intercession, or, at the very least, recognition that something fundamentally intolerable could happen, was happening, to other human beings. Instead we saw but one more token of the isolation in which doctors often operate. They do not know how their business offices work and, we suspect, they do not want to know, because knowledge implies responsibility. Ignorance conveniently narrows the focus and enables them to legitimize the disowning of painful problems. Someone else will pay.

What happened at Pediatric Hospital has had a final bitter psychological cost: we have been robbed of the opportunity to grieve at the death of our child. We have friends whose baby son, brain-damaged and unable to breathe on his own, died a day after birth in a community hospital. No respirators were available to prolong the suffering of everyone concerned, and the family was able to grieve for the baby in a normal way. The baby is buried in an old country cemetery where the parents, their older child, and their year-old normal, healthy son gather now and then to think of the child who might have been.

There can be no such scene for Andrew. By the time he was finally permitted to die, the death itself could bring only feelings of profound relief: relief that Andrew's pain, as well as our own, was finished at last; relief that we had all escaped the clutches of Pediatric Hospital at last.

We have taken the money that might have gone under different circumstances for a graveside marker and committed it to the only memorial which can have any meaning for us now: to the sponsorship of a living child, an impoverished child whose only problem at birth was that he was born into an affluent society that does not choose to put his well-being at very high priority. For we believe Andrew's case raises broad and difficult questions which the medical profession in particular and society as a whole must face up to.

What sort of memories or thoughts could we have of Andrew? By the time he was allowed to die, the technology being used to "salvage" him had produced not so much a human life as a grotesque caricature of a human life, a "person" with a stunted, deteriorating brain and scarcely an undamaged vital organ in his body, who existed only as an extension of a machine. This is the image left to us for the rest of our lives of our son, Andrew.

Sincerely yours . . .

How did the hospital reply?

The administration agreed to drop the $2100 charge and think about ways of improving parent-staff relations, but Mr. Clark's response did not address seriously any of the issues Andrew's case raised. The official reply cited the progress in infant survival that had come about "because of perseverance in units such as ours," and regretted that we had interpreted Dr. Farrell's behavior as offensive. His "very behavior reflects the hospital's mission of providing tertiary care," Mr. Clark explained.

No one can deny that there has been progress in saving premature infants, and we are happy for the children and families who can benefit from the experimentation that made this possible. But there will always be a frontier to challenge neonatologists—an "Andrew" of 600 grams, or 300; of 20 weeks, or 16, or 12. Success even at these levels may someday be possible, but as doctors press onward they will inflict pain and heavy costs on tiny subjects and their families.

Who will set the limits? Can society afford to pay? If research must proceed, can't we at least limit it to consenting families?

We referred Andrew's case to the hospital's patient care committee, but without apparent result. We sent twenty copies of our letter to people involved in Andrew's life and death and asked most for a response, but only two replied.

Aren't these issues of interest? Shouldn't we all be discussing them? If there are others who do not wish to deal with hospitals whose mission is to act as Pediatric Hospital did, they must make their wishes known.

U.S. DEPARTMENT OF HEALTH AND HUMAN SERVICES, OFFICE OF HUMAN DEVELOPMENT SERVICES

Child Abuse and Neglect Prevention and Treatment

§ 1340.15   Services and treatment for disabled infants.

(a) *Purpose.* The regulations in this section implement certain provisions of the Child Abuse Amendments of 1984, including section 4(b)(2)(K) of the Child Abuse Prevention and Treatment Act governing the protection and care of disabled infants with life-threatening conditions.

(b) *Definitions.* (1) The term "medical neglect" means the failure to provide adequate medical care in the context of the definitions of "child abuse and neglect" in section 3 of the Act and § 1340.2(d) of this part. The term "medical neglect" includes, but is not limited to, the withholding of medically indicated treatment from a disabled infant with a life-threatening condition.

(2) The term "withholding of medically indicated treatment" means the failure to respond to the infant's life-threatening conditions by providing treatment (including appropriate nutrition, hydration, and medication) which, in the treating physician's (or physicians') reasonable medical judgment, will be most likely to be effective in ameliorating or correcting all such conditions, except that the term does not include the failure to provide treatment (other than appropriate nutrition, hydration, or medication) to an infant when, in the treating physician's (or physicians') reasonable medical judgment any of the following circumstances apply:

(i) The infant is chronically and irreversibly comatose;

(ii) The provision of such treatment would merely prolong dying, not be effective in ameliorating or correcting all of the infant's life-threatening conditions, or otherwise be futile in terms of the survival of the infant; or

Reprinted from *Federal Register* 50 (April 15, 1985), pp. 14887–14888.

(iii) The provision of such treatment would be virtually futile in terms of the survival of the infant and the treatment itself under such circumstances would be inhumane.

(3) Following are definitions of terms used in paragraph (b)(2) of this section:

(i) The term "infant" means an infant less than one year of age. The reference to less than one year of age shall not be construed to imply that treatment should be changed or discontinued when an infant reaches one year of age, or to affect or limit any existing protections available under State laws regarding medical neglect of children over one year of age. In addition to their applicability to infants less than one year of age, the standards set forth in paragraph (b)(2) of this section should be consulted thoroughly in the evaluation of any issue of medical neglect involving an infant older than one year of age who has been continuously hospitalized since birth, who was born extremely prematurely, or who has a long-term disability.

(ii) The term "reasonable medical judgment" means a medical judgment that would be made by a reasonably prudent physician, knowledgeable about the case and the treatment possibilities with respect to the medical conditions involved. . . .

J O H N   C .   M O S K O P   A N D
R I T A   L .   S A L D A N H A

The Baby Doe Rule: Still a Threat

On April 15, 1985, the Department of Health and Human Services published a final rule entitled "Child Abuse and Neglect Prevention and Treatment Program," its fifth attempt in two years to formulate regulations regarding medical treatment of severely handicapped newborns. Like its predecessors, all of which were either struck down in the courts or revised in response to public comments . . . this latest "Baby Doe" rule has serious weaknesses.

The final regulations may indeed represent the best compromise achievable in the current political atmosphere. There remains, however, a major question: Should physicians feel confident that the new regulations will allow them to provide appropriate care for handicapped infants in all circumstances? We will argue that they should not.

Reprinted by permission of the authors and reproduced by permission. © The Hastings Center, from *Hastings Center Report*, Vol. 16, No. 2 (April 1986), pp. 8–14.

The intent of the current policy can be summarized in a single phrase from the rule: to prevent "the withholding of medically indicated treatment from a disabled infant with a life-threatening condition" by making such withholding an instance of medical neglect. The key term "withholding of medically indicated treatment" is further defined as ". . . the failure to respond to the infant's life-threatening conditions by providing treatment . . . which, in the treating physician's . . . reasonable medical judgment, will be most likely to be effective in ameliorating or correcting all such conditions." According to this policy, if there is a treatment that can ameliorate or correct an infant's life-threatening condition, that treatment must be provided.

The regulations go on to recognize three specific exceptions to this policy, that is, three circumstances in which treatment is not required. These exceptions are: (1) when "the infant is chronically and irreversibly comatose"; (2) when "treatment would merely prolong dying, not be effective in ameliorating or correcting all of the infant's life-threatening conditions, or otherwise be futile in terms of the survival of the infant''; and (3) when "treatment would be virtually futile in terms of the survival of the infant and the treatment itself under such circumstances would be inhumane."

HOW WILL DOCTORS REACT?

Several discussions of the April 15 final Baby Doe rule have offered a benign interpretation. One striking example of this view was expressed by Thomas Murray, . . . who argues that the rule is mainly symbolic and will have minimal impact on medical practice.[1]

This appraisal strikes us as extremely optimistic for several reasons. First of all, Murray takes certain liberties with the language of the rule. Nowhere does the rule say that inhumane treatments in and of themselves are not mandatory, as Murray claims; rather it makes an exception for treatments whose provision "would be virtually futile in terms of the survival of the infant *and* . . . would be inhumane." Thus, a treatment judged "inhumane" may be withheld only if it is also "virtually futile" in terms of survival.

Second, the rule does not state that any "reasonable medical opinion" is to be respected, as Murray suggests; rather it requires physicians to use "reasonable medical judgment" in deciding which (if any) treatment will be most likely to be effective in ameliorating or correcting an infant's life-threatening condition(s) and in deciding whether one of the three exceptions applies. In other words, physicians are expected to use reasonable medical judgment in applying the rule, but they may not appeal to medical judgment to justify a decision to ignore or violate this rule.

Finally, Murray claims that the maximum sanction for violating the rule would be the withholding of federal child abuse funding from states. He acknowledges, however, that there is a "faint possibility" that physicians or parents might be charged under state child abuse and neglect statutes. But is this possibility so faint, when the regulation explicitly defines withholding treatment from handicapped infants (except in three specific circumstances) as an instance of medical neglect and requires state child protection agencies to have procedures for identifying and investigating such instances?

In today's malpractice-wary climate, will physicians choose to ignore the rule or to interpret its exceptions very broadly so as to include almost all infants for whom withholding treatment is contemplated? In our opinion, physicians (and perhaps infant care review committees as well) are far more likely to react by treating aggressively in all but the most clearly hopeless cases so as to avoid the real possibility of criminal and civil liability for medical neglect. Such a reaction would surely be understandable, if not exactly praiseworthy, in the already high-risk fields of obstetrics and neonatology. We believe that the final Baby Doe rule, like its predecessors, will continue to have a significant chilling effect on decisions not to treat handicapped infants.

This is particularly true, as Murray acknowledges, with respect to withholding nutrition and fluids. The rule explicitly states that "appropriate nutrition, hydration, and medication" must be provided to all infants without exception, thus leaving almost no room for medical judgment about their advisability.

Because the final rule still requires treatment in all but a very few extreme circumstances, we maintain that basic federal policy has not changed significantly from the first "Baby Doe" regulations proposed in March 1983, although it is more carefully and extensively explicated. The procedures for reviewing treatment decisions and protecting endangered infants have been significantly modified, however, and the new review mechanisms included in the regulations can be very useful. Infant care review committees, for example, may help physicians make decisions in difficult cases, support physicians in those decisions, and obviate the need for external review or investigation. Likewise, state child protective services may well be the most appropriate oversight agencies in these cases. Nevertheless, both infant care review committees and child protective service agencies must abide by the substantive federal policy regarding treatment of disabled infants stated in the DHHS final rule. This is the policy we find most problematic.

The goal of this policy, namely, to protect handicapped infants from medical neglect, is surely important, and the policy may result in long-term benefits for some infants who would otherwise have died for lack of treatment. Despite the highly publicized Bloomington "Baby Doe" case, however, it is not clear that very many infants in recent years have been harmed by withholding or withdrawing medical care. In fact, largely *because* of widespread scholarly criticism of an earlier decision to withhold treatment from an infant with Down syndrome and duodenal atresia, the

1971 Johns Hopkins case,[2] and a widely distributed film dramatization of this case called "Who Should Survive?" which was produced by the Joseph P. Kennedy, Jr. Foundation, such neglect probably occurred infrequently. In contrast to its 1983 warnings of widespread physician neglect of handicapped infants, DHHS now argues that its most recent regulations will affect the care of so few infants that no regulatory impact analysis is required.

Thus, there may not have been a compelling need for new federal regulation in this area, especially since the current policy has at least three significant drawbacks. First, though it may prevent harm to some infants, the current policy threatens the significant harm of unjustified prolongation of life to other seriously handicapped infants. Second, because of the harm it would cause, the policy would force physicians to violate their traditional and fundamental obligation to do no harm without compensating benefit. Third, the policy may exacerbate existing problems or create new problems in the distribution of health care. These three problems will be examined in turn.

UNJUSTIFIED PROLONGATION OF LIFE

Current federal policy threatens to create significant harms of unjustified prolongation of life to some seriously handicapped infants. In requiring that any infant whose life can be more than temporarily prolonged must be treated (provided that the infant is not irreversibly comatose), the policy comes close to supporting the principle of "vitalism"; namely, as Father John Paris describes it, that "life is the ultimate value, and something that is to be preserved regardless of prognosis, regardless of cost, and regardless of social considerations."[3] The policy's only departures from this principle are its statements that infants who are permanently comatose, who are in the process of dying, or who are highly unlikely to survive need not be treated.

The policy assumes, in other words, that noncomatose, nonterminal life is always preferable to nonexistence; it expressly prohibits consideration of the future quality of life of the infant. This, however, is not a plausible assumption; there are conditions other than irreversible coma or death in the near future in which people would overwhelmingly choose a shorter span of life over a longer life of very poor quality. Treatment policies for adult patients recognize this possibility by requiring that physicians ordinarily obtain the informed consent of the patient even for life-saving or life-prolonging treatment.[4]

An obvious difficulty in determining the value of life-prolonging care for infants is that infants cannot express preferences regarding the continuation of their lives; indeed, they do not have any such preferences. But this incapacity does not require that we doom some infants to longer lives of significant suffering. Where treatment has a high probability of causing significant pain and suffering and a low probability of preserving a life valuable to the patient, should we not permit a decision to withhold it?

In requiring that seriously handicapped infants be treated in almost all circumstances, the policy departs from a growing trend to allow legal guardians or next of kin in many circumstances to authorize the withholding or withdrawal of life-prolonging treatment that is not in the best interests of incompetent patients. The use of family contracts in extended care facilities and durable power of attorney designations for health care are examples of this trend.[5]

Infants whose conditions are severe enough to raise questions about the wisdom of aggressive treatment are fairly common in neonatal intensive care units (NICUs). Among such conditions are extreme prematurity, severe intracranial hemorrhage, severe asphyxia, trisomy 13 and 18, and multiple severe congenital anomalies (such as high-lesion meningomyelocele with hydrocephalus, quadriplegia, scoliosis, and incontinence). Sophisticated life-support systems make it possible to sustain the lives of infants with these conditions, at least for a time, but technology frequently cannot ameliorate the severe underlying handicaps. Neither do life support systems prevent life-threatening complications associated with prematurity, such as bronchopulmonary dysplasia (chronic lung disease), necrotizing enterocolitis (gangrene of the intestines), and severe intracranial hemorrhage.

DO NO HARM

In view of the suffering and uncertain prognosis of many of these infants, parents and health care professionals have found it extremely difficult to make decisions about withholding or withdrawing aggressive treatment. We recognize this difficulty and do not believe that a set of moral or technical criteria can be developed that would provide simple and clear solutions in all cases. We are concerned, however, that current federal policy significantly restricts the circumstances in which physicians and parents can act on their own considered judgments about what would be in the infant's best interests; instead it substitutes a hard and fast rule—whenever current technology can prolong life (that is, can prolong noncomatose life beyond the "near future"), it must be employed.

Admittedly, this policy greatly simplifies treatment decisions; parents and professionals need not, indeed may not, consider the "salvageable" infant's life prospects, no matter how harmful they may appear. A graphic illustration of the potential for harm in the treatment of a handicapped infant is provided by Robert and Peggy Stinson's account of their son Andrew, who was born on December 17, 1976 at a gestational age of 24 1/2 weeks and a weight of 800 grams. He was placed on a respirator against his parents' wishes and without their consent on January 13, and remained dependent on the respirator until June 14, when he was finally permitted to die.

The sad list of Andrew's afflictions, almost all of which were iatrogenic, reveals how disastrous this hospitalization was. Andrew had a months-long, unresolved case of bronchopulmonary dysplasia, sometimes referred to as "respirator lung syndrome." He was "saved" by the respirator to endure countless episodes of bradycardia and cyanosis, countless suctionings and tube insertions and blood samplings and blood transfusions, "saved" to develop retrolental fibroplasia, numerous infections, demineralized and fractured bones, an iatrogenic cleft palate, and, finally, as his lungs became irreparably diseased, pulmonary artery hypertension and seizures of the brain. He was, in effect "saved" by the respirator to die five long, painful, and expensive months later of the respirator's side effects.[6]

We grant that this case may represent one of the worst treatment outcomes neonatologists could expect and that some of the elder Stinsons' problems may have been due to a poor relationship with their son's physicians. Nevertheless, as we understand the current policy, aggressive treatment of Andrew would be required until a judgment could be made that continued treatment was highly unlikely to prevent his death in the near future or that he was irreversibly comatose, that is, probably not before the last few weeks (or months) of his life.

How common is Andrew Stinson's plight? This is difficult to estimate. The medical literature is not rife with similar case reports; physicians are understandably reluctant to dwell on the details of their failures. There are, however, statistical data on mortality and morbidity for very small infants like Andrew. Infants who fall into the lowest birth weight category of 500 to 1000 grams (between 1.1 and 2.2 pounds) are only a small percentage of total births (3.4 to 4 per 1000 live births in one study[7]), but a significant percentage of the patient population of neonatal intensive care units. Over the last twenty years, neonatal intensive care has significantly improved their prospects for survival. Nevertheless, mortality rates for infants in this category remain very high; using somewhat different inclusion criteria, three recently published studies report mortality rates of 48 to 66 percent.[8] Some of these infants will exhibit uncorrectable lethal conditions or irreversible coma at birth or shortly thereafter. Many very low birthweight infants, however, will not, or at least not immediately, satisfy the Baby Doe exception criteria, despite poor longer term survival prospects and the expectation of significant morbidity associated with painful aggressive treatment and with severe mental and physical handicaps. Because the Baby Doe rule does not allow physicians and parents even to take the latter criteria into account in making treatment decisions, it threatens harmful overtreatment for at least some of these infants.

If Mr. and Mrs. Stinson are correct in their judgment that aggressive treatment significantly harmed their son without the prospect of greater compensating benefits, then the physicians who treated him violated an ancient and honored Hippocratic principle of professional ethics, "*Primum non nocere*," "First, do no harm." In an era in which powerful treatments often produce significant harms as well as benefits, this principle requires interpretation. One obvious interpretation is that, absent special circumstances such as a patient's specific request, treatments that promise greater overall harm than benefit to the patient ought not be provided. As already noted, determining when prolonging treatment constitutes a harm to the patient is not a simple matter, but neither is it impossible or purely arbitrary. At some point, the harms of painful and disabling treatment must surely outweigh the benefit of some chance at survival with a much diminished quality of life. At that point, providing further treatment violates the physician's commitment to do no harm.

A SHORTAGE OF BEDS?

What about the impact of this federal policy regarding treatment of handicapped infants on the distribution of health care? As a high-technology, labor-intensive area of medical care, neonatal intensive care is very expensive. One 1980 study put the total annual cost of neonatal intensive care at $1.5 billion for 150,000 patients, for an average of $10,000 per patient.[9] Another study cited by DHHS reports an average cost per patient at over $20,000.[10] Charges vary widely depending on the severity of the case; Andrew Stinson's bill for six months of hospitalization in 1977 amounted to $104,403. A Canadian study calculated the cost in 1978 dollars of neonatal intensive care at $52,182 per survivor for newborns weighing 1000 to 1499 grams and $89,892 per survivor for newborns weighing 500 to 999 grams.[11]

Infants of poor families are disproportionately represented in NICUs, probably due to their mothers' poorer overall health status, younger age, and limited use of prenatal care. Because many poor families lack health insurance and are unable to pay for their infants' care, hospitals are naturally reluctant to expand NICUs and assume a greater risk of financial losses. Dr. Arthur Kopelman, director of the NICU at East Carolina University School of Medicine, described the situation *before* the publication of the current federal policy in these terms:

To be blunt, there are inadequate resources available to provide optimal care for every sick infant. The resources available reflect federal and state funding decisions. Intensive care nurseries often run out of space to admit more infants, but somehow we have always found a place for each infant at some center within our State. Our situation is neither unique nor the worst; sick neonates have on occasion been transferred to us who were born in hospitals several states distant because bed space was unavailable any closer. This is the best we can do under the circumstances, but it is not optimal. Because time is critical for these sick neonates, it would be better and much safer if they could be admitted to an intensive care unit close to where they are born.[12]

Current federal policy requiring treatment under almost all circumstances can only intensify this problem. NICUs will likely have to devote a larger and larger proportion of their beds to the most severely and chronically disabled infants, infants like Andrew Stinson who will have very lengthy stays in intensive care, some with limited prospects of ever leaving the unit. As this occurs it will become more and more difficult to provide intensive care promptly for all those infants with acute but completely reversible life-threatening conditions. Such infants may need to be transported long distances to secure care; occasionally their condition may deteriorate or they may die while they are waiting for a bed to become available.

This shortage of neonatal intensive care beds could be ameliorated by special programs to support NICUs or by increasing reimbursement through programs like Medicaid and Crippled Children's Services, for which a significant number of such infants may qualify. Instead, however, current budget proposals seek to make further deep cuts in health care programs, along with most other domestic programs.

Fear of potential legal liability and financial losses may also prompt smaller hospitals to engage in "dumping." Hospitals that formerly accepted some handicapped infants may now invariably transfer such infants to tertiary care centers, further worsening the NICU bed shortage and creating severe and perhaps unnecessary financial and emotional stresses on families. Paradoxically, then, a policy designed to protect infants from medical neglect may, by prolonging the lives of a small but increasing number of the most compromised infants, result in higher overall morbidity and mortality for all those infants needing intensive care.

Recent and proposed cuts in federal health care and social welfare programs also jeopardize continuing care for those infants who finally leave intensive care units with severe disabilities. Does current policy "save" these infants from medical neglect in the neonatal period only to neglect their continuing substantial needs? Whether life will be of value for a handicapped infant obviously depends to some extent on what resources are available to help the infant develop his or her potentialities and meet future crises. A strong network of services providing custodial, medical, habilitative, and educational support for handicapped infants bolsters claims that such infants will benefit from neonatal intensive care. Current federal policies, however, mandate such care while seeking to dismantle many of the services on which handicapped individuals will later depend.[13]

WHY SINGLE OUT INFANTS?

Finally, if this federal policy is justified in order to prevent the medical neglect of handicapped infants, then presumably we could justify a similar policy to protect all incompetent patients who cannot protect their own interests. As a final test of the soundness of this policy, then, consider whether aggressive treatment should be required for all incompetent patients unless death will occur in the near future or the patient is irreversibly comatose.

Is it always in the best interest of the elderly senile patient with advanced cancer to receive chemotherapy or radiation therapy until he is highly unlikely to survive beyond the near future? Should the severely debilitated (but not comatose) stroke victim be resuscitated an indefinite number of times until respiration cannot be restored by any means? Providing treatment in such circumstances seems to us clearly not always in the best interests of such patients. There comes a point at which further prolongation of one's life simply does not make up for the burden of continued aggressive treatment, especially if the quality of life prolonged is diminished by suffering and incapacity. If it would be cruel to prolong the life of adult patients under these circumstances, then it must also be cruel to prolong the life of handicapped infants under comparable circumstances.

Potential cruelty to patients would not be the only problem of such a policy; finding the resources to support a greatly increased reliance on sophisticated medical care would also be extremely difficult. Recent studies have suggested that a very large percentage of health care costs are incurred by patients in the last two years of life.[14] Requiring that all potentially life-prolonging treatments be provided would increase this percentage significantly. Because such last-ditch efforts for seriously ill patients often fail, our policy would then likely place us in the curious position of requiring those treatments which will have the least favorable cost-benefit ratio. We would then be forced either to pay much more for health care than we do today or to cut back on effective treatments for conditions that are not life-threatening.

Neither alternative seems wise. The former, providing unlimited funds for life-prolonging care, would represent a capitulation to the technological imperative. Do we, for example, want to try to provide an artificial heart for all of the 140,000 potential candidates for this procedure, at a cost of $3 to $5 billion annually?[15] Since this treatment does appear to have the potential to prolong life, there would be tremendous pressure to make it widely available under a policy that required the provision of all life-prolonging treatments. The latter alternative, cutting back on treatment for nonlife-threatening conditions, would sacrifice quality of life and long-term life expectancy to short-term prolongation of life. It thus seems highly undesirable to apply the current policy regarding treatment of handicapped infants to all incompetent patients. Why then single out infants and require that they alone receive aggressive treatment?

For all the above reasons, the threat of unjustified prolongation of life, the violation of the physician's duty to do no harm, and undesirable effects on the distribution of health care, the continuing attempt to enforce treatment by federal regulation is an ill-advised response to the problem of caring sensitively for severely compromised infants. We should be proud that our health care system is able to care for very sick newborns, but also recognize that there are limits to our powers. In medicine as elsewhere, advanced technology cannot cure all the ills to which we are heir. And, as the power of any technology increases, so does its potential for harm.

NOTES

1. Thomas H. Murray, "The Final, Anticlimactic Rule on Baby Doe," *Hastings Center Report* 15:3 (1985), 5–9.

2. See, e.g., James M. Gustafson, "Mongolism, Parental Desires and the Right to Life," *Perspectives in Biology and Medicine* 16 (1973), 529–57.

3. John J. Paris, "Terminating Treatment for Newborns: A Theological Perspective," *Law, Medicine, and Health Care* 10 (1983), 120–24.

4. Virginia Abernethy and Keith Lundin, "Competency and the Right to Refuse Medical Treatment," in *Frontiers in Medical Ethics*, edited by Virginia Abernethy (Cambridge: Ballinger, 1980), pp. 79–98.

5. For a discussion of durable powers of attorney, see President's Commission for the Study of Ethical Problems in Medicine and Biomedical and Behavioral Research, *Deciding to Forego Life-Sustaining Treatment* (Washington, 1983), pp. 145–53.

6. Robert Stinson and Peggy Stinson, "On the Death of a Baby," *Atlantic Monthly* (July 1979), pp. 64–65.

7. Sargent P. Horwood et al., "Mortality and Morbidity of 500- to 1499-Gram Birth Weight Infants Live-born to Residents of a Defined Geographic Region Before and After Neonatal Intensive Care," *Pediatrics* 69 (1982), 616.

8. Sharon Buckwald, et al., "Mortality and Follow-Up Data for Neonates Weighing 500 to 800 g at Birth," *American Journal of Diseases of Children* 138 (1984), 779–82; William Kitchen and Laurence J. Murton, "Survival Rates of Infants with Birth Weight Between 501 and 1000 g," *AJDC*, 139 (1985), 470–71; Ernest Kraybill et al., "Infants with Birth Weights Less Than 1001 g," *AJDC*, 138 (1984), 837–42.

9. Peter P. Budetti et al., *The Cost Effectiveness of Neonatal Intensive Care* (Washington: Office of Technology Assessment, 1980), cited in Andrew T. Griffin and David C. Thomasma, "Triage and Critical Care of Children," *Theoretical Medicine* 4 (1983), 157.

10. Department of Health and Human Services, "Child Abuse and Neglect Prevention and Treatment Program," *Federal Register* 50 (1985), 14873–92.

11. Michael H. Boyle et al., "Economic Evaluation of Neonatal Intensive Care of Very-Low-Birthweight Infants," *New England Journal of Medicine* 308 (1983), 1330–37.

12. Arthur E. Kopelman, "Dilemmas in the Neonatal Intensive Care Unit," in *Ethics and Mental Retardation*, edited by Loretta Kopelman and John C. Moskop (Dordrecht: D. Reidel, 1984), p. 243.

13. See, for example, Peter P. Budetti et al., "Federal Health Program Reforms: Implications for Child Health Care," *Milbank Memorial Fund Quarterly* 60 (1982), 155–181, and Mary O. Mundinger, "Health Service Funding Cuts and the Declining Health of the Poor," *New England Journal of Medicine* 313 (1985), 44–47.

14. See, for example, Steven A. Schroeder et al., "Survival of Adult High-Cost Patients," *Journal of the American Medical Association* 245 (1981), 1446–1449, and Christopher J. Zook and Francis D. Moore, "High-Cost Users of Medical Care," *New England Journal of Medicine* 302 (1980), 996–1002.

15. Penelope Rowlands, "Bionic Bill's Heart: Critics Say Deficient," *Medical News and International Report* 9:3 (Feb. 4, 1985), 9.

The Role of Hospital Ethics Committees

NORMAN FOST AND RONALD E. CRANFORD

Hospital Ethics Committees: Procedural Aspects

The custom of physicians making decisions about life and death in private with relatives is becoming an anachronism. While that custom may persist in some hospitals and particularly when patients die at home, such events increasingly occur in referral hospitals,[1] with the involvement or scrutiny of innumerable consultants, residents, nurses, social workers, students, and other personnel. As the privacy of these decisions has diminished, public awareness and interest have increased. A growing catalogue of controversial court cases,[2-7] statutes,[8] and regulations[9-11] marks the beginning of a search for principles to guide conduct in a way that can attract consensus. These changes have not occurred in a vacuum. They are part of the response to practices that have aroused concern. Laws are generally not written until there is a perception that an important moral principle has been broken.

Proposals for regulating decisions about life-sustaining medical care fall into two major categories: substantive guidelines, specifying what kinds of patients may permissibly have treatment withdrawn or withheld and for what reasons, and procedural guidelines. Among the latter are so-called ethics committees—hospital-based interdisciplinary groups that would classify,[12] prognosticate,[2] consult,[13-17] or possibly even make decisions.[18] The nation's experience with such committees is too limited to justify strong approval or opposition. It is clear, however, that they have attracted increasing interest as a possible response to a growing dilemma in health care.[11,19,20] The American Medical Association House of Delegates has adopted a resolution supporting such committees.[21] Federal regulations strongly encouraged the formation of such committees to review decisions regarding handicapped infants.[11] While these regula-

This article was originally published as "Hospital Ethics Committees: Administrative Aspects," and is reprinted by permission of the authors and publisher from the *Journal of the American Medical Association* 253 (May 1985), pp. 2687–2692. © 1985, American Medical Association.

tions were subsequently declared invalid by a federal court, the number of hospitals with such committees has grown rapidly, and it is likely that similar committees will be involved in decisions regarding other kinds of patients. It is therefore timely and important to review some administrative and legal issues that need to be addressed in their formation and operation.

COMMITTEES FOR RESOLVING ETHICAL CONTROVERSIES

Hospital committees for resolving or preventing ethical problems are not new. The best-known example would be the Institutional Review Boards (IRBs), which are multidisciplinary groups formed for the purpose of protecting human subjects from unethical research. They were mandated by the US Department of Health, Education, and Welfare in 1966 in response to increasing evidence that protection was needed.[22] They have come to be accepted as contributing to substantial resolution of the problem without undue interference with legitimate research goals.[23] Tissue committees, which review surgical specimens, can be thought of as addressing what is primarily an ethical question: was the potential benefit sufficient to justify exposing a patient to the risk of surgery? While similar committees could be used to address a variety of ethical problems and controversies in a hospital, we will focus on the application of greatest current interest—consultation for decisions regarding termination of life-sustaining treatment.

The word *committee* is offensive to many physicians, suggesting an unwelcome bureaucratization of what should be personal and private decisions. The word may be misleading since such groups, as currently operating and proposed, do not usually have the regulatory or decision-making roles typical of other hospital committees. A better term might be *ethics consultation group*. Nonetheless, terms such as *hospital ethics committee* (HEC) and *infant bioethics committee* have come into use.[24] We have had experience in establishing such committees in our own hospitals and consulting in the formation of others.

THE RATIONALE FOR A CLINICAL ETHICS COMMITTEE

Collaborative decision making is not a new idea. Physicians commonly seek opinions of others when making difficult decisions. This collaboration is sometimes required by law or regulation, as in the case of IRBs.[25]

Decisions regarding termination of care are fundamentally ethical, not medical. Sound judgments will obviously depend on accurate medical information—good ethics starts with good facts—but the crucial question is usually an ethical one: Is it right to deliberately shorten a patient's life by withholding or withdrawing life-sustaining treatment? Physicians ordinarily consider themselves able to make sound ethical judgments, sometimes claiming a special ability to make good ethical decisions.[26] Even for those inclined to seek second opinions on ethical matters, expert opinion is not widely available and may be difficult to define even when it is close at hand.

Making better ethical decisions does not necessarily depend on ethical expertise, although people trained in ethics are increasingly recognized as useful colleagues in clinical settings.[27,28] Some have found a justification for ethics committees in "ideal observer theory,"[29] which states that ethically correct decisions should be approvable by an observer whose qualities include omniscience, disinterest, and dispassion. Since no individual can possess these virtues, it suggests that a broadening of the decision-making process be required.[30,31] Institutional Review Boards for the review of proposed research involving human subjects, tumor boards, and even juries are, in part, reflections of a belief that diverse viewpoints often lead to better decisions. Ethics committees, according to this view, may be more likely than individual physicians to arrive at decisions that, in retrospect, will withstand ethical scrutiny and legal challenge.

A 1982 survey of 602 hospitals revealed only 3% with committees that had the potential to become involved in decision making in specific cases.[37] A 1984 survey suggests that over 50% of hospitals now have such committees, and most of the remaining hospitals are considering establishing them. Even in those hospitals where they have been established for several years, they review only a small percentage of decisions involving termination of care.

The much-publicized "Baby Doe Regulations," issued by the US Department of Health and Human Services in response to the death of a baby in Bloomington , Ind,[9,11] probably had an effect in stimulating the formation of infant bioethics committees. The original regulations, which featured roving "Baby Doe Squads," were widely criticized[33-35] and struck down by a federal district court.[36] The rules were revised and in their final form offered institutions the alternative of forming local review committees, implicitly as a way of avoiding federal investigators. These, too, were invalidated by a federal court.[37] It is likely that federal involvement helped to stimulate some medical organizations to propose alternatives, including ethics committees, but others had recommended similar approaches before the Baby Doe regulations.[29,38,39] The New Jersey Supreme Court, in its decision approving withdrawal of life support from Karen Quinlan,[2] stipulated that such decisions *must* be approved by a hospital "ethics committee," but this was a misnomer. What they clearly intended was a neurological consultation committee: a group of persons expert in the medical, and particularly neurological, prognosis of the patient. . . .

PURPOSES OF ETHICS COMMITTEES

Hospitals contemplating formation of such committees should consider which of several purposes they hope to achieve: improvement of intrainstitutional or extrainstitutional public relations, education, development of policy and guidelines, or consultation for active decisions. All could be accomplished, but political considerations might argue for beginning with functions that are perceived by physicians as less intrusive and threatening.

Educational activities are usually, but not always, unobjectionable. One hospital director, when asked if the chiefs of staff would welcome an ethics committee, replied with noticeable restraint: "I am sure the clinical chiefs would welcome any activity which would help them better understand the principles which will enable them to make better decisions." Another hospital experienced a short but intense crisis when a weekly conference on ethical issues was shut down by a powerful clique, some of whom objected to such issues being discussed in public. Most hospitals, however, welcome new and interesting educational programs, and most physicians express an interest in learning more about ethical dimensions of practice.

Development of guidelines on such issues as do-not-resuscitate orders may be the most difficult and exacting function of an ethics committee. Several groups have prepared such guidelines,[40,42] and it is probably not necessary for every hospital to reinvent this wheel. Modifications of existing guidelines can be made to meet local needs and institutional realities. One important function of such documents is to define the limits of ethically acceptable and legally permissible behavior. They can alert physicians to those decisions that are, in the opinion of the ethics committee and hospital attorney, within the range of permissible behavior and those that are likely to involve moral controversy and legal hazards. While legal limits do not always reflect morally correct decisions, they are a reasonable starting point for reflection.

The most controversial role of an ethics committee is as a consulting group for urgent decisions about withholding, withdrawing, or continuing life-sustaining medical care. The remainder of our comments will address problems involved in this function. While some might advocate investing decision-making authority in such committees, there has been little experience with such a role. The majority of existing ethics committees surveyed by the President's Commission did not view themselves as primary decision makers.[31] This has also been our experience as we have worked with at least 20 HECs around the country. The majority have emphasized their consultative, advisory, informational, and consensus-development roles rather than primary decision making. The discussion will therefore be predicated on the assumption that such a committee's involvement in live cases will be consultative rather than decision making.

ADMINISTRATIVE AUTHORITY AND MEMBERSHIP

Even if a committee were consultative and had no decision-making authority, it needs to be legitimized by the hospital leadership. If it were not mandatory to consult the committee, it need not be part of the hospital by-laws, but if one purpose of consulting a committee was to provide partial protection from later charges of negligence, it would be helpful if the committee had official status. Whether it should be constituted by the medical or administrative staff would depend on its primary purpose.[15] If the major purpose is to provide consultation to physicians, it is appropriate that it be formed by and responsive to the medical staff, rather than the administrative staff or governing board, although administration should be represented. If its purpose is to set hospital policy and guidelines, it would be constituted by the governing board. If its purpose were purely as a prognosis committee, the qualifications for membership would be primarily medical and particularly neurological. Finally, such committees could conceivably be formed primarily for the purpose of psychological counseling and support, in which case the qualifications would include competence in such fields as counseling, group process, and psychotherapy. It would seem desirable for committees to have the potential for all these functions, in which case membership would have to be authorized by the agency responsible for setting hospital policy and forming committees. The confidentiality of committee records may depend on whether the committee is under the administration or medical board, but this will vary among states.

In performing a consultative function, it is desirable that committee membership fill the need for *expertise* as well as *representation* of various factions. Expert information is needed on complex medical and psychosocial issues, including prognosis; alternative treatments; likely benefits and risks; the realities of handicapped life for patients and families with similar conditions, as well as this particular patient and family; rapidly evolving legal concepts and court decisions; financial considerations; and religious and ethical considerations. Persons with a special interest in the disposition include the patient and family, the attending physician, nurses directly involved, and the community, including, in some cases, groups with a special concern for the handicapped. A typical committee embodying these considerations would include a physician, nurse, social worker, attorney, member of the hospital administration, clergyperson, community member, advocate for the handicapped, and medical ethicist. For individual cases, persons directly involved could be invited, including family members or their representative; the attending physician and primary nurse; and the clergyperson who best knows the patient. Each hospital will obviously have to tailor its membership to its own needs and resources. In the beginning, a smaller group is more likely to work together constructively, but this will have to be balanced with the need for specific competencies and viewpoints.

In addition to the specific needs outlined above, it is desirable that all members acquire and develop competence in the ethical and legal questions that recurrently arise in decisions involving critically ill patients. This can be accomplished in part through hospitalwide educational programs, for the benefit of the entire hospital community as well as the committee. There are also extensive reading materials available as well as national and regional conferences on ethics committees and related issues.

It is possible that hospital personnel may feel excessive loyalty, deference, or obligation to the attending physician and be reluctant to ask hard questions and make unwelcome suggestions. Our experience with institutional review boards and clinical ethics committees suggests that this problem is not insurmountable. With appropriate leadership, both from clinical chiefs not serving on the committee and from the committee chair, members can and have become responsible to the task at hand. This is not to say that covert issues or outside loyalties can be eliminated, but only that vigorous debate can occur and the ultimate decision makers will benefit from such discussion.

As with IRBs, it is desirable that the group be broadly based, representing diverse viewpoints, including at least one "community" member—a person with no vested interest in or connection with the hospital. Intragroup leadership, as with all small groups, is vital but will be of no avail if the hospital leadership, including the medical director and the chiefs of staff, is opposed.

The remaining membership question is whether patients and families should participate in such group discussions. The family's wishes, resources, and religious orientation are obviously of major importance. The question is whether this information should be presented directly by them or presented to the committee by someone else. While many physicians have paternalistic impulses on this subject, the great majority of patients[43] and parents[44] resent being excluded from discussions about management of a critically or terminally ill patient. When competent patients are under discussion, it is fundamental in American law that "every human being of adult years has a right to determine what shall be done with his own body."[45] Assumptions that relatives cannot tolerate candid discussions or that they will experience long-term guilt are not supported by existing data.[46]

The question, therefore, is not whether to include patient and family in such discussions but whether that involvement should include direct discussion with a group of strangers. In some cases it will be appropriate for relatives to join the discussion (e.g., when they insist on it), but that should not preclude the group having an opportunity to discuss the issues among themselves, free of the inhibition that would accompany the presence of patients or relatives. In other cases, family involvement may be unnecessary and/or unwanted by the family. If the primary function of the group is to be advisory to the attending physician, apologies should not be needed for the physician's desire to have a free and uninhibited consultation. A flexible policy would be to invite family members to present their views but not require it.

It is unclear whether physicians could consult such committees without explicit permission from the patient or family. Anyone making such a claim would have to provide some justification for overriding the usual duty to maintain confidentiality. It is possible that a federal or state regulation requiring such consultation could provide this justification, but the matter has not been tested as yet. Considering the profound importance and sensitivity of this area, it would seem prudent, if not required by law, to obtain permission from the patient or family.

As with all committees, the entire membership will not be available for all meetings. There will be times when a majority will not be available. As long as the committee has no regulatory role, there would be no compelling need to formalize quorum requirements. Some HECs provide for consultation with the chairman or any available member of the committee. That person can activate a subcommittee of available members. While every case is unique, as with all areas of medicine there are recurring themes and syndromes, and in some cases the experienced committee person may be able to anticipate a committee consensus accurately. If and when such committees are mandated, such problems as quorum requirements will have to be addressed.

OPEN VS. CLOSED MEETINGS, RECORDS, AND ACCOUNTABILITY

The educational functions of ethics committees would be better served if they were open to all interested persons, both for the audience's benefit and so the committee members could get ideas, feelings, and feedback from peers and the community. Many institutional review boards open their meetings to the public, but it is obviously unknown whether such scrutiny has a net positive or negative effect on the quality of review. Case conferences can be developed to promote this purpose, using semifictional data to protect confidential information. Discussion of current cases, however, would be necessarily closed to those who are not officially members of or consultants to the committee. Patient rights of confidentiality would require this, as well as the need for candid discussion.

A related question is whether the substance of discussion in such meetings should be recorded and whether such records should be publicly available in the form of tape recordings, transcripts, minutes, summaries, or notes in the medical record. It is important for there to be accountability for crucial decisions about life and death, and there is broad consensus among medicolegal experts that the basis for a decision to withdraw life-sustaining treatment should be documented in the medical record.[40] This can be accomplished by a note in the chart by the attending physician documenting that a consultation was obtained and summarizing the key points in that discussion.

Maintaining a permanent, detailed record of the committee's discussion has advantages and disadvantages. On the one hand, it allows for greater accountability, provides a valuable teaching resource, and reduces the possibility for misunderstanding. If one purpose is to provide legal protection for the physician and hospital, it would be essential to have a record of the content of the discussion. On the other hand, there is the risk of inhibiting discussion and possibly increasing the legal liability for members. Such discussions could conceivably be construed as conspiracy to commit homicide,[47] although no such charges have ever been brought. Whether or not records could be protected from discovery proceedings or subpoena in a malpractice or criminal trial is unclear. The need to prepare minutes could unintentionally push the committee toward voting or directing a plan of action rather than confining itself to the more acceptable roles of consultation and advice.

ACCESS AND INDICATIONS FOR CONVENING THE COMMITTEE

The most controversial question confronting an institution considering formation of an ethics committee is the definition of access and jurisdiction. The slow growth of ethics committees nationally, and the modest use of them in institutions where they have had some success, is partly due to resistance and opposition from the medical staff. An extreme view would prohibit or oppose the formation of such committees, usually on the grounds that such a group is less likely to make a good decision than a wise clinician or sensitive family.[48] Others tolerate the existence of such a committee, so long as they are free not to consult it. At the other extreme, some would propose defining cases for which consultation would be mandatory.[49]

At present, most physicians appear unlikely to consult such a group of their own volition, even with the understanding that the committee would have no authority to make decisions. This resistance suggests that hospitals should initially establish a policy of voluntary consultation, with no decision-making authority in the committee. Informal discussion and consensus development may encourage consultation until such review becomes standard through custom or by legal requirement. While mandatory consultation with such committees might be necessary if they are to become an important part of decision making in hospitals, there is no such mandate at present.

It is undesirable for such a committee to be faced with a large volume of cases in the beginning. It is important for the committee to discover and define its own rules, for the members to become comfortable with each other, and for it to gain some early success and esteem in the institution. Consultation on a voluntary basis will minimize the load and allow this development to occur with less pressure.

If a hospital establishes a voluntary committee—with consultation available on an optional basis—there remains the question of access by persons other than the attending physician. While this is in part a political issue to be resolved within the personalities and traditions of each hospital, one purpose of a committee—to minimize the probability of a decision that, in retrospect, may be difficult to justify—would be served by facilitating access to its views. If a house officer, nurse, student, patient, or family member feels sufficiently concerned about a patient's management and cannot obtain satisfaction from discussions with the attending physician, an ethics committee offers a mechanism for intrainstitutional resolution of a potential dispute. Whistle blowers are usually frustrated by the inadequacy of internal review or appeal processes. The celebrated cases involving criminal charges for withholding treatment[50-54] (*California Magazine*, November 1982, pp. 79–81, 164–175) were triggered by reports from nurses who thought physicians were making hasty or improper decisions and who felt an inability to seek support within the institution.

While the general policy of the committee might be one of optional consultation, there may be exceptions, cases for which mandatory review would seem prudent. One such category might be handicapped newborns who are not terminally ill but whose interests seem best served by withdrawal of life support. It is this class of patients that has provoked the greatest controversy and stimulated governmental intrusion. Mandatory review would not imply that it is improper to withhold or withdraw treatment from such patients but only that it is a sufficiently weighty decision to justify consultation to reduce the probability of error. There may be no legal authority for mandating review

over the objections of the patient or family, although the recent federal statute and subsequent regulations might provide such authority. A proposed statute, which includes standards for jurisdiction, is available in the report of the President's Commission for the Study of Ethical Problems in Medicine.[55]

In summary, consultation can be optional or mandatory with regard to which cases are brought to the committee, and the committee's deliberations can be optional or mandatory with regard to whether they are advisory or action forcing. . . .

While many correctly point out that a committee cannot be convened at moments of crisis, it is our experience that this concern is overdrawn. The great majority of decisions regarding withdrawal of care can be anticipated days, and often weeks, before a moment of crisis. In truly unexpected emergencies, if there is ambiguity about whether to resuscitate or otherwise treat a dying patient, the prudent course is to avoid making irreversible decisions based on inadequate data or reflection; i.e., to maintain life until consultation is available. There will usually be other opportunities to withdraw treatment, if that appears to be the correct course, although it must be conceded that emergency resuscitation sometimes leads to long life, which, in retrospect, should not have been prolonged. Some emergency crises involve situations that are sufficiently similar to allow development of policies before the moment of crisis. Examples include the extremely small, nonviable premature infant; live abortuses; anencephalic newborns; and newborns with Down's syndrome. Guidelines do not necessarily dictate behavior in all cases, but they can identify behaviors that are permissible, those that should be forbidden, and those that are sufficiently controversial to warrant consultation.[56] Even in those cases that do not allow for consultation or development of guidelines, post hoc discussion—a "clinical-ethical conference"—can be useful in guiding conduct in future cases.

EFFECT ON LIABILITY

Consultation with an HEC has potential risks and benefits for the hospital and its personnel. Physicians, nurses, and others who participate in decisions to withhold life-sustaining teatment could be charged with civil or criminal offenses, such as negligence and homicide.[7,38,47,50-54] Committee discussion could be construed as conspiracy to commit homicide.[47] Committee members and records of the meeting could be subpoenaed, and a disgruntled member could testify against the attending physician.

We would not view these concerns as arguments discouraging to an attending physician, as they do not present risks different from those that exist without committee consultation. As mentioned earlier, prosecutions can be triggered by disgruntled employees in any case and might be more likely when internal mechanisms for discussion are unavailable. With or without committee consultation, an attending physician must be accountable for a decision to withdraw life-support, which requires, at least, a statement in the chart summarizing the reasons for the decision. We believe the use of a committee is more likely to reduce the risk of litigation and/or prosecution. It provides reassurance and evidence that due care was used in arriving at a decision, and the substance of the consultation is likely to reduce the chance of a decision that would invite legal attention.

Committee members might incur liability for decisions that they have little ability to affect. They could be liable under child abuse laws for failing to report neglect, although many such statutes only require reporting for patients under the care of the reporter. Such questions may be resolved in part by institutional insurance coverage and assurances that legal services would be provided, but that may not be consoling for the individual involved. If a prosecution were brought, it would most likely be for an egregious case, but a committee member may feel powerless to affect what he considers an egregious decision. We would not consider these risks to be significantly greater than the risks of collaborative care in general. Individuals with serious concerns about liability can obviously choose not to participate in such committees.

CONCLUSIONS

Hospital ethics committees are increasingly becoming a part of decision making involving life support in critically ill patients. Such committees can help promote ethically defensible decisions in three ways: through education, establishment of hospital policies, and consultation and review.

There is adequate experience to justify some optimism in the feasibility and usefulness of such committees, providing they have competent, diverse membership and effective leadership and are supported by opinion leaders in the hospital. It would be desirable for ethics committees to be formed voluntarily, before they are required by law, while the flexibility exists to try alternative procedures. Given the present inexperience and the complex and highly charged cases with which they would deal, it is probable that a mandate for their formation would be associated with unwelcome side effects.

John Robertson and Dan Wikler made many helpful comments and suggestions.

NOTES

1. Brim OG, Freeman HE, Levine S, et al: *The Dying Patient*, New York, Russell Sage Foundation, 1970, pp 20–26.

2. *In re* Quinlan, 70 NJ 10, 355 A2d 647, *cert denied*, 429 US 922 (1976).

3. *Superintendent of Belchertown State School v Saikewicz*, 370 NE2d 417 (Mass 1977).

4. *In re* Spring, 405 NE2d 115 (Mass 1980).

5. *Eichner v Dillon*, 426 NYS2d 527 (App Div 1980).

6. *In re* Storar, 420 NE2d 64 (NY 1981), *rev'g in re* Storar, 433 NYS2d 388 (App Div 1980).

7. Robertson JA: *The Rights of the Critically Ill*. New York, Bantam Books Inc, 1983.

8. Arizona HB 2209, July 27, 1983.

9. Donnelly TR Jr: Nondiscrimination on the basis of handicap, Interim Final Rule (45 CFR 84). *Federal Register* 1983;48 (March 17):9630–9632.

10. Heckler MM: Nondiscrimination on the basis of handicap relating to health care for handicapped infants: Proposed rules (45 CFR 84). *Federal Register* 1983;48(July 5):30846–30852.

11. Nondiscrimination on the basis of handicap: Procedure and guidelines relating to health care for handicapped infants. *Federal Register* (45 CFR 84). 1984;49:1622–1654.

12. Optimum care for hopelessly ill patients: A report of the Clinical Care Committee of the Massachusetts General Hospital. *N Engl J Med* 1976;295:362–364.

13. Cohen C: Interdisciplinary consultation on the care of the critically ill and dying: The role of one hospital ethics committee. *Crit Care Med* 1982;10:776–784.

14. Levine C: Hospital ethics committees: A guarded prognosis. *Hastings Center Rep* 1977;7:28–30.

15. Veatch R: Hospital ethics committees: Is there a role? *Hastings Center Rep* 1977;7:22–25.

16. Bader D: Medical-moral committees: Guarding values in an ambivalent society. *Hosp Prog* 1982, pp 80–83.

17. Esqueda K: Hospital ethics committees: Four case studies. *Hosp Med Staff* 1978, pp 26–31.

18. President's Commission for the Study of Ethical Problems in Medicine and Biomedical and Behavioral Research: *Deciding to Forego Life-Sustaining Treatment*. Government Printing Office, 1983, p 164.

19. President's Commission for the Study of Ethical Problems in Medicine and Biomedical and Behavioral Research: *Deciding to Forego Life-Sustaining Treatment*. Government Printing Office, 1983, pp 160–170, 224–228.

20. Committee on Bioethics, American Academy of Pediatrics: Treatment of critically ill newborns. *Pediatrics* 1983;72:565–566.

21. Bioethics committees in hospitals, substitute resolution 70. Adopted by the American Medical Association House of Delegates, Annual Meeting, Chicago, June 17–21, 1984.

22. Beecher HK: *Research and the Individual*. Boston, Little Brown & Co, 1970.

23. National Commission for the Protection of Human Subjects in Biomedical and Behavioral Research: *Institutional Review Boards*. Government Printing Office, 1978, p 74.

24. American Academy of Pediatrics Task Force on Infant Bioethics Committees: Guidelines for infant bioethics committees. *Pediatrics* 1984;72:306–310.

25. 45 CFR 46.

26. Veatch RM: Generalization of expertise. *Hastings Center Studies* 1973;1:29–40.

27. Ruddick W (ed): *Philosophers in Medical Centers*. New York, The Society for Philosophy and Public Affairs, 1980.

28. Delgado R, McAllen P: The moralist as expert witness. *Boston Univ Law Rev* 1982;62:869–926.

29. Fost N: Ethical problems in pediatrics. *Curr Probl Pediatr* 1976;6:1–31.

30. Fost N: Proxy consent for seriously ill newborns, in Smith D (ed): *No Rush to Judgment: Essays on Medical Ethics*. Bloomington, Ind, Poynter Center, 1977, pp 1–17.

31. Fost N: How decisions are made: A physician's view, in Swinyard C (ed): *Decision Making and the Defective Newborn: Proceedings of a Conference on Spina Bifida and Ethics*. Springfield, Ill, Charles C Thomas Publisher, 1978, pp 220–230.

32. Youngner SJ, Jackson DL, Coulton C, et al: A national survey of hospital ethics committees, in President's Commission for the Study of Ethical Problems in Medicine and Biomedical and Behavioral Research: *Deciding to Forego Life-Sustaining Treatment*, appendix F. Government Printing Office, 1983, pp. 443–449.

33. Fost N: Putting hospitals on notice. *Hastings Center Rep* 1982;12:5–8.

34. Annas GJ: Disconnecting the Baby Doe hotline. *Hastings Center Rep* 1983;13:14–16.

35. Strain JE: The decision to forego life-sustaining treatment for seriously ill newborns. *Pediatrics* 1983;72:572–573.

36. *American Academy of Pediatrics v Heckler*, No. 83–0774 (D DC April 14, 1983).

37. *AHA v Heckler*, 585 F Suppl 541 (SDNY 1984).

38. Robertson JA, Fost N: Passive euthanasia of defective newborn infants: Legal considerations. *J Pediatr* 1976;88:883.

39. Relman AS: The Saikewicz decision: A medical viewpoint. *Am J Law Med* 1978;4:233–242.

40. Orders against resuscitation: Selected policy statements, appendix I in President's Commission for the Study of Ethical Problems in Medicine and Biomedical and Behavioral Research: *Deciding to Forego Life-Sustaining Treatment*, Government Printing Office, 1983.

41. Hospitals and physicians at risk: The need for formal policies for the care of terminally ill patients. *Issues Health Care Technol* 1981, pp 1–5.

42. Miles SH, Cranford R, Schultz AL: The do-not-resuscitate order in a teaching hospital: Considerations and a suggested policy. *Ann Intern Med* 1982;96:660–664.

43. Gilbertsen VA, Wangensteen OH: Should the doctor tell the patient the disease is cancer? in *The Physician and the Total Care of the Cancer Patient*. New York, American Cancer Society, 1961.

44. Ellis HL: Parental involvement in the decision to treat spina bifida cystica. *Br Med J* 1974;1:369–372.

45. *Schloendorff v Society of New York Hospital*, 105 NE 92 (NY 1914).

46. Benfield DG, Leib SA, Vollman JH: Grief responses of parents to neonatal death and parent participation in deciding care. *Pediatrics* 1978;62:171.

47. Robertson JA: Involuntary euthanasia of defective newborns: Legal considerations. *Stanford Law Rev* 1975;27:213.

48. Duff RS: Counseling families and deciding care in severely defective children: A way of coping with 'medical Vietnam.' *Pediatrics* 1981;67:315–320.

49. President's Commission for the Study of Ethical Problems in Medicine and Biomedical and Behavioral Research: *Deciding to Forego Life-Sustaining Treatment*. Government Printing Office, 1983, pp 227–228.

50. Robertson JA: After Edelin: Little guidance. *Hastings Center Rep* 1977;7:15–17.

51. Robertson JA: Dilemma in Danville. *Hastings Center Rep* 1981;11:5–8.

52. Towers B: Irreversible coma and withdrawal of life support: Is it murder if the IV line is disconnected? *J Med Ethics* 1982;8:203–205.

53. Breo DL, Lefton D, Rust ME: MDs face unprecedented murder charge. *Am Med News* 1983; pp 1,13–19,21–22.

54. Barber v. Sup. Court for the State of California. Court of Appeals, 2nd Appellate District, Division Two, Sup Ct. #A025586, October 12, 1983.

55. Hospital ethics committees: Proposed statute and national survey, appendix F in President's Commission for the Study of Ethical Problems in Medicine and Biomedical and Behavioral Research: *Deciding to Forego Life-Sustaining Treatment*. Government Printing Office, 1983.

56. University of Wisconsin Hospital and Clinics: Guidelines regarding decisions to give, withhold or terminate care, appendix I in President's Commission for the Study of Ethical Problems in Medicine and Biomedical and Behavioral Research: *Deciding to Forego Life-Sustaining Treatment*. Government Printing Office, 1983, pp 513–517.

ROBERT M. VEATCH

An Ethical Framework for Hospital Ethics Committees

Institutional ethics committees deal with ethics. They are created to confront some of the most difficult ethical questions faced by patients and their agents in hospitals and other health care facilities. They often participate in ethical dilemmas faced by physicians, nurses, and other health professional decision makers as well. What quickly becomes apparent to any participant in a hospital ethics committee is that the committees themselves pose ethical questions.

The idea of hospital ethics committees has been with us for over a decade.[1] After this period of development, it makes sense that we pause to see if we can gain some understanding of the ethical mandate that governs these committees and the ethical problems they may confront in bearing out their mission. This, then, is the beginning of an ethic for ethics committees. . . .

ETHICAL PRINCIPLES FOR HOSPITAL ETHICS COMMITTEES

Anyone analyzing the nature of an ethical framework within which an ethics committee might operate faces an immediate problem. Some people working in medical ethics have begun with the assumption that a professional group may generate its own code of ethics or ethical principles. This presents serious problems, however. Professional groups may well hold unique positions on the ethics of professional obligation that are not shared by laypeople with whom the profes-

This article was originally published as "The Ethics of Institutional Ethics Committees" and is reprinted by permission of the publisher from Ronald E. Cranford and A. Edward Doudera, eds., *Institutional Ethics Committees and Health Care Decision Making* (Health Administration Press, 1984), pp. 35, 37–39, 42–45, 46–50.

sionals will be interacting. Any unilateral imposition of a code or set of principles may disenfranchise the patient population, the very group that will be most affected by the ethical code being adopted. Moreover, a philosopher or professional analyst of ethical systems is not in a much better position to articulate a code or set of principles for the lay-professional relation. He or she may also be part of a special tradition or hold special commitments. This has forced many to the conclusion that the structure of the ethical framework for a medical ethic must be generated by a complex process involving the active participation of both laypeople and health professionals. It must be the result of an understanding, a contract, or a covenant between laypeople and professionals established in three different stages.[2] It must begin with an understanding about the most basic moral commitments operating in our community. At the second stage, there has to be an understanding between laypeople and professionals about the nature of the roles that each party will assume; and, finally, there must be room for maneuvering at the level of individual decision making where both the layperson and the professional are given maximum freedom to be guided by their own consciences. This means that in principle I will not be able to set out one set of ethical principles that will be definitive for all hospital ethics committees. I would assume, for example, that the ethics committee at the local Catholic hospital might operate on a moral mandate that differed somewhat from that of the city hospital or the Jewish hospital. Still, given our general knowledge of ethical theory as it has evolved over the last decade, we can say something about the general content of any set of ethical principles governing the work of a hospital ethics committee.

It seems clear that any such set of principles will include the recognition that the health care team, including the ethics committee, should strive to serve the welfare of the patient. This is simply good old-fashioned Hippocratic ethics.[3] What is new in research work in medical ethics in the last decade, however, is the recognition that the old Hippocratic ethic of benefiting the patient must be placed within severe constraints. Two important kinds of ethical constraints have emerged. First, if the only moral mandate were to serve the welfare of the individual isolated patient, several important medical activities would immediately be immoral. Research medicine, where the objective is to serve the welfare of society more generally, would be ethically unacceptable. The institutional review board for the protection of human subjects must be an example of a kind of hospital-based ethics committee that supplements the old Hippocratic ethic with a more general principle of beneficence that takes into account the welfare of others in the society.

There is a second, more substantial, kind of limit to be placed on the old Hippocratic ethic of patient benefit. We have increasingly recognized in medical ethics that even in cases where there is no potential conflict between the welfare of the individual and the welfare of society, moral limits must be placed on the idea that health care professionals should always benefit their patients. To paraphrase the opening of a now famous book by Robert Nozick, patients have rights and there are certain things that health care professionals and hospital ethics committees cannot do to them without violating their rights.[4] Increasingly, a consensus is emerging that there is a small set of ethical principles that must supplement—indeed, take precedence over—the principle that we must serve the welfare of the individual and the welfare of society in individual cases. The *Belmont Report* of the National Commission for the Protection of Human Subjects is the only official public document at the federal level ever to endorse a set of ethical principles. In addition to beneficence, it acknowledges respect for persons, including autonomy, as a second principle, and justice in the distribution of resources as a third principle.[5] A number of other people would add the principles of truth telling and promise keeping—notions that the National Commission apparently includes under the rubric of respect for persons.[6] Finally, I have argued elsewhere that the principle of avoiding killing human beings has to be understood as an additional independent principle of medical morality.[7]

There will be some debate at the edges about precisely which principles should show up on any such list. Controversy will continue over the exact content of the list. What is striking, however, is that there is a substantial and very broad consensus that some such list is the basis for medical morality. Moreover, that list includes beneficence, doing good for people and avoiding evil, but it also includes certain other important moral considerations such as autonomy and justice—and probably truth telling, promise keeping, and avoiding killing.

There is also continuing disagreement about why these items are chosen and exactly what function they serve. Some people, now referred to in the jargon as rule utilitarians, say that these principles are fundamental characteristics of actions that deserve high claim on us because they tend to produce good consequences.[8] The deontologists among us say that these are inherently right-making characteristics of actions, whether or not they produce good consequences. That tension can and probably will remain in the future of debate in medical ethical theory. What is important is that both camps agree on some such short list. They must also agree that these considerations be given substantial weight in any medical ethical deliberation. To shift language somewhat, they suggest correlative rights claims that people have that are to be given substantial independent ethical weight. None of these considerations can be overridden by mere ad hoc situational claims that the consequences for the patient or for society would be better if these rights were overlooked in a particular case.

While not everyone will accept this kind of framework for an ethic for ethics committees, the notion that there are basic ethical principles and rights derived from them is a view held very widely in our society. It is, in effect, the moral framework used by just about everyone writing in medical ethics today. It is the framework used by our courts when they adjudicate disputes about the rights of patients, health care professionals, and society. It is also the framework used in all of the relevant American codes of health professional ethics. Such a framework has been the basis of the American Nurses' Association code for many years.[9] In June of 1980, when the American Medical Association revised its principles of ethics, it also abandoned its more traditional framework and began using rights language and referring to autonomy, honesty, and other core ethical principles as if they were to be given this fundamental independent status.[10] When a hospital ethics committee decides to adopt a basic set of ethical principles for its deliberations, when it consults with patients, health care professionals, and members of the community for guidance about what its core ethical framework ought to be, it will adopt this kind of set of ethical principles. The real question then becomes, what does this set of ethical principles mean when an institutional ethics committee sits down to work? . . .

AUTONOMY AND INDIVIDUAL PATIENT DECISIONS

No matter how much we would like to escape it, it is clear that the first task people think of for an institutional ethics committee is participation in individual patient care decisions. The usual problem is that of a terminally ill patient where the ethical question is whether it is appropriate to stop or continue treatment. Exactly the same moral structure would apply for any other kind of individual-case-oriented clinical decision. The early suggestions for hospital ethics committees, such as those made by Karen Teel and by the Massachusetts General Hospital Committee, saw the committees participating in clinical decisions, either making the actual decision or providing advice and counsel to the decision makers.[11] In the simple and straightforward case these are fundamentally patient-centered problems. We want to know not only how to promote the welfare of the patient, but also how to do right by the patient. If we begin by considering the competent patient or the formerly competent patient whose wishes are known, these are fundamentally problems of autonomy and the related ethical principles needed to preserve autonomy—that is, truth telling and promise keeping. If there is an ethical problem at all, it is whether the health care professional or anyone else is ever justified in infringing upon the autonomy of the individual patient as a decision maker about his own health care. I am for the moment not considering cases where we might want to restrict medical care for purposes of conserving scarce resources, but only those cases where the welfare of the patient is the decisive consideration. The ethical problem is one of whether some other decision maker might, on paternalistic grounds, attempt to promote the welfare of the patient in violation of the patient's own autonomy. I take it as a conclusion of both law

and ethics resulting from the last decade's debate that there is considerable agreement now that in such a simple case the principle of autonomy must dominate. The competent patient has the right to consent to treatment or refuse treatment on any grounds whatsoever, provided that treatment is offered for the patient's own good.[12] Thus, one possible ethical mandate for a committee is to be patient-centered, not focusing exclusively on the welfare of the patient in Hippocratic fashion, but on the rights of the patient, as well as on helping the patient preserve his or her autonomy in decision making.

The implications for an institutional ethics committee are radical. If the principle of autonomy is the dominant ethical principle, and the patient is the primary decision maker, then the institutional ethics committee for this kind of case must be accountable to the patient and must function as the agent of the patient, helping the patient clarify available alternatives and the ethical justifications for and against the treatment alternatives under consideration.

Several implications follow immediately from this conceptualization of the task as one of promoting autonomy. First, any committee that enters a patient's case without the knowledge of the patient is surely in violation of its mandate. If the health care professional, the physician, nurse, chaplain, or social worker, believes that the case is complex enough to require assistance from an ethics committee, that individual should approach the patient and ask the patient for permission to bring the committee in contact with the patient.

Second, the composition of the committee should be governed by the task at hand. People should be placed on the committee for their skills in counseling and analyzing ethical alternatives and in clarifying to the patient the medical and social implications of alternative therapies. Since patients are unique and operate with quite distinctive systems of beliefs and values, a standing committee at the hospital may discover that some of its members should step aside to be replaced by trusted counselors and advisors whom the patient might introduce to the committee. For example, if the standing committee included the hospital chaplain, it might be appropriate for the chaplain to step aside in favor of the patient's own clergyperson so that the spiritual counsel received could be based upon the patient's religious heritage.

Third, insofar as the promotion of autonomy is the ethical mission of the institutional ethics committee, it should be clear that in principle it is not possible to create a protocol that would provide substantive guidance for hospital staff about when to treat or when to stop treatment. The old Massachusetts General Hospital scheme that would classify all patients in four treatment groups solely on the basis of diagnosis and prognosis makes no sense.[13] Attempting to classify all patients solely on the basis of medical criteria violates the autonomy of the patient. Likewise, any protocol to decide which patients should be resuscitated would be ethically unacceptable if that protocol attempted to make substantive judgments based solely on the medical criteria of diagnosis and prognosis. Any guidelines created for institutional ethics committees, insofar as they are performing the task of promoting the autonomy of the patient, will necessarily be procedural. The guidelines might indicate who should be consulted, at what points patients should be asked to consent or refuse to consent to DNR and "no-code" orders, and so on. The guidelines should never, however, spell out substantively which patients to treat and which patients not to treat.

JUSTICE, SOCIAL ETHICS, AND RESOURCE ALLOCATION DECISIONS

A second, radically different task is sometimes envisioned for an institutional ethics committee. It requires the abandonment of the exclusively patient-centered perspective. The second kind of ethical constraint on the Hippocratic ethic of benefiting the patient grows out of social considerations of the welfare of others in the society and the promotion of justice in the distribution of goods. A committee at New Britain, Connecticut, General Hospital was formed on the basis of these concerns.[14] Suppose, for example, that a hospital needed to decide whether to spend a large bequest to build an expanded intensive care unit or to open a walk-in, holistic preventive medicine clinic. This is the kind of question that raises ethical issues that might be referred to an institutional ethics committee. It is obvious, however, that the ethical principle of autonomy will not get us very far. Presumably, patients who are candidates for an ICU would favor the intensive care unit, whereas those in the local community who are active promoters of holistic health care would autonomously decide for the preventive medicine clinic. An institutional ethics committee that takes on these kinds of questions is functioning in the realm of the ethical principles of justice and social welfare.

The same kind of ethical question arises when a committee is asked to participate in decisions about allocation of scarce medical beds or to create guidelines about such allocation. These questions cannot be answered by asking individual patients and by assisting them in expressing their autonomous decisions. It is important to realize that this ethical mandate, rooted in the principles of justice and social welfare, would not necessarily limit a committee to larger questions of hospital policy and macro-allocation. A justice problem would arise if an ethics committee were asked to participate in policy-making decisions about when to limit expensive but marginal medical care for a terminally ill patient. For example, whether to permit a 93-year-old comatose patient in end-stage renal failure to be dialyzed is not a question to be answered under the rubric of the principle of autonomy; it is a problem of justice. The problem for an ethics committee is whether it can take on the patient-centered tasks of promoting the rights and welfare of the patient and simultaneously be expected to make social ethics judgments based on justice and social welfare in which the rights and welfare of the individual patients must be compromised. It is sometimes maintained that individuals can operate from time to time under two different moral mandates, shifting hats, as it were, as the role dictates. A physician may, for example, be patient-centered while delivering clinical care and then abandon the patient-centered perspective when administering a clinic or research program. Others have argued that it is extremely difficult psychologically for individuals to shift moral mandates in this way. It is, in fact, impossible to act faithfully on both mandates at the same time.

If it is difficult for an individual to shift ethical principles, it is even more difficult for a committee—a corporate person—to do so. If an ethics committee is to take on these questions of justice and social welfare, it must be accountable to a much larger social unit. It needs to be accountable to the hospital as an institution and, ultimately, to the moral community to whom the hospital itself is accountable, that is, to a government or church or other sponsoring agency.

An ethics committee that is to take on these questions of justice and social welfare will require skills different from those required of a committee whose ethical mandate is to further patient autonomy. The committee will need not only expertise in the technical aspects of medicine and nursing involved in the decision, but also the capacity to represent the ethical and other values of the group to which the committee is accountable—the government, church, or other sponsoring community. By contrast, a committee whose purpose is to facilitate autonomous patient choice has much less reason to be so representative of the sponsoring group. In fact, for choices rooted in the moral principle of autonomy we could say that if the committee successfully reflects the moral consensus of the community and thereby entices the patient into a choice based on that consensus, then it has failed. The committee charged with the responsibility of basing choices on justice and social welfare, on the other hand, may not want to simply mirror the community values; rather, the committee must be very conscious of those values and should articulate its sense of what is just when communicating with the community.

I am forced to the conclusion that it is extremely difficult, if not impossible, for one committee to work under the conflicting mandates of promoting patient-centered rights and promoting justice in the distribution of resources. At the very least, if the committee sees as its task the placing of limits on patients' rights and welfare in cases where justice requires devoting scarce resources to others, the patient has to be informed that that is the committee's conception of its task. . . .

INCOMPETENTS AND PATIENT-CENTERED BENEFICENCE COMMITTEES

This drives us to a rather startling conclusion. There is virtually no area of work for which a committee should take as its mandate making a choice that will most benefit the patient. Promotion of patient autonomy is one legitimate ethical mandate. Much committee education work will be justified under this rubric, as will be counseling with patients and families as well as with health professionals. Promotion of justice and social welfare is also a legitimate ethical mandate for some institutional ethics committees. Neither of these types of committees, however, should see itself as making substantive decisions to benefit individual patients.

There is, however, one type of committee involvement where patient-centered welfare might appear to be the real ethical mission. This occurs in cases where someone has to make individual patient care decisions and the patient is simply incompetent to participate as an autonomous decision maker: where the patient is too sick, too young, or too senile. Here someone else must make a decision. In those cases where we have no idea what the patient would prefer—when the patient

has not expressed himself or herself while competent—the only basis for the decision is what someone else considers to be best for the welfare of the patient. Is it here, finally, that the institutional ethics committee is able to act on the classical Hippocratic principle of doing what it can to try to benefit the patient? Perhaps here it finally can, but only in a most attenuated way.

Normally, someone is designated to be the agent of an incompetent patient. By a law just passed in the state of Virginia, any competent person may designate someone for this role.[15] By law in several jurisdictions, the next of kin is the presumed agent in cases where no one has been so designated. In other cases, such as that of a parent of a minor child, there is a presumption of guardianship whereby the agent—but not necessarily an ethics committee—has the task of attempting to make a decision that will serve the interest of the patient. This patient agent, however, does not have unlimited discretion. As in the case of the Jehovah's Witness parent attempting to refuse to consent to a life-saving blood transfusion, any interested party has the right to seek judicial review to determine if the agent is being reasonable. Physicians or hospital administrators often take on this task, not by acting directly on what they determine to be the patient's best interest, but by attempting to get court authorization to have someone else legitimated to give the consent.

The present arrangement is admittedly a bit chaotic. Anyone may seek review. If an individual physician chooses not to do so, however, there has been no due process and his or her judgment may be idiosyncratic. It might be good to have a committee responsible specifically for determining whether or not to seek judicial review. In such a role the committee would at least indirectly be acting out the ethical principle of promoting the welfare of the patient. It would not have the authority to authorize reversal of the agent's decision, but it would have formal responsibility for taking the first step to see whether the courts would reverse it. The committee might appear to be making this decision on the basis of the ethical principle of attempting to promote the incompetent patient's welfare. That is certainly the ethical charge to the parent or other agent who is the initial decision maker. While the committee would evaluate the case in terms of the patient's welfare, it is clear that it would not want to seek judicial review at every point at which the agent's decision appeared to deviate from the best interest of the patient. The deviation would have to appear to be substantial; it would have to be intolerable. Otherwise, we would have committees, and eventually courts, second-guessing parents on every decision they make. The agent's decision would have to appear to be beyond the realm of reason.[16] Thus, while the agent for the patient would strive to choose what is in the patient's best interest, a committee (or an individual health professional) would seek to initiate review only if the agent's decision appeared to be beyond the limits of reason.

A related question is whether the committee could be given quasi-judicial authority to overrule the agent or to affirm the agent's decision, thus granting legal protection against charges of neglect. While such an arrangement may appear attractive, it poses some problems. The committee at best will reflect the moral consensus of the institution and its sponsors. That may not be the same, however, as the moral consensus of the broader community. In fact, it is conceivable that a small minority of physicians could become aligned with a small minority of parents and other agents in approving decisions that most reasonable people would take to be seriously contrary to the patient's interest. If those physicians were clustered in a small number of hospitals, it is possible that a committee (even if it were representative of the medical staff) would also express deviant moral judgments. If even a dozen hospitals nationally had committees that routinely approved grossly deviant decisions, and if agents and professionals favoring grossly deviant decisions were clustered together at those hospitals, serious ethical infringement on the rights and welfare of patients could occur.

If the committee were so constituted that it could reflect the reasonable judgment of the community, a judgment by the committee not to have an agent's decision reviewed by the court could be taken as supportive evidence that the parents were acting within the realm of reason. Here at last the committee might begin to approach the ethical mission of making a decision based on concern for the welfare of the patient.

CONCLUSION

Here, then, we might have the beginnings of an ethic for ethics committees. Such an ethic will not only have to deal with more mundane problems of euthanasia, confidentiality, and committee integrity, but will also have to determine whether it is dealing with decisions that raise problems primarily of autonomy, of justice and social welfare, or of patient benefit. For the most part the traditional committee involved in terminal care clinical cases will have as its ethical responsibility the promotion of patient autonomy. In other cases the ethical issues will concern justice and social welfare. Only in those rare cases where the patient is incompetent and the patient's agent appears to have exceeded the limits of reason will a committee possibly find for itself a limited role in making a decision to try to benefit the patient. Even here it will not be to directly overrule the patient's agent, but to determine whether the hospital should initiate a formal judicial review of that decision. To remain clear about these diverging ethical responsibilities, institutional ethics committees ought to begin thinking about adopting a set of ethical principles to guide their work, and they ought to determine which of those principles should govern the particular tasks they are undertaking.

NOTES

1. Veatch, R. M., *Choosing Not to Prolong Dying*, MEDICAL DIMENSIONS (December 1972) at 8, 10; R. M. Veatch, DEATH, DYING AND THE BIOLOGICAL REVOLUTION: OUR LAST QUEST FOR RESPONSIBILITY (Yale University Press, New Haven, Connecticut) (1976) at 60–61, 173–76; Veatch, R. M., *Hospital Ethics Committees: Is There a Role?* HASTINGS CENTER REPORT 7(3):22–25 (June 1977).

2. See R. M. Veatch, *A Theory of Medical Ethics* (Basic Books, New York) (1981), pp. 108–38.

3. The Oath of Hippocrates states, "I will follow that method of treatment which, according to my ability and judgement, I consider for the benefit of my patients, and abstain from whatever is deleterious and mischievous."

4. Robert Nozick's formulation of this idea is as follows: "Individuals have rights, and there are things no person or group may do to them [without violating their rights]." R. Nozick, *Anarchy, State, and Utopia* (Basic Books, New York) (1974) at ix.

5. The National Commission for the Protection of Human Subjects of Biomedical and Behavioral Research, *The Belmont Report: Ethical Principles and Guidelines for the Protection of Human Subjects of Research* (U.S. Gov't Printing Office, Washington, D.C.) (1978) at 4–10.

6. Veatch, *supra* note 2, at 179–84, 214–22.

7. *Id.* at 227–49.

8. T. L. Beauchamp, J. F. Childress, *Principles of Biomedical Ethics*, 2d ed. (Oxford University Press, New York) (1983), pp. 30–33.

9. American Nurses' Association, *Code for Nurses with Interpretive Statements* (Kansas City, Missouri) (1976) at 1, 4, 6.

10. Beauchamp, Childress, *supra* note 8 at 331–32.

11. Teel, K., *The Physician's Dilemma—A Doctor's View: What the Law Should Be*, BAYLOR LAW REVIEW 27:6, 9 (Winter 1975); Critical Care Committee of the Massachusetts General Hospital, *Optimum Care for Hopelessly Ill Patients*, NEW ENGLAND JOURNAL OF MEDICINE 295(7):362–64 (August 12, 1976) [hereinafter referred to as Critical Care Committee].

12. Stephenson, S. A., *The Right to Die: A Proposal for Natural Death Legislation*, UNIVERSITY OF CINCINNATI LAW REVIEW 49: 228–43 (1980); Cantor, N. L., *A Patient's Decision to Decline Life-Saving Medical Treatment: Bodily Integrity versus the Preservation of Life*, RUTGERS LAW REVIEW 26:228–64 (1973).

13. *See* Critical Care Committee, *supra* note 11. For similar criteria of New York's Mount Sinai Hospital, *see* Kirchner, M., *How Far to Go Prolonging Life: One Hospital's System*, MEDICAL ECONOMICS 53:70 (July 12, 1976).

14. Esqueda, K., *Hospital Ethics Committees: Four Case Studies*, THE HOSPITAL MEDICAL STAFF 7:30 (November 1978).

15. "Natural Death Act of Virginia" signed into law by Governor Robb on March 28, 1983. Virginia Code, Section 54–325.8:1 (1983) states: "[T]he General Assembly hereby declares that the laws of the Commonwealth of Virginia shall recognize the right of a competent adult to make an oral or written declaration instructing his physician to withhold or withdraw life-prolonging procedures or to designate another to make the treatment decision for him, in the event such person is diagnosed as suffering from a terminal condition."

16. For a development of the "limits of reason" concept and its role in overriding agent decisions, see Veatch, R. M., *The Limits of Guardian Treatment Refusal: The Standard of Reasonableness*, AMERICAN JOURNAL OF LAW & MEDICINE 9(4): 427 (Winter 1984); President's Commission for the Study of Ethical Problems in Medicine and Biomedical and Behavioral Research, *Deciding to Forego Life-Sustaining Treatment: Ethical, Medical and Legal Issues in Treatment Decisions* (U.S. Gov't Printing Office, Washington, D.C.) (1983) at 136. The Commission concluded that in situations in which no consensus as to decision exists, the surrogate should "retain discretion to choose among a range of acceptable choices."

SUGGESTED READINGS FOR CHAPTER 6

GENERAL ISSUES

Annas, George J. "Whose Space Is This Anyway?" *Hastings Center Report* 16 (April 1986), 24–25.

Anonymous. "It's Over, Debbie." *Journal of the American Medical Association*, Vol. 259, No. 2 (January 8, 1988), 272.

Areen, Judith, King, Patricia, Goldberg, Steven, and Capron, Alexander Morgan. "Death and Dying." In their *Law, Science and Medicine*. Mineola, N.Y.: Foundation Press, 1984, pp. 1063–1235.

Barnard, Christian. "The Need for Euthanasia." In Downing, A. B., and Smoker, Barbara, eds. *Voluntary Euthanasia: The Experts Debate the Right to Die* (London: Peter Owen, 1986), 173–183.

Bayles, Michael D., and High, Dallas M., eds. *Medical Treatment of the Dying: Moral Issues*. Cambridge, Mass.: Schenkman, 1978.

Beauchamp, Tom L. "The Moral Justification for Withholding Heroic Procedures." In Bell, Nora K., ed. *Who Decides? Conflicts of Rights in Health Care*. Clifton, N.J.: Humana Press, 1982.

———, and Childress, James F. *Principles of Biomedical Ethics*. New York: Oxford University Press, 1979. Chaps. 4 and 7.

———, and Davidson, Arnold I. "The Definition of Euthanasia." *Journal of Medicine and Philosophy* 4 (September 1979), 294–312.

———, and Perlin, Seymour, eds. *Ethical Issues in Death and Dying*. Englewood Cliffs, N.J.: Prentice-Hall, 1978.

Behnke, John A., and Bok, Sissela, eds. *The Dilemma of Euthanasia*. Garden City, N.Y.: Doubleday Anchor, 1975.

Bok, Sissela. "Personal Directions for Care at the End of Life." *New England Journal of Medicine* 295 (August 12, 1976), 367–369.

———. "Death and Dying: Euthanasia and Sustaining Life: Ethical Views." In Reich, Warren T., ed. *Encyclopedia of Bioethics*. New York: Free Press, 1978. Vol. 1, pp. 268–278.

Brock, Dan W. "Taking Human Life." *Ethics* 95 (July 1985), 851–865.

Canada, Law Reform Commission. *Euthanasia, Aiding Suicide and Cessation of Treatment*. Ottawa: LRCC, 1983.

Cantor, Norman. "A Patient's Decision to Decline Life-Saving Medical Treatment: Bodily Integrity Versus the Preservation of Life." *Rutgers Law Review* 26 (Winter 1972), 228–264.

A Children's Physician. "Non-Treatment of Defective Newborn Babies." *Lancet* 2 (November 24, 1979), 1123–1124.

Childress, James F. "To Live or Let Die." In his *Priorities in Biomedical Ethics*. Philadelphia: Westminster Press, 1981, pp. 34–50.

Childress, James F., and Dalle Mura, Steven L. "Caring for Patients and Caring for Symbols: Reflections on Artificial Nutrition and Hydration." In Childress, James F., and Gaare, Ruth D., eds. *BioLaw, Volume II*. Frederick, Md.: University Publications, 1986, pp. S:1–S:8.

Coburn, Robert C. "Morality and the Defective Newborn." *Journal of Medicine and Philosophy* 5 (December 1980), 340–357.

Devine, Philip E. *The Ethics of Homicide*. Ithaca, N.Y.: Cornell University Press, 1978.

Downing, A. B., ed. *Euthanasia and the Right to Die*. New York: Humanities Press, 1978.

Duff, Raymond S., and Campbell, A. G. M. "Moral and Ethical Dilemmas in the Special-Care Nursery." *New England Journal of Medicine* 289 (October 25, 1973), 890–894.

Dyck, Arthur. "An Alternative to the Ethic of Euthanasia." In Williams, Robert H., ed. *To Live and To Die: When, Why, and How*. New York: Springer-Verlag, 1973, pp. 98–112.

Eisendrath, Stuart J., and Jonsen, Albert R. "The Living Will: Help or Hindrance?" *Journal of the American Medical Association* 249 (April 1983), 2054–2058.

Feinberg, Joel. "Voluntary Euthanasia and the Inalienable Right to Life." *Philosophy and Public Affairs* 7 (Winter 1978), 93–123.

———. "The Choice of Death." In his *The Moral Limits of the Criminal Law, Vol. 3: Harm to Self*. New York: Oxford University Press, 1986, pp. 344–374, 409–412.

Fletcher, George P. "Prolonging Life: Some Legal Considerations." *Washington Law Review* 42 (1967), 999–1016.

Fletcher, Joseph. "Ethics and Euthanasia." In Williams, Robert H., ed. *To Live and To Die: When, Why, and How*. New York: Springer-Verlag, 1973, pp. 113–122.

Foot, Philippa. "Euthanasia." *Philosophy and Public Affairs* 6 (Winter 1977), 85–112.

Gevers, J. K. M. "Legal Developments Concerning Active Euthanasia." *Bioethics* 1 (April 1987), 156–162.

Glover, Jonathan. *Causing Death and Saving Lives*. New York: Penguin Books, 1977.

Grisez, Germain, and Boyle, Joseph M. *Life and Death with Liberty and Justice: A Contribution to the Euthanasia Debate*. Notre Dame, Ind.: University of Notre Dame Press, 1979.

Hare, R. M. "Euthanasia: A Christian View." *Philosophic Exchange* 2 (Summer 1975), 43–52.

Horan, Dennis J., and Mall, David, eds. *Death, Dying, and Euthanasia*. Washington, D.C.: University Publications of America, 1977.

Jonsen, Albert R. "Dying *Right* in California: The Natural Death Act." *Clinical Research* 26 (February 1978), 55–60.

Jonsen, Albert R., and Garland, Michael J., eds. *Ethics of Newborn Intensive Care*. Berkeley, Calif.: University of California, Institute of Governmental Studies, 1976.

Kluge, Eike-Henner W. *The Practice of Death*. New Haven, Conn.: Yale University Press, 1975.

Kohl, Marvin, ed. *Beneficent Euthanasia*. Buffalo, N.Y.: Prometheus Books, 1975.

———, ed. *Infanticide and the Value of Life*. Buffalo, N.Y.: Prometheus Books, 1978.

Kuhse, Helga. "Active and Passive Euthanasia—Ten Years into the Debate." *Euthanasia Review* 1 (Summer 1986), 108–119.

———. "The Case for Active Voluntary Euthanasia." *Law, Medicine, and Health Care* 14 (September 1986), 145–148.

Kuhse, Helga, and Singer, Peter. *Should the Baby Live? The Problem of Handicapped Newborns*. New York: Oxford University Press, 1985.

Ladd, John, ed. *Ethical Issues Relating to Life and Death*. New York: Oxford University Press, 1979.

Lavin, Michael. "Ulysses Contracts." *Journal of Applied Philosophy* 3 (March 1986), 89–101.

Lynn, Joanne, ed. *By No Extraordinary Means: The Choice to Forgo Life-Sustaining Food and Water*. Bloomington, Ind.: Indiana University Press, 1986.

McCormick, Richard A. "To Save or Let Die: The Dilemma of Modern Medicine." *Journal of the American Medical Association* 229 (July 8, 1974), 172–176.

Meilaender, Gilbert. "On Removing Food and Water: Against the Stream." *Hastings Center Report* 14 (December 1984), 11–13.

New York State Task Force on Life and the Law. *Life-Sustaining Treatment: Making Decisions and Appointing a Health Care Agent*. New York: The Task Force, 1987.

President's Commission for the Study of Ethical Problems in Medicine and Biomedical and Behavioral Research. *Deciding to Forego Life-Sustaining Treatment*. Washington, D.C.: U.S. Government Printing Office, 1983.

Rachels, James. "Euthanasia." In Regan, Tom, ed. *Matters of Life and Death*. New York: Random House, 1980, pp. 28–66.

———. *The End of Life: Euthanasia and Morality*. New York: Oxford University Press, 1986.

Ramsey, Paul. *The Patient as Person*. New Haven, Conn.: Yale University Press, 1970. Chap. 3.

———. *Ethics at the Edges of Life: Medical and Legal Intersections*. New Haven, Conn.: Yale University Press, 1978.

Redleaf, Diane L., et al. "The California Natural Death Act: An Empirical Study of Physicians' Practices." *Stanford Law Review* 31 (May 1979), 913–945.

Robertson, John A., and Fost, Norman. "Passive Euthanasia of Defective Newborn Infants: Legal Considerations." *Journal of Pediatrics* 88 (May 1976), 883–889.

Samek, Robert. "Euthanasia and Law Reform." *Ottawa Law Review* 17 (1984), 86–115.

Society for the Right to Die. *Handbook of Living Will Laws: 1987 Edition*. New York: SRD, 1987.

Steinbrook, Robert, and Lo, Bernard. "The Case of Elizabeth Bouvia: Starvation, Suicide, or Problem Patient?" *Archives of Internal Medicine* 146 (January 1986), 161–164.

Strong, Carson. "Euthanasia: Is the Concept Really Nonevaluative?" *Journal of Medicine and Philosophy* 5 (December 1980), 313–325.

Suckiel, Ellen K. "Death and Benefit in the Permanently Unconscious Patient: A Justification of Euthanasia." *Journal of Medicine and Philosophy* 3 (March 1978), 38–52.

Swinyard, Chester A., ed. *Decision Making and the Defective Newborn*. Springfield, Ill.: Thomas, 1978.

Tooley, Michael. "Infants: Infanticide: A Philosophical Perspective." In Reich, Warren T., ed. *Encyclopedia of Bioethics*. New York: Free Press, 1978. Vol. 2, pp. 742–751.

U.S. Congress, Office of Technology Assessment. *Life-Sustaining Technologies and the Elderly*. Washington, D.C.: OTA, July 1987.

Veatch, Robert M. *Death, Dying and the Biological Revolution: Our Last Quest for Responsibility*. New Haven, Conn.: Yale University Press, 1976.

Weir, Robert F., ed. *Ethical Issues in Death and Dying*. New York: Columbia University Press, 1977.

Williams, Peter C. "Rights and the Alleged Right of Innocents to Be Killed." *Ethics* 87 (July 1977), 383–394.

KILLING AND LETTING DIE

Atkinson, Gary M. "Killing and Letting Die: Hidden Value Assumptions." *Social Science and Medicine* 17 (1983), 1915–1925.

Benjamin, Martin. "Moral Agency and Negative Acts in Medicine." In Robison, Wade L., and Pritchard, Michael S., eds. *Medical Responsibility: Paternalism, Informed Consent, and Euthanasia*. Clifton, N.J.: Humana Press, 1979, pp. 169–180.

Gillon, Raanan. "Acts and Omissions, Killing and Letting Die." *British Medical Journal* 292 (January 1986), 126–127.

Menzel, Paul T. "Are Killing and Letting Die Morally Different in Medical Contexts?" *Journal of Medicine and Philosophy* 4 (September 1979), 159–171.

Reichenbach, Bruce R. "Euthanasia and the Active-Passive Distinction." *Bioethics* 1 (January 1987), 51–73.

Singer, Peter. "Taking Life: Euthanasia." In his *Practical Ethics*. Cambridge: Cambridge University Press, 1979, 127–157.

Trammell, Richard L. "The Presumption Against Taking Life." *Journal of Medicine and Philosophy* 3 (March 1978), 53–67.

THE ROLE OF HOSPITAL ETHICS COMMITTEES

American Academy of Pediatrics. "Guidelines for Infant Bioethics Committees." *Pediatrics* 74 (August 1984), 306–310.

American Medical Association, Judicial Council. "Guidelines for Ethics Committees in Health Care Institutions." *Journal of the American Medical Association* 253 (May 1985), 2698–2699.

Cranford, Ronald E., and Doudera, A. Edward, eds. *Institutional Ethics Committees and Health Care Decision Making*. Ann Arbor, Mich.: Health Administration Press, 1984.

Fleischman, Alan R., and Murray, Thomas H. "Ethics Committees for Infants Doe?" *Hastings Center Report* 13 (December 1983), 5–9.

Siegler, Mark. "Ethics Committees: Decision by Bureaucracy." *Hastings Center Report* 16 (June 1986), 22–24.

BIBLIOGRAPHIES

Goldstein, Doris Mueller. *Bioethics: A Guide to Information Sources*. Detroit: Gale Research Company, 1982. See under "Death and Dying," "Euthanasia," "Prolongation of Life and Refusal of Treatment," and "Treatment of Defective Newborns and Infanticide."

Lineback, Richard H., ed. *Philosopher's Index*. Vols. 1– . Bowling Green, Ohio: Bowling Green State University. Issued quarterly. See under "Active Euthanasia," "Death," "Dying," "Euthanasia," "Killing," and "Letting Die."

Walters, LeRoy, and Kahn, Tamar Joy, eds. *Bibliography of Bioethics*. Vols. 1– . Washington, D.C.: Kennedy Institute of Ethics, Georgetown University. Issued annually. See under "Allowing to Die," "Ethics Committees," "Euthanasia," "Infanticide," "Killing," "Terminal Care," and "Treatment Refusal." (The information contained in the annual *Bibliography of Bioethics* can also be retrieved from BIOETHICSLINE, an online database of the National Library of Medicine.)

Part IV

THE PATIENT-
PROFESSIONAL
RELATIONSHIP

7.
Patients' Rights and Professional Responsibilities

That the practice of medicine is an applied science none would deny. But it also involves the common human transactions of contracts and services. Interesting professional responsibilities and patients' rights emerge from this human side of medical practice. Professional obligations have long been recognized in medical codes, but only recently has much systematic thought been given to the moral and legal rights of patients. In this chapter both the traditional conceptions of and the emerging problems in the professional-patient relationship are explored.

PROFESSIONAL CODES
The three codes of ethics included in this chapter are samples of numerous codes that have been developed by health professionals in both ancient and modern times. The Hippocratic Oath took the form of a series of religious vows. More recent codes, including those of the American Medical Association and the American Nurses' Association, generally contain secular statements of moral rules. The central affirmation of such codes is that, in treating the (frequently vulnerable) patient, the health professional will not exploit his or her position of relatively controlling power and influence.

A comparison of the "Principles of Medical Ethics" adopted in 1980 by the American Medical Association and the 1976 code of the American Nurses' Association reveals several striking differences in emphasis. For example, the primary focus in the AMA code is on the physician's duty to benefit the patient. In contrast, the Code for Nurses begins by vigorously affirming the "self-determination of the clients." Each code is sufficiently nuanced to mention the theme emphasized by the other; however, a clear difference in accent is evident. The two codes also take divergent approaches to the questions of health care delivery. In the AMA principles, the right of each physician to choose which patients he or she will serve is reaffirmed, except, of course, in emergency situations. By contrast, the Code for Nurses asserts a rather sweeping welfare right—the right to quality health care—for all citizens. (See Chapter 11 for a detailed discussion of issues in health care allocation.)

Two questions arise concerning the status of these codes of conduct: (1) What is their relation to law? and (2) What is their relation to general ethical principles? The codes, though quasi-legal in form, are self-legislative documents developed by particular professions. As such, they have only the force that the profession chooses to attribute to them. In most professions, including medicine and nursing, professional self-discipline or self-policing has usually been less vigorous.

Two possible relationships between codes of professional ethics and general ethical principles can be envisioned. Professional codes may constitute autonomous, self-contained systems of ethics that are unrelated to external validating principles. On the other hand, the codes may be viewed as specific applications of universal ethical principles. According to the latter conception, the codes consist primarily of moral rules that implicitly appeal to general ethical principles, and perhaps even to particular ethical theories. On this view, the same canons of logical coherence and consistency that are applied to any other system of moral rules can also be employed in the critical evaluation of the professional codes. (See the discussion of moral rules and moral justification in Chapter 1.)

PROFESSIONAL OBLIGATIONS

In addition to being formulated in brief codes, the moral obligations of health professionals—and especially of physicians and nurses—have been explored more discursively by commentators from numerous disciplines. Central to most essays on professional obligations is the relationship between physicians or nurses and the patients in their care. But, as we shall see in the final section of this chapter, obligations to third parties may and often do intrude into the primary relationship between patients and professionals.

A focus on the moral *obligations* of health professionals is not the only possible approach to the moral evaluation of the patient-professional relationship. In his essay in this chapter Edmund Pellegrino distinguishes among three standards by which professional behavior might be judged. The first standard is the least stringent: It asks, "Has the professional violated any legal rules or administrative regulations in his or her treatment of the patient?" The second standard is the one employed in most essays in this chapter—and indeed in this book. This standard evaluates professional performance on the basis of its conformity with widely accepted ethical principles and moral rules, such as the principle of respect for the autonomy of persons. The third and most stringent standard is one that requires professionals not only to fulfill their moral obligations but to be virtuous as well. In what ways does virtue go beyond mere conformity with moral rules? First, a virtuous person performs morally right actions for the right reasons, as an expression of his or her genuine concern for the welfare of others. Second, in some cases a virtuous person will behave in a self-sacrificial way, going beyond the obligations that are imposed, for example, by the usual requirements of justice. Pellegrino is under no illusion that all health professionals are necessarily virtuous persons. However, he recommends the cultivation of character as an important adjunct to the clarification of moral concepts and the development of coherent theories of moral obligation.

Gerald Winslow's essay illustrates how a dominant metaphor can be correlated with, and perhaps even influence, one's conception of virtue and moral obligation. In an earlier era, it was widely thought that the nursing profession should exhibit the virtue of loyalty and adhere to the norm of obedience to superiors. This character trait and this kind of strict discipline in behavior were considered essential to medicine's war on disease, especially infectious disease. By the 1960s and 1970s the military metaphor began to give way to a legal metaphor, the metaphor of advocacy. This new image, which permeates the ANA Code for Nurses discussed above, called for the exercise of a new virtue—courage—and was closely correlated with the nurse's obligation to defend patients against threatened infringements of their rights.

PATIENTS' RIGHTS

Most health-related codes of professional ethics—with the notable exception of the ANA Code—emphasize the duties of professionals rather than the rights of patients. However, in the 1970s explicit declarations of patients' rights began to be formulated. Perhaps the best-known and most widely distributed of these declarations is the American Hospital Association's "Patient's Bill of Rights," which was first formulated in 1972. This Bill of Rights can be interpreted as a statement of the moral rights that ought to be enjoyed by hospital patients. Some of the asserted rights are negative or noninterference rights, for example, the right to privacy and the right to refuse treatment. Other rights included in the Bill of Rights require positive action on the part of hospitals or health professionals; for example, patients have the right to "considerate and respectful care" or the right to various kinds of information. (See the detailed discussions of rights in Chapter 1 and of positive and negative rights in Chapter 11.)

The Patient's Bill of Rights provides an interesting test of the thesis that most rights of individuals and duties to individuals are correlative. (See Chapter 1.) One can envision how the assertion of patients' *rights* in the bill could be translated without substantive loss into statements concerning the *obligations* of hospitals and/or health professionals to patients. For example, the assertion that "the patient has the right to considerate and respectful care" could also be formulated as "the hospital has the obligation to provide the patient decent and respectful care." Why the authors of the AHA statement preferred the rhetoric of rights to the more traditional language of duty is not entirely clear. However, the patients' rights approach of the AHA document may reflect the consumer participation—by representatives of the National Welfare Rights Organization—that occurred during the drafting process.

George Annas sketches the intellectual context for rights language in the moral and legal philosophy of the 1970s, then argues that patient rights like those enumerated in the "Patient's Bill of Rights" are currently under attack. In his view, not only should the AHA statement be observed in health care practice, but new and more extensive rights should be guaranteed to patients. Among these are the right to open access to one's own medical record and the right to an effective patient advocate. Paul Chodoff, a psychiatrist, questions whether the emphasis on patients' rights has not been carried too far by civil liberties lawyers and their allies in the health professions. In the context of mental illness, and in cases involving persons of questionable competence to care for themselves, an overly zealous respect for the rights of patients may, in Chodoff's view, lead to unmitigated disaster.

CONFLICTS OF OBLIGATIONS

At first glance, it might seem that the primary moral obligation of health professionals is always to promote the welfare (or respect the autonomy) of their patients. However, even at a purely descriptive level, we know that physicians and nurses must make decisions about how to allocate time among the multiple patients for whom they almost always bear responsibility. Further, both patients and health professionals live in complex webs of interrelationships outside the health care setting. There is no easy way for either patients or professionals to avoid taking these extra-medical relationships into account in their decision making.

Tom Beauchamp and Laurence McCullough focus their attention on the role of physicians and argue that physicians have a moral duty at least to consider third-party interests in their encounters with patients. In some cases the third parties are identifiable individuals or institutions, for example, a child of the patient or the patient's spouse, employer, or insurance company. In other cases, a vague entity often described as "the wider society" is the intended beneficiary of actions that involve the patient—medical education, biomedical research, and the reporting of communicable disease. (Note that substantial sections of Chapters 9 through 12 deal with these broader dimensions of the patient-professional relationship.) According to Beauchamp and McCullough, one cannot stipulate in advance whether the moral obligations of physicians to patients will be stronger than, equivalent to, or weaker than their obligations to third parties.

The remaining essays in this chapter illustrate various facets of the conflict-of-obligations theme. Stephen Toulmin surveys some of the historical and social factors that, in his view, lead to morally ambiguous relationships between professionals and patients in the contemporary U.S. health care system. The competing obligations of health professionals to pregnant women and the fetuses they are carrying are the central focus of the Annas essay on forced cesarean deliveries. In Annas's view, the legal right of a pregnant woman to refuse surgery should always take precedence over any asserted moral obligation of health professionals to rescue the fetus she is carrying. Arnold Relman identifies what he considers to be morally objectionable practices of some physicians that tend to undermine confidence in the medical profession. Unlike Edmund Pellegrino, who assigns a central role to virtue in the restoration of public trust, Relman seems ready to rely on moral education and the development of new and more detailed codes of professional conduct.

L. W.

Professional Codes

The Hippocratic Oath

I swear by Apollo Physician and Asclepius and Hygieia and Panaceia and all the gods and goddesses, making them my witnesses, that I will fulfill according to my ability and judgment this oath and this covenant:

To hold him who has taught me this art as equal to my parents and to live my life in partnership with him, and if he is in need of money to give him a share of mine, and to regard his offspring as equal to my brothers in male lineage and to teach them this art—if they desire to learn it—without fee and covenant; to give a share of precepts and oral instruction and all the other learning to my sons and to the sons of him who

Reprinted with permission of the publisher from "The Hippocratic Oath," in Ludwig Edelstein, *Ancient Medicine*, edited by Oswei Temkin and C. Lillian Temkin (Baltimore: Johns Hopkins University Press, 1967).

has instructed me and to pupils who have signed the covenant and have taken an oath according to the medical law, but to no one else.

I will apply dietetic measures for the benefit of the sick according to my ability and judgment; I will keep them from harm and injustice.

I will neither give a deadly drug to anybody if asked for it, nor will I make a suggestion to this effect. Similarly I will not give to a woman an abortive remedy. In purity and holiness I will guard my life and my art.

I will not use the knife, not even on sufferers from stone, but will withdraw in favor of such men as are engaged in this work.

Whatever houses I may visit, I will come for the benefit of the sick, remaining free of all intentional injustice, of all mischief and in particular of sexual relations with both female and male persons, be they free or slaves.

What I may see or hear in the course of the treatment or even outside of the treatment in regard to the life of men, which on no account one must spread abroad, I will keep to myself holding such things shameful to be spoken about.

If I fulfill this oath and do not violate it, may it be granted to me to enjoy life and art, being honored with fame among all men for all time to come; if I transgress it and swear falsely, may the opposite of all this be my lot.

AMERICAN MEDICAL ASSOCIATION

Principles of Medical Ethics (1980)

PREAMBLE

The medical profession has long subscribed to a body of ethical statements developed primarily for the benefit of the patient. As a member of this profession, a physician must recognize responsibility not only to patients, but also to society, to other health professionals, and to self. The following Principles adopted by the American Medical Association are not laws, but standards of conduct which define the essentials of honorable behavior for the physician.

PRINCIPLES

I. A physician shall be dedicated to providing competent medical service with compassion and respect for human dignity.

II. A physician shall deal honestly with patients and colleagues, and strive to expose those physicians deficient in character or competence, or who engage in fraud or deception.

From *American Medical News*, August 1/8, 1980, p. 9. Reprinted with permission of the American Medical Association.

III. A physician shall respect the law and also recognize a responsibility to seek changes in those requirements which are contrary to the best interests of the patient.

IV. A physician shall respect the rights of patients, of colleagues, and of other health professionals, and shall safeguard patient confidences within the constraints of the law.

V. A physician shall continue to study, apply and advance scientific knowledge, make relevant information available to patients, colleagues, and the public, obtain consultation, and use the talents of other health professionals when indicated.

VI. A physician shall, in the provision of appropriate patient care, except in emergencies, be free to choose whom to serve, with whom to associate, and the environment in which to provide medical services.

VII. A physician shall recognize a responsibility to participate in activities contributing to an improved community.

AMERICAN NURSES' ASSOCIATION

Code for Nurses (1976)

POINT 1

The nurse provides services with respect for human dignity and the uniqueness of the client unrestricted by considerations of social or economic status, personal attributes, or the nature of health problems.

1.1 SELF-DETERMINATION OF CLIENTS

Whenever possible, clients should be fully involved in the planning and implementation of their own health care. Each client has the moral right to determine what will be done with his/her person; to be given the information necessary for making informed judgments; to be told the possible effects of care; and to accept, refuse, or terminate treatment. These same rights apply to minors and others not legally qualified and must be respected to the fullest degree permissible under the law. The law in these areas may differ from state to state; each nurse has an obligation to be knowledgeable about and to protect and support the moral and legal rights of all clients under state laws and applicable federal laws, such as the 1974 Privacy Act.

The nurse must also recognize those situations in which individual rights to self-determination in health care may temporarily be altered for the common good. The many variables involved make it imperative that each case be considered with full awareness of the need to provide for informed judgments while preserving the rights of clients.

1.2 SOCIAL AND ECONOMIC STATUS OF CLIENTS

The need for nursing care is universal, cutting across all national, ethnic, religious, cultural, political, and economic differences, as does nursing's responses to this fundamental need. Nursing care should be determined solely by human need, irrespective of background, circumstances, or other indices of individual social and economic status.

1.3 PERSONAL ATTRIBUTES OF CLIENTS

Age, sex, race, color, personality, or other personal attributes, as well as individual differences in background, customs, attitudes, and beliefs, influence nursing practice only insofar as they represent factors the nurse must understand, consider, and respect in tailoring care to personal needs and in maintaining the individual's self-respect and dignity. Consideration of individual value systems and lifestyles should be included in the planning of health care for each client.

1.4 THE NATURE OF HEALTH PROBLEMS

The nurse's respect for the worth and dignity of the individual human being applies irrespective of the nature of the health problem. It is reflected in the care given the person who is disabled as well as the normal; the patient with the long-term illness as well as the one with the acute illness, or the recovering patient as well as the one who is terminally ill or dying. It extends to all who require the services of the nurse for the promotion of health, the prevention of illness, the restoration of health, and the alleviation of suffering.

The nurse's concern for human dignity and the provision of quality nursing care is not limited by personal attitudes or beliefs. If personally opposed to the delivery of care in a particular case because of the nature of the health problem or the procedures to be used, the nurse is justified in refusing to participate. Such refusal should be made known in advance and in time for other appropriate arrangements to be made for the client's nursing care. If the nurse must knowingly enter such a case under emergency circumstances or enters unknowingly, the obligation to provide the best possible care is observed. The nurse withdraws from this type of situation only when assured that alternative sources of nursing care are available to the client. If a client requests information or counsel in an area that is legally sanctioned but contrary to the nurse's personal beliefs, the nurse may refuse to provide these services but must advise the client of sources where such service is available.

1.5 THE SETTING FOR HEALTH CARE

The nurse adheres to the principle of non-discriminatory, non-prejudicial care in every employment setting or situation and endeavors to promote its acceptance by others. The nurse's readiness to accord respect to clients and to render or obtain needed services should not be limited by the setting, whether nursing care is given in an acute care hospital, nursing home, drug or alcoholic treatment center, prison, patient's home, or other setting.

1.6 THE DYING PERSON

As the concept of death and ways of dealing with it change, the basic human values remain. The ethical problems posed, however, and the decision-making responsibilities of the patient, family, and professional are increased.

The nurse seeks ways to protect these values while working with the client and others to arrive at the best decisions dictated by the circumstances, the client's rights and wishes, and the highest standards of care. The measures used to provide assistance should enable the client to live with as much comfort, dignity, and freedom from anxiety and pain as possible. The client's nursing care will determine to a great degree how this final human experience is lived and the peace and dignity with which death is approached.

POINT 2

The nurse safeguards the client's right to privacy by judiciously protecting information of a confidential nature.

2.1 DISCLOSURE TO THE HEALTH TEAM

It is an accepted standard of nursing practice that data about the health status of clients be accessible, communicated, and recorded. Provision of quality health services requires that such data be available to all members of the health team. When knowledge gained in confidence is relevant or essential to others involved in planning or implementing the client's care, professional judgment is used in sharing it. Only information pertinent to a client's treatment and welfare is disclosed and only to those directly concerned with the client's care. The rights, well-being, and safety of the individual client should be the determining factors in arriving at this decision.

2.2 DISCLOSURE FOR QUALITY ASSURANCE PURPOSES

Patient information required to document the appropriateness, necessity, and quality of care that is required for peer review, third party payment, and other quality assurance mechanisms must be disclosed only under rigidly defined policies, mandates, or protocols. These written guidelines must assure that the confidentiality of client information is maintained.

2.3 DISCLOSURE TO OTHERS NOT INVOLVED IN THE CLIENT'S CARE

The right of privacy is an inalienable right of all persons, and the nurse has a clear obligation to safeguard any confidential information about the client acquired from any source. The nurse-client relationship is built on trust. This relationship could be destroyed and the client's welfare and reputation jeopardized by injudicious disclosure of information provided in confidence. Since the concept of confidentiality has legal as well as ethical implications, an inappropriate breach of confidentiality may also expose the nurse to liability.

2.4 DISCLOSURE IN A COURT OF LAW

Occasionally, the nurse may be obligated to give testimony in a court of law in relation to confidential information about a client. This should be done only under proper authorization or legal compulsion. Privilege in relation to the disclosure of such information is a legal right that only the patient or his representative may claim or waive. The statutes governing privilege and the exceptions to them vary from state to state, and the nurse may wish to consult legal counsel before testifying in court to be fully informed about professional rights and responsibilities.

2.5 ACCESS TO RECORDS

If, in the course of providing care, there is need for access to the records of persons not under the nurse's care, as may be the case in relation to the records of the mother of a newborn, the person should be notified and permission first obtained whenever possible. Although records belong to the agency where collected, the individual maintains the right of control over the information provided by him, his family, and his environment. Similarly, professionals may exercise the right of control over information generated by them in the course of health care.

If the nurse wishes to use a client's treatment record for research or nonclinical purposes in which confidential information may be identified, the client's consent must first be obtained. Ethically, this insures the client's right to privacy; legally, it serves to protect the client against unlawful invasion of privacy and the nurse against liability for such action.

POINT 3

The nurse acts to safeguard the client and the public when health care and safety are affected by incompetent, unethical, or illegal practice of any person.

ROLE OF ADVOCATE

The nurse's primary commitment is to the client's care and safety. Hence, in the role of client advocate, the nurse must be alert to and take appropriate action regarding any instances of incompetent, unethical, or illegal practice(s) by any member of the health care team or the health care system itself, or any action on the part of others that is prejudicial to the client's best interests. To function effectively in the role, the nurse should be fully aware of the state laws governing practice in the health care field and the employing institution's policies and procedures in relation to incompetent, unethical, or illegal practice.

• • •

POINT 4

The nurse assumes responsibility and accountability for individual nursing judgments and actions.

• • •

POINT 5

The nurse maintains competence in nursing.

• • •

POINT 6

The nurse exercises informed judgment and uses individual competence and qualifications as criteria in seeking consultation, accepting responsibilities, and delegating nursing activities to others.

• • •

POINT 7

The nurse participates in activities that contribute to the ongoing development of the profession's body of knowledge.

7.1 THE NURSE AND RESEARCH

Every profession must engage in systematic inquiry to identify, verify, and continually enlarge the body of knowledge which forms the foundations for its practice. A unique body of verified knowledge provides both framework and direction for the profession in all of its activities and for the practitioner in the provision of nursing care. The accrual of knowledge promotes the advancement of practice and with it the well-being of the profession's clients. Ongoing research is thus indispensable to the full discharge of a profession's obligations to society. Each nurse has a role in this area of professional activity, whether involved as an investigator in the furthering of knowledge, as a participant in research, or as a user of research results.

7.2 GENERAL GUIDELINES FOR PARTICIPATING IN RESEARCH

Before participating in research the nurse has an obligation:

1. To ascertain that the study design has been approved by an appropriate body.
2. To obtain information about the intent and the nature of the research.
3. To determine whether the research is consistent with professional goals.

Research involving human subjects should be conducted only by scientifically qualified persons or under such supervision. The nurse who participates in research in any capacity should be fully informed about both nurse and client rights and responsibilities as set forth in the publication *Human Rights Guidelines for Nurses in Clinical and Other Research* prepared by the ANA Commission on Nursing Research.

7.3 THE PROTECTION OF HUMAN RIGHTS IN RESEARCH

The individual rights valued by society and by the nursing profession have been fully outlined and discussed in *Human Rights Guidelines for Nurses in Clinical and Other Research*; namely, the right to freedom from intrinsic risks of injury and the rights of privacy and dignity. Inherent in these rights is respect for each individual to exercise self-determination, to choose to participate, to have full information, to terminate participation without penalty.

It is the duty of both the investigator and the nurse participating in research to maintain vigilance in protecting the life, health, and privacy of human subjects from unanticipated as well as anticipated risks. The subjects' integrity, privacy, and rights must be especially safeguarded if they are unable to protect themselves because of incapacity or because they are in a dependent relationship to the investigator. The investigation should be discontinued if its continuance might be harmful to the subject.

7.4 THE PRACTITIONER'S RIGHTS AND RESPONSIBILITIES IN RESEARCH

Practitioners of nursing providing care to clients who serve as human subjects for research have a special need to clearly understand in advance how the research can be expected to affect treatment and their own moral and legal responsibilities to clients. Here, as in other problematic situations, the practitioner has the right not to participate or to withdraw under the circumstances described in paragraph 1.4 of this document. More detailed guidance about the rights and responsibilities of nurses in relation to research activities may be found in *Human Rights Guidelines for Nurses in Clinical and Other Research*.

POINT 8

The nurse participates in the profession's efforts to implement and improve standards of nursing.

· · ·

POINT 9

The nurse participates in the profession's efforts to establish and maintain conditions of employment conducive to high quality nursing care.

· · ·

POINT 10

The nurse participates in the profession's effort to protect the public from misinformation and misrepresentation and to maintain the integrity of nursing.

· · ·

POINT 11

The nurse collaborates with members of the health professions and other citizens in promoting community and national efforts to meet the health needs of the public.

11.1 QUALITY HEALTH CARE AS A RIGHT

Quality health care is mandated as a right to all citizens. Availability and accessibility to quality health services for all citizens require collaborative planning by health providers and consumers at both the local and national level. Nursing care is an integral part of quality health care, and nurses have a responsibility to help ensure that citizens' rights to health care are met.

11.2 RESPONSIBILITY TO THE CONSUMER OF HEALTH CARE

The nurse is a member of the largest group of health providers, and therefore the philosophies and goals of the nursing profession should have a significant impact on the consumer of health care. An effective way of ensuring that nurses' views regarding health care and nursing service are properly represented is by involvement of nurses in political decision making.

11.3 RELATIONSHIPS WITH OTHER DISCIPLINES

The complexity of the delivery of health care service demands an interdisciplinary approach to delivery of health services as well as strong support from allied health occupations. The nurse should actively seek to promote collaboration needed for ensuring the quality of health services to all persons.

11.4 RELATIONSHIP WITH MEDICINE

The interdependent relationship of the nursing and medical professions requires collaboration around the need of the client. The evolving role of the nurse in the health delivery system requires joint practice as col-leagues, deliberations in determining functional relationships, and differentiating areas of practice between the two professions.

11.5 CONFLICT OF INTEREST

Nurses who provide public service and who have financial or other interests in health care facilities or services should avoid a conflict of interest by refraining from casting a vote on any deliberation affecting the public's health care needs in those areas.

Professional Obligations

EDMUND D. PELLEGRINO

The Virtuous Physician, and the Ethics of Medicine

Consider from what noble seed you spring: You were created not to live like beasts, but for pursuit of virtue and of knowledge.

Dante, *Inferno* 26, 118–120

THE VIRTUOUS PERSON, THE VIRTUOUS PHYSICIAN

Virtue implies a character trait, an internal disposition, habitually to seek moral perfection, to live one's life in accord with the moral law, and to attain a balance between noble intention and just action. Perhaps C. S. Lewis has captured the idea best by likening the virtuous man to the good tennis player: "What you mean by a good player is the man whose eye and muscles and nerves have been so trained by making innumerable good shots that they can now be relied upon. . . . They have a certain tone or quality which is there even when he is not playing. . . . In the same way a man who perseveres in doing just actions gets in the end a certain quality of character. Now it is that quality rather than the particular actions that we mean when we talk of virtue" [1].

On almost any view, the virtuous person is someone we can trust to act habitually in a 'good' way—courageously, honestly, justly, wisely, and temperately. He is committed to *being* a good person and to the pursuit of perfection in his private, professional and communal life. He is someone who will act well even when there is no one to applaud, simply because to act otherwise is a violation of what it is to be a good person. No civilized society could endure without a significant number of citizens committed to this con-

Reprinted from Earl E. Shelp (ed.), *Virtue and Medicine: Exploration in the Character of Medicine* (Philosophy and Medicine Series, No. 17), pp. 243–255. © 1985 by D. Reidel Publishing Company. Reprinted by permission of Kluwer Academic Publishers.

cept of virtue. Without such persons no system of general ethics could succeed, and no system of professional ethics could transcend the dangers of self interest. That is why, even while rights, duties, obligations may be emphasized, the concept of virtue has 'hovered' so persistently over every system of ethics.

Is the virtuous physician simply the virtuous person practicing medicine? Are there virtues peculiar to medicine as a practice? Are certain of the individual virtues more applicable to medicine than elsewhere in human activities? Is virtue more important in some branches of medicine than others? How do professional skills differ from virtue? These are pertinent questions propadeutic to the later questions of the place of virtue in professional medical ethics.

I believe these questions are best answered by drawing on the Aristotelian-Thomist notion of virtues and its relationship to the ends and purposes of human life. The virtuous physician on this view is defined in terms of the ends of medicine. To be sure, the physician, before he is anything else, must be a virtuous person. To be a virtuous physician he must also be the kind of person we can confidently expect will be disposed to the right and good intrinsic to the practice he professes. What are those dispositions?

To answer this question requires some exposition of what we mean by the good in medicine, or more specifically the good of the patient—for that is the end the patient and the physician ostensibly seek. Any theory of virtue must be linked with a theory of the good because virtue is a disposition habitually to do the good. Must we therefore know the nature of the good the virtuous man is disposed to do? As with the definition of virtue we are caught here in another perennial philosophical question—what is the nature of the Good? Is the good whatever we make it to be or does it have validity independent of our desires or interest? Is the good one, or many? Is it reducible to riches, honors, pleasures, glory, happiness, or something else?

I make no pretense to a discussion of a general theory of the good. But any attempt to define the virtuous physician or a virtue-based ethic for medicine must offer some definition of the good of the patient. The patient's good is the end of medicine, that which shapes the particular virtues required for its attainment. That end is central to any notion of the virtues peculiar to medicine as a practice.

I have argued elsewhere that the architectonic principle of medicine is the good of the patient as ex-

pressed in a particular right and good healing action [2]. This is the immediate good end of the clinical encounter. Health, healing, caring, coping are all good ends dependent upon the more immediate end of a right and good decision. On this view, the virtuous physician is one so habitually disposed to act in the patient's good, to place that good in ordinary instances above his own, that he can reliably be expected to do so.

But we must face the fact that the 'patient's good' is itself a compound notion. Elsewhere I have examined four components of the patient's good: (1) clinical or biomedical good; (2) the good as perceived by the patient; (3) the good of the patient as a human person; and (4) the Good, or ultimate good. Each of these components of patient good must be served. They must also be placed in some hierarchical order when they conflict within the same person, or between persons involved in clinical decisions [3].

Some would consider patient good, so far as the physician is concerned, as limited to what applied medical knowledge can achieve in *this* patient. On this view the virtues specific to medicine would be objectivity, scientific probity, and conscientiousness with regard to professional skill. One could perform the technical tasks of medicine well, be faithful to the skills of good technical medicine per se, but without being a virtuous person. Would one then be a virtuous physician? One would have to answer affirmatively if technical skill were all there is to medicine.

Some of the more expansionist models of medicine—like Engel's biopsychosocial model, or that of the World Health Organization (total well-being) would require compassion, empathy, advocacy, benevolence, and beneficence, i.e., an expanded sense of the affective responses to patient need [4]. Some might argue that what is required, therefore, is not virtue, but simply greater skill in the social and behavioral sciences applied to particular patients. On this view the physician's habitual dispositions might be incidental to his skills in communication or his empathy. He could achieve the ends of medicine without necessarily being a virtuous person in the generic sense.

It is important at this juncture to distinguish the virtues from technical or professional skills, as MacIntyre and, more clearly, Von Wright do. The latter defines a skill as 'technical goodness'—excellence in some particular activity—while virtues are not tied to any one activity but are necessary for "the good of man" ([5], pp. 139–140). The virtues are not "characterized in terms of their results" ([6], p. 141). On this view, the technical skills of medicine are not virtues and could be practiced by a non-virtuous person. Aristotle held *techne* (technical skills) to be one of the five intellectual virtues but not one of the moral virtues.

The virtues enable the physician to act with regard to things that are good for man, when man is in the specific existential state of illness. They are dispositions always to seek the good intent inherent in healing. Within medicine, the virtues do become in MacIntyre's sense acquired human qualities ". . . the possession and exercise of which tends to enable us to achieve those goods which are internal to practices and the lack of which effectively prevents us from achieving any such goods" ([7], p. 178).

We can come closer to the relationships of virtue to clinical actions if we look to the more immediate ends of medical encounters, to those moments of clinical truth when specific decisions and actions are chosen and carried out. The good the patient seeks is to be healed—to be restored to his prior, or to a better, state of function, to be made 'whole' again. If this is not possible, the patient expects to be helped, to be assisted in coping with the pain, disability or dying that illness may entail. The immediate end of medicine is not simply a technically proficient performance but the use of that performance to attain a good end—the good of the patient—his medical or biomedical good to the extent possible but also his good as he the patient perceives it, his good as a human person who can make his own life plan, and his good as a person with a spiritual destiny if this is his belief [8]. It is the sensitive balancing of these senses of the patient's good which the virtuous physician pursues to perfection.

To achieve the end of medicine thus conceived, to practice medicine virtuously, requires certain dispositions: conscientious attention to technical knowledge and skill to be sure, but also compassion—a capacity to feel something of the patient's experience of illness and his perceptions of what is worthwhile; beneficence and benevolence—doing and wishing to do good for the patient; honesty, fidelity to promises, perhaps at times courage as well—the whole list of virtues spelled out by Aristotle: ". . . justice, courage, temperance, magnificence, magnanimity, liberality, placability, prudence, wisdom" (*Rhetoric*, 1, c, 13666, 1–3).

Not every one of these virtues is required in every decision. What we expect of the virtuous physician is that he will exhibit them when they are required and that he will be so habitually disposed to do so that we can depend upon it. He will place the good of the patient above his own and seek that good unless its pursuit imposes an injustice upon him, or his family, or requires a violation of his own conscience.

While the virtues are necessary to attain the good internal to medicine as a practice, they exist independently of medicine. They are necessary for the practice of a good life, no matter in what activities that life may express itself. Certain of the virtues may become duties in the Stoic sense, duties because of the nature of medicine as a practice. Medicine calls forth benevolence, beneficence, truth telling, honesty, fidelity, and justice more than physical courage, for example. Yet even physical courage may be necessary when caring for the wounded on battlefields, in plagues, earthquakes, or other disasters. On a more ordinary scale courage is necessary in treating contagious diseases, violent patients, or battlefield casualties. Doing the right and good thing in medicine calls for a more regular, intensive, and selective practice of the virtues than many other callings.

A person who is a virtuous person can cultivate the technical skills of medicine for reasons other than the good of the patient—his own pride, profit, prestige, power. Such a physician can make technically right decisions and perform skillfully. He could not be depended upon, however, to act against his own self-interest for the good of his patient.

In the virtuous physician, explicit fulfillment of rights and duties is an outward expression of an inner disposition to do the right and the good. He is virtuous not because he has conformed to the letter of the law, or his moral duties, but because that is what a good person does. He starts always with his commitment to be a certain kind of person, and he approaches clinical quandaries, conflicts of values, and his patient's interests as a good person should.

Some branches of medicine would seem to demand a stricter and broader adherence to virtue than others. Generalists, for example, who deal with the more sensitive facets and nuances of a patient's life and humanity must exercise the virtues more diligently than technique-oriented specialists. The narrower the specialty the more easily the patient's good can be safeguarded by rules, regulations, rights and duties; the broader the specialty the more significant are the physician's character traits. No branch of medicine, however, can be practiced without some dedication to some of the virtues [9].

Unfortunately, physicians can compartmentalize their lives. Some practice medicine virtuously, yet are guilty of vice in their private lives. Examples are common of physicians who appear sincerely to seek the good of their patients and neglect obligations to family or friends. Some boast of being 'married' to medicine and use this excuse to justify all sorts of failures in their own human relationships. We could not call such a person virtuous. Nor could we be secure in, or trust, his disposition to act in a right and good way even in medicine. After all, one of the essential virtues is balancing conflicting obligations judiciously.

As Socrates pointed out to Meno, one cannot really be virtuous in part:

Why did not I ask you to tell me the nature of virtue as a whole? And you are very far from telling me this; but declare every action to be virtue which is done with a part of virtue; as though you had told me and I must already know the whole of virtue, and this too when frittered away into little pieces. And therefore my dear Meno, I fear that I must begin again, and repeat the same question: what is virtue? For otherwise, I can only say that every action done with a part of virtue is virtue; what else is the meaning of saying that every action done with justice is virtue? Ought I not to ask the question over again; for can any one who does not know virtue know a part of virtue? (*Meno*, 79)

VIRTUES, RIGHTS AND DUTIES IN MEDICAL ETHICS

Frankena has neatly summarized the distinctions between virtue-based and rights- and duty-based ethics as follows:

In an ED (ethics of duty) then, the basic concept is that a certain kind of external act (or doing) ought to be done in certain circumstances; and that of a certain disposition being a virtue is a dependent one. In an EV (ethics of virtue) the basic concept is that of a disposition or way of being— something one has, or if not does—as a virtue, as morally good; and that of an action's being virtuous or good or even right, is a dependent one [10].

There are some logical difficulties with a virtue-based ethic. For one thing, there must be some consensus on a definition of virtue. For another there is a circularity in the assertion that virtue is what the good man habitually does, and that at the same time one becomes virtuous by doing good. Virtue and good are defined in terms of each other and the definitions of both may vary among sincere people in actual practice when there is no consensus. A virtue-based ethic is difficult to defend as the sole basis for normative judgments.

But there is a deficiency in rights- and duty-ethics as well. They too must be linked to a theory of the good. In contemporary ethics, theories of good are rarely explicitly linked to theories of the right and good. Von Wright, commendably, is one of the few contemporary authorities who explicitly connects his theory of good with his theory of virtue. . . .

In most professional ethical codes, virtue- and duty-based ethics are intermingled. The Hippocratic Oath, for example, imposes certain duties like protection of confidentiality, avoiding abortion, not harming the patient. But the Hippocratic physician also pledges: ". . . in purity and holiness I will guard my life and my art." This is an exhortation to be a good person and a virtuous physician, in order to serve patients in an ethically responsible way.

Likewise, in one of the most humanistic statements in medical literature, the first century A.D. writer, Scribonius Largus, made *humanitas* (compassion) an essential virtue. It is thus really a role-specific duty. In doing so he was applying the Stoic doctrine of virtue to medicine [11].

The latest version (1980) of the AMA 'Principles of Medical Ethics' similarly intermingles duties, rights, and exhortations to virtue. It speaks of 'standards of behavior', 'essentials of honorable behavior', dealing 'honestly' with patients and colleagues and exposing colleagues 'deficient in character'. The *Declaration of Geneva*, which must meet the challenge of the widest array of value systems, nonetheless calls for practice 'with conscience and dignity' in keeping with 'the honor and noble traditions of the profession'. Though their first allegiance must be to the Communist ethos, even the Soviet physician is urged to preserve 'the high title of physician', 'to keep and develop the beneficial traditions of medicine' and to 'dedicate' all his 'knowledge and strength to the care of the sick'.

Those who are cynical of any protestation of virtue on the part of physicians will interpret these excerpts as the last remnants of a dying tradition of altruistic benevolence. But at the very least, they attest to the recognition that the good of the patient cannot be fully protected by rights and duties alone. Some degree of supererogation is built into the nature of the relationship of those who are ill and those who profess to help them.

This too may be why many graduating classes, still idealistic about their calling, choose the Prayer of Maimonides (not by Maimonides at all) over the more deontological Oath of Hippocrates. In that 'prayer' the physician asks: ". . . may neither avarice nor miserliness, nor thirst for glory or for a great reputation engage my mind; for the enemies of truth and philanthropy may easily deceive me and make me forgetful of my lofty aim of doing good to thy children." This is an unequivocal call to virtue and it is hard to imagine even the most cynical graduate failing to comprehend its message.

All professional medical codes, then, are built of a three-tiered system of obligations related to the special roles of physicians in society. In the ascending order of ethical sensitivity they are: observance of the laws of the land, then observance of rights and fulfillment of duties, and finally the practice of virtue.

A legally based ethic concentrates on the minimum requirements—the duties imposed by human laws which protect against the grosser aberrations of personal rights. Licensure, the laws of torts and contracts, prohibitions against discrimination, good Samaritan laws, definitions of death, and the protection of human subjects of experimentation are elements of a legalistic ethic.

At the next level is the ethics of rights and duties which spells out obligations beyond what law defines. Here, benevolence and beneficence take on more than their legal meaning. The ideal of service, of responsiveness to the special needs of those who are ill, some degree of compassion, kindliness, promise-keeping, truth-telling, and non-maleficence and specific obligations like confidentiality and autonomy, are included. How these principles are applied, and conflicts among them resolved in the patient's best interests, are subjects of widely varying interpretation. How sensitively these issues are confronted depends more on the physician's character than his capability at ethical discourse or moral casuistry.

Virtue-based ethics goes beyond these first two levels. We expect the virtuous person to do the right and the good even at the expense of personal sacrifice and legitimate self-interest. Virtue ethics expands the notions of benevolence, beneficence, conscientiousness, compassion, and fidelity well beyond what strict duty might require. It makes some degree of supererogation mandatory because it calls for standards of ethical performance that exceed those prevalent in the rest of society [12].

At each of these three levels there are certain dangers from over-zealous or misguided observance. Legalistic ethical systems tend toward a justification for minimalistic ethics, a narrow definition of benevolence or beneficence, and a contract-minded physician-patient relationship. Duty- and rights-based ethics may be distorted by too strict adherence to the letter of ethical principles without the modulations and nuances the spirit of those principles implies. Virtue-based ethics, being the least specific, can more easily lapse into self-righteous paternalism or an unwelcome over-involvement in the personal life of the patient. Misapplication of any moral system even with good intent converts benevolence into maleficence. The virtuous person might be expected to be more sensitive to these aberrations than someone whose ethics is more deontologically or legally flavored.

The more we yearn for ethical sensitivity the less we lean on rights, duties, rules, and principles, and the more we lean on the character traits of the moral agent. Paradoxically, without rules, rights, and duties specifically spelled out, we cannot predict what form a particular person's expression of virtue will take. In a pluralistic society, we need laws, rules, and principles to assure a dependable minimum level of moral conduct. But that minimal level is insufficient in the complex and often unpredictable circumstances of decision-making, where technical and value desiderata intersect so inextricably.

The virtuous physician does not act from unreasoned, uncritical intuitions about what feels good. His dispositions are ordered in accord with that 'right reason' which both Aristotle and Aquinas considered essential to virtue. Medicine is itself ultimately an exercise of practical wisdom—a right way of acting in difficult and uncertain circumstances for a specific end, i.e., the good of a particular person who is ill. It is when the choice of a right and good action becomes more difficult, when the temptations to self-interest are most insistent, when unexpected nuances of good and evil arise and no one is looking, that the differences between an ethics based in virtue and an ethics based in law and/or duty can most clearly be distinguished.

Virtue-based professional ethics distinguishes itself, therefore, less in the avoidance of overtly immoral practices than in avoidance of those at the margin of moral responsibility. Physicians are confronted, in today's morally relaxed climate, with an increasing number of new practices that pit altruism against self-interest. Most are not illegal, or, strictly speaking, immoral in a rights- or duty-based ethic. But they are not consistent with the higher levels of moral sensitivity that a virtue-ethics demands. These practices usually involve opportunities for profit from the illness of others, narrowing the concept of service for personal convenience, taking a proprietary attitude with respect to medical knowledge, and placing loyalty to the profession above loyalty to patients.

Under the first heading, we might include such things as investment in and ownership of for-profit hospitals, hospital chains, nursing homes, dialysis units, tie-in arrangements with radiological or laboratory services, escalation of fees for repetitive, high-volume procedures, and lax indications for their use, especially when third party payers 'allow' such charges.

The second heading might include the ever decreasing availability and accessibility of physicians, the diffusion of individual patient responsibility in group practice so that the patient never knows whom he will see or who is on call, the itinerant emergency room physician who works two days and skips three with little commitment to hospital or community, and the growing over-indulgence of physicians in vacations, recreation, and 'self-development'.

The third category might include such things as 'selling one's services' for whatever the market will bear, providing what the market demands and not necessarily what the community needs, patenting new procedures or keeping them secret from potential competitor-colleagues, looking at the investment of time, effort, and capital in a medical education as justification for 'making it back', or forgetting that medical knowledge is drawn from the cumulative experience of a multitude of patients, clinicians, and investigators.

Under the last category might be included referrals on the basis of friendship and reciprocity rather than skill, resisting consultations and second opinions as affronts to one's competence, placing the interest of the referring physician above those of the patients, looking the other way in the face of incompetence or even dishonesty in one's professional colleagues.

These and many other practices are defended today by sincere physicians and even encouraged in this era of competition, legalism, and self-indulgence. Some can be rationalized even in a deontological ethic. But it would be impossible to envision the physician committed to the virtues assenting to these practices. A virtue-based ethic simply does not fluctuate with what the dominant social mores will tolerate. It must interpret benevolence, beneficence, and responsibility in a way that reduces self-interest and enhances altruism. It is the only convincing answer the profession can give to the growing perception clearly manifest in the legal commentaries in the FTC ruling that medicine is nothing more than business and should be regulated as such.

A virtue-based ethic is inherently elitist, in the best sense, because its adherents demand more of themselves than the prevailing morality. It calls forth that extra measure of dedication that has made the best physicians in every era exemplars of what the human spirit can achieve. No matter to what depths a society may fall, virtuous persons will always be the beacons that light the way back to moral sensitivity; virtuous physicians are the beacons that show the way back to moral credibility for the whole profession.

Albert Jonsen, rightly I believe, diagnoses the central paradox in medicine as the tension between self-interest and altruism [13]. No amount of deft juggling of rights, duties, or principles will suffice to resolve that tension. We are all too good at rationalizing what we want to do so that personal gain can be converted from vice to virtue. Only a character formed by the virtues can feel the nausea of such intellectual hypocrisy.

To be sure, the twin themes of self-interest and altruism have been inextricably joined in the history of medicine. There have always been physicians who reject the virtues or, more often, claim them falsely. But, in addition, there have been physicians, more often than the critics of medicine would allow, who have been truly virtuous both in intent and act. They have been, and remain, the leaven of the profession and the hope of all who are ill. They form the sea-wall that will not be eroded even by the powerful forces of commercialization, bureaucratization, and mechanization inevitable in modern medicine.

We cannot, need not, and indeed must not, wait for a medical analogue of MacIntyre's 'new St. Benedict' to show us the way. There is no new concept of virtue waiting to be discovered that is peculiarly suited to the dilemmas of our own dark age. We must recapture the courage to speak of character, virtue, and perfection in living a good life. We must encourage those who are willing to dedicate themselves to a "higher standard of self effacement" [14].

We need the courage, too, to accept the obvious split in the profession between those who see and feel the altruistic imperatives in medicine, and those who do not. Those who at heart believe that the pursuit of private self-interest serves the public good are very different from those who believe in the restraint of self-interest. We forget that physicians since the beginnings of the profession have subscribed to different values and virtues. We need only recall that the Hippocratic Oath was the Oath of physicians of the Pythagorean school at a time when most Greek physicians followed essentially a craft ethic [15]. A perusal of the Hippocratic Corpus itself, which intersperses ethics and etiquette, will show how differently its treatises deal with fees, the care of incurable patients, and the business aspects of the craft.

The illusion that all physicians share a common devotion to a high-flown set of ethical principles has done damage to medicine by raising expectations some members of the profession could not, or will not, fulfill. Today, we must be more forthright about the differences in value commitment among physicians. Professional codes must be more explicit about the relationships between duties, rights, and virtues. Such explicitness encourages a more honest relationship between physicians and patients and removes the hypocrisy of verbal assent to a general code, to which an individual physician may not really subscribe. Explicitness enables patients to choose among physicians on the basis of their ethical commitments as well as their reputations for technical expertise.

Conceptual clarity will not assure virtuous behavior. Indeed, virtues are usually distorted if they are the subject of too conscious a design. But conceptual clarity will distinguish between motives and provide criteria for judging the moral commitment one can expect from the profession and from its individual members. It can also inspire those whose virtuous inclinations need re-enforcement in the current climate of commercialization of the healing relationship.

To this end the current resurgence of interest in virtue-based ethics is altogether salubrious. Linked to a theory of patient good and a theory of rights and duties, it could provide the needed groundwork for a reconstruction of professional medical ethics as that work matures. Perhaps even more progress can be made if we take Shakespeare's advice in *Hamlet*: "Assume the virtue if you have it not. . . . For use almost can change the stamp of nature."

NOTES

1. Lewis, C.: 1952, *Mere Christianity*, MacMillan Co., New York.

2. Pellegrino, E.: 1983, 'The Healing Relationship: The Architectonics of Clinical Medicine', in E. Shelp (ed.), *The Clinical Encounter*, D. Reidel, Dordrecht, Holland, pp. 153–172.

3. Pellegrino, E.: 1983, 'Moral Choice, The Good of the Patient and the Patient's Good', in J. Moskop and L. Kopelman (eds.), *Moral Choice and Medical Crisis*, D. Reidel, Dordrecht, Holland.

4. Engel, G.: 1980, 'The Clinical Application of the Biopsychosocial Model', *American Journal of Psychiatry* 137: 2, 535–544.

5. Von Wright, G.: 1965, *The Varieties of Goodness*, The Humanities Press, New York.

6. Ibid.

7. MacIntyre, A.: 1981, *After Virtue*, University of Notre Dame Press, Notre Dame, Indiana.

8. Pellegrino, E.: 1979, 'The Anatomy of Clinical Judgments: Some Notes on Right Reason and Right Action', in H. T. Engelhardt, Jr., *et al.* (eds.), *Clinical Judgment: A Critical Appraisal*, D. Reidel, Dordrecht, Holland, pp. 169–194. Pellegrino, E.: 1979, 'Toward a Reconstruction of Medical Morality: The Primacy of the Act of Profession and the Fact of Illness', *Journal of Medicine and Philosophy* 4: 1, 32–56.

9. May, W.: Personal communication, 'Virtues in a Professional Setting', unpublished.

10. Frankena, W.: 1982, 'Beneficence in an Ethics of Virtue', in E. Shelp (ed.), *Beneficence and Health Care*, D. Reidel, Dordrecht, Holland, pp. 63–81.

11. Cicero: 1967, *Moral Obligations*, J. Higginbotham (trans.), University of California Press, Berkeley and Los Angeles. Pellegrino, E.: 1983, '*Scribonius Largus* and the Origins of Medical Humanism', address to the American Osler Society.

12. Reeder, J.: 1982, 'Beneficence, Supererogation, and Role Duty', in E. Shelp (ed.), *Beneficence and Health Care*, D. Reidel, Dordrecht, Holland, pp. 83–108.

13. Jonsen, A.: 1983, 'Watching the Doctor', *New England Journal of Medicine* 308: 25, 1531–1535.

14. Cushing, H.: 1929, *Consecratio Medici and Other Papers*, Little, Brown and Co., Boston.

15. Edelstein, L.: 1967, 'The Professional Ethics of the Greek Physician', in O. Temkin (ed.), *Ancient Medicine: Selected Papers of Ludwig Edelstein*, Johns Hopkins University Press, Baltimore.

GERALD R. WINSLOW

From Loyalty to Advocacy:
A New Metaphor for Nursing

Nurses are by far the largest group of health care professionals, numbering well over one million in the United States today. They are often the professionals with whom patients have the most sustained contact. And because of the profession's perceived tradition of holism and "care more than cure," nursing is often upheld as a hopeful paradigm for the future.

But the paradigm is changing. For over a decade, professional nursing has been engaged in profound revision of its ethic. The evidence is abundant: revised codes of ethics, new legal precedents, a flood of books and articles on nursing ethics, and, what may be more significant than any other attestation, a shift in the central metaphors by which nursing structures its own self-perception.

The metaphors associated with nursing are numerous. Two examples that have received considerable attention recently are the nurse as traditional-mother substitute and the nurse as professional contractor.[1] As substitute mother, the nurse cares for sick children (patients) and follows the orders of the traditional father (the physician). As professional contractor, the nurse negotiates a plan for the care of clients (patients) and consults with other contractors (other health care professionals).

Such metaphors are not mere niceties of language. Rather, they interact with the more explicit features of nursing ethics, such as stated rules and principles, in ways that tend to be either mutually supportive or productive of change. The power of metaphors is due in part to their capacity to focus attention on some aspects of reality while concealing others.[2] For example, thinking of the nurse as a parent may highlight certain functions, such as nurture, protection, and domination, while hiding the patient's responsibility for decisions about his or her own care. The metaphor has the ability to create a set of expectations and make some forms of behavior seem more "natural" than others. Thus, if both nurse and patient begin to use the metaphor of nurse as contractor and its associated forms of expression, such as "negotiations," they may come to expect actions in keeping with a "business-like" relationship.

This article examines the developing changes in nursing ethics by considering two basic metaphors and the norms and virtues consonant with them. The first is nursing as military effort in the battle against disease, a metaphor that permeates many of the early discussions of nursing ethics. It is associated with virtues such as loyalty and norms such as obedience to those of "higher rank" and the maintenance of confidence in authority figures. The second metaphor is nursing as advocacy of patient rights, an essentially legal metaphor that has pervaded much of the literature on nursing ethics within the past decade. The metaphor of advocacy is associated with virtues such as courage and norms such as the defense of the patient against infringements of his or her rights. I did not select these two metaphors for analysis randomly, but, in part, because they have played a prominent role in the formation of ethics within nursing's own literature. More than most others, these metaphors have been espoused by the leaders of nursing, and have had obvious effects on nursing education and practice. Metaphors such as the nurse as surrogate parent, nun, domestic servant, or "handmaiden of the physician"

Reprinted by permission of the author and reproduced by permission. © The Hastings Center, from *Hastings Center Report* 14 (June 1984), pp. 32–39.

have often been discussed. But these discussions have been almost entirely intended to reject such metaphors and not to uphold them as representative of nursing ideals. Indeed, such metaphors have been used most often to serve as foils for images considered more adequate. On the other hand, the military metaphor, with its language of loyalty and obedience, and the legal metaphor, with its language of advocacy and rights, have served as basic models of ideal nursing practice as proposed in nursing literature.

THE MILITARY METAPHOR

It would be surprising if professional nursing had *not* early adopted the metaphor of military service. Modern nursing is generally acknowledged to have begun with the work of Florence Nightingale, superintendent of nurses in British military hospitals during the Crimean War in the 1850s.[3] Upon her return to England, she continued her work with the military and was instrumental in founding the British Army Medical School. Whatever else Nightingale was, she most certainly was a practitioner and proponent of strict military discipline. And though some have criticized Nightingale's work, the idealization of the "Lady with the Lamp" continues, with rare exceptions, in professional nursing to this day. As two nurses very recently declared: "We think of ourselves as Florence Nightingale—tough, canny, powerful, autonomous, and heroic."[4]

Not only was modern nursing born in a military setting, it also emerged at a time when medicine was appropriating the military metaphor: medicine as war.[5] It has now become difficult to imagine a more pervasive metaphor in contemporary medicine (unless, perhaps, it is medicine as economic enterprise).[6] Disease is the *enemy*, which threatens to *invade* the body and overwhelm its *defenses*. Medicine *combats* disease with *batteries* of tests and *arsenals* of drugs. And young staff physicians are still called house *officers*. But what about nurses?

Perhaps even more than medicine, nursing explicitly chose the military metaphor. It was used to engender a sense of purpose and to explain the training and discipline of the nurse. In the fledgling *American Journal of Nursing*, Charlotte Perry, an early leader, described the education required to produce the "nursing character." Upon entering training, wrote Perry,

the student "soon learns the military aspect of life—that it is a life of toil and discipline. . . ." Such discipline, the author asserted, is part of the "ethics of nursing," and it should be evidenced in the "look, voice, speech, walk, and touch" of the trained nurse. The nurse's "whole being bristles with the effect of the military training she has undergone and the sacrifices she has been called upon to make. A professional manner is the result."[7]

The goal of the military discipline was to produce trained nurses with many of the qualities of good soldiers. The military imagery was neither subtle nor unusual, as a passage from an early book on nursing ethics illustrates:

[An] excellent help to self devotion is the love a nurse has for the stern strife of her constant battle with sickness. . . . "The stern joy which warriors feel, in foemen worthy of their steel," should inspirit the valiant heart of the nurse as it does the heart of the brave soldier who bears long night watches, weary marches, dangerous battles, for the love of the conflict and the keen hope of victory. The soldier in a just war is upheld by this keen joy of battle. So will the nurse be spurred on to devotion by the love of conflict with disease.[8]

The moral force of the metaphor is obvious. Nurses should be prepared for the hardships of night duty, personal danger, weary walking, and so forth. And there can be little doubt that the military metaphor supported a number of nursing behaviors. A minor example is the uniform. Early discussions of nursing ethics almost always included sections on propriety regarding dress. The uniforms of different schools had characteristic differences, reminiscent of the differences signifying various military units. And as nurses progressed up the ranks, stripes were added to their caps and insignia pins to their uniforms. The uniform was always to be worn while "on duty" but never while "off duty." And ordinary clothing was even referred to as "civilian dress."[9]

Some traits are more important to good soldiers than the proper wearing of uniforms. More central, for example, is suitable respect for those of higher rank. Such respect is evidenced both in obedience and in various symbolic gestures of deference. Commenting on nursing ethics, Perry urged her fellow nurses to have proper respect for rank:

Carrying out the military idea, there are ranks in authority. . . . "Please" and "Thank you" are phrases which may be exchanged between those of equal rank. The military command is couched in no uncertain terms. Clear, explicit directions are given, and are received with unquestioning obedience.

Later, Perry added that there are "necessary barriers" between those of different ranks and "familiarity" should not be allowed to dismantle these barriers.[10] The ideal of military obedience was applied often to the nurse's work with physicians. Physicians were the commanding officers. In a published lecture to nurses, one physician did not hesitate to use the military metaphor in explaining why there must be discipline in the hospital "just as in the regiment, [where] we have the captains, the lieutenants, and the sergeants. . . . Obedience to one's superiors is an essential duty of all." The author acknowledged that some of the rules are bound to "appear captious and unfair." Nevertheless, they must be obeyed. And such obedience should be not in a spirit of fear but rather in a spirit of "loyalty."[11]

Loyalty was one of the key virtues of the ideal nurse. In the words of the Nightingale Pledge: "With loyalty will I endeavor to aid the physician in his work. . . ."[12] Nearly every early discussion of nursing ethics includes a major section on loyalty, and the link between loyalty and the military metaphor was strong. For example, the physician just quoted reminded nurses of their obligation: "As in the hospital loyalty to her superior officers is the duty of the nurse, so in private nursing she must be loyal to the medical man who is in attendance on her patient."[13] This sentiment is echoed in Charlotte Aikens's 1916 book on nursing ethics, a standard text for over twenty years:

Loyalty to the physician is one of the duties demanded of every nurse, not solely because the physician is her superior officer, but chiefly because the confidence of the patient in his physician is one of the important elements in the management of his illness, and nothing should be said or done that would weaken this faith or create doubts as to the character or ability or methods of the physician. . . .[14]

What, then, did it mean for the "trained nurse" to be loyal? It meant, to be sure, faithful and self-sacrificial care of patients. But most of the discussions of loyalty were occupied more with another concern: the protection of confidence in the health care effort. Loyalty meant refusal to criticize the nurse's hospital or training school, fellow nurses, and most importantly, the physician under whom the nurse worked.

Ideally, all these loyalties should harmonize. And nurses were often reminded that being loyal to the physician by preserving the patient's confidence was the same as being loyal to the patient. As one doctor put it: "[L]oyalty to the physician means faithfulness to the patient, even if the treatment is not always in line with what [the nurse] has been taught in the training school. . . . Loyalty to the physician and faithfulness to the patient do not form a twofold proposition, but a single one."[15] The reasoning was supposed to be obvious: the patient's recovery could be aided powerfully by trust in the doctor and the prescribed regimen. Worry over the doctor's competence was likely to worsen the patient's condition not only because of the wasted energy but also because of the lost power of suggestion and the patient's failure to comply with the treatment. The author of a text on nursing ethics summed up the idea:

Confidence and skepticism are both contagious, and we know very well how important it often is for a patient's cure that he should have the attitude of faith and confidence in his physician. . . . [It] is unkind indeed to destroy a confidence which is so beneficent and comforting.[16]

The moral power of this reasoning should not be overlooked. Nurses accepted as their solemn obligation assisting in the patient's recovery. And nurses were taught repeatedly that the "*faith* that people have in a physician is as much a healing element as is any medicinal treatment."[17] Thus, even if the physician blundered, the patient's confidence should usually be maintained at all costs. To quote an early nursing text:

If a mistake has been made in treating a patient, the patient is not the person who should know it if it can be kept from him, because the anxiety and lack of confidence that he would naturally feel might be injurious to him and retard his recovery.[18]

But what if the nurse finally concluded that the confidence in the physician simply was not merited? It is one of the myths of a later generation that nurses of the past never questioned loyalty to the physician. In speeches, journals, and books, leading nurses complained that loyalty to the physician often was not deserved and even more often was not returned in kind.[19] And the difficult moral dilemmas faced by nurses were usually discussed in terms of conflicts of loyalties. For example, in an earlier editorial titled "Where Does Loyalty End?" the author claimed that many letters from nurses asked essentially the same questions: "Where does the nurse's loyalty to the doctor end? And is she required to be untruthful or to practice deceit in order to uphold the reputation of the physician at her own expense or that of the patient?"[20]

The published letters revealed the kinds of cases troubling nurses. One told how a physician inserted a catheter too far into the patient's bladder—a mistake that, according to the nurse, required surgery to correct. The nurse reported that she was blamed in order to protect the doctor's reputation. Another nurse told how a physician failed to remove a surgical sponge, causing the patient great suffering and near-death. When the problem became apparent, the nurse was unable to keep the truth from the family. Later, the doctor chastised the nurse for failure to conceal the truth. The writer claimed that "nurses are taught that they must stand by the doctor whether he is right or wrong." But, she concluded, if this means lying to the patient in order "to defend the doctor then I don't care for the profession. . . ."[21]

Such letters (and many similar discussions in early nursing literature) indicate that conflicts of loyalties tended to focus on two main issues: truth-telling and physicians' competency. Obviously, these two were often linked. Nurses felt obliged to protect doctors even if the care seemed deficient and the truth suffered. But in many cases the truth was concealed because physicians did not want their patients to know their diagnoses. In her text on ethics, Aikens complained: "From the beginning of her career [the nurse] is impressed with the idea that . . . it is an unpardonable sin to lie to a doctor about a patient but perfectly pardonable, and frequently very desirable, to lie to a patient about his own condition."[22] So, although lying was often roundly condemned, clearly it was often the "order" of the day. Dissonance was the inevitable result. Nurses were pleased, as Lena Dietz put it, to "enjoy a confidence such as is placed in no other women in the world. . . . The fact that they are nurses is accepted as an unquestionable guarantee of honesty."[23] But, at times, loyalty to the "superior officers" left the guarantee more than a little tattered.

In all likelihood loyal protection of the physician often was motivated, in no small measure, by the nurse's desire for self-protection. In the early years of nursing, the goal of most graduate nurses was to leave the hospital and become "private duty nurses."[24] The names of those available for this work were obtained from the local "registry" (kept variously by hospitals, nurses' associations, or medical associations) or simply by word of mouth. Technically, such nurses were hired directly by the patient. But in reality the attending physician was highly influential in the selection of the private nurse and, if need be, in the nurse's dismissal. Understandably, this arrangement led at times to conflicting interests and loyalties. One doctor grumbled: "Paid by the patient, or someone close to him, and not by the physician, [the nurse] sometimes seems to think that it is safest to 'stand in' with the patient, and actually obey him, rather than the physician."[25] The patient paid the wages of the nurse, but the doctor was supposed to be in charge. The financial implications of this arrangement were not lost on nurses. Aikens wrote: "Not infrequently, a nurse is torn between her desire to be loyal to the patient's interests, and not disloyal to the doctor, who has it in his power to turn calls in her direction, and influence other doctors to do the same, or the reverse."[26]

Troubled at times by conflicting loyalties and worried about employment, nurses advocated a number of strategies for coping with some doctors' apparent ineptitude. Of these strategies, four stand out.

First, the nurse could faithfully obey all orders and simply assume that the doctor knew best. Isabel Robb, in the first American book on nursing ethics, wrote: "Apart from the fact that [the nurse] may be quite wrong in her opinions, her sole duty is to obey orders, and so long as she does this, she is not to be held responsible for untoward results."[27] On this, the prevailing view, the nurse was supposed to be absolved from guilt so long as she followed orders. The doctrine of *respondeat superior* generally did offer nurses legal protection. But moral protection is not always so easily secured, hence the additional strategies.

Second, the nurse could gently question the doctor's orders. Sara Parsons suggested to her nursing colleagues that when the nurse "becomes sufficiently experienced to detect a mistake, she will, of course, call [the doctor's] attention to it by asking if her understanding of the order is correct."[28] This approach of nurses making what amounts to recommendations in the form of questions is apparently long-lived. Recent work indicates that it is still an expected part of the "doctor-nurse game."[29]

A third maneuver was consultation with some other authority figure.[30] In the hospital, the nursing supervisor was the most likely candidate. But the private duty nurse had no such recourse. This difficulty led one author to propose that the nurse call the family's "religious advisor" in a confidential attempt to engineer a change of physicians.[31]

Finally, the nurse could withdraw from the case, or refuse the physician's patients from the beginning. If the doctor was intolerably deficient, Robb counseled, the nurse could "always find some means of refusing to take charge of the nursing of his patients. . . ." Robb added, however, "[O]nce having put herself under [the doctor], let her remain loyal and carry out his orders to the letter."[32] And in his lecture to nurses, a physician put the same point bluntly: "Better to be an honest deserter than a traitor in the camp."[33]

Better than deserter or traitor, however, was the nurse as loyal soldier. Then the world changed. Or at least the metaphors did.

THE LEGAL METAPHOR

It would be foolish to set a date to the changing of nursing's self-image. The process has been gradual, the way tortuous. As was noted earlier, nurses' criticism of the "one-sided loyalty" expected of them dates back nearly to the beginning of the profession. And by 1932, Annie Warburton Goodrich, an acknowledged leader, could speak of nursing's "militarism, that splendid drilling in subordination of self to the machine" as a feature that the profession was attempting to "modify, if not abolish."[34]

Even if the abolition has come slowly, some major events can be identified. For example, a significant blow to nursing's ethic of military loyalty occurred in an unlikely place in 1929. In Manila, a newly graduated nurse, Lorenza Somera, was found guilty of manslaughter, sentenced to a year in prison, and fined one thousand pesos because she followed a physician's order. The physician had mistakenly called for the preparation of cocaine injections (he meant procaine) for a tonsillectomy patient. Witnesses agreed that the physician ordered the cocaine, that Somera verified that order, and that the physician administered the injections. But the physician was acquitted and Somera found guilty because she failed to *question* the orders. The Supreme Court upheld the lower court's decision.[35]

Nurses around the world (and especially in the United States, because the Philippine Islands were under U.S. jurisdiction) were at first stunned and then incensed. A successful protest campaign was organized, and Somera was pardoned before serving a day of her sentence. But the whole affair left an enduring impression on nurses. The doctrine of *respondeat superior* turned out to be thin security. Never again could nurses be taught simply to follow doctors' orders. Even now, over fifty years later, nursing texts still refer to *Somera* as proof of nurses' independent accountability.[36]

But, despite *Somera* and later similar cases, the tradition of loyalty to the physician retained considerable power. This strength was illustrated by the first codes of nursing ethics. Nurses had been calling for a code of ethics before the turn of the century. But not until 1926 was the first "suggested code" for nurses proposed. By present standards this proposed code must be judged remarkably enlightened. It speaks of broad principles and, with regard to nurses' relationship to physicians, it says that "neither profession can secure complete results without the other." When the proposed code discusses loyalty, it says that "loyalty to the motive which inspires nursing should make the nurse fearless to bring to light any serious violation of the ideals herein expressed." Perhaps not surprisingly, the code failed to gain acceptance.[37] The next attempt came in 1940. This proposal was much more similar to what later became the accepted tenets.[38] Obligations to the physicians were central. For example, the code adopted by the American Nurses' Association (ANA) called for nurses to verify and carry out the physician's orders, sustain confidence in the physician, and report incompetency or unethical conduct "only to the proper authority."[39] A similar code, approved by the International Council of Nurses in 1953, spelled out the nurse's obligation to follow the physician's orders "loyally" and to maintain confidence in the physician.[40]

In the 1960s and 1970s the image of the loyal nurse began to be significantly revised. The forces for change in health care delivery during the past two decades are too numerous and complex to analyze here. In his social history of medicine, Paul Starr describes the "stunning loss of confidence" sustained by medicine during the 1970s. The formerly unquestioned mandate of the "sovereign profession" was challenged with increased frequency. Consumerism was strengthening. And the ever-higher costs of medical care along with the perceived arrogance of many in the medical profession irritated large numbers of consumers. Moreover, medicine was viewed increasingly as a large, impersonal institution, a privileged and protected castle constantly resisting needed modifications. For nursing, a profession populated almost entirely by women, the growth of feminism also proved a highly important development. These forces, and many others, achieved sharp focus in the patients' rights movement which, in Starr's words, "went beyond traditional demands for more medical care and challenged the distribution of power and expertise."[41] Few in the health care system seemed more eager for the challenge to succeed than nurses. It was hardly surprising, therefore, that leaders of the patients' rights movement turned to nurses in the search for "patient advocates." For example, George Annas, an attorney and author of *The Rights of Hospital Patients*, called for nurses to accept the new role of patient advocacy.[42] It is worthy of note that Annas prefaced his appeal to nurses by explicitly attacking the military metaphor. Nurses who accepted such traditional images would be poorly equipped to be patient advocates. At times, orders would have to be challenged. But, Annas argued, properly retrained nurses had the potential to play a "key role" in patient advocacy.[43]

In rejecting the metaphor of nurse as loyal soldier, Annas offered a replacement—the nurse as courageous advocate. The image was essentially legal. As a significant part of their retraining, for example, nurses needed "some clear understanding of the law" relating to patients' rights. "*The powers of the advocate would be precisely the legal powers of the patient*." Acceptance of the advocacy role entailed a readiness to enter disputes. Patients needed assurance that their advocate was "someone who could be trusted to fight for their rights." Included in Annas's list of rights are those that became the standards of the patients' rights movement: the right to adequate information about proposed medical procedures, the right to refuse or accept any or all such procedures, the right to full information about prognosis and diagnosis, the right to leave the hospital, and so forth. To these canons, Annas added the right of the patient to around-the-clock access to a patients' rights advocate. Clearly, the assumptions were that patients' rights were often being threatened and someone was needed continually to contend for patients. Annas hoped that nurses would

be among those to take up the fight. He was not to be disappointed—not, that is, if the volume of nursing literature promoting the role of nurse as patient advocate is a measure of success.

From the mid-1970s to the present, literally scores of nursing books and articles have appeared advocating advocacy.[44] It is now not at all uncommon for nurses to argue, as one recently did, that "the nurse is the ideal patient advocate!"[45] And at least two thoughtful nurse-philosophers have argued that the concept of advocacy is the most appropriate philosophical foundation for the nursing profession.[46] After all, nurses usually have the most regular contact with the patient. And more than any other health care professionals, nurses tend to be concerned with the well-being of the *whole* patient. Moreover, nurses have a long tradition of educating patients, so it is entirely natural for nurses to accept responsibility for assuring that patients are properly informed. Finally, nurses and patients should make obvious and genuine allies since both groups have often suffered the indignities of powerlessness in the modern health care system. Who, then, could function better as a patient advocate than a nurse?

So the arguments go. And, the result has been more than a flurry of words. The metaphor has had a way of "working into life." For example, one school of nursing now requires all of its advanced students to devise and carry out an "Advocacy Project."[47] A student might discover, for instance, that elderly patients in a nursing home feel a need for legal advice. The student would develop a plan for securing such advice and then attempt to put the plan into action.

During the 1970s, the concept of advocacy was also incorporated into nursing's codes of ethics. In its 1973 revision, the International Council of Nurses' code dropped all mention of loyal obedience to the physician's orders.[48] Instead, the code said that the "nurse's primary responsibility is to those people who require nursing care," and the "nurse takes appropriate action to safeguard the individual when his care is endangered by a co-worker or any other person." Even more striking, in some respects, are the 1976 revisions of the ANA code. The revised code requires nurses to protect "the client" from the "incompetent, unethical, or illegal practice of any person."[49] In the interpretive statements on this point, the code makes explicit use of the language of advocacy: "[I]n the role of client advocate, the nurse must be alert to and take appropriate action regarding any instances of incompetent, unethical, or illegal practice(s) by any member of the health care team or the health care system itself, or any action on the part of others that is prejudicial to the client's best interests." The revised ANA code is revealing not only because of this addition but also because of its subtractions. Gone are the rules obliging nurses to maintain confidence in physicians or obey their orders. In fact, "physician" does not even appear in the revised code.

Nursing's adoption of the ethic of advocacy has brought to life a whole new genre of nursing literature: the nurse-as-advocate short story. In a recent example, a nurse detailed her attempts to become an "advocate for the clients." While employed as director of nursing in a county health department, she became aware of the very poor record of maternity care at one hospital. The postpartum infection rate was nearly three times higher than the national average. And the Apgar scores of many newborns were lower than should have been expected statistically. But the hospital resented having the problems called to public attention and resisted any suggested changes. For her efforts, the nurse was ostracized by the health care community. Finally, she resigned before she could be fired. In her view, the theories about advocacy were fine, but "the problem lies in putting these theories into action."[50] Unfortunately, this account is typical of most published nurse-as-advocate stories.[51] They usually describe a nurse's attempt to defend a patient or group of patients against mistreatment. Most often, the endeavor fails because the system overpowers the nurse. The patient suffers or dies. The nurse gets fired or resigns in outrage. The system goes on. As literature, the stories tend to have the features of tragedy (though the flaw is in the character of the system rather than the advocate).

Of such stories, none has been more widely publicized as an example of patient advocacy than the case of Jolene Tuma.[52] In March 1976, Tuma, a clinical instructor of nursing, was asked by a cancer patient about alternatives to chemotherapy. The patient was apprehensive about the therapy. She did not want to question her physician further, however, because he had already indicated his conviction that chemotherapy was the only acceptable treatment. Tuma knew that discussing options with the patient would be risky. In fact, she told the patient that such a conversation would not be "exactly ethical." Nevertheless, Tuma proceeded to discuss a number of alternatives about which the patient had questions, including nutritional

therapy and Laetrile. The patient then decided to continue chemotherapy. But, in spite of the efforts, she died two weeks later. One of the patient's children informed the attending physician about Tuma's discussion with the patient. The physician protested to Tuma's employing college and to the Board of Nurse Examiners of Idaho. As a result, Tuma lost her job and her nursing license. The state's nursing board concluded that Tuma had interfered unethically with the physician-patient relationship. During the conflict, Tuma wrote to a nursing journal and described her predicament:

Does the nurse have the right to assist the patient toward full and informed consent? Litigation against nurses already shows us we have the responsibility when we do not properly inform the patient. But do we have the authority to go along with this responsibility as the patient's advocate?[53]

Tuma's case might have ended like so many other nurse-as-advocate stories except for the fact that she appealed the state board's ruling. Three years later, the Supreme Court of Idaho ruled that the nursing board had been wrong in suspending Tuma's license.[54] It is difficult, however, to assess the extent of Tuma's victory. She did not regain her teaching position, she suffered through three years of legal appeals, and it was too late to change the outcome for the patient. Certainly, the physician and at least some of the patient's family were displeased by her actions. Still, Tuma believes that her actions were justified. She feels that her personal sacrifice has been repaid not only by the assurance that the patient's rights were defended but also by the public attention directed toward the rightful role of nurses as patient advocates.[55] And a recently published poll of 12,500 nurses reveals that Tuma has strong support from her colleagues. Over 80 percent of the respondents agreed that a nurse who acted as Tuma did would be doing the "right thing."[56]

The response of nurses to the Tuma case is a clear indication of the profession's changing self-perception. The new metaphor of nurse as advocate has risen to power. Indeed, if the profession's literature during the past decade is taken as primary evidence, then it can be said safely that no other symbol has so captured imagination or won acceptance within nursing as that of the advocate.

ASSESSING THE ADVOCACY METAPHOR

It is generally easier to criticize the metaphors of an earlier age than to evaluate those now regnant. But further criticism of the military metaphor is hardly in order. The nurse as loyal soldier is dead. Among nurses, mourners of the metaphor's passage are either nonexistent or well hidden. Meanwhile, the metaphor of nurse as patient advocate has nearly achieved the status of a slogan. Criticism of patient advocacy in nursing literature is virtually unknown.[57]

But those who hope that the rise of advocacy is a positive sign of a maturing profession (and I am among them) should give careful attention to the ambiguities and potential criticisms of the advocacy role. I mention only five:

1. *The meaning of advocacy needs clarification.* Metaphors tend to be unruly. Part of their richness is their capacity to generate new and at times surprising perspectives. Thus, referring to nurses as advocates opens apparently boundless possibilities for new understandings. And, as might be expected, a survey of the nursing literature on advocacy soon reveals that the metaphor is invoked in a variety of ways, some of which may be incompatible. At times, advocacy is construed so broadly that it seems to mean something like "doing the best for the patient." But most supporters of advocacy have in mind more specific actions such as helping the patient to obtain needed health care, assuring the quality of health care, defending the patient's rights (such as the right of informed consent), serving as a liaison between the patient and health care professionals, and counseling the patient in order to alleviate fear.

In one of the few thorough discussions, Sally Gadow proposes a model of "existential" advocacy. In her view, the ideal is "that individuals be *assisted* by nursing to *authentically* exercise their freedom of self-determination."[58] Gadow argues for a type of advocacy that avoids paternalistic manipulation of the patient on the one hand and reduction of the nurse to a mere technician who is unwilling to recommend alternatives on the other hand. Whether most nurses would agree entirely with Gadow's interpretation, most discussions of the nurse as advocate would benefit both from Gadow's example of careful analysis and from her thesis. In my view, the central, moral significance of the advocacy metaphor lies in its power to shape actions intended to protect and enhance the personal autonomy of patients. Further clarification of this significance is essential if the metaphor is to rise above the level of a simple slogan.

2. *The states' nurse practice acts need revision.* Since 1971, states have been revising practice acts to allow for newly expanded nursing roles.[59] But changes in the laws generally have not kept pace with nursing's adoption and understanding of advocacy. And, as *Tuma* illustrates, the legal limits are often unclear. What does it mean, for example, to interfere with the physician-patient relationship? Does unacceptable interference include suggesting a second medical opinion? What about recommending a change of physicians? As a result of such uncertainties, nurses who set out to be patient advocates may find themselves needing a lawyer. One nurse recently reported just such an experience. She was present when a surgical resident botched a tracheotomy and severed the patient's carotid artery. The patient bled to death. The nurse decided that for the sake of other patients she should report the resident. But the medical director cautioned the nurse not to pursue the matter unless she hired an attorney. As the nurse put it: "Dr. X kills the patient and I need a lawyer."[60] The threat of retaliation and the loss of professional and economic security are bound to have a chilling effect on nurses' willingness to function as patient advocates.

To be effective, the calls for nurses to become patient advocates must be accompanied by political action aimed at needed revision of the states' laws. But when it comes to politics, a more apt metaphor for nursing might be that of slumbering giant. Nursing's status as the largest health care profession generally has not translated into commensurate political strength. As the profession has adopted the ethic of advocacy, however, nurses have begun to pay more attention to the need for political action.[61] We should hope that the effect of such action will be to make patient advocacy a less dangerous activity.

3. *Patients (or their families) are often unprepared to accept the nurse as advocate.* In at least one important respect, nurses are unlike many other professionals whom the patient might engage for services. The patient is usually free to accept or reject the efforts of, say, a physician or an attorney. But in most instances the patient is not involved in the selection of his or her nurse. Thus, the nurse who functions as a patient advocate usually does so for one who has not chosen the nurse's services and who does not *expect* the nurse to serve as an advocate.

There is abundant evidence that society generally accepts a more traditional role for nurses. On this subject, nursing literature is peppered with analyses, laments, and calls for change.[62] But old metaphors die hard. And it is a frustrating fact that vestigial images of the nurse as loyal soldier, substitute parent, assistant physician, or even handmaiden will probably remain in the minds of the public long after most nurses have rejected them. For patient advocacy to be fully successful, further attention must be given to the mechanisms for appropriate public education.

4. *Advocacy is frequently associated with controversy.* It would be a rare advocacy story that did not include a measure of discord. The patient who needs an advocate is often being mistreated by someone's action or inaction. The nurse accepts the responsibility of contending for the rights of the patient, work that may involve conflict.

Some people may thrive on controversy. Many do not. Nursing educators who share the ethic of advocacy must ask how well the nursing curriculum prepares nurses to cope with the potential conflicts. They should also ask how an ethic that makes advocacy central avoids the risk of being *unduly* contentious.

5. *As advocate, the nurse is bound to be torn, at times, by conflicting interests and loyalties.* Metaphors can conceal as well as reveal facets of reality. The advocacy metaphor may hide the depths of potential conflicts by leaving the impression that only loyalty to the patient counts. But as Susan Thollaug, a nurse interested in patient advocacy, put it: "We can easily underestimate the difficulty of being a patient advocate, forgetting how divided our loyalties tend to be."[63] Patients come and go; the nurse's employing institution and professional colleagues tend to remain. To admit this is not merely to say that nurses may be tempted, along with other mortals, to place self-interest ahead of professional or moral obligations. The issue is more complicated morally. Most of us would acknowledge loyalty to associates as a virtue. An unwillingness to expose a colleague's shortcomings to public view and a desire to preserve confidence in one's institution are among the characteristic features of loyalty. Deeming such loyalty a vice would be a mistake likely to produce detrimental results for both the health care providers and their patients. The obvious difficulty is deciding when the role of advocacy must take precedence over the legitimate concerns of loyalty. Borderline cases, which bring us to the edges of our ability to reason morally, are inevitable. But no ethic of advocacy could be called adequate without a place for the virtue of loyalty.

These five concerns illustrate the impediments that must be overcome if nursing's new ethic of advocacy is to be most effective. But my discussion of these difficulties is in no way intended to suggest that nursing's adoption of advocacy is meaningless, undesirable, or impossible. I believe that nursing's change of images is a hopeful sign for a developing profession. Of course, no metaphor can convey fully the complexities of the profession's moral virtues and obligations. But the season for the nurse as advocate has arrived. Nursing is still a relatively new profession, and one that has often experienced the indignities of powerlessness. The language of advocacy provides a new way to express a growing sense of professional responsibility and power. Once an ethic of "good soldiers," with loyal obedience at its core, made sense to nurses. But nursing has been moving away from a heteronomous morality of constraint and toward a more autonomous morality of cooperation. An ethic of advocacy, with a concern for rights and the virtue of courage at its center, is an important development in this process of change.

NOTES

1. See, for example, Sheri Smith, "Three Models of the Nurse-Patient Relationship," in *Nursing: Images and Ideals*, Stuart F. Spicker and Sally Gadow, eds. (New York: Springer Publishing Company, 1980), pp. 176–88.

2. I am thinking of the work of George Lakoff and Mark Johnson, "Conceptual Metaphor in Everyday Language," *The Journal of Philosophy* 78 (August 1980), 453–86. See also the same authors' book, *Metaphors We Live By* (Chicago: University of Chicago Press, 1980).

3. Richard H. Shryock, *The History of Nursing* (Philadelphia: W. B. Saunders Company, 1959), pp. 273–84. For an interesting and recent discussion of Nightingale's work see Irene Palmer, "From Whence We Came," in *The Nursing Profession: A Time to Speak Out*, Norma L. Chaska, ed. (New York: McGraw-Hill Book Company, 1983), pp. 1–28.

4. Claire Fagin and Donna Diers, "Nursing as Metaphor," *The New England Journal of Medicine* 309 (July 14, 1983), 117.

5. Susan Sontag, *Illness as Metaphor* (New York: Farrar, Straus and Giroux, 1978). Sontag suggests that medicine adopted the military metaphor in the late nineteenth century about the time germ theory was accepted. My thoughts on medicine's use of the military metaphor have also been influenced by an unpublished paper by Virginia Warren, "Medicine as War," and by James Childress, *Who Should Decide? Paternalism in Health Care* (New York: Oxford University Press, 1982), p. 7.

6. Rashi Fein has recently complained that medicine is now being corrupted by "the language of the marketplace." "What Is Wrong with the Language of Medicine?" *The New England Journal of Medicine* 306 (April 8, 1982), 863–64.

7. Charlotte M. Perry, "Nursing Ethics and Etiquette," *The American Journal of Nursing* 6 (April 1906), 450–51.

8. Edward Francis Garsche, *Ethics and the Art of Conduct for Nurses* (Philadelphia: W. B. Saunders, 1929), p. 189.

9. Isabel Hampton Robb, *Nursing Ethics: For Hospital and Private Use* (Cleveland: E. C. Koeckert Publishing, 1900), p. 118.

10. Perry, "Nursing Ethics," p. 452.

11. T. Percy, C. Kirkpatrick, *Nursing Ethics* (Dublin: Dublin University Press, 1917), p. 24.

12. The Nightingale Pledge was first used by Farrand Training School, Harper Hospital, Detroit in 1893. For the text of the pledge, see Anne J. Davis and Mila A. Aroskar, *Ethical Dilemmas and Nursing Practice* (New York: Appleton-Century-Crofts, 1978), pp. 12–13.

13. Kirkpatrick, *Nursing Ethics*, p. 35.

14. Charlotte Albina Aikens, *Studies in Ethics for Nurses* (Philadelphia: W. B. Saunders Company, 1916), p. 44.

15. Thomas E. Satterthwaite, "Private Nurses and Nursing: With Recommendations for Their Betterment," *New York Medical Journal* 91 (January 15, 1910), 109.

16. Garesche, *Ethics and Conduct for Nurses*, p. 234.

17. Lena Dixon Dietz, *Professional Problems of Nurses*, 3rd. ed. rev. (Philadelphia: F. A. Davis Company, 1939), p. 165.

18. Sara E. Parsons, *Nursing Problems and Obligations* (Boston: Whitcomb and Barrows, 1916), p. 32. Parsons later allows for informing the patient about a mistake, after the patient has recovered sufficiently.

19. See for example Aikens, *Ethics for Nurses*, p. 297. See also S. H. Cabiniss, "Ethics," *The American Journal of Nursing* 3 (August 1903), 875–79. Cabiniss wrote: "What of the ingratitude . . . of physicians who accept all courtesy and loyalty and give none in return?" p. 878.

20. "Where Does Loyalty End?" (editorial) *The American Journal of Nursing* 10 (January 1910), 230–31.

21. "Where Does Loyalty to the Physician End?" (letters) *The American Journal of Nursing* 10 (January 1910), 274, 276.

22. Aikens, *Ethics for Nurses*, p. 192.

23. Dietz, *Professional Problems*, p. 162.

24. Susan Reverby, "Re-forming the Hospital Nurse: The Management of American Nursing," in *The Sociology of Health and Illness: Critical Perspectives*, Peter Conrad and Rochelle Kern, eds. (New York: St. Martin's Press, 1981), pp. 220–33. See also Jo Ann Ashley, *Hospitals, Paternalism, and the Role of the Nurse* (New York: Teachers College Press, 1976).

25. Satterthwaite, "Private Nurses," p. 109.

26. Aikens, *Ethics for Nurses*, p. 297.

27. Robb, *Nursing Ethics*, p. 250.

28. Parsons, *Nursing Problems*, p. 58.

29. L. I. Stein, "The Doctor-Nurse Game," *Archives of General Psychiatry* 16 (1967), 699–703. See also Sandra Weiss and Naomi Remen, "Self-Limiting Patterns of Nursing Behavior within a Tripartite Context Involving Consumers and Physicians," *Western Journal of Nursing Research* 5 (Winter 1983), 77–89.

30. Dietz, *Professional Problems*, p. 163.

31. Garesche, *Ethics and Conduct for Nurses*, p. 233.

32. Robb, *Nursing Ethics*, p. 251.

33. Kirkpatrick, *Nursing Ethics*, p. 24.

34. Annie Warburton Goodrich, *The Social Significance of Nursing* (New York: Macmillan, 1932), p. 167.

35. *Somera Case*, G. R. 31693 (Philippine Islands, 1929).

36. See, for example, Janine Fiesta, *The Law and Liability: A Guide for Nurses* (New York: John Wiley and Sons, 1983), p. 181.

37. For the entire text see "A Suggested Code," *The American Journal of Nursing* 26 (August 1926), 599–601.

38. See "A Tentative Code," *The American Journal of Nursing* 40 (September 1940), 977–80.

39. "A Code for Nurses," *The American Journal of Nursing* 50 (April 1950), 196.

40. "International Code of Nursing Ethics," *The American Journal of Nursing* 53 (September 1953), 1070.

41. Paul Starr, *The Social Transformation of American Medicine* (New York: Basic Books, 1982), pp. 379, 389.

42. George Annas, "The Patient Rights Advocate: Can Nurses Effectively Fill the Role?" *Supervisor Nurse* 5 (July 1974), 21–25. For another, similar work see George Annas and Joseph Healey, "The Patient Rights Advocate," *Journal of Nursing Administration* 4 (May–June 1974), 25–31.

43. Annas, "Patient Rights Advocate: Can Nurses Effectively Fill the Role?" p. 23.

44. Here is but a small sample: Jane E. Chapman and Harry Chapman, *Behavior and Health Care: A Humanistic Helping Process* (St. Louis: C. V. Mosby, 1975). This was one of the first works to set forth an "advocacy model" for health care delivery. Although it was not directed specifically to nurses, it had an obvious impact on subsequent nursing literature. M. Patricia Donahue, "The Nurse: A Patient Advocate?" *Nursing Forum* 17 (1978), 143–51. Corinne Sklar, "Patient's Advocate—A New Role for the Nurse?" *The Canadian Nurse* 75 (June 1979), 39–41. Mary Elizabeth Payne, "The Nurse as Patient Advocate in the Rehab Setting," *ARN* (The Official Journal of the Association of Rehabilitation Nurses) 4 (September–October 1979), 9–11. Mary Kohnke, "The Nurse as Advocate," *The American Journal of Nursing* 80 (November 1980), 2038–40. Ruth Purtilo and Christine Cassel, "Professionalism and Advocacy," in *Ethical Dimensions in the Health Professions* (Philadelphia: W. B. Saunders, 1981). Sally H. Durel, "Advocacy: A Function of the Community Mental Health Nurse," *Virginia Nurse* 49 (Spring 1981), 33–36. Marzena Laszewski, "Patient Advocacy in Primary Nursing," *Nursing Administration Quarterly* 5 (Summer 1981), 28–30. M. Josephine Flaherty, "This Nurse *Is* a Patient Advocate," *Nursing Management* 12 (September 1981), 12–13. George Castledine, "The Nurse as the Patient's Advocate: Pros and Cons," *Nursing Mirror* 153 (November 11, 1981), 38–40. H. Terri Brower, "Advocacy: What It Is," *Journal of Gerontological Nursing* 8 (March 1982), 141–43.

45. Payne, "The Nurse as Patient Advocate," p. 9.

46. Leah L. Curtin, "The Nurse as Advocate: A Philosophical Foundation for Nursing," *ANS* (Advances in Nursing Science) 1 (April 1979), 1–10. Sally Gadow, "Existential Advocacy: Philosophical Foundation of Nursing," in *Nursing: Images and Ideals*, pp. 79–101. Both authors wish to distinguish the concept of advocacy that they present as the philosophical basis for nursing from the concept of advocacy associated with the patient rights movement. But it is clear that most of their nursing colleagues who have written on the subject of advocacy have either failed to appreciate the distinction or rejected it.

47. M. Jo Namerow, "Integrating Advocacy into the Gerontological Nursing Major," *Journal of Gerontological Nursing* 8 (March 1982), 149–51.

48. International Council of Nurses, "Code for Nurses," reprinted in Davis and Aroskar, *Ethical Dilemmas*, pp. 13–14.

49. American Nurses' Association, *Code for Nurses with Interpretive Statements* (Kansas City: American Nurses' Association, 1976), p. 8.

50. Christine Spahn Smith, "Outrageous or Outraged: A Nurse Advocate Story," *Nursing Outlook* 28 (October 1980), 624–25.

51. See for example Flaherty, "This Nurse *Is* a Patient Advocate."

52. Of the many accounts of this case, the one I find most thorough and perceptive is in Purtilo and Cassel, *Ethical Dimensions*, pp. 126–137.

53. Jolene Tuma, Letter to the Editor, *Nursing Outlook* 25 (September 1977), 846.

54. *In re Tuma*. Supreme Court of the State of Idaho. 1977 Case 12587.

55. Purtilo and Cassel report this to be Tuma's position on the basis of personal communication. See *Ethical Dimensions*, p. 136.

56. Ronni Sandroff, "Protecting the M.D. or the Patient: Nursing's Unequivocal Answer," *RN* 44 (February 1981), 28–33.

57. I know of only one significant essay that is critical of nurses' adoption of the advocacy role: Natalie Abrams, "A Contrary View of the Nurse as Patient Advocate," *Nursing Forum* 17 (1978), 258–67. I have drawn on the thoughts in this essay in my discussion of the difficulties associated with the nurse as advocate.

58. Gadow, "Existential Advocacy," p. 85. In addition to this essay and the one by Curtin (note 46), a very helpful discussion appears in James L. Muyskens, *Moral Problems in Nursing: A Philosophical Investigation* (Totowa, NJ: Rowman and Littlefield, 1982).

59. For a helpful article on the developments in the states' nurse practice acts see Bonnie Bullough, "The Relationship of Nurse Practice Acts to the Professionalization of Nursing," in *The Nursing Profession: A Time to Speak*, pp. 609–633.

60. Patricia Murphy, "Deciding to Blow the Whistle," *The American Journal of Nursing* 81 (September 1981), 1691.

61. Sarah Archer and Patricia Goehner, *Speaking Out: The Views of Nurse Leaders* (New York: National League for Nursing, 1981).

62. See for example Linda Hughes, "The Public Image of the Nurse," *ANS* (Advances in Nursing Science) 2 (April 1980), 55–72.

63. Susan Thollaug, "The Nurse as Patient Advocate," *Imprint* 37 (December 1980), 37.

Patients' Rights

AMERICAN HOSPITAL ASSOCIATION

A Patient's Bill of Rights

The American Hospital Association presents a Patient's Bill of Rights with the expectation that observance of these rights will contribute to more effective patient care and greater satisfaction for the patient, his physician, and the hospital organization. Further, the Association presents these rights in the expectation that they will be supported by the hospital on behalf of its patients, as an integral part of the healing process. It is recognized that a personal relationship between the physician and the patient is essential for the provision of proper medical care. The traditional physician-patient relationship takes on a new dimension when care is rendered within an organizational structure. Legal precedent has established that the institution itself also has a responsibility to the patient. It is in recognition of these factors that these rights are affirmed.

1. The patient has the right to considerate and respectful care.

2. The patient has the right to obtain from his physician complete current information concerning his diagnosis, treatment, and prognosis in terms the patient can be reasonably expected to understand. When it is not medically advisable to give such information to the patient, the information should be made available to an appropriate person in his behalf. He has the right to know, by name, the physician responsible for coordinating his care.

3. The patient has the right to receive from his physician information necessary to give informed consent prior to the start of any procedure and/or treatment. Except in emergencies, such information for informed consent should include but not necessarily be limited to the specific procedure and/or treatment, the medically significant risks involved, and the probable duration of incapacitation. Where medically significant alternatives for care or treatment exist, or when the patient requests information concerning medical alternatives, the patient has the right to such information. The patient also has the right to know the name of the person responsible for the procedures and/or treatment.

4. The patient has the right to refuse treatment to the extent permitted by law and to be informed of the medical consequences of his action.

5. The patient has the right to every consideration of his privacy concerning his own medical care program. Case discussion, consultation, examination, and treatment are confidential and should be conducted discreetly. Those not directly involved in his care must have the permission of the patient to be present.

6. The patient has the right to expect that all communications and records pertaining to his care should be treated as confidential.

7. The patient has the right to expect that within its capacity a hospital must make reasonable response to the request of a patient for services. The hospital must provide evaluation, service, and/or referral as indicated by the urgency of the case. When medically permissible, a patient may be transferred to another facility only after he has received complete information and explanation concerning the needs for and alternatives to such a transfer. The institution to which the patient is to be transferred must first have accepted the patient for transfer.

8. The patient has the right to obtain information as to any relationship of his hospital to other health care and educational institutions insofar as his care is concerned. The patient has the right to obtain information as to the existence of any professional relationships among individuals, by name, who are treating him.

9. The patient has the right to be advised if the hospital proposes to engage in or perform human experimentation affecting his care or treatment. The patient has the right to refuse to participate in such research projects.

10. The patient has the right to expect reasonable continuity of care. He has the right to know in advance what appointment times and physicians are available and where. The patient has the right to expect that the hospital will provide a mechanism whereby he is informed by his physician or a delegate of the physician of the patient's continuing health care requirements following discharge.

11. The patient has the right to examine and receive an explanation of his bill regardless of source of payment.

12. The patient has the right to know what hospital rules and regulations apply to his conduct as a patient.

No catalog of rights can guarantee for the patient the kind of treatment he has a right to expect. A hospital has many functions to perform, including the prevention and treatment of disease, the education of both health professionals and patients, and the conduct of clinical research. All these activities must be conducted with an overriding concern for the patient, and, above all, the recognition of his dignity as a human being. Success in achieving this recognition assures success in the defense of the rights of the patient.

GEORGE J. ANNAS

The Emerging Stowaway:
Patients' Rights in the 1980s

At one point in Edgar Allan Poe's *Narrative of Arthur Gordon Pym of Nantucket*, Pym, who has stowed away in the hold of a whaling vessel, believes he has been abandoned and that the hold will be his tomb. He expressed sensations of "extreme horror and dismay," and "the most gloomy imaginings, in which the dreadful deaths of thirst, famine, suffocation, and premature interment, crowded in as the prominent disasters to be encountered."

It is probably uncommon for hospitalized patients to feel as gloomy as Pym. Nevertheless, installed in a strange institution, separated from friends and family, forced to wear a degrading costume, confined to bed, and attended to by a variety of strangers who may or may not keep the patient informed of what they are doing, the average patient is intimidated and disoriented. Such an environment encourages dependence and discourages the assertion of individual rights.

As the physician-director of Boston's Beth Israel Hospital has warned: "today's hospital stands increasingly to become a jungle, whose pathways to the uninitiated are poorly marked and fraught with danger. . . ."[1] In this jungle the notion that patients have rights that demand respect is often foreign.

The movement for enhanced patients' rights is based on two premises: (1) citizens possess certain rights that are not automatically forfeited by entering into a relationship with a physician or a health care facility; and (2) most physicians and health care facilities fail to recognize these rights, fail to provide for their protection or assertion, and limit their exercise without recourse.[2]

Reprinted by permission of the publisher from *Law, Medicine, and Health Care* 10 (February 1982), pp. 32–45, 46.

The primary argument against patients' rights is that patients have "needs" and that defining these needs in terms of rights leads to the creation of an unhealthy adversary relationship.[3] It is not, however, the creation of rights, but the disregard of them, that produces adversaries. When provider and patient work together in an atmosphere of mutual trust and understanding, the articulation of rights can only enhance their relationship.

Many issues, however, cannot be resolved entirely within the provider-patient relationship. Providers not only have formal relationships with their patients but also have relationships with other providers, health care institutions, and numerous governmental agencies. A provider's relationship with these institutions and individuals is often a very complex one, and providers often find themselves confused and therefore submissive in cases where they do not understand their own rights or those of their patients.

RIGHTS IN HEALTH CARE

In most instances, both the health care provider *and* the patient will be better off if the status of the law regarding both patient *and* provider rights is understood, and the means of change or challenge well delineated.[4] I would go even further. An understanding of the law can be as important to the proper care of patients as an understanding of emergency medical procedures or proper drug dosages. But how are rights to be understood, and how does a person know that he or she has a "right" to something?

There is a formidable amount of literature on rights in the archives of philosophy and jurisprudence. Rather than review it, let me note briefly the thoughts of two relatively recent entrants who have written with great insight. The first is John Rawls. In expounding his *Theory of Justice*,[5] he imagines that a group of men and women come together to form a social contract. These individuals all have ordinary tastes, talents, ambitions, and convictions, but each is temporarily unaware of his own personality and best interests and must agree to the terms of the contract before his awareness of his own identity is restored. The theory postulates that under such circumstances all will agree to two principles: (1) each person shall enjoy the most extensive liberty, compatible with a like liberty for others; and (2) inequalities in wealth and power should exist only where they work to the benefit of the worst-off members of society. One could develop an entire system of patients' rights that rests on these premises. Such a document would be strongly pro-patient since this group is currently the one that generally lacks rights and is always the group that will be viewed as "worst-off" in the health care setting.

A second approach is suggested by the writings of Ronald Dworkin in his book of essays *Taking Rights Seriously*.[6] Dworkin notes the great confusion in "rights language," generally created by attributing to it different meanings in different contexts: "In most cases when we say that someone has a right to something, we imply that it would be wrong to interfere with his doing it, or at least that some special grounds are needed for justifying an interference." An example is the right to spend one's money the way one pleases. This is, of course, different from saying that the way one spends one's money, *e.g.*, gambling it away, is the "right" thing to do, or that there is nothing "wrong" with it. When we speak of patients' rights, this distinction may be critical to understanding what we are talking about. For example, a woman may have a legal right to have an abortion, but such a decision may still be considered "wrong" by her.

Dworkin argues further that there are some rights that can be said to be fundamental in the sense that the government is bound to recognize and protect them. Such rights, which we often denote as "legal rights," and less frequently as "constitutional rights," are generally spelled out in statutes and court decisions. By respecting such rights, the government guarantees to the weakest members of the society that they will not be trampled on by the strongest. In Dworkin's words:

The bulk of the law—that part which defines and implements social, economic, and foreign policy—cannot be neutral. It must state, in its greatest part, the majority's view of the common good. The institution of rights is therefore crucial, because it represents the majority's promise to the minorities that their dignity and equality will be respected. When the divisions among the groups are most violent, then this gesture, if law is to work, must be most sincere . . . taking individual rights seriously is the one feature that distinguishes law from ordered brutality.[7]

Without going too far afield, one can apply Dworkin's notion directly to health care and note that rights can form a useful means of guaranteeing to defenseless patients that they will be treated with human dignity and respect. While the health care provider often has the power to deny certain rights almost at will, he or she does this only at the peril of jeopardizing the integrity of the health care system itself.

THE AHA BILL OF RIGHTS

It must strike most as ironic that the first major health care organization to put forward a patients' bill of rights was the American Hospital Association, an organization composed primarily of hospital administrators. One would not expect landlords to pen a bill of rights for tenants, police for suspects, or wardens for prisoners. Nor would one reasonably expect that the hospital administrator's view on rights for patients would be the same as either the patient's or society's. Nevertheless, physicians and nurses should be ashamed that the administrators were out in front on this issue. Even though it leaves much to be desired in terms of completeness, specificity, and enforceability the AHA Bill has tremendous symbolic value in legitimizing the notion of rights in the health care institution.[8] On the other hand, fewer than half of all AHA-member hospitals have formally adopted even this bill, and the symbolic victory of the 1970s is currently under attack.

THE ATTACK ON PATIENT RIGHTS

Physicians, who perhaps value their own professional autonomy more than any other group, nevertheless devalue it for their own patients. Instead, paternalism is the norm with the majority of physicians who believe that the health and continued life of their patients is much more important than their patients' right to self-determination. This belief system not only leads to conflicts with individual patients about their own care, but also to a general view that patients' rights are a luxury item in medicine rather than a necessity.

A few examples illustrate the point. Two particular rights of patients have recently come under attack in the medical literature: access to medical records and informed consent. In an attack on "record reading," four psychiatrists at Peter Bent Brigham Hospital in Boston, Massachusetts, interviewed the 11 out of 2,500 patients at that hospital who, in a one year period, asked to see their medical records.[9] It is doubtful that anything of general importance about a patient's reactions to reading their charts can be learned from an uncontrolled, non-blind, clinically impressionistic study of those few individuals who, for whatever reason, buck a system which routinely fails to inform them of their right of access to their records. Nonetheless, the authors' conclusion that such patients have a variety of personality defects, usually manifesting themselves in mistrust of and hostility toward the hospital staff, should not be permitted to go uncontested. In a setting where trusting patients are not routinely told of their right to access, it seems reasonable to assume that only the least trusting or most angry will ask to see their records. To locate the source of mistrust in the patient's personality or in the stress of illness and hospitalization is to forget, as Dr. Lipsett perceptively suggests, that "the doctor-patient relationship cannot be understood simply in terms of the patient's side of the equation."[10] Altman, et al., thus fall into what Professor Robert Burt, of Yale Law School, has referred to as "the conceptual trap of attempting to transform two-party relationships, in which mutual self-delineations are inherently confused and intertwined, by conceptually obliterating one party. . . ."[11] Thus, it would seem that the ten women who asked to read their charts "to confirm the belief that the staff harbored negative personal attitudes toward them . . ." were correct in their belief; the psychiatrists labelled them "of the hysterical type with demanding, histrionic behavior and emotional over-involvement with the staff."

Altman, et al., also seem unaware of the wide variety of settings in which patients have *benefitted* from routine record access; and incorrectly assert that there were no strikingly beneficial effects in the two studies they do cite. In the first study, for example, two patients expressed their unfounded fear that they had cancer only after their records were reviewed with them, and one pregnant patient noted an incorrect Rh typing that permitted Rho-Gam to be administered at the time of delivery.[12] In the other study they cite, 50 percent of the patients made some factual correction in their records.[13]

In short, the study seems to have been done and published for the primary purpose of proving that the right to access one's medical record is unimportant since it is only exercised by "mentally disturbed" people who are not improved by reading their charts. The study fails to prove this, and even if it succeeded, I would still be unwilling to deprive the other 2,489 patients at that hospital of their right to access in the future.

If we believe in individual freedom and the concept of self-determination, we must give all citizens the right to make their *own* decisions and to have access to the same information that is widely available to those making decisions about them. It is as irrelevant in this connection that 2,489 patients at the Brigham did not ask to see their records as it is that more than 200 million Americans never have had to exercise their right to remain silent when arrested. Rights serve us all, whether we exercise them or not.

The attack on informed consent, which many physicians have long considered a "legal fiction,"[14] more recently surfaced in a study designed to prove that informed consent was not an important practice because patients could not remember what they were informed of.[15] The methodology involved interviewing 200 consecutive cancer patients who had consented to chemotherapy, surgery, or radiation therapy for their cancers within 24 hours after they had signed consent forms. Upon questioning, most could not recall the procedure consented to, its major risks, or the alternatives to it. From this the authors conclude that the process is not working and that informed consent itself is suspect. While this may seem a reasonable conclusion (although an alternative one is simply that patients have poor recall), it turns out that the authors presumed their major premise. Approximately two-thirds of their sample group (66 percent) opted for radiation therapy. That group signed a consent form that said "the procedure, its risks and benefits and alternatives have been explained to me." Maybe they were, but maybe they weren't. The authors did not know, so their entire study was based on a premise that was unsubstantiated. Such a poorly designed study, it seems to me, could only be published if the editors agreed so strongly with the conclusion that they did not even review the methodology.

A perhaps more interesting part of the study asked the patients some general questions about informed consent. The first was "What are consent forms for?" Approximately 80 percent responded: "To protect the physicians' rights." The authors were upset at this response, but the patients, of course, were correct. That *is* the primary function of *forms*. If one wants these forms also to protect the patient, three simple steps are necessary: (1) the forms must be complete; (2) they must be in lay language; and (3) the patients must be given a copy of the form and time to think over the information it contains.[16] The reason none of these is usually done is clear: informed consent is not taken seriously in the hospital setting. It is, like a record access, a luxury which is secondary to caring for the medical "needs" of the patient, and besides, it really does not matter anyway because patients cannot remember anything they've been told.

Other significant findings indicate the extent to which patients understand and appreciate the consent process: 80 percent thought the forms were necessary; 76 percent thought they contained just the right amount of information; 84 percent understood all or most of the information; 75 percent thought the explanations given were important; and 90 percent said they would try to remember the information contained on the forms. To me, this suggests that the patients surveyed understood and appreciated the informed consent process much better than the researchers did. While their data is certainly not flawless, one can conclude from it just the opposite of what the researchers did: for almost all patients, informed consent is very important.

Related to this general attack on rights is an attack on the patient population itself. The notion is that the major problems with the health care delivery system are not problems with providers, but with patients. We eat too much, smoke too much, don't exercise, take too many risks, etc., and so what do we expect when we get sick? Not only must the American health care enterprise deal with a bad class of patients, but now they want some say in what kind of care is provided! As Lewis Thomas has put it in a related vein: this is becoming "folk doctrine about disease. You become ill because of not living right. If you get cancer it is, somehow or other, your own fault. If you didn't cause it by smoking or drinking, or eating the wrong things, it came from allowing yourself to persist with the wrong kind of personality in the wrong environment."[17]

This attitude would be humorous if it was not so pervasive and did not affect patient care so profoundly. Martha Lear has given us some excellent and telling examples in her deeply moving book, *Heartsounds*, that chronicles the final four years of life of her physician-husband who goes through eight operations and

eleven hospitalizations during that period. Together they identify the "it's your fault ploy" which means that no matter what goes wrong in the hospital setting, it is the fault of the patient, not the health care system:

> Why did the operation take so long?
> Because you lost so much blood.
> *Not:* Because the surgeon blew it.
> Why do you keep making these tests?
> Because you have a very stubborn infection.
> *Not:* Because I can't diagnose your case.
> Why did I get sick again?
> Because you were very weak.
> *Not:* Because I did not treat you competently the first time.[18]

Dr. Lear is constantly asking himself if he treated patients that way, and usually admits that he did. He suggests that every physician be required to spend at least a week per year in a hospital bed: "That would change some things in a hurry."

AN AGENDA FOR THE '80s

Since patients *do* have rights and *do* want to exercise them, and since the major attacks on the notion of patients' rights have been based on sloppy studies and false premises, the patients' rights movement is likely to gain momentum. Indeed, the 1970s can be most properly viewed as a decade in which the existence of patients' rights became legitimized through basic education of the health care providers. I suggest that the 1980s will be a decade in which the primary thrust will be working on ways to directly enhance the status of patients in the hospital as a means of humanizing the hospital environment so that patients can have a greater voice in how they are treated.

I suggest the following five point "agenda for the '80s:"

Patients' Rights Agenda

1. No Routine Procedures
2. Open Access to Medical Records
3. Twenty-Four-Hour-a-Day Visitor Rights
4. Full Experience Disclosure
5. Effective Patient Advocate

1. *No Routine Procedures:* It is all too common for nurses and others to respond to the question, "Why is this being done?" with, "Don't worry, it's routine." This should not be an acceptable response. No procedure should *ever* be performed on a patient because it is routine; it should only be performed if it is *specifi-*

cally indicated for that patient. Thus routine admission tests, routine use of johnnies, routine use of wheelchairs for in-hospital transportation, routine use of sleeping pills, to name a few notable examples, should be abolished. Use of these procedures means patients are treated as fungible robots rather than as individual human beings. Moreover, these procedures are often demeaning and unnecessary.

2. *Open Access to Medical Records:* While currently provided for by federal law and many state statutes and regulations, open access to medical records by patients remains difficult, and a patient often asserts his right to see his record at the peril of being labeled "distrustful" or a "troublemaker." The information in the hospital chart is about the patient and properly belongs to the patient. The patient must have access to it, both to enhance his own decision-making ability and to make it clear that the hospital is an "open" institution that is not trying to hide things from the patient. Surely if hospital personnel make decisions about the patient on the basis of information in the chart, the patient also deserves access to the information.

3. *Twenty-Four-Hour-a-Day Visitor Rights:* One of the most important ways both to humanize the hospital and to enhance patient autonomy is to assure the patient that at least one person of his choice has unlimited access to him or her at any time of the day or night. This person should also be permitted to stay with the patient during any procedure (*e.g.*, childbirth or induction of anesthesia) so long as the person does not interfere with the care of other patients.

4. *Full Experience Disclosure:* The most important gain of the past decade has been the almost universal acknowledgement of the need for the patient's informed consent. Nevertheless, some information that is material to the patient's decision is still withheld: the experience of the person doing the procedure.[19] Patients have a right to know if the person asking permission to draw blood, take blood gases, do a bone marrow aspiration, or do a spinal tap has ever performed the procedure before, and if so, what the person's complication rate is. This applies not only to medical students and student nurses, but also to board certified surgeons—we all do things for the first time, and not every patient wants to take such an active role in our education.

5. *An Effective Patient Advocate:* While a patients' bill of rights is necessary, it is not sufficient. Rights are not self-actualizing. Patients are sick and desire relief from pain and discomfort more than they demonstrate

a desire to exercise their rights; they are also anxious, and may hold back complaints for fear of retaliation. It is critical that patients have access to a person whose job it is to work *for the patient* to help the patient exercise the rights outlined in the institution's bill of rights. This person should sit in on all major hospital committees that deal with patient care, have authority to obtain medical records for patients, call consultants, launch complaints directly with all members of the hospital, medical, nursing, and administrative staff, and be able to delay discharges. While there appear to be some successful "patient representatives" that are hired by the hospitals, it is not fair to give them this title since they must represent their employer—the hospital. It is likely that ultimately effective representation can only be obtained by someone who is hired by a consumer group or governmental agency outside the hospital in which the representative works.

CONCLUSION

We have made a beginning in the long journey toward humanizing the hospital and promoting patients' self-determination. But more specific measures are needed before patients will be assured that they can effectively exercise their rights in institutional settings.

Like Poe's Arthur Gordon Pym, the notion that patients have rights has survived the days of darkness, isolation, and starvation. Patients' rights are now generally accepted (although sporadically attacked) and it is up to patients and providers alike to see to it that these rights become a reality for every citizen.

NOTES

1. Rabkin, M., *quoted in* Annas, G. J., *The Hospital: A Patient Rights Wasteland*. CIVIL LIBERTIES REVIEW (Fall 1974) at 11.

2. *See generally* G. J. Annas, *The Rights of Hospital Patients* (Avon Books, New York) (1975).

3. Margolis, E. G., *Conceptual Aspects of a Patient's Bill of Rights*, CONNECTICUT MEDICINE SUPPLEMENT 43:9 (October 1979). *See also* Ladd, *Legalism and Medical Ethics*, in Davis, Hoffmaster, Shorten, eds., CONTEMPORARY ISSUES IN BIOMEDICAL ETHICS (Humana Press, New Jersey) (1978).

4. Examples of patient abuse based on providers' misunderstandings of the law after the *Saikewicz* case in Massachusetts are cited in Annas, G. J., *Reconciling* Quinlan *and* Saikewicz: *Decision Making for the Terminally Ill Incompetent*, AMERICAN JOURNAL OF LAW & MEDICINE 4(4):367, 387 (Winter 1979).

5. J. Rawls, *A Theory of Justice* (Harvard Univ. Press, Cambridge, Mass.) (1971).

6. R. Dworkin, *Taking Rights Seriously* (Harvard Univ. Press, Cambridge, Mass.) (1977).

7. *Id.* at 205.

8. Reprinted in Annas, *supra* note 1, at 25–27.

9. Altman, J. H., *et al.*, *Patients Who See Their Medical Record*, NEW ENGLAND JOURNAL OF MEDICINE 302(3):169 (January 17, 1980).

10. Lipsett, D., *Editorial*, NEW ENGLAND JOURNAL OF MEDICINE 302(3):167 (January 17, 1980).

11. R. Burt, *Taking Care of Strangers: The Rule of Law in Doctor-Patient Relations* (Free Press, New York) (1979) at 43.

12. Stevens, D. P., Stagg, R., MacKay, I., *What Happens When Hospitalized Patients See Their Own Records*, ANNALS OF INTERNAL MEDICINE 86:474, 476 (1977). For a more complete discussion of this issue, including additional studies of patients given routine access to their records, *see* G. J. Annas, L. H. Glantz, B. F. Katz, *The Rights of Doctors, Nurses and Allied Health Professionals* (Avon Books, New York) (1981) at 159–61.

13. Golodetz, A., Ruess, J., Milhous, R., *The Right to Know: Giving the Patient His Medical Record*, ARCHIVES OF PHYSICAL MEDICINE AND REHABILITATION 57:78, 80 (1976). Experience under the new record access regulation enacted by the Massachusetts Board of Registration in Medicine indicates that patients want access to their records for a variety of reasons. In the period from October 13, 1978 (when the regulation went into effect) to January 31, 1980, the Board received more phone calls from consumers asking about the medical records regulation (approximately ten per month) than about any other single issue dealt with by the Board. There were also 33 formal complaints filed concerning record access during this period. Of this number, almost half (16) needed help from the Board to get their physician to forward a copy of their records directly to another physician. Of the remaining 17, six needed information for insurance purposes, six wanted to personally review the records for various reasons, one alleged negligence, one wanted the record sent to a school nurse, one was moving to another state, one wanted a second opinion, and one wanted her contact lens prescription. (Statistics compiled by Judy Miller, a student at Boston College Law School.)

14. *See, e.g.*, Laforet, E. G., *The Fiction of Informed Consent*, JOURNAL OF THE AMERICAN MEDICAL ASSOCIATION 235:1579 (April 12, 1976).

15. Cassileth, B. R., *et al.*, *Informed Consent—Why Are Its Goals Imperfectly Realized?* NEW ENGLAND JOURNAL OF MEDICINE 302(16):896 (April 17, 1980).

16. *See generally* chapter on *Informed Consent* in G. J. Annas, L. H. Glantz, B. F. Katz, THE RIGHTS OF DOCTORS, NURSES AND ALLIED HEALTH PROFESSIONALS (Avon Books, New York) (1981); and G. J. Annas, L. H. Glantz, B. F. Katz, *Informed Consent to Human Experimentation: The Subject's Dilemma* (Ballinger, Cambridge, Mass.) (1977). *See also* Rennie, D., *Informed Consent by "Well-Nigh Abject" Adults*. NEW ENGLAND JOURNAL OF MEDICINE 302(16):916 (April 17, 1980). "I suggest that the physician accept far more than simply the duty to improve consent forms. . . . They should accept education of the patient through the process of consent as a worthwhile therapeutic goal. To deny the possibility of informed consent is to ensure that it will never be achieved—an attitude that is immoral and . . . illegal." *Id.* at 918.

17. Thomas, L., *On Magic in Medicine*, NEW ENGLAND JOURNAL OF MEDICINE 299:461, 462 (August 31, 1978).

18. M. L. Lear, *Heartsounds* (Simon & Schuster, New York) (1980) at 47.

19. Annas, G. J., *The Care of Private Patients in Teaching Hospitals: Legal Implications*, BULLETIN OF NEW YORK ACADEMY OF MEDICINE 56(4):403–11 (May 1980).

PAUL CHODOFF

The Case for Involuntary Hospitalization of the Mentally Ill

I will begin this paper with a series of vignettes designed to illustrate graphically the question that is my focus: under what conditions, if any, does society have the right to apply coercion to an individual to hospitalize him against his will, by reason of mental illness?

Case 1. A woman in her mid 50s, with no previous overt behavioral difficulties, comes to believe that she is worthless and insignificant. She is completely preoccupied with her guilt and is increasingly unavailable for the ordinary demands of life. She eats very little because of her conviction that the food should go to others whose need is greater than hers, and her physical condition progressively deteriorates. Although she will talk to others about herself, she insists that she is not sick, only bad. She refuses medication, and when hospitalization is suggested she also refuses that on the grounds that she would be taking up space that otherwise could be occupied by those who merit treatment more than she.

Case 2. For the past 6 years the behavior of a 42-year-old woman has been disturbed for periods of 3 months or longer. After recovery from her most recent episode she has been at home, functioning at a borderline level. A month ago she again started to withdraw from her environment. She pays increasingly less attention to her bodily needs, talks very little, and does not respond to questions or attention from those about her. She lapses into a mute state and lies in her bed in a totally passive fashion. She does not respond to other people, does not eat, and does not void. When her arm is raised from the bed it remains for several

minutes in the position in which it is left. Her medical history and a physical examination reveal no evidence of primary physical illness.

Case 3. A man with a history of alcoholism has been on a binge for several weeks. He remains at home doing little else than drinking. He eats very little. He becomes tremulous and misinterprets spots on the wall as animals about to attack him, and he complains of "creeping" sensations in his body, which he attributes to infestation by insects. He does not seek help voluntarily, insists there is nothing wrong with him, and despite his wife's entreaties he continues to drink.

Case 4. Passersby and station personnel observe that a young woman has been spending several days at Union Station in Washington, D.C. Her behavior appears strange to others. She is finally befriended by a newspaper reporter who becomes aware that her perception of her situation is profoundly unrealistic and that she is, in fact, delusional. He persuades her to accompany him to St. Elizabeths Hospital, where she is examined by a psychiatrist who recommends admission. She refuses hospitalization and the psychiatrist allows her to leave. She returns to Union Station. A few days later she is found dead, murdered, on one of the surrounding streets.

Case 5. A government attorney in his late 30s begins to display pressured speech and hyperactivity. He is too busy to sleep and eats very little. He talks rapidly, becomes irritable when interrupted, and makes phone calls all over the country in furtherance of his political ambitions, which are to begin a campaign for the Presidency of the United States. He makes many purchases, some very expensive, thus running through

Reprinted with permission of the author and the publisher from *American Journal of Psychiatry*, Vol. 133, No. 5 (May 1976), pp. 496–501. Copyright 1976, the American Psychiatric Association.

a great deal of money. He is rude and tactless to his friends, who are offended by his behavior, and his job is in jeopardy. In spite of his wife's pleas he insists that he does not have the time to seek or accept treatment, and he refuses hospitalization. This is not the first such disturbance for this individual; in fact, very similar episodes have been occurring at roughly 2-year intervals since he was 18 years old.

Case 6. Passersby in a campus area observe two young women standing together, staring at each other, for over an hour. Their behavior attracts attention, and eventually the police take the pair to a nearby precinct station for questioning. They refuse to answer questions and sit mutely, staring into space. The police request some type of psychiatric examination but are informed by the city attorney's office that state law (Michigan) allows persons to be held for observation only if they appear obviously dangerous to themselves or others. In this case, since the women do not seem homicidal or suicidal, they do not qualify for observation and are released.

Less than 30 hours later the two women are found on the floor of their campus apartment, screaming and writhing in pain with their clothes ablaze from a self-made pyre. One woman recovers; the other dies. There is no conclusive evidence that drugs were involved.[1]

Most, if not all, people would agree that the behavior described in these vignettes deviates significantly from even elastic definitions of normality. However, it is clear that there would not be a similar consensus on how to react to this kind of behavior and that there is a considerable and increasing ferment about what attitude the organized elements of our society should take toward such individuals. Everyone has a stake in this important issue, but the debate about it takes place principally among psychiatrists, lawyers, the courts, and law enforcement agencies.

Points of view about the question of involuntary hospitalization fall into the following three principal groups: the "abolitionists," medical model psychiatrists, and civil liberties lawyers.

THE ABOLITIONISTS

Those holding this position would assert that in none of the cases I have described should involuntary hospitalization be a viable option because, quite simply, it should never be resorted to under any circumstances. As Szasz[2] has put it, "we should value liberty more

highly than mental health no matter how defined" and "no one should be deprived of his freedom for the sake of his mental health." Ennis[3] has said that the goal "is nothing less than the abolition of involuntary hospitalization."

Prominent among the abolitionists are the "antipsychiatrists,"who, somewhat surprisingly, count in their ranks a number of well-known psychiatrists. For them mental illness simply does not exist in the field of psychiatry.[4] They reject entirely the medical model of mental illness and insist that acceptance of it relies on a fiction accepted jointly by the state and by psychiatrists as a device for exerting social control over annoying or unconventional people. The anti-psychiatrists hold that these people ought to be afforded the dignity of being held responsible for their behavior and required to accept its consequences. In addition, some members of this group believe that the phenomena of "mental illness" often represent essentially a tortured protest against the insanities of an irrational society.[5] They maintain that society should not be encouraged in its oppressive course by affixing a pejorative label to its victims.

Among the abolitionists are some civil liberties lawyers who both assert their passionate support of the magisterial importance of individual liberty and react with repugnance and impatience to what they see as the abuses of psychiatric practice in this field—the commitment of some individuals for flimsy and possibly self-serving reasons and their inhuman warehousing in penal institutions wrongly called "hospitals."

The abolitionists do not oppose psychiatric treatment when it is conducted with the agreement of those being treated. I have no doubt that they would try to gain the consent of the individuals described earlier to undergo treatment, including hospitalization. The psychiatrists in this group would be very likely to confine their treatment methods to psychotherapeutic efforts to influence the aberrant behavior. They would be unlikely to use drugs and would certainly eschew such somatic therapies as ECT*. If efforts to enlist voluntary compliance with treatment failed, the abolitionists would not employ any means of coercion. Instead, they would step aside and allow social, legal, and community sanctions to take their course. If a human being should be jailed or a human life lost as a result of this attitude, they would accept it as a necessary evil to be tolerated in order to avoid the greater evil of unjustified loss of liberty for others.[6]

*Ed. note: Electroconvulsive therapy.

I use this admittedly awkward and not entirely accurate label to designate the position of a substantial number of psychiatrists. They believe that mental illness is a meaningful concept and that under certain conditions its existence justifies the state's exercise, under the doctrine of *parens patriae*, of its right and obligation to arrange for the hospitalization of the sick individual even though coercion is involved and he is deprived of his liberty. I believe that these psychiatrists would recommend involuntary hospitalization for all six of the patients described earlier.

THE MEDICAL MODEL

There was a time, before they were considered to be ill, when individuals who displayed the kind of behavior I described earlier were put in "ships of fools" to wander the seas or were left to the mercies, sometimes tender but often savage, of uncomprehending communities that regarded them as either possessed or bad. During the Enlightenment and the early nineteenth century, however, these individuals gradually came to be regarded as sick people to be included under the humane and caring umbrella of the Judeo-Christian attitude toward illness. This attitude, which may have reached its height during the era of moral treatment in the early nineteenth century, has had unexpected and ambiguous consequences. It became overextended and partially perverted, and these excesses led to the reaction that is so strong a current in today's attitude toward mental illness.

However, reaction itself can go too far, and I believe that this is already happening. Witness the disastrous consequences of the precipitate dehospitalization that is occurring all over the country. To remove the protective mantle of illness from these disturbed people is to expose them, their families, and their communities to consequences that are certainly maladaptive and possibly irreparable. Are we really acting in accordance with their best interests when we allow them to "die with their rights on"[1] or when we condemn them to a "preservation of liberty which is actually so destructive as to constitute another form of imprisonment"[7]? Will they not suffer "if [a] liberty they cannot enjoy is made superior to a health that must sometimes be forced on them"?[8]

Many of those who reject the medical model out of hand as inapplicable to so-called "mental illness" have tended to oversimplify its meaning and have, in fact, equated it almost entirely with organic disease. It is necessary to recognize that it is a complex concept and that there is a lack of agreement about its meaning. Sophisticated definitions of the medical model do not require only the demonstration of unequivocal organic pathology. A broader formulation, put forward by sociologists and deriving largely from Talcott Parsons' description of the sick role,[9] extends the domain of illness to encompass certain forms of social deviance as well as biological disorders. According to this definition, the medical model is characterized not only by organicity but also by being negatively valued by society, by "non-voluntariness," thus exempting its exemplars from blame, and by the understanding that physicians are the technically competent experts to deal with its effects.[10]

Except for the question of organic disease, the patients I described earlier conform well to this broader conception of the medical model. They are all suffering both emotionally and physically, they are incapable by an effort of will of stopping or changing their destructive behavior, and those around them consider them to be in an undesirable sick state and to require medical attention.

Categorizing the behavior of these patients as involuntary may be criticized as evidence of an intolerably paternalistic and antitherapeutic attitude that fosters the very failure to take responsibility for their lives and behavior that the therapist should uncover rather than encourage. However, it must also be acknowledged that these severely ill people are not capable at a conscious level of deciding what is best for themselves and that in order to help them examine their behavior and motivation, it is necessary that they be alive and available for treatment. Their verbal message that they will not accept treatment may at the same time be conveying other more covert messages—that they are desperate and want help even though they cannot ask for it.[11]

Although organic pathology may not be the only determinant of the medical model, it is of course an important one and it should not be avoided in any discussion of mental illness. There would be no question that the previously described patient with delirium tremens is suffering from a toxic form of brain disease. There are a significant number of other patients who require involuntary hospitalization because of organic brain syndrome due to various causes. Among those who are not overtly organically ill, most of the candidates for involuntary hospitalization suffer from schizophrenia or one of the major affective disorders. A growing and increasingly impressive body of evidence points to the presence of an important genetic-biological factor in these conditions; thus, many of them qualify on these grounds as illnesses.

Despite the revisionist efforts of the anti-psychiatrists, mental illness *does* exist. It does not by any means include all of the people being treated by psychiatrists (or by nonpsychiatrist physicians), but it does encompass those few desperately sick people for whom involuntary commitment must be considered. In the words of a recent article, "The problem is that mental illness is not a myth. It is not some palpable falsehood propagated among the populace by power-mad psychiatrists, but a cruel and bitter reality that has been with the human race since antiquity."[12]

CRITERIA FOR INVOLUNTARY HOSPITALIZATION

Procedures for involuntary hospitalization should be instituted for individuals who require care and treatment because of diagnosable mental illness that produces symptoms, including marked impairment in judgment, that disrupt their intrapsychic and interpersonal functioning. All three of these criteria must be met before involuntary hospitalization can be instituted.

1. Mental Illness. This concept has already been discussed, but it should be repeated that only a belief in the existence of illness justifies involuntary commitment. It is a fundamental assumption that makes aberrant behavior a medical matter and its care the concern of physicians.

2. Disruption of Functioning. This involves combinations of serious and often obvious disturbances that are both intrapsychic (for example, the suffering of severe depression) and interpersonal (for example, withdrawal from others because of depression). It does not include minor peccadilloes or eccentricities. Furthermore, the behavior in question must represent symptoms of the mental illness from which the patient is suffering. Among these symptoms are actions that are imminently or potentially dangerous in a physical sense to self or others, as well as other manifestations of mental illness such as those in the cases I have described. This is not to ignore dangerousness as a criterion for commitment but rather to put it in its proper place as one of a number of symptoms of the illness. A further manifestation of the illness, and indeed, the one that makes involuntary rather than

voluntary hospitalization necessary, is impairment of the patient's judgment to such a degree that he is unable to consider his condition and make decisions about it in his own interests.

3. Need for Care and Treatment. The goal of physicians is to treat and cure their patients; however, sometimes they can only ameliorate the suffering of their patients and sometimes all they can offer is care. It is not possible to predict whether someone will respond to treatment; nevertheless, the need for treatment and the availability of facilities to carry it out constitute essential preconditions that must be met to justify requiring anyone to give up his freedom. If mental hospital patients have a right to treatment, then psychiatrists have a right to ask for treatability as a front-door as well as a back-door criterion for commitment.[7] All of the six individuals I described earlier could have been treated with a reasonable expectation of return to a more normal state of functioning.

I believe that the objections to this formulation can be summarized as follows:

1. The whole structure founders for those who maintain that mental illness is a fiction.

2. These criteria are also untenable to those who hold liberty to be such a supreme value that the presence of mental illness per se does not constitute justification for depriving an individual of his freedom; only when such illness is manifested by clearly dangerous behavior may commitment be considered. For reasons to be discussed later, I agree with those psychiatrists[13,14] who do not believe that dangerousness should be elevated to primacy above other manifestations of mental illness as a *sine qua non* for involuntary hospitalization.

3. The medical model criteria are "soft" and subjective and depend on the fallible judgment of psychiatrists. This is a valid objection. There is no reliable blood test for schizophrenia and no method for injecting grey cells into psychiatrists. A relatively small number of cases will always fall within a grey area that will be difficult to judge. In those extreme cases in which the question of commitment arises, competent and ethical psychiatrists should be able to use these criteria without doing violence to individual liberties and with the expectation of good results. Furthermore, the possible "fuzziness" of some aspects of the medical model approach is certainly no greater than that of the supposedly "objective" criteria for dangerousness, and there is little reason to believe that lawyers and judges are any less fallible than psychiatrists.

4. Commitment procedures in the hands of psychiatrists are subject to intolerable abuses. Here, as Peszke said, "It is imperative that we differentiate between the principle of the process of civil commitment and the practice itself."[13] Abuses can contaminate both the medical and the dangerousness approaches, and I believe that the abuses stemming from the abolitionist view of no commitment at all are even greater. Measures to abate abuses of the medical approach include judicial review and the abandonment of indeterminate commitment. In the course of commitment proceedings and thereafter, patients should have access to competent and compassionate legal counsel. However, this latter safeguard may itself be subject to abuse if the legal counsel acts solely in the adversary tradition and undertakes to carry out the patient's wishes even when they may be destructive.

COMMENT

The criteria and procedures outlined will apply most appropriately to initial episodes and recurrent attacks of mental illness. To put it simply, it is necessary to find a way to satisfy legal and humanitarian considerations and yet allow psychiatrists access to initially or acutely ill patients in order to do the best they can for them. However, there are some involuntary patients who have received adequate and active treatment but have not responded satisfactorily. An irreducible minimum of such cases, principally among those with brain disorders and process schizophrenia, will not improve sufficiently to be able to adapt to even a tolerant society.

The decision of what to do at this point is not an easy one, and it should certainly not be in the hands of psychiatrists alone. With some justification they can state that they have been given the thankless job of caring, often with inadequate facilities, for badly damaged people and that they are now being subjected to criticism for keeping these patients locked up. No one really knows what to do with these patients. It may be that when treatment has failed they exchange their sick role for what has been called the impaired role,[15] which implies a permanent negative evaluation of them coupled with a somewhat less benign societal attitude. At this point, perhaps a case can be made for giving greater importance to the criteria for dangerousness and releasing such patients if they do not pose a threat to others. However, I do not believe that the release into the community of these severely malfunctioning individuals will serve their interests even though it may satisfy formal notions of right and wrong.

It should be emphasized that the number of individuals for whom involuntary commitment must be considered is small (although, under the influence of current pressures, it may be smaller than it should be). Even severe mental illness can often be handled by securing the cooperation of the patient, and certainly one of the favorable effects of the current ferment has been to encourage such efforts. However, the distinction between voluntary and involuntary hospitalization is sometimes more formal than meaningful. How "voluntary" are the actions of an individual who is being buffeted by the threats, entreaties, and tears of his family?

I believe, however, that we are at a point (at least in some jurisdictions) where, having rebounded from an era in which involuntary commitment was too easy and employed too often, we are now entering one in which it is becoming very difficult to commit anyone, even in urgent cases. Faced with the moral obloquy that has come to pervade the atmosphere in which the decision to involuntarily hospitalize is considered, some psychiatrists, especially younger ones, have become, as Stone[16] put it, "soft as grapes" when faced with the prospect of committing anyone under any circumstances.

THE CIVIL LIBERTIES LAWYERS

I use this admittedly inexact label to designate those members of the legal profession who do not in principle reject the necessity for involuntary hospitalization but who do reject or wish to diminish the importance of medical model criteria in the hands of psychiatrists. Accordingly, the civil liberties lawyers, in dealing with the problem of involuntary hospitalization, have enlisted themselves under the standard of dangerousness, which they hold to be more objective and capable of being dealt with in a sounder evidentiary manner than the medical model criteria. For them the question is not whether mental illness, even of disabling degree, is present, but only whether it has resulted in the probability of behavior dangerous to others or to self. Thus they would scrutinize the cases previously described for evidence of such dangerousness and would make the decision about involuntary hospitalization accordingly. They would probably feel that commitment is not indicated in most of these cases, since they were selected as illustrative of severe mental illness in which outstanding evidence of physical dangerousness was not present.

The dangerousness standard is being used increasingly not only to supplement criteria for mental illness but, in fact, to replace them entirely. The recent Supreme Court decision in *O'Connor v. Donaldson*[17] is certainly a long step in this direction. In addition, "dangerousness" is increasingly being understood to refer to the probability that the individual will inflict harm on himself or others in a specific physical manner rather than in other ways. This tendency has perhaps been carried to its ultimate in the *Lessard v. Schmidt* case[18] in Wisconsin, which restricted suitability for commitment to the "extreme likelihood that if the person is not confined, he will do immediate harm to himself or others." (This decision was set aside by the U.S. Supreme Court in 1974.) In a recent Washington, D.C., Superior Court case[19] the instructions to the jury stated that the government must prove that the defendant was likely to cause "substantial physical harm to himself or others in the reasonably foreseeable future."

For the following reasons, the dangerousness standard is an inappropriate and dangerous indicator to use in judging the conditions under which someone should be involuntarily hospitalized. Dangerousness is being taken out of its proper context as one among other symptoms of the presence of severe mental illness that should be the determining factor.

1. To concentrate on dangerousness (especially to others) as the sole criterion for involuntary hospitalization deprives many mentally ill persons of the protection and treatment that they urgently require. A psychiatrist under the constraints of the dangerousness rule, faced with an out-of-control manic individual whose frantic behavior the psychiatrist truly believes to be a disguised call for help, would have to say, "Sorry, I would like to help you but I can't because you haven't threatened anybody and you are not suicidal." Since psychiatrists are admittedly not very good at accurately predicting dangerousness to others, the evidentiary standards for commitment will be very stringent. This will result in mental hospitals becoming prisons for a small population of volatile, highly assaultive, and untreatable patients.[14]

2. The attempt to differentiate rigidly (especially in regard to danger to self) between physical and other kinds of self-destructive behavior is artificial, unrealistic, and unworkable. It will tend to confront psychiatrists who want to help their patients with the same kind of dilemma they were faced with when justification for therapeutic abortion on psychiatric grounds depended on evidence of suicidal intent. The advocates of the dangerousness standard seem to be more comfortable with and pay more attention to the factor of dangerousness to others even though it is a much less frequent and much less significant consequence of mental illness than is danger to self.

3. The emphasis on dangerousness (again, especially to others) is a real obstacle to the right-to-treatment movement since it prevents the hospitalization and therefore the treatment of the population most amenable to various kinds of therapy.

4. Emphasis on the criterion of dangerousness to others moves involuntary commitment from a civil to a criminal procedure, thus, as Stone[14] put it, imposing the procedures of one terrible system on another. Involuntary commitment on these grounds becomes a form of preventive detention and makes the psychiatrist a kind of glorified policeman.

5. Emphasis on dangerousness rather than mental disability and helplessness will hasten the process of deinstitutionalization. Recent reports[20,21] have shown that these patients are not being rehabilitated and reintegrated into the community, but rather, that the burden of custodialism has been shifted from the hospital to the community.

6. As previously mentioned, emphasis on the dangerousness criterion may be a tactic of some of the abolitionists among the civil liberties lawyers[22] to end involuntary hospitalization by reducing it to an unworkable absurdity.

DISCUSSION

It is obvious that it is good to be at liberty and that it is good to be free from the consequences of disabling and dehumanizing illness. Sometimes these two values are incompatible, and in the heat of the passions that are often aroused by opposing views of right and wrong, the partisans of each view may tend to minimize the importance of the other. Both sides can present their horror stories—the psychiatrists, their dead victims of the failure of the involuntary hospitalization process, and the lawyers, their Donaldsons. There is a real danger that instead of acknowledging the difficulty of the problem, the two camps will become polarized, with a consequent rush toward extreme and untenable solutions rather than working toward reasonable ones.

The path taken by those whom I have labeled the abolitionists is an example of the barren results that ensue when an absolute solution is imposed on a complex problem. There are human beings who will suffer greatly if the abolitionists succeed in elevating an abstract principle into an unbreakable law with no exceptions. I find myself oppressed and repelled by their position, which seems to stem from an ideological rigidity which ignores that element of the contingent immanent in the structure of human existence. It is devoid of compassion.

The positions of those who espouse the medical model and the dangerousness approaches to commitment are, one hopes, not completely irreconcilable. To some extent these differences are a result of the vantage points from which lawyers and psychiatrists view mental illness and commitment. The lawyers see and are concerned with the failures and abuses of the process. Furthermore, as a result of their training, they tend to apply principles to classes of people rather than to take each instance as unique. The psychiatrists, on the other hand, are required to deal practically with the singular needs of individuals. They approach the problem from a clinical rather than a deductive stance. As physicians, they want to be in a position to take care of and to help suffering people whom they regard as sick patients. They sometimes become impatient with the rules that prevent them from doing this.

I believe we are now witnessing a pendular swing in which the rights of the mentally ill to be treated and protected are being set aside in the rush to give them their freedom at whatever cost. But is freedom defined only by the absence of external constraints? Internal physiological or psychological processes can contribute to a throttling of the spirit that is as painful as any applied from the outside. The "wild" manic individual without his lithium, the panicky hallucinator without his injection of fluphenazine hydrochloride and the understanding support of a concerned staff, the sodden alcoholic—are they free? Sometimes, as Woody Guthrie said, "Freedom means no place to go."

Today the civil liberties lawyers are in the ascendancy and the psychiatrists on the defensive to a degree that is harmful to individual needs and the public welfare. Redress and a more balanced position will not come from further extension of the dangerousness doctrine. I favor a return to the use of medical criteria by psychiatrists—psychiatrists, however, who have been chastened by the buffeting they have received and

are quite willing to go along with even strict legal safeguards as long as they are constructive and not tyrannical.

NOTES

1. Treffert, D. A.: "The practical limits of patients' rights." *Psychiatric Annals* 5(4):91–96, 1971.

2. Szasz, T.: *Law, Liberty and Psychiatry.* New York, Macmillan Co., 1963.

3. Ennis, B.: *Prisoners of Psychiatry.* New York, Harcourt Brace Jovanovich, 1972.

4. Szasz, T.: *The Myth of Mental Illness.* New York, Harper & Row, 1961.

5. Laing, R.: *The Politics of Experience.* New York, Ballantine Books, 1967.

6. Ennis, B.: "Ennis on 'Donaldson.'" *Psychiatric News*, Dec. 3, 1975, pp. 4, 19, 37.

7. Peele, R., Chodoff, P., Taub, N.: "Involuntary hospitalization and treatability. Observations from the DC experience." *Catholic University Law Review* 23:744–753, 1974.

8. Michels, R.: "The right to refuse psychotropic drugs." *Hastings Center Report*, Hastings-on-Hudson, NY, 1973.

9. Parsons, T.: *The Social System.* New York, Free Press, 1951.

10. Veatch, R. M.: "The medical model: its nature and problems." *Hastings Center Studies* 1(3):59–76, 1973.

11. Katz, J.: "The right to treatment–an enchanting legal fiction?" *University of Chicago Law Review* 36:755–783, 1969.

12. Moore, M. S.: "Some myths about mental illness." *Arch Gen Psychiatry* 32:1483–1497, 1975.

13. Peszke, M. A.: "Is dangerousness an issue for physicians in emergency commitment?" *Am J Psychiatry* 132:825–828, 1975.

14. Stone, A. A.: "Comment on Peszke, M.A.: Is dangerousness an issue for physicians in emergency commitment?" *Ibid.*, 829–831.

15. Siegler, M., Osmond, H.: *Models of Madness, Models of Medicine.* New York, Macmillan Co., 1974.

16. Stone, A.: Lecture for course on The Law, Litigation, and Mental Health Services. Adelphi, Md., Mental Health Study Center, September 1974.

17. O'Connor v Donaldson, 43 USLW 4929 (1975).

18. Lessard v Schmidt, 349 F Supp 1078, 1092 (ED Wis 1972).

19. In re Johnnie Hargrove. Washington, D.C., Superior Court Mental Health number 506–75, 1975.

20. Rachlin, S., Pam, A., Milton, J.: "Civil liberties versus involuntary hospitalization." *Am J Psychiatry* 132:189–191, 1975.

21. Kirk, S. A., Therrien, M. E.: "Community mental health myths and the fate of former hospitalized patients." *Psychiatry* 38:209–217, 1975.

22. Dershowitz, A. A.: "Dangerousness as a criterion for confinement." *Bulletin of the American Academy of Psychiatry and the Law* 2:172–179, 1974.

TOM L. BEAUCHAMP AND LAURENCE B. McCULLOUGH

Third-Party Interests

. . . The rule that the patient always comes first has undoubted intuitive appeal, as well as the weight of medical tradition. On closer examination, however, this principle rests on the dubious, indeed indefensible, assumption that the patient-physician relationship never involves primary obligations to third parties. The physician's professional relationships are multileveled. It is not uncommon for a physician's initial contact with a patient to come through a third party, and the relationship may encompass several other levels. For example, a woman may request health care services from the family physician for her seriously ill husband. After examining the patient and assessing his needs, the physician in turn may contact a local visiting nurse, who visits the home to provide required services. In addition, the physician's fees, as well as those of the nurse, are often paid by third parties. Private insurance, health maintenance organizations, and publicly funded programs such as Medicare and Medicaid may place restrictions on payment for certain services.

There are compelling moral reasons why the physician must consider the interests of such third parties. For example, third parties such as spouses, parents, and guardians often have rights and responsibilities that cannot be ignored. They may be the patient's fiduciary no less than the physician, and they may have legal authority to act to benefit the patient. At the same time, these parties may be significantly harmed if the physician acts in the best interests of the patient alone. The parents of a seriously ill infant may, for example, suffer

overwhelming emotional, psychological, and financial consequences if their child is aggressively treated.[1]

Third parties also shape the physician's responsibilities because of the many roles the physician plays in contemporary medicine, particularly institutional roles. For example, the physician may be a research investigator or have public health responsibilities. Promoting the best interests of a patient—under the directives of the beneficence and autonomy models—may threaten or even harm the best interests of others the physician is expected to serve in these roles—for example, future patients and the local community. In these circumstances the general philosophical *principle* of beneficence (though not the beneficence *model*) directs the physician to promote the interests of third parties,[2] and this may generate obligations that conflict with or even override the physician's obligations to a patient.

Because they focus exclusively on the best interests of patients, the beneficence and autonomy models of moral responsibility in medicine are, by themselves, unable to take into account such obligations to third parties. At most, the two models have the moral power to determine that the physician must, *as a prima facie duty*, put the patient's best interests first. They do not tell the physician how to weigh the requirements of the models against a competing principle that would put some third party's best interests first. There is, therefore, no *a priori* ground for asserting that third-party obligations cannot be primary.

As a consequence, we argue in this [essay] that "The health of my patient will be my first consideration" is but *one* prima facie valid principle. It must yield on occasion to a more complex account of conflicts between obligations to patients and obligations to

Reprinted with permission of the publisher from *Medical Ethics: The Moral Responsibilities of Physicians* (Englewood Cliffs, N.J.: Prentice-Hall, 1984), pp. 133–137, 138–140, 141–145, 148–154, 158–159, 164.

third parties. We shall see in this [essay] that these conflicts are resolvable in one of three ways: (1) In some instances obligations to patients justifiably override those to third parties. (2) In other instances the obligations owed to patients and third parties are equal in weight, and the physician faces a genuine moral dilemma—that is, a circumstance involving a conflict of obligations, where inevitably an outcome of great value will be lost by pursuing one obligation at the expense of another. (3) Finally, in still other cases, the weight of morality shifts in favor of third-party interests, and obligations owed to third parties override those owed to patients. . . .

THIRD PARTIES WITH FIDUCIARY OBLIGATIONS: PARENTS AND GUARDIANS

We begin with an analysis of the physician's conflicting obligations to patients and to their fiduciaries—in particular, parents and guardians. A physician must sometimes abide by the decisions of parents and guardians, and sometimes must accept them even if he or she believes the decisions are not in the best interests of the child. Indeed, some have argued that the *child* is the third party in such circumstances, because the physician's contract is with the fiduciary parents, a view we reject.[3] Such a context is rife with the potential for moral conflict. For example, parents sometimes make poor and even disastrous decisions for children, including circumstances of neglect and unjustified decisions to allow newborn infants to die. But the reverse may also be true: Adolescents may make disastrous decisions that they wish to shield from their parents—for example, decisions about sexual activity that eventuate in a need for medical care. The physician can have powerful obligations to both parents and children in such circumstances and may be trapped between competing obligations. As one court recently put it, there can be agonizing conflict between the "parental rights doctrine" and the "doctrine of the best interests of the child."[4]

We narrow our investigation here to conflicts involving the treatment of life-threatening conditions of infants and conflicts involving the control of confidential information about adolescent minors in sexual matters. Because the fiduciary—the parent or guardian—is expected to act to benefit the patient, we shall consider the obligations of the parent or guardian to protect the patient as well as the potential harm that may result if those obligations are discharged in certain ways. Our goal in each case is to determine whether the physician's obligations to avoid harm to the patient or to respect the rights of the patient outweigh conflicting obligations to avoid harm to the fiduciary or to respect the rights of the fiduciary.

CHILDREN WITH LIFE-THREATENING CONDITIONS

Raymond Duff and A. G. M. Campbell have reported that fourteen percent of the deaths recorded in the special-care nursery of the Yale–New Haven Hospital from January 1, 1970 through June 30, 1972, were associated with refusal, withholding, discontinuance, or withdrawal of treatment. The parents' decision was usually the decisive consideration, and Drs. Duff and Campbell view these parental decisions as generally legitimate.[5] By contrast, some institutions, such as Children's Hospital in Philadelphia, have a reputation for being much more aggressive.[6] They rarely discontinue or withhold treatment, irrespective of parental desires. Despite variations from institution to institution and physician to physician, questions remain about how the physician should respond if parents refuse permission for treatment of their seriously ill infant. This is but one instance of the more general problem of how the physician should weigh the interests of parents in determining his or her moral responsibilities. . . .

We begin our analysis with the following case: A baby girl is born with trisomy 21 (Down's syndrome), a genetic defect that involves varying and, at birth, unpredictable levels of mental retardation. The baby also has a life-threatening defect, an esophogeal-tracheal fistula, an opening between the baby's airway and passage to the stomach. The danger of this anatomical malformation is that her lungs can become infected or even blocked as a result of contact with food regurgitated from her stomach into her lungs. As a consequence, this infant cannot be fed by mouth. If the defect is not corrected by surgical intervention to close the opening, or if the baby is not supplied with nutrients by artificial means, she will die by dehydration. In addition, if her anatomical malformation is not corrected, she is at risk of contracting aspiration pneumonia, which, if not treated, will take her life— probably before dehydration. The parents, George and Sandra Breckner, already have three children, ages two, five, and seven. Together they earn a moderate wage. They refuse treatment on the grounds that it would not be worth the effort and ultimate costs— neither for the child's sake nor for theirs. The baby will be mentally retarded, they note, and raising a handicapped child would impose psychological, emotional, and serious financial burdens on them and their other children. . . .

In what respects, if any, do the interests of parents (and perhaps other family members) determine the physician's obligations in cases like that of baby girl Breckner?

To answer this question, we first need an understanding of parental obligations and interests. What obligations do Mr. and Mrs. Breckner have regarding the treatment of their infant? Are they morally free to refuse treatment for any reason they regard as sufficient? To the latter question the answer is decisively negative. From the legal as well as the moral point of view, the responsibility of parents toward their children is defined as that of the fiduciary: They are to act in the best interests of the child. While the common-law tradition treats children as chattels (personal property) of their parents, owing obedience to their dictates about education and medical intervention, it is also assumed in law that parents, as fiduciaries, always act in their children's best interests. The state is not to interfere until it and the parents disagree regarding some decision with potentially serious consequences for the child. For this reason, the state—which has fiduciary responsibilities it may assert in a petition for guardianship—has often intervened in cases like that presented by the Breckner baby.

The state traditionally has had the right to seize authority to act in the best interests of children, and incompetents generally, in order to protect them from serious harm that parents or guardians might cause or permit.[7] When the best interests test is applied by the courts to the parent as decisionmaker, the test sometimes has been treated in a highly malleable fashion, taking into account intangible factors of questionable importance. For example, in cases where parents seek court permission for a kidney transplant from an incompetent minor to a competent sibling, the best interests of the donor have occasionally taken into account projected psychological trauma resulting from the death of the sibling and psychological benefits of the unselfish act of donation.[8] Consideration of such factors can easily lead to abuse, and the safest application of the best interests standard should require reference to *tangible* factors, such as demonstrable and significant physical, financial, and psychological risks.

The Breckners, then, are bound by certain obligations that constitute the parental role, namely to see to

it that their daughter's best interests are promoted by her physicians. Following the principle of beneficence (not, of course, the beneficence model), and assuming normal circumstances, their obligation is to authorize the required surgery. The obligations of the Breckners and the attending physicians coincide in protecting their daughter's best interests through vigorous medical intervention. Accordingly, it seems reasonably clear that this child's interests in medical treatment ought to override the interests of the parents, and if the parents reach an unacceptable decision, the physician should attempt to overrule it. The physician's obligation in such cases is primarily to the patient. However, this conclusion can be escaped if it is genuinely in the best interests of the child *not* to have the surgery, as it is in some cases of very severe abnormalities and problems. This could be the case if the treatment is futile because death is imminent or the patient is irreversibly dying, or if the burdens of treatment clearly outweigh the benefits to the patient.[9] . . .

In sum, we have seen in this section that in cases involving life-threatening conditions of children the physician faces conflicting obligations. In those cases in which it is in the patient's best interests to be treated, parents usually have an obligation to authorize treatment, an obligation that tends to override personal interests they might have. In such circumstances, the "weight of morality" resides with the normal obligation of the physician to provide treatment. We also saw that decisions for or against treatment are not the whole of the matter in cases involving life-threatening conditions. If treatment is provided, other obligations may have to be determined, especially regarding the continued care and support of the child. The physician faces genuine dilemmas, in some cases between obligations to the child and obligations to parents, and in still other cases the obligations to parents justifiably override what the physician recognizes to be the patient's best interests.

ADOLESCENT SEXUALITY AND PRIVACY

Conflicts between the patient's interests and those of the parents increase in complexity when older children are involved. In recent years older children have ever more frequently been recognized as developing in autonomy and not as mere chattels of their parents (or the state, in the case of wards). These children are now acknowledged as having legal and moral rights (and responsibilities) unimagined in earlier times. There is currently a legal trend toward the explication and expansion of children's rights, some of which are referred to as "rights of self-determination." Similarly, many child psychologists view autonomy on a sliding scale from no autonomy to more or less full autonomy, as the child develops from birth to late adolescence.[10] The problem is how full an older child's autonomy must be before the child's decisions and the obligations they create override obligations to respect the decisions of their parents or guardians.

This problem is especially difficult in cases where minor children seek medical treatment without their parents' knowledge or consent. Ordinarily, parental decisions for the benefit of their children require access to information in the sole possession of their children's physician. Obligations to maintain a very young child's confidentiality are usually not given overriding authority, but as autonomy grows in presence and importance, obligations to maintain the child's privacy and confidentiality also increase in weight.

These autonomy-based considerations are given additional weight from the perspective of the beneficence model. Irresponsible parents—for example, those who drink heavily and abuse the child—create grounds for protecting the child's confidentiality that are not otherwise present. Also, young people may not trust the physician without assurances of confidentiality. With such assurances, the adolescent patient is more likely to be open and honest, a key condition in the pursuit of the goods highlighted in the beneficence model. These reasons underlie laws in virtually every state in the U.S. allowing physicians to treat venereal disease in adolescents without parental consent.[11] At some point, the parent loses all rights of special access. But at what point?

Leading cases emerged in *Planned Parenthood of Central Missouri v. Danforth* and *Bellotti v. Baird*,[12] where the United States Supreme Court invalidated state statutes requiring parental consent, consultation, or notification in cases of abortions for minors. The Court ruled that the statutes were impermissible because they restricted the *competent* minor's constitutional rights of privacy and imposed an undue burden on the right to seek an abortion. The Court, however, did not set out a relevant test for "competence"—a major consideration, especially if legal and moral demands of informed consent are pertinent. . . . Other medical interventions that some minors may request without parental consent include treatment for venereal disease, addiction, pregnancy, consultation for contraception, treatment for psychological disturbance, blood donation, treatment for emergency, "necessary services," and treatment for reportable disease. Legal accessibility to these treatments varies from state to state, and moral views are no less settled than the legal situation.

If *Danforth* and *Bellotti* were accepted as the final word, one might be tempted to draw the following conclusion: In the case of adolescents and their autonomous decisions about their own sexuality (not merely a choice for abortion), "Put the patient's interests first" is an absolute principle, one that in every case overrides the principle that the parents' interests in their child should come first. This view is consistent with the demands of both models, which seem to converge on a strong obligation of confidentiality. It is not difficult, however, to imagine circumstances in which this obligation of confidentiality to the adolescent patient is weaker. This obligation would clearly be weakened if a profound threat to health or life were present, but it would be weakened in less dramatic cases as well.

Suppose that an adolescent requesting an abortion is deeply and perhaps irrationally fearful of her parents' possibly negative reaction to her decision. The physician may detect that the patient in these circumstances takes this view primarily because of the views of her friends and not because she has made a thoughtful assessment of her parents' likely response. In addition, the physician may know her parents and have good reason to believe that while they would not necessarily accept her choice or the values it expresses, they would be concerned to help her reach an autonomous decision. If her parents are excluded from helping her reach a thoughtful decision, the relationship between them may be damaged, especially if the parents discover the truth later. In short, the patient's choice for an abortion may reflect a degree of reduced autonomy, her parents might be an invaluable resource for an autonomous decision, and her parents might be harmed by being excluded.

Because the interests of the parents coincide with the patient's best interest, it would be unreasonable to exclude her parents altogether. To be sure, including them might unduly influence the patient, and in such circumstances the physician might be faced with a genuine dilemma. However, consider the following case: The young woman's parents know that she is pregnant. She believes that they want her to have an abortion, but the physician has spoken with them and knows that they do not. The young woman very much wants to keep her baby and tells the physician that she thinks her parents do not understand her at all and are wrong and insensitive to want her to have an abortion. In the physician's judgment, the patient's growing bitterness and anger toward her parents could severely damage an otherwise positive relationship with them. The only way to avoid damaging the relationship irreparably would be to involve the parents in the patient's decisions about her pregnancy, even if she did not believe that doing so would be in her best interests.[13]

The physician, then, must carefully weigh all competing obligations when dealing with conflicts between obligations to minors who are patients and obligations to their parents. Broad declarations of parents' rights or of children's rights do a disservice, rather than a service, and may unnecessarily squeeze the physician into an untenable position. Distinctive virtues such as compassion or tact may serve the physician more steadily than moral principles of duty or assertions of rights. If the adolescent's confidentiality merits rigid protection, considerable tact and compassion may be demanded, because the physician may have to deflect well-intended—and very direct—parental inquiries concerning the source and nature of the child's problem.

THIRD PARTIES WITH NONFIDUCIARY OBLIGATIONS

The physician has potentially conflicting obligations to third parties other than fiduciaries such as parents and guardians. Some of these third parties—e.g., health care institutions and employers—may have some limited fiduciary obligations to the patient. But they also have competing obligations and interests. Unlike parents, whose *primary* charge is to act as the patient's fiduciary, these third parties have primary responsibilities that are sometimes remote from serving the patient's interests. In this section we explore how the physician should weigh obligations based in such interests.

HEALTH CARE INSTITUTIONS

Physicians practice ever less frequently in the solo style of one patient–one physician. Increasingly, they provide care to patients in institutional settings such as group practices, clinics, health maintenance organizations (HMOs), private (nonprofit and profit) hospitals, nursing homes, and hospices. In a group practice, for example, a patient is seen primarily by one physician but also, on occasion, by other physicians in the group,

especially in multi-specialty group practices. In clinics and HMOs the physician practices alongside many health care professionals, and in hospitals the patient is seen and treated by a sometimes bewildering train of physicians, nurses, and other health care professionals, including medical students and physicians in training. As the number of highly specialized practitioners increases, the individual responsibilities they have for patients tend to decrease. Sometimes the patient may not have a single physician in charge of the case—and no one to turn to for information and comfort.

The institutional organization of medical care has expanded in novel directions in order to provide a quantity and quality of care that the individual physician cannot provide.[14] While health care institutions are committed to the well-being of patients, their large scale and complexity generate commitments to other values as well. These tend to cluster around considerations of efficiency, with special emphasis on cost-effectiveness and cost-reduction, and, increasingly, profit. Goods and harms understood from the perspective of medicine can conflict with broader, though related, institutional perspectives. The patient, too, may not accept such an institutional perspective, and this produces conflicts between obligations based in beneficence generally and obligations based in the autonomy model. . . .

MEDICAL RESEARCH AND EDUCATION

A major goal of medicine is to provide for medical care to future generations of patients by training physicians and by producing new knowledge, skills, medicines, and technologies. These enterprises, however, can be a source of conflict of obligations for clinicians engaged in both patient care and research or teaching.

Medical Research. Consider the role of the clinician-researcher. He or she has a dual responsibility that easily produces a conflict of obligations: The physician is obligated to act in the patient's best interests and is also obligated to carry out research according to strict canons of scientific methodology. Controlled clinical trials require accurate confirmation of a scientific hypothesis. They can involve the random assignment of therapies and even placebos to patients, as well as other maneuvers intended to eliminate bias in the research. While in theory patients do not receive treatments that are known to be less safe or less effective than other available treatments, preliminary data occasionally indicate an increased efficacy of one therapy, and animal studies sometimes indicate efficacy prior to initiation of the trial.

In any event, it would be inconsistent with the beneficence model to *randomly* select a treatment for a patient *unless* he or she were involved in a clinical trial. As Arthur Schafer puts it, ''regardless of whether a patient benefits from agreeing to become a research subject, the physician who attempts to combine the traditional role of healer with the modern role of scientist places himself in a situation that contains a potential conflict of values. His commitment can no longer be exclusively and unequivocally to promote the interests of his patients.''[15] To preserve the integrity of the research protocol, physicians involved in clinical research would be obligated to make recommendations about care that the nonresearch physician would not make. How should the physician weigh these competing obligations?

To illustrate these concerns, consider the following case. Gloria Wallace is an eighteen-year-old woman with Hodgkin's disease, a form of cancer. She is presently at stage II of the disease, for which the standard therapy is radiation. This treatment carries the risk of secondary cancer. An alternative treatment, still in the experimental stage, is ''combined therapy'': narrowly focused radiation (to reduce the secondary risk of cancer) combined with chemotherapy. The latter causes nausea and in some cases hair loss. Gloria's physician is part of a multisite research project that is examining the relative efficacy of this treatment, as compared with standard radiation treatment, in a randomized clinical trial. When presented with the information that she might receive combined therapy in the clinical trial if she should choose to participate in the project as a research subject, Gloria elects not to participate. Her reason is that she does not want to be disfigured.

If the role of the physician in this case is regarded as that of clinician alone, matters are unclouded: Ms. Wallace has been offered and has accepted the standard therapy. She has exercised her autonomy in an informed decision. . . . Moreover, she has chosen a mode of treatment known to be effective for her disease. Thus, the physician's obligation to Ms. Wallace, based in both models of moral responsibility, is explicit. For the clinician who is also a research scientist, however, matters are more complex. The research in which Ms. Wallace is invited to participate is based on a morally justified goal—to develop for patients with

her disease a form of therapy that possibly will reduce the risks of secondary cancer, while maintaining as much or greater efficacy in treating the disease than radiation alone.

This consideration is not irrelevant to the clinician's role: Without the new therapy, he or she will have no choice but to treat future patients by standard radiation therapy, which for some patients results in yet another form of cancer. The risk of secondary cancer is not eliminated with combined therapy, but it is hoped that its frequency will be reduced. When the two modes of treatment are viewed from the perspective of the beneficence model, the new, combined therapy—*if* shown to be as effective in combating the primary disease as the standard therapy—is the one that should be used, because it presents a lower level of risk. Here the dual roles of clinician and researcher produce a genuine moral dilemma. On the one hand, the physician as *clinician* is obligated to provide treatment that serves the patient's best interests, as directed by the beneficence and autonomy models. This obligation is most satisfactorily discharged by use of standard therapy because the experimental therapy has not yet been shown to be of equal or greater benefit. On the other hand, the principle of beneficence generates an obligation for the physician as *researcher* to benefit future patients with effective therapies that carry the lowest possible risks. The investigator also has institutional obligations to perform the research. He or she will not be able to discharge these obligations unless sufficient numbers of present patients participate in the experimental protocol. This might not occur if the physician were to act exclusively in the best interests of the patient. The physician in the dual role of clinician *and* researcher thus faces equally compelling claims on the part of present patients and those of future patients.[16] . . .

Medical Education. A similar range of conflicts is present in medical education. Patients who receive their medical care in clinics and hospitals that are teaching institutions are seen by medical students and physicians-in-training, as well as by practicing physicians. When so informed by their physician, some patients adamantly insist that they be examined and treated by their physician alone. Based on the autonomy model, it would seem that the physician's obligation is to respect the patient's wishes. The physician engaged in medical education, however, has the additional responsibility of assisting in the education of the next generation of physicians in order to serve the interests of future patients. If patients do not consent to be "teaching material" for students and others new to medical "practice," this important goal cannot be realized. The consequence might be that levels of care now enjoyed by patients will not be available to future patients. Thus, the academic physician faces a conflict of equally compelling interests: those of the patient presently in his or her care, and those of future patients who will be cared for by the students and physicians-in-training for whose education he or she also is responsible.

Consider the following case. Dr. Sean O'Malley is chief of cardiology in a university teaching hospital. In his educational role, Dr. O'Malley is responsible for the training of medical residents—physicians who have completed their medical degrees and are taking specialty training. Among the procedures that they must learn is how to thread a catheter (a hollow tube) into a patient's heart as part of a complex diagnostic procedure. This diagnostic intervention poses significant risk, even when performed by a physician with many years of experience. These risks increase if a relatively inexperienced resident performs the procedure. Dr. O'Malley is also the physician in charge of the care of patients who become "teaching material" for the residents. As the patient's physician, Dr. O'Malley would not be justified in placing the patient in a position where the risks involved when a resident performs catheterization fall below a minimally acceptable level of professional skill. As residents learn, incurring the possibility of such risk is inevitable. Yet if residents are not given the opportunity to learn, they will not be as competent to benefit future patients as they would be as the result of many such learning opportunities.

Ordinarily, this problem is handled by providing close supervision of physicians-in-training and medical students. At best, this approach reduces increased risk to the patients, but it does not always reduce risk to an acceptable minimum level.[17] Such risk is justifiably incurred, however, in the interests of future patients. If physicians are not provided with adequate training, they may well subject their patients to risks higher than those that present patients encounter at the hands of their physicians—an unacceptable balancing of goods and harms under the principle of beneficence.

Obligations to such patients override those of present patients, who are themselves the beneficiaries of former teaching exercises on other patients.

Problems of Persuasion and Manipulation. Institutional commitment to teaching and research facilities can also raise subtle questions about the limits of persuasion and manipulation as means to gain the cooperation of patients in medical research and education. Concerns about manipulation are of course ubiquitous in life—as testified by popular debates about whether or not various forms of advertising are manipulative. These are usually concerns about whether we are being played upon by devious or unfair techniques—whether or not that is the intention of the manipulator. Problems of manipulation and perhaps even coercion can be of importance in medicine because patients are often abnormally weak, dependent, and surrender-prone. Influences that can normally be resisted might become irresistible.

Dr. Franz Ingelfinger argued that "some element of coercion" is present in virtually every circumstance in which a physician asks a patient to join an experimental investigation. Ingelfinger characterized what he took to be a *typical* situation of influence as follows: "Incapacitated and hospitalized because of illness, frightened by strange and impersonal routines, and fearful for his health and perhaps life, the patient is far from exercising a free power of choice when the person to whom he anchors all his hopes asks, 'Say, you wouldn't mind, would you, if you joined some of the other patients on this floor and helped us to carry out some very important research we are doing?' . . . Here the thumb screws of coercion are . . . relentlessly applied . . . to the patient with disease."[18] The point to be extracted from such examples is that the physician could compel compliance both in education and in research by playing upon desperation, anxiety, boredom, hope, and a wide variety of human emotions so poignantly present in the life of the hospitalized or seriously ill patient. Thus, what the physician regards as an attempt at truly rational persuasion may have the effect of irrational persuasion or manipulation because of the way in which the words tug at such patients' vulnerabilities.[19]

Education, advertising, and propaganda (to take some distant analogies) can certainly be used as rationally persuasive and quite acceptable techniques, but they can also easily glide into unjustifiable means of "persuasion," especially if a powerful authority figure employs them. Similarly, the influence of a physician may be welcomed by the patient and may be perfectly appropriate—up to a limiting point. Just as educators, advertising agencies, and propagandists can inadvertently (or advertently) move from persuasion to manipulation to coercion, so can physicians. It can be agonizingly difficult to pinpoint the conditions under which a surrender-prone patient, desperately needing an authority, willingly submits to the physician's authority, as distinct from the conditions under which a physician uses authority for undue, even exploitative, advantage.

It does not follow from these problems of medical practice that physicians *do* routinely manipulate or exploit the psychological vulnerabilities of patients. It follows only that patients are vulnerable to such forms of influence and that due care must be taken to cultivate virtues of restraint and compassion that avoid or minimize manipulation and coercion, especially in implementing obligations based on third-party interests in medical research and education.[20]

EMPLOYERS

The third-party interests discussed thus far have generally not been altogether remote from those of serving the patient's interests. The patient's health and well-being are expectably at the forefront, even if they are not always foremost for health care, research, and academic institutions. Some third-party interests, however, diverge sharply from those of the patient. This is commonly the case in some dimensions of occupational medicine. For example, physicians who contract to examine job applicants or employees, physicians who are employed in industry, prisons, and the military to provide medical care for employees, or physicians who are employed to develop health-education and preventive-medicine programs regularly confront conflicts between the individual worker's best interests and the interests of an employer to whom the physician owes a contractual obligation.

The employer's best interests are not captured by the objectives of the beneficence model. Efficiency, cost-reduction, and profitability are among the employer's primary interests; maintaining the health and welfare of employees may often be a remote interest. The contract between physician and employer may, for example, require disclosure to the employer and records open to the company (and sometimes to unions). The occupational physician's obligation to disclose to

employees the nature of health hazards that may exist in their workplace can be in direct conflict with these contractual commitments. . . .

THE LOCAL COMMUNITY AND THE STATE

Physicians have long accepted obligations to protect the health and welfare of the communities in which they reside. The first *Code of Ethics* of the American Medical Association, for example, contains a lengthy section on the obligations of physicians to "the public," including the care of those who are sick and poor, as well as general public health responsibilities.[21] This position had been defended in the previous century by Johann Peter Frank, a German physician who held high posts in government and academia. His view of the physician's obligations to the community stems from a strong general principle of beneficence directed toward public health: "Medical police [Frank's term for the public health role of physicians] . . . is an art of defense, a model of protection of people and their animal helpers against the deleterious consequences of dwelling together in large numbers, but especially of promoting their physical well-being so that people will succumb as late as possible to their eventual fate from the many physical illnesses to which they are subject."[22] In a more recent article in the *New England Journal of Medicine*, Dr. Fitzhugh Mullan similarly argues that primary care and community medicine should be united in what he terms "community-oriented primary care."[23] Under this proposal, the physician is obligated not only to care for his or her patients but to attend to "the overall problems of the community," including activities to "promote health and prevent disease."[24] . . .

CONCLUSION

We conclude that the principle, "The best interests of my patient come first" is not absolute. It is a rebuttable presumption that must sometimes give way to the principle, "The interests of third parties come first." Although there is no well-developed *model* of moral responsibility to third parties, any adequate account of the physician's moral responsibilities must accommodate interests of parties such as the family, health care institutions, medical education and research, future generations of patients, employers, the local community, and the state. For each, a range of conflicts is present for the physician. Some forms of conflict are best resolved in favor of the patient, others present genuine dilemmas, and still others are best resolved in favor of the third party. . . .

NOTES

1. See Natalie Abrams, "Scope of Beneficence in Health Care," in *Beneficence and Health Care*, ed. Earl Shelp (Boston: D. Reidel, 1982), p. 194. For a compelling account of these issues from the parental perspective, see Robert and Peggy Stinson, *The Long Dying of Baby Andrew* (Boston: Atlantic–Little, Brown, 1983).

2. Others have analyzed the physician's moral conflict differently. Robert Veatch, for example, insists on a lexical order that places a principle of justice over that of beneficence. This leads him to a quite different account of how conflicts based in third-party interests might be resolved. See his *A Theory of Medical Ethics* (New York: Basic Books, 1982), Chapters 6, 12, and 13.

3. In "Involuntary Euthanasia of Defective Newborns: A Legal Analysis," *Stanford Law Review* 27 (1975), John Robertson argues that the infant is effectively a third-party beneficiary by virtue of the parents' contract with the physicians.

4. *Guardianship of Becker*, Superior Court of Santa Clara, California, 1981, no. 101981, p. 1. This wardship case involves a Down's child with an at-birth ventricular septal defect of the heart and possible need for life-prolonging surgery. The court asserts that the case has "floundered on the rock of parental rights."

5. R. S. Duff and A. G. M. Campbell, "Moral and Ethical Dilemmas in the Special Care Nursery," *The New England Journal of Medicine* 289 (1973): 890–94. See also "On Deciding the Care of Severely Handicapped or Dying Persons with Particular Reference to Infants," *Pediatrics* 57 (1976): 487–93; and "Counselling Families and Deciding Care of Severely Defective Children," *Pediatrics* 67 (1981): 315–20. This perspective has clearly been influential in American medicine. See *Current Opinions of the Judicial Council of the A.M.A.*, Article 2. 10 (Chicago: American Medical Association, 1982).

6. See D. C. Drake, "Keeping Infants Alive Is Only Half the Battle," *Philadelphia Inquirer* (September 24, 1978): 16.

7. Every state in the U.S. requires parents to provide necessary medical assistance, and any failure to do so that causes death may result in prosecution for manslaughter or murder. Many forms of medical neglect may result in criminal charges. A physician who accepts such a parental decision may also be criminally liable, because he or she, too, has breached a legal duty of care. See John A. Robertson and Norman Fost, "Passive Euthanasia of Defective Newborn Infants: Legal Considerations," *Journal of Pediatrics* 88 (1976): 883–89.

8. The precedent case for many later cases is *Strunk v. Strunk*, 445 S.W.2d 145 (Ky. 1969). See also *Hart v. Brown*, 289 A2d 386 (Conn. 1972). Contrast *Lausier v. Pescinski*, 67 Wis. 2d 4, 226 N.W.2d 180 (1975). See also John A. Robertson, "Organ Donations by Incompetents and the Substituted Judgment Doctrine," *Columbia Law Review* 76 (1976), esp. pp. 57–65.

9. These justifying conditions are explored in detail in Tom L. Beauchamp and James Childress, *Principles of Biomedical Ethics*, 2d ed. (New York: Oxford University Press, 1983), Chapter 4. For important related arguments, see Terrence F. Ackerman, "Meningomyelocele and Parental Commitment: A Policy Proposal Regarding Selection for Treatment," *Man and Medicine* 5 (1980): 291ff.; "The Limits of Beneficence," *Hastings Center Report* 10

(August 1980): 13–18; Albert R. Jonsen and Michael J. Garland, "A Moral Policy for Life/Death Decisions in the Intensive Care Nursery," in *Ethics of Newborn Intensive Care*, ed. Albert R. Jonsen and Michael J. Garland (Berkeley: University of California, Institute of Governmental Studies, 1976); H. Tristram Engelhardt, Jr., "Ethical Issues in Aiding the Death of Young Children," in *Beneficent Euthanasia*, ed. Marvin Kohl (Buffalo, N.Y.: Prometheus Books, 1975); R. B. Zachary, "Ethical and Social Aspects of Treatment of Spina Bifida," *Lancet* 2 (3 August 1968): 274–76; John M. Freeman, "To Treat or Not to Treat: Ethical Dilemmas of Treating the Infant with a Myelomeningocele," *Clinical Neurosurgery* 20 (1973): 134–46; John Lorber, "Selective Treatment of Myelomeningocele: To Treat or Not to Treat?" *Pediatrics* 53 (1974): 307–8; several articles in Chester Swinyard, ed., *Decision Making and the Defective Newborn* (Springfield, Ill.: Charles C Thomas, 1978); and President's Commission for the Study of Ethical Problems in Medicine and Biomedical and Behavioral Research, *Deciding to Forego Life-Sustaining Treatment* (Washington, D.C.: U.S. Government Printing Office, 1983), pp. 6–8 and 197–229. These problems are often discussed in law and ethics alike in terms of the confusing distinction between withholding ordinary means and withholding extraordinary means.

10. See Lucy Rau Ferguson, "The Competence and Freedom of Children to Make Choices Regarding Participation in Biomedical and Behavioral Research," in *Research Involving Children, Appendix* (Washington, D.C.: DHHS for the National Commission for the Protection of Human Subjects, 1977), pp. 4–1 to 4–42.

11. See H. F. Pilpel, "Minors' Rights to Medical Care," *Albany Law Review* 36 (1972): 462ff.

12. *Planned Parenthood of Central Missouri v. Danforth*, 428 U.S. 52 (1976) and *Bellotti v. Baird*, 443 U.S. 622 (1979). See also *Carey v. Population Services Int'l.*, 431 U.S. 678 (1977)—a contraception case—and contrast *H.L. v. Matheson*, 101 S.Ct. 1164 (1981) to all three of the above.

13. A convincing case of an 11-year-old girl whose confidentiality about venereal disease was not broken, but probably should have been, is found in Norman Fost, "Ethical Problems in Pediatrics," *Current Problems in Pediatrics* 6 (October 1976): 25. Fost argues that "an unnecessary and often harmful isolation from the parents" can be created by rules of confidentiality.

14. For an important analysis of the impact of the institutionalization of medicine, see Paul Starr, *The Social Transformation of American Medicine* (New York: Basic Books, 1982).

15. Arthur Schafer, "The Ethics of the Randomized Clinical Trial," *New England Journal of Medicine* 307 (16 September 1982): 720.

16. A similar problem is identified by D. Mark Mahler et al. regarding research on medical cost containment. See D. Mark Mahler, Robert M. Veatch, and Victor W. Seidel, "Ethical Issues in Informed Consent: Research on Medical Cost Containment," *Journal of the American Medical Association* 247 (22–29 January 1982): 481–85.

17. For a moving account of how important it was to one leukemia patient to have the intravenous nurse-team draw blood, see Morris B. Abram, *The Day Is Short* (New York: Harcourt Brace Jovanovich, 1982), p. 209.

18. Franz J. Ingelfinger, "Informed (But Uneducated) Consent," *New England Journal of Medicine* 288 (31 August 1972): 465–66. See also Henry W. Riecken and Ruth Ravich, "Informed Consent to Biomedical Research in Veterans' Administration Hospitals," *Journal of the American Medical Association* 248 (16 July 1982): 344–48.

19. A complicating factor here—and elsewhere in medical practice—is conflict of interest for the physician. Thus, for exam-

ple, the young clinical-researcher seeking tenure and other signs of recognition may allow ambition to override his or her moral responsibilities. The topic of conflicts of interests in medicine is a large one and, unfortunately, beyond the scope of this [essay].

20. For concrete recommendations, see President's Commission for the Study of Ethical Problems in Medicine and Biomedical and Behavioral Research, *Making Health Care Decisions* (Washington, D.C.: U.S. Government Printing Office, 1982), Chapter 6, pp. 129–49.

21. American Medical Association, "Code of Ethics," in *Proceedings of the National Medical Convention, 1846–1847*, reprinted in *Ethics in Medicine*, ed. Stanley Reiser et al. (Cambridge: MIT Press, 1977), pp. 33–34.

22. Johann Peter Frank, *A System of Complete Medical Police*, trans. Erna Lesky (Baltimore: Johns Hopkins University Press, 1976), p. 12.

23. Fitzhugh Mullan, "Community-Oriented Primary Care," *New England Journal of Medicine* 307 (21 October 1982): 1076–78.

24. Ibid., 1077.

S T E P H E N   T O U L M I N

Divided Loyalties and Ambiguous Relationships

Professionals in any field of service face moral conflicts of several different kinds, ranging from simple conflicts of obligation, through multiple and ambiguous relationships to outright divisions of loyalty; and many of these are illustrated in the material presented in this set of articles. I shall here begin by drawing a first distinction, between the two extremes: namely, *conflicts of obligation* and *divisions of loyalty*.

The efforts involved in facing and overcoming normal moral conflicts of obligation (I argue) may, but need not, give rise to issues of loyalty also. As a result, the serious moral issue is under what circumstances, and on what conditions, something that began as a simple internal conflict, within the proper exercise of professional responsibilities, may escalate into a larger question of divided loyalties or fiduciary ambiguities.

Within the practice of any profession, situations must often be faced and dealt with which involve straightforward ethical conflicts: situations in which any professional, whether doctor or teacher, journalist or computer engineer, is subject to two or more concurrent obligations, which pull him in different ways. This happens in two kinds of case. In one kind, the professional ('he' for short) finds himself torn between the demands of his professional situation and other, *outside* claims, e.g. those of family. He must then use his judgment in deciding, for instance, at what point personal duties, arising (say) from the fact that his father is dying, are so grave as to override his professional duties toward a client in need, and so justify him in pleading a 'crisis' and suspending his practice. But, in another kind of case, he may find himself, instead, pulled two ways between different types of claim both of which arise *within* his practice.

The possibility of such internal conflicts of obligation has been built into the practice of medicine ever since the time of Hippocrates, whose oath had the physician swear to serve, not merely his immediate patient, but also 'the art.' At the present time, this second kind of conflict shows up most strikingly in the moral quandaries attending the conduct of random clinical trials. (At the stage at which the effectiveness of a novel, life saving treatment is approaching the point of appearing 'proven,' but has not yet met the fullest and most rigorous demands of statistical demonstration, the physicians conducting the trials may be torn between the respective claims of the art, which require continuing the experiment to the point of 'proper proof,' and of those research subjects/patients who are on the placebo and may be 'condemned to death' if the experiment is not suspended.) But it can arise in less

Reprinted by permission of the publisher from *Social Science and Medicine* 23 (1986), pp. 783–787.

critical or dramatic ways, also. A patient's symptoms may be ambiguous, in ways that would call for alternative but incompatible modes of treatment; a patient may, quite innocently, make requests to the physician which offend against his professional conscience; or a physician may, without any pretence or deceit, have obligations to an alternative client (e.g. an insurance company) whose claims may run counter to the true needs of the subject under examination.

About these straightforward *conflicts of obligation*, only two philosophical points need making here. First: ever since Socrates, clear headed moral analysts have recognized that no *single* obligation of this kind imposes on our conduct anything more than a presumptive, all-other-things-being-equal claim. This is the point that Sir David Ross had in mind when he wrote of ethical rules as carrying only *prima facie* obligation; and the point is not much affected by claiming that the rules or obligations in question are 'absolute;' for absoluteness can be claimed on behalf of more than one such rule or obligation, and it is only a matter of time before a situation arises in which the two absolute rules pull in opposite ways. (In traditional moral theology, indeed, the term 'absolute' itself meant simply 'leaving aside the unavoidable exceptions,' i.e. the same as Ross's *'prima facie.'*)

In the second place, it does little good either in theory or in practice to shut our eyes to these conflicts of obligation, or pretend that they can always be resolved without someone or something coming out the loser. Some philosophers are determined to demonstrate, against the evidence of (e.g.) Aristotle's *Nicomachean Ethics*, that ethical problems may be resolved by the use of some algorithm, or criterion, which will always give us unambiguous answers, however ambiguous the circumstances at first appear. To argue in this way, however, is to deny the very possibility of moral tragedies; and that in turn is to trivialize the actual course of human life, by destroying its potential for moral depth. So all such philosophical theories are open to the challenge that they are self discrediting, in that they deny some of the most evident features of the very problems that they profess to explain. A similar tendency exists in the practical realm, equally: some writers are determined to demonstrate that no actual working situation can ever involve the professional in a true conflict of obligation. This claim has been made many times, e.g. for occupational medicine, or in the case of medical research. Yet although, in general

terms, the problems facing practitioners in such fields need involve no *formal* conflicts of intention, their actual conduct in particular cases may still have to steer a way between conflicting *substantial* demands.

So much, then, about conflicts of obligation, by way of introduction to the thornier issues, of loyalty and trust: to make the transition easier, let me begin by underlining a first crucial point. I asserted at the outset that professional conflicts of obligation *may* escalate into issues of loyalty, but *need not* do so. What makes the difference, in this respect, is the degree of mutual understanding between physician and patient or, more generally, between professional and client. Where the patient wholly trusts the physician's *bona fides* and devotion to his concerns, the fact that he is faced by serious and difficult conflicts of obligation need not be a source of any distrust or anxiety. On the contrary: to the extent that the physician has rightly won that trust, the patient will rely on him to exercise his discretion *equitably*, i.e. to apply his ability and conscience as best he knows how, in dealing honestly with the situation, and finding the least damaging way to resolve the conflicts.

Why should this rather simple point be open to any doubt or misunderstanding? A number of reasons may be suggested, of somewhat different kinds. To begin with, as Alasdair MacIntyre and Sam Gorovitz have argued, many people approach physicians nowadays with unrealistic ideas and exaggerated expectations. Having failed to grasp that an element of fallibility cannot be avoided, even in the most conscientious of medical practice, they assume that the doctor is *guaranteeing* to alleviate their complaint, i.e. that the maxim *prima non nocere* amounts, at the very least, to an implicit contract never to injure a patient, however tricky his case may be. Such false expectations, of course, affect the quality of the mutual trust and understanding between the patient and the physician; and, faced with the unhappy consequences that can sometimes flow in actual fact from the best exercise of a scrupulous and fully informed medical judgment, the patient may infer that his trust in the physician had been misplaced. Perhaps the physician did not have his mind on the job; perhaps he was simply out for 'the quick buck;' perhaps he advertised himself as having competences he did not really possess; or perhaps his loyalties were really directed elsewhere . . . in any event, *Medical Malpractice!*

But (I suspect) other more complex issues are also involved, which call for a more careful look at the idea of 'loyalties' in general, and particularly at the circumstances in which we would say that loyalties were 'divided.' In the most typical case of divided loyalties, an individual's previously legitimate and compatible relationships, either to *two or more individuals*, or to *two or more institutions*, become irreconcilable in ways that force him to choose between them. In the years 1910 to 1913, for example, there were hundreds of people in Britain and Germany who had one parent from the other country, and many of them even held dual citizenship. The outbreak of the First World War in August 1914 placed these individuals in the proto-typical position, of having their loyalties divided as between their two parents' respective native countries; and this division had the effect of subjecting them to irreconcilable demands *at the same time*, and *in the same respect*.

Notice that, in the typical case of divided loyalties, more is involved than the simple fact that some individual stands in multiple relationships to different individuals or institutions. Life rarely allows us the luxury of standing in one-and-only-one relationship to one-and-only-one person or institution. Most of us live in multiple relationships, to family, to profession, to church and so on, without this automatically landing us in trouble; and the few exceptions to that general statement (e.g. a hermit) are untypical enough to be set aside. Nor is it enough that these multiple relationships subject us to several specific and temporary demands, between which we must find some way of arbitrating, as in the case of 'conflicts of obligation.' Our loyalties are 'divided' only where the demands of the various relationships are *fully and generally* irreconcilable, because the continuing claims to which some of them expose us require us to *abjure* those of the others.

Straightforward everyday conflicts of obligation, and deeper longterm divisions of loyalty, are however only the extremes of a spectrum; and some of the notions that are most relevant to the present discussion fall in between these extremes. Here, we should look at two of these in particular: that of *multiple* loyalties, and that of *ambiguous* loyalties. Indeed (I would argue) one of the central issues that we should be addressing is the question:

On what conditions do multiple loyalties become also ambiguous loyalties? And what precautions should we take to guard against the risks of such ambiguity?

Once again, there are those who would like to believe that, either in theory or in practice (or both) ambiguous or divided loyalties can be either eliminated, or ruled out. In their view, multiple loyalties can always be reconciled, and can be prevented from subjecting us to irreconcilable demands, still less forcing us to make an outright choice between rival institutions.

In an ideal world, no doubt, all our working institutions, and the whole society, would command the loyalties of individuals unambiguously. In that case, the problems of balancing off and reconciling the multiple loyalties to which people would remain subject, even there, could safely be left to their personal discretions, in accordance with Burke's maxim about the demands of ethics—"what humanity, reason and justice tell me I ought to do." In short, there would be no occasion for loyalties to be divided, or for the peculiar difficulties that divided loyalties create.

But this remains an ideal or aspiration, not a statement about the world we actually live in: still less, about the way in which ethical problems actually arise for people within institutions whose modes of operation are something less than ideal. Actual societies, by contrast, may fail to command our loyalties clearly enough for our courses of moral action to be clear and whole hearted. Even the life and career of Edmund Burke himself was testimony to this fact: Oliver Goldsmith described him as a man:

Who, born for the Universe, narrow'd his mind. And to *party* gave up what was meant for *mankind*.

Nor is this problem a new one created by the complexity of modern industrial society, as Sophocles' *Antigone* reminds us. Rather, Creon puts forward on behalf of the State claims whose moral authority Antigone cannot accept, since bowing to them would require her to 'narrow her mind' in a way incompatible with proper regard for family piety and obligations.

In our present context, the issue of *moral ambiguity* thus faces us with two central problems. These are, first, to explain how, and under what circumstances, the demands of less-than-perfect institutions may make relations between a physician and a patient—particularly, the loyalty of the physician to the patient—morally ambiguous; and, second, to consider how we can best minimize the resulting difficulties. The two issues are connected. In any context, things remain ambiguous only for so long as they are *left* ambiguous: where there are initial ambiguities, these can be *cleared up*. Suppose, for example, that I go to a physician for medical tests in connection with an insurance application, and I am tempted to take advantage of the situation to ask him for advice; he can then explain to me that, in this context, his business is to advise the insurers, not me, and I will do better to consult my usual doctor.

Similarly, in the wartime military, there is usually no real ambiguity, and little real problem. Only the very naive would suppose that a doctor in military uniform, working in a field hospital or dressing station like those depicted in M*A*S*H, was in just the same position as a family physician in peacetime, civilian life. So long as an army doctor does not pretend to be a normal civilian M.D., therefore, all may be well. But this requirement is sometimes more easily stated than satisfied. In a peacetime base, the medical corps keeps its hand in by providing regular medical service, not merely to the serving personnel, but also to their families; and this can create understandable problems.

We encountered similar ambiguities, and similar problems, in the case of sports teams. Still, a professional player should not be confused about the position of the team physician, or make the mistake of treating him *in every respect* as a normal private physician. If he does so, he may well end up in a problematical position; but he will do so by his own fault. When he finds himself, as a result, in trouble over (say) his contract or his use of illegal drugs, it will *at that stage* be too late—and also quite unfair—for him to complain that the physician's position was ambiguous. Everyone involved knows that a football team physician has multiple loyalties to deal with; and that, on occasion, the team's standing and performance may well be a 'higher loyalty,' which justifies his treating a player's confessions with a somewhat lesser degree of confidentiality than is demanded in a normal family practice. So what else is new?

About problems of these kinds, two general things can be said. In the first place, all of them are human problems of a quite familiar kind: they are the problems that always arise in close knit communities, within which people interact in multiple ways. In such a context, one person may well have occasion to ask another: "In speaking to me as you are doing—about how I decide who to sell my house to—are you talking as a personal friend, as my minister of religion, or as chairman of the zoning commission?" These issues are best dealt with by clarifying them; and, in this case, once we know where we stand, there is no longer any reason for complaint. The only people whose conduct can then leave us with *standing* reasons for complaint are those people—surely not unknown—who exploit their multiple roles and duties to manipulate their neighbors, in the interest of their own self aggrandizement.

This brings us to the second general point. The key issue is well stated in Robert Gellman's article, when he writes about 'fair information practices,' i.e. the requirement that anyone who gives information, in conditions where the confidence is only qualified or partial, should have a chance to know how his confidences are liable to be used. (The basis for this argument can be found in Aristotle's remarks in the *Ethics*, on the subject of *philia*—a term whose full sense is not well captured by the usual translation, 'friendship.' Our ethical obligations arise always within the human relationships in which we find ourselves. There is no general way of defining what anybody 'ought' to do in particular cases, regardless of how he stands in relation to all the other parties involved: on the contrary, those relationships are the heart of the matter.) So, in our own discussion, the term 'ambiguity' is a well chosen one: moral problems are created, chiefly, by *leaving in ambiguity* things about the human relationships involved that would be better sorted out, and cleared out of the way.

Are there any circumstances, then, in which it is *impossible* to sort out, and resolve ambiguities about, the loyalties of professional practitioners; or, at the very least, to indicate how, and why, they can quite properly have multiple loyalties? Clearly enough, the answer to that question is, *yes*. We do, indeed, know of such circumstances; and the question is whether, at the present time, professional physicians in the United States are *systematically* placed in situations that expose them to such irresoluble ambiguities.

Irresolubly divided or ambiguous loyalties are, of course, no accident: rather, they reflect divided or ambiguous social or historical situations. So the best—perhaps, the only—way of elucidating our question is through a case by case analysis, given in terms drawn from social history. Here, I can only outline a few sample instances in which this difficulty is, or has recently been, a special problem for American doctors.

(1) To begin with, it is not for nothing that many of the moral questions raised by bioethics became particularly acute during the Vietnam War. In the Second World War, there was little ambiguity about loyalties. Leaving aside the special problems of conscience that

affected a few Americans of German or Japanese origin, most Americans shared both a common repugnance for Hitler and Tojo, and a common conviction that they had to be defeated; and this consensus served to define 'higher' loyalties which everyone could recognize without difficulty. So, when a military physician in World War II patched up a wounded soldier and sent him back into action, he did not have to explain the basis for his actions: both he and the soldier were 'in this thing together,' and understood what had to be done. No such happy consensus, by contrast, united either Americans in Vietnam, or their civilian counterparts back home. When a country becomes caught up in what is widely perceived as 'an unjust war,' people inevitably find their loyalties torn and ambiguous; and physicians and other professionals are, in this respect, in no different a situation from anyone else. So if, in Vietnam, there were occasions when doctors on active duty found themselves in more serious moral conflict than their World War II counterparts, e.g. over how to handle the individuals who passed through their hands, that fact was just one more consequence of the wider ambiguity over the entire American involvement in the Vietnam conflict.

(2) A similar ambiguity currently affects relations between children and parents in this country. We live in a time when ideas about those relations are in flux, and people from varied regions and backgrounds have quite different ideas about the age at which growing children are entitled to full autonomy and confidentiality in dealing with their personal lives. Such questions are professionally important for, e.g. doctors involved in providing psychiatric services to students in universities, or those who may be approached by young women clients for birth control and abortion counselling. Issues of this kind are made only the more acute and contentious by the lack of any public consensus about the ages of adolescence and maturity, or about the extent to which the law can be asked to protect the rights and duties of parents to retain control over, and responsibility for, the conduct of their children. In this respect, the physicians are simply 'caught in the middle.'

(3) To some extent, this is also the fate of occupational physicians. In their case, however, we might expect the differences between different industries and regions of the country to be even more marked. The tone of relations between labor and management has for a long time differed strikingly, as between the basic mining and extraction industries of U.M.W. country in the Appalachians, whose workers are largely of British origin; the secondary manufacturing industries in the Midwest with many German and East European workers, typified by the auto workers; and the newer electronics plants on the West Coast, whose very mixed labor force is still largely unorganized. (These variations arise from the histories of the regions and industries concerned, from differences in the nature of the actual work, and possibly from other factors, about which social historians do not fully agree.)

So, the relationships and roles that are open to any cadre of professionals whose work places them between the two millstones of management and labor, as happens to occupational physicians, may also be expected to vary greatly depending on where, and in what kind of industry, those professionals are employed; and with them the character and acuteness of the ethical problems to which their work exposes them. It is one thing to keep your conscience and reputation clear—to reconcile your proper loyalties to all parties, and to be *seen* to do so—if you are a factory doctor in Silicon Valley; but, if you work in the West Virginia minefields and are answerable to both Consolidated Coal and the United Mine Workers, that is quite another story.

(4) Meanwhile, physicians are also affected by the general bureaucratization of modern society. Living in the Prussian state, Max Weber foresaw the growth of those large administrative structures that have come to dominate our lives; and he foresaw also the ethical problems that would be created as a result. In dealing with these structures, citizens—now renamed 'consumers' to mark their diminished social function—are afflicted by an impotence which undermines their confidence in the *bona fides* of the authorities, in their role as 'providers.'

Notoriously, contemporary medicine had been taking the same road. The individual patient or 'health care consumer' who turns up in a hospital emergency room, and is sent from clinic to clinic for diagnosis and treatment, is barely aware of being a party to any 'human relationship.' Instead, Alasdair MacIntyre remarks, he feels like a package; while the clerks who check him into and out of each clinic, and confirm that he possesses the documents needed for the hospital's 'reimbursement,' behave toward him in just the same way as any Weberian functionary. This is not to *criticize* the clerks, physicians, or anyone else involved. As Weber knew, 'routinizing' administration at first increases its efficiency: this is true of modern hospitals also. But, as Weber also knew, a price has to be paid for that increase in efficiency; and this price is largely paid in the corrosion of human relations and the ethical problems so created.

(5) Aside from general factors that affect all modern societies, some special ones are particularly relevant to the United States today. Let me mention three of these briefly in conclusion. First, of course, there is the standing contrast in institutions and traditions between America and Japan; all of the major problems in medical ethics are refracted through this contrast. Even in straightforward patient-physician situations (I am told) much less attention is paid in Japan to questions of informed consent and the like—by placing himself in the hands of a doctor, a Japanese patient gives *trust* which is expected to be unquestioning—so it would be highly instructive to have a Japanese commentary on the moral ambiguities involved in the practice of (say) occupational medicine or sports medicine.

Secondly, the profession of medicine is not immune to the *racial* issues that have played so large a part in recent American history; nor are those issues irrelevant to current discussions in philosophical ethics. On the contrary, John Rawls' emphasis on a 'compensatory' element in the theory of justice arguably represents less a timeless contribution to the analysis of a perennial concept than it does a timely amendment to our ethical conceptions, in response to the problems of mid-twentieth century America. Furthermore, those racial issues are part of a larger change, that has affected the whole temper of the American social and political debate since the mid 1960s. Before 1965, or thereabouts, we were still living in the time of *consensus* politics, of which Lyndon Johnson was the last great master; and nobody was embarrassed to hear political issues discussed in terms of phrases like 'national goals.' Since the late sixties, we have moved into a phase of *adversary* politics, in which the 'goals' of political action are defined, rather, in sectional, particularistic terms—as the goals of Blacks, or women, or the handicapped, or the Grey Panthers. This element, too, has helped to undermine people's trust in any authority, including the authority of physicians; and so aggravates the moral choices and decisions facing the doctor in the course of his practice.

Finally, let me grasp a disagreeable but unavoidable nettle. One last factor also has aggravated *all* of the medical profession's ethical problems, and this must be put on the record. Doctors complain about a miasma of public mistrust, to which they feel unjustly exposed; and their natural convictions about their own good intentions make this response understandable. Without any commentary or judgment, it has to be said that some of their clients regard these 'good intentions' as hypocrisy. They are strongly aware of the wide disparities of income that separate physicians—and some other professionals—from most of their clientele; and they notice how much energy such professional organizations as the A.M.A. give to the task of 'protecting' the economic interests of the profession.

In this connection, I will make just one closing remark. Aristotle argued, in the *Nicomachean Ethics*, that a full and open moral relationship was possible only between two people who were on a sufficiently equal level. There was, in his view, no way in which *un*equals—whether master and slave, Greek and Barbarian, or father and son—could enter into a relationship of the kind that was possible for two 'large spirited human beings' of the same rank and status. And there is little doubt that he would have been prepared to say the same thing about rich and poor.

Economic disparities tend to have the same corrosive effect on personal relationships as social inequalities; and, in doing so, they undermine the chances of any full and equal moral relations. Justly or unjustly, the efforts of the A.M.A. to promote the *financial* position of its members may thus be having the unwanted side effect of undercutting their *moral* position. If that is so, the problems of 'divided loyalties,' 'conflicting obligations,' and notably that of 'ambiguous relationships,' are liable to be afflicting the medical profession for some time to come.

GEORGE J. ANNAS

Forced Cesareans: The Most Unkindest Cut of All

About three years ago, four Israeli obstetricians suggested that when women in labor refuse surgical intervention recommended to save the life of their fetuses, "It is probably that the patient hopes to be freed in this way of an undesired pregnancy . . . because it is an unplanned pregnancy, the woman is divorced or widowed, the pregnancy is an extramarital one, there are inheritance problems, etc." (J.R. Leiberman et al., "The Fetal Right to Live," *Obstetrics and Gynecology* 53 [1979], 515).

The view that women who refuse cesarean sections are in some way willfully abusing their fetuses seems prevalent and deeply held, at least by some male obstetricians and judges. It is reflected in two recent cases in which Georgia and Colorado judges ordered women who were refusing surgical interventions during labor to undergo them.* This [essay] reviews the Georgia and Colorado cases and argues that the law is and should remain that a pregnant woman has a right to refuse surgery recommended for the sake of her fetus.

THE GEORGIA CASE

Jessie Mae Jefferson was due to deliver her child in about four days when the hospital in which she would be attended sought a court order authorizing it to perform a cesarean section and any necessary blood transfusions should she enter the hospital and refuse. She had previously notified the hospital that it was her religious belief that the Lord had healed her body and

whatever happened to the child was the Lord's will. At an emergency hearing conducted at the hospital, her examining physician testified that she had complete placenta previa with a 99 percent certainty that her child would not survive vaginal delivery and a 50 percent chance that she herself would not survive it. On this basis, the court decided that the "unborn child" merited legal protection and authorized the administration of "all medical procedures deemed necessary by the attending physician to preserve the life of the defendant's unborn child."

The next day a public agency petitioned for temporary custody in the same court, alleging that the unborn child was "a deprived child without proper parental care" and seeking an order requiring the mother to submit to a cesarean section. The odds that the unborn child would die if a vaginal birth was attempted were put at 99 to 100 percent by the physician. The court granted the petition, on the basis that the "State has an interest in the life of this unborn, living human being [and] the intrusion involved . . . is outweighed by the duty of the state to protect a living, unborn human being from meeting his or her death before being given the opportunity to live."

The parents immediately petitioned the Georgia Supreme Court to stay the order; and on the evening of the same day as the hearing, that Court denied their motion, with a two-sentence conclusory opinion, citing *Roe* v. *Wade*, *Raleigh Fitkin*, and *Strunk* v. *Strunk* as authority (Jefferson v. Griffin Spalding Co. Hospital Authority, 247 Ga. 86, 274 S.E. 2d 457 [1981]). A few days later, Mrs. Jefferson uneventfully delivered a healthy baby without surgical intervention.

THE COLORADO CASE

The pregnant woman in the Colorado case was unmarried, and had previously given birth to twins. She was described as obese, angry, and uncooperative. An

---

*A similar case has been reported in Chicago, in which a juvenile court judge gave a hospital lawyer temporary custody of a fetus after a mother refused for religious reasons to consent to a cesarean section. Her three other children had been born by cesarean. After birth, custody reverted to the parents (*American Medical News*, Feb. 19, 1982, p. 11).

Reprinted by permission of the author and publisher. © The Hastings Center, from *Hastings Center Report* 10 (June 1982), pp. 16–17, 45.

internal fetal heart monitor suggested fetal hypoxia, and a cesarean section was recommended. Because of the patient's fear of surgery, she refused. Her mother, sister, and the father of her child attempted unsuccessfully to change her mind. A psychiatric consultant concluded she was neither delusional nor mentally incompetent.

The hospital administration was notified, and a decision was made to request court intervention. The hospital staff petitioned the juvenile court to find the unborn baby a dependent and neglected child and order a cesarean section to safeguard its life. An emergency hearing was convened in the patient's room, following which the court granted the petition and ordered the surgery. The cesarean section was performed, resulting in a healthy child without complication for the mother. Since more than nine hours elapsed between the external fetal heart monitor tracings that indicated distress (and six hours from internal tracings) and the delivery, the physician was surprised that the outcome was not poor. He indicated that the case "simply underscores the limitations of continuous fetal heart monitoring as a means of predicting neonatal outcome" (W.A. Bowes, and B. Selgestad, "Fetal versus Maternal Right: Medical and Legal Perspectives," *American Journal of Obstetrics and Gynecology* 58 [1981], 209–14).

Both cases hold that a woman can be forced to undergo a cesarean section if her physicians determine it necessary to safeguard the life of her fetus. These are remarkable rulings from geographically and politically diverse areas of the country. But both were decided within hours after they were argued, without time for thoughtful judicial consideration, and neither court made any attempt to analyze the rights of the pregnant woman. At least three questions arise: what is the state of the law? What should the role of the judiciary be in labor room disputes? What position should physicians and hospitals take when confronted with a woman who refuses cesarean section against medical advice?

THE STATE OF THE LAW

Both cases lack an analysis of the precedents, and place heavy and primary reliance upon: *Raleigh Fitkin* and *Roe* v. *Wade*. The courts should at least have considered the severe limitations of these two cases. *Raleigh Fitkin* involved a woman who was approximately eight months pregnant. Physicians believed that at some time before giving birth she would hemor-

rhage severely and both she and her unborn child would die if she did not submit to blood transfusions which she refused because she was a Jehovah's Witness. The trial court upheld her refusal, and the hospital appealed to the New Jersey Supreme Court. In the meantime the woman had left the hospital, against medical advice, and the case was moot. Nevertheless, the court proceeded to determine that the unborn child was "entitled to the law's protection" and that blood transfusions could be administered to the woman "if necessary to save her life or the life of her child, as the physician in charge at the time may determine" (*Raleigh Fitkin-Paul Morgan Memorial Hospital* v. *Anderson*, 201 A. 2d 537, 538 [N.J. 1964]).

This opinion is of limited value because: first, no one was forced to do anything as a result, i.e. no transfusion was actually performed, and no police were dispatched to apprehend the woman and return her to the hospital. Second, it was a one-page opinion, with little policy discussion. Third, the extent of bodily invasion involved in a blood transfusion is much less than that involved in a cesarean, major abdominal surgery. And fourth, the case was decided eight years before the U.S. Supreme Court decision in *Roe* v. *Wade* and more than a decade before the same New Jersey court decided the case of Karen Ann Quinlan. One question posed (and not yet resolved), for example, is: would the parents of Karen Ann Quinlan have been permitted to remove her from the respirator if she had been pregnant?

The second case, *Roe* v. *Wade*, does stand for the proposition that the state has a compelling interest in preserving the life of viable fetuses. But it does *not* have such an interest if "the life or health of the mother" is endangered by carrying the child to term. The question that needs to be discussed is the relevance of the additional danger (physical or mental) to the mother of undergoing a cesarean section where its purpose is to protect the health of the fetus. In the Colorado case, for example, it was noted that excessively obese patients are "generally considered at increased risk of anesthetic and surgical complications." When do such increased risk factors outweigh the child's right to be born via cesarean? And what would happen if, despite a court order, the patient refused to submit to the cesarean? The physician in the Colorado case cautions that "had the patient steadfastly refused it might not have been either safe or possible to administer anesthesia to a struggling, resistant woman who weighed in excess of 157.5 kg." Surely nothing in *Roe* v. *Wade* gives either judges or physicians the right to favor the life or health of the fetus over that of the pregnant woman.

No mother has ever been legally required to undergo surgery or general anesthesia (e.g., bone marrow or kidney transplant) to save the life of her dying child. It would be ironic, to say the least, if she could be forced to submit to more invasive surgical procedures for the sake of her fetus than for her child. It is premature to label the conclusions of two quickly decided cases that lack any meaningful analysis "the law."

COURTS IN THE HOSPITAL

Judges are not terribly good at making emergency decisions. Perhaps the most famous example is the opinion of Judge Skelly Wright in the *Georgetown College* case (Application of the President and Directors of Georgetown College, 331 F. 2d 1000 [1964]). That case involved an emergency petition to permit blood transfusions to a Jehovah's Witness to save her life. A lower court judge refused to issue such an order, but Judge Wright did, less than an hour-and-a-half after he was approached by counsel for the hospital. He went to the hospital and interviewed the woman and her husband. The woman, a twenty-five-year-old with a seven-month-old child, was "not in a mental condition to make a decision." Her husband refused; but said if the judge ordered it, it would not be his responsibility. Because the judge believed that the woman's reasoning would be similar, he ordered the transfusions.

The full bench of the U.S. Circuit Court of Appeals refused to review the case, but some of the members dissented from this refusal, and noted their concerns (331 F 2d 1010). Judge Miller, for example, noted that Judge Wright was

impelled, I am sure, by humanitarian impulses and doubtless was himself under considerable strain . . . In the interval of about an hour and twenty minutes between the appearance of the attorney at his chambers and the signing of the order at the hospital, the judge had no opportunity for research as to the substantive legal problems and procedural questions involved. He should not have been asked to act in these circumstances.

Judge Warren Burger, now Chief Justice of the U.S. Supreme Court, quoted Cardozo on judicial restraint:

The judge, even when he is free, is still not wholly free. He is not to innovate at pleasure. He is not a knight-errant, roaming at will in pursuit of his own ideal of beauty or of

goodness. He is to draw his inspiration from consecrated principles. He is not to yield to spasmodic sentiment, to vague and unregulated benevolence.

It is inappropriate for judges to act impulsively, without benefit of reflection on past precedent and the likely future impact of their opinions. Both the cesarean section cases discussed in this article suffer from lack of reflection. Obviously the delivery room is not conducive to such reflection, and judges probably do not belong there at all in such circumstances.

WHAT SHOULD THE LAW BE?

The law can take one of two paths, neither completely satisfactory. The first is to follow the lead of the Georgia and Colorado cases, and require women to submit to cesarean sections when their physicians deem them necessary to protect their fetuses. The problems with this approach are illustrated by these two cases. First, physician prediction of fetal harm is not very accurate. Indeed, in both of these cases serious errors were made. In the first, a 99 percent certainty turned out to be wrong; the supposed 1 percent reality occurred. And in the Colorado case, the fetal heart monitor significantly overstated the amount of damage to the fetus from delayed delivery. So permitting physicians to judge when fetuses are in danger may simply be giving them a license to perform cesarean sections whenever they want to, without regard to the pregnant woman's desires.

But suppose 100 percent accuracy. We may still want to permit women to refuse surgery, to protect their liberty as well as that of all competent adults. Practical considerations also support the woman over the fetus. Women may take matters into their own hands and not deliver in hospitals. Other interventions they might consent to will be unavailable at home, and an opportunity to try to change their minds will be lost. The question of what to do with a woman who continues to refuse in the face of a court order remains. Do we really want to restrain, forcibly medicate, and operate on a competent, refusing adult? Such a procedure may be "legal," especially when viewed from the judicial perspective that the woman is irrational, hysterical, and evil-minded; but it is certainly brutish and not what one generally associates with medical care. It also encourages an adversarial relationship between the obstetrician and the patient, and gives the obstetrician a weapon to bully women he views as irrational into submission. Attempts at vaginal deliveries after one birth by cesarean section, for example, may fall victim to such a rule.

Could the case be distinguished from other medical interventions, including fetal surgery, if and when it becomes accepted medical procedure, or would women be forced to consent to these as well? And if one can lawfully force surgery, one should certainly be able to restrain the liberty of a woman for the sake of her fetus, e.g., by confining her during all or part of her pregnancy. It seems wrong to say that patients have the right to be wrong in all cases except pregnancy—in that case, why should only doctors have the right to be wrong?

The second alternative is to honor the rare case of a woman's refusal. I assume this is general practice at the vast majority of hospitals in the country, and I believe it is the proper practice ethically and legally. This may seem callous to the rights of fetuses since some fetuses that might be salvaged may die or be born defective. This will be tragic, but it is likely to be rare. It is the price society pays for protecting the rights of all competent adults, and preventing forcible, physical violations of women by coercive obstetricians and judges. The choice between fetal health and maternal liberty is laced with moral and ethical dilemmas. The force of law will not make them go away.

A R N O L D S . R E L M A N

Dealing with Conflicts of Interest

The medical profession in this country has always had its entrepreneurs and hustling businessmen, but until recently they were on the fringe and in a small minority. Most practicing physicians concentrated on providing or supervising services to their patients, and their professional income was largely limited to the fees or salaries paid for such services.

Lately, however, a new entrepreneurial fever has begun to affect the profession, and what was formerly on the fringe seems to be moving into the mainstream. More and more practitioners are seeking profits from business arrangements with hospitals, equipment manufacturers, and most recently, companies providing ambulatory health care services. Practicing physicians now have financial interests in diagnostic laboratories, radiologic imaging centers, walk-in clinics, ambulatory surgery centers, dialysis units, physical therapy centers, and other such facilities. In most of these business ventures, the investing physicians' profits

depend, at least in part, on referral of patients to these facilities or on other decisions they make in the care of their patients.

A few examples will illustrate the conflicts of interest involved in such arrangements. Consider, first, the various ways some enterprising surgeons are augmenting their professional income through business connections with the facilities in which they operate on their patients. Free-standing investor-owned ambulatory surgical centers are springing up everywhere. To increase the use of their facilities, which are often in competition with similar units in the community hospitals, these companies offer local surgeons a share in the profits. Some ambulatory surgical centers are owned by the surgeons who use the facility, and they share in the profits from its use. A few investor-owned hospitals have also offered profit-sharing deals to surgeons. According to public statements made by its management, one large hospital chain substantially increased the use of its operating rooms by sharing the profits with its staff surgeons. In each of these examples, surgeons have benefited financially not only from

Reprinted by permission of *The New England Journal of Medicine*, Vol. 313, No. 12.

providing professional services but from referring their patients to a facility in which they have an interest.

Free-standing radiologic imaging centers (usually featuring CAT scanners and magnetic resonance imaging units) are another recent phenomenon that is attracting increasing entrepreneurial interest from physicians. Radiologists and nonradiologists are now investing in these centers, often in partnership with venture capitalists. For the nonradiologist investors, such arrangements constitute an economic incentive to refer their own patients to the imaging center and to use radiologic procedures. The radiologist investors in such centers may have less opportunity for self-referral than their nonradiologist partners, but since they are acting as radiologic consultants, they can recommend follow-up studies. In any case, their entrepreneurial interests in the financial success of the center may be even more compelling than their partners', because they benefit twice—once as professional supervisors and interpreters of the diagnostic procedure, and again as investors in the facility.

Another kind of business arrangement was in the news recently when a congressional committee investigating Medicare payments for cataract surgery[1] reported that some ophthalmologists accept inducements from manufacturers of intraocular lens implants, which are intended to persuade the physician to use a particular brand of lens. These include quantity discounts, cash rebates, shares of stock in the company, and a variety of gifts, such as free vacations, the use of a yacht, and expensive office equipment. The ophthalmologist makes a profit beyond the professional fee for doing the operation by charging Medicare a large markup on the implanted lens, in addition to whatever consideration he or she receives from the manufacturer for using the product.

Many other examples could be cited to demonstrate that entrepreneurialism among physicians is a widespread and rapidly growing phenomenon that is creating conflicts of interest in almost all sectors of the medical profession. Considering the manifold forces now moving medical practice in the direction of commerce,[2] this is hardly surprising. But is it in the best interests of society and the profession? And, if it is not, what if anything can be done to change the trend?

Defenders of the marketplace approach to health care say there is nothing wrong with physicians acting as entrepreneurs. They argue that fee-for-service practice is essentially a business anyway and the economic conflicts of interest that arise when physicians make financial arrangements with health care businesses are

in principle not much different from those already existing in private practice.

There is something to be said for that latter point, particularly when practitioners benefit financially from special tests or procedures that they have recommended for their patients and that they themselves then supervise or carry out. However, this argument ignores the basic social role of the physician, which is to be an agent and trustee for the patient. Physicians are ethically bound to place the medical care needs of their patients before their own financial interests—an obligation that clearly sets the practice of medicine apart from business. Conflicts of interest may be inherent in the fee-for-service system, but ethical practitioners minimize them by avoiding self-referral whenever possible, by conservative use of tests and procedures, and by conscientiously attempting to meet their fiduciary responsibilities to their patients. Furthermore, whatever conflicts of interest may exist in the fee-for-service relation between doctor and patient are clearly visible to all concerned and have long been accepted by society. When patients have any doubts, they are free to seek other advice.

The situation is different when physicians seek income beyond fee for service and make business arrangements with other providers of services to their patients. Such arrangements introduce a new and unnecessary conflict, which strains the physician's fiduciary commitment to the patient. Unlike the conflicts of interest in the fee-for-service system, these new arrangements are usually not fully disclosed to the patient, and therefore are more difficult to control.

The new entrepreneurialism among physicians is beginning to attract legislative attention. The state of Michigan now prohibits physicians from referring their patients to any facility in which the practitioner has a financial interest. Pennsylvania has recently enacted a similar law, but it applies only to patients receiving state medical assistance. California law currently requires that physicians disclose any financial interests in free-standing diagnostic facilities to which they refer their patients, but the legislature is now considering a bill (AB 1325) that would prohibit such referrals regardless of disclosure.

State laws dealing with this issue are likely to multiply as the commercialization of our medical care system becomes ever more pervasive and public concern mounts. In my view, however, legal measures alone are not the answer. There can be no really satisfactory solution until the medical profession itself faces up to the threat of entrepreneurialism and decides to take a firm stand in defense of professional ethics. That is why I have been pleased to see the American Medical Association (AMA) debate this subject at its last few meetings and attempt to develop policy guidelines. The AMA has quite properly reminded physicians that "medicine is a profession, a calling, and not a business . . . ,"[3] and it has reaffirmed that physicians must put the needs of their patients above economic self-interest. But it has also said that physicians may ethically invest in facilities and share profits with hospitals or pharmaceutical or equipment manufacturers, provided that the arrangements are lawful, do not lead to overutilization or improper care of patients, are disclosed in advance to patients, and do not involve profit sharing with institutions being paid under the Medicare system of diagnosis-related groups (DRGs).[4,5] At its recent annual meeting, the AMA vigorously denounced a chain of investor-owned hospitals that has been sharing profits with its medical staff as a means of inducing the staff to reduce expenditures on Medicare patients.[6]

The AMA thus seems to be drawing a distinction between profit sharing in the traditional reimbursement system (ethically permissible if certain conditions are met) and profit sharing in the Medicare DRG-based prospective payment system (ipso facto unethical, a form of "kickback"). It is a distinction that defies logic, however, and I doubt that it will withstand further reflection and discussion. If profit sharing with hospitals under a DRG system is unethical (and I agree that it is), then so is profit sharing under a charge reimbursement system, since there are possibilities for abuse and exploitation of patients in both systems and profit sharing by physicians in either system creates temptations that may be difficult to resist. Withholding or skimping on needed services (the possible abuse in the prospective payment system) is no more reprehensible than providing unneeded or inappropriate service (the possible abuse in the charge reimbursement system). Financial arrangements that tempt physicians in either direction ought to be avoided.

The AMA's present position has an even more troublesome aspect. In admitting that business deals create conflicts of interest for physicians, but arguing that we need be concerned only about arrangements that demonstrably lead to bad practice, the AMA's statements ignore the damage done to the public trust in the medical profession by even the *appearance* of conflicts of interest. That, after all, is a major problem with conflicts of interest. Full disclosure might help prevent that loss of trust, but there is already a strong popular sense that physicians are too interested in exploiting the financial advantages of their position, and disclosure is not likely to do much to change that. The continued unchecked growth of entrepreneurialism will only strengthen public suspicion and give further impetus to the kinds of legislative action now being taken in some states.

I would therefore hope that the current position of the AMA on this issue is in transition and that, after further deliberation, a stronger policy statement will emerge. The American College of Physicians, in its recently issued Ethics Manual, has taken such a position.[7] It says, "The physician must avoid any personal commercial conflict of interest that might compromise his loyalty and treatment of the patient." A similarly firm and unequivocal statement of conscience from all the important sectors of organized medicine in the United States would be salutary. Of course, we will need much more than a statement of conscience to reverse the trend, but it is a good way to begin. We cannot expect to take any practical steps in defense of our professionalism until we publicly agree that physicians serve their patients' interests best when they divorce themselves from financial interests in the medical marketplace.

NOTES

1. Cataract surgery: fraud, waste, and abuse: a report by the Chairman of the Subcommittee on Health and Long-Term Care of the Select Committee on Aging of the House of Representatives, Ninety-Ninth Congress, July 19, 1985. Washington, D.C.: Government Printing Office, 1985. (Committee publication no. 99-506).

2. Relman AS. The future of medical practice. Health Affairs 1983; 2(2): 5–19.

3. House of Delegates of the American Medical Association. Commercialism in the practice of medicine: report of the Board of Trustees of the American Medical Association, June 1983.

4. House of Delegates of the American Medical Association. Conflict of interest—guidelines: report of the Judicial Council of the American Medical Association, December 1984.

5. House of Delegates of the American Medical Association. Ethical implications of hospital-physician risk-sharing arrangements under DRGs: report of the Judicial Council of the American Medical Association, December 1984.

6. Kickback plan by hospital hit. American Medical News, 28–July 5, 1985:1, 34.

7. Ad Hoc Committee on Medical Ethics of the American College of Physicians. American College of Physicians ethics manual. Part I. History of medical ethics, the physician and the patient, the physician's relationship to other physicians, the physician and society. Ann Intern Med 1984; 101:129–37.

GENERAL ISSUES

Annas, George J. *The Rights of Hospital Patients*. New York: Avon Books, 1975.

Beauchamp, Tom L., and McCullough, Laurence B. *Medical Ethics: The Moral Responsibilities of Physicians*. Englewood Cliffs, N.J.: Prentice-Hall, 1984.

Benjamin, Martin, and Curtis, Joy. *Ethics in Nursing*. New York: Oxford University Press, 1981.

Bloom, Samuel W. Therapeutic Relationship: Sociohistorical Perspectives." In Reich, Warren T., ed. *Encyclopedia of Bioethics*. New York: Free Press, 1978. Vol. 4, pp. 1663–1668.

Bowie, Norman. "'Role' as a Moral Concept in Health Care." *Journal of Medicine and Philosophy* 7 (February 1982), 57–63.

Branson, Roy. "The Secularization of American Medicine." *Hastings Center Studies*, Vol. 1, No. 2 (1973), 17–28.

Brecher, Robert, and Cannell, Hugh. "Striking Responsibilities." *Journal of Medical Ethics* 11 (June 1985), 66–69.

Brett, Allan S., and McCullough, Laurence B. "When Patients Request Specific Interventions: Defining the Limits of the Physician's Obligation." *New England Journal of Medicine* 315 (November 1986), 1347–1351.

Daly, Michael E. "Towards a Phenomenology of Caregiving: Growth in the Caregiver Is a Vital Component." *Journal of Medical Ethics* 13 (March 1987), 34–39.

Davis, Anne J., and Aroskar, Mila A. *Ethical Dilemmas and Nursing Practice*. New York: Appleton-Century-Crofts, 1978.

Doudera, Edward A. "Decisionmaking and Patients' Rights." *Journal of the American Health Care Association* 11 (May 1985), 5–8.

Downie, Robert S. "Collective Responsibility in Health Care." *Journal of Medicine and Philosophy* 7 (February 1982), 43–56.

Ennis, Bruce J., and Emery, Richard D. *The Rights of Mental Patients*. New York: Avon Books, 1978.

Etziony, M. B., comp. *The Physician's Creed: An Anthology of Medical Prayers, Oaths and Codes of Ethics Written and Recited by Medical Practitioners Through the Ages*. Springfield, Ill.: Thomas, 1973.

Gass, Ronald S. "Appendix: Codes and Statements Related to Medical Ethics." In Reich, Warren T., ed. *Encyclopedia of Bioethics*. New York: Free Press, 1978. Vol. 4, pp. 1721–1815.

Gillon, Raanan. "Doctors and Patients." *British Medical Journal* 296 (February 1985), 466–469.

Gorovitz, Samuel, and MacIntyre, Alasdair. "Toward a Theory of Medical Fallibility." *Journal of Medicine and Philosophy* 1 (March 1976), 51–71.

Jameton, Andrew. "The Nurse: When Roles and Rules Conflict." *Hastings Center Report* 7 (August 1977), 22–23.

Kass, Leon. "Ethical Dilemmas in the Care of the Ill." *Journal of the American Medical Association* 244 (October 17 and 24/31, 1980), 1811–1816, 1946–1949.

Margolis, Joseph. "Conceptual Aspects of a Patient's Bill of Rights." *Journal of Value Inquiry* 11 (Summer 1977), 126–135.

Masters, Roger D. "Is Contract an Adequate Basis for Medical Ethics?" *Hastings Center Report* 5 (December 1975), 24–28.

May, William F. "Code, Covenant, Contract, or Philanthropy." *Hastings Center Report* 5 (December 1975), 29–38.

Mechanic, David. *Future Issues in Health Care: Social Policy and the Rationing of Medical Services*. New York: Free Press, 1979. Chap. 9.

Muyskens, James L. "Nurses' Collective Responsibility and the Strike Weapon." *Journal of Medicine and Philosophy* 7 (February 1982), 101–112.

Ramsey, Paul. *The Patient as Person*. New Haven, Conn.: Yale University Press, 1970.

Stanley, Theresa. "Nursing." In Reich, Warren T., ed. *Encyclopedia of Bioethics*. New York: Free Press, 1978. Vol. 3, pp. 1138–1146.

Theis, E. Charlotte. "Ethical Issues: A Nursing Perspective." *New England Journal of Medicine* 315 (November 1986), 1222–1224.

Veatch, Robert M. "Models for Ethical Medicine in a Revolutionary Age." *Hastings Center Report* 2 (June 1972), 5–7.

———. *Case Studies in Medical Ethics*. Cambridge, Mass.: Harvard University Press, 1977.

———. "Professional Medical Ethics: The Grounding of Its Principles." *Journal of Medicine and Philosophy* 4 (March 1979), 1–19.

———. *A Theory of Medical Ethics*. New York: Basic Books, 1981.

Veatch, Robert M., and Fry, Sara T. *Case Studies in Nursing Ethics*. Philadelphia, Pa.: Lippincott, 1987.

CONFLICTS OF INTEREST

Levine, Robert J. "The Physician-Researcher: Role Conflicts." In Melnick, Vijaya et al., eds. *Alzheimer's Dementia: Dilemmas in Clinical Research*. Clifton, N.J.: Humana Press, 1985, pp. 41–50.

Murray, Thomas H. "Divided Loyalties for Physicians: Social Context and Moral Problems." *Social Science and Medicine* 23 (1986), 827–832.

Sieghart, Paul. "Professions as the Conscience of Society." *Journal of Medical Ethics* 11 (September 1985), 117–122.

Silver, George. "Whom Do We Serve?" *Lancet* 1 (February 1986), 315–316.

INVOLUNTARY COMMITMENT

Bazelon, David. "Institutionalization, Deinstitutionalization, and the Adversary Process." *Columbia Law Review* 75 (June 1975), 897–912.

Brock, Dan W. "Involuntary Commitment of the Mentally Ill: Some Moral Issues." In Davis, John W. et al., eds. *Contemporary Issues in Biomedical Ethics*. Clifton, N.J.: Humana Press, 1978, pp. 213–226.

Culver, Charles M., and Gert, Bernard. "The Morality of Involuntary Hospitalization." In Spicker, Stuart F. et al., eds. *The Law-Medicine Relation: A Philosophical Exploration*. Boston: D. Reidel, 1981, pp. 159–175.

Kittrie, Nicholas N. *The Right to Be Different: Deviance and Enforced Therapy*. Baltimore, Md.: Johns Hopkins University Press, 1971.

Szasz, Thomas. *Law, Liberty, and Psychiatry: An Inquiry into the Social Uses of Mental Health Practices*. New York: Macmillan, 1963.

———. *Psychiatric Slavery*. New York: Free Press, 1977.

BIBLIOGRAPHIES

American Nurses' Association, Committee on Ethics. *Ethics in Nursing: References and Resources*. Kansas City, Mo.: American Nurses' Association, 1979.

Goldstein, Doris Mueller. *Bioethics: A Guide to Information Sources*. Detroit: Gale Research Company, 1982. See under "Codes of Ethics," Professional-Patient Relationship," and "Behavior Control."

Lineback, Richard H., ed. *Philosopher's Index*. Vols. 1– . Bowling Green, Ohio: Philosophy Documentation Center, Bowling Green State University. Issued quarterly. See under "Codes," "Physicians," "Rights," and "Therapy."

Walters, LeRoy, and Kahn, Tamar Joy, eds. *Bibliography of Bioethics*. Vols. 1– . Washington, D.C.: Kennedy Institute of Ethics, Georgetown University. Issued annually. See under "Involuntary Commitment," "Medical Ethics," "Nursing Ethics," "Patient Care," "Patients' Rights," "Professional-Patient Relationship," and "Voluntary Admission." (The information contained in the annual *Bibliography of Bioethics* can also be retrieved from BIOETHICSLINE, an online database of the National Library of Medicine.)

8.
The Management of Medical Information

In Chapter 7 we examined professional obligations and patients' rights. In this chapter we extend this discussion to the disclosure and confidentiality of information. The primary problems are those of determining the conditions under which patients and related parties should have control over information about their health status and how professionals should manage and protect information in the medical setting.

Several pioneers in the history of medical ethics have explored issues of justifiable nondisclosure and confidentiality. These figures include classical historical documents such as the Hippocratic writings (fifth to fourth century, B.C.), Thomas Percival's *Medical Ethics* (1803), and the authors of the first *Code of Ethics* (1846–1847) of the American Medical Association. In these traditional codes and writings, moral concerns for the *autonomy* of patients are not found. By contrast, a major feature of the contemporary discussion is whether and, if so, to what extent respect for autonomy requires *more* disclosure, consultation, mutual decision making, and protection of confidential information than has traditionally been deemed prudent or required.

TRUTHFULNESS

In modern medicine the nature and quality of the physician-patient relationship may vary with the duration of prior contact, the mental or physical state of the patient, the style the physician chooses for relating to the family, and problems of patient-family interaction. The patient's right to know the truth and the physician's obligation to tell it have often been thought to be contingent on these and other factors in the relationship. Many physicians believe that pressing circumstances or encounters with strangers justify departures from the general principle of truth telling. Very few writers on medical ethics have regarded truth telling as an absolute obligation, especially if telling the truth would in the circumstances cause a patient's delicate condition of health to deteriorate or collapse. Nevertheless, almost everyone now agrees that there is some duty of veracity in medicine and that it derives from the respect we owe to autonomous persons.

Many physicians—represented by Alexander Guiora in this chapter—view truthfulness through the Hippocratic principle that they should do no harm to patients by revealing an upsetting condition. If disclosure of a diagnosis of cancer, for example, would cause the patient anxiety or lead to an act of self-destruction, good medical ethics requires the physician to withhold the information that would cause the harm. A common thesis is that where risks of harm from nondisclosure are low and benefits of nondisclosure to the patient substantial, a physician may legitimately lie, deceive, or underdisclose. A physician might decide, for example, that the use of a placebo would be in a patient's best interest, even though the patient would not consent. Similarly, a physician might decide it is necessary to withdraw medication used to control pain, whereas the patient would not agree to a gradual withdrawal.

Deception that does not involve lying is commonly believed less difficult to justify than lying, because deception does not so deeply threaten the relationship of trust; and underdisclosure and nondisclosure are thought even less difficult to justify, in many contexts. Those who share this perspective argue that it is important not to conflate duties of not to lie, not to deceive, and to disclose. They argue that much of the literature on truth telling mistakenly treats these duties as if they were a single duty of veracity.

A contrasting view is that (except for patients who do not want to know the truth) all intentional suppression of pertinent information violates a patient's autonomy rights and violates fundamental duties of the health professional. The duty of veracity is here conceived as derivative from obligations of respect for persons. Kant (as quoted by Henry Sidgwick in this chapter) condemns lying in these terms. A less severe thesis is that lying is prima facie wrong, but sometimes it is permissible and even right. From this perspective, the obligation of veracity can, like all moral principles, conflict with other valid principles. The question then becomes, "What are the limits of justified deception and nondisclosure?"

In this chapter, this question is addressed in the context of clinical medicine by Guiora, who argues that it is "part and parcel of the therapeutic process" to balance the type and amount of information to be provided to patients. Immediately before his contribution are two classic articles on the subject of truthfulness, one by a physician and the other by a philosopher. The selection by Worthington Hooker is from his 1849 work entitled *Physician and Patient*. Hooker begins with a discussion of truth and beneficence in the work of his predecessor Thomas Percival, who argued in favor of benevolent deception in medicine. Hooker extols the importance of the benevolent physician, but he rejects benevolent deception insofar as it includes "real falsehood." Hooker characterizes his book as an attack on medical quackery and on all who "unjustly cast aspersions" on the medical profession. He is at the same time determined to attack abuses by physicians "with an unsparing hand." His article, above all others in the history of medical ethics, is an uncompromising denunciation of lying and deception in medicine, insisting that physicians should concentrate on the patient's sense of a need for information.

The selection that follows Hooker is by the moral philosopher Henry Sidgwick, a near contemporary of Hooker. Sidgwick argues: "Where deception is designed to benefit the person deceived, Common Sense seems to not hesitate to concede that it may sometimes be right." His essay illustrates how simplistic it would be to suppose that philosophers necessarily have a bias favoring respect for autonomy while physicians necessarily have a bias toward the principle of beneficence. Indeed, the greatest British moral philosophers of the period in which Hooker and Sidgwick were writing (including Francis Hutcheson, who is quoted by both Percival and Hooker) tended to recognize the legitimacy of benevolent deception and were locked in moral harmony with figures in medical ethics such as Percival. The juxtaposition of the nineteenth-century views of Hooker and Sidgwick captures what is still today the central issue about the ethics of truth telling. Both see the issue as that of the conditions (if there are any) under which utility validly overrides the obligation of veracity.

INFORMED CONSENT

It is now widely believed that the physician has a moral obligation not only to make it possible for patients to know the truth but also to help patients decide about important matters that affect their health. This ability to "make a decision" is dependent upon the availability of truthful information and a capacity in the patient to handle the information. Hence, it is often said that before a physician performs a medical procedure on a competent patient, he or she has an obligation to obtain the patient's informed consent and to engage in mutual decision making with the patient. In recent years this principle has become virtually an axiom of medical ethics, but it remains conceptually and morally unclear how this axiom is to be formulated without overtaxing the medical system's capacity for supplying information.

The practice of obtaining informed consent has its history predominantly in medicine and medical research, where the disclosure and the withholding of information are daily events. But the history of informed consent is not ancient. The term "informed consent" never appeared in any literature until 1957, and discussions of the concept, as it is used today, began only around 1972. Concomitantly, a revolution was occurring in the traditional conception of the patient-physician interaction—a revolution that has increasingly moved from a narrow focus on the physician's obligation to *disclose* information to the quality of a patient's or subject's *understanding* and *consent*.

Because of the considerable vagueness around the term "informed consent," some writers have been interested in tightening the concept so that its meaning is as clear as possible. Jay Katz, one of the authors in this chapter, has been at the forefront of this effort. He analyzes informed consent by using a model of "shared decision making" between doctor and patient, so that "informed consent" and "shared decision making" are treated as virtually synonymous terms. The selection by the President's Commission for the Study of Ethical Problems generally follows Katz's analysis. By contrast, Ruth Faden and Tom Beauchamp argue that although there is a historical relationship in clinical medicine between medical decision making and informed consent, it is confusing to treat informed consent and shared decision making as *synonymous*. They argue that even in clinical contexts the personal dynamics and informational interactions through which medical interventions are selected should be distinguished from a subject's or patient's act of autonomously authorizing the intervention, that is, giving an informed consent. They argue, in addition, that there are two distinct concepts of informed consent, only one of which approximates the analysis by Katz.

It has been widely agreed in legal, philosophical, regulatory, medical, and psychological literatures that informed consent can be analyzed in terms of conditions such as the following: (1) disclosure, (2) comprehension, (3) voluntariness, (4) competence, and (5) consent. The idea is that one gives an informed consent to an intervention if and only if one receives a thorough disclosure about it, one comprehends the disclosure, one acts voluntarily, one is competent to act, and one consents to the intervention. But the agreement that these conditions are necessary for an informed consent hides a considerable disagreement about how to explicate each one of these five conditions. In this chapter Katz and also Faden and Beauchamp concentrate on (1), (2), and (5). The President's Commission concentrates on (3) and touches on (4).

One of the most crucial questions addressed in each of the readings on informed consent is whether a true informed consent can be given if a patient or subject does *not* autonomously authorize an intervention. All four articles in this chapter tend to answer "No" to this question. Yet most of the "consents" obtained in health care institutions at the present time probably do not constitute autonomous authorizations, in the sense of autonomy discussed in Chapter 1. That is, it is doubtful that in these acts of "consent" a subject or a patient substantially understands the circumstances, decides in substantial absence of control by others, and intentionally authorizes a professional to proceed with a medical or research intervention. This possibility opens up a range of questions about the adequacy of the ideas and practices of consent actually at work in contemporary medicine and research.

Another problem addressed in these articles concerns adequate standards of disclosure in informed consent contexts. These standards are not at present well articulated in either biomedical ethics or case law, despite their origin and development in law. Legal history reveals an evolving legal doctrine of informed consent—from the 1767 case (*Slater* v. *Baker and Stapleton*) of a failure to adhere to customary professional standards of disclosure to the 1972 *Canterbury* v. *Spence* case (and its aftermath) discussed in this chapter.

This case was the first and most influential of the recent landmark informed consent cases and led to a shift of focus on the problem of a standard for disclosure.

In law, litigation occurs over the *absence* of informed consent because of an alleged civil injury to a person that is intentionally or negligently inflicted by a physician's failure to disclose and that must be measured in terms of, and compensated by, money damages. In *Canterbury* a form of surgery on the back (laminectomy) and a subsequent accident in the hospital led to an injury and unexpected paralysis, the possibility of which had not been disclosed. Judge Spottswood Robinson's opinion focuses on the needs of the reasonable person and the right to self-determination: "The root premise is the concept, fundamental in American jurisprudence, that '[e]very human being of adult years and sound mind has a right to determine what shall be done with his own body.' . . ." True consent is held in this case to be contingent upon the informed exercise of a choice, and thus the physician's disclosure must provide the patient an opportunity to assess available options and attendant risks. As for sufficiency of information, the court holds: "The patient's right of self-decision shapes the boundaries of the duty to reveal. That right can be effectively exercised only if the patient possesses enough information to enable an intelligent choice."

In case law two general standards or rules for defining adequate disclosures are in competition as a result of this case and the history of cases that preceded it: the "professional practice standard" and the "reasonable person standard." In addition, a third alternative standard has been proposed, commonly called the "subjective standard," or sometimes the "individual standard." These standards deserve careful scrutiny because so much in contemporary law and ethics turns on which of them is accepted. Katz delivers a blistering attack on the development of these standards in the precedent legal cases, especially the Canterbury case.

The first standard holds that adequate disclosure is determined by the customary rules or traditional practices of a professional community—for example, a community of physicians, psychologists, or anthropologists. The custom in a profession establishes both the topics to be discussed and the amount and kinds of information to be disclosed about each topic. In the aftermath of *Canterbury*, a "reasonable person standard" arose to compete with this first standard. According to this newer standard, information to be disclosed is determined by reference to a hypothetical reasonable person, and the materiality of a piece of information is measured by the significance a reasonable person would attach to a risk in deciding whether to submit to a procedure. Proponents of the reasonable person standard believe that considerations of autonomy generally outweigh those of beneficence and that (all things considered) the reasonable person standard better serves the individual than does the professional practice standard.

Many have challenged whether either of these standards is adequate for clinical ethics (as distinct from a standard in law). Katz argues that no broad duty of disclosure follows from either of the first two standards. If one takes this view, the alternative would seem to be a more subjective standard that pays attention to how individual information needs can differ and how far physicians must go to anticipate individual needs for information and counseling. Both Katz and the President's Commission adopt this perspective as appropriate for ethics. However, critics of this view have objected that it is too onerous on the health care professional. They hold that the worthy ideal of informed consent would be out of control under this standard, requiring much more discussion and disclosure than the medical system can afford or meaningfully provide.

It remains undecided in contemporary writings which of these three proposed standards will ultimately prevail—or whether they should somehow be combined into a different standard that includes components from each. It is a promising thesis that at the present time law and ethics are interacting to produce different standards. The authors in this chapter, with the possible exception of Judge Robinson, would not be disturbed by this eventuality.

CONFIDENTIALITY

Unlike informed consent, which is a relatively recent topic in codes of professional ethics, confidentiality played a significant role in some of the earliest codes, including the Hippocratic Oath. There the physician vowed: "What I may see or hear in the course of treatment or even outside of the treatment in regard to the life of men, . . . I will keep to myself. . . ." Rules of confidentiality are as prominently mentioned today in medicine as in the traditional codes. Here confidentiality is understood as a means of controlling access to sensitive information that one party has disclosed to another party with the understanding that the information will be kept in confidence.

Despite its venerable history and status, a question raised by Mark Siegler in this chapter is whether confidentiality is now a "decrepit" concept of more symbolic than real value. Siegler maintains that traditional medical confidentiality is a relic of the past that has been systematically compromised in the course of modern bureaucratic health care and data storage systems. He and other critics argue that infringements of confidentiality have become routine parts of medical practice—the rule rather than the exception. Medical confidentiality, in this argument, lacks credibility and needs a reconstruction into a more viable form if it is to be anything more than a myth. Although Raanan Gillon denies, in his contribution, that confidentiality is a decrepit concept in modern medicine, he agrees that it needs reconstituting in a more serious form.

In assessing these arguments, we need to ask why we care so much about confidentiality and what would justify a practice of maintaining confidentiality in a profession where access to vital information may mean the difference between life and death. Two general types of justifications have been proposed for the confidentiality principle in health care relationships. The first type of justification appeals to the principle of respect for autonomy. This argument is that the health professional does not show proper respect for the patient's autonomy and privacy if he or she does not uphold the confidentiality of the professional-patient relationship. A variant of this approach asserts that there is an implied promise of confidentiality inherent in the professional-patient relationship, whether the professional explicitly recognizes the promise or not. The claim is that in the absence of an explicit acknowledgment that confidentiality does *not* hold, the patient is always entitled to assume that it does hold.

A second type of justification is that violations of confidentiality will make patients unwilling to reveal sensitive information to health professionals; this unwillingness will render diagnosis and cure more difficult and will, in the long run, be detrimental to the health of patients. The assumption of the argument is that the physician-patient relationship rests on a basis of trust that would be imperiled if physicians were not under an obligation to maintain confidence. Without the proper disclosures by patients, physicians could not practice proper medicine because sensitive information would be suppressed.

This second form of justification appeals to the positive *consequences* of confidentiality practices for a justification of rules of confidentiality, whereas the first looks to a moral violation that would be wrong irrespective of the kinds of consequences envisaged in the second form of justification. That is, the first set of arguments maintains that breaches of trust, broken promises, and failures to keep contractual obligations are themselves wrong, whereas the second argument looks not to what is intrinsically wrong but instead to whether the consequences on balance support maintaining confidentiality. As we might expect, criticisms have been made of both arguments. Both have been challenged, for example, by the argument that there is a duty to warn those who might be harmed if confidentiality were maintained.

Whatever its justification, if one holds that the rule of medical confidentiality expresses a duty, there remains the question of whether it states an absolute duty, and if not, under what conditions it is permissible to reveal otherwise confidential information. Many who support a *firm* rule of confidentiality do not support an *absolute* rule, because they recognize a range of exceptions under which disclosure of clearly confidential information is permitted. One example of this problem is found in the contemporary discussion of the conditions under which confidential information about AIDS patients may be disclosed. This is the primary subject of the essay in this chapter by Gillon.

A classic case of conflict between the obligation of confidentiality and the obligation to protect others from harm occurred in *Tarasoff* v. *Regents of the University of California*. In this case a patient confided to his psychologist that he intended to kill a third party. The psychologist then faced the choice of preserving the confidentiality of the patient or of infringing the principle of confidentiality to warn a young woman that her life might be in danger. The logic of the reasoning in this case is that confidentiality is a prima facie duty but not an absolute duty. The psychologist therefore must weigh a peril to the public that a patient discloses in confidence against the disvalue of infringing confidentiality. However, this court and the courts generally have left open precisely *which duties* legitimately override obligations of confidentiality. In some countries the law requires that abortions be reported. But whatever the regional variations, almost every jurisdiction has recognized a core set of justified infringements of confidentiality. These requirements include the reporting of contagious diseases, child abuse, gunshot wounds, epilepsy (to a motor vehicles department), and the like.

Not all examples of the problem of confidentiality are so dramatic or socially significant. More troublesome and pervasive problems concern such questions as how much of a patient's medical record can be fed into a widely accessed "public" data bank, how much information about a patient's genetic makeup may be revealed to a sexual partner if there is a substantial likelihood of the couple's producing genetically handicapped children, how information about an irresponsible and publicly dangerous AIDS patient is to be handled, what information employers and insurance companies should and should not receive, and to whom in a family the full range of test results in genetic screening should be disclosed. In each case, we also need to determine what counts as an actual *infringement* of confidentiality and not a mere loss of privacy. Often these questions involve whether the explicit informed consent of the patient is the only condition that would validate release of the information.

The readings in this chapter provide only a few samples of the rich literature on the management of information in the relationship between patients and health professionals. In the past, this literature was generally written by health professionals for health professionals. It therefore highlighted their conception of *obligations to patients*. In the foreseeable future, it seems likely that much of the literature on this topic will continue the current trend of emphasizing *the rights of patients*, especially autonomy rights. Perhaps we would do best to place an equal emphasis on the two perspectives.

T.L.B.

WORTHINGTON HOOKER

Truth in Our Intercourse with the Sick

On the question, whether strict veracity should be adhered to, in every case and under all circumstances, in our intercourse with the sick, there is very great difference of opinion, as well among medical men, as in the community at large. Some are most scrupulously strict in their regard to truth; others, while they are generally so, make some few occasional exceptions in cases of great emergency and necessity; while others still (and I regret to say that they are very numerous) give themselves great latitude in their practice, if they do not in their avowed opinions.

In examining this subject, it is not so much my intention to discuss the abstract question, as to present the many practical considerations that present themselves, illustrating them, so far as is necessary, by facts and cases.

In order to introduce the subject, I will here quote a passage from Percival's Medical Ethics, which presents the views of those who are in favor of an occasional departure from truth, where the necessity of the case seems to demand it.

"Every practitioner must find himself occasionally in circumstances of very delicate embarrassment, with respect to the contending obligations of veracity and professional duty; and when such trials occur, it will behoove him to act on fixed principles of rectitude, derived from previous information and serious reflection. Perhaps the following brief considerations, by which I have conscientiously endeavored to govern my own conduct, may afford some aid to his decision. Moral truth, in a professional view, has two references; one to the party to whom it is delivered, and another to the individual by whom it is uttered. In the first it is a *relative duty*, constituting a branch of justice, and may properly be regulated by the divine rule of equity prescribed by our Saviour, *to do unto others as we would*, all circumstances duly weighed, *they should do unto us*. In the second it is a relative duty, regarding solely the sincerity, the purity and the probity of the physician himself. To a patient, therefore, perhaps the father of a numerous family, or one whose life is of the highest importance to the community, who makes inquiries, which, if faithfully answered, might prove fatal to him, it would be a gross and unfeeling wrong to reveal the truth. His right to it is suspended, and even annihilated; because its beneficial nature being reversed, it would be deeply injurious to himself, to his family, and to the public. And he has the strongest claim, from the trust reposed in his physician, as well as from the common principle of humanity, to be guarded against whatever would be detrimental to him. In such a situation, therefore, the only point at issue is, whether the practitioner shall sacrifice that delicate sense of veracity, which is so ornamental to, and indeed forms a characteristic excellence of the virtuous man, to this claim of professional justice and social duty. Under such a painful conflict of obligations, a wise and good man must be governed by those which are the most imperious, and will, therefore, generously relinquish any consideration referable only to himself. Let him be careful, however, not to do this but in cases of real emergency, which, happily, seldom occur, and to guard his mind sedulously against the injury it may sustain by such violations of the native love of truth." . . .

The question that presents itself is not, let it be understood, whether the truth shall in any case be *withheld*, but whether, in doing this, real falsehood is justifiable, in any form, whether direct or indirect, whether palpable or in the shape of equivocation.

From *Physician and Patient*, 1849.

And we may also remark, that the question is not, whether those who practice deception upon the sick are guilty of a criminal act. This depends altogether on the motive which prompts it, and it is certainly often done from the best and kindest motives. The question is stripped of all considerations of this nature, and comes before us as a simple practical question— whether there are any cases in which, for the sake of benefitting our fellow men, perhaps even to the saving of life, it is proper to make an exception to the great general law of truth.

The considerations which will bring us to a clear and undoubted decision of this question, are not all to be drawn from the preciousness of the principle of truth, as an unbroken, invariable, and ever-present principle, the soul of all order, and confidence, and happiness, in the wide universe. But the principle of expediency also furnishes us with some considerations that are valuable in confirming our decision, if not in leading us to it. In truth, expediency and right always correspond, and would be seen to do so, if we could always see the end from the beginning.

I will remark upon each of the considerations as I present them.

First. It is erroneously assumed by those who advocate deception, that the knowledge to be concealed from the patient would, if communicated, be essentially injurious to him. Puffendorf remarks in relation to this point, that "when a man is desirous, and it is his duty, to do a piece of service, he is not bound to take measures that will *certainly* render his attempts unsuccessful." The certainty of the result, thus taken for granted, is far from being warranted by facts. Even in some cases where there was a strong probability (and this is all we can have in any case) that the effect would be hurtful, it has been found not to be so. I might here narrate some cases to prove the truth of this assertion, but it is not necessary. Suffice it to say, that it is confirmed by the experience of every physician who has pursued a frank and candid course in his intercourse with the sick.

Secondly. It is also erroneously assumed that concealment can always or generally be effectually carried out. There are so many ways by which the truth can be betrayed, even where concerted plans are laid, guarded at every point, that failure is much more common than success, so far as my observation has extended. Some unguarded expression or act, even on the part of those who are practising the concealment,

or some information communicated by those who are not in the secret, perhaps by children, or some evidence casually seen, very often either reveals the truth, or awakens suspicion and prompts inquiry which the most skilful equivocation may not be able to elude. The very air that is assumed in carrying on the deception often defeats the object. In one instance where this was the case, the suspecting patient said very significantly, "How strangely you all seem—you act as if something dreadful had happened that you mean to keep from me." . . .

Thirdly. If the deception be discovered or suspected, the effect upon the patient is much worse than a frank and full statement of the truth can produce. If disagreeable news, for example, be concealed from him, there is very great danger that it will in some way be revealed to him so abruptly and unexpectedly, as to give him a severe shock, which can for the most part be avoided when the communication is made voluntarily. And then, too, the very fact that the truth has been withheld, increases, for obvious reasons, this shock. . . .

[Fourthly.] . . . The momentary good which occasionally results to *individual* cases from deception, is not to be put in comparison, for one moment, with the vast and permanent evils of a *general* character, that almost uniformly proceed from a breach of the great law of truth. And there is no warrant to be found for shutting our eyes to these general and remote results, in our earnestness to secure a particular and present good, however precious that good may be—a plain principle, and yet how often it is disregarded.

[Fifthly.] If it be adopted by the community as a common rule, that the truth may be sacrificed in urgent cases, the very object of the deception will be defeated. For why is it that deception succeeds in any case? It is because the patient supposes that all who have intercourse with him deal with him truthfully— that no such common rule has been adopted. There is even now, while the policy on this subject is unsettled and matter of dispute, enough distrust produced to occasion trouble. And if it should become a settled policy under an acknowledged common rule, the result would be *general* distrust, of course defeating deception at every point. And yet if it be proper to deceive, then most clearly is it proper to proclaim it as an adopted principle of action. Else we are driven to the absurd proposition, that while it is right to practice deception, it is wrong to say to the world that it is right.

It is in vain to say that the evil result which would attend this adoption of occasional deception, as the settled policy of the medical profession, would find a correction in the very terms of the rule which should be adopted, viz. that the case must be an urgent one to warrant deception, and there must be a fair prospect that it can be carried through without discovery. For every patient, that was aware of the adoption of such a rule, might and often probably would suspect that his own case is considered as coming within the terms of the rule.

[Sixthly.] Once open the door for deception, and you can prescribe for it no definite limits. Every one is to be left to judge for himself. And as present good is the object for which the truth is to be sacrificed, the amount of good, for which it is proper to do it, can not be fixed upon with any exactness. Each one is left to make his own estimate, and the limit is in each one's private judgment, in each one's individual case as it arises. And the limit, which is at first perhaps quite narrow, is apt to grow wider, till the deception may get to be of the very worst and most injurious character. . . .

The uncertainty of our knowledge of the circumstances of each case prevents then our defining any limits, within which deception shall be bounded. We can make no accurate distinctions, which will enable us to say, that it can be beneficially employed in one case, while in another it will be inexpedient.

I have now finished the examination of the various considerations which have been suggested to my mind in relation to this subject. And I think that they settle the question as to the expediency of deception beyond all doubt. I think it perfectly evident, that the good, which may be done by deception in a *few* cases, is almost as nothing, compared with the evil which it does in *many* cases, when the prospect of its doing good was just as promising as it was in those in which it succeeded. And when we add to this the evil which would result from a *general* adoption of a system of deception, the importance of a strict adherence to truth in our intercourse with the sick, even on the ground of expediency, becomes incalculably great.

In the passage, which I quoted in the beginning of this article from Percival's Medical Ethics, the writer makes, I conceive, a false issue on the question under consideration. He assumes that the injury, which results from a sacrifice of the truth for the good of the sick, comes upon him who practices the deception, and that in doing it, "he generously relinquishes every consideration referable only to himself." But the considerations that I have presented show, that the injury is very far from being thus confined. Often the very person intended to be benefited is injured, perhaps

deeply, in some cases even fatally. And then the indirect effects can not be estimated.

There are many illustrations, used by those who advocate deception, which are plausible but fallacious. I will cite a single example. Dr. Hutcheson of Glasgow, as quoted by Dr. Percival, in remarking on the maxim, that we must not do evil that good may come, says, "Must one do nothing for a good purpose, which would have been evil without this reference? It is evil to hazard life without a view of some good; but when it is necessary for a public interest, it is very lovely and honorable. It is criminal to expose a good man to danger for nothing; but it is just even to force him into the greatest dangers for his country. It is criminal to occasion any pain to innocent persons, without a view to some good; but for restoring of health we reward chirurgeons for scarifyings, burnings, and amputations."

I would remark on this that the infliction of pain is not in itself a moral act, but the purpose for which it is done gives it all the moral character that it has. Aside from this, it affects no moral principle, as the infliction of an injury upon truth certainly does, independent of the object for which it is done. The infliction of pain then for a good purpose can not be said to be doing evil that good may come—it is doing good.

The sacrifice of life which the writer speaks of, is the sacrifice of a less good for a greater one simply, and not the sacrifice of any principle. But when the truth is sacrificed for what is deemed to be a greater good, it is in fact the sacrifice of a greater good, for not only a less, but an uncertain good—a sacrifice of the eternal principle, which binds together the moral universe in harmony, for a mere temporary good, which after all may prove to be a shadow instead of a reality.

I can not leave this subject without making some explanations of a few points, in order to guard against some erroneous inferences to which the sentiments that I have advanced might otherwise be liable.

I wish not to be understood as saying that we should never take pains to withhold knowledge from the sick, which we fear might be injurious to them. There are cases in which this should be done. All that I claim is this—that in withholding the truth no deception should be practised, and that if sacrifice of the truth be the necessary price for obtaining the object, no such sacrifice should be made. In the passage which I have quoted from Dr. Percival, he states a case in which he very properly says, that the patient's right to the truth is suspended; but I do not agree with him, that in withholding the truth we have the right to *put absolute falsehood in its place*.

It is always a question of expediency simply, whether the truth ought to be withheld. And it is a question that depends, for its proper decision, upon a variety of considerations in each individual case. It is very often decided injudiciously. There is generally too great a readiness to adopt an affirmative decision. It is too easily taken for granted, that the knowledge in question will do harm to the patient if it be communicated to him. The obvious rule on this subject is this—that the truth should not be withheld unless there be a reasonable prospect of effectually preventing a discovery of it, and that too by fair and honest means.

H E N R Y   S I D G W I C K

Benevolence and Veracity

§ 1. It may easily seem that when we have discussed Benevolence, Justice, and the observance of Law and Contract, we have included in our view the whole sphere of social duty, and that whatever other maxims we find accepted by Common Sense must be subordinate. . . .

One of the most important [duties] is Veracity: and the affinity in certain respects of this duty—in spite of fundamental differences—to the duty of Good Faith or Fidelity to Promises renders it convenient to examine the two in immediate succession. Under either head a certain correspondence between words and facts is prescribed: and hence the questions that arise when we try to make the maxims precise are somewhat similar in both cases. For example, just as the duty of Good Faith did not lie in conforming our acts to the *admissible* meaning of certain words, but to the meaning which we knew to be put on them by the promisee; so the duty of Truthspeaking is not to utter words which *might*, according to common usage, produce in other minds beliefs corresponding to our own, but words which we believe will have this effect on the persons whom we address. And this is usually a very simple matter, as the natural effect of language is to convey our beliefs to other men, and we commonly know quite well whether we are doing this or not. . . .

§ 2. In the first place, it does not seem clearly agreed whether Veracity is an absolute and independent duty, or a special application of some higher principle. We find (*e.g.*) that Kant regards it as a duty owed to oneself to speak the truth, because "a lie is an abandonment or, as it were, annihilation of the dignity of man." And this seems to be the view in which lying is prohibited by the code of honour, except that it is not thought (by men of honour as such) that the dignity of man is impaired by *any* lying: but only that lying for selfish ends, especially under the influence of fear, is mean and base. In fact there seems to be circumstances under which the code of honour prescribes lying. Here, however, it may be said to be plainly divergent from the morality of Common Sense. Still, the latter does not seem to decide clearly whether truth-speaking is absolutely a duty, needing no further justification: or whether it is merely a general right of each man to have truth spoken to him by his fellows, which right however may be forfeited or suspended under certain circumstances. Just as each man is thought to have a natural right to personal security generally, but not if he is himself attempting to injure others in life and property: so if we may even kill in defence of ourselves and others, it seems strange if we may not lie, if lying will defend us better against a palpable invasion of our rights: and Common Sense does not seem to prohibit this decisively. And again, just as the orderly and

From *The Methods of Ethics*, 1907.

systematic slaughter which we call war is thought perfectly right under certain circumstances, though painful and revolting: so in the word-contests of the law-courts, the lawyer is commonly held to be justified in untruthfulness within strict rules and limits: for an advocate is thought to be over-scrupulous who refuses to say what he knows to be false, if he is instructed to say it. Again, where deception is designed to benefit the person deceived, Common Sense seems to concede that it may sometimes be right: for example, most persons would not hesitate to speak falsely to an invalid, if this seemed the only way of concealing facts that might produce a dangerous shock: nor do I perceive that any one shrinks from telling fictions to children, on matters upon which it is thought well that they should not know the truth. But if the lawfulness of benevolent deception in any case be admitted, I do not see how we can decide when and how far it is admissible, except by considerations of expediency; that is, by weighing the gain of any particular deception against the imperilment of mutual confidence involved in all violation of truth.

The much argued question of religious deception ("pious fraud") naturally suggests itself here. It seems clear, however, that falsehoods may rightly be told in the interests of religion. But there is a subtler form in which the same principle is still maintained by moral persons. It is sometimes said that the most important truths of religion cannot be conveyed into the minds of ordinary men, except by being enclosed, as it were, in a shell of fiction; so that by relating such fictions as if they were facts, we are really performing an act of substantial veracity. Reflecting upon this argument, we see that it is not after all so clear wherein Veracity consists. For from the beliefs immediately communicated by any set of affirmations inferences are naturally drawn, and we may clearly foresee that they will be drawn. And though commonly we intend that both the beliefs immediately communicated and the inferences drawn from them should be true, and a person who always aims at this is praised as candid and sincere: still we find relaxation of the rule prescribing this intention claimed in two different ways by at least respectable sections of opinion. For first, as was just now observed, it is sometimes held that if a conclusion is true and important, and cannot be satisfactorily communicated otherwise, we may lead the mind of the hearer to it by means of fictitious premises. But the exact reverse of this is perhaps a commoner view: viz. that it is only an absolute duty to make our actual affirmations true: for it is said that though the ideal condition of human converse involves perfect sincerity and candour, and we ought to rejoice in exhibiting these virtues where we can, still in our actual world concealment is frequently necessary to the well-being of society, and may be legitimately effected by any means short of actual falsehood. Thus it is not uncommonly said that in defence of a secret we may not indeed *lie*, *i.e.* produce directly beliefs contrary to fact; but we may "turn a question aside," *i.e.* produce indirectly, by natural inference from our answer, a negatively false belief. . . .

On the whole, then, reflection seems to show that the rule of Veracity, as commonly accepted, cannot be elevated into a definite moral axiom: for there is no real agreement as to how far we are bound to impart true beliefs to others: and while it is contrary to Common Sense to exact absolute candour under all circumstances, we yet find no self-evident secondary principle, clearly defining when it is not to be exacted.

ALEXANDER Z. GUIORA

Freedom of Information vs. Freedom from Information

Not too surprisingly perhaps, I am likely to approach the problem [of a right to know] from a perspective other than [a philosopher's]. . . . Instead, I wish to offer the observations of a clinician, a clinician much sobered by a rich experience of poor judgment calls.

First of all, I would suggest that the conceptual framework as posited in . . . "the right of the patient to know" is the wrong question. As a matter of fact it is worse than that, it is a bad question. And, once you are willing to answer a bad question, you are being led down the garden path of somebody else's choosing. Accordingly, I don't intend to address the question of the "right of the patient to know," and certainly not in the conceptual frame of reference created by the freedom of information act. Rather, I shall argue that information relating to the process of illness and recovery is very much part of that very process, influencing it significantly. It is not an entity independent of it. Consequently, information is to be conceived as part and parcel of the medical intervention, and has to be examined using the same criteria one would in scrutinizing any other aspect of the medical intervention equation.

Now, I believe that many practitioners of the healing arts, experienced in the ways of patients, would not disagree with this position, especially if they stop to think of their own actual clinical behaviors. The traditionally and formally articulated position however is quite another matter. This traditional response treats the patient in the most patronizing fashion, reinforcing dependence and regression, if you will. The illness, in this view, is not the patient's business, it is the proprietary domain of the physician. The sick person must

not intrude himself into this relationship either by his conduct or by his curiosity. Doctor will take care of everything, patient has only to follow orders. You don't tell the patient anything, he wouldn't understand, and he needs to know nothing anyway; all he needs is the reassuring hand of the physician. There are entire medical cultures subscribing to this view and to this set.

On the other hand, you have another extreme response, couched in the language of freedom of information, holding that the patient has the right to all knowledge about him (it is his property as it were), and it is the duty of the physician to share all he knows (as if he and the patient were discussing something outside of the situation).

Both extreme positions are very convenient for the physician: they represent socially sanctioned freedom from decision making.

What I am suggesting here is that neither of these positions is correct. Information is medicine, very potent medicine indeed, that has to be titrated, properly dosaged based on proper diagnosis. Diagnosis, of course, in this context means an assessment of how information will affect the course of illness, how much and what kind of information is the most therapeutic in face of the patient's preferred modes of coping. The plea I am making here parenthetically is for the physician to include a rudimentary (but not just intuitive) personality assessment in the total intervention equation.

Now let me illustrate my point, using a hypothetical clinical situation of the kind that I am most familiar with. Let us take a daily occurrence in the emergency room. Somebody is brought in by friends or relatives, in an obviously agitated, perhaps even in a violent state. He is telling about experiences that do not seem reasonable. He is hearing voices that you the examin-

From *Ethics, Humanism, and Medicine*, ed. Marc D. Basson (New York: Alan R. Liss, Inc., 1980), pp. 31–34. Reprinted by permission.

ing physician cannot hear. He presents you with a system of logic that you, brought up in the Aristotelian tradition, cannot share. In short, you have a patient who is hallucinating and has delusions. All evidence seems to point to an acute psychotic state. Now what do you tell him? Are you going to tell him, in keeping with the simplistic interpretation of freedom of information, that the voices he is hearing are in his head, he is hearing them because he is crazy? Are you going to tell him that no electricity is coming out of the wall, and he has those strange notions only because he is sick in the head, or are you considering what is most conducive to the patient's well-being? If so, then I suggest that you make a therapeutic decision and tell him something like, "you seem to be upset, you seem to be experiencing all kinds of things that you are not entirely in control of, and I think it would be a good idea for you to stay here now for a while, until things straighten themselves out." The idea, of course, is that information, what, how much, and when, is part and parcel of the therapeutic process.

Some of you might argue that I had set up a straw man, in the above example, only to knock it down. Some of you might say that in the case of an obviously deranged person, the freedom of information concept doesn't apply. I could respond, of course, that "obviously deranged" is a matter of judgment, but will not press the point for the moment.

Let's take another example, when there is no suspicion of psychosis, where the patient is clearly in "possession of his faculties." Let us take the patient who comes in a state of extreme agitation. He is tense, anxious, ready to climb the wall. After a careful and patient assessment you come to the conclusion that the patient is in an acute homosexual panic. Homosexual panic means that the person is in the throes of acute panic that he might become a practicing homosexual. Now, what do you tell him? The simplistic advocates of the "freedom of information" concept would un-

doubtedly argue that it is his truth, and you must share it with him. The rigid adherents of the paternalistic medical tradition will tell you that it is none of the patient's business, your task is to reassure him, to reduce his anxiety. I would suggest that they are both wrong. What you tell this hypothetical patient is part of the therapeutic process based on clinical judgment. In some cases confrontation might be the most therapeutic course, in others careful circumlocution, in still others outright withholding. The point is that whatever you do and say must have a good, defensible therapeutic reason.

I would like to conclude with a final illustration taken from my daily work. The reference is to uncovering psychotherapy and the role of the interpretive process in it. Uncovering, insight oriented, or psychoanalytic psychotherapy is a delicate and slow process, in the course of which connections are made between past and present, the conscious and the unconscious, symptom and conflict, behavior and motivation. A delicate and intensive process, in which the therapist is usually ahead of the patient in making connections, in discovering the link-ups. This moment of discovery and the sharing of it with the patient is what we call interpretation. The very curative process in psychotherapy rests on a system of *properly* timed interpretations. I always tell my residents it is not enough for an interpretation to be correct, it must be right, because if it is not timed right it can be more harmful than helpful. Here, perhaps more than in any other clinical circumstance, the absolute irrelevance of both the freedom of information position and the traditional paternalistic position is clearly demonstrated.

It is my suggestion that the interpretive process in psychotherapy can serve as a paradigm for all clinical situations regarding information disclosure and withholding.

UNITED STATES COURT OF APPEALS

Canterbury v. Spence

SPOTTSWOOD W. ROBINSON, III,
Circuit Judge

Suits charging failure by a physician adequately to disclose the risks and alternatives of proposed treatment are not innovations in American law. They date back a good half-century, and in the last decade they have multiplied rapidly. There is, nonetheless, disagreement among the courts and the commentators on many major questions, and there is no precedent of our own directly in point. For the tools enabling resolution of the issues on this appeal, we are forced to begin at first principles.

The root premise is the concept, fundamental in American jurisprudence, that "[e]very human being of adult years and sound mind has a right to determine what shall be done with his own body. . . ." True consent to what happens to one's self is the informed exercise of a choice, and that entails an opportunity to evaluate knowledgeably the options available and the risks attendant upon each. The average patient has little or no understanding of the medical arts, and ordinarily has only his physician to whom he can look for enlightenment with which to reach an intelligent decision. From these almost axiomatic considerations springs the need, and in turn the requirement, of a reasonable divulgence by physician to patient to make such a decision possible.

. . .

Once the circumstances give rise to a duty on the physician's part to inform his patient, the next inquiry

No. 22099, U.S. Court of Appeals, District of Columbia Circuit, May 19, 1972. 464 Federal Reporter, 2nd Series, 772.

is the scope of the disclosure the physician is legally obliged to make. The courts have frequently confronted this problem, but no uniform standard defining the adequacy of the divulgence emerges from the decisions. Some have said "full" disclosure,[1] a norm we are unwilling to adopt literally. It seems obviously prohibitive and unrealistic to expect physicians to discuss with their patients every risk of proposed treatment—no matter how small or remote—and generally unnecessary from the patient's viewpoint as well. Indeed, the cases speaking in terms of "full" disclosure appear to envision something less than total disclosure,[2] leaving unanswered the question of just how much.

The larger number of courts, as might be expected, have applied tests framed with reference to prevailing fashion within the medical profession. Some have measured the disclosure by "good medical practice," others by what a reasonable practitioner would have bared under the circumstances, and still others by what medical custom in the community would demand. We have explored this rather considerable body of law but are unprepared to follow it. The duty to disclose, we have reasoned, arises from phenomena apart from medical custom and practice. The latter, we think, should no more establish the scope of the duty than its existence. Any definition of scope in terms purely of a professional standard is at odds with the patient's prerogative to decide on projected therapy himself. That prerogative, we have said, is at the very foundation of the duty to disclose, and both the patient's right to know and the physician's correlative obligation to tell him are diluted to the extent that its compass is dictated by the medical profession.

In our view, the patient's right of self-decision shapes the boundaries of the duty to reveal. That right can be effectively exercised only if the patient possesses enough information to enable an intelligent choice. The scope of the physician's communications to the patient, then, must be measured by the patient's need, and that need is the information material to the decision. Thus the test for determining whether a particular peril must be divulged is its materiality to the patient's decision: all risks potentially affecting the decision must be unmasked. And to safeguard the patient's interest in achieving his own determination on treatment, the law must itself set the standard for adequate disclosure.

Optimally for the patient, exposure of a risk would be mandatory whenever the patient would deem it significant to his decision, either singly or in combination with other risks. Such a requirement, however, would summon the physician to second-guess the patient, whose ideas on materiality could hardly be known to the physician. That would make an undue demand upon medical practitioners, whose conduct, like that of others, is to be measured in terms of reasonableness. Consonantly with orthodox negligence doctrine, the physician's liability for nondisclosure is to be determined on the basis of foresight, not hindsight; no less than any other aspect of negligence, the issue of nondisclosure must be approached from the viewpoint of the reasonableness of the physician's divulgence in terms of what he knows or should know to be the patient's informational needs. If, but only if, the factfinder can say that the physician's communication was unreasonably inadequate is an imposition of liability legally or morally justified.

Of necessity, the content of the disclosure rests in the first instance with the physician. Ordinarily it is only he who is in a position to identify particular dangers; always he must make a judgment, in terms of materiality, as to whether and to what extent revelation to the patient is called for. He cannot know with complete exactitude what the patient would consider important to his decision, but on the basis of his medical training and experience he can sense how the average, reasonable patient expectably would react. Indeed, with knowledge of, or ability to learn, his patient's background and current condition, he is in a position superior to that of most others—attorneys, for example—who are called upon to make judgments on pain of liability in damages for unreasonable miscalculation.

From these considerations we derive the breadth of the disclosure of risks legally to be required. The scope of the standard is not subjective as to either the physician or the patient; it remains objective with due regard for the patient's informational needs and with suitable leeway for the physician's situation. In broad outline, we agreed that "[a] risk is thus material when a reasonable person, in what the physician knows or should know to be the patient's position, would be likely to attach significance to the risk or cluster of risks in deciding whether or not to forgo the proposed therapy."[3]

The topics importantly demanding a communication of information are the inherent and potential hazards of the proposed treatment, the alternatives to that treatment, if any, and the results likely if the patient remains untreated. The factors contributing significance to the dangerousness of a medical technique are, of course, the incidence of injury and the degree of the harm threatened. A very small chance of death or serious disablement may well be significant; a potential disability which dramatically outweighs the potential benefit of the therapy or the detriments of the existing malady may summon discussion with the patient.

There is no bright line separating the significant from the insignificant; the answer in any case must abide a rule of reason. Some dangers—infection, for example—are inherent in any operation; there is no obligation to communicate those of which persons of average sophistication are aware. Even more clearly, the physician bears no responsibility for discussion of hazards the patient has already discovered, or those having no apparent materiality to patients' decision on therapy. The disclosure doctrine, like others marking lines between permissible and impermissible behavior in medical practice, is in essence a requirement of conduct prudent under the circumstances. Whenever nondisclosure of particular risk information is open to debate by reasonable-minded men, the issue is for the finder of the facts.

Two exceptions to the general rule of disclosure have been noted by the courts. Each is in the nature of a physician's privilege not to disclose, and the reasoning underlying them is appealing. Each, indeed, is but a recognition that, as important as is the patient's right to know, it is greatly outweighed by the magnitudinous circumstances giving rise to the privilege. The first comes into play when the patient is unconscious or otherwise incapable of consenting, and harm from a failure to treat is imminent and outweighs any harm threatened by the proposed treatment. When a genuine emergency of that sort arises, it is settled that the impracticality of conferring with the patient dispenses with need for it. Even in situations of that character the physician should, as current law requires, attempt to secure a relative's consent if possible. But if time is too short to accommodate discussion obviously the physician should proceed with the treatment.

The second exception obtains when risk-disclosure poses such a threat of detriment to the patient as to become unfeasible or contraindicated from a medical point of view. It is recognized that patients occasionally become so ill or emotionally distraught on disclosure as to foreclose a rational decision, or complicate or hinder the treatment, or perhaps even pose psychological damage to the patient. Where that is so, the cases have generally held that the physician is armed with a privilege to keep the information from the patient, and we think it clear that portents of that type may justify the physician in action he deems medically warranted. The critical inquiry is whether the physician responded to a sound medical judgment that communication of the risk information would present a threat to the patient's well-being.

The physician's privilege to withhold information for therapeutic reasons must be carefully circumscribed, however, for otherwise it might devour the disclosure rule itself. The privilege does not accept the paternalistic notion that the physician may remain silent simply because divulgence might prompt the patient to forgo therapy the physician feels the patient really needs. That attitude presumes instability or perversity for even the normal patient, and runs counter to the foundation principle that the patient should and ordinarily can make the choice for himself. Nor does the privilege contemplate operation save where the patient's reaction to risk information, as reasonably foreseen by the physician, is menacing. And even in a situation of that kind, disclosure to a close relative with a view to securing consent to the proposed treatment may be the only alternative open to the physician.

NOTES

1. *E.g.*, Salgo v. Leland Stanford Jr. Univ. Bd. of Trustees, 154 Cal. App. 2d 560, 317 P.2d 170, 181 (1975); Woods v. Brumlop, *supra* note 13 [in original text], 377 P.2d at 524–525.

2. See, Comment, Informed Consent in Medical Malpractice, 55 Calif. L. Rv. 1396, 1402–03 (1967).

3. Waltz and Scheuneman, Informed Consent to Therapy, 64, Nw. U.L. Rev. 628, 640 (1970).

J A Y   K A T Z

Physicians and Patients: A History of Silence

Reprinted by permission of the author.

Disclosure and consent, except in the most rudimentary fashion, are obligations alien to medical thinking and practice. Disclosure in medicine has served the function of getting patients to "consent" to what physicians wanted them to agree to in the first place. "Good" patients follow doctor's orders without question. Therefore, disclosure becomes relevant only with recalcitrant patients. Since they are "bad" and "ungrateful," one does not need to bother much with them. Hippocrates once said, "Life is short, the Art long, Opportunity fleeting, Experiment treacherous, Judgment difficult. The physician must be ready, not only to do his duty himself, but also to secure the cooperation of the patient, of the attendants and of externals." These were, and still are, the lonely obligations of physicians: to wrestle as best they can with life, art, opportunity, experiment and judgment. Sharing with patients the vagaries of available opportunities, however perilous or safe, or the rationale underlying judgments, however difficult or easy, is not part of the Hippocratic task. For doing that, the Art is too long and Life too short.

Physicians have always maintained that patients are only in need of caring custody. Doctors felt that in order to accomplish that objective they were obligated to attend to their patients' physical and emotional needs and to do so on their own authority, without consulting with their patients about the decisions that needed to be made. Indeed, doctors intuitively believed that such consultations were inimical to good patient care. The idea that patients may also be entitled to liberty, to sharing the burdens of decision with their doctors, was never part of the ethos of medicine. Being unaware of the idea of patient liberty, physicians did not address the possible conflict between notions of custody and liberty. When, however, in recent decades courts were confronted with allegations that professionals had deprived citizen-patients of freedom of choice, the conflict did emerge. Anglo-American law has, at least in theory, a long-standing tradition of preferring liberty over custody; and however much judges tried to sidestep law's preferences and to side with physicians' traditional beliefs, the conflict remained and has ever since begged for a resolution. . . .

The legal doctrine remained limited in scope, in part, because judges believed or wished to believe that their pronouncements on informed consent gave legal force to what good physicians customarily did; therefore they felt that they could defer to the disclosure practices of "reasonable medical practitioners." Judges did not appreciate how deeply rooted the tradition of silence was and thus did not recognize the revolutionary, alien implications of their appeal for patient "self-determination." In fact, precisely because of the appeal's strange and bewildering novelty, physicians misinterpreted it as being more far-reaching than courts intended it to be.

Physicians did not realize how much their opposition to informed consent was influenced by suddenly encountering obligations divorced from their history, their clinical experience, or medical education. Had they appreciated that even the doctrine's modest appeal to patient self-determination represented a radical break with medical practices, as transmitted from teacher to student during more than two thousand years of recorded medical history, they might have been less embarrassed by standing so unpreparedly, so nakedly before this new obligation. They might then perhaps have realized that their silence had been until most recently a historical necessity, dictated not only by the inadequacy of medical knowledge but also by physicians' incapacity to discriminate between therapeutic

effectiveness based on their actual physical interventions and benefits that must be ascribed to other causes. They might also have argued that the practice of silence was part of a long and venerable tradition that deserved not to be dismissed lightly. . . .

When I speak of silence I do not mean to suggest that physicians have not talked to their patients at all. Of course, they have conversed with patients about all kinds of matters, but they have not, except inadvertently, employed words to invite patients' participation in sharing the burden of making joint decisions. . . .

Judges have made impassioned pleas for patient self-determination, and then have undercut them by giving physicians considerable latitude to practice according to their own lights, exhorting them only to treat each patient with the utmost care. Judges could readily advance this more limited plea because generally doctors do treat their patients with solicitude. The affirmation of physicians' commitment to patients' physical needs, however, has failed to address physicians' lack of commitment to patients' decision making needs. These tensions have led judges to fashion a doctrine of informed consent that has secured for patients the right to better custody but not to liberty—the right to choose how to be treated. . . .

CANTERBURY V. SPENCE (1972)

Judge Robinson, of the D.C. Court of Appeals, who authored the . . . last landmark informed consent decision, also had good intentions. . . . The lesson to be learned from a study of Canterbury [is that]: The strong commitment to self-determination at the beginning of the opinion gets weaker as the opinion moves from jurisprudential theory to the realities of hospital and courtroom life. By the end, the opinion has only obscured the issue it intended to address: the nature of the relationship between the court's doctrine of informed consent, as ultimately construed, and its root premise of self-determination. . . .

Respect for the patient's right of self-determination on particular therapy demands a standard set by law for physicians rather than one which physicians may or may not impose upon themselves.

For this apparently bold move, Canterbury has been widely celebrated, as well as followed in many jurisdictions.

The new rule of law laid down in *Canterbury*, however, is far from clear. Judge Robinson, returning to basic principles of expert testimony, simply said that there is "no basis for operation of the special medical standard where the physician's activity does not bring his medical knowledge and skills peculiarly into play," and that ordinarily disclosure is not such a situation. But he left room for such situations by adding: "When medical judgment enters the picture and for that reason the special standard controls, prevailing medical practice must be given its *just due*." He did not spell out the meaning of "*just due*."

Both standards tend to confuse the need for *medical knowledge* to elucidate the risks of and alternatives to a proposed procedure in the light of professional experience with the need for *medical judgment* to establish the limits of appropriate disclosure to patients. The difference is crucial to the clarification of the law of informed consent. In *Natanson* and many subsequent cases, judges lumped the two together uncritically, relying solely on current medical practice to resolve the question of reasonableness of disclosure. In *Canterbury*, the distinction was formally recognized. The plaintiff was required to present expert evidence of the applicable medical knowledge, while the defendant had to raise the issue of medical judgment to limit disclosure in defense. But even *Canterbury* did not undertake a detailed judicial analysis of the nature of medical judgment required, precisely because judges were hesitant to make rules in an area that doctors strongly believed was solely the province of medicine.

In *Canterbury*, Dr. Spence claimed that "communication of that risk (paralysis) to the patient is not good medical practice because it might deter patients from undergoing needed surgery and might produce adverse psychological reactions which could preclude the success of the operation." Such claims will almost invariably be raised by physicians since they are derived from deeply held tenets of medical practice. Judge Robinson's enigmatic phrase of "just due" certainly suggests that the medical professional standard would be applicable in such a case, raising profound questions about the extent to which the novel legal standard has been swallowed up by the traditional and venerable medical standard.

In fact, medical judgment was given its "just due" twice. It could also be invoked under the "therapeutic privilege" not to disclose, which Judge Robinson retained as a defense to disclosure:

It is recognized that patients occasionally become so ill or emotionally distraught on disclosure as to foreclose a rational decision, or complicate or hinder the treatment, or perhaps even pose psychological damage to the patient. . . . The critical inquiry is whether the physician responded to a sound medical judgment that communication of the risk information would present a threat to the patient's well-being.

The therapeutic privilege not to disclose is merely a procedurally different way of invoking the professional standard of care. . . .

Since the court wished to depart from medical custom as the standard, it had to give some indication as to the information it expected physicians to disclose. The court said that "the test for determining whether a particular peril must be divulged is its materiality to the patient's decision: all risks potentially affecting the decision must be unmasked." It added that physicians must similarly disclose alternatives to the proposed treatment and the "results likely if the patient remains untreated."

But then the court chose to adopt an "objective" test for disclosure of risks and alternatives—"what a [reasonable] *prudent* person in the patient's position would have decided if suitably informed"—and rejected a "subjective" test of materiality—"what an *individual* patient would have considered a significant risk." In opting for an "objective" standard, self-determination was given unnecessarily short shrift. The whole point of the inquiry was to safeguard the right of *individual* choice, even where it may appear idiosyncratic. Although law generally does not protect a person's right to be unreasonable and requires reasonably prudent conduct where injury to another may occur, it remains ambiguous about the extent to which prudence can be legally enforced where the potential injury is largely confined to the individual decision maker. For example, courts have split on the question of whether society may require the wearing of motorcycle helmets and whether an adult patient may be compelled to undergo unwanted blood transfusions.

The "objective" standard for disclosure contradicts the right of each individual to decide what will be done with his or her body. The belief that there is one "reasonable" or "prudent" response to every situation inviting medical intervention is nonsense, from the point of view of both the physician and the patient. The most cursory examination of medical practices demonstrates that what is reasonable to the internist may appear unreasonable to the surgeon or even to other internists and, more significantly, that the value preferences of physicians may not coincide with those of their patients. For example, doctors generally place a higher value on physical longevity than their patients do. But physical longevity is not the only touchstone of prudence. Why should not informed consent law countenance a wide range of potentially reasonable responses by patients to their medical condition based on other value preferences? . . .

Ascertaining patients' informational needs is difficult. Answers do not lie in guessing or "sensing" patients' particular concerns or in obliterating the "subjective" person in an "objective" mass of persons. The "objective" test of materiality only tempts doctors to introduce their own unwarranted subjectivity into the disclosure process. It would have been far better if the court had not committed itself prematurely to the labels "objective" and "subjective." Instead it should have considered more the patients' plight and required physicians to learn new skills: how to inquire openly about their patients' *individual* informational needs and patients' concerns, doubts, and misconceptions about treatment—its risks, benefits, and alternatives. Safeguarding self-determination requires assessing whether patients' informational needs have been satisfied by asking them whether they understand what has been explained to them. Physicians should not try to "second-guess" patients or "sense" how they will react. Instead, they need to explore what questions require further explanation. Taking such unaccustomed obligations seriously is not easy. . . .

SUMMING UP

The legal life of "informed consent," if quality of human life is measured not merely by improvements in physical custody but also by advancement of liberty, was over almost as soon as it was born. Except for the . . . law promulgated in a handful of jurisdictions and the more generally espoused dicta about "self-determination" and "freedom of choice," this is substantially true. Judges toyed briefly with the idea of patients' right to self-determination and largely cast it aside. . . .

Treatment decisions are extremely complex and require a more sustained dialogue, one in which patients are viewed as participants in medical decisions affecting their lives. This is not the view of most physicians, who believe instead that patients are too ignorant to make decisions on their own behalf, that disclosure increases patients' fears and reinforces "foolish" decisions, and that informing them about the uncertainties of medical interventions in many instances seriously undermines faith so essential to the success of therapy. Therefore, physicians asserted that they must be the ultimate decision makers. Judges did not probe these contentions in depth but were persuaded to refrain from interfering significantly with traditional medical practices.

I have not modified my earlier assessment of law's informed consent vision:

[T]he law of informed consent is substantially mythic and fairy tale-like as far as advancing patients' rights to self-decisionmaking is concerned. It conveys in its dicta about such rights a fairy tale-like optimism about human capacities for "intelligent" choice and for being respectful of other persons' choices; yet in its implementation of dicta, it conveys a mythic pessimism of human capacities to be choice-makers. The resulting tensions have had a significant impact on the law of informed consent which only has made a bow toward a commitment to patients' self-determination, perhaps in an attempt to resolve these tensions by a belief that it is "less important that this commitment be total than that we believe it to be there."

Whether fairy tale and myth can and should be reconciled more satisfactorily with reality remains to be seen. If judges contemplate such a reconciliation, they must acquire first a more profound understanding and appreciation of medicine's vision of patients and professional practice, of the capacities of physicians and patients for autonomous choice, and of the limits of professional knowledge. Such understanding cannot readily be acquired in courts of law, during disputes in which inquiry is generally constrained by claims and counter-claims that seek to assure victory for one side.

The call to liberty, embedded in the doctrine of informed consent, has only created an atmosphere in which freedom has the potential to survive and grow. The doctrine has not as yet provided a meaningful blueprint for implementing patient self-determination. The message . . . is this: Those committed to greater patient self-determination can, if they look hard enough, find inspiration in the common law of informed consent, and so can those, and more easily, who seek to perpetuate medical paternalism. Those who look for evidence of committed implementation will be sadly disappointed. The legal vision of informed consent, based on *self-determination*, is still largely a mirage. Yet a mirage, since it not only deceives but also can sustain hope, is better than no vision at all. . . .

PRESIDENT'S COMMISSION FOR THE STUDY OF ETHICAL PROBLEMS IN MEDICINE AND BIOMEDICAL AND BEHAVIORAL RESEARCH

Informed Consent as Active, Shared Decisionmaking

In the past quarter-century, American courts, supported by legal and ethical commentary, have articulated a legal doctrine of "informed consent" that requires health care practitioners not simply to seek the consent of their patients, but also, through a process of disclosure and discussion between practitioners and patients, to make such consents "informed." Thus, the law requiring informed consent has become an important means by which society regulates relationships between patients and health care professionals. . . .

Current requirements for informed consent owe much to the legal system, but the values underlying these requirements are not merely legal artifacts. Rather, they are deeply embedded in American culture and the American character; they transcend partisan ideologies and the politics of the moment. Fundamentally, informed consent is based on respect for the individual, and, in particular, for each individual's capacity and right both to define his or her own goals and to make choices designed to achieve those goals. But in defining informed consent (and its exceptions) the law has tempered this right of self-determination with respect for other values, such as promotion of well-being in the context of an expert-layperson relationship. . . .

From *Making Health Care Decisions*. Vol. 1. Washington, D.C.: Government Printing Office, 1982.

LAW, ETHICS, AND MEDICAL PRACTICE

The realities of court decisions on informed consent . . . fall short of the law's professed commitment to the value of self-determination. Since "the courts imposed primarily a duty-to-warn on physicians," thereby avoiding a judicial recognition of the proposition that patients have a decisive role to play in the medical decisionmaking process, they have merely reinforced "physicians' traditional monologue of talking *at* and not *with* patients."[1] As a result they have missed the opportunity to move toward what is needed: "a new and unaccustomed dialogue between physicians and their patients . . . in which both, appreciative of their respective inequalities, make a genuine effort to voice and clarify their uncertainties and then to arrive at a mutually satisfactory course of action."[2]

The Commission, while recognizing the difficulty of the task, believes that "shared decisionmaking" is the appropriate ideal for patient-professional relationships that a sound doctrine of informed consent should support. The Commission doubts that this will occur, however, if primary reliance is placed on the courts. This is not to say that present legal requirements for informed consent should be abandoned or reduced in scope. Current law serves the important purpose of encouraging health care professionals to disclose important facts to patients and not to proceed with medical interventions unless patients have consented. The law also serves a critical moral and educative role in proclaiming (even if not always fully enforcing) the value of self-determination. These functions can and should continue. The Commission's skepticism relates solely to the likelihood that an expansion of the existing law could control ever more minutely the relationships of patients and health care professionals. . . .

The Commission concludes that considerable flexibility should be accorded to patients and professionals to define the terms of their own relationships. The resolution favored by the Commission is a presumption that certain fundamental types of information should be made available to patients and that all patients competent to do so have a right to accept or reject medical interventions affecting them. Similarly, a professional who has been as flexible about possible avenues of treatment as his or her beliefs and standards allow is not generally obligated to accede to the patient in a way that violates the bounds of acceptable medical practice or the provider's own deeply held moral beliefs.

Nevertheless, in light of the disparities between the positions of the parties, the interaction should, at a minimum, provide the patient with a basis for effective participation in sound decisionmaking regardless of the particular form of the accommodation. It will usually consist of discussions between professional and patient that bring the knowledge, concerns, and perspective of each to the process of seeking agreement on a course of treatment.[3] Simply put, this means that the physician or other health professional invites the patient to participate in a dialogue in which the professional seeks to help the patient understand the medical situation and available courses of action, and the patient conveys his or her concerns and wishes.[4] This does not involve a mechanical recitation of abstruse medical information, but should include disclosures that give the patient an understanding of his or her condition and an appreciation of its consequences.

The Commission encourages, to perhaps a greater degree than is explicitly recognized by current law, the ability of patients and health care professionals to vary the style and extent of discussion from that mandated by this general presumption. Such variations might take any of several directions: in one relationship, the patient might prefer not to be burdened by detailed discussion of risks unlikely to arise or to affect the decision; in another relationship, a patient might request unusually detailed information on unconventional alternative therapies; in a third, a patient with a longstanding and close relationship of trust with a particular physician might ask that physician to proceed as he or she thinks best, choosing the course of therapy and revealing any information that the physician thinks would best serve the interests of the patient. Inherent in allowing such variations is the difficulty of ensuring they are genuinely agreeable to both parties and do not themselves arise out of an imbalance in status or bargaining power.

The health professional's expert knowledge, focused through the particular diagnosis and prognosis for the patient, usually confers on that person the natural role of leader and initiator in building this shared understanding. The patient, on the other hand, is especially well placed to assess the overall effects of the medical condition and possible treatments, in light of his or her own particular goals and values. Thus each party brings to the relationship special knowledge and perspectives that can help to clarify for both parties what is actually at issue in any decision to be reached.

The Commission is aware that its description of mutual participation and shared decisionmaking sets a high ideal. Both professional and patient in this dialogue are liable to misunderstandings and confusions, false hope or despair, unvoiced fears, anxiety, and questions. Even when each is sensitive to the presence of these barriers to full understanding and seeks to surmount them in the interest of agreeing on their common venture—that is, treating the patient successfully—difficulties will persist. Yet it remains a goal worth striving toward. . . .

VOLUNTARINESS IN DECISIONMAKING

[One] requirement for informed consent is that the patient's participation in the decisionmaking process and ultimate decision regarding care must be voluntary. A choice that has been coerced, or that resulted from serious manipulation of a person's ability to make an intelligent and informed decision, is not the person's own free choice. This has long been recognized in law: a consent forced by threats or induced by fraud or misrepresentation is legally viewed as no consent at all. From the perspective of ethics, a consent that is substantially involuntary does not provide moral authorization for treatment because it does not respect the patient's dignity and may not reflect the aims of the patient.

Of course, the facts of disease and the limited capabilities of medicine often constrict the choices available to patient and physician alike. In that sense, the condition of illness itself is sometimes spoken of as "coercive" or involuntary. But the fact that no available alternative may be desirable in itself, and that the preferred course is, at best, only the least bad among a bad lot, does not render a choice coerced in the sense employed here. No change in human behavior or institutional structure could remove this limitation. Such constraints are merely facts of life that should not be regarded as making a patient's choice involuntary.

Voluntariness is best regarded as a matter of degree, rather than as a quality that is wholly present or absent in particular cases. Forced treatment—the embodiment of coercive, involuntary action—appears to be rare in the American health care system. Health care professionals do, however, make limited intrusions on voluntary choice through subtle, or even overt, manipulations of patients' wills when they believe that patients would otherwise make incorrect decisions.

Forced Treatment. The most overt forms of involuntariness in health care settings involve interventions forced on patients without their consent (and sometimes over their express objection) and those based on coerced consent. Although rare in mainstream American health care, such situations do arise in certain special settings, and therefore require brief discussion. Society currently legitimates certain forced medical interventions to serve important social goals such as promoting the public health (with, for example, compulsory vaccination laws), enforcing the criminal law (removing bullets needed as evidence for criminal prosecutions), or otherwise promoting the well-being of others (sedating uncontrollable inmates of mental institutions on an emergency basis, for example, to protect other inmates or staff).

Although it is typically not viewed as forced treatment, a good deal of routine care in hospitals, nursing homes, and other health care settings is provided (usually by health professionals such as nurses) without explicit and voluntary consent by patients. The expectation on the part of professionals is that patients, once in such a setting, will simply go along with such routine care. However, the Commission's study of treatment refusals found that in a hospital setting it was the routine tests that were most likely to be refused. At least some patients expected that participation was

voluntary and refused tests and medications ordered without their knowledge until adequate information was provided about the nature, purpose, and risks of these undertakings. Lack of information in such cases may not only preclude voluntary participation but also raise questions about a patient's rationality, and hence competence.

When a situation offers the patient an opportunity to refuse care, then patient compliance or acquiescence may be viewed as implicit consent. But when the tacit communication accompanying such care is that there is no choice for the patient to make, and compliance is expected and enforced (at least in the absence of vigorous objections), the treatment can be properly termed "forced." The following conversation between a nurse and a patient regarding postoperative care, obtained in one of the Commission's observational studies, illustrates forced treatment that follows routinely from another decision (surgery) that was made voluntarily.

Nurse: Did they mention anything about a tube through your nose?

Patient: Yes, I'm gonna have a tube in my nose.

Nurse: You're going to have the tube down for a couple of days or longer. It depends. So you're going to be NPO, nothing by mouth, and also you're going to have IV fluid.

Patient: I know. For three or four days they told me that already. I don't like it, though.

Nurse: You don't have any choice.

Patient: Yes, I don't have any choice, I know.

Nurse: Like it or not, you don't have any choice. (laughter) After you come back, we'll ask you to do a lot of coughing and deep breathing to exercise your lungs.

Patient: Oh, we'll see how I feel.

Nurse: (Emphasis) No matter how you feel, you have to do that!

The interview ended a few minutes later with the patient still disputing whether he was going to cooperate with the postoperative care.

Coerced Treatment. Unlike forced treatment, for which no consent is given, coerced treatment proceeds on the basis of a consent that was not freely given. As used in this sense, a patient's decision is coerced when the person is credibly threatened by another individual, either explicitly or by implication, with unwanted and avoidable consequences unless the patient accedes to the specified course of action. Concern about coercion is accordingly greatest when a disproportion in power or other significant inequality between a patient and another individual lends credibility to the threat of harm and when the perceived interests of the individuals diverge.

The disparity in power between patient and health care professional may be slight or substantial, depending on the nature of the patient's illness, the institutional setting, the personalities of the individuals involved, and several other factors. In nonemergency settings, a patient typically can change practitioners or simply forego treatment, thus avoiding the potential for coercion. Further, although health care professionals do have interests distinct from and sometimes in conflict with those of their patients, strong social and professional norms usually ensure that priority is accorded to patients' welfare. To be sure, coercion can be exercised with benevolent motives if practitioner and patient differ in their assessments of how the patient's welfare is best served. Nonetheless, there is little reason to believe that blatant forms of coercion are a problem in mainstream American health care. When isolated instances of abuse do arise, the law provides suitable remedies.

A patient's family and other concerned persons may often play a useful role in the decisionmaking process. Sometimes, however, they may try to coerce a particular decision, either because of what they perceive to be in the patient's best interests or because of a desire to advance their own interests. In such instances, since the health care professional's first loyalty is to the patient, he or she should attempt to enhance the patient's ability to make a voluntary, uncoerced decision and to overcome any coercive pressures.

Manipulation. Blatant coercion may be of so little concern in professional-patient relationships because, as physicians so often proclaim, it is so easy for health professionals to elicit a desired decision through more subtle means. Indeed, some physicians are critical of the legal requirement for informed consent on the grounds that it must be mere window dressing since "patients will, if they trust their doctor, accede to almost any request he cares to make."[5] On some occasions, to be sure, this result can be achieved by rational persuasion, since the professional presumably has good reasons for preferring a recommended course of action. But the tone of such critics suggests they have something else in mind: an ability to package and present the facts in a way that leaves the patient with no real choice. Such conduct, capitalizing on disparities in knowledge, position, and influence, is manipulative in character and impairs the voluntariness of the patient's choice.

Manipulation has more and less extreme forms. At one end of the spectrum is behavior amounting to misrepresentation or fraud. Of particular concern in health care contexts is the withholding or distortion of information in order to affect the patient's beliefs and decisions. The patient might not be told about alternatives to the recommended course of action, for example, or the risks or other negative characteristics of the recommended treatment might be minimized. Such behavior is justly criticized on two grounds: first, that it interferes with the patient's voluntary choice (and thus negates consent) and, second, that it interferes with the patient's ability to make an informed decision. At the other end of the spectrum are far more subtle instances: a professional's careful choice of words or nuances of tone and emphasis might present the situation in a manner calculated to heighten the appeal of a particular course of action.

It is well known that the way information is presented can powerfully affect the recipient's response to it. The tone of voice and other aspects of the practitioner's manner of presentation can indicate whether a risk of a particular kind with a particular incidence should be considered serious. Information can be emphasized or played down without altering the content. And it can be framed in a way that affects the listener—for example, "this procedure succeeds most of the time" versus "this procedure has a 40 percent failure rate." Health professionals who are aware of the effects of such minor variations can choose their language with care; if, during discussions with a patient, they sense any unintended or confused impressions being created, they can adjust their presentation of information accordingly.

Because many patients are often fearful and unequal to their physicians in status, knowledge, and power, they may be particularly susceptible to manipulations of this type. Health care professionals should, therefore, present information in a form that fosters understanding. Patients should be helped to understand the prognosis for their situation and the implications of different courses of treatment. The difficult distinction, both in theory and in practice, is between acceptable forms of informing, discussion, and rational persuasion on the one hand, and objectionable forms of influence or manipulation on the other.

Since voluntariness is one of the foundation stones of informed consent, professionals have a high ethical obligation to avoid coercion and manipulation of their patients. The law penalizes those who ignore the requirements of consent or who directly coerce it. But it can do little about subtle manipulations without incurring severe disruptions of private relationships by intrusive policing, and so the duty is best thought of primarily in ethical terms.

NOTES

1. Jay Katz, *Disclosure and Consent: In Search of Their Roots*, in Aubrey Milunsky and George J. Annas, eds., GENETICS AND THE LAW II, Plenum Press, New York (1980) at 122.

2. *Id.*

3. The Commission's focus in this discussion on the process of reaching agreement is quite deliberate. For perhaps understandable reasons, much of the scholarly legal and philosophical literature concentrates on the "hard case," the case in which no agreement can be reached: when it comes to the crunch, who ultimately has the power to decide? Although such questions cannot be ignored, the Commission's effort in this Report is to readjust the balance toward fuller consideration of those less dramatic issues that arise routinely in the day-to-day practice of responsible medicine and nursing but that have received less attention and emphasis.

4. This image of reaching out to a patient is captured well in the following: "The skillful doctor, metaphorically speaking, throws out a rope to the patient drowning in illness and by encouraging the patient to hold on furthers the healing process."

5. Henry K. Beecher, *Some Guiding Principles for Clinical Investigation*, 195 J.A.M.A. 1135, 1135 (1966). *See also* Norman Fost, *A Surrogate System for Informed Consent*, 233 J.A.M.A. 800 (1975).

RUTH R. FADEN AND TOM L. BEAUCHAMP

The Concept of Informed Consent

What is an informed consent? Answering this question is complicated because there are two common, entrenched, and starkly different meanings of "informed consent." That is, the term is analyzable in two profoundly different ways—not because of mere subtle differences of connotation that appear in different contexts, but because two different *conceptions* of informed consent have emerged from its history and are still at work, however unnoticed, in literature on the subject.

In one sense, which we label *sense₁*, "informed consent" is analyzable as a particular kind of action by individual patients and subjects: an autonomous authorization. In the second sense, *sense₂*, informed consent is analyzable in terms of the web of cultural

and policy rules and requirements of consent that collectively form the social practice of informed consent in institutional contexts where *groups* of patients and subjects must be treated in accordance with rules, policies, and standard practices. Here, informed consents are not always *autonomous* acts, nor are they always in any meaningful respect *authorizations*.

SENSE₁: INFORMED CONSENT AS AUTONOMOUS AUTHORIZATION

The idea of an informed consent suggests that a patient or subject does more than express agreement with, acquiesce in, yield to, or comply with an arrangement or a proposal. He or she actively *authorizes* the proposal in the act of consent. John may *assent* to a treatment plan without authorizing it. The assent may be a mere submission to the doctor's authoritative order, in which case John does not call on his *own* authority in order to give permission, and thus does not authorize the plan. Instead, he acts like a child who submits, yields, or assents to the school principal's spanking and in no way gives permission for or authorizes the spanking. Just as the child merely submits to an authority in a system where the lines of authority are quite clear, so often do patients.

Accordingly, an informed consent in sense$_1$ should be defined as follows: An informed consent is an autonomous action by a subject or a patient that authorizes a professional either to involve the subject in research or to initiate a medical plan for the patient (or both). We can whittle down this definition by saying that an informed consent in sense$_1$ is given if a patient or subject with (1) substantial understanding and (2) in substantial absence of control by others (3) intentionally (4) authorizes a professional (to do intervention I).

All substantially autonomous acts satisfy conditions 1–3; but it does not follow from that analysis alone that all such acts satisfy 4. The fourth condition is what distinguishes informed consent as one *kind* of autonomous action. (Note also that the definition restricts the kinds of authorization to medical and research contexts.) A person whose act satisfies conditions 1–3 but who refuses an intervention gives an *informed refusal*. The conditions of this latter kind of action are identical to 1–4 above, except that the fourth condition is the converse, a nonauthorization or refusal to authorize.

The Problem of Shared Decisionmaking. This analysis of informed consent in sense$_1$ is deliberately silent on the question of how the authorizer and the agent(s) being authorized *arrive at an agreement* about the performance of "I." Recent commentators on informed consent in clinical medicine, notably Jay Katz and the President's Commission, have tended to equate the idea of informed consent with a model of "shared decisionmaking" between doctor and patient. The President's Commission titles the first chapter of its report on informed consent in the patient-practitioner relationship "Informed Consent as Active, Shared Decision Making," while in Katz's work "the idea of informed consent" and "mutual decisionmaking" are treated as virtually synonymous terms.[1]

There is of course an historical relationship in clinical medicine between medical decisionmaking and informed consent. The emergence of the legal doctrine of informed consent was instrumental in drawing attention to issues of decisionmaking as well as authority in the doctor-patient relationship. Nevertheless, it is a

confusion to treat informed consent and shared decisionmaking as anything like *synonymous*. For one thing, informed consent is not restricted to clinical medicine. It is a term that applies equally to biomedical and behavioral research contexts where a model of shared decisionmaking is frequently inappropriate. Even in clinical contexts, the social and psychological dynamics involved in selecting medical interventions should be distinguished from the patient's *authorization*.

We endorse Katz's view that effective communication between professional and patient or subject is often instrumental in obtaining informed consents (sense$_1$), but we resist his conviction that the idea of informed consent entails that the patient and physician "share decisionmaking," or "reason together," or reach a consensus about what is in the patient's best interest. This is a manipulation of the concept from a too singular and defined moral perspective on the practice of medicine that is in effect a moral program for changing the practice. Although the patient and physician *may* reach a decision together, they need not. It is the essence of informed consent in sense$_1$ only that the patient or subject *authorizes autonomously*; it is a matter of indifference where or how the proposal being authorized originates.

For example, one might advocate a model of shared decisionmaking for the doctor-patient relationship without simultaneously advocating that every medical procedure requires the consent of patients. Even relationships characterized by an ample slice of shared decisionmaking, mutual trust, and respect would and should permit many decisions about routine and low-risk aspects of the patient's medical treatment to remain the exclusive province of the physician, and thus some decisions are likely always to remain subject exclusively to the physician's authorization. Moreover, in the uncommon situation, a patient could autonomously authorize the physician to make *all* decisions about medical treatment, thus giving his or her informed consent to an arrangement that scarcely resembles the sharing of decisionmaking between doctor and patient.

Authorization. Because authorization is central to our account of informed consent in sense$_1$, it seems appropriate that we provide an analysis of the notion of authorization. Because to do so with thoroughness would require its own volume, our analysis must be brief: In authorizing, one both assumes responsibility for what one has authorized and transfers to another one's authority to implement it. There is no informed consent unless one *understands* these features of the act and *intends* to perform that act. That is, one must understand that one is assuming responsibility and warranting another to proceed.

To say that one assumes responsibility does not quite locate the essence of the matter, however, because a *transfer* of responsibility as well as of authority also occurs. One's authorization gives another both permission to proceed and the responsibility for proceeding. Depending on the social circumstances, X's having authorized Y to do I generally signifies either that X and Y *share* responsibility for the consequences of I or that the responsibility is entirely X's (assuming, of course, that Y executes I in a non-negligent and responsible fashion). Thus, the crucial element in an authorization is that the person who authorizes uses whatever right, power, or control he or she possesses in the situation to endow another with the right to act. In so doing, the authorizer assumes some responsibility for the actions taken by the other person. Here one could either authorize *broadly* so that a person can act in accordance with general guidelines, or *narrowly* so as to authorize only a particular, carefully circumscribed procedure.

SENSE$_2$: INFORMED CONSENT AS EFFECTIVE CONSENT

By contrast to sense$_1$, sense$_2$, or *effective* consent, is a policy-oriented sense whose conditions are not derivable solely from analyses of autonomy and authorization, or even from broad notions of respect for autonomy. "Informed consent" in this second sense does not refer to *autonomous* authorization, but to a legally or institutionally *effective* (sometimes misleadingly called *valid*) authorization from a patient or a subject. Such an authorization is "effective" because it has been obtained through procedures that satisfy the rules and requirements defining a specific institutional practice in health care or in research.

The social and legal practice of requiring professionals to obtain informed consent emerged in institutional contexts, where conformity to operative rules was and still is the sole necessary and sufficient condition of informed consent. Any consent is an informed consent in sense$_2$ if it satisfies whatever operative rules apply to the practice of informed consent. Sense$_2$ requirements for informed consent typically do not focus on the autonomy of the act of giving consent (as sense$_1$ does), but rather on regulating the behavior of the *consent-seeker* and on establishing *procedures and rules* for the context of consent. Such requirements of professional behavior and procedure are obviously more readily monitored and enforced by institutions.

However, because formal institutional rules such as federal regulations and hospital policies govern whether an act of authorizing is effective, a patient or subject can autonomously authorize an intervention, and so give an informed consent in sense$_1$, and yet *not effectively authorize* that intervention in sense$_2$.

Consider the following example. Carol and Martie are nineteen-year-old, identical twins attending the same university. Martie was born with multiple birth defects, and has only one kidney. When both sisters are involved in an automobile accident, Carol is not badly hurt, but her sister is seriously injured. It is quickly determined that Martie desperately needs a kidney transplant. After detailed discussions with the transplant team and with friends, Carol consents to be the donor. There is no question that Carol's authorization of the transplant surgery is substantially autonomous. She is well informed and has long anticipated being in just such a circumstance. She has had ample opportunity over the years to consider what she would do were she faced with such a decision. Unfortunately, Carol's parents, who were in Nepal at the time of the accident, do not approve of her decision. Furious that they were not consulted, they decide to sue the transplant team and the hospital for having performed an unauthorized surgery on their minor daughter. (In this state the legal age to consent to surgical procedures is twenty-one.)

According to our analysis, Carol gave her informed consent in sense$_1$ to the surgery, but she did not give her informed consent in sense$_2$. That is, she autonomously authorized the transplant and thereby gave an informed consent in sense$_1$ but did not give a consent that was effective under the operative legal and institutional policy, which in this case required that the person consenting be a legally authorized agent. Examples of other policies that can define sense$_2$ informed consent (but not sense$_1$) include rules that consent be witnessed by an auditor or that there be a one-day waiting period between solicitation of consent and implementation of the intervention in order for the person's authorization to be effective. Such rules can and do vary, both within the United States by jurisdiction and institution, and across the countries of the world.

Medical and research codes, as well as case law and federal regulations, have developed models of informed consent that are delineated entirely in a sense$_2$ format, although they have sometimes attempted to justify the rules by appeal to something like sense$_1$. For example, disclosure conditions for informed consent are central to the history of "informed consent" in sense$_2$, because disclosure has traditionally been a *necessary* condition of effective informed consent (and sometimes a *sufficient* condition!). The legal doctrine of informed consent is primarily a law of disclosure; satisfaction of disclosure rules virtually consumes "informed consent" in law. This should come as no surprise, because the legal system needs a generally applicable informed consent mechanism by which injury and responsibility can be readily and fairly assessed in court. These disclosure requirements in the legal and regulatory contexts are not conditions of "informed consent" in sense$_1$; indeed disclosure may be entirely irrelevant to giving an informed consent in sense$_1$. If a person has an adequate *understanding* of relevant information without benefit of a disclosure, then it makes no difference whether someone *disclosed* that information.

Other sense$_2$ rules besides those of disclosure have been enforced. These include rules requiring evidence of adequate comprehension of information and the aforementioned rules requiring the presence of auditor witnesses and mandatory waiting periods. Sense$_2$ informed consent requirements generally take the form of rules focusing on disclosure, comprehension, the minimization of potentially controlling influences, and competence. These requirements express the present-day mainstream conception in the federal government of the United States. They are also typical of international documents and state regulations, which all reflect a sense$_2$ orientation.

THE RELATIONSHIP BETWEEN SENSE$_1$ AND SENSE$_2$

A sense$_1$ "informed consent" can fail to be an informed consent in sense$_2$ by a lack of conformity to applicable rules and requirements. Similarly, an informed consent in sense$_2$ may not be an informed consent in sense$_1$. The rules and requirements that determine sense$_2$ consents need not result in autonomous authorizations at all in order to qualify as informed consents.

Such peculiarities in informed consent law have led Jay Katz to argue that the legal doctrine of "informed consent" bears a "name" that "promises much more

than its construction in case law has delivered." He has argued insightfully that the courts have, in effect, imposed a mere duty to warn on physicians, an obligation confined to risk disclosures and statements of proposed interventions. He maintains that "This judicially imposed obligation must be distinguished from the *idea* of informed consent, namely, that patients have a decisive role to play in the medical decision-making process. The idea of informed consent, though alluded to also in case law, cannot be implemented, as courts have attempted, by only expanding the disclosure requirements." By their actions and declarations, Katz believes, the courts have made informed consent a "cruel hoax" and have allowed "the idea of informed consent . . . to wither on the vine."[2]

The most plausible interpretation of Katz's contentions is through the sense$_1$/sense$_2$ distinction. If a physician obtains a consent under the courts' criteria, then an informed consent (sense$_2$) has been obtained. But it does not follow that the courts are using the *right* standards, or *sufficiently rigorous* standards in light of a stricter autonomy-based model—or "idea" as Katz puts it—of informed consent (sense$_1$).[3] If Katz is correct that the courts have made a mockery of informed consent and of its moral justification in respect for autonomy, then of course his criticisms are thoroughly justified. At the same time, it should be recognized that people can proffer legally or institutionally effective authorizations under prevailing rules even if they fall far short of the standards implicit in sense$_1$.

Sense$_1$ as a Model for Sense$_2$. Despite the differences between sense$_1$ and sense$_2$, a definition of informed consent need not fall into one or the other class of definitions. It may conform to both. Many definitions of informed consent in policy contexts reflect at least a strong and definite reliance on informed consent in sense$_1$. Although the conditions of sense$_1$ are not logically necessary conditions for sense$_2$, we take it as morally axiomatic that they *ought* to serve—and in fact have served—as the benchmark or model against which the moral adequacy of a definition framed for sense$_2$ purposes is to be evaluated. This position is, roughly speaking, Katz's position.

A defense of the moral viewpoint that policies governing informed consent in sense$_2$ *should* be formulated to conform to the standards of informed consent in sense$_1$ is not hard to express. The goal of informed consent in medical care and in research—that is, the purpose behind the obligation to obtain informed consents—is to enable potential subjects and patients to make autonomous decisions about whether to grant or refuse authorization for medical and research interventions. Accordingly, embedded in the reason for having the social institution of informed consent is the idea that institutional requirements for informed consent in sense$_2$ *should* be intended to maximize the likelihood that the conditions of informed consent in sense$_1$ will be satisfied.

A major problem at the policy level, where rules and requirements must be developed and applied in the aggregate, is the following: The obligations imposed to enable patients and subjects to make authorization decisions must be evaluated not only in terms of the demands of a set of abstract conditions of "true" or sense$_1$ informed consent, but also in terms of the impact of imposing such obligations or requirements on various institutions with their concrete concerns and priorities. One must take account of what is fair and reasonable to require of health care professionals and researchers, the effect of alternative consent requirements on efficiency and effectiveness in the delivery of health care and the advancement of science, and—particularly in medical care—the effect of requirements on the welfare of patients. Also relevant are considerations peculiar to the particular social context, such as proof, precedent, or liability theory in case law, or regulatory authority and due process in the development of federal regulations and IRB consent policies.

Moreover, at the sense$_2$ level, one must resolve not only which requirements will define effective consent; one must also settle on the rules stipulating the conditions under which effective consents must be obtained.

In some cases, hard decisions must be made about whether requirements of informed consent (in sense$_2$) should be imposed at all, even though informed consent (in sense$_1$) *could* realistically and meaningfully be obtained in the circumstances and could serve as a model for institutional rules. For example, should there be any consent requirements in the cases of minimal risk medical procedures and research activities?

This need to balance is not a problem for informed consent in sense$_1$, which is not policy oriented. Thus, it is possible to have a *morally acceptable* set of requirements for informed consent in sense$_2$ that deviates considerably from the conditions of informed consent in sense$_1$. However, the burden of moral proof rests with those who defend such deviations since the primary moral justification of the obligation to obtain informed consent is respect for autonomous action.

NOTES

1. President's Commission, *Making Health Care Decisions*, Vol. 1, 15 and Jay Katz, *The Silent World of Doctor and Patient* (New York: The Free Press, 1984), 87 and "The Regulation of Human Research—Reflections and Proposals," *Clinical Research* 21 (1973): 785–91. Katz does not provide a sustained analysis of joint or shared decisionmaking, and it is unclear precisely how he would relate this notion to informed consent. At times, Katz links informed consent to individual self-determination and the (implicit) decisionmaking authority of patients (see *The Silent World*, xvii, 85ff, 99, and 102), and at times he mentions the role of authorization; but more frequently the notion of shared authority or decisionmaking serves as virtually the sole criterion. See, for example, *The Silent World*, 86 and 87: "Yet, the idea of informed consent demands joint decision making between physician and patient, a sharing of authority. . . . The idea of informed consent—of mutual decision making—remains severely compromised."

2. Jay Katz, "Disclosure and Consent," in A. Milunsky and G. Annas, eds., *Genetics and the Law II* (New York: Plenum Press, 1980), 122, 128.

3. We have already noted that Katz's "idea" of informed consent—as the active involvement of patients in the medical decision-making process—is different from our sense$_1$.

CALIFORNIA SUPREME COURT

Tarasoff v. Regents of the University of California

TOBRINER, Justice.

On October 27, 1969, Prosenjit Poddar killed Tatiana Tarasoff. Plaintiffs, Tatiana's parents, allege that two months earlier Poddar confided his intention to kill Tatiana to Dr. Lawrence Moore, a psychologist employed by the Cowell Memorial Hospital at the University of California at Berkeley. They allege that on Moore's request, the campus police briefly detained Poddar, but released him when he appeared rational. They further claim that Dr. Harvey Powelson, Moore's superior, then directed that no further action be taken to detain Poddar. No one warned plaintiffs of Tatiana's peril.

• • •

We shall explain that defendant therapists cannot escape liability merely because Tatiana herself was not their patient. When a therapist determines, or pursuant to the standards of his profession should determine, that his patient presents a serious danger of violence to another, he incurs an obligation to use reasonable care to protect the intended victim against such danger. The discharge of this duty may require the therapist to take one or more of various steps, depending upon the nature of the case. Thus it may call for him to warn the intended victim or others likely to apprise the victim of the danger, to notify the police, or to take whatever other steps are reasonably necessary under the circumstances.

• • •

131 California Reporter 14. Decided July 1, 1976. All footnotes and numerous references in the text of the decision and a dissent have been omitted.

1. PLAINTIFFS' COMPLAINTS

Plaintiffs, Tatiana's mother and father, filed separate but virtually identical second amended complaints. The issue before us on this appeal is whether those complaints now state, or can be amended to state, causes of action against defendants. We therefore begin by setting forth the pertinent allegations of the complaints.

Plaintiffs' first cause of action, entitled "Failure to Detain a Dangerous Patient," alleges that on August 20, 1969, Poddar was a voluntary outpatient receiving therapy at Cowell Memorial Hospital. Poddar informed Moore, his therapist, that he was going to kill an unnamed girl, readily identifiable as Tatiana, when she returned home from spending the summer in Brazil. Moore, with the concurrence of Dr. Gold, who had initially examined Poddar, and Dr. Yandell, assistant to the director of the department of psychiatry, decided that Poddar should be committed for observation in a mental hospital. Moore orally notified Officers Atkinson and Teel of the campus police that he would request commitment. He then sent a letter to Police Chief William Beall requesting the assistance of the police department in securing Poddar's confinement.

Officers Atkinson, Brownrigg, and Halleran took Poddar into custody, but, satisfied that Poddar was rational, released him on his promise to stay away from Tatiana. Powelson, director of the department of psychiatry at Cowell Memorial Hospital, then asked the police to return Moore's letter, directed that all copies of the letter and notes that Moore had taken as therapist be destroyed, and "ordered no action to place Prosenjit Poddar in 72-hour treatment and evaluation facility."

Plaintiffs' second cause of action, entitled "Failure to Warn On a Dangerous Patient," incorporates the allegations of the first cause of action, but adds the assertion that defendants negligently permitted Poddar to be released from police custody without "notifying the parents of Tatiana Tarasoff that their daughter was in grave danger from Prosenjit Poddar." Poddar persuaded Tatiana's brother to share an apartment with him near Tatiana's residence; shortly after her return from Brazil, Poddar went to her residence and killed her.

• • •

2. PLAINTIFFS CAN STATE A CAUSE OF ACTION AGAINST DEFENDANT THERAPISTS FOR NEGLIGENT FAILURE TO PROTECT TATIANA

The second cause of action can be amended to allege that Tatiana's death proximately resulted from defendants' negligent failure to warn Tatiana or others likely to apprise her of her danger. Plaintiffs contend that as amended, such allegations of negligence and proximate causation, with resulting damages, establish a cause of action. Defendants, however, contend that in the circumstances of the present case they owed no duty of care to Tatiana or her parents and that, in the absence of such duty, they were free to act in careless disregard of Tatiana's life and safety.

In analyzing this issue, we bear in mind that legal duties are not discoverable facts of nature, but merely conclusory expressions that, in cases of a particular type, liability should be imposed for damage done. As stated in *Dillion v. Legg* (1968): "The assertion that liability must . . . be denied because defendant bears no 'duty' to plaintiff 'begs the essential question— whether the plaintiff's interests are entitled to legal protection against the defendant's conduct . . . [Duty] is not sacrosanct itself, but only an expression of the sum total of those considerations of policy which lead the law to say that the particular plaintiff is entitled to protection.' (Prosser, Law of Torts [3d ed. 1964] at pp. 332–333.)"

In the landmark case of *Rowland v. Christian* (1968), Justice Peters recognized that liability should be imposed "for an injury occasioned to another by his want of ordinary care or skill" as expressed in section 1714 of the Civil Code. Thus, Justice Peters, quoting from *Heaven v. Pender* (1883) stated: " 'whenever one person is by circumstances placed in such a position with regard to another . . . that if he did not use ordinary care and skill in his own conduct . . . he would cause danger of injury to the person or property of the other, a duty arises to use ordinary care and skill to avoid such danger.' "

We depart from "this fundamental principle" only upon the "balancing of a number of considerations"; major ones "are the foreseeability of harm to the plaintiff, the degree of certainty that the plaintiff suffered injury, the closeness of the connection between the defendant's conduct and the injury suffered, the moral blame attached to the defendant's conduct, the policy of preventing future harm, the extent of the burden to the defendant and consequences to the community of imposing a duty to exercise care with resulting liability for breach, and the availability, cost and prevalence of insurance for the risk involved."

The most important of these considerations in establishing duty is foreseeability. As a general principle, a "defendant owes a duty of care to all persons who are foreseeably endangered by his conduct, with respect to all risks which make the conduct unreasonably dangerous."

As we shall explain, however, when the avoidance of foreseeable harm requires a defendant to control the conduct of another person, or to warn of such conduct, the common law has traditionally imposed liability only if the defendant bears some special relationship to the dangerous person or to the potential victim. Since the relationship between a therapist and his patient satisfies this requirement, we need not here decide whether foreseeability alone is sufficient to create a duty to exercise reasonable care to protect a potential victim of another's conduct.

Although, as we have stated above, under the common law, as a general rule, one person owed no duty to control the conduct of another, . . . nor to warn those endangered by such conduct, the courts have carved out an exception to this rule in cases in which the defendant stands in some special relationship to either the person whose conduct needs to be controlled or in a relationship to the foreseeable victim of that conduct. Applying this exception to the present case, we note that a relationship of defendant therapists to either Tatiana or Poddar will suffice to establish a duty of care; as explained in section 315 of the Restatement Second of Torts, a duty of care may arise from either "(a) a special relation . . . between the actor and the third person which imposes a duty upon the actor to control the third person's conduct, or (b) a special relation . . . between the actor and the other which gives to the other a right of protection."

Although plaintiffs' pleadings assert no special relation between Tatiana and defendant therapists, they establish as between Poddar and defendant therapists the special relation that arises between a patient and his doctor or psychotherapist. Such a relationship may support affirmative duties for the benefit of third persons. Thus, for example, a hospital must exercise reasonable care to control the behavior of a patient which may endanger other persons. A doctor must also warn a patient if the patient's condition or medication renders certain conduct, such as driving a car, dangerous to others.

Although the California decisions that recognize this duty have involved cases in which the defendant stood in a special relationship *both* to the victim and to the person whose conduct created the danger, we do not think that the duty should logically be constricted to such situations. Decisions of other jurisdictions hold that the single relationship of a doctor to his patient is sufficient to support the duty to exercise reasonable care to protect others against dangers emanating from the patient's illness. The courts hold that a doctor is liable to persons infected by his patient if he negligently fails to diagnose a contagious disease, or, having diagnosed the illness, fails to warn members of the patient's family.

Since it involved a dangerous mental patient, the decision in *Merchants Nat. Bank & Trust Co. of Fargo v. United States* (1967) comes closer to the issue. The Veterans Administration arranged for the patient to work on a local farm, but did not inform the farmer of the man's background. The farmer consequently permitted the patient to come and go freely during nonworking hours; the patient borrowed a car, drove to his wife's residence and killed her. Notwithstanding the lack of any "special relationship" between the Veterans Administration and the wife, the court found the Veterans Administration liable for the wrongful death of the wife.

In their summary of the relevant rulings Fleming and Maximov conclude that the "case law should dispel any notion that to impose on the therapists a duty to take precautions for the safety of persons threatened by a patient, where due care so requires, is in any way opposed to contemporary ground rules on the duty relationship. On the contrary, there now seems to be sufficient authority to support the conclusion that by entering into a doctor-patient relationship the therapist becomes sufficiently involved to assume some responsibility for the safety, not only of the patient himself, but also of any third person whom the doctor knows to be threatened by the patient." (Fleming & Maximov, *The Patient or His Victim: The Therapist's Dilemma* [1974] 62 Cal.L.Rev. 1025, 1030.)

Defendants contend, however, that imposition of a duty to exercise reasonable care to protect third persons is unworkable because therapists cannot accurately predict whether or not a patient will resort to violence. In support of this argument amicus representing the American Psychiatric Association and other professional societies cites numerous articles which indicate that therapists, in the present state of the art, are unable reliably to predict violent acts; their forecasts, amicus claims, tend consistently to overpredict violence, and indeed are more often wrong than right. Since predictions of violence are often erroneous, amicus concludes, the courts should not render rulings that predicate the liability of therapists upon the validity of such predictions.

The role of the psychiatrist, who is indeed a practitioner of medicine, and that of the psychologist who performs an allied function, are like that of the physician who must conform to the standards of the profession and who must often make diagnoses and predictions based upon such evaluations. Thus the judgment of the therapist in diagnosing emotional disorders and in predicting whether a patient presents a serious danger of violence is comparable to the judgment which doctors and professionals must regularly render under accepted rules of responsibility.

We recognize the difficulty that a therapist encounters in attempting to forecast whether a patient presents a serious danger of violence. Obviously we do not require that the therapist, in making that determination, render a perfect performance; the therapist need only exercise "that reasonable degree of skill, knowledge, and care ordinarily possessed and exercised by members of [that professional specialty] under similar circumstances." Within the broad range of reasonable practice and treatment in which professional opinion and judgment may differ, the therapist is free to exercise his or her own best judgment without liability; proof, aided by hindsight, that he or she judged wrongly is insufficient to establish negligence.

In the instant case, however, the pleadings do not raise any question as to failure of defendant therapists to predict that Poddar presented a serious danger of violence. On the contrary, the present complaints allege that defendant therapists did in fact predict that Poddar would kill, but were negligent in failing to warn.

Amicus contends, however, that even when a therapist does in fact predict that a patient poses a serious danger of violence to others, the therapist should be absolved of any responsibility for failing to act to protect the potential victim. In our view, however, once a therapist does in fact determine, or under applicable professional standards reasonably should have determined, that a patient poses a serious danger of violence to others, he bears a duty to exercise reasonable care to protect the foreseeable victim of that danger. While the discharge of this duty of due care will necessarily vary with the facts of each case, in each instance the adequacy of the therapist's conduct must be measured against the traditional negligence standard of the rendition of reasonable care under the circumstances. As explained in Fleming and Maximov, *The Patient or His Victim: The Therapist's Dilemma* (1974) 62 Cal.L.Rev. 1025, 1967: ". . . the ultimate question of resolving the tension between the conflicting interests of patient and potential victim is one of social policy, not professional expertise. . . . In sum, the therapist owes a legal duty not only to his patient, but also to his patient's would-be victim and is subject in both respects to scrutiny by judge and jury."

Contrary to the assertion of amicus, this conclusion is not inconsistent with our recent decision in *People v. Burnick* (1975). Taking note of the uncertain character of therapeutic prediction, we held in *Burnick* that a person cannot be committed as a mentally disordered sex offender unless found to be such by proof beyond a reasonable doubt. The issue in the present context, however, is not whether the patient should be incarcerated, but whether the therapist should take any steps at all to protect the threatened victim; some of the alternatives open to the therapist, such as warning the victim, will not result in the drastic consequences of depriving the patient of his liberty. Weighing the uncertain and conjectural character of the alleged damage done the patient by such a warning against the peril to the victim's life, we conclude that professional inaccuracy in predicting violence cannot negate the therapist's duty to protect the threatened victim.

The risk that unnecessary warnings may be given is a reasonable price to pay for the lives of possible victims that may be saved. We would hesitate to hold that the therapist who is aware that his patient expects to attempt to assassinate the President of the United States would not be obligated to warn the authorities because the therapist cannot predict with accuracy that his patient will commit the crime.

Defendants further argue that free and open communication is essential to psychotherapy, that "Unless a patient . . . is assured that . . . information [revealed to him] can and will be held in utmost confidence, he will be reluctant to make the full disclosure upon which diagnosis and treatment . . . depends." The giving of a warning, defendants contend, constitutes a breach of trust which entails the revelation of confidential communications.

We recognize the public interest in supporting effective treatment of mental illness and in protecting the rights of patients to privacy, and the consequent public importance of safeguarding the confidential character of psychotherapeutic communication. Against this interest, however, we must weigh the public interest in safety from violent assault. The Legislature has undertaken the difficult task of balancing the countervailing concerns. In Evidence Code section 1014, it established a broad rule of privilege to protect confidential communications between patient and psychotherapist. In Evidence Code section 1024, the Legislature created a specific and limited exception to the psychotherapist-patient privilege: "There is no privilege . . . if the psychotherapist has reasonable cause to believe that the patient is in such mental or emotional condition as to be dangerous to himself or to the person or property of another and that disclosure of the communication is necessary to prevent the threatened danger."

We realize that the open and confidential character of psychotherapeutic dialogue encourages patients to express threats of violence, few of which are ever executed. Certainly a therapist should not be encouraged routinely to reveal such threats; such disclosures could seriously disrupt the patient's relationship with his therapist and with the persons threatened. To the contrary, the therapist's obligations to his patient require that he not disclose a confidence unless such disclosure is necessary to avert danger to others, and even then that he do so discreetly, and in a fashion that would preserve the privacy of his patient to the fullest extent compatible with the prevention of the threatened danger.

The revelation of a communication under the above circumstances is not a breach of trust or a violation of professional ethics; as stated in the Principles of Medical Ethics of the American Medical Association (1957), section 9: "A physician may not reveal the confidence entrusted to him in the course of medical attendance . . . *unless he is required to do so by law or unless it becomes necessary in order to protect the welfare of the individual or of the community*." (Emphasis added.) We conclude that the public policy favoring protection of the confidential character of patient-psychotherapist communications must yield to the extent to which disclosure is essential to avert danger to others. The protective privilege ends where the public peril begins.

Our current crowded and computerized society compels the interdependence of its members. In this risk-infested society we can hardly tolerate the further exposure to danger that would result from a concealed knowledge of the therapist that his patient was lethal. If the exercise of reasonable care to protect the threatened victim requires the therapist to warn the endangered party or those who can reasonably be expected to notify him, we see no sufficient societal interest that would protect and justify concealment. The containment of such risks lies in the public interest. For the foregoing reasons, we find that plaintiffs' complaints can be amended to state a cause of action against defendants Moore, Powelson, Gold, and Yandell and against the Regents as their employer, for breach of a duty to exercise reasonable care to protect Tatiana.

• • •

CLARK, Justice (dissenting).

Until today's majority opinion, both legal and medical authorities have agreed that confidentiality is essential to effectively treat the mentally ill, and that imposing a duty on doctors to disclose patient threats to potential victims would greatly impair treatment. Further, recognizing that effective treatment and society's safety are necessarily intertwined, the Legislature has already decided effective and confidential treatment is preferred over imposition of a duty to warn.

The issue of whether effective treatment for the mentally ill should be sacrificed to a system of warnings is, in my opinion, properly one for the Legislature, and we are bound by its judgment. Moreover, even in the absence of clear legislative direction, we must reach the same conclusion because imposing the majority's new duty is certain to result in a net increase in violence.

• • •

COMMON LAW ANALYSIS

Entirely apart from the statutory provisions, the same result must be reached upon considering both general tort principles and the public policies favoring effective treatment, reduction of violence, and justified commitment.

Generally, a person owes no duty to control the conduct of another. Exceptions are recognized only in limited situations where (1) a special relationship exists between the defendant and injured party, or (2) a special relationship exists between defendant and the active wrongdoer, imposing a duty on defendant to control the wrongdoer's conduct. The majority does not contend the first exception is appropriate to this case.

Policy generally determines duty. Principal policy considerations include foreseeability of harm, certainty of the plaintiff's injury, proximity of the defendant's conduct to the plaintiff's injury, moral blame attributable to defendant's conduct, prevention of future harm, burden on the defendant, and consequences to the community.

Overwhelming policy considerations weigh against imposing a duty on psychotherapists to warn a potential victim against harm. While offering virtually no benefit to society, such a duty will frustrate psychiatric treatment, invade fundamental patient rights and increase violence.

The importance of psychiatric treatment and its need for confidentiality have been recognized by this court. "It is clearly recognized that the very practice of psychiatry vitally depends upon the reputation in the community that the psychiatrist will not tell." (Slovenko, *Psychiatry and a Second Look at the Medical Privilege* (1960) 6 Wayne L.Rev. 175, 188.)

Assurance of confidentiality is important for three reasons.

DETERRENCE FROM TREATMENT

First, without substantial assurance of confidentiality, those requiring treatment will be deterred from seeking assistance. It remains an unfortunate fact in our society that people seeking psychiatric guidance tend to become stigmatized. Apprehension of such stigma—apparently increased by the propensity of people considering treatment to see themselves in the worst possible light—creates a well-recognized reluctance to seek aid. This reluctance is alleviated by the psychiatrist's assurance of confidentiality.

FULL DISCLOSURE

Second, the guarantee of confidentiality is essential in eliciting the full disclosure necessary for effective treatment. The psychiatric patient approaches treatment with conscious and unconscious inhibitions against revealing his innermost thoughts. "Every person, however well-motivated, has to overcome resistances to therapeutic exploration. These resistances seek support from every possible source and the possibility of disclosure would easily be employed in the service of resistance." (Goldstein & Katz, 36 Conn. Bar J. 175, 179.) Until a patient can trust his psychiatrist not to violate their confidential relationship, "the unconscious psychological control mechanism of repression will prevent the recall of past experiences." (Butler, *Psychotherapy and Griswold: Is Confidentiality a Privilege or a Right?* (1971) 3 Conn.L.Rev. 599, 604.)

SUCCESSFUL TREATMENT

Third, even if the patient fully discloses his thoughts, assurance that the confidential relationship will not be breached is necessary to maintain his trust in his psychiatrist—the very means by which treatment is effected. "[T]he essence of much psychotherapy is the contribution of trust in the external world and ultimately in the self, modelled upon the trusting relationship established during therapy." (Dawidoff, *The Malpractice of Psychiatrists*, 1966 Duke L.J. 696, 704.) Patients will be helped only if they can form a trusting relationship with the psychiatrist. All authorities appear to agree that if the trust relationship cannot be developed because of collusive communication between the psychiatrist and others, treatment will be frustrated.

Given the importance of confidentiality to the practice of psychiatry, it becomes clear the duty to warn imposed by the majority will cripple the use and effectiveness of psychiatry. Many people, potentially violent—yet susceptible to treatment—will be deterred from seeking it; those seeking it will be inhibited from making revelations necessary to effective treatment; and, forcing the psychiatrist to violate the patient's trust will destroy the interpersonal relationship by which treatment is effected.

VIOLENCE AND CIVIL COMMITMENT

By imposing a duty to warn, the majority contributes to the danger to society of violence by the mentally ill and greatly increases the risk of civil commitment—the total deprivation of liberty—of those who should not be confined. The impairment of treatment and risk of improper commitment resulting from the new duty to warn will not be limited to a few patients but will extend to a large number of the mentally ill. Although under existing psychiatric procedures only a relatively few receiving treatment will ever present a risk of violence, the number making threats is huge, and it is the latter group—not just the former—whose treatment will be impaired and whose risk of commitment will be increased.

Both the legal and psychiatric communities recognize that the process of determining potential violence in a patient is far from exact, being fraught with complexity and uncertainty. In fact precision has not even been attained in predicting who of those having already committed violent acts will again become violent, a task recognized to be of much simpler proportions.

This predictive uncertainty means that the number of disclosures will necessarily be large. As noted above, psychiatric patients are encouraged to discuss all thoughts of violence, and they often express such thoughts. However, unlike this court, the psychiatrist does not enjoy the benefit of overwhelming hindsight in seeing which few, if any, of his patients will ultimately become violent. Now, confronted by the majority's new duty, the psychiatrist must instantaneously calculate potential violence from each patient on each visit. The difficulties researchers have encountered in accurately predicting violence will be heightened for the practicing psychiatrist dealing for brief periods in his office with heretofore nonviolent patients. And, given the decision not to warn or commit must always be made at the psychiatrist's civil peril, one can expect most doubts will be resolved in favor of the psychiatrist protecting himself.

Neither alternative open to the psychiatrist seeking to protect himself is in the public interest. The warning itself is an impairment of the psychiatrist's ability to treat, depriving many patients of adequate treatment. It is to be expected that after disclosing their threats, a significant number of patients, who would not become violent if treated according to existing practices, will engage in violent conduct as a result of unsuccessful treatment. In short, the majority's duty to warn will not only impair treatment of many who would never become violent but worse, will result in a net increase in violence.

The second alternative open to the psychiatrist is to commit his patient rather than to warn. Even in the absence of threat of civil liability, the doubts of psychiatrists as to the seriousness of patient threats have led psychiatrists to overcommit to mental institutions. This overcommitment has been authoritatively documented in both legal and psychiatric studies. This practice is so prevalent that it has been estimated that "as many as twenty harmless persons are incarcerated for every one who will commit a violent act." (Steadman & Cocozza, *Stimulus/Response: We Can't Predict Who Is Dangerous* (Jan. 1975) 8 Psych. Today 32, 35.)

Given the incentive to commit created by the majority's duty, this already serious situation will be worsened, contrary to Chief Justice Wright's admonition "that liberty is no less precious because forfeited in a civil proceeding than when taken as a consequence of a criminal conviction."

MARK SIEGLER

Confidentiality in Medicine—A Decrepit Concept

Medical confidentiality, as it has traditionally been understood by patients and doctors, no longer exists. This ancient medical principle, which has been included in every physician's oath and code of ethics since Hippocratic times, has become old, worn-out, and useless; it is a decrepit concept. Efforts to preserve it appear doomed to failure and often give rise to more problems than solutions. Psychiatrists have tacitly acknowledged the impossibility of ensuring the confidentiality of medical records by choosing to establish a separate, more secret record. The following case illustrates how the confidentiality principle is compromised systematically in the course of routine medical care.

A patient of mine with mild chronic obstructive pulmonary disease was transferred from the surgical intensive-care unit to a surgical nursing floor two days after an elective cholecystectomy. On the day of transfer, the patient saw a respiratory therapist writing in his medical chart (the therapist was recording the results of an arterial blood gas analysis) and became concerned about the confidentiality of his hospital records. The patient threatened to leave the hospital prematurely unless I could guarantee that the confidentiality of his hospital record would be respected.

This patient's complaint prompted me to enumerate the number of persons who had both access to his hospital record and a reason to examine it. I was amazed to learn that at least 25 and possibly as many as

100 health professionals and administrative personnel at our university hospital had access to the patient's record and that all of them had a legitimate need, indeed a professional responsibility, to open and use that chart. These persons included 6 attending physicians (the primary physician, the surgeon, the pulmonary consultant, and others); 12 house officers (medical, surgical, intensive-care unit, and "covering" house staff); 20 nursing personnel (on three shifts); 6 respiratory therapists; 3 nutritionists; 2 clinical pharmacists; 15 students (from medicine, nursing, respiratory therapy, and clinical pharmacy); 4 unit secretaries; 4 hospital financial officers; and 4 chart reviewers (utilization review, quality assurance review, tissue review, and insurance auditor). It is of interest that this patient's problem was straightforward, and he therefore did not require many other technical and support services that the modern hospital provides. For example, he did not need multiple consultants and fellows, such specialized procedures as dialysis, or social workers, chaplains, physical therapists, occupational therapists, and the like.

Upon completing my survey I reported to the patient that I estimated that at least 75 health professionals and hospital personnel had access to his medical record. I suggested to the patient that these people were all involved in providing or supporting his health-care services. They were, I assured him, working for him. Despite my reassurances the patient was obviously distressed and retorted, "I always believed that

Reprinted by permission of *The New England Journal of Medicine*, Vol. 307. © 1982 Massachusetts Medical Society.

medical confidentiality was part of a doctor's code of ethics. Perhaps you should tell me just what you people mean by 'confidentiality'!''

TWO ASPECTS OF MEDICAL CONFIDENTIALITY

CONFIDENTIALITY AND THIRD-PARTY INTERESTS

Previous discussions of medical confidentiality usually have focused on the tension between a physician's responsibility to keep information divulged by patients secret and a physician's legal and moral duty, on occasion, to reveal such confidences to third parties, such as families, employers, public-health authorities, or police authorities. In all these instances, the central question relates to the stringency of the physician's obligation to maintain patient confidentiality when the health, well-being, and safety of identifiable others or of society in general would be threatened by a failure to reveal information about the patient. The tension in such cases is between the good of the patient and the good of others.

CONFIDENTIALITY AND THE PATIENT'S INTEREST

As the example above illustrates, further challenges to confidentiality arise because the patient's personal interest in maintaining confidentiality comes into conflict with his personal interest in receiving the best possible health care. Modern high-technology health care is available principally in hospitals (often, teaching hospitals), requires many trained and specialized workers (a "health-care team"), and is very costly. The existence of such teams means that information that previously had been held in confidence by an individual physician will now necessarily be disseminated to many members of the team. Furthermore, since health-care teams are expensive and few patients can afford to pay such costs directly, it becomes essential to grant access to the patient's medical record to persons who are responsible for obtaining third-party payment. These persons include chart reviewers, financial officers, insurance auditors, and quality-of-care assessors. Finally, as medicine expands from a narrow, disease-based model to a model that encompasses psychological, social, and economic problems, not only will the size of the health-care team and medical costs increase, but more sensitive information (such as one's personal habits and financial condition) will now be included in the medical record and will no longer be confidential.

The point I wish to establish is that hospital medicine, the rise of health-care teams, the existence of third-party insurance programs, and the expanding limits of medicine all appear to be responses to the wishes of people for better and more comprehensive medical care. But each of these developments necessarily modifies our traditional understanding of medical confidentiality.

THE ROLE OF CONFIDENTIALITY IN MEDICINE

Confidentiality serves a dual purpose in medicine. In the first place, it acknowledges respect for the patient's sense of individuality and privacy. The patient's most personal physical and psychological secrets are kept confidential in order to decrease a sense of shame and vulnerability. Secondly, confidentiality is important in improving the patient's health care—a basic goal of medicine. The promise of confidentiality permits people to trust (i.e., have confidence) that information revealed to a physician in the course of a medical encounter will not be disseminated further. In this way patients are encouraged to communicate honestly and forthrightly with their doctors. This bond of trust between patient and doctor is vitally important both in the diagnostic process (which relies on an accurate history) and subsequently in the treatment phase, which often depends as much on the patient's trust in the physician as it does on medications and surgery. These two important functions of confidentiality are as important now as they were in the past. They will not be supplanted entirely either by improvements in medical technology or by recent changes in relations between some patients and doctors toward a rights-based, consumerist model.

POSSIBLE SOLUTIONS TO THE CONFIDENTIALITY PROBLEM

First of all, in all nonbureaucratic, noninstitutional medical encounters—that is, in the millions of doctor–patient encounters that take place in physicians' offices, where more privacy can be preserved—meticulous care should be taken to guarantee that patients' medical and personal information will be kept confidential.

Secondly, in such settings as hospitals or large-scale group practices, where many persons have opportunities to examine the medical record, we should aim to provide access only to those who have "a need to know." This could be accomplished through such administrative changes as dividing the entire record into several sections—for example, a medical and financial section—and permitting only health professionals access to the medical information.

The approach favored by many psychiatrists—that of keeping a psychiatric record separate from the general medical record—is an understandable strategy but one that is not entirely satisfactory and that should not be generalized. The keeping of separate psychiatric records implies that psychiatry and medicine are different undertakings and thus drives deeper the wedge between them and between physical and psychological illness. Furthermore, it is often vitally important for internists or surgeons to know that a patient is being seen by a psychiatrist or is taking a particular medication. When separate records are kept, this information may not be available. Finally, if generalized, the practice of keeping a separate psychiatric record could lead to the unacceptable consequence of having a separate record for each type of medical problem.

Patients should be informed about what is meant by "medical confidentiality." We should establish the distinction between information about the patient that generally will be kept confidential regardless of the interest of third parties and information that will be exchanged among members of the health-care team in order to provide care for the patient. Patients should be made aware of the large number of persons in the modern hospital who require access to the medical record in order to serve the patient's medical and financial interests.

Finally, at some point most patients should have an opportunity to review their medical record and to make informed choices about whether their entire record is to be available to everyone or whether certain portions of the record are privileged and should be accessible only to their principal physician or to others designated explicitly by the patient. This approach would rely on traditional informed-consent procedural standards and might permit the patient to balance the personal value of medical confidentiality against the personal value of high-technology, team health care. There is no reason that the same procedure should not be used with psychiatric records instead of the arbitrary system now employed, in which everything related to psychiatry is kept secret.

AFTERTHOUGHT: CONFIDENTIALITY AND INDISCRETION

There is one additional aspect of confidentiality that is rarely included in discussions of the subject. I am referring here to the wanton, often inadvertent, but avoidable exchanges of confidential information that occur frequently in hospital rooms, elevators, cafeterias, doctors' offices, and at cocktail parties. Of course, as more people have access to medical information about the patient the potential for this irresponsible abuse of confidentiality increases geometrically.

Such mundane breaches of confidentiality are probably of greater concern to most patients than the broader issue of whether their medical records may be entered into a computerized data bank or whether a respiratory therapist is reviewing the results of an arterial blood gas determination. Somehow, privacy is violated and a sense of shame is heightened when intimate secrets are revealed to people one knows or is close to—friends, neighbors, acquaintances, or hospital roommates—rather than when they are disclosed to an anonymous bureaucrat sitting at a computer terminal in a distant city or to a health professional who is acting in an official capacity.

I suspect that the principles of medical confidentiality, particularly those reflected in most medical codes of ethics, were designed principally to prevent just this sort of embarrassing personal indiscretion rather than to maintain (for social, political, or economic reasons) the absolute secrecy of doctor–patient communications. In this regard, it is worth noting that Percival's Code of Medical Ethics (1803) includes the following admonition: "Patients should be interrogated concerning their complaint in a tone of voice which cannot be overheard."* We in the medical profession frequently neglect these simple courtesies.

CONCLUSION

The principle of medical confidentiality described in medical codes of ethics and still believed in by patients no longer exists. In this respect, it is a decrepit concept. Rather than perpetuate the myth of confidentiality and invest energy vainly to preserve it, the public and the profession would be better served if they devoted their attention to determining which aspects of the original principle of confidentiality are worth retaining. Efforts could then be directed to salvaging those.

---

*Leake CD, ed. Percival's medical ethics. Baltimore: Williams & Wilkins, 1927.

RAANAN GILLON

AIDS and Medical Confidentiality

Consultants in sexually transmitted disease clinics dealing with patients with the acquired immune deficiency syndrome (AIDS) or positive for the human immunodeficiency virus (HIV) "are being over-protective of confidentiality," a general practitioner and member of the British Medical Association's central ethical committee is reported to have said.[1] On the other hand, the BMA in its third and most recent statement on AIDS says, "The traditional confidentiality of the doctor-patient relationship must be upheld in the case of patients suffering from AIDS and HIV seropositive individuals."[2]

Clearly, the advice from the BMA is disputed by many general practitioners. The Leicestershire Local Medical Committee, representing 400 general practitioners, wrote to the BMA complaining that its guidelines were "very wrong"; as with any other serious illness general practitioners should be informed by specialists who discovered important medical information about their patients, including infection with HIV.[3] In a straw poll three out of the four general practitioners questioned by a medical newspaper on this issue are reported to have opposed the BMA's policy and to have stated that general practitioners should be told.[4] At the BMA's annual representative meeting this year a variety of motions demand that they shall be told.[5] But in an excellent debate last week the annual conference of local medical committees, which represents all National Health Service general practitioners, rejected by 156 votes to 109 a proposal that family doctors had a right to be told if a patient was found to be positive for HIV and decided that patients were entitled to normal standards of confidentiality (p 1707).

Reprinted by permission of *British Medical Journal* from *BMJ* 294 (June 27, 1987).

The problem arises when people are found to be positive for HIV in a clinic for sexually transmitted diseases and refuse permission for the information to be passed on, despite advice about why it would be preferable for their general practitioner to be informed. The main justifications stated or implied in favour of breaking confidentiality in such circumstances are (1) that it is normal medical practice; (2) that it is in the interests of the patient by leading to better medical care; (3) that it is in the interests of the general practitioner and associated staff by reducing their risks of accidentally acquiring HIV infection; (4) that it may be in the interests of other patients who might risk becoming infected by the patient; and (5) that it is in the interests of society in general by helping to reduce the spread of the AIDS epidemic.

NORMAL MEDICAL PRACTICE?

Two questions need to be answered. Firstly, Is it normal medical practice to pass on medical information to other doctors against patients' wishes? Secondly, If it is, what follows?

To agree that specialists normally pass on information to patients' general practitioners in no way means that they normally do so *when the patient refuses to allow such transfer of information about him or her.* The fact that it is normal for specialists to pass on information to general practitioners surely only reflects the fact that in most cases patients agree, or can be reasonably assumed to agree, that it is in their interests for such information to be passed on. But when patients do not agree, or can reasonably be expected not to agree, then is it not also entirely "normal medical practice" for doctors to respect their patients' wishes? The two most obvious categories of such medical behaviour are when a patient is receiving psychotherapy or when a sexually transmitted disease has been diagnosed; the latter instance offers the most clearly relevant example in which it is precisely *not* normal medical practice for specialists to pass on medical information to general practitioners against the patient's wishes.

In any case, even if it were normal medical practice to pass on medical information against patients' wishes what would follow from this? Certainly not that the practice is therefore right. For it to be accepted as right independent justification would be required, and the example of AIDS, as in so many other contexts, provides a stimulus for re-examining our normal practices. Some might argue (especially perhaps in other European countries) that to urge the breaking of confidentiality in cases of HIV positivity is a regrettable indication of how far we have already travelled down the slippery slope away from the absolute requirement of medical confidentiality demanded in the World Medical Association's international code of medical ethics[6] and also apparently, but equivocally, in the new European guide to medical ethics[7] (equivocally because as well as requiring a guarantee to the patient of complete confidentiality the guide also provides for exceptions "where national law provides for exceptions"). The claim that medical confidentiality is an absolute requirement has been thoroughly presented by one contemporary European medical writer[8] and in the face of erosions undoubtedly has its attractions. But, though I have argued previously that such absolutism is in the end untenable,[9] medical confidentiality clearly remains a strong medicomoral principle and should be broken only if yet stronger moral reasons prevail. A mere claim that overriding confidentiality has become normal medical practice, even if it were true, would not provide moral justification for doing so.

IS DISCLOSURE IN THE INTERESTS OF THE PATIENT?

Given that a patient, because he perceives his own interests to be best served by confidentiality, rejects the view of a clinician in a sexually transmitted diseases clinic that it would be preferable to tell his general practitioner of his disease, it would surely be unusually arrogant for a doctor to persist in assuming that "doctor knows best" and that disclosure is in the patient's best interests. A vital aspect of the medical objective of doing good for one's patients is to discount one's own perception of what is good for them in favour of their own, autonomous beliefs about what is good for them. Even in cases in which we believe that there is a clear discrepancy between what the patient

autonomously desires and what is in the patient's best interests we have to be extremely careful in justifying imposing our beliefs on our patients in their interests when they explicitly reject such "help." A poignant example of reluctance to do so, even when death will be the outcome, was given by Sir Richard Bayliss, the patient being a Christian Scientist who refused medical treatment for thyrotoxicosis.[10] Can justification "in the patient's best interests" be offered in this particular context of overriding confidentiality against the patient's will?

Three reported justifications are that if the general practitioner does not know of the patient's HIV positivity he may make wrong diagnoses, not treat the patient properly, or order potentially risky diagnostic tests.[3] Of course there is a higher chance of wrong diagnosis and inappropriate treatment, but patients who are positive for HIV tend to maintain a continuing therapeutic relationship with the clinician at the clinic for sexually transmitted diseases who made the original diagnosis; thus even if the general practitioner does not pick up disorders related to AIDS the clinician at the clinic is likely to do so and treat them appropriately. As for potentially harmful diagnostic tests, I wonder which ones and in what sorts of circumstances. Thinking of the typical diagnostic tests in general practice that I request, such as radiography, blood tests, and urine tests, it is not clear to me how, if the tests were clinically in the patient's interests without my knowing about his HIV positivity, they would be transformed into being against his interests if I did know. In any case patients who did not wish me to know about their HIV positivity would probably consult their clinician at the sexually transmitted diseases clinic before undergoing special tests recommended by me such as contrast radiography. Thus it seems unlikely, from the point of view of the patient's best interests, that diagnostic tests would be a problem, and the problems of imperfect diagnosis and treatment by the general practitioner are likely to be compensated for by the continuing care of the specialist in sexually transmitted diseases.

Like most general practitioners I would regret such lack of confidence by the patient in me, but I do not believe that overriding his wishes for confidentiality is likely to improve matters or to be in his best interests. Even if I did I can certainly see no general justification in "the patient's best interests" for imposing such transfer of information to me against his will.

INSURANCE MEDICALS AND PATIENTS' BEST INTERESTS

In the context of best interests it is worth recalling that benefiting one's patients should also be considered in the context of the harm that a proposed benefit risks: it is net benefit over harm that counts. A patient's interests are not confined to strictly medical interests, and a proposed medical benefit may result in non-medical harms. A single example should suffice to demonstrate this. It is usually the general practitioner who is contacted for medical information when patients want life and health insurance. If the general practitioner knows about his patient's HIV positivity he must, presumably, in honestly and professionally answering the relevant question disclose this information. If, however, the general practitioner does not know he can honestly say so. Thus in some cases it may well be in the patient's best interests for the general practitioner not to know.

Here, incidentally, is another example in which our current medical norms—those concerning insurance medicals—are called into stark relief by the AIDS epidemic. It seems clear that when we complete an insurance medical form we use information gathered in the course of a therapeutic relationship for an essentially commercial purpose, and this commercial purpose is in some cases likely to conflict with the best interests of the patient. It is of course done with consent, but the sort of consent that the patient in many cases would prefer not to have to give. Perhaps we ought to change our norms so that in all cases in which there is any doubt in the general practitioner's mind about whether completing an insurance medical questionnaire would be in the patient's best interests (1) the patient should be consulted and (2) if the patient prefers the general practitioner should return the insurance medical form uncompleted. The company could then arrange for an independent and explicitly "non-therapeutic" medical assessment. In addition, the choice of having an independent medical assessment should perhaps be explicitly offered by insurance companies to all applicants for insurance right from the start.

IS DISCLOSURE IN THE INTERESTS OF GENERAL PRACTITIONERS AND OTHER MEMBERS OF THE PRIMARY CARE TEAM?

This is essentially the argument that confidentiality is too dangerous for general practitioners and other primary care health workers including nurses to respect in cases of HIV positivity. I considered the arguments of danger in a previous article about refusal to treat patients with AIDS and those positive for HIV.[11] In summary, I argued (1) that the medical profession (including "the greater medical profession") accepted a certain degree of risk as part of its professional norms and (2) that the extensive empirical evidence currently available showed that the probability of accidental transmission of HIV to medical staff and families and other close contacts of patients positive for HIV or with AIDS was very low, given normal care with blood and other body fluids.

IS DISCLOSURE IN THE INTERESTS OF OTHER POSSIBLE PATIENTS?

I find this the most difficult of the arguments in favour of breaking confidentiality, though at most it seems to justify disclosure against a patient's will only in exceptional circumstances. Thus if either a clinician in a sexually transmitted diseases clinic or a general practitioner knows or has strong reason to believe that a patient positive for HIV intends to have sexual intercourse with a new and uninfected partner or partners without telling the partner(s), and efforts to persuade the patient to tell have been rejected and there is a reasonable prospect of preventing the event(s), then efforts to inform such contacts do seem justifiable in order to try to prevent them from being infected with what is likely to be a fatal virus. This seems particularly clearly justified if the previously uninfected contact is also a patient of the doctor concerned (because of the special obligations doctors have to their patients), but it might also apply, for example, in the context of tracing contacts of patients with sexually transmitted diseases as part of a general concern to protect others from potentially fatal diseases.

Even against this very limited justification of breach of confidentiality, however, it might be argued, as I do below, that it is still better not to break confidentiality. Thus by being known to maintain a very strict level of confidentiality the medical profession has a better chance of maintaining the trust of high risk groups; it will therefore be better able to influence them and more effectively protect the health of others in general. Although I would agree that it is almost always likely in practice that preserving confidentiality will be the better course for precisely such consequentialist justification I find it impossible to rule out circumstances in which I, at any rate, would believe it right to break confidentiality. I can imagine, for example, a "psychopath" positive for HIV who makes it clear that he or she does not care about transmitting the virus to others, and indeed intends to do so, and when I know that another of my patients, probably uninfected with HIV, is a likely new partner.

The possible existence of such rare exceptions (for most patients positive for HIV like most other patients and people in general are not psychopaths and do care about others) is simply evidence for my earlier claim that medical confidentiality should not be an absolute requirement, only a very strong one. In the context of a just society strong evidence of likely and preventable death or severe injury to others can afford justification for overriding confidentiality, including the passing on of information between doctors and to new contacts. But such circumstances will be extremely rare. In most cases the probability of preventing death or severe injury by breaking medical confidentiality about HIV state will be low—and every time a doctor does break such confidentiality he or she will further reduce a trust in the profession that while it exists can itself be reasonably expected to help reduce the spread of the disease.

IS DISCLOSURE IN THE INTERESTS OF SOCIETY?

The final argument sometimes offered for passing on information about patients positive for HIV is that it is in the interests of society by helping to reduce the spread of AIDS. Justice, it might be added, requires doctors to take into account not only the interests of their individual patients of the moment but of society in general. Though the desire to minimize the spread of AIDS is doubtless shared by all sane people, and though the claim that doctors must include the interests of society in their medicomoral reasoning is one that I would strongly support, it does not follow that overriding the traditional norms of medical practice in the context of AIDS is the best way to achieve those objectives. I hope to return to this theme in a subsequent paper, but, in brief, the spread of AIDS seems most likely to be curtailed and the interests of society best served if the trust and cooperation of those at greatest risk can be obtained and maintained. Thus the consequentialist objective of minimizing the spread of AIDS fortunately seems to point in the same direction as the traditional rules of medical deontology, including the norms of medical confidentiality. In the context of this paper it seems particularly implausible to argue that the spread of AIDS will be curtailed if specialists in sexually transmitted diseases are routinely required to break medical confidentiality by passing on to gen-

eral practitioners information about patients' HIV positivity against those patients' wishes. On the contrary, it seems far more probable that the interests of society will be best served if the medical profession in general, and perhaps specialists in sexually transmitted diseases in particular, can preserve their reputation, especially among those most at risk of infection, for conforming to a very strong—though not absolute—principle of medical confidentiality.

SUMMARY

In summary, I have argued that the arguments offered or hinted at in favour of doctors' breaking medical confidentiality by passing on information about their patients' HIV state to others, including other doctors, when this is against the patient's considered wishes are generally unconvincing. Although in highly exceptional cases there may be justifications for overriding confidentiality, the requirement of medical confidentiality is a very strong, though not absolute, obligation. Patients, their contacts, doctors and their staff, and the common good are most likely to be best served if that tradition continues to be honoured.

NOTES

1. Duncan N. GPs demand to be told results of AIDS tests. *Pulse* 1987; Jan 3:1.

2. British Medical Association. *Third BMA statement on AIDS*. London: BMA, 1986.

3. Beecham L. Support for confidentiality for AIDS patients. *Br Med J* 1987; 294:1177.

4. Kennard N. Should GPs be told AIDS test results? *Pulse* 1987; Jan 17:25.

5. British Medical Association. Agenda of the British Medical Association's annual representative meeting 1987, motions 359–374. *Br Med J* 1987; 294 (insert in issue of 6 June).

6. British Medical Association. *Handbook of medical ethics*. London: BMA, 1984; 70–1.

7. Anonymous. European guide to medical ethics. *IME Bulletin* 1987; No 25:3–7.

8. Kottow MH. Medical confidentiality: an intransigent and absolute obligation. *J Med Ethics* 1986; 12:117–22.

9. Gillon R. Confidentiality. *Br Med J* 1985; 291:1634–6.

10. Bayliss R. A health hazard. *Br Med J* 1982; 285:1824–5.

11. Gillon R. Refusal to treat AIDS and HIV positive patients. *Br Med J* 1987; 294:1332–3.

SUGGESTED READINGS FOR CHAPTER 8

TRUTH TELLING

Bok, Sissela. *Lying: Moral Choice in Public and Private Life*. New York: Pantheon Books, 1978.

————. "Truth-Telling: Ethical Aspects." In Reich, Warren T., ed. *Encyclopedia of Bioethics*. New York: Free Press, 1978. Vol. 4, pp. 1682–1688.

Cabot, Richard C. "The Use of Truth and Falsehood in Medicine," as edited by Jay Katz from the 1909 version. *Connecticut Medicine* 42 (1978), 189–194.

Cousins, Norman. "A Layman Looks at Truth Telling in Medicine." *Journal of the American Medical Association* 244 (October 24, 1980), 1929–1930.

Gillon, Raanan. "Telling the Truth and Medical Ethics." *British Medical Journal* 291 (November 30, 1985), 1556–1557.

Horn, Sheila E. "What's in a Name?" *Journal of Medical Humanities and Bioethics* 6 (Fall/Winter 1985), 99–108.

Schöne-Seifert, Bettina, and Childress, James F. "How Much Should the Patient Know and Decide?" *CA-A Cancer Journal for Clinicians* 36 (March–April 1986), 85–94.

VanDeVeer, Donald. "The Contractual Argument for Withholding Medical Information." *Philosophy and Public Affairs* 9 (Winter 1980), 198–205.

Veatch, Robert M. *Case Studies in Medical Ethics*. Cambridge, Mass.: Harvard University Press, 1977. Chaps. 6 and 12.

Weir, Robert. "Truthtelling in Medicine." *Perspectives in Biology and Medicine* 24 (Autumn 1980), 95–112.

INFORMED CONSENT

Appelbaum, Paul S., Lidz, Charles W., and Meisel, Alan. *Informea Consent: Legal Theory and Clinical Practice*. New York: Oxford University Press, 1987.

Beauchamp, Tom L., and Childress, James F. *Principles of Biomedical Ethics*. 3rd edition. New York: Oxford University Press, 1989. Chap. 3.

Canada Law Reform Commission. *Consent to Medical Care*. A monograph prepared by Margaret A. Somerville. Ottawa: Canadian Government Publication, 1979.

Childress, James F. *Who Should Decide? Paternalism in Health Care*. New York: Oxford University Press, 1982.

Curran, William J. "Informed Consent in Malpractice Cases: A Turn Toward Reality." *New England Journal of Medicine* 314 (February 13, 1986), 429–431.

Engelhardt, H. Tristram, Jr. *The Foundations of Bioethics*. New York: Oxford University Press, 1986. Chap. 7.

Faden, Ruth R., and Beauchamp, Tom L. *A History and Theory of Informed Consent*. New York: Oxford University Press, 1986.

Hull, Richard T. "Informed Consent: Patient's Right or Patient's Duty?" *Journal of Medicine and Philosophy* 10 (May 1985), 183–197.

Katz, Jay. "Informed Consent—A Fairy Tale?: Law's Vision." *University of Pittsburgh Law Review* 39 (Winter 1977), 137–174.

————. *The Silent World of Doctor and Patient*. New York: Free Press, 1984.

Kopelman, Loretta. "Consent and Randomized Clinical Trials: Are There Moral or Design Problems?" *Journal of Medicine and Philosophy* 11 (November 1986), 317–345.

Lidz, Charles W., et al. *Informed Consent: A Study of Decisionmaking in Psychiatry*. New York: Guilford Press, 1984.

McNeil, Barbara, et al. "On the Elicitation of Preferences for Alternative Therapies." *New England Journal of Medicine* 306 (May 27, 1982), 1259–1262.

Meisel, Alan, and Roth, Loren H. "Toward an Informed Discussion of Informed Consent: A Review and Critique of the Empirical Studies." *Arizona Law Review* 25 (1983), 265–346.

Miller, Leslie J. "Informed Consent: I, II, III, IV." *Journal of the American Medical Association* 244 (November 7, 1980–December 12, 1980), 2100–2103, 2347–2350, 2556–2558, 2661–2662.

President's Commission for the Study of Ethical Problems in Medicine and Biomedical and Behavioral Research. *Making Health Care Decisions*. Vols. 1–3. Washington: Government Printing Office, 1982.

Rosoff, Arnold. *Informed Consent*. Rockville, Md.: Aspen Systems Corporation, 1981.

Veatch, Robert M. *The Patient as Partner: A Theory of Human-Experimentation Ethics*. Bloomington: Indiana University Press, 1987. Chaps. 3 and 12.

Weisbard, Alan J. "Informed Consent: The Law's Uneasy Compromise with Ethical Theory." *Nebraska Law Review* 65 (1986), 749–767.

CONFIDENTIALITY AND PRIVACY

Appelbaum, Paul S., et al. "Researchers' Access to Patient Records: An Analysis of the Ethical Problems." *Clinical Research* 32 (October 1984), 399–403.

Beauchamp, Tom L., and Childress, James F. *Principles of Biomedical Ethics*. 3rd edition. New York: Oxford University Press, 1989. Chaps. 3 and 7.

Bok, Sissela. *Secrets: On the Ethics of Concealment and Revelation*. New York: Pantheon Books, 1983.

Cranford, Ronald E., et al. "Institutional Ethics Committees: Issues of Confidentiality and Immunity." *Law, Medicine, and Health Care* 13 (April 1985), 52–60.

Curran, William J. "Protecting Confidentiality in Epidemiologic Investigations by the Centers for Disease Control." *New England Journal of Medicine* 314 (April 17, 1986), 1027–1028.

Everstine, Louis, et al. "Privacy and Confidentiality in Psychotherapy." *American Psychologist* 35 (September 1980), 828–840.

Gillon, Raanan. "Confidentiality." *British Medical Journal* 291 (December 7, 1985), 1634–1636.

Gordis, Leon, and Gold, Ellen. "Privacy, Confidentiality, and the Use of Medical Records in Research." *Science* 207 (January 11, 1980), 153–156.

Havard, John. "Medical Confidence." *Journal of Medical Ethics* 11 (March 1985), 8–11.

Kelsey, Jennifer L. "Privacy and Confidentiality in Epidemiological Research Involving Patients." *IRB: A Review of Human Subjects Research* 3 (February 1981), 1–4.

Kottow, Michael H. "Medical Confidentiality: An Intransigent and Absolute Obligation." *Journal of Medical Ethics* 12 (September 1986), 117–122.

Miller, Randolph A., et al. "Ethical and Legal Issues Related to the Use of Computer Programs in Clinical Medicine." *Annals of Internal Medicine* 102 (April 1985), 529–536.

Perkins, Henry S., and Jonsen, Albert R. "Conflicting Duties to Patients: The Case of a Sexually Active Hepatitis B." *Annals of Internal Medicine* 94 (April 1981), 523–530.

Schmid, Donald, et al. "Confidentiality in Psychiatry: A Study of the Patient's View." *Hospital and Community Psychiatry* 34 (April 1983), 353–355.

U.S. Congress. House Committee on the Judiciary, Subcommittee on Civil and Constitutional Rights. *Unauthorized Access to*

Individual Medical Records. Washington, D.C.: Government Printing Office, 1986.

Wexler, David B. "Patients, Therapists, and Third Parties: The Victimological Virtues of Tarasoff." *International Journal of Law and Psychiatry* 2 (1979), 1–28.

Winston, Morton, and Landesman, Sheldon H. "AIDS and a Duty to Protect." *Hastings Center Report* 17 (February 1987), 22–23.

BIBLIOGRAPHIES

Goldstein, Doris Mueller. *Bioethics: A Guide to Information Sources.* Detroit: Gale Research Company, 1982. See under "Physician-Patient Communication and Truth-Telling," "Confidentiality," "Informed Consent," and "Refusal of Treatment."

Lineback, Richard H., ed. *Philosopher's Index.* Vols. 1– . Bowling Green, Ohio: Philosophy Documentation Center, Bowling Green State University. Issued quarterly. See under "Coercion," "Deception," "Informed Consent," "Lie(s)," "Lying," and "Paternalism."

Walters, LeRoy, and Kahn, Tamar Joy, eds. *Bibliography of Bioethics.* Vols. 1–14. Washington, D.C.: Kennedy Institute of Ethics, Georgetown University. Issued annually. See under "Confidentiality," "Disclosure," "Informed Consent," "Patient Care," "Patients' Rights," "Physician-Patient Relationship," and "Treatment Refusal." (The information contained in the annual *Bibliography of Bioethics* can also be retrieved from BIOETHICSLINE, an online database of the National Library of Medicine.)

Part V

BIOMEDICAL RESEARCH AND TECHNOLOGY

9.

Research with Human and Animal Subjects

This chapter is closely related to several earlier chapters in this book. Chapter 4 considered the question of personhood and the extent of our moral obligations to nonhuman animals. Chapters 7 and 8 surveyed a series of general issues in the clinical care of patients by health professionals. The present chapter analyzes general problems that arise in the context of biomedical research, both research involving human subjects and research involving animals.

CONCEPTUAL QUESTIONS

The definition of "research" can perhaps be best approached by way of considering the concepts of "therapy" and "research." In the biomedical and behavioral fields, "therapy" refers to a class of activities designed solely to benefit an individual or the members of a group. Therapy may take several forms: It may be a treatment for a disease, or it may consist of diagnostic procedures or even preventive measures. In contrast, "research" refers to a class of scientific activities designed to develop or contribute to generalizable knowledge. Examples of research are the comparative study of alternative methods for training pigeons, the search for the best among alternative drug therapies, and the laboratory analysis of a chemical reaction.

Two subtypes of research involving human or animal subjects can be identified. Research can be combined with therapy or the prevention of illness; that is, it can be aimed directly toward discovering better methods of treating the illness or condition from which human or animal patients are suffering or toward preventing disease in susceptible humans or animals. These kinds of inquiry are often designated as *clinical research*. Randomized clinical trials are an important subtype of clinical research. On the other hand, research can be unrelated (or at least not directly related) to the illness or susceptibility of the subjects involved. For example, healthy human volunteers can be involved in studies that examine how long a new drug remains in the body of people who receive a certain dose of the drug. Similarly, healthy nonhuman animals are frequently involved in research that aims to understand disease processes in human beings. Thus, coronary arteries may be obstructed in canine subjects so that researchers can better understand what happens to the human heart in a myocardial infarction (heart attack). There is no simple or widely accepted term that applies to all the various kinds of nonclinical research. In some cases it is called "toxicology testing," in others "the development of animal models." What unites the various kinds of nonclinical research is that the experimental procedures are not intended to provide direct benefit for the subjects of the research.

RESEARCH INVOLVING HUMAN SUBJECTS

THE MORAL JUSTIFICATION

In the literature on human research, including codes of research ethics, surprisingly little attention is paid to the general justification for involving human subjects in research. This silence at the most general level of justification is particularly striking when one considers that the traditional ethic of medicine has been exclusively a patient-benefit ethic. The motto *primum non nocere* (do no harm) has generally been interpreted to mean "Do nothing that is not intended for the direct benefit of the patient." We must ask, then, whether good reasons can be given for deviating in any way from therapy, as that term was defined above.

The primary argument in favor of human research appeals to the principle of beneficence (as was briefly noted in Chapter 1). It asserts that the social benefits to be gained from such research are substantial and that the harms resulting from the cessation of such investigations would be exceedingly grave. In his essay in this chapter, Leon Eisenberg advances such claims. He notes that the therapeutic value of many reputed "therapies" is in fact unknown; indeed, these treatments may be no more useful than the bloodletting technique so much in vogue during the eighteenth and early nineteenth centuries. On this view, the only alternative to a perpetual plague of medically induced illness is the vigorous pursuit of biomedical research, particularly research involving human subjects.

A second approach to the justification of human research is based on a joint appeal to the principles of beneficence and justice. According to this view, beneficence requires that each of us make at least a modest positive contribution to the good of our fellow citizens or the society as a whole. If our participation in research promises significant benefit to others, at little or no risk to ourselves, then such participation may become a duty of beneficence. In addition, if we fail to fulfill this modest duty while most of our contemporaries perform it, we may be acting unjustly, since we are not performing our fair share of a communal task. Eisenberg advances a qualified version of this argument.

The justice argument can be further elaborated by reference to the past. Every person currently alive is the beneficiary of earlier subjects' involvement in research. To be specific, the willingness of past human volunteers to take part in studies of antibiotics (such as penicillin) and vaccines (such as polio vaccine) has contributed to the health of us all. Accordingly, it seems unfair for us to reap the benefits of already performed research without making a reciprocal contribution to the alleviation of disability and disease.

Hans Jonas vigorously challenges both of these approaches to the general justification of human research. In answer to the consequential argument advanced by Eisenberg, Jonas asserts that while human research generally contributes to medical progress, most research involving human subjects is not *essential* to the well-being or survival of the human species. According to Jonas, progress, even medical progress, is "an optional goal, not an unconditional commitment." On this view, only a national health emergency or a similar "clear and present danger" would provide a sufficient justification for nontherapeutic human research.

Implicit in Jonas's characterization of most human research as optional is a rejection of the thesis of a general moral duty to participate in such research. Thus, there is no injustice involved in our not volunteering to take part in nontherapeutic studies. In Jonas's view, most volunteers of the past, including investigators involved in self-experimentation, performed acts of altruism and moral heroism. If we of the present owe any debt to the past, it is a debt of gratitude to these bygone heroes, not an obligation to society required by a reciprocity principle of justice.

A presupposition of Jonas's position on the general justification of human research is that autonomy rights—for example, the right to be free from invasions of one's body and the right to consent—are supremely important. Jonas also regards all nontherapeutic research involving human subjects as an infringement of the individual's "primary inviolability"; in Kantian terms, he objects to the use of a person as a means rather than an end. Because of this primary commitment to protecting the rights, dignity, and inviolability of the individual, Jonas is unwilling to accept either ordinary social benefits or the notion of universal duties to society as sufficient justification for human research.

But the principle of autonomy can be taken in another direction, as well. One additional justification, not explicitly mentioned by either Eisenberg or Jonas, is sometimes advanced in support of research involving human subjects. Investigators, it is asserted, should be free to decide what kinds of research they will perform and how they wish to conduct that research. According to this view, the freedom of scientific inquiry should be protected from outside interference, unless there are strong reasons for overriding the presumption of freedom. Thus, if an investigator can find human subjects who are willing to take part in some proposed research, he or she should generally be allowed to proceed with the research. Critics of this freedom-of-inquiry position reply that there is a significant difference between the freedom to do research and the freedom to involve human subjects in research. For example, there may be a qualitative distinction between analyzing the properties of a chemical compound, on the one hand, and soliciting the participation of human subjects in a research project, on the other. In addition, critics of the freedom-of-inquiry viewpoint argue that the knowledge differential between most investigators and most subjects is so great that some intervention by society is justified, if only to ensure that the consent of prospective subjects is adequately informed.

THE DESIGN

One important mode of clinical research is the randomized prospective controlled trial. In this type of research, subjects who fulfill the inclusion criteria are assigned at random, or by chance, to the various treatment groups of the study. The primary rationale for randomized controlled trials is that the randomization procedure helps to balance out unknown and therefore uncontrollable variables among the treatment groups. In some cases neither the investigators conducting the trial nor the patients participating in the trial know to which treatment group patients have been assigned. Such a study is called "double-blind."

Commentators on the ethics of research with human subjects have raised questions about several aspects of randomized controlled trials. They note first that leaving the choice of therapy to chance may seem to undermine the usual patient-professional relationship, in which the choice of therapy is made in the best interests of the patient. Further, the informed consent transaction is more complicated when the patient, and in many cases the professional, does not know what the treatment actually is. The monitoring of data emerging from the trial, the informing of patients and investigators about the interim data, and the appropriate criteria for prematurely terminating a trial are additional matters of dispute. Several of these issues are discussed in the Arthur Schafer essay included in this chapter.

RESEARCH INVOLVING ANIMALS

Perhaps the first question to be clarified in any discussion of animal research is: Which animals are to be included within the scope of consideration? Books and articles on the ethics of animal research have devoted surprisingly little attention to this question. One can usually infer from these writings that nonhuman mammals—such as monkeys, dogs, and rats—are to be included in the protected group. Indeed, Tom Regan explicitly limits his argument to "all species of mammalian animals." A somewhat broader class would be all vertebrates, that is, mammals plus birds, reptiles, amphibians, and fish. In the discussion that follows, it is assumed that the term "animals" refers to nonhuman vertebrates, although the question of research involving invertebrates may also deserve ethical analysis in its own right. (The "International Guiding Principles for Biomedical Research Involving Animals" focus their attention on vertebrate animals.)

Two primary issues can be identified in the animal research debate: (1) the consequences of the research and (2) the moral status of animals. Proponents of animal research usually advance arguments that appeal rather straightforwardly to the principle of beneficence. The weak form of the argument can be formulated as follows: Good consequences are achieved through the use of animals in research. A somewhat stronger thesis is that at least some of these good consequences can be achieved *only* by means of animal reseach; that is, no alternative (nonhuman) means to the desired end exist. In his essay in this chapter, H. J. McCloskey seems prepared to defend this stronger thesis.

The empirical background for the strong claim by proponents of animal research is that intact, live animals respond to research interventions in complex ways that cannot be simulated through any other research technique involving nonanimal systems. For example, administering a drug to a dog or presenting a learning stimulus to a rat may produce a complex reaction that affects multiple physiological systems. At present, such a response simply cannot be duplicated through the manipulation of cells in tissue culture or even through the use of sophisticated computer simulations. In theory at least, human subjects could be substituted for animal subjects and would be capable of producing the same kinds of complex response. However, given the painful, invasive, and even lethal character of much animal research, the use of humans in such research would itself pose serious ethical problems.

Critics of animal research can also appeal to the principle of beneficence. In response to the weak form of the proponents' argument, the critics urge that alternatives to animal research be more vigorously explored and actively employed. The strong form of the proponents' argument presents a more formidable challenge, however. If animal research is the only means for achieving a desirable consequence, the critic can respond by insisting on a conscientious weighing of research benefits against harm to animals. Indeed, reformers like Regan recommend the use of precisely this kind of calculus.

A complicating factor in any such effort to assess consequences is the problem of animal sentience, or sensitivity to pain. The notion of sentience raises both conceptual and empirical issues. A broad construal of the concept of sentience might conceivably include primitive "avoidance" reactions to aversive stimuli, for example, a paramecium's response to a toxic chemical or a rabbit's reaction to cold. However, a narrower construal of sentience might require the presence of anticipatory or retrospective psychological states such as fear or regret. Even if one were able to agree on a definition of sentience, there would remain the formidable empirical problem of measuring exactly how much pain is being inflicted upon, or in some sense being experienced by, animal subjects.

The second major issue in the animal research debate is the moral status of animals. This issue closely parallels the problem of personhood and the question of fetal status. In an influential essay reprinted in part in Chapter 4, Joel Feinberg argues that animals can have rights because they have, or can have, interests. Among the rights ascribed to animals by Feinberg is the right to be treated humanely. In his view, such treatment is owed to animals as their due and therefore involves the principle of justice. In the present chapter, Regan adopts a similar position, arguing that animals have rights because they are conscious beings that have interests in certain kinds of welfare. According to Regan, mammalian animals can even be said to have a certain kind of autonomy. H. J. McCloskey disputes Regan's thesis that nonhuman mammals have genuine preference autonomy and vigorously rejects the notion that nonhuman animals have moral rights. Tom Beauchamp regards the debate about the moral status of animals as an as-yet-unresolved "metaphysical dispute about the universe of values." Without committing himself to the language of rights, Beauchamp clearly believes that we have a strong moral obligation to prevent unnecessary suffering in animals, even if the fulfillment of that obligation results in the forgoing of otherwise achievable benefits for human beings.

ETHICAL REVIEW OF RESEARCH

Since its modest beginnings in 1966, a robust and increasingly international system for prior review of research with human subjects has evolved. In the 1980s a parallel development occurred in the realm of animal research. The responsible committees have been assigned various names in various countries, such as "ethics committees," "institutional review boards," "animal research committees," and "institutional animal care and use committees." What is common to all committees is that a body comprised of at least four or five people, usually from more than one academic discipline and often including one or more so-called "laypeople," provides external review of research involving humans or animals. While each committee is likely to employ local or national standards for research review, there is a near-consensus internationally on the moral rules that should govern human research and a gradual evolution toward international guidelines on research with animals. In their essays in this chapter, Robert Veatch, Peter Williams, and Lawrence Finsen discuss the appropriate roles of research review committees and indicate some of the pitfalls encountered by these innovative social institutions. (For a discussion of analogous bodies in clinical medicine, especially in the hospital context, see the concluding section of Chapter 6.)

L. W.

Codes of Research Ethics

The Nuremberg Code

The great weight of the evidence before us is to the effect that certain types of medical experiments on human beings, when kept within reasonably well-defined bounds, conform to the ethics of the medical profession generally. The protagonists of the practice of human experimentation justify their views on the basis that such experiments yield results for the good of society that are unprocurable by other methods or means of study. All agree, however, that certain basic principles must be observed in order to satisfy moral, ethical and legal concepts.

1. The voluntary consent of the human subject is absolutely essential.

This means that the person involved should have legal capacity to give consent; should be so situated as to be able to exercise free power of choice, without the intervention of any element of force, fraud, deceit, duress, overreaching, or other ulterior form of constraint or coercion; and should have sufficient knowledge and comprehension of the elements of the subject matter involved as to enable him to make an understanding and enlightened decision. This latter element requires that before the acceptance of an affirmative decision by the experimental subject there should be made known to him the nature, duration, and purpose of the experiment; the method and means by which it is to be conducted; all inconveniences and hazards reasonably to be expected; and the effects upon his health or person which may possibly come from his participation in the experiment.

The duty and responsibility for ascertaining the quality of the consent rests upon each individual who initiates, directs or engages in the experiment. It is a personal duty and responsibility which may not be delegated to another with impunity.

2. The experiment should be such as to yield fruitful results for the good of society, unprocurable by other methods or means of study, and not random and unnecessary in nature.

3. The experiment should be so designed and based on the results of animal experimentation and a knowledge of the natural history of the disease or other problems under study that the anticipated results will justify the performance of the experiment.

4. The experiment should be so conducted as to avoid all unnecessary physical and mental suffering and injury.

5. No experiment should be conducted where there is an *a priori* reason to believe that death or disabling injury will occur; except perhaps, in those experiments where the experimental physicians also serve as subjects.

6. The degree of risk to be taken should never exceed that determined by the humanitarian importance of the problem to be solved by the experiment.

7. Proper preparations should be made and adequate facilities provided to protect the experimental subject against even remote possibilities of injury, disability, or death.

8. The experiment should be conducted only by scientifically qualified persons. The highest degree of skill and care should be required through all stages of the experiment of those who conduct or engage in the experiment.

9. During the course of the experiment the human subject should be at liberty to bring the experiment to an end if he has reached the physical or mental state where continuation of the experiment seems to him to be impossible.

10. During the course of the experiment the scientist in charge must be prepared to terminate the experiment at any stage, if he has probable cause to believe, in the exercise of the good faith, superior skill and careful judgment required of him that a continuation of the experiment is likely to result in injury, disability, or death to the experimental subject.

From *Trials of War Criminals Before the Nuremberg Military Tribunals Under Control Council Law No. 10*. Vol. II, Nuremberg, October 1946–April 1949.

WORLD MEDICAL ASSOCIATION

Declaration of Helsinki

Recommendations guiding physicians in biomedical research involving human subjects

Adopted by the 18th World Medical Assembly, Helsinki, Finland, June 1964, amended by the 29th World Medical Assembly, Tokyo, Japan, October 1975, and the 35th World Medical Assembly, Venice, Italy, October 1983

INTRODUCTION

It is the mission of the physician to safeguard the health of the people. His or her knowledge and conscience are dedicated to the fulfillment of this mission.

The Declaration of Geneva of the World Medical Association binds the physician with the words, "The health of my patient will be my first consideration," and the International Code of Medical Ethics declares that, "A physician shall act only in the patient's interest when providing medical care which might have the effect of weakening the physical and mental condition of the patient." The purpose of biomedical research involving human subjects must be to improve diagnostic, therapeutic and prophylactic procedures and the understanding of the aetiology and pathogenesis of disease.

In current medical practice most diagnostic, therapeutic or prophylactic procedures involve hazards. This applies especially to biomedical research.

Medical progress is based on research which ultimately must rest in part on experimentation involving human subjects.

In the field of biomedical research a fundamental distinction must be recognized between medical research in which the aim is essentially diagnostic or therapeutic for a patient, and medical research the essential object of which is purely scientific and without implying direct diagnostic or therapeutic value to the person subjected to the research.

Special caution must be exercised in the conduct of research which may affect the environment, and the welfare of animals used for research must be respected.

Because it is essential that the results of laboratory experiments to be applied to human beings to further scientific knowledge and to help suffering humanity, the World Medical Association has prepared the following recommendations as a guide to every physician in biomedical research involving human subjects. They should be kept under review in the future. It must be stressed that the standards as drafted are only a guide to physicians all over the world. Physicians are not relieved from criminal, civil and ethical responsibilities under the law of their own countries.

I. BASIC PRINCIPLES

1. Biomedical research involving human subjects must conform to generally accepted scientific principles and should be based on adequately performed laboratory and animal experimentation and on a thorough knowledge of the scientific literature.

2. The design and performance of each experimental procedure involving human subjects should be clearly formulated in an experimental protocol which should be transmitted to a specially appointed independent committee for consideration, comment and guidance.

3. Biomedical research involving human subjects should be conducted only by scientifically qualified persons and under the supervision of a clinically competent medical person. The

responsibility for the human subject must always rest with a medically qualified person and never rest on the subject of the research, even though the subject has given his or her consent.

4. Biomedical research involving human subjects cannot legitimately be carried out unless the importance of the objective is in proportion to the inherent risk to the subject.

5. Every biomedical research project involving human subjects should be preceded by careful assessment of predictable risks in comparison with foreseeable benefits to the subject or to others. Concern for the interests of the subject must always prevail over the interests of science and society.

6. The right of the research subject to safeguard his or her integrity must always be respected. Every precaution should be taken to respect the privacy of the subject and to minimize the impact of the study on the subject's physical and mental integrity and on the personality of the subject.

7. Physicians should abstain from engaging in research projects involving human subjects unless they are satisfied that the hazards involved are believed to be predictable. Physicians should cease any investigation if the hazards are found to outweigh the potential benefits.

8. In publication of the results of his or her research, the physician is obliged to preserve the accuracy of the results. Reports of experimentation not in accordance with the principles laid down in this Declaration should not be accepted for publication.

9. In any research on human beings, each potential subject must be adequately informed of the aims, methods, anticipated benefits and potential hazards of the study and the discomfort it may entail. He or she should be informed that he or she is at liberty to abstain from participation in the study and that he or she is free to withdraw his or her consent to participation at any time. The physician should then obtain the subject's freely given informed consent, preferably in writing.

10. When obtaining informed consent for the research project the physician should be particularly cautious if the subject is in a dependent relationship to him or her or may consent under duress. In that case the informed consent should be obtained by a physician who is not engaged in the investigation and who is completely independent of this official relationship.

11. In case of legal incompetence, informed consent should be obtained from the legal guardian in accordance with national legislation. Where physical or mental incapacity makes it impossible to obtain informed consent, or when the subject is a minor, permission from the responsible relative replaces that of the subject in accordance with national legislation. Whenever the minor child is in fact able to give a consent, the minor's consent must be obtained in addition to the consent of the minor's legal guardian.

12. The research protocol should always contain a statement of the ethical considerations involved and should indicate that the principles enunciated in the present declaration are complied with.

II. MEDICAL RESEARCH COMBINED WITH PROFESSIONAL CARE
(Clinical research)

1. In the treatment of the sick person, the physician must be free to use a new diagnostic and therapeutic measure, if in his or her judgement it offers hope of saving life, reestablishing health or alleviating suffering.

2. The potential benefits, hazards and discomfort of a new method should be weighed against the advantages of the best current diagnostic and therapeutic methods.

3. In any medical study, every patient—including those of a control group, if any—should be assured of the best proven diagnostic and therapeutic method.

4. The refusal of the patient to participate in a study must never interfere with the physician-patient relationship.

5. If the physician considers it essential not to obtain informed consent, the specific reasons for this proposal should be stated in the experimental protocol for transmission to the independent committee (1, 2).

6. The physician can combine medical research with professional care, the objective being the acquisition of new medical knowledge, only to the extent that medical research is justified by

its potential diagnostic or therapeutic value for the patient.

III. NON-THERAPEUTIC BIOMEDICAL RESEARCH INVOLVING HUMAN SUBJECTS
(Non-clinical biomedical research)

1. In the purely scientific application of medical research carried out on a human being, it is the duty of the physician to remain the protector of the life and health of that person on whom biomedical research is being carried out.

2. The subjects should be volunteers—either healthy persons or patients for whom the experimental design is not related to the patient's illness.
3. The investigator or the investigating team should discontinue the research if in his/her or their judgement it may, if continued, be harmful to the individual.
4. In research on man, the interest of science and society should never take precedence over considerations related to the well-being of the subject.

COUNCIL FOR INTERNATIONAL ORGANIZATIONS OF MEDICAL SCIENCES

International Guiding Principles for Biomedical Research Involving Animals

PREAMBLE

Experimentation with animals has made possible major contributions to biological knowledge and to the welfare of man and animals, particularly in the treatment and prevention of diseases. Many important advances in medical science have had their origins in basic biological research not primarily directed to practical ends as well as from applied research designed to investigate specific medical problems. There is still an urgent need for basic and applied research that will lead to the discovery of methods for the prevention and treatment of diseases for which adequate control methods are not yet available—notably the noncommunicable diseases and the endemic communicable diseases of warm climates.

Past progress has depended, and further progress in the foreseeable future will depend, largely on animal experimentation which, in the broad field of human medicine, is the prelude to experimental trials on human beings of, for example, new therapeutic, prophylactic, or diagnostic substances, devices, or procedures.

There are two international ethical codes intended principally for the guidance of countries or institutions that have not yet formulated their own ethical requirements for human experimentation: The Tokyo revision of the *Declaration of Helsinki* of the World Medical Association (1975); and the *Proposed International Guidelines for Biomedical Research Involving Human Subjects* of the Council for International Organizations of Medical Sciences and the World Health Organization (1982). These codes recognize that while experiments involving human subjects are a *sine qua non* of medical progress, they must be subject to strict ethical requirements. In order to ensure that such ethical requirements are observed, national and institutional ethical codes have also been elaborated with a view to the protection of human subjects involved in biomedical (including behavioural) research.

A major requirement both of national and international ethical codes for human experimentation, and of

Reprinted with permission of the Council for International Organizations of Medical Sciences, *International Guiding Principles for Biomedical Research Involving Animals* (Geneva: CIOMS, 1985), pp. 17–19.

national legislation in many cases, is that new substances or devices should not be used for the first time on human beings unless previous tests on animals have provided a reasonable presumption of their safety.

The use of animals for predicting the probable effects of procedures on human beings entails responsibility for their welfare. In both human and veterinary medicine animals are used for behavioural, physiological, pathological, toxicological, and therapeutic research and for experimental surgery or surgical training and for testing drugs and biological preparations. The same responsibility toward the experimental animals prevails in all of these cases.

Because of differing legal systems and cultural backgrounds there are varying approaches to the use of animals for research, testing, or training in different countries. Nonetheless, their use should be always in accord with humane practices. The varying approaches in different countries to the use of animals for biomedical purposes, and the lack of relevant legislation or of formal self-regulatory mechanisms in some, point to the need for international guiding principles elaborated as a result of international and interdisciplinary consultations.

The guiding principles proposed here provide a framework for more specific national or institutional provisions. They apply not only to biomedical research but also to all uses of vertebrate animals for other biomedical purposes, including the production and testing of therapeutic, prophylactic, and diagnostic substances, the diagnosis of infections and intoxications in man and animals, and to any other procedures involving the use of intact live vertebrates.

BASIC PRINCIPLES

I. The advancement of biological knowledge and the development of improved means for the protection of the health and well-being both of man and of animals require recourse to experimentation on intact live animals of a wide variety of species.

II. Methods such as mathematical models, computer simulation and *in vitro* biological systems should be used wherever appropriate.

III. Animal experiments should be undertaken only after due consideration of their relevance for human or animal health and the advancement of biological knowledge.

IV. The animals selected for an experiment should be of an appropriate species and quality, and the minimum number required to obtain scientifically valid results.

V. Investigators and other personnel should never fail to treat animals as sentient, and should regard their proper care and use and the avoidance or minimization of discomfort, distress, or pain as ethical imperatives.

VI. Investigators should assume that procedures that would cause pain in human beings cause pain in other vertebrate species, although more needs to be known about the perception of pain in animals.

VII. Procedures with animals that may cause more than momentary or minimal pain or distress should be performed with appropriate sedation, analgesia, or anesthesia in accordance with accepted veterinary practice. Surgical or other painful procedures should not be performed on unanesthetized animals paralysed by chemical agents.

VIII. Where waivers are required in relation to the provisions of article VII, the decisions should not rest solely with the investigators directly concerned but should be made, with due regard to the provisions of articles IV, V, and VI, by a suitably constituted review body. Such waivers should not be made solely for the purposes of teaching or demonstration.

IX. At the end of, or, when appropriate, during an experiment, animals that would otherwise suffer severe or chronic pain, distress, discomfort, or disablement that cannot be relieved should be painlessly killed.

X. The best possible living conditions should be maintained for animals kept for biomedical purposes. Normally the care of animals should be under the supervision of veterinarians having experience in laboratory animal science. In any case, veterinary care should be available as required.

XI. It is the responsibility of the director of an institute or department using animals to ensure that investigators and personnel have appropriate qualifications or experience for conducting procedures on animals. Adequate opportunities shall be provided for in-service training, including the proper and humane concern for the animals under their care. . . .

Issues in Human Research

LEON EISENBERG

The Social Imperatives of Medical Research

Peculiar to this time[1] is the need to restate a proposition that, a decade ago, would have been regarded as self-evident, namely, that fostering excellence in medical research is in the public interest. Contemporary news accounts and learned journals alike have announced as exposé what always has been true: that doctors are fallible, that researchers are not all noble, and that what appeared to be true in the light of yesterday's evidence proves false by tomorrow's. The sins committed in the name of medical research are stressed in entire disproportion to the human gains that continue to flow from the enterprise. That a significant amount of funded research will inevitably fail to yield the expected answers is taken as a sign of boondoggling, because the nature of science is not understood. We are asked for guarantees of absolute safety as if this were an attainable goal.

Some of the specific criticism has been just and instructive, some of it merely misinformed, some of it completely irrelevant. A constructive response to the criticism of medical research would have been easier had not distrust been aroused at the same time by the misapplications of technical knowledge (the spread of weapons systems, wire tapping, computerization, nuclear wastes) and the use of technical devices by government against its own people. Those of us who argue for the necessity of scientific research in medicine are too often regarded as if we were indifferent to misuses of it and as though we were apologists for the Establishment. I know of no remedy other than to redouble our effort to explain the nature and the justification of well-designed medical research, the calculus of risk and benefit that is an integral part of it, and the design of methods to maximize its potential for gain. If we permit it to be circumscribed with a bureaucracy of regulation so cumbersome as to impede its progress, we incur a risk to society from the restriction of medical science that will far outweigh the aggregate risk to all the subjects in experimental studies.

MEDICAL PRACTICE AND MEDICAL RESEARCH

One source of misunderstanding is the confusion of what is usual and customary in medical practice with what is safe and useful. The critics of research are often exquisitely aware of the dangers in an experiment (indeed, the responsible investigator is at pains to spell them out as precisely as he or she can). At the same time, these critics, surprisingly naive about the extent to which medical practice rests on custom rather than evidence, fail to appreciate the necessity for controlled trials to determine whether what is traditional does harm rather than good.

Consider, for example, the fact that about 1 million tonsillectomies and adenoidectomies are done each year in the United States; T and A's make up 30 percent of all surgery on children. Set aside budgetary considerations, even though the outlay—about $500 million—represents a significant "opportunity cost" in resources lost to more useful medical care.[2] During the 1950s, T and A's resulted in some 200 to 300 deaths per year.[3] Current mortality has been estimated at one death per 16,000 operations.[4] Yet this procedure (whose origins are lost in antiquity) continues at epidemic rates though there is no evidence that it is effective[5] except for a few uncommon conditions.[6] Doctors disagree so widely about the "indications" for T and A that within one state (Vermont) there is a fivefold variation by area of residence in the probability that a person will have his or her tonsils removed

From *Science* 198 (December 16, 1977), 1105–1110. Copyright © 1977 by the American Association for the Advancement of Science. Reprinted with permission of the author and the publisher.

by age 20.[7] Thus, we have a procedure of dubious value employed at high frequency despite significant mortality and dollar costs. Why? It is done because doctors and parents believe in it; having become usual and customary, it is not subject to the systematic scrutiny of an experimental design.

Compare the human cost from this single routine and relatively minor procedure to the risk to human subjects in nontherapeutic and therapeutic research. Cardon and his colleagues[8] surveyed investigators conducting research on 133,000 human subjects over the past 3 years. In nontherapeutic research, which involved some 93,000 subjects, there was not one fatality, there was only one instance of permanent disability (0.001 percent), and there were 37 cases of temporary disability (0.04 percent). In therapeutic research (that is, clinical research carried out on sick people who stood to benefit directly from the knowledge gained), among 39,000 patients, 43 died (0.1 percent) and 13 suffered permanent disability (0.03 percent). (Most of the deaths were of patients on cancer chemotherapy.) The risk to experimental subjects in nontherapeutic research is comparable to the rates for accidental injury in the general population (when one makes appropriate calculation for days of risk per year). Tonsillectomy, a relatively minor surgical procedure, produces more deaths per 100,000 each year than the total from all nontherapeutic research! If we add into our calculation the deaths resulting from major surgical procedures that may be performed more often than is warranted—for example, the current rate of 647 hysterectomies per 100,000 females projects to loss of the uterus for half the female population by age 65[9]—and from excessive and injudicious prescription of powerful drugs, it becomes clear that the gain in public safety from exacting scrutiny of medical practice by means of controlled trials would far outweigh any possible gain from the most restrictive approach to medical research. Let me not be misunderstood: I do not deny the necessity for surveillance of the ethics of the research community; the point I stress is that medical research, applied to medical practice, stands alone in its ability to avert unnecessary human suffering and death.

THE SOURCES OF MEDICAL ERROR

Among the reasons given for the persistence of medical error are venality on the part of physicians, professional incompetence, and lack of commitment to the public weal. There are venal physicians; we need look no further than the exposure of Medicaid mills to find them. But that hardly accounts for the overprescription of surgery when we recognize that surgery is performed on physicians' families even more often than it is on the general public[10]; physicians as consumers follow the advice they proffer as providers. There are incompetent doctors, and we still lack adequate methods for weeding them out; but anesthetic and surgical deaths occur in the best of hands because of the risks inherent in the procedures. Not all doctors are actuated by the public interest, but this hardly explains what concerns us about physician behavior. Although these factors contribute to wrongheadedness in medical practice, a far more important source is simply the doctor's conviction that what he or she does is for the patient's welfare. When good evidence is lacking, the best and most dedicated of us do wrong in the utter conviction of being right.

BLOODLETTING AS PANACEA

Let me offer a historical illustration from the career of a man with many admirable qualities, a leading U.S. physician of the late 18th century. Benjamin Rush was uncommon among his peers in having a university degree in medicine (from Edinburgh); he was appointed professor of chemistry at the College of Philadelphia (soon to become the Medical School of the University of Pennsylvania, the first medical school in America) and later professor of the institute and practices of medicine. He was among the most steadfast of patriots, a signer of the Declaration of Independence, a member of the Pennsylvania delegation that voted to adopt the Constitution of the United States, and a founder of the first antislavery society.[11] His book *Medical Inquiries and Observations upon the Diseases of the Mind* was the first comprehensive American treatise on mental illness.[12] Thus, we have a physician with as good an education as his time could provide, a leading member of the faculty of the premier school of medicine, and a man dedicated to the public interest.

In 1793, a severe epidemic of yellow fever fell upon the city of Philadelphia.[13] It is estimated that more than one-third of its population of 50,000 fled the city and that more than 4,000 lives were lost. Panic beset the medical community, and doctors were among those who took flight to escape the pestilence. From illness and defection at the height of the epidemic, only three physicians were available to treat more than 6,000 patients. Rush dispatched his wife and children to the safety of the countryside and remained behind to fulfill his medical responsibility.

Rush was an adherent of the Brunonian system of medicine, according to which febrile illnesses resulted from an excess of stimulation and a corresponding excitement of the blood. In keeping with this theory, he ministered to his patients by vigorous bleeding and purging, the latter to "divert the force of the fever to [the bowels] and thereby save the liver and brains from a fatal and dangerous congestion." Rush went from patient to patient, letting blood copiously and purging with vigor. His desperate remedies, contemporary critics contended, were more dangerous than the disease, a criticism history has borne out.

His beliefs were not something he reserved for others. He himself was taken with a violent fever. He instructed his assistant to bleed him "plentifully" and give him "a dose of the mercurial medicine." From illness and treatment combined, he almost died; his convalescence was prolonged. That he did recover persuaded him that his methods were correct. Thus, when the epidemic subsided, he wrote: "Never before did I experience such sublime joy as I now felt on contemplating the success of my remedies. . . . The conquest of a formidable disease was through the triumph of a principle in medicine."[14] Neither dedication so great that he risked his life to minister to others, nor willingness to treat himself as he treated others, nor yet the best education to be had in his day was sufficient to prevent Rush from committing grievous harm in the name of doing good. Convinced of the correctness of his theory of medicine and lacking a means for the systematic study of treatment outcome, he attributed each new instance of improvement to the efficacy of his treatment and each new death that occurred despite it to the severity of the disease.

INTRODUCTION OF THE NUMERICAL METHOD

Bloodletting continued to be a widely used medical remedy until the middle of the 19th century. According to Osler,[15] it was finally abandoned because of the introduction into American medicine of the "numerical method" of the French physician Pierre Charles Alexandre Louis. Louis had been disenchanted with his medical education and his experience as a practitioner. He withdrew from practice to devote himself to study. As one contemporary commented:[15]

He consecrated the whole of his time and talent to rigorous, impartial observation. All private practice was relinquished

and he allowed no considerations of personal emolument to interfere with the resolution he had formed. For some time, his extreme minuteness in inquiry and accuracy of description were the subjects of sneering and ridicule, and "to what end?" was not infrequently and tauntingly asked.

One result of his study, an essay on bloodletting, appeared in Paris in 1835.[16] Within a year, it was translated into English by G. C. Putnam.[17] In a preface to the volume James Jackson, physician to the Massachusetts General Hospital, wrote:[18]

If anything may be regarded as settled in the treatment of diseases, it is that bloodletting is useful in the class of diseases called inflammatory; and especially in inflammation of the thoracic viscera. To this general opinion or belief on this subject, M. Louis gives support by his observations; but the result of these observations is that the benefits derived from bleeding in the diseases, which he has here examined, are not so great and striking as they had been represented by many teachers. If the same methods should be obtained by others, after making observations as rigorous as M. Louis, many of us will be forced to modify our former opinions. . . . The author does not pretend that the questions, here discussed, are decided forever. He makes a valuable contribution to the evidence, on which they must be decided; he points out the mode, in which this evidence should be collected, and in which its material should be analyzed; seeking truth only, he calls on others to adduce facts, which, being gathered from various quarters, may show us, with a good degree of exactness, the precise value of the remedy in question.

Louis himself began his monograph with the comment:[19]

The results of my researches on the effects of bloodletting in inflammation are so little in accord with the general opinion, that it is not without a degree of hesitation I have decided to publish them. After having analyzed the facts, which relate to them, for the first time, I thought myself deceived, and began my work anew; but having again from this new analysis, obtained the same results, I could no longer doubt their correctness.

He was led to conclude:

We infer that bloodletting has had very little influence on the progress of pneumonitis . . . ; that its influence has not been more evident in the cases bled copiously and repeatedly, than in those bled only once and to a small amount; that we do not at once arrest inflammations, as is too often finally imagined;

that, in cases where it appears to be otherwise, it is undoubtedly owing, either to an error in diagnosis, or to the fact that the bloodletting was practiced at an advanced period of the disease, when it had nearly run its course.

Yet, so strong was the power of authority, that he was moved to comment:[20]

I will add that bloodletting, notwithstanding its influence is limited, should not be neglected in inflammations which are severe and are seated in an important organ.

Louis's precise observations, his stress on the importance of studying series of cases, and his insistence on reexamining standard belief were to have an enormous influence. Many American physicians went to Paris to become his pupils and returned to these shores persuaded of the value of his method. Insofar as it can be said that any single contribution led to the abandonment on this continent of bloodletting as a panacea, it was Louis's numerical method. It had its roots in the earlier applications of elementary statistics to public health and became far more powerful as a method when the concepts of probability statistics were applied to its simple tabulations.[21] From these beginnings stems much of the progress in medical science.

IMPORTANCE OF CLINICAL DESCRIPTION AND CLASSIFICATION

I have thus far stressed the contributions of the controlled clinical trial[22] to the provision of more effective remedies and to the elimination of harmful ones. But before physicians can treat, they must be able to discriminate disorders one from another. Here, careful delineation of disease patterns, both immediate and longitudinal, and attention to ways in which patients resemble and differ from each other provide the necessary groundwork for identifying the underlying pathophysiology. The process begins with the report of a puzzling and hitherto undescribed group of cases. Initially attention is directed at differentiating the new syndrome from superficially similar conditions. Some decades pass during which doctors disagree on the diagnosis and include or exclude a penumbra of cases which markedly affect the reported outcome. Next a fundamental pathogenic lesion is discovered, and confirmed by other workers, to be present in "typical" cases. As the mechanism of the disease is clarified, the disease itself is redefined in terms of the underlying

pathology. Now new and variant clinical forms can be identified, cases that would not have met the original criteria. Let me illustrate this by an example from hematology.

In 1925 Cooley and Lee separated out from the group of childhood anemias (known as von Jaksch's anemia) five cases with hepatosplenomegaly, skin pigmentation, thick bones, and oddly shaped red cells with decreased osmotic fragility. Cooley's anemia was renamed thalassemia in 1932 by Whipple and Bradford, who noted that the children came from families of Mediterranean origin. The genetic basis of thalassemia was established by Wintrobe in 1940 in a paper which distinguished thalassemia minor (the heterozygous state) from thalassemia major (the homozygous state). Fifteen years later Kunkel discovered the normal minor hemoglobin component hemoglobin A_2 and found it to be elevated in individuals with thalassemia minor.[23] A subsequent explosion of research on the hemoglobin molecule has led to the recognition of some 50 combinations of genetic errors which can produce the clinical picture of thalassemia. . . .

BASIC RESEARCH AND DISEASE PREVENTION

Hand in hand with the controlled clinical trial and with the continuing search for diagnostic precision must go fundamental research in basic biology. Much of our armamentarium for the treatment and prevention of disease is at the level of what Lewis Thomas[24] has called "halfway technology," measures which, though useful, only partly reverse the disease process, are costly, and are toxic. Consider the situation this nation faced not long ago in coping with poliomyelitis. Each year it took 2,000 lives and left 3,000 persons with severe paralysis. The hospital cost for acute and chronic care, the iron lung, the wet pack, and physiotherapy exceeded $1 billion a year. For an investment of $40 million in the basic research which led to Ender's method of cultivating the polio virus in the chick embryo, and not more than several hundred million dollars for applied technology and population trials, an enormous human and financial loss has been averted.[25]

The psychiatrist today is in the position of the pediatrician a generation ago. Chemotherapy aborts acute psychotic episodes, but recurrence is common, permanent disability frequent, and drug toxicity considerable. We have strong evidence for familial predisposition but cannot specify modes of inheritance or what is inherited, or distinguish the potential patient before illness occurs. The hope of prevention must rest upon increased support for fundamental research in neurobiology, genetics, and epidemiology.[26] The problem is not a gap in the application of knowledge but a gap in knowledge itself.

Basic research does not begin and end with molecular biology. Vaccination provides a model for infectious diseases and perhaps even for neoplasms; it is simply irrelevant to behavior-linked health problems: the consequences of smoking, overeating, drinking, drugging, and reckless driving. Belloc and Breslow have shown that seven personal health habits sum to a powerful prediction of morbidity[27] and mortality[28] for middle-aged adults. To recognize that cultural patterns, social forces, and idiosyncratic personal behaviors have major effects on health[29] is not equivalent to knowing how to alter them. It does, however, argue for the urgency of research in the social as well as the biological sciences if physicians are to learn how to intervene effectively.[30]

THE RESTRICTION OF RISK
AND THE RISK OF RESTRICTION

Health will be held hazard to custom until the current preoccupation with the dangers of research is placed in the appropriate context: namely, weighing in the very same scales the dangers of not doing research. Surveillance of research ethics requires simultaneous assessment of the scientific and the ethical soundness of the protocols themselves. "A poorly or improperly designed study involving human subjects—one that could not possibly yield scientific facts (that is, reproducible observations) relevant to the question under study—is by definition unethical."[31] Commendation for a high rate of rejection of research proposals implies that the proper goal for a research review committee is blocking human studies. To the contrary, the systematic imposition of impediments to significant therapeutic research is itself unethical because an important benefit is being denied to the community.

This is not a call for unrestricted rights for medical researchers. If I do not accept the view that medical researchers are worse than lawyers or philosophers, I will not argue that they are better. They are simply human; that is to say, fallible. As in the case of all professional activity, social controls are necessary. But in establishing those controls, it is necessary to weigh fully the possible resultant losses. The decision not to do something poses as many ethical quandaries as the decision to do it. Not to act is to act.[32]

Important ethical issues in medical research have been overlooked in the preoccupation with ethical ab-

solutes. Consider, for example, the clear social class bias in the likelihood of being a subject in a medical experiment. For that there can be no justification. Even if risk in research be inevitable, inequity in exposure because of caste or class need not be. The patients on whom clinical research is most often done are clinic patients, those who by reason of economic circumstance and education are the least able to assert their rights against medical authority.

It was not long ago, to our shame, that this practice was explicitly justified on the ground that the poor paid society back for the "privilege" of receiving charitable care by being suitable clinical material for research and teaching. Few would defend that position in so callous a way today. Yet the practice continues, less by plan than by fallout from our two-track medical care system. Researchers are located in teaching hospitals. Teaching hospitals are a major medical resource for the poor. The poor become the patients on whom studies are done because of their convenience as a study population and our insensitivity to the injustice of the practice. It is not enough to say that we now offer explanation and choice and obtain informed consent. Indeed, we do. But the quality of consent is not the same when the social position of doctor and patient are disparate as it is when they are more nearly equals.

Enhancing the human quality of the community in which we live is the responsibility of every citizen; one way to meet that responsibility is by sharing in the risks of the search to diminish human suffering. Richard Titmuss[33] has pointed to the health benefits to the United Kingdom from a public policy based on a voluntary blood donor system [but see Sapolsky and Finkelstein for a contrary view[34]]. I suggest that there will be moral gain as well as health gain to the United States to the extent that we succeed in creating a community of shared responsibility for health research.

INFORMED CONSENT IN THE
ABSENCE OF INFORMATION

What does "informed" consent mean in the real world of medical practice? When risks are specifiable so that it is possible to make a rational decision by weighing alternatives, it is clearly the physician's duty to inform the patient fully. That has long been a hallmark of good medical practice and sound clinical investigation; it is no contemporary discovery. But what does "informed" mean when what is available to the physician, let alone the patient, is not information but noise? In what sense is there a choice to be made between treatment A and treatment B if there is no proof that either works or that one is superior to the other? What right have I lost if, in a national health scheme, I am assigned to a randomized trial without being asked my preference, when that preference can only be capricious? The very justification for a randomized trial is that there is insufficient information to permit a rational, that is, informed, choice. In a free society we will reserve the right for any citizen to opt out. But when we respect the privilege to be guided by superstition, astrology, or simple orneriness, let us drop the adjective "informed" and speak only of "consent."

DO WE NEED MEDICAL RESEARCH?

A major undercurrent in the criticism of medical research is a growing belief that it is basically irrelevant to contemporary human needs. The argument runs something like this: what doctors do has only marginal effects on health; anyway, what researchers learn, when it does add to knowledge, doesn't get into practice; besides, from a higher moral view, what really matters is learning to live with the existential realities of pain and dying and not to permit technical iatrogenesis to alienate man from his nature.[35] To what extent is this credible?

There is good evidence for the proposition that the increase in longevity over the past century in industrialized nations has been principally the result of social forces: better nutrition, better hygiene, and changed behavior.[36] An instructive example is the striking decline in mortality from tuberculosis over the last 100 years, with only a small additional decrement visible after the introduction of streptomycin. But there is no assurance that further social change will eliminate the residual cases. Moreover, chemotherapy is decisive in the treatment of the tuberculosis that is still with us; the lack of a prominent effect on aggregate mortality statistics reflects the lesser prevalence of the disease as a public health problem, not the ineffectiveness of treatment. But the major defect of the proposition, as a general indictment of medical care, is at a more fundamental level. Doctors, at best, postpone death; death itself is inevitable. Most of what doctors do is to mitigate discomfort and pain and to enhance function in the presence of chronic disease, an effect that is not registered in mortality tables.[37] Sole reliance on longevity and mortality leaves unmeasured the benefits most patients consult doctors for and the major benefits they have always derived from them.[38] Morbidity rates, and the consequent demand for medical resources,[39] cannot be predicted from mortality data.[40]

The second theme, the failure to translate research into practice, . . . is grossly exaggerated. Lag undoubtedly occurs in the transfer of medical skills from highly specialized centers to rural areas; the much more troublesome problem is the indiscriminate introduction into practice of new drugs and surgical innovations well before their indications and limitations are clear, often in such ways as to compromise their usefulness. The major barriers to the treatment of life-threatening disease stem not from failing to use what we know but from not knowing what to use.

Eighty percent of the deaths in this country are caused by cardiovascular, neoplastic, cerebrovascular, and renal disease.[24] For the very great majority of the specific disorders within these categories the treatments we have are only palliatives. Palliatives are important, and certainly they should be distributed fairly; but the most evenhanded and prompt distribution of all available remedies would have only a small effect on death rates. As to resource allocation, the percentage of the health dollar (well under 2 percent) devoted to applied and basic medical research in toto is so small a part of total health costs that complete diversion of those funds would have negligible effects on health care delivery. The one clear result would be to end all prospect for improving the quality of the care delivered.

The idea that pain and dying are integral parts of man's fate, though put forth as a truism, is in fact a theological view of the human condition.[35] To comprehend its meaning, it is necessary to ask: How much pain? Death at what age? Whose pain and whose death? By what standards: today's or a century ago's, white American or black American, Indian or African? Perhaps, with a life expectancy exceeding the Biblical threescore and ten, affluent white Americans can afford the luxury of wondering whether medical research makes much sense in view of the risks and costs it entails. That is, we can if we mistake our fate for man's fate, ourselves for all of humankind.

A THIRD WORLD PERSPECTIVE ON RESEARCH

The armchair view of medical research as fun and games undergoes radical transformation from the standpoint of the third world, where infant mortality may be as high as 20 percent and life expectancy no more than 30 years. "People are sick because they are poor, they become poorer because they are sick and they become sicker because they are poorer."[41] Six infectious diseases that are almost unknown on our shores plague Africa, Asia, and Latin America: Malaria afflicts an estimated quarter billion; the mosquito that spreads it is becoming resistant to the standard pesticides and the plasmodium to chloroquin. Trypanosomiasis afflicts perhaps 20 million; we lack effective weapons against either the vector or the parasite; the treatment in use can be more dangerous than the disease. Leishmaniasis claims some 12 million; there is no known treatment. Filariasis and onchocerciasis infect 300 million; treatment is ineffective. Schistosomiasis afflicts 250 million; as nations attempt to improve their agricultural productivity through irrigation, the snail vector multiplies. Finally, there are 12 to 15 million lepers in the world; the current treatment requires 7 years; drug-resistant lepra bacilli have begun to appear.

In the face of all this, there is a clear moral imperative in developed nations for medical research in tropical diseases, to seek to permit two-thirds of the world's population to share in the freedom from pain and untimely death we have achieved for ourselves. In the forceful words of Barry Bloom:[41]

Discourse about medicine and ethics has focused almost entirely on problems of a wealthy society, and relatively little attention has been given to those affecting the vast majority of people in the world. There is a preponderant concern with individualism and individual rights, most recently reflected in the enormous preoccupation with death and dying. Imagine the impact of the anguished disquisitions about the Karen Quinlan case on the reader in Bangladesh or Upper Volta. The public agitation over "pulling the plug" on a single machine seems almost perverse when juxtaposed against the unmet health needs, the desperate struggle for survival of millions of people around the globe. I do not deny that there are serious problems of individual liberty at stake or that the Quinlan case may serve as a model for delimiting the role of the family, physician, or state in authorizing medical treatment for those unable to speak for themselves. But when the model so fills the horizon as to obscure the reality, then all perspective is lost.

• • •

M. PASTEUR'S RESEARCH

Because science is incomplete, reason imperfect, and both can be put to damaging uses, some would abandon science and reason in favor of mysticism, hermeneutics, and transcendental rapture. It is not knowledge but ignorance that assures misery. It is not science but its employment for inhuman purposes that threatens our survival. The fundamental ethical questions of science are political questions:[42] Who shall control its products? For what purposes shall they be employed?

Four years after the community protests against the dangers of [Louis Pasteur's] research, the citizens of France, by public subscriptions in gratitude for his contribution to human welfare, erected the Pasteur Institute. In the ceremony of dedication, Pasteur, overcome by his feelings, asked his son to read his remarks, which concluded:[43]

Two opposing laws seem to be now in contest. The one, a law of blood and of death, ever imagining new means of destruction, forces nations always to be ready for battle. The other, a law of peace, work and health, ever evolving means of delivering man from the scourges which beset him. The one seeks violent conquests, the other the relief of humanity. The one places a single life above all victories, the other sacrifices hundreds of thousands of lives to the ambition of a single individual. The law of which we are the instruments strives even in the midst of carnage to cure the wounds due to the law of war. Treatment by our antiseptic methods may save the lives of thousands of soldiers. Which of these two laws will ultimately prevail, God alone knows. But this we may assert: that French science will have tried, by obeying the law of Humanity, to extend the frontiers of life.

NOTES

1. A. Etzioni and C. Nunn, *Daedalus* 103, 191 (1974).

2. H. H. Hiatt, *N. Engl. J. Med.* 293, 235 (1975).

3. H. Bakwin, *J. Pediatr.* 52, 339 (1958).

4. L. W. Pratt, *Trans. Am. Acad. Ophthalmol. Otolaryngol.* 74, 1146 (1970).

5. W. Shaikh, E. Vayda, W. Feldman, *Pediatrics* 57, 401 (1976).

6. C. Guilleminault, F. L. Eldridge, F. B. Simons, W. C. Dement, *ibid.* 58, 23 (1976).

7. J. Wennberg and A. Gittelsohn, *Science* 182, 1102 (1973).

8. P. V. Cardon, F. W. Dommel, R. R. Trumble, *N. Engl. J. Med.* 295, 650 (1976).

9. J. Bunker, V. C. Donahue, P. Cole, M. Notman, *ibid.*, p. 264.

10. J. Bunker and B. Brown, *ibid.*, 290, 1051 (1974).

11. G. W. Corner, *The Autobiography of Benjamin Rush* (Princeton Univ. Press, Princeton, N.J., 1948).

12. B. Rush, *Medical Inquiries and Observations Upon the Diseases of the Mind* (Kimber & Richardson, Philadelphia, 1812; reprinted by Hafner, New York, 1962).

13. W. S. Middleton, *Ann. Med. Hist.* 10, 434 (1928).

14. *Ibid.*, p. 442.

15. W. Osler, *Bull. Johns Hopkins Hosp.* 8, 161 (1897).

16. W. J. Gaines and H. G. Langford, *Arch. Intern. Med.* 106, 571 (1960).

17. P. C. A. Louis, *Researches on the Effects of Bloodletting in Some Inflammatory Diseases and on the Influence of Tartarized Antimony and Vesication in Pneumonitis*, translated by C. G. Putnam with preface and appendix by J. Jackson (Hilliard, Gray, Boston, 1836).

18. *Ibid.*, pp. v–vi.

19. *Ibid.*, p. 1.

20. *Ibid.*, p. 22.

21. G. Rosen, *Bull. Hist. Med.* 29, 27 (1955).

22. A. L. Cochrane, *Effectiveness and Efficiency: Random Reflections on Health Services* (Nuffield Provincial Hospitals Trust, London, 1972).

23. D. J. Weatherall, *Johns Hopkins Med. J.* 139, 194 (1976).

24. L. Thomas, *Daedalus* 106, 35 (1977).

25. H. H. Fudenberg, *J. Invest. Dermatol.* 61, 321 (1973).

26. L. Eisenberg, *Bull. N.Y. Acad. Med.* 51, 118 (1975).

27. N. B. Belloc and L. Breslow, *Prev. Med.* 1, 409 (1972).

28. ———, *ibid.* 2, 67 (1973).

29. L. Eisenberg, *N. Engl. J. Med.* 296, 903 (1977).

30. A. Kleinman, L. Eisenberg, B. Good, *Ann. Intern. Med.* 88, 251 (1978).

31. D. D. Rutstein, *Daedalus* 98, 523 (1969).

32. L. Eisenberg, *J. Child Psychol. Psychiatr.* 16, 93 (1975).

33. R. Titmuss, *The Gift Relationship: From Human Blood to Social Policy* (Pantheon, New York, 1971).

34. H. M. Sapolsky and S. N. Finkelstein, *Public Interest* (Winter 1977), p. 15.

35. I. Illich, *Medical Nemesis: The Expropriation of Health* (Calder & Boyars, London, 1975).

36. T. McKeown, *The Role of Medicine: Dream, Mirage or Nemesis?* (Nuffield Provincial Hospitals Trust, London, 1976).

37. W. McDermott, *Daedalus* 106, 135 (1977).

38. L. Eisenberg, in *Research and Medical Practice* (Ciba Foundation Symposium 44, Elsevier/Excerpta Medica/North-Holland, Amsterdam, 1976), pp. 3–23.

39. A. Barr and R. F. L. Logan, *Lancet* 1977-I, 994 (1977).

40. D. P. Forster, *ibid.*, p. 997.

41. B. R. Bloom, *Hastings Center Rep.* 6, 9 (1976).

42. L. Eisenberg, *J. Med. Philos.* 1, 318 (1976).

43. R. Vallery-Radot, *The Life of Pasteur* (Doubleday, Page, Garden City, N.Y., 1923), p. 444.

HANS JONAS

Philosophical Reflections on Experimenting with Human Subjects

Experimenting with human subjects is going on in many fields of scientific and technological progress. It is designed to replace the overall instruction by natural, occasional experience with the selective information from artificial, systematic experiment which physical science has found so effective in dealing with inanimate nature. Of the new experimentation with man, medical is surely the most legitimate; psychological, the most dubious; biological (still to come),

Reprinted with permission of George Braziller, Inc. from *Experimentation with Human Subjects* by Paul A. Freund (ed.). Copyright © 1969, 1970 by the American Academy of Arts and Sciences. This essay is included, on pp. 105–131, in a 1980 reedition of Jonas's *Philosophical Essays: From Current Creed to Technological Man*, published by the University of Chicago Press.

the most dangerous. I have chosen here to deal with the first only, where the case *for* it is strongest and the task of adjudicating conflicting claims hardest. . . .

THE PECULIARITY OF HUMAN EXPERIMENTATION

Experimentation was originally sanctioned by natural science. There it is performed on inanimate objects, and this raises no moral problems. But as soon as animate, feeling beings become the subjects of experiment, as they do in the life sciences and especially in medical research, this innocence of the search for knowledge is lost and questions of conscience arise. The depth to which moral and religious sensibilities can become aroused over these questions is shown by the vivisection issue. Human experimentation must sharpen the issue as it involves ultimate questions of personal dignity and sacrosanctity. One profound difference between the human experiment and the physical (besides that between animate and inanimate, feeling and unfeeling nature) is this: The physical experiment employs small-scale, artificially devised substitutes for that about which knowledge is to be obtained, and the experimenter extrapolates from these models and simulated conditions to nature at large. Something deputizes for the "real thing"—balls rolling down an inclined plane for sun and planets, electric discharges from a condenser for real lightning, and so on. For the most part, no such substitution is possible in the biological sphere. We must operate on the original itself, the real thing in the fullest sense, and perhaps affect it irreversibly. No simulacrum can take its place. Especially in the human sphere, experimentation loses entirely the advantage of the clear division between vicarious model and true object. Up to a point, animals may fulfill the proxy role of the classical physical experiment. But in the end man himself must furnish knowledge about himself, and the comfortable separation of noncommittal experiment and definitive action vanishes. An experiment in education affects the lives of its subjects, perhaps a whole generation of schoolchildren. Human experimentation for whatever purpose is always *also* a responsible, nonexperimental, definitive dealing with the subject himself. And not even the noblest purpose abrogates the obligations this involves.

This is the root of the problem with which we are faced: Can both that purpose and this obligation be satisfied? If not, what would be a just compromise? Which side should give way to the other? The question is inherently philosophical as it concerns not merely pragmatic difficulties and their arbitration, but a genuine conflict of values involving principles of a high order. May I put conflict in these terms. On principle, it is felt, human beings *ought* not to be dealt with in that way (the "guinea pig" protest); on the other hand, such dealings are increasingly urged on us by considerations, in turn appealing to principle, that claim to override those objections. Such a claim must be carefully assessed, especially when it is swept along by a mighty tide. Putting the matter thus, we have already made one important assumption rooted in our "Western" cultural tradition: The prohibitive rule is, to that way of thinking, the primary and axiomatic one; the permissive counter-rule, as qualifying the first, is sec-

ondary and stands in need of justification. We must justify the infringement of a primary inviolability, which needs no justification itself; and the justification of its infringement must be by values and needs of a dignity commensurate with those to be sacrificed.

•   •   •

HEALTH AS A PUBLIC GOOD

The cause invoked [for medical experimentation] is health and, in its more critical aspect, life itself—clearly superlative goods that the physician serves directly by curing and the researcher indirectly by the knowledge gained through his experiments. There is no question about the good served or about the evil fought—disease and premature death. But a good to whom and an evil to whom? Here the issue tends to become somewhat clouded. In the attempt to give experimentation the proper dignity (on the problematic view that a value becomes greater by being "social" instead of merely individual), the health in question or the disease in question is somehow predicated on the social whole, as if it were society that, in the persons of its members, enjoyed the one and suffered the other. For the purposes of our problem, public interest can then be pitted against private interest, the common good against the individual good. Indeed, I have found health called a national resource, which, of course it is, but surely not in the first place.

In trying to resolve some of the complexities and ambiguities lurking in these conceptualizations, I have pondered a particular statement, made in the form of a question, which I found in the *Proceedings* of the earlier *Daedalus* conference: "Can society afford to discard the tissues and organs of the hopelessly unconscious patient when they could be used to restore the otherwise hopelessly ill, but still salvageable individual?" And somewhat later: "A strong case can be made that society can ill afford to discard the tissues and organs of the hopelessly unconscious patient; they are greatly needed for study and experimental trial to help those who can be salvaged."[1] I hasten to add that any suspicion of callousness that the "commodity" language of these statements may suggest is immediately dispelled by the name of the speaker, Dr. Henry K. Beecher, for whose humanity and moral sensibility there can be nothing but admiration. But the use, in all innocence, of this language gives food for thought. Let me, for a moment, take the question literally. "Discarding" implies proprietary rights—nobody can discard what does not belong to him in the first place. Does society then own my body? "Salvaging" implies the same and, moreover, a use-value to the owner. Is the life-extension of certain individuals then a public interest? "Affording" implies a critically vital level of such an interest—that is, of the loss or gain involved. And "society" itself—what is it? When does a need, an aim, an obligation become social? Let us reflect on some of these terms.

WHAT SOCIETY CAN AFFORD

"Can Society afford . . .?" Afford what? To let people die intact, thereby withholding something from other people who desperately need it, who in consequence will have to die too? These other, unfortunate people indeed cannot afford not to have a kidney, heart, or other organ of the dying patient, on which they depend for an extension of their lease on life; but does that give them a right to it? And does it oblige society to procure it for them? What is it that *society* can or cannot afford—leaving aside for the moment the question of what it has a *right* to? It surely can afford to lose members through death; more than that, it is built on the balance of death and birth decreed by the order of life. This is too general, of course, for our question, but perhaps it is well to remember. The specific question seems to be whether society can afford to let some people die whose death might be deferred by particular means if these were authorized by society. Again, if it is merely a question of what society can or cannot afford, rather than of what it ought or ought not to do, the answer must be: Of course, it can. If cancer, heart disease, and other organic, noncontagious ills, especially those tending to strike the old more than the young, continue to exact their toll at the normal rate of incidence (including the toll of private anguish and misery), society can go on flourishing in every way.

Here, by contrast, are some examples of what, in sober truth, society cannot afford. It cannot afford to let an epidemic rage unchecked; a persistent excess of deaths over births, but neither—we must add—too great an excess of births over deaths; too low an average life expectancy even if demographically balanced by fertility, but neither too great a longevity with the necessitated correlative dearth of youth in the social body; a debilitating state of general health; and things

of this kind. These are plain cases where the whole condition of society is critically affected, and the public interest can make its imperative claims. The Black Death of the Middle Ages was a *public* calamity of the acute kind; the life-sapping ravages of endemic malaria or sleeping sickness in certain areas are a public calamity of the chronic kind. Such situations a society as a whole can truly not "afford," and they may call for extraordinary remedies, including, perhaps, the invasion of private sacrosanctities.

This is not entirely a matter of numbers and numerical ratios. Society, in a subtler sense, cannot "afford" a single miscarriage of justice, a single inequity in the dispensation of its laws, the violation of the rights of even the tiniest minority, because these undermine the moral basis on which society's existence rests. Nor can it, for a similar reason, afford the absence or atrophy in its midst of compassion and of the effort to alleviate suffering—be it widespread or rare—one form of which is the effort to conquer disease of any kind, whether "socially" significant (by reason of number) or not. And in short, society cannot afford the absence among its members of *virtue*, with its readiness for sacrifice beyond defined duty. Since its presence—that is to say, that of personal idealism—is a matter of grace and not of decree, we have the paradox that society depends for its existence on intangibles of nothing less than a religious order, for which it can hope, but which it cannot enforce. All the more must it protect this most precious capital from abuse.

For what objectives connected with the medicobiological sphere should this reserve be drawn upon—for example, in the form of accepting, soliciting, perhaps even imposing the submission of human subjects to experimentation? We postulate that this must be not just a worthy cause, as any promotion of the health of anybody doubtlessly is, but a cause qualifying for transcendent social sanction. Here one thinks first of those cases critically affecting the whole condition, present and future, of the community we have illustrated. Something equivalent to what in the political sphere is called "clear and present danger" may be invoked and a state of emergency proclaimed, thereby suspending certain otherwise inviolable prohibitions and taboos. We may observe that averting a disaster always carries greater weight than promoting a good. Extraordinary danger excuses extraordinary means. This covers human experimentation, which we would like to count, as far as possible, among the extraordinary rather than the ordinary means of serving the common good under public auspices. Naturally, since foresight and responsibility for the future are of the essence of institutional society, averting disaster extends into long-term prevention, although the lesser urgency will warrant less sweeping licenses.

SOCIETY AND THE CAUSE OF PROGRESS

Much weaker is the case where it is a matter not of saving but of improving society. Much of medical research falls into this category. As stated before, a permanent death rate from heart failure or cancer does not threaten society. So long as certain statistical ratios are maintained, the incidence of disease and of disease-induced mortality is not (in the strict sense) a "social" misfortune. I hasten to add that it is not therefore less of a human misfortune, and the call for relief issuing with silent eloquence from each victim and all potential victims is of no lesser dignity. But it is misleading to equate the fundamentally human response to it with what is owed to society: it is owed by man to man—and it is thereby owed by society to the individuals as soon as the adequate ministering to these concerns outgrows (as it progressively does) the scope of private spontaneity and is made a public mandate. It is thus that society assumes responsibility for medical care, research, old age, and innumerable other things not originally of the public realm (in the original "social contract"), and they become duties toward "society" (rather than directly toward one's fellow man) by the fact that they are socially operated.

Indeed, we expect from organized society no longer mere protection against harm and the securing of the conditions of our preservation, but active and constant improvement in all the domains of life: the waging of the battle against nature, the enhancement of the human estate—in short, the promotion of progress. This is an expansive goal, one far surpassing the disaster norm of our previous reflections. It lacks the urgency of the latter, but has the nobility of the free, forward thrust. It surely is worth sacrifices. It is not at all a question of what society can afford, but of what it is committed to, beyond all necessity, by our mandate. Its trusteeship has become an established, ongoing, institutionalized business of the body politic. As eager beneficiaries of its gains, we now owe to "society," as its chief agent, our individual contributions toward its *continued pursuit*. I emphasize "continued pursuit." Maintaining the existing level requires no more than the orthodox means of taxation and enforcement of professional standards that raise no problems. The

more optional goal of pushing forward is also more exacting. We have this syndrome: Progress is by our choosing an acknowledged interest of society, in which we have a stake in various degrees; science is a necessary instrument of progress; research is a necessary instrument of science; and in medical science experimentation on human subjects is a necessary instrument of research. Therefore, human experimentation has come to be a societal interest.

The destination of research is essentially melioristic. It does not serve the preservation of the existing good from which I profit myself and to which I am obligated. Unless the present state is intolerable, the melioristic goal is in a sense gratuitous, and this not only from the vantage point of the present. Our descendants have a right to be left an unplundered planet; they do not have a right to new miracle cures. We have sinned against them, if by our doing we have destroyed their inheritance—which we are doing at full blast; we have not sinned against them if by the time they come around arthritis has not yet been conquered (unless by sheer neglect). And generally, in the matter of progress, as humanity had no claim on a Newton, a Michelangelo, or a St. Francis to appear, and no right to the blessings of their unscheduled deeds, so progress, with all our methodical labor for it, cannot be budgeted in advance and its fruits received as a due. Its coming-about at all and its turning out for good (of which we can never be sure) must rather be regarded as something akin to grace.

THE MELIORISTIC GOAL, MEDICAL RESEARCH, AND INDIVIDUAL DUTY

Nowhere is the melioristic goal more inherent than in medicine. To the physician, it is not gratuitous. He is committed to curing and thus to improving the power to cure. Gratuitous we called it (outside disaster conditions) as a *social* goal, but noble at the same time. Both the nobility and the gratuitousness must influence the manner in which self-sacrifice for it is elicited, and even its free offer accepted. Freedom is certainly the first condition to be observed here. The surrender of one's body to medical experimentation is entirely outside the enforceable "social contract."

Or can it be construed to fall within its terms—namely, as repayment for benefits from past experimentation that I have enjoyed myself? But I am indebted for these benefits not to society, but to the past "martyrs," to whom society is indebted itself, and society has no right to call in my personal debt by way of adding new to its own. Moreover, gratitude is not an enforceable social obligation; it anyway does not mean that I must emulate the deed. Most of all, if it was wrong to exact such sacrifice in the first place, it does not become right to exact it again with the plea of the profit it has brought me. If, however, it was not exacted, but entirely free, as it ought to have been, then it should remain so, and its precedence must not be used as a social pressure on others for doing the same under the sign of duty.

• • •

THE "CONSCRIPTION" OF CONSENT

. . . The mere issuing of the appeal, the calling for volunteers, with the moral and social pressures it inevitably generates, amounts even under the most meticulous rules of consent to a sort of *conscripting*. And some soliciting is necessarily involved. . . . And this is why "consent," surely a nonnegotiable minimum requirement, is not the full answer to the problem. Granting then that soliciting and therefore some degree of conscripting are part of the situation, who may conscript and who may be conscripted? Or less harshly expressed: Who should issue appeals and to whom?

The naturally qualified issuer of the appeal is the research scientist himself, collectively the main carrier of the impulse and the only one with the technical competence to judge. But his being very much an interested party (with vested interests, indeed, not purely in the public good, but in the scientific enterprise as such, in "his" project, and even in his career) makes him also suspect. The ineradicable dialectic of this situation—a delicate incompatibility problem—calls for particular controls by the research community and by public authority that we need not discuss. They can mitigate, but not eliminate the problem. We have to live with the ambiguity, the treacherous impurity of everything human.

SELF-RECRUITMENT OF THE COMMUNITY

To whom should the appeal be addressed? The natural issuer of the call is also the first natural addressee: the physician-researcher himself and the scientific confraternity at large. With such a coincidence—indeed, the noble tradition with which the whole business of human experimentation started—almost all of the associated legal, ethical, and metaphysical problems vanish. If it is full, autonomous identification of the subject with the purpose that is required for the dignifying of his serving as a subject—here it is; if strongest motivation—here it is; if fullest understanding—here it is; if freest decision—here it is; if greatest integration with the person's total, chosen pursuit—here it is. With the fact of self-solicitation the issue of consent in all its insoluble equivocality is bypassed per se. Not even the condition that the particular purpose be truly important and the project reasonably promising, which must hold in any solicitation of others, need be satisfied here. By himself, the scientist is free to obey his obsession, to play his hunch, to wager on chance, to follow the lure of ambition. It is all part of the "divine madness" that somehow animates the ceaseless pressing against frontiers. For the rest of society, which has a deep-seated disposition to look with reverence and awe upon the guardians of the mysteries of life, the profession assumes with this proof of its devotion the role of a self-chosen, consecrated fraternity, not unlike the monastic orders of the past, and this would come nearest to the actual, religious origins of the art of healing.

• • •

"IDENTIFICATION" AS THE PRINCIPLE OF RECRUITMENT IN GENERAL

If the properties we adduced as the particular qualifications of the members of the scientific fraternity itself are taken as general criteria of selection, then one should look for additional subjects where a maximum of identification, understanding, and spontaneity can be expected—that is, among the most highly motivated, the most highly educated, and the least "captive" members of the community. From this naturally scarce resource, a descending order of permissibility leads to greater abundance and ease of supply, whose use should become proportionately more hesitant as the exculpating criteria are relaxed. An inversion of normal "market" behavior is demanded here—namely, to accept the lowest quotation last (and excused only by the greatest pressure of need); to pay the highest price first.

The ruling principle in our considerations is that the "wrong" of reification can only be made "right" by such authentic identification with the cause that it is the subject's as well as the researcher's cause—whereby his role in its service is not just permitted by him, but *willed*. That sovereign will of his which embraces the end as his own restores his personhood to the otherwise depersonalizing context. To be valid it must be autonomous and informed. The latter condition can, outside the research community, only be fulfilled by degrees; but the higher the degree of the understanding regarding the purpose and the technique, the more valid becomes the endorsement of the will. A margin of mere trust inevitably remains. Ultimately, the appeal for volunteers should seek this free and generous endorsement, the appropriation of the research purpose into the person's own scheme of ends. Thus, the appeal is in truth addressed to the one, mysterious, and sacred source of any such generosity of the will—"devotion," whose forms and objects of commitment are various and may invest different motivations in different individuals. The following, for instance, may be responsive to the "call" we are discussing: compassion with human suffering, zeal for humanity, reverence for the Golden Rule, enthusiasm for progress, homage to the cause of knowledge, even longing for sacrificial justification (do not call that "masochism," please). On all these, I say, it is defensible and right to draw when the research objective is worthy enough; and it is a prime duty of the research community (especially in view of what we called the "margin of trust") to see that this sacred source is never abused for frivolous ends. For a less than adequate cause, not even the freest, unsolicited offer should be accepted.

THE RULE OF THE "DESCENDING ORDER" AND ITS COUNTERUTILITY SENSE

We have laid down what must seem to be a forbidding rule to the number-hungry research industry. Having faith in the transcendent potential of man, I do not fear that the "source" will ever fail a society that does not destroy it—and only such a one is worthy of the blessings of progress. But "elitistic" the rule is (as is the enterprise of progress itself), and elites are by nature small. The combined attribute of motivation and information, plus the absence of external pressures, tends to be socially so circumscribed that strict adherence to the rule might numerically starve the research process. This is why I spoke of a descending order of permissibility, which is itself permissive, but where the realization that it is a *descending* order is not without pragmatic import. Departing from the august norm, the appeal must needs shift from idealism to docility, from high-mindedness to compliance, from judgment to trust. Consent spreads over the whole

spectrum. I will not go into the casuistics of this penumbral area. I merely indicate the principle of the order of preference: The poorer in knowledge, motivation, and freedom of decision (and that, alas, means the more readily available in terms of numbers and possible manipulation), the more sparingly and indeed reluctantly should the reservoir be used, and the more compelling must therefore become the countervailing justification.

Let us note that this is the opposite of a social utility standard, the reverse of the order by "availability and expendability": The most valuable and scarcest, the least expendable elements of the social organism, are to be the first candidates for risk and sacrifice. It is the standard of *noblesse oblige*; and with all its counter-utility and seeming "wastefulness," we feel a rightness about it and perhaps even a higher "utility," for the soul of the community lives by this spirit.[2] It is also the opposite of what the day-to-day interests of research clamor for, and for the scientific community to honor it will mean that it will have to fight a strong temptation to go by routine to the readiest sources of supply—the suggestible, the ignorant, the dependent, the "captive" in various senses.[3] I do not believe that heightened resistance here must cripple research, which cannot be permitted; but it may indeed slow it down by the smaller numbers fed into experimentation in consequence. This price—a possibly slower rate of progress—may have to be paid for the preservation of the most precious capital of higher communal life.

EXPERIMENTATION ON PATIENTS

So far we have been speaking on the tacit assumption that the subjects of experimentation are recruited from among the healthy. To the question "Who is conscriptable?" the spontaneous answer is: Least and last of all the sick—the most available of all as they are under treatment and observation anyway. That the afflicted should not be called upon to bear additional burden and risk, that they are society's special trust and the physician's trust in particular—these are elementary responses of our moral sense. Yet the very destination of medical research, the conquest of disease, requires at the crucial stage trial and verification on precisely the sufferers from the disease, and their total exemption would defeat the purpose itself. In acknowledging this inescapable necessity, we enter the most sensitive area of the whole complex, the one most keenly felt and most searchingly discussed by the practitioners themselves. No wonder, it touches the heart of the doctor-patient relation, putting its most solemn obligations to the test. There is nothing new in what I have to say about the ethics of the doctor-patient relation, but for the purpose of confronting it with the issue of experimentation some of the oldest verities must be recalled.

THE FUNDAMENTAL PRIVILEGE OF THE SICK

In the course of treatment, the physician is obligated to the patient and to no one else. He is not the agent of society, nor of the interests of medical science, nor of the patient's family, nor of his co-sufferers, nor of future sufferers from the same disease. The patient alone counts when he is under the physician's care. By the simple law of bilateral contract (analogous, for example, to the relation of lawyer to client and its "conflict of interest" rule), the physician is bound not to let any other interest interfere with that of the patient in being cured. But manifestly more sublime norms than contractual ones are involved. We may speak of a sacred trust; strictly by its terms, the doctor is, as it were, alone with his patient and God.

There is one normal exception to this—that is, to the doctor's not being the agent of society vis-à-vis the patient, but the trustee of his interests alone: the quarantining of the contagious sick. This is plainly not for the patient's interest, but for that of others threatened by him. (In vaccination, we have a combination of both: protection of the individual and others.) But preventing the patient from causing harm to others is not the same as exploiting him for the advantage of others. And there is, of course, the abnormal exception of collective catastrophe, the analogue to a state of war. The physician who desperately battles a raging epidemic is under a unique dispensation that suspends in a nonspecifiable way some of the structures of normal practice, including possibly those against experimental liberties with his patients. No rules can be devised for the waiving of rules in extremities. And as with the famous shipwreck examples of ethical theory, the less said about it the better. But what is allowable there and may later be passed over in forgiving silence cannot serve as a precedent. We are concerned with non-extreme, non-emergency conditions where the voice of principle can be heard and claims can be adjudicated free from duress. We have conceded that there are such claims, and that if there is to be medical advance at all, not even the superlative privilege of the suffering and the sick can be kept wholly intact from the intrusion of its needs. About this least palatable, most disquieting part of our subject, I have to offer only groping, inconclusive remarks.

THE PRINCIPLE OF "IDENTIFICATION" APPLIED TO PATIENTS

On the whole, the same principles would seem to hold here as are found to hold with "normal subjects": motivation, identification, understanding on the part of the subject. But it is clear that these conditions are peculiarly difficult to satisfy with regard to a patient. His physical state, psychic preoccupation, dependent relation to the doctor, the submissive attitude induced by treatment—everything connected with his condition and situation makes the sick person inherently less of a sovereign person than the healthy one. Spontaneity of self-offering has almost to be ruled out; consent is marred by lower resistance or captive circumstance, and so on. In fact, all the factors that make the patient, as a category, particularly accessible and welcome for experimentation at the same time compromise the quality of the responding affirmation that must morally redeem the making use of them. This, in addition to the primacy of the physician's duty, puts a heightened onus on the physician-researcher to limit his undue power to the most important and defensible research objectives and, of course, to keep persuasion at a minimum.

Still, with all the disabilities noted, there is scope among patients for observing the rule of the "descending order of permissibility" that we have laid down for normal subjects, in vexing inversion of the utility order of quantitative abundance and qualitative "expendability." By the principle of this order, those patients who most identify with and are cognizant of the cause of research—members of the medical profession (who after all are sometimes patients themselves)—come first; the highly motivated and educated, also least dependent, among the lay patients come next; and so on down the line. An added consideration here is seriousness of condition, which again operates in inverse proportion. Here the profession must fight the tempting sophistry that the hopeless case is expendable (because in prospect already expended) and therefore especially usable; and generally the attitude that the poorer the chances of the patient, the more justifiable his recruitment for experimentation (other than for his own benefit). The opposite is true.

Then there is the case where ignorance of the subject, sometimes even of the experimenter, is of the essence of the experiment (the "double blind"-control group-placebo syndrome). It is said to be a necessary element of the scientific process. Whatever may be said about its ethics in regard to normal subjects, especially volunteers, it is an outright betrayal of trust in regard to the patient who believes that he is receiving treatment. Only supreme importance of the objective can exonerate it, without making it less of a transgression. The patient is definitely wronged even when not harmed. And ethics apart, the practice of such deception holds the danger of undermining the faith in the *bona fides* of treatment, the beneficial intent of the physician—the very basis of the doctor-patient relationship. In every respect, it follows that concealed experiment on patients—that is, experiment under the guise of treatment—should be the rarest exception, at best, if it cannot be wholly avoided.

This has still the merit of a borderline problem. The same is not true of the other case of necessary ignorance of the subject—that of the unconscious patient. Drafting him for nontherapeutic experiments is simply and unqualifiedly impermissible; progress or not, he must never be used, on the inflexible principle that utter helplessness demands utter protection.

When preparing this paper, I filled pages with a casuistics of this harrowing field, but then scrapped most of it, realizing my dilettante status. The shadings are endless, and only the physician-researcher can discern them properly as the cases arise. Into his lap the decision is thrown. The philosophical rule, once it has admitted into itself the idea of a sliding scale, cannot really specify its own application. It can only impress on the practitioner a general maxim or attitude for the exercise of his judgment and conscience in the concrete occasions of his work. In our case, I am afraid, it means making life more difficult for him.

It will also be noted that, somewhat at variance with the emphasis in the literature, I have not dwelt on the element of "risk" and very little on that of "consent." Discussion of the first is beyond the layman's competence; the emphasis on the second has been lessened because of its equivocal character. It is a truism to say that one should strive to minimize the risk and to maximize the consent. The more demanding concept of "identification," which I have used, includes "consent" in its maximal or authentic form, and the assumption of risk is its privilege.

NO EXPERIMENTS ON PATIENTS UNRELATED TO THEIR OWN DISEASE

Although my ponderings have, on the whole, yielded points of view rather than definite prescriptions, premises rather than conclusions, they have led me to a few unequivocal yeses and noes. The first is the emphatic rule that patients should be experimented upon, if at all, *only* with reference to *their disease*. Never should there be added to the gratuitousness of the experiment as such the gratuitousness of service to an unrelated cause. This follows simply from what we have found to be the *only* excuse for infracting the special exemption of the sick at all—namely, that the scientific war on disease cannot accomplish its goal without drawing the sufferers from disease into the investigative process. If under this excuse they become subjects of experiment, they do so *because*, and only because, of *their* disease.

This is the fundamental and self-sufficient consideration. That the patient cannot possibly benefit from the unrelated experiment therapeutically, while he might from experiment related to his condition, is also true, but lies beyond the problem area of pure experiment. I am in any case discussing nontherapeutic experimentation only, where *ex hypothesi* the patient does not benefit. Experiment as part of therapy—that is, directed toward helping the subject himself—is a different matter altogether and raises its own problems but hardly philosophical ones. As long as a doctor can say, even if only in his own thought: "There is no known cure for your condition (or: You have responded to none); but there is promise in a new treatment still under investigation, not quite tested yet as to effectiveness and safety; you will be taking a chance, but all things considered, I judge it in your best interest to let me try it on you"—as long as he can speak thus, he speaks as the patient's physician and may err, but does not transform the patient into a subject of experimentation. Introduction of an untried therapy into the treatment where the tried ones have failed is not "experimentation on the patient."

Generally, and almost needless to say, with all the rules of the book, there is something "experimental" (because tentative) about every individual treatment, beginning with the diagnosis itself; and he would be a poor doctor who would not learn from every case for the benefit of future cases, and a poor member of the profession who would not make any new insights gained from his treatments available to the profession at large. Thus, knowledge may be advanced in the treatment of any patient, and the interest of the medical art and all sufferers from the same affliction as well as the patient himself may be served if something happens to be learned from his case. But his gain to knowledge and future therapy is incidental to the *bona fide* service to the present patient. He has the right to expect that the doctor does nothing to him just in order to learn.

In that case, the doctor's imaginary speech would run, for instance, like this: "There is nothing more I can do for you. But you can do something for me. Speaking no longer as your physician but on behalf of medical science, we could learn a great deal about future cases of this kind if you would permit me to perform certain experiments on you. It is understood that you yourself would not benefit from any knowledge we might gain; but future patients would." This statement would express the purely experimental situation, assumedly here with the subject's concurrence and with all cards on the table. In Alexander Bickel's words: "It is a different situation when the doctor is no longer trying to make [the patient] well, but is trying to find out how to make others well in the future."[4]

But even in the second case, that of the nontherapeutic experiment where the patient does not benefit, at least the patient's own disease is enlisted in the cause of fighting that disease, even if only in others. It is yet another thing to say or think: "Since you are here—in the hospital with its facilities—anyway, under our care and observation anyway, away from your job (or, perhaps, doomed) anyway, we wish to profit from your being available for some other research of great interest we are presently engaged in." From the standpoint of merely medical ethics, which has only to consider risk, consent, and the worth of the objective, there may be no cardinal difference between this case and the last one. I hope that the medical reader will not think I am making too fine a point when I say that from the standpoint of the subject and his dignity there is a cardinal difference that crosses the line between the permissible and the impermissible, and this by the same principle of "identification" I have been invoking all along. Whatever the rights and wrongs of any experimentation on any patient—in the one case, at least that residue of identification is left him that it is his own affliction by which he can contribute to the conquest of that affliction, his own kind of suffering which he helps to alleviate in others; and so in a sense it is his own cause. It is totally indefensible to rob the unfortunate of this intimacy with the purpose and make his misfortune a convenience for the furtherance of alien concerns.

• • •

CONCLUSION

. . . I wish only to say in conclusion that if some of the practical implications of my reasonings are felt to work out toward a slower rate of progress, this should not cause too great dismay. Let us not forget that progress is an optional goal, not an unconditional commitment, and that its tempo in particular, compulsive as it may become, has nothing sacred about it. Let us also remember that a slower progress in the conquest of disease would not threaten society, grievous as it is to those who have to deplore that their particular disease be not yet conquered, but that society would indeed be threatened by the erosion of those moral values whose loss, possibly caused by too ruthless a pursuit of scientific progress, would make its most dazzling triumphs not worth having. Let us finally remember that it cannot be the aim of progress to abolish the lot of mortality. Of some ill or other, each of us will die. Our mortal condition is upon us with its harshness but also its wisdom—because without it there would not be the eternally renewed promise of the freshness, immediacy, and eagerness of youth; nor would there be for any of us the incentive to number our days and make them count. With all our striving to wrest from our mortality what we can, we should bear its burden with patience and dignity.

NOTES

1. *Proceedings of the Conference on the Ethical Aspects of Experimentation on Human Subjects*, November 3–4, 1967 (Boston, Massachusetts; hereafter called *Proceedings*), pp. 50–51.

2. Socially, everyone is expendable relatively—that is, in different degrees; religiously, no one is expendable absolutely: The "image of God" is in all. If it can be enhanced, then it is not by anyone being expended, but by someone expending himself.

3. This refers to captives of circumstance, not of justice. Prison inmates are, with respect to our problem, in a special class. If we hold to some idea of guilt, and to the supposition that our judicial system is not entirely at fault, they may be held to stand in a special debt to society, and their offer to serve—from whatever motive—may be accepted with a minimum of qualms as a means of reparation.

4. *Proceedings*, p. 33.

ARTHUR SCHAFER

The Ethics of the Randomized Clinical Trial

The ethics of medical experimentation on human subjects has attracted much attention in recent years. There has, however, been rather less attention paid to the special ethical problems and dilemmas posed by the randomized clinical trial.

The sheer number of such trials, the risks and costs that they involve, and the dangers that are posed both by permitting and by restricting their use would seem to warrant further ethical analysis of the randomized clinical trial.

This article attempts to distinguish some of the major ethical problems posed by the randomized clinical trial, to set out some of the principal considerations that militate in favor of and against permitting such trials, and to suggest some tentative ethical criteria for medical researchers involved with them.

THE AMBIGUITIES OF MEDICAL EXPERIMENTATION

There is a sense of the term "experimentation" in which it would be true to say that physicians have been experimenting on their patients since time immemorial. From earliest times, when a patient has presented unusual symptoms or a condition that fails to respond to conventional treatment, doctors have experimented with new therapies. This ad hoc, empirical approach to medical knowledge—trying out new treatments and procedures and then carefully observing the results—was the dominant method in Western medical science until well into the present century. Physicians were able to learn from their patients while they were treating them, with little or no conflict of values and obligations.

Reprinted by permission of the *New England Journal of Medicine*. Originally published in *NEJM* 307 (September 16, 1982), 719–724.

There are medical scientists who appear to believe that nothing has changed notably with the introduction of the randomized clinical trial:

Medical experimentation on human beings, in its broadest meaning and for the good of the individual patient, takes place continually in every doctor's office. Hence the general question of human experimentation is one of degrees rather than of kind. Deliberate experimentation on a group of cases with adequate controls rather than on individual patients is merely an efficient and convenient means of collecting and interpreting data that would otherwise be dispersed and inaccessible.[1]

Against this claim, I would contend that modern clinical investigation is an altogether different sort of enterprise from the medical experimentation of previous times. What is now referred to as medical experimentation involves the designing of procedures that systematically manipulate subjects, and the use of controls for the purpose of gaining knowledge.

The employment of properly controlled clinical trials in medical experimentation has been of vital importance in the progress of medical science. But this new form of experimentation has also generated some of our most difficult and perplexing moral dilemmas.

CONFLICT OF OBLIGATIONS

When a physician, responsible for the medical treatment of a particular patient and bound by a moral oath (typically, some contemporary version of the Hippocratic oath) to hold the interests of that person as paramount, enrolls the patient as an experimental subject in a clinical trial, the physician inevitably puts himself in the morally ambiguous position of having two distinct and potentially conflicting roles. In his traditional role of healer, the physician's commitment is exclusively to his patient. By contrast, in his modern role of scientific investigator, the physician engaged in medical research or experimentation has a commitment to promote the acquisition of scientific knowledge.

Since each of these roles—that of scientist on the one hand and personal physician on the other—defines itself by reference to a different primary purpose, the possibility of conflict is an ever-present danger.

One should note in passing that this is not, of course, the only conflict of obligations faced by the physician. The physician's obligation of confidentiality to his patient may conflict, for example, with his legal obligation to report gunshot wounds or certain infectious diseases. This example is but one of many possible value conflicts, all of which arise from the fact that the physician has a plurality of responsibilities—to society, to future generations, to the legal system (the state), and to his own career and self-interest—in addition to his obligation to his patients. These responsibilities and obligations will, on occasion, run afoul of each other and even when there is no outright conflict, there may be difficult tensions.

Having drawn a clear-cut distinction between therapy and experimentation, one must admit that in practice this distinction is often blurred by the large number of gradations between the experimental and the therapeutic ends of the spectrum. A good deal of research is carried out by physicians on subjects who are simultaneously patients—their own or those of some other doctor. In many cases the patient himself is intended to benefit directly from the experiment; that is part of its purpose, but not its whole purpose. One of the essential aims underlying so-called therapeutic experimentation is to contribute to medical knowledge. In pursuit of this objective, procedures may be undertaken that are not strictly necessary for the treatment or cure of a particular patient. Systems of treatment are chosen partly with a view to curing the patient and partly with a view to testing new procedures or comparing the efficacy of various established procedures. The patient who is also a research subject may thereby be exposed to added hazards, discomforts, or inconveniences. Despite these disadvantages, it will sometimes be to the direct and immediate benefit of a patient to become a research subject. For example, by agreeing to participate in an experiment, a patient may gain access to a new and promising drug that is being tried out in a limited way. Alternatively, or additionally, the patient may benefit indirectly by receiving especially careful

attention and care from an elite group of highly trained specialists.

The point that needs to be emphasized, however, is that regardless of whether a patient benefits from agreeing to become a research subject, the physician who attempts to combine the traditional role of healer with the modern role of scientist places himself in a situation that contains a potential conflict of values. His commitment can no longer be exclusively and unequivocally to promote the interests of his patient. He is fortunate indeed when his scientific and personal obligations overlap or coincide, but when they conflict, as they often must (for reasons explained below), serious ethical dilemmas must be faced and priorities assigned.

THE NEED TO SACRIFICE INDIVIDUALIZED TREATMENT

The first of the special moral problems raised by the randomized clinical trial is the potential conflict between the goals of therapy and the goals of experimentation. Although a patient who has been enrolled as a research subject in a randomized clinical trial may benefit from the therapeutic effects of the treatment being tested, the fact that the treatment cannot be entirely tailored to that patient's special needs seems to violate the physician's obligation of unqualified fidelity to his patient's health. Fried asks the key question in this regard: "[i]s it ever likely to be the case that in a complex medical situation the balance of harms and benefits discounted by their appropriate probabilities really does appear on the then available evidence to be in equipoise? Or even approximately enough in equipoise to make the argument go through?"[2]

The morally troubling doubt concerns the likelihood that physicians may be able to recruit a statistically significant number of volunteers for randomized clinical trials only by neglecting the particular circumstances of individual patients. When all the patient's circumstances, including his attitudes and value system, are brought into the equation, it seems doubtful that the risks and benefits of the treatment alternatives will often be in perfect (or even rough) equilibrium.

Consider for illustrative purposes the situation facing a woman with breast cancer who is being asked by her physician to participate in a randomized clinical trial designed to test the relative efficacy of radical as opposed to conservative mastectomy. It is likely that one would find considerable variations in the priorities assigned by the women involved to such factors as the prolongation of life and esthetic disfigurement. Some patients would have, as their overriding priority, the reduction of the risk of mortality. Others would opt as strongly for the procedure involving the least disfigurement. Still others would adopt intermediate positions, trading off risks and benefits or harms according to their concept of self and self-image.

Here is the dilemma: if the physician recommends that his patient enter a randomized clinical trial as a research subject without a detailed inquiry about whether this would be the best plan from the patient's point of view—taking all the patient's relevant attitudes and values into consideration—then the physician would seem to be guilty of sacrificing the interests of the patient to the interests of science or humanity. On the other hand, if the physician conducts such an inquiry, there is the risk of introducing bias into the selection of subjects or eliminating too many from the study.

There might seem to be a quick and easy solution to this dilemma. After all, it is the patient who must give informed consent to becoming a research subject. The physician's role is merely to explain the nature of the experiment and to offer a recommendation. The difficulty with this as a solution, however, is that it flies in the face of sociologic data indicating that patients generally rely heavily on the advice of their physicians with respect to value trade-offs.[3] This is especially the case when the patient is acutely ill. Such patients are typically in a weakened physical state, perhaps in pain or drugged, often emotionally upset, and likely to feel dependent on and submissive toward those charged with their care and treatment. This submissive deference can be easily exploited (consciously or unconsciously) by physicians who are engaged in scientific research and who solicit patients to participate in a research program. Although there may be no question of force, fraud, or deceit, the circumstances surrounding serious illness may be thought to constitute a kind of duress.

What are the implications of all this for the physician-researcher who wishes to recruit his (or a colleague's) patients for a randomized clinical trial? The physician's traditional obligation of unqualified fidelity to his patient's well-being may be somewhat compromised by his desire, as a clinical investigator, to enlist the cooperation of patients as participants in a randomized trial. Unless the trial includes an adequately large sample of research subjects, its scientific value will be undermined. But close attention to the individual circumstances, attitudes, and values of each patient-subject may create a major obstacle to the recruitment of such an adequate sample.

The moral question at issue, then, is this: When, if ever, is it morally justifiable to sacrifice the patient's right to completely individualized treatment for the benefit of scientific progress? The dilemma that must be confronted arises from the fact that the moral point of view requires that "therapeutic" measures be investigated thoroughly before they become widely used and, at the same time, places serious obstacles in the path of those who would carry out such investigations. To the extent that formal design is sacrificed to individually tailored treatment, scientific rigor will be lost. This course, too, has ethical costs: a therapeutic trial that is inconclusive owing to a poor design will yield questionable results, possible harm to future patients, and a need to repeat the entire experimental process with a new set of subjects and proper controls.

This point was made concisely by Sackett in the *Journal*:

The intervention trial of greatest benefit to patients satisfies three objectives: validity (its results are true), generalizability (its results are widely applicable), and efficiency (the trial is affordable and resources are left over for patient care and for other health research). The first objective, validity, has become a nonnegotiable demand; hence the ascendancy of the randomized trial.[4]

One clear tenet of what we might label "the ethics of design" is that by ensuring validity a properly designed experiment will protect us from a false conclusion of efficacy or failure.

Even here, however, there is a troubling dilemma, for our desire to avoid false conclusions of efficacy may come into conflict with a second desire: to provide the medical community with promising early results of uncontrolled clinical trials. By a happy coincidence, the same issue of the *Journal* cited above, in which scientific validity is declared by Sackett to be a "nonnegotiable demand," contains two letters on the same subject, one upholding and one challenging the position expressed by Sackett.

Hollenberg, Dzau, and Williams had published what they considered to be "promising" results of an initial, open, uncontrolled trial of a new therapy.[5] The ethics of conducting such uncontrolled studies and publishing the ensuing results was challenged by Sacks,

Kupfer, and Chalmers.[6] Sacks declared that the therapeutic study conducted by Dzau and his colleagues should not have been approved by an ethically vigilant human experimentation committee or carried out by ethically conscientious investigators, and that its results should not have been submitted for publication nor, once submitted, published.

The argument in support of these conclusions, briefly, is this: that without adequate controls, the results of such a study lack validity; that to report merely anecdotal experience from uncontrolled and unblinded studies is to risk seriously misleading other investigators and their patients about the effectiveness of a new drug for a life-threatening condition; that once investigators become convinced or persuaded, on scientifically invalid grounds, of the efficacy of a drug, they will then mistakenly consider themselves ethically bound to administer such a drug to their patients and will, accordingly, be unable to enroll their patients in a properly randomized trial; and finally, that when sick patients are placed at risk in the course of experimentation with new drugs, such risks cannot be justified unless rigorous scientific design ensures statistical validity.

Dzau and his colleagues rejected these conclusions, and counterposed an alternative set of values that may override a mechanical insistence on employing randomized clinical trials for all therapeutic research. Their argument can be summarized as follows. It is unethical to undertake the enormous cost and demands of a large, controlled clinical trial until one has collected "some preliminary evidence of efficacy"; moreover, it is impractical to carry out full-scale randomized clinical trials without such preliminary data because of the difficulty of recruiting patients in the absence of favorable preliminary indications; and, when preliminary uncontrolled trials produce dramatic evidence of therapeutic benefit, the medical community is entitled to receive notice of this evidence so that it can consider enrolling appropriate patients in subsequent controlled trials. From this it follows that it is not only ethically permissible but ethically mandatory that such uncontrolled studies be undertaken and that their results, at least in certain circumstances, be published.

I do not believe that this conflict of values can be easily resolved, but it can perhaps be reduced to some extent by the introduction of some additional restricting qualifications. The availability of resources will inevitably operate as a constraining factor, but every clinician is under an obligation to conduct therapeutic trials with as much statistical and methodologic rigor as possible. Patients who are invited to participate in clinical trials should be apprised (at least in some general manner) of the degree of rigor built into the experimental design. When an uncontrolled clinical trial produces results so dramatic and noteworthy that it is deemed essential to present preliminary data to the medical community, those who release such speculations are under a stringent obligation to issue clear and unmistakable warnings about the unproved status of their results. The advantages to the medical community of receiving such early notice must be set against the dangers that either the medical community itself or the general public (which is usually less sophisticated in these matters) may place unwarranted and potentially harmful constructions on the data.

One is faced here with the need for some kind of judicious balancing act. Broad guidelines appear to be more appropriate than rigid rules. Risks and benefits must be weighed and assessed on a case-by-case basis. Both the costs of undertaking scientifically ill-founded studies and the harm from publishing unreliable speculations are worryingly high. But any blanket prohibition against such research and publication would itself impose an unnecessarily high cost—namely, the loss of certain very considerable benefits, at least in some circumstances.

INFORMED CONSENT

Closely related to the foregoing is a moral problem, raised by randomized clinical trials, that involves the requirement of informed consent. The patient who is invited to become a research subject is clearly entitled to know that he is taking part in an experiment; and he has a right to know that he may decline to participate. He is clearly entitled to know also that the treatment used in his case is one whose efficacy has not yet been established. The issue becomes more problematic, however, when one asks whether the patient also always has a right to be informed that his therapy is being selected by a randomizing device.

There is some reason to fear that such full disclosure would be an insuperable obstacle to recruitment of volunteers in sufficient numbers and would thereby make it impossible to perform further randomized clinical trials. Since such trials are of great importance to medical advances, it might be contended by some researchers that when there is nothing to choose between the treatments, the patient-subject need not be informed of the method (randomization) by which his particular treatment will be chosen.

It is ethically unnecessary to disclose the fact of randomization, so the argument goes, so long as the patient knows everything a reasonable person would need to know to reach a decision. To resolve this issue one must decide whether the fact of randomization is "materially relevant." This is a requirement both of law and of morality. But how are we to interpret the requirement in this instance?

Every potential research subject is legally and morally entitled to undertake his own evaluation of the risks and benefits and to bring to bear his own attitudes and values in reaching a decision. He is entitled to have the opportunity to view himself and to be viewed by the investigator as a joint venturer or a partner in the enterprise, rather than as raw material. (Some physicians would insist that this should also be the norm, the paradigm, for the nonexperimental doctor-patient relationship.) Consent makes this relationship possible, and represents the duties of fidelity and loyalty owed to each other by research and subject.[7]

Of course, the moral legitimacy of an experiment requires more than simple consent. If a person agrees to become a research subject without first having been given adequate information in a form that he can understand, then he has not really had an opportunity to decide his own fate. He has been used as a guinea pig, treated as an object or thing, rather than as a person or co-adventurer.

Since the purpose of the doctrine of informed consent is to make meaningful the research subject's right to autonomy, the patient is entitled to receive all the information relating to his choice that will facilitate his deliberations. All risks potentially affecting the decision must be unmasked.

Those who favor withholding from patients the information that, once they become research subjects, their treatment will be chosen according to a randomizing formula rather than according to the individual judgment of their physician can argue that no disclosure is necessary because there is nothing material to disclose. So long as no "better treatment" is known—and this will be the case until the results from the experiment are in—the patient cannot legitimately complain. No material information has been withheld.

Against this view, I would argue that information is material and ought to be disclosed, even if it would not influence a reasonable person, when it is known that it would (or might) influence the potential subject. It seems likely that many patients would be influenced by knowing that selection of treatment was to be randomized. Indeed, it is because of the fear that many patients would be (unreasonably) influenced that some investigators would like to withhold the information. Whether or not it is rational for potential subjects to be influenced by such information (and I agree that it is not entirely rational), it is their right to have it. To withhold from the subject information relating to the process by which the treatment method is to be selected would be, in effect, to usurp the subject's right to autonomy. I conclude, therefore, that it is unethical to solicit consent from prospective subjects for a randomized clinical trial without informing them of the manner in which their treatment will be selected.

THE PROBLEM OF TREATMENT PREFERENCE

It is widely accepted that physicians have an ethical obligation to provide the best treatment available for their patients and that this obligation generally overrides such competing goals as the desire to promote scientific knowledge. The recruitment of patients as research subjects for randomized clinical trials is nevertheless held to be morally permissible because, before such trials are completed, we do not actually know which is the best treatment. Consequently, the randomized clinical trial is not inconsistent with the physician's duty to provide the best possible treatment for his patient.

There is, however, a difficulty with this line of reasoning. It is true that before scientific testing of various treatment alternatives is completed, physicians cannot know which is the best treatment for any given patient. But it is also true that most physicians will have from the outset some sort of treatment preference based on incomplete scientific evidence. Such a treatment preference (for conservative as opposed to radical mastectomy, let us say) on the part of the physician falls well short of knowledge and might even be labeled a bias or hunch. The point is, however, that physicians will seldom be truly indifferent to the alternatives being tested. If the physician informs the patient of an intuitive preference, is it likely that the patient will then consent to participate in a clinical trial in which, because of the randomized nature of treatment selection, he may receive a treatment different from the one preferred by the physician? Will the patient readily distinguish a merely intuitive preference on the part of the physician from a scientifically based preference? The fear harbored by many medical scientists is that once patients learn that the physician has a preference with respect to available treatments, they will decline to participate in any clinical trial in which an alternative treatment may be substituted. The adverse effects of such reactions on medical experimentation are potentially severe.

At this point in the argument, one may opt for any of several alternative ethical positions. One could, for example, reject the initial assumption that physicians have an absolute ethical obligation to provide the best treatment for their patients. One could, that is, invoke such competing values as the advancement of medical knowledge and the benefit of humanity (including future generations) to justify withholding from patients the information that their doctor has a treatment preference. In support of this position, it might be noted that for the many centuries before the advent of the randomized clinical trial, a period in which medical progress depended on ad hoc clinical judgments, medical interventions were typically inefficacious when they were not positively dangerous to the health of the patient. If a study of the history of medicine reveals anything, it reveals that clinical judgment without the check of scientific controls is a highly fallible compass.

A critic may object, however, that the utility of the randomized clinical trial is not really in dispute. One could readily concede that the preference of a physician, unsupported by adequate scientific evidence, is relatively unreliable, but one might nevertheless insist that patients are entitled to know of such preferences (accompanied by appropriate warnings as to their merely intuitive nature). For a physician to withhold such information would be to violate his patient's right to the best possible care. This is an important right, a fundamental part of the implied contract between doctor and patient. It would be quite wrong to violate it lightly. But this is not necessarily to confer on it an absolute status. There may be circumstances in which other, competing values are entitled to an even higher priority. The truly difficult task for society, in cooperation with medical scientists, is to identify such circumstances with sufficient care so that what should be an unusual and infrequent violation of a basic right does not expand to become a common and frequent occurrence.

Let us suppose that a physician has obtained consent from his patient to participate in a randomized clinical trial. The contract for experimentation is based, at least in part, on the patient's understanding that the physician has no present treatment preference. Let us further suppose, however, that as the early data from the trial become available for interpretation, a trend seems to be developing that favors one treatment over another. Is the physician then morally obligated to withdraw his patient from the trial? If not, is the physician morally obligated to convey this information to the patient so that the patient can choose whether to continue or to withdraw?

From the medical researchers' point of view, such withdrawals, if they were to become numerous, could well vitiate the scientific value of their work. The medical scientists might argue that it would often be scientifically inappropriate to rush to judgment on the basis of early data. Long-term as well as short-term effects may be important, and in any case, proper treatment decisions should not generally be based on a single clinical trial, however rigorous and well conducted. Moreover, such decisions should not generally be based on incomplete early data. Efficacy and safety can be adequately assessed only on the basis of a large body of data and only by those with proper scientific training. Again, the history of medicine provides us with innumerable cases of hasty judgments that were later modified or reversed in the light of subsequent studies and clinical experience.

The conclusion of this line of reasoning is that physicians should not, in general, withdraw their patients from clinical trials because of a treatment preference based on incomplete data, nor should they inform their patients that they have changed from being indifferent to the method of treatment to having a preference. Patients are not in a good position to assess the strength of the scientific evidence, and numerous patient withdrawals would have potentially disastrous effects on medical research.

One must, I think, concede the force and plausibility of this line of argument. But its conclusion is worrying. Can it really be proper for physicians to permit patients committed to their care to receive treatment that appears—on the basis of the available evidence—to be less than the best? What does this do to the physician's oath, "The health and life of my patients shall be my first consideration"?

Such a practice, if it were to become widespread, would represent an important shift from a patient-centered to a social-welfare-centered ethic. Perhaps such a shift is overdue and should be welcomed. Critics of the medical profession have been suggesting for some time that modern medicine is too individualistic. A wider social focus might be considered ethically preferable.

Those who would accept such a change of ethical orientation by the medical profession ought nevertheless to be concerned about the element of betrayal of trust that is involved. The implicit contract on which the doctor-patient relationship now rests commits doctors to place the highest priority on their patients' health and to provide patients with all the information they need to give informed consent. To sacrifice (or to risk sacrificing) the patient's best interests by withholding from him information that might well lead to his withdrawal from a randomized clinical trial violates that contract.

On the other hand, perhaps there are ways to avoid such a violation of trust. The patient could be informed from the outset that one of the ground rules of a particular randomized clinical trial required that the physician not act on trends emerging from incomplete data, not even to apprise the patient of such early results. The patient would then be in a position to take this into account in making the decision to become a research subject. Having been given this information, the patient would not be able to complain later that he had been duped or deceived. The advantages of participation in randomized clinical trials might still outweigh those of refusal, so the interests of science would be protected equally with the right of the patient to know where he stood.

CONCLUSION

In this discussion I have canvassed arguments relating to a number of ethical problems associated with randomized clinical trials. Several conclusions have emerged, albeit tentatively, from the discussion.

The physician who enlists his patient in a randomized trial faces at least the possibility of a conflict of obligations. In many cases the tension between the physician's traditional role as healer and his modern role as scientific investigator can be resolved without serious cost either to the patient or to science. In other cases, however, the tension may reach the level of outright contradiction. The Hippocratic principle of exclusive commitment to patient welfare, with its corollary of totally individualized treatment, may sometimes properly be modified so as to permit randomized clinical trials to proceed with a statistically significant sample of subjects. The circumstances in which it is ethically permissible to abrogate the Hippocratic principle are in need of careful definition.

It is generally unethical to solicit consent from prospective subjects for a randomized trial without telling them how their treatment will be selected. It may, in some circumstances, be ethically permissible for a physician to withhold the information that he has an intuitive treatment preference. But again, some carefully worked out criteria are needed to define when it is and when it is not appropriate to withhold such information from the potential research subject.

Finally, the physician whose judgment concerning competing treatments undergoes a change in the course of a randomized clinical trial may keep his patients in the trial and may withhold the interim adverse data from the patient, but only if the patient has given antecedent consent to such a procedure. Without the patient's consent, such a practice would constitute an unethical violation of the patient's rights and would risk undermining the trust on which the doctor-patient relationship rests.

NOTES

1. Shimkin MB. The problem of experimentation on human beings. I. The research worker's point of view. Science. 1953; 117:205–7.

2. Fried C. Medical experimentation: personal integrity and social policy. In: Bearn AG, Black DAK, Hiatt HH, eds. Clinical studies. Vol. 5. New York: Elsevier Press, 1974.

3. Gray BH. Human subjects in medical experimentation: a sociological study of the conduct and regulation of clinical research. New York: John Wiley, 1975.

4. Sackett DL. The competing objectives of randomized trials. N Engl J Med. 1980; 303:1059–60.

5. Hollenberg NK, Dzau VJ, Williams GH. Are uncontrolled clinical studies ever justified? N Engl J Med. 1980; 303:1067.

6. Sacks H, Kupfer S, Chalmers TC. Are uncontrolled clinical studies ever justified? N Engl J Med. 1980; 303:1067.

7. Ramsey P. The patient as person: explorations in medical ethics. New Haven: Yale University Press, 1970.

TOM REGAN

The Case Against Animal Research

THE AUTONOMY OF ANIMALS

Autonomy can be understood in different ways. On one interpretation, which finds its classic statement in Kant's writings, individuals are autonomous only if they are capable of acting on reasons they can will that any other similarly placed individual can act on. For example, if I am trying to decide whether I morally ought to keep a promise, I must, Kant believes, ask whether I could will that everyone else who is similarly placed (i.e., who has made a promise) can act as I do for the same reasons as I have. In asking what I ought to do, in other words, I must determine what others can do, and it is only if I have the ability to think through and reflectively evaluate the merits of acting in one way or another (e.g., to decide to keep the promise or to break it), and, having done this, to make a decision on the basis of my deliberations, that I can be viewed as an autonomous individual.

It is highly unlikely that any animal is autonomous in the Kantian sense. To be so animals would have to be able to reason at a quite sophisticated level indeed, bringing to bear considerations about what other animals (presumably those who belong to their own species) can or ought to do in comparable situations, a process that requires assessing the merits of alternative acts from an impartial point of view. Not only is it doubtful that animals could have the requisite abilities to do this; it is doubtful that we could confirm their possession of these abilities if they had them. . . .

But the Kantian sense of autonomy is not the only one. An alternative view is that individuals are autono-

Reprinted with permission of the University of California Press, from Tom Regan, *The Case for Animal Rights.* © 1983 The Regents of the University of California Press, pp. 84–86, 327–328, 376–383, 384–385, 387–394, 416.

mous if they have preferences and have the ability to initiate action with a view to satisfying them. It is not necessary, given this interpretation of autonomy (let us call this *preference autonomy*), that one be able to abstract from one's own desires, goals, and so on, as a preliminary to asking what any other similarly placed individual ought to do; it is enough that one have the ability to initiate action because one has those desires or goals one has and believes, rightly or wrongly, that one's desires or purposes will be satisfied or achieved by acting in a certain way. Where the Kantian sense requires that one be able to think impartially if one is to possess autonomy, the preference sense does not.

Both the Kantian and the preference sense of autonomy obviously exclude some of the same individuals from the class of autonomous beings. Rocks, clouds, rivers, and plants, for example, lack autonomy given either sense. But the preference sense includes some individuals excluded by the Kantian sense, most notably many animals. . . . [M]ammalian animals, at least, are reasonably viewed as creatures meeting the requirements for possession of preference autonomy. These animals are reasonably viewed as possessing the cognitive prerequisites for having desires and goals; they perceive and remember, and have the ability to form and apply general beliefs. From this it is a short step to acknowledging that these animals are reasonably viewed as being capable of making preferential choices.

Two types of cases illustrate the propriety of viewing these animals in this way. The first involves cases where they regularly behave in a given way when given the opportunity to do one thing or another. For example, if, when Fido is both hungry and has not recently had an opportunity to run outdoors, he regularly opts for eating when given the choice between food or the outdoors, we have adequate behavioral grounds for saying that the dog prefers eating to running in such cases and so acts (i.e., chooses) accordingly. A second type of case involves situations where there is no regular behavioral pattern because of the novelty of a given set of circumstances. If Fido is hungry, if we place before him both a bowl of his regular food and a bowl of boiled eggplant, and if, as is predictable, Fido opts for his regular food, then we again have adequate behavioral grounds for saying that the dog prefers his normal food to the eggplant and so acts (i.e., chooses) accordingly. And this we may reasonably contend even if this is the only time Fido is presented with the choice in question.

When autonomy is understood in the preference sense, the case can be made for viewing many animals as autonomous. Which animals it is reasonable to view as autonomous will turn, first, on whether we have reasonable grounds for viewing them as having preferences, understood as desires or goals, and, second, on whether we find that how they behave in various situations is intelligibly described and parsimoniously explained by making reference to their preferences and the choices they make because of the preferences they have. Like other comparable issues, where one draws the line is certain to be controversial. But at least in the case of normal mammalian animals, aged one or more—even if not in the case of any others—the conclusions reached in the previous two chapters, including the need to view their behavior holistically, underwrite the reasonableness of ascribing preference autonomy to them.

We have, then, two senses of autonomy—the Kantian and the preference sense—each differing significantly from the other. If it could be shown that the Kantian sense is the only true sense of autonomy or that the preference sense is silly, or muddled, or worse, then one could rightfully claim that animals lack autonomy. But none of these options hold any promise. The Kantian interpretation of autonomy does not give us a condition that must be met if one is to be autonomous in any sense. It provides a condition that must be met if one is to be an autonomous *moral agent*—that is, an individual who can be held morally accountable for the acts he performs or fails to perform, one who can rightly be blamed or praised, criticized or condemned. Central to the Kantian sense of autonomy is the idea that autonomous individuals can rise above thinking about their individual preferences and think about where their moral duty lies by bringing impartial reasons to bear on their deliberations. These two ideas

(that of individual preferences, on the one hand, and, on the other, one's moral duty) are distinct. Just because I prefer your death or public shame, for example, it does not follow that either I or anyone else has a moral duty to terminate your life or bring about your public disgrace, and there are many things I might be morally obligated to do that I personally do not prefer doing (e.g., keeping a promise). Suppose it is agreed that one must be autonomous in the Kantian sense to have the status of a moral agent. . . . It does not follow that one must be autonomous in *this* sense to be autonomous in *any* sense. So long as one has the ability to act on one's preferences, the ascription of autonomy is intelligible and attributions of it are confirmable. Though normal mammalian animals aged one or more are not reasonably viewed as moral agents because they are not reasonably viewed as autonomous in the Kantian sense, they are reasonably viewed as autonomous in the preference sense.

• • •

THE RIGHTS OF ANIMALS

. . . [A]ll moral agents and patients have certain basic moral rights. To say that these individuals possess basic (or unacquired) moral rights means that (1) they possess certain rights independently of anyone's voluntary acts, either their own or those of others, and independently of the position they happen to occupy in any given institutional arrangement; (2) these rights are universal—that is, they are possessed by all relevantly similar individuals, independently of those considerations mentioned in (1); and (3) all who possess these rights possess them equally. Basic moral rights thus differ *both* from acquired moral rights (e.g., the right of the promisee against the promisor) because one acquires these rights as a result of someone's voluntary acts or one's place in an institutional arrangement *and* from legal rights (e.g., the right to vote) since legal rights, unlike basic moral rights, are not equal or universal. . . .

The principal basic moral right possessed by all moral agents and patients is the right to respectful treatment. . . . [A]ll moral agents and patients are intelligibly and nonarbitrarily viewed as having a distinctive kind of value (inherent value) and as having this value equally. All moral agents and patients must always be treated in ways that are consistent with the recognition of their equal possession of value of this kind. These individuals have a basic moral right to respectful treatment because the claim made to it is (a) a valid claim-against assignable individuals (namely, all moral agents) and (b) a valid claim-to, the validity of the claim-to resting on appeal to the respect principle, . . . The basic moral right to respectful treatment prohibits treating moral agents or patients as if they were mere receptacles of intrinsic values (e.g., pleasure), lacking any value of their own, since such a view of these individuals would allow harming some (e.g., by making them suffer) on the grounds that the aggregate consequences for all those other "receptacles" affected by the outcome would be "the best." . . . [A]ll moral agents and patients [also] have a prima facie basic moral right not to be harmed. . . .

TOXICOLOGY

. . . Some humans are harmed . . . as a result of a variety of pathological conditions, and many more will be harmed if we fail to investigate the causes, treatments, and cures of these conditions. Indeed, some will today lose their lives as a result of these maladies, and many more will lose theirs in the future if we fail to investigate their causes and cures. Now, one thing we must do, it may be claimed, is reduce the risk that the treatment prescribed for a given malady will make patients worse-off than they otherwise would have been, and this will require establishing the toxic properties of each new drug before, not after, humans take them. Thus arises the need to test the toxicity of each new drug on test animals. If we do not test the toxicity of all new drugs on animals, humans who use these drugs will run a much greater risk of being made worse-off as a result of using them than they would if these drugs were pretested on animals. In the nature of the case, we cannot say which drugs are toxic for humans *in advance* of conducting tests on animals (if we could, there would be no need to do the test in the first place). Indeed, we cannot even eliminate all risks *after* the drug has been extensively pretested on animals (thalidomide is a tragic example). The best we can do is minimize the risks humans who use drugs face, as best we can, and that requires testing for their toxicity on animals.

The rights view rejects this defense of these tests. *Risks are not morally transferable to those who do not voluntarily choose to take them in the way this defense assumes.* If I hang-glide, then I run certain risks, including the possibility of serious head injury, and I shall certainly, if I am prudent, want to minimize my risks by wearing a protective helmet. You, who do not hang-glide, have no duty to agree to serve in tests that establish the safety of various helmet designs so that hang-gliders might reduce their risks, and hang-gliders, or those who serve the interests of these enthusiasts, would violate your rights if they coerced or forced you to take part in such tests. *How much* you would be harmed is not decisive. What matters is that you would be *put at risk of harm, against your will*, in the name of reducing the risks that others voluntarily undertake and so can voluntarily decide *not* to undertake by the simple expedient of choosing not to run them in the first place (in this case, by choosing not to hang-glide). That tests on you would make it possible for those who hang-glide to lessen the risk of being made worse-off goes no way toward justifying placing you at risk of harm. As hang-gliders are the ones who stand to benefit from participation in this sport, they are the ones who must run the risks involved in participating. They may do all that they can to reduce the risks they run, but only so long as they do not coerce others to find out what these risks are or how to reduce them.

It would be a mistake to suppose that what is true in the case of high-risk activity is not true in the case of low-risk activity. Whenever I plug in my toaster, take an elevator, drink water from my faucet or from a clear mountain stream, I take some risks, though not of the magnitude of those who, say, sky-dive or canoe in turbid waters. But even in the case of my voluntarily taking minor risks, others have no duty to volunteer to establish or minimize my risks for me, and anyone who would be made to do this, against her will, would have her rights unjustifiably overridden. For example, the risks I run when I drive my car could be minimized by the design and manufacture of the most effective seat belts and the most crash-proof automobile. But it does not follow that anyone else has a duty to take part in crash tests in the name of minimizing my risks, and anyone who was coerced to do so, whether injured or not, would have every reason to claim that her rights had been violated or, if the test subject is incapable of making the claim, others would have every reason to make this claim on the subject's behalf. "No harm done" is no defense in circumstances such as these.

To minimize the risks humans who use new drugs would run by testing them on animals is morally no different. Anyone who elects to take a drug voluntarily chooses to run certain risks, and the risks we choose to run or, as in the case of moral patients for whom we choose, the risks we elect to allow them to run are not morally transferable to others. Coercively to harm others or to put others, whether human or animal, at risk of harm in order to identify or minimize the risks of those who voluntarily choose to run them, is to violate the rights of the humans or animals in question. It is not *how much* the test subjects are harmed (though the greater the harm, the worse the offense). What matters is that they are coercively used to establish or minimize risks for others. To place these animals at risk of harm so that others who voluntarily choose to run certain risks, and who thus can voluntarily choose not to run them, may minimize the risks they run, is to fail to treat the test animals with that respect they are due as possessors of inherent value. As is true of toxicity tests on new products, similar tests of new drugs on animals involve treating them as *even less* than receptacles, as if their value were reducible to their possible utility relative to the interests of others— in this case, relative to the interests humans who voluntarily take drugs have in minimizing their risks. Laboratory animals, to borrow an apt phrase from the Harvard philosopher Robert Nozick, "are distinct individuals who are not resources for others."[1] To utilize them so that we might establish or minimize our risks, especially when it is within our power to decide not to take these risks in the first place, *is* to treat them as if they were "resources for others," most notably for us, and to defend these tests on the grounds that animals sometimes are not harmed is as morally lame as defending fox hunting on the grounds that the fox sometimes gets away.

The rights view is not in principle opposed to efforts to minimize the risks involved in taking new drugs. Toxicity tests are acceptable, so long as they violate no one's rights. To use human volunteers, persons who do not suffer from a particular malady but who give their informed consent as a test subject, is, though possible, not generally to be encouraged. To tie the progress of pharmacology and related sciences to the availability of healthy, consenting human subjects itself runs significant risks, including the risk that some may use deceptive or coercive means to secure participation. Moreover, few, if any, volunteers from the affluent classes are likely to step forward; the ranks of volunteers would likely be comprised of the poor, the uneducated, and those human moral patients whose relatives lack sufficient "sentimental interests"

to protect them. There is a serious danger that the least powerful will be exploited. More preferable by far is the development of toxicity tests that harm no one— that is, tests that harm neither moral agents nor patients, whether humans or animals. Even at this date promising alternatives are being developed.[2] To validate them scientifically is no small challenge, but it is the challenge that must be met if we continue to desire or require that new drugs be tested for their toxicity prior to being made available on the market. To test them on healthy human volunteers is dangerous at best; to test them coercively on healthy animals and human moral patients is wrong. The moral alternative that remains is: find valid alternatives.

A number of objections can be anticipated. One claims that there are risks and then there are risks. If we stopped testing new drugs for their toxicity, think of the risks people would run if they took them! Who could say what disastrous consequences would result? The rights view agrees. People would run greater risks if drugs were not pretested. But (a) the rights view does not oppose all pretesting (only those tests that coercively utilize some so that others may reduce those risks they may choose to run or choose not to run), and (b) those who had the choice to use an untested drug, assuming it was available, could *themselves* choose not to run the risks associated with taking it by deciding not to take it. Indeed, prudence would dictate acting in this way, except in the direst circumstances.

Of course, if untested drugs were allowed on the market and if people acted prudently, sales of new (untested) drugs would fall off, and we can anticipate that those involved in the pharmaceutical industry, people who, in addition to their chosen vocation of serving the health needs of the public, also have an economic interest in the stability and growth of this industry, might look with disfavor on the implications of the rights view. Four brief replies must suffice in this regard. First, whatever financial losses these companies might face if they were not permitted to continue to do toxicity tests on animals carry no moral weight, since the question of overriding basic moral rights is at issue. That these companies might lose money if the rights of animals are respected is one of the risks they run. Second, there is mounting evidence that these companies could save, rather than lose, money if nonanimal tests were used. Animals are an expensive proposition. They must be bred or purchased, fed and watered, their living quarters must be routinely cleaned, their environment controlled (otherwise one runs the scientific risk of an uncontrolled variable), and so forth. This requires employing trained personnel, in adequate numbers, as well as a large and continued outpouring of capital for initial construction, expansion, and maintenance. Tissue and cell cultures, for example, are cheaper by far. So the economic interests of commercial pharmaceutical firms are not necessarily at odds with the changes that will have to be made, as the rights of laboratory animals are respected. Third, anyone who defends present toxicological practice *merely* by claiming that these tests are required by the involved regulatory agencies (e.g., the Food and Drug Administration) would miss the essential moral point: though these agencies have yet to recognize nonanimal tests as meeting their regulations, these agencies themselves do not require that any pharmaceutical firm manufacture any new drug. That is a moral decision each company makes on its own and for which each must bear responsibility. Fourth, appeals to what the laws require can have no moral weight if we have good reason to believe that the laws in question are unjust. And we have good reasons in the present case. Laboratory animals are not a "resource" whose moral status in the world is to serve human interests. They are themselves the subjects-of-a-life that fares better or worse for them as individuals, logically independently of any utility they may or may not have relative to the interests of others. They share with us a distinctive kind of value—inherent value—and whatever we do to them must be respectful of this value as a matter of strict justice. To treat them *as if* their value were reducible to their utility for human interests, even important human interests, is to treat them unjustly; to utilize them so that humans might minimize the risks we voluntarily take (and that we can voluntarily decide not to take) is to violate their basic moral right to be treated with respect. That the laws require such testing, when they do, does not show that these tests are morally tolerable; what this shows is that the laws themselves are unjust and ought to be changed.

One can also anticipate charges that the rights view is antiscientific and antihumanity. This is rhetoric. The rights view is not antihuman. We, as humans, have an equal prima facie right not to be harmed, a right that the rights view seeks to illuminate and defend; but we do not have any right coercively to harm others, or to put them at risk of harm, so that we might minimize the risks we run as a result of our own voluntary decisions. That violates their rights, and that is one thing no one has a right to do. Nor is the rights view antiscientific. It places the *scientific* challenge before pharmacologists and related scientists: find scientifically valid ways that serve the public interest without violating individual rights. The overarching goal of pharmacology should be to reduce the risks of those who use drugs without harming those who don't. Those who claim that this cannot be done, in advance of making a concerted effort to do it, are the ones who are truly antiscientific.

Perhaps the most common response to the call for elimination of animals in toxicity testing is the benefits argument:

1. Human beings and animals have benefited from toxicity tests on animals.
2. Therefore, these tests are justified.

Like all arguments with missing premises, everything turns on what that premise is. If it read, "These tests do not violate the rights of animals," then we would be on our way to receiving an interesting defense of toxicity testing. Unfortunately for those who countenance these tests, however, and even more unfortunately for the animals used in them, that premise is not true. These tests do violate the rights of the test animals, for the reasons given. The benefits these tests have for others are irrelevant, according to the rights view, since the tests violate the rights of the individual animals. As in the case of humans, so also in the case of animals: overriding their rights cannot be defended by appealing to "the general welfare." Put alternatively, the benefits *others* receive count morally only if no *individual's* rights have been violated. Since toxicity tests of new drugs violate the rights of laboratory animals, it is morally irrelevant to appeal to how much others have benefited.[3]

A further objection is conceptual in nature. "Animals cannot volunteer or refuse to volunteer to take part in toxicity tests," it may be claimed, "and so cannot be forced or coerced to take part in them either. Thus the rights view's opposition to using them is fatuous." Now it is true that, unlike *some* humans, animals cannot give or withhold their informed consent, relative to participation in a toxicity test. But this is because they cannot be informed in the relevant way.

It is no good trying to inform them about pH factors or carcinogens. They *will not* understand because they *cannot* understand; but it does not follow from this that animals cannot be forced or coerced to do something they do not want to do. Because these animals are intelligibly viewed as having preference-autonomy, . . . we are able intelligibly to say, and confirm statements made about, what they want, desire, prefer, aim at, intend, and so forth. We can, therefore, give a perfectly clear sense to saying that they are being forced or coerced to do something they do not want to do. Beyond any doubt, those animals used in the LD50 test,* for example, are not doing what they want to do, and those who use them in these tests do so by means of force or coercion.

To establish the scientific validity of nonanimal toxicity tests is a difficult challenge certainly, one that can only be met by scientists. No moral philosophy can do this. What a moral philosophy can do is articulate and defend the morally permissible means of conducting science. If the rights view has the best reasons on its side, this is the view we ought to use to assess what is and what is not permissible in the case of toxicity testing. And the implications of this view are clear. *Toxicity tests of new products and drugs involving animals are not morally justified. These tests violate the rights of these animals. They are not morally tolerable. All ought to cease.*

SCIENTIFIC RESEARCH

One can imagine someone accepting the arguments advanced against toxicity tests on animals but putting his foot down when it comes to scientific research. To deny science use of animals in research is, it might be said, to bring scientific and allied medical progress to a halt, and that is reason enough to oppose it. The claim that progress would be "brought to a halt" is an exaggeration certainly. It is not an exaggeration to claim that, given its present dominant tendency, the rights view requires massive redirection of scientific research. The dominant tendency involves routinely harming animals. It should come as no surprise that the rights view has principled objections to its continuation.

A recent statement of the case for unrestricted use of animals in neurobiological research contrasts sharply with the rights view and will serve as an introduction to the critical assessment of using animals in basic research. The situation, as characterized by C. R. Gallistel, a psychologist at the University of Pennsylvania, is as follows:[4] "Behavioral neurobiology tries to establish the manner in which the nervous system mediates behavioral phenomena. It does so by studying the behavioral consequences of one or more of the following procedures: (a) destruction of a part of the nervous system, (b) stimulation of a part, (c) administration of drugs that alter neural functioning. These three techniques are as old as the discipline. A recent addition is (d) the recording of electrical activity. All four cause the animal at least temporary distress. In the past they have frequently caused intense pain, and they occasionally do so now. Also, they often impair an animal's proper functioning, sometimes transiently, sometimes permanently."[5] The animals subjected to these procedures are, in a word, harmed. When it comes to advancing our knowledge in neurobiology, however, "there is no way to establish the relation between the nervous system and behavior without some experimental surgery," where by "experimental surgery" Gallistel evidently means to include the four procedures just outlined. The issue, then, in Gallistel's mind, is not whether to allow such surgery or not; it is whether any restrictions should be placed on the use made of animals. Gallistel thinks not.

In defense of unrestricted use of animals in research, Gallistel claims that "most experiments conducted by neurobiologists, *like scientific experiments generally*, may be seen in retrospect to have been a waste of time, in the sense that they did not prove or yield any new insight." But, claims Gallistel, "there is no way of discriminating in advance the waste-of-time experiments from the illuminating ones with anything approaching certainty."[6] The logical upshot, so Gallistel believes, is that "restricting research on living animals is certain to restrict the progress in our understanding of the nervous system and behavior. Therefore," he concludes, "one should advocate such restrictions only if one believes that the moral value of this scientific knowledge and of the many human and humane benefits that flow from it cannot outweigh the suffering of a rat," something that, writing autobiographically, Gallistel finds "an affront to my ethical sensibility."[7] . . .

[T]he rights view rejects Gallistel's approach at a fundamental level. On the rights view, we cannot

---

*Tests in which 50% of the animals die due to the toxicity of the dose of a substance to which they are exposed.

justify harming a single rat *merely* by aggregating "the many human and humane benefits" that flow from doing it, since, as stated, this is to assume that the rat has value only as a receptacle, which, on the rights view, is not true. Moreover, . . . [n]ot even a single rat is to be treated as if that animal's value were reducible to his *possible utility* relative to the interests of others, which is what we would be doing if we intentionally harmed the rat on the grounds that this *just might* "prove" something, *just might* "yield" a "new insight," *just might* produce "benefits" for others. . . .

If we are seriously to challenge the use of animals in research, we must challenge the *practice* itself, not only individual instances of it or merely the liabilities in its present methodology. The rights view issues such a challenge. Routine use of animals in research assumes that their value is reducible to their possible utility relative to the interests of others. The rights view rejects this view of animals and their value, as it rejects the justice of institutions that treat them as renewable resources. They, like us, have a value of their own, logically independently of their utility for others and of their being the object of anyone else's interests. To treat them in ways that respect their value, therefore, requires that we *not* sanction practices that institutionalize treating them as if their value was reducible to their possible utility relative to our interests. Scientific research, when it involves routinely harming animals in the name of possible "human and humane benefits," violates this requirement of respectful treatment. Animals are not to be treated as mere receptacles or as renewable resources. Thus does the practice of scientific research on animals violate their rights. Thus ought it to cease, according to the rights view. It is not enough first conscientiously to look for nonanimal alternatives and then, having failed to find any, to resort to using animals.[8] Though that approach is laudable as far as it goes, and though taking it would mark significant progress, it does not go far enough. It assumes that it is all right to allow practices that use animals as if their value were reducible to their possible utility relative to the interests of others, provided that we have done our best not to do so. The rights view's position would have us go further in terms of "doing our best." *The best we can do in terms of not using animals is not to use them.* Their inherent value does not disappear just because we have failed to find a way to avoid harming them in pursuit of our chosen

goals. Their value is independent of these goals and their possible utility in achieving them. . . .

The rights view does not oppose using what is learned from conscientious efforts to treat a sick animal (or human) to facilitate and improve the treatment tendered other animals (or humans). In *this* respect, the rights view raises no objection to the "many human and humane benefits" that flow from medical science and the research with which it is allied. What the rights view opposes are practices that cause intentional harm to laboratory animals (for example, by means of burns, shock, amputation, poisoning, surgery, starvation, and sensory deprivation) preparatory to "looking for something that just might yield some human or humane benefit." Whatever benefits happen to accrue from such a practice are irrelevant to assessing its tragic injustice. Lab animals are not our tasters; we are not their kings.

The tired charge of being antiscientific is likely to fill the air once more. It is a moral smokescreen. The rights view is not against research on animals, if this research does not harm these animals or put them at risk of harm. It is apt to remark, however, that this objective will not be accomplished merely by ensuring that test animals are anaesthetized, or given postoperative drugs to ease their suffering, or kept in clean cages with ample food and water, and so forth. For it is not only the pain and suffering that matters—though they certainly matter—but it is the *harm* done to the animals, including the diminished welfare opportunities they endure as a result of the deprivations caused by the surgery, *and* their untimely death. It is unclear whether a *benign* use of animals in research is possible or, if possible, whether scientists could be persuaded to practice it. That being so, and given the serious risks run by relying on a steady supply of human volunteers, research should take the direction away from the use of any moral agent or patient. If nonanimal alternatives are available, they should be used; if they are not available, they should be sought. That is the moral challenge to research, given the rights view, and it is those scientists who protest that this "can't be done," in advance of the scientific commitment to try—not those who call for the exploration—who exhibit a lack of commitment to, and belief in, the scientific enterprise—who are, that is, antiscientific at the deepest level. Like Galileo's contemporaries, who would not look through the telescope because they had already convinced themselves of what they would see and thus saw no need to look, those scientists who have convinced themselves that there can't be viable scientific alternatives to the use of whole animals in research (or toxicity tests, etc.) are captives of mental habits that true science abhors.

The rights view, then, is far from being antiscientific. On the contrary, as is true in the case of toxicity tests, so also in the case of research: it calls upon scientists *to do science* as they redirect the traditional practice of their several disciplines away from reliance on "animal models" toward the development and use of nonanimal alternatives. All that the rights view prohibits is science that violates individual rights. If that means that there are some things we cannot learn, then so be it. There are also some things we cannot learn by using humans, if we respect their rights. The rights view merely requires moral consistency in this regard.

The rights view's position regarding the use of animals in research cannot be fairly criticized on the grounds that it is antihumanity. The implications of this view in this regard are those that a rational human being should expect, especially when we recall that nature neither respects nor violates our rights. . . . Only moral agents do; indeed, only moral agents *can*. And nature is not a moral agent. We have, then, no basic right against nature not to be harmed by those natural diseases we are heir to. And neither do we have any basic right against humanity in this regard. What we do have, at this point in time at least, is a right to fair treatment on the part of those who have voluntarily decided to offer treatment for these maladies, a right that will not tolerate the preferential treatment of some (e.g., Caucasians) to the detriment of others (e.g., Native Americans). The right to fair treatment of our naturally caused maladies (and the same applies to mental and physical illnesses brought on by human causes, e.g. pollutants) is an *acquired right* we have against those moral agents who acquire the duty to offer fair treatment because they voluntarily assume a role within the medical profession. Both those in this profession, as well as those who do research in the hope that they might improve health care, are not morally authorized to override the *basic rights* of others in the process—rights others have, that is, independently of their place in any institutional arrangement and independently of any voluntary act on the part of anyone. . . . And yet that is what is annually done to literally millions of animals whose services, so to speak, are enlisted in the name of scientific research, including that research allied with medical

science. For this research treats these animals as if their value is reducible to their possible utility relative to the interests of others. Thus does it routinely violate their basic right to respectful treatment. Though those of us who today are to be counted among the beneficiaries of the human benefits obtained from this research in the past might stand to lose some future benefits, at least in the short run, if this research is stopped, the rights view will not be satisfied with anything less than its total abolition. Even granting that we face greater prima facie harm than laboratory animals presently endure if future harmful research on these animals is stopped, and even granting that the number of humans and other animals who stand to benefit from allowing this practice to continue exceeds the number of animals used in it, this practice remains wrong because unjust.

A further objection has a distinctively contractarian flavor. As a society, it might be claimed, we have decided that the use of animals for scientific purposes, even their harmful use, is permissible. Anyone who becomes a scientist in a nation that supports science by the use of public funds *acquires the duty to serve the public will*, and the public has a right against scientists to do so. Since the harmful use of animals in pursuit of scientific purposes is necessary if science is to fulfill the terms of its contract with society, the existence of this contract is a special consideration that justifies the continued use of animals in science.

The rights view is not unsympathetic to appeals to contracts and other voluntary arrangements as a basis for validating acquired duties and correlative rights. . . . [H]owever, the moral validity of a contract or other voluntary arrangement is not shown just by establishing that certain individuals voluntarily entered into a given agreement. Moral validity depends upon the respectful treatment of all those involved, not just those who enter into the agreement. A slave-trader does not do what is right by supplying his client with a promised slave, and he has no valid moral duty to do so, despite his promising to do so. Since the institution of slavery treats slaves with a lack of respect, promises made in the name of the perpetuation of this institution are morally null and void. The same is true regarding society's "contract" with science and the supposed duty of scientists to carry out their end of the agreement by harming some animals so that others, both humans and animals, might benefit. This "contract" has no moral validity, according to the rights view, because it fails to treat lab animals with the respect they are due. That science that routinely harms animals in pursuit of its goals is morally corrupt, because unjust at its core, something that no appeal to the "contract" between society and science can alter. What is required is a new contract, one that takes account of, and respects, those currently exploited by the existing one, a contract that, if it cannot be drawn up and enforced by education and opinion, will have to take the form of law. Only then will society's contract with science constitute a valid special consideration. . . .

A final objection urges that the rights view cannot have any principled objection to using mammalian animals for scientific purposes generally, or in research in particular, before these animals attain the degree of physical maturity that makes it reasonable to view them as subjects-of-a-life, in the sense that is central to the rights view. . . . For example, use of newly born mammalian animals must stand outside the scope of the proscriptions issued by the rights view.

This objection is half right. *If certain conditions are met*, the rights view could sanction the scientific use of mammalian animals at certain stages of their physical development. As has been remarked on more than one occasion in the preceding, however, where one draws the line, both as regards what species of animals contain members who are subjects-of-a-life and as regards when a given animal acquires the abilities necessary for being such a subject, is controversial. We simply do not know, with anything approaching certainty, exactly where to draw the line in either case. Precisely because we are so palpably ignorant about a matter so fraught with moral significance, we ought to err on the side of caution, not only in the case of humans but also in the case of animals. Though during the earliest stages of development it is most implausible to regard a fetal mammalian animal as conscious, sentient, and so on, it becomes increasingly less implausible as the animal matures physically, acquiring the physical basis that underlies consciousness, perception, sentience, and the like. Although throughout the present [essay] attention has been for the most part confined to normal mammalian animals, aged one or more, it does not follow that animals less than one year of age may be treated in just any way we please. Because we do not know exactly where to draw the line, it is better to give the benefit of the doubt to mammalian

animals less than one year of age who have acquired the physical characteristics that underlie one's being a subject-of-a-life. The rights view's position concerning those animals, then, is against their use for scientific purposes.

There are Kantian-like grounds that strengthen the case against using newborn and soon-to-be-born mammalian animals in science. To allow the routine use of these animals for scientific purposes would most likely foster the attitude that animals are just "models," just "tools," just "resources." Better to root out at the source, than to allow to take root, attitudes that are inimical to fostering respect for the rights of animals. Just as in the analogous areas of abortion and infanticide in the case of humans, . . . therefore, the rights view favors policies that foster respect for the rights of the individual animal, even if the creation of these attitudes requires that we treat some animals who may not have rights as if they have them.

Finally, even in the case of mammalian animals in the earliest stages of fetal development, the rights view does not issue a blank check for their use in science. For though, on the rights view, we do not owe a duty of justice to these fetuses, we do owe justice to those animals who would be enlisted to produce them in the number researchers are likely to desire. Were mature animals used as "fetal machines" and, as a result, were they housed in circumstances conducive to their reproducing at the desired rate, it is most unlikely that the rights of these mature animals would be respected. For example, it is very unlikely that *these* animals would be provided with a physical environment conducive to the exercise of their preference autonomy, or one that was hospitable to their social needs; and it is equally unlikely that they would avoid having their life brought to an untimely end, well in advance of their having reached a condition where killing them could be defended on grounds of preference-respecting or paternalistic euthanasia. Once they had stopped reproducing, they would likely be killed. To the extent that we have reason to believe that these mature mammals would be treated as if they had value only relative to human purposes, to that extent the rights view would oppose the scientific use of fetal mammalian animals, not because these latter have rights that would be violated, but because this would be true in the case of the mature animals used as breeders. Those who would use mammalian animals in the earliest stages of their fetal development, then, may do so, according to the rights view, but only if they ensure *both* that (1) the lab animals used to produce the fetuses are treated with the respect they are due *and* that (2) reliance on mammalian fetuses does not foster beliefs and attitudes that encourage scientists to use mature mammalian animals for scientific purposes, including research. It is unclear that science could institute policies that satisfied the first condition. It is clear that a policy could be introduced that satisfied the second. This would be for science to cease using mammalian animals who are subjects-of-a-life in ways that harm them directly, or that put them at risk of harm, or that foster an environment in which their harm is allowed. That is a policy the rights view could allow, but one science has yet to adopt.

ANIMALS IN SCIENCE, UTILITARIANISM, AND ANIMAL RIGHTS

The fundamental differences between utilitarianism and the rights view are never more apparent than in the case of the use of animals in science. For the utilitarian, whether the harm done to animals in pursuit of scientific ends is justified depends on the balance of the aggregated consequences for all those affected by the outcome. If the consequences that result from harming animals would produce the best aggregate balance of good over evil, then harmful experimentation is obligatory. If the resulting consequences would be at least as good as what are otherwise obtainable, then harmful experimentation is permissible. Only if harmful experimentation would produce less than the best consequences would it be wrong. For a utilitarian to oppose or support harmful experimentation on animals, therefore, requires that he have the relevant facts—who will be benefited or harmed, how much, and so on. *Everyone's* interests, including the interests of those who do the tests or conduct the research, their employers, the dependents of these persons, the retailers and wholesalers of cages, animal breeders, and others, must be taken into account and counted equitably. For utilitarians, such *side effects count*. The animals used in the test have no privileged moral status. Their interests must be taken into account, to be sure, but not any more than anybody else's interests.

As is "almost always" the case, utilitarians simply fail to give us what is needed—the relevant facts, facts that we must have, given their theory, to determine whether use of animals in science is or is not justified. Moreover, for a utilitarian to claim or imply that there must be something wrong with a given experiment, if the experimenter would not be willing to use a less intelligent, less aware human being but would be will-

ing to use a more intelligent, more aware animal, simply lacks a utilitarian basis. For all we know, and for all the utilitarian has thus far told us, the consequences of using such an animal, all considered, might be better than those that would result from using the human being. It is not *who* is used, given utilitarian theory, that matters; it is *the consequences* that do.

The rights view takes a very different stand. No one, whether human or animal, is ever to be treated as if she were a mere receptacle, or as if her value were reducible to her possible utility for others. We are, that is, never to harm the individual merely on the grounds that this will or just might produce "the best" aggregate consequences. To do so is to violate the rights of the individual. That is why the harm done to animals in pursuit of scientific purposes is wrong. The benefits derived are real enough; but some gains are ill-gotten, and all gains are ill-gotten when secured unjustly.

So it is that the rights view issues its challenge to those who do science: advance knowledge, work for the general welfare, but not by allowing practices that violate the rights of the individual. These are, one might say, the terms of the new contract between science and society, a contract that, however belatedly, now contains the signature of those who speak for the rights of animals. *Those who accept the rights view, and who sign for animals, will not be satisfied with anything less than the total abolition of the harmful use of animals in science—in education, in toxicity testing, in basic research.* But the rights view plays no favorites. No scientific practice that violates human rights, whether the humans be moral agents or moral patients, is acceptable. And the same applies to those humans who, for reasons analogous to those advanced in the present [essay] in regard to nonhumans, should be given the benefit of the doubt about having rights because of the weight of our ignorance—the newly born and the soon-to-be born. Those who accept the rights view are committed to denying any and all access to these "resources" on the part of those who do science. And we do this not because we oppose cruelty (though we do), nor because we favor kindness (though we do), but because justice requires nothing less. . . .

NOTES

1. Robert Nozick, *Anarchy, State, and Utopia* (New York: Basic Books, 1974), p. 33. Nozick does not have animals in mind when he says this.

2. Richard D. Ryder, *Victims of Science: The Use of Animals in Research* (London: Davis-Poynter, 1975); and Dallas Pratt, *Alternatives to Pain in Experiments on Animals* (New York: Argus Archives, 1980).

3. The benefit argument sometimes is advanced, especially by veterinarians, in defense of testing for the toxicity of drugs on some animals in the hope that *other animals* might benefit. It is true that some animals have benefited because these tests have been done on others, but this does not provide a moral justification of these tests. Just as animals used in the laboratory are not resources to be used in the name of obtaining *human* benefits, so they are not to be viewed as a resource to be used in pursuit of benefits for *other animals*.

4. C. R. Gallistel, "Bell, Magendie, and the Proposal to Restrict the Use of Animals in Neurobehavioral Research," *American Psychologist* (April 1981), pp. 357–360.

5. Ibid., p. 357.

6. Ibid., p. 358.

7. Ibid., p. 360.

8. This is the view recommended in Dale Jamieson and Tom Regan, "On the Ethics of the Use of Animals in Science" [in *And Justice for All*, ed. Tom Regan and Donald VanDeVeer (Totowa, N.J.: Rowman and Littlefield, 1982), 169–196]. In disassociating myself from this earlier view, I speak only for myself. I am in no position to speak for Professor Jamieson.

H. J. McCLOSKEY

The Moral Case for Experimentation on Animals

The moral case for experimentation on animals rests both on the goods to be realized, the evils to be avoided thereby, and on the duty to respect persons and to secure them in the enjoyment of their natural moral rights. Some experimentation on animals presents no problems of justification as it involves no harm at all to the animals which are the subject of experiments and is such as to seek to achieve an advance in knowledge. Experiments on non-sentient animals, like those on plant life, may harm the subjects but in ways that in themselves need raise no morally significant issues. Moral issues may arise if the subjects of experiments are members of an endangered species and for like reasons but not simply on account of the harm caused by the experiment to the subjects. Other experimentation on animals is to be justified solely in terms of its benefit to animals, even though it involves harm to the animals upon which experiments are performed. There are many poisons and diseases to which animals and not human beings are exposed which give rise to the need for experiments to determine effective therapies, treatments, or other remedies. Examples include annual rye grass toxicity, foot-and-mouth disease, the many fowl diseases, and so on. Human beings commonly have an interest in successfully experimenting to find effective remedies, either a financial interest as with farm animals, race horses and the like, amusement interest as with pets, or a concern not to have a species or variety become extinct. The moral case for such experiments may be strengthened by reference to such interests if they in turn have a moral basis, but generally it does not depend for its validity on this. Other experimentation that harms the animals involved is to be justified in terms of the benefits to be realized and evils lessened for persons by the knowledge and the use of the knowledge gained, where the knowledge is used to secure the enjoyment of their moral rights by persons. Much experimentation benefits both persons, contributing to the securing of their enjoyment of their moral rights, and animals which do not possess moral rights, and is to be morally justified on both counts. Obviously a great amount of experimentation occurs today which does not admit of justification along any of these lines, and hence, is such that it must be condemned as being morally wrong.

The experimentation that is to be considered in this [essay] relates to determining the toxicity of materials that may be harmful to animals and/or man, and the testing of possible antidotes and remedies, and to the investigation of substances, drugs, vaccines, thera-

Reprinted with permission of the publisher from *The Monist* 70(1), January 1987, pp. 64–72, 73–76, 79–81, 82.

pies, treatments that may also be beneficial or harmful to animals and/or man.

The ethical basis of the view developed here is that there is a prima facie duty to maximize the balance of good over evil, where pleasure and pain are among the important goods and evils, and that among the other basic prima facie duties that hold of persons is the duty to respect persons, to treat persons as persons, as beings to be respected, and not simply as means to ends. (Other humanly oriented duties are those of honesty and justice, these holding of persons in respect of persons.) Persons as morally autonomous beings possess moral rights by virtue of their nature as persons, that is, as morally autonomous, rational, sentient, affective beings, the rights including the rights to life, health, bodily integrity, respect as a person and all that that implies, moral autonomy and integrity, self-development and education as dictated by that and other rights, and knowledge and true belief. There are obvious difficulties in the way of providing a justification of such an ethic. The principle of maximizing the balance of good over evil is exposed to the problem that it involves a rejection of the distinction between acts of supererogation and duties proper. However, for the purposes of this [essay], it is not essential that this problem be met as it is the causing of avoidable suffering without good cause that is of central importance here. There is a general acknowledgement and acceptance of the duty not unnecessarily to cause or allow to continue unnecessary suffering. Objections may be urged against the claims that persons ought to be respected, and that, as persons with the nature they possess, they possess as rights of recipience the rights noted above. Here, as also with the principle relating to maximizing the balance of good over evil, appeal must ultimately be made to the self-evidence of the principles and of the possession of these rights by persons.[1]

It is important now to examine the nature of the moral justification of those experiments on animals for the good of animals that are justified. The experiments must be such that the knowledge sought from them cannot be obtained by means that are morally less costly. They must so be planned and structured as to minimize such pain and loss of pleasure as will occur, such scientifically and morally indefensible overtesting as by LD50* tests being avoided, and the pain being lessened where possible by the use of anaesthe-

sia and/or analgesia, and terminated as soon as possible in terms of the completion of the experiment. Such suffering and distress as may be caused by confinement before and after the experiment, and by the confinement and transporting of animals is to be minimized by care in ensuring satisfactory accommodation and conditions of transportation. Experiments so-called which cause hurt or harm to the animals and which merely duplicate past experiments and this not by way of seeking necessary confirmation of past results are such as not to admit of moral justification.

It is not possible to lay down in detail necessary and sufficient conditions for ethically justifiable experiments. This is due in part to the great differences between animals in respect of their capacity to experience pain. All that can be done here is to indicate general guidelines and what practices can have no moral basis. Experiments must be constructed so as to minimize suffering and not use scientifically unnecessary over-testing, overkill methods. More important, animals that may experience pain should be used only when the relevant information sought can be obtained only through them or human beings and not by experiments on non-sentient animals. Further, it is essential, when well-thought-out ethical codes of conduct of animal experiments are laid down, it be ensured that experimentation conform with the required standards. Experimenters, whether they be experimenters on humans or on animals, notoriously fail to conform with the ethical standards laid down for experimentation in the absence of effective controls and supervision.

It is possible to ground a justification of experimentation on animals for the good of animals which conforms with sound ethical criteria of the kind indicated here when it is *experimentation in general* as a scientific tool used to gain knowledge about drugs, toxins, antidotes, and the like, that it is sought to justify, as the use of such a tool overall may be seen to lead to the greatest balance of good over evil. However there are problems in justifying specific, ethically and scientifically well-planned experiments which involve great suffering which it is hoped will produce results beneficial to animals, and which produce no useful outcome, no useful knowledge, and whose value seems to lie simply in the intrinsic value of this knowledge. Yet, in advance of the experiment, it is impossible to know which experiments will provide useful knowledge and useful outcomes. Even after an experiment, the knowledge that is gained may at that time appear to be of no

---

Ed. note: Tests in which 50% of the animals die due to the toxicity of the dose of a substance to which they are exposed.

value, and only much later come to be seen to be of great value. This suggests that it is experimentation as a whole activity, ethically and scientifically well-planned experimentation, not individual experiments as such, that admits of ethical justification by reference to the principle of maximizing the balance of good over evil.

The general justification of experimentation on animals for the sake of persons alone or of persons and animals together is to be set out by reference to the principle of maximizing the balance of good over evil and that of respecting persons. Clearly not to lessen unnecessary, avoidable pain and suffering, vast amounts of pain and suffering of very many persons as by producing and testing drugs, vaccines (these being produced using animals and animal experimentation), therapies to combat diseases such as smallpox, cholera, malaria, poliomyelitis, tuberculosis, and the like, is to act immorally both because it is thereby to fail to lessen preventable suffering of persons, and to show serious lack of respect for persons as persons. To respect the moral rights of persons is to seek to prevent suffering, disablement, degeneration of their bodies, and death that such diseases can bring. Consider the evils that would now be besetting mankind had animal experimentation never occurred in respect of antibiotics, vaccines, and such like, and the evils that would befall mankind if such experimentation were to be stopped today. Without animal experimentation in the past we should still be afflicted by such diseases on a vast scale, we should still be incapable of checking the ravages of septicaemia, gangrene, diabetes and a host of other diseases. Without continued experimentation we shall be exposed to the new strains and new diseases that continue to emerge, golden staphylococcal infection, Legionnaire's disease, AIDS, and the very many other diseases that are emerging.

What distinguishes attempts to justify animal experimentation by reference to respect for persons and for human rights by contrast with maximizing the balance of good over evil is that lack of success in any specific experiment constitutes no problem, as respect for persons dictates not necessarily successful endeavour but endeavour that is rationally based. Much is made by critics of animal experimentation of the difficulty of extrapolating the results of animal experiments as they apply to human beings. There are of course problems here, but they lessen as the animals experimented upon are closer to man. Hence the use of mammals in so many important, productive experiments, experiments beneficial to man.

Those who are morally critical of animal experimentation argue that a vast amount of animal experimentation is unnecessary because it relates to inessentials that could be dispensed with, without loss, cosmetics in particular getting a very bad press on many counts, not least because of the scientifically unnecessary, morally indefensible use of over-testing as in the use of LD50 tests. Clearly a great deal of experimentation relating to substances such as cosmetics is unnecessary because we already have the relevant knowledge. Nonetheless, that cosmetics are inessentials is not in itself a reason for not testing them although it may be a reason for seeking to ban the production and sale of any new, untested cosmetics. However, as long as we have cosmetics in use, testing of their toxicity and their other effects in respect of causing diseases, will continue to be morally important and necessary. Cosmetics as inessentials do not constitute the very special kind of case it is suggested they do. There are many other inessentials such as tobacco, cannabis, the various hallucinatory drugs, addictive drugs such as alcohol, cocaine, and heroin, for example, which need not be used by persons but which are so used, even when their use is prohibited by states, the effects of which it is important to determine. In so far as animal experimentation can help to reveal their effects, and help in the search for counter-measures, antidotes, and the like, to that extent at least animal experimentation has a moral justification provided of course the experiments conform with the kinds of ethical criteria noted above. Not to seek to extend our knowledge of the effects of such substances and of ways of counteracting them, given the difficulty of checking their use, is to show serious disrespect for persons.

It is useful now to consider possible alternatives to the testing of substances, drugs, therapies, treatments that may harmfully affect or benefit mankind by the use of experimentation on animals.

(i) It has been suggested that we could opt immediately to stop animal experimentation, to develop no new substance, drugs, materials by and in industry, treatments, therapies, and to use only those substances we now use and which have been tested up to the present time. So to act would be both foolish and immoral. We do not know all the properties, all the effects, harmful or otherwise, of substances, drugs, therapies used today. It has taken a very long time to gain the very limited knowledge we now have. Consider how long it has taken to learn of many of the important, harmful effects of smoking tobacco, using asbestos, the carcinogenic and other harmful effects of substances and drugs so long unsuspected of having any adverse effects. Very many new substances, pesticides, fertilizers, complex compounds, preservatives, food dyes, sweeteners, thickeners, drugs, antibiotics, have come into use since World War II, such that we know little about their effects today. Our knowledge of the effects of such familiar substances as alcohol, cannabis, heroin, cocaine is very limited; much knowledge remains to be gained, and this in part at least by and through animal experimentation. New poisons are becoming important in our ecosystems because of new interactions, through industrial waste, pollution, the spread of plants to new areas with new climates, and so on. Consider the serious problems that annual rye grass toxicity, industrial waste seeping into river and bay ecosystems, and atmospheric pollution are causing in Australia. It is therefore essential that we extend our knowledge using animal experimentation. Further, bacteria and their hosts, and the hosts of viruses, are continually developing resistance to antibiotics, pesticides, such that new antibiotics and pesticides are continually needed if we are not to be ravaged by new strains of old diseases and old diseases carried by resistant hosts. Golden staphylococcal infection, the spread of malaria after the near conquest of malaria, and like phenomena, bring out the nature of the problem. These new strains create the need for new tests for new drugs and pesticides. Further, new diseases such as AIDS and genital herpes are developing or moving into new populations in such a way as to call for further research using animals where possible, and this, perhaps, in order to develop vaccines as our knowledge increases. It is quite unrealistic to speak as if it is overall possible and desirable to opt to use only those substances now in use. The growing world population, the increased use of resources that must come if the standard of living of those in the Third World is to improve, necessitate the use of new substances and the finding of new uses for substances already in use, with new problems arising, many of which cannot satisfactorily be tackled or solved without resort to experimentation on animals.

There is a school of ethical thought, one which I reject, to the effect that it is immoral to make use of knowledge gained by seriously immoral means, and hence that it is immoral to use such knowledge as that gained by the Nazis in their experiments on inmates of concentration camps. If that reasoning were to be accepted by those opposed to animal experimentation,

they would need to put aside all that we know of substances, drugs, therapies, by means of animal experimentation. They would in addition need to abandon the production and use of vaccines produced using animals whether or not such vaccines were discovered via animal experimentation. So to act would be to opt for vast epidemics, for a vast increase in human suffering, and untimely deaths for untold numbers of persons. So to act would be to opt for a course of blatant immorality.

(ii) Alternatively or complementary to the course advocated in (i), it is suggested that knowledge be sought and that it can be gained using avenues other than experimentation on animals. This suggestion is little short of irresponsible. Our knowledge of physics, chemistry, bio-sciences, is much too limited for us to be able to determine by reference to them what substances in what quantities will be toxic to animals and humans, what will be safe antidotes, which will cause chromosome damage, impairments, which cancer, and the like, and which drugs and treatments will be beneficial. Some of the alternatives to animal experimentation which could if morally available have a limited use are experiments on aborted live human foetuses, human embryos, 'brain dead' human beings—more could be done by way of experiments on such organisms if human body banks where the bodies were kept functioning on support machines were to be instituted—themselves raise significant moral issues which need to be resolved. It is morally vital that those methods of gaining knowledge that involve the least moral cost be used if other things are equal. However it is extremely misleading to suggest that more than an almost insignificant amount of relevant knowledge that is now gained using experiments on animals could at present be obtained by means of morally acceptable methods of other kinds.

(iii) Another approach might be that of relying on observations of effects of substances on humans and animals by way of post-mortems as well as in life, where the substances are those that are encountered or used by some in the course of their lives, for example, in respect of pollutants such as leaded petrol, DDT and other pesticides, addictive drugs used by addicts, and in respect of other materials and drugs, using also observations of the reactions of persons who volunteer to be subjects of experiments where they give free and informed consent to the experiments. Alternatively, it might be suggested that some persons, criminals, incompetents, or the like, be conscripted to be subjects of such experiments. Most accounts of the ethics of human experimentation insist, rightly, that experiments on human beings are morally desirable only if embarked upon after all the relevant preliminary animal experiments have been carried out. To forbid experimentation on animals but to permit experimentation on human conscripts and/or human volunteers who are made necessary because animal experimentation is outlawed, is morally outrageous.

(iv) It might be urged that new drugs, vaccines, therapies, treatments, food dyes, fertilizers, materials used in industry, be used without any testing at all by means of animal experimentation. This is distinct from position (i). There the suggestion is that we opt not to use new substances and processes. Here the proposal is that we use new substances and processes and in effect engage in inefficient testing by observing their effects on humans and animals. Since such haphazard testing would be even more costly in terms of human welfare and human life, and human and animal suffering than would be controlled experiments on a limited number of human beings—conscripts and/or volunteers—and since it would amount to having involuntary subjects of the experiments, it is morally completely unacceptable as an alternative to animal experimentation.

T. Regan in *The Case for Animal Rights* offers no objections of principle to such a contention as the above concerning experimentation on animals other than mammals provided they lack the valued attributes he claims to be possessed by mammals.[2] Non-mammalian animals morally seem to be cast either into a moral limbo or onto a moral scrapheap as having no moral significance in themselves, all Regan's arguments against animal experimentation and research using animals focusing on mammals, and this by reference to the capacities and traits mammals possess which constitute the basis for ascribing them inherent value and possession of rights. By contrast, the foregoing argument implies that if it could and were to be discovered that non-mammals suffered pain, but lacked Regan's other valued capacities experimenting on them would need serious moral justification.

Regan argues that mammals have beliefs, desires, perception, memory, intentions, a sense of the future, self-consciousness *from the age one* on. From this he argues that they are in an important sense autonomous, that they possess what he calls "preference autonomy", the capacity to act on the basis of their preferences. They have interests in two senses, that of preference-satisfaction, and that of having a welfare; they want, desire, prefer various things, and various things are in their interests, biological, social, and psychological. Mammals admit of being harmed. They are claimed to have a psychophysical identity over time. Against the claims of hedonistic utilitarians, Regan stresses that not all harms hurt, where it is morally wrong not only or primarily to hurt, but rather to harm. He distinguishes between moral agents, those beings like man who can act on the basis of their moral beliefs, who possess moral autonomy, and moral patients, mammals other than human beings, beings who are the objects of direct duties, in particular, the duty not to harm, where death, not simply the infliction of suffering, constitute harm. . . .

Regan seeks to show that both moral patients and moral agents, that is all those who meet the subject-of-a-life criterion by reference to his contention that justice dictates the principle of respect, that is that those who possess inherent value, must be treated in ways that respect their inherent value. Possessors of inherent value must in justice be given their due, where their due may be assistance from moral agents. The rights theory is developed as the reverse side of the respect principle, it being explained that possessors of inherent value have a prima facie moral right to respect, this right encompassing the prima facie right not to be harmed. Regan does not seek to explain his theory of moral rights in terms of a list of more specific moral rights of possessors of inherent value. It seems that he sees the rights to life, freedom from harm, to liberty, and the like, where they hold, to be either elements of the basic right to respect or as rights that follow in determinate situations from that right. The principle of respect imposes a duty to help, hence the right to respect is seen as a right of recipience, a right to be helped and not simply not to be harmed or treated without respect.

Moral rights are explained as valid moral claims, where the claims are claims against assignable individuals who owe a duty to the bearer of the rights by virtue of valid principles of direct duties. The basic moral right to respectful treatment is said to be possessed equally as is inherent value by all possessors of inherent value. The assignable individuals against whom the rights claims hold are *all the moral agents*, where the relevant principle validating the rights is the respect principle which prohibits treating moral agents and patients as mere receptacles of intrinsic value as is enjoined by utilitarianism and various other ethical theories. The rights are said to be prima facie in the sense that they may be overridden but only on the basis of an appeal to valid moral principles that override the right in the specific case. . . .

Regan rejects the use of mammals in toxicology on many grounds, the most important being that their use is to treat possessors of inherent value as mere receptacles and thereby to violate their rights. Backup arguments relate to the alleged lack of moral necessity to develop new products. As has already been noted, such a contention cannot be sustained. Toxicity tests continue to be needed for substances long in use, and this because of limitations of our knowledge and the new contexts in which the substances come to be encountered. In any case it is impossible in our politico-socioeconomic conditions to opt to use no new substances. Regan notes but backs away from the possibility of using human volunteers and instead puts his faith in the ultimate development of toxicity tests that are not dependent on the use of humans and mammals, even though the present state of development of scientific knowledge gives no solid grounds for such faith. The problem of determining by tests not involving mammals whether substances are carcinogenic, or harmful in other ways to such organisms and/or their off-spring is even greater, scientists investigating such effects having no alternative other than to experiment on mammals and/or man if they are to enlarge their knowledge. Not to do so would be to opt to allow due to our ignorance very many substances to cause avoidable harm to humans and animals. . . .

[M]ammals other than man, ought not on the basis of our present knowledge of them, to be ascribed possession of natural moral rights by virtue of their alleged possession of inherent value such as to be objects of respect. Rather, our duties towards such mammals are what Regan calls indirect duties, duties *concerning* mammals, rather than duties *to* them. The duties that govern the morality of experimentation on mammals are those of not causing unnecessary, pointless suffering, not needlessly to destroy beautiful animals, and duties so to use such mammals as may be appropriate to seek to reduce animal and human suffering and death, and thereby to show respect for persons. Further . . . even were it the case that mammals other than man possessed natural moral rights, it would still be right and obligatory to perform various experiments

on them in order to respect the natural rights of recipience of persons and other mammalian rights-holders.

. . . [I]t is impossible here for reasons of space to do more than register my belief that Regan's arguments do not establish his claims that mammals (from the age of 1 year) are capable of having (whether to the same extent or degree or not) beliefs, desires, intentions in a core sense of intention, that they are self-conscious in a full sense of self-conscious, having awareness of self-identity over time. The claim that mammals are capable of autonomy, preference autonomy, is more easily exposed as unsound, no convincing argument being offered for the view that autonomy is possessed by all mammals in the primary sense of 'autonomy', that of being able to choose or form one's preferences and choose whether or not to act on the basis of them. The control over both motivation and action that is central to the concept of autonomy needs to be shown to hold of mammals before special value is to be attributed to them by virtue of their possession of autonomy. That Regan acknowledges that such mammals are not moral agents, simply moral patients, beings incapable of moral autonomy—and this because they lack the capacity both to have moral concepts, and to make and act on the basis of moral judgments, that is, because they lack moral autonomy—brings out the very misleading nature of the claim that such mammals possess autonomy, albeit preference autonomy.

On the basis of the many capacities ascribed to mammals it is claimed that they possess what is characterised as inherent value, where inherent value is distinguished from intrinsic value. Two objections arise, here. The one relates to whether there is any sound basis for ascribing any value to such beings. The second concerns whether a concept of inherent value as distinct from intrinsic value has meaning. By way of an extension of Kant's discussion of persons as morally autonomous beings, as ends in themselves possessed of worth, where worth is represented as being distinct from intrinsic value and incommensurably greater than intrinsic value, Regan ascribes to mammals other than man a special value by virtue of their attributes. However there are problems in the way of explaining and justifying Kant's talk about the worth of persons as a kind of value distinct from intrinsic value. Kant more felicitously sought also to express his claim in terms of persons being ends in themselves, where that concept is explained in turn in terms of persons meriting respect. Things have value; persons are to be respected. Regan offers no satisfactory reasons for extending to mammals possessing the capacities he indicates the respect to be attributed to persons, i.e., for attributing to them as the basis of this respect, the idea that they are ends in themselves. The concept of being worthy of respect that Kant sought to catch by speaking of ends in themselves as possessors of worth has no relevance to beings possessed only of the capacities Regan attributes to mammals which he sees as having inherent value and as being moral patients. The dog, cat, rat, cow *qua* possessors of these capacities, do not evidently merit respect. . . .

. . . [O]nly moral agents and potential moral agents who can be represented by guardians may possess moral rights, as the exercise of moral rights involves the capacity for moral judgments, namely, moral awareness of the extent of the liberty the right confers, the entitlements to aids and services that can properly be demanded, and the ability to decide morally whether to insist on or waive that to which one has a right. A guardian may represent a non-moral being in respect of its interests in so far as the guardian can determine what is for that being's good. However it is impossible for a guardian to read or to anticipate the moral mind of a non-moral being in respect of its exercise of its rights. Without a moral capacity, actually or potentially, there can be no moral entitlement, no moral authority, no moral exercise or waiving of a moral right, and hence no moral rights possessed by mammals that lack moral autonomy, actually and potentially.

Regan makes two important claims about moral rights: namely, that similar beings similar in relevant respects have the same rights and that those who possess the same rights possess them equally (p. 267). The right to respect is said to be the basic right, a right held by all rights holders, equally. The rights not to be harmed, not to be killed, are simply elements of that basic right, and therefore ought also to be held by all rights holders, equally. They are all seen by Regan to be prima facie rights. Both of the former claims can be questioned by reference to the rights of promisors, creditors, and children *vis-a-vis* their parents. However here it is more important to discuss the second claim, that rights are held equally by their possessors, and this by reference to Regan's discussion of the right

to life that rightly implies the opposed view. The right to life on Regan's account is not a mere derivative conditional duty, to be derived from the right to respectful treatment; it is an element in that right. Yet Regan explicitly and rightly argues that the right to life of a lesser being, a moral patient, is a less stringent right than is the right to life of a higher being, a moral agent. Thus it is that Regan argues:

"Now the harm that death is, is a function of the opportunities for satisfaction it forecloses, and no reasonable person would deny that the death of any of the four humans would be a greater prima facie loss, and thus a greater prima facie harm, than would be true in the case of the dog." (p. 324)

"Let the number of dogs be as large as one likes; suppose they number a million; and suppose the lifeboat will support only four survivors. Then the rights view still implies that, special considerations apart, the million dogs should be thrown overboard and the four humans saved." (p. 325)

What is true of rights being held equally is that those natural rights that are possessed by virtue of one's nature are possessed equally by those who have their nature in common. Thus if dogs could and did possess natural rights to life, health, etc., it would be on the basis of a different nature from that of persons, and hence would be a different right, with a different stringency from that of the corresponding right of persons. This fact is of importance in determining how conflicts of rights are to be resolved. Basic natural rights are prima facie rights. If all mammals possessed rights such as that to respectful treatment including all its elements, it would be necessary to weigh up the conflicting rights with their different stringencies, as Regan in effect does, in respect of the rights to life of persons and dogs. However it is not only the right to life of persons that may outweigh the right to life of a dog. The rights to health, to bodily integrity, to self-development of persons, as rights of recipience, may outweigh the rights of mammals such as dogs to life, and freedom from suffering. That is to say, once it is acknowledged as it is by Regan that the rights of mammals, if they possess rights, are prima facie rights of recipience, the flood-gates are opened to justify animal experimentation that is scientifically and ethically well-planned, to secure for persons the enjoyment of the more stringent rights of persons, at the expense of the less stringent rights of mammals. In most cases the experimentation will be directed at saving human and animal lives without wrongly calling on persons to be subjects of unnecessary experiments. This use of animals would be comparable with the resort to a fair system of conscription of persons to be combatants who will be exposed to death and injury in a just war. Just as it is wrong to speak of those who are conscripted to serve in a just war as persons who are being treated as mere receptacles, so too if mammals possessed moral rights, it would be wrong to speak of those conscripted to be subjects of harmful, dangerous experiments as a result of a just resolution of a conflict of prima facie rights, as beings who are treated as mere receptacles. Indeed, the moral calculus, to be a morally sound calculus, would necessarily take full account of their possession of natural moral rights, where the rights involved in the conflict are prima facie natural *rights of recipience*. . . .

NOTES

1. For a defence of the ethic sketched in here see my *Meta-Ethics and Normative Ethics* (The Hague: Martinus Nijhoff, 1969), chs. 6, 7, 9, *Ecological-Ethics and Politics* (Totowa: NJ: Rowman and Littlefield, 1983), pp. 70–80 and "The Right to Life," *Mind*, LXXXIV, 1975, pp. 403–25.

2. Tom Regan, *The Case for Animal Rights* (Berkeley and Los Angeles: University of California Press, 1983).

T O M   L .   B E A U C H A M P

Problems in Justifying Research on Animals

For two decades we have witnessed a vibrant discussion of the moral and legal issues presented by research involving *human* subjects. Some of the issues that plagued NIH Director James Shannon and Surgeon General Luther Terry in the mid-1960's, and later Director Robert Marston and Senators such as Jacob Javits and Edward Kennedy in the early 1970's, eventuated in the passage of the National Research Act in 1974, with a provision creating a national commission to examine predominantly ethical issues. After two national commissions, thousands of scholarly publications, and continuous planning and monitoring at NIH, my impression is that we now have a fairly firm hold on the nature of the issues, appropriate regulatory activity, procedures for IRB's, and the like. A decade ago no comparable claim could have been sustained. At that time we were reeling with hesitation under blows inflicted by critics in such cases as Tuskegee,

Willowbrook, and the Jewish Chronic Disease Hospital and on such issues as research with fetuses, prisoners, children, and the mentally infirm.

It would be instructive to compare the history of developments over the last 20 years in the ethics of research involving human subjects with the history during the same period of ethical issues in research with animal subjects. I have little doubt that such an investigation would reveal major advances in treating ethical issues in research with humans, but comparatively minor and sporadic advances in understanding and resolving ethical issues in research with animals. A plausible hypothesis is that in the ethics of animal research we are now no further along than we were in the 1971-72 period when the *Institutional Guide* or "Yellow Book"[1] was first issued and Jay Katz's encyclopedic anthology on experimentation was published.[2] We have some broad ideals, no consensus, some tentative but promising regulations, and a fragmentary collection of scholarly publications; but, for all that, little serious work on the specific subject of ethical issues in

From National Institutes of Health, *National Symposium on Imperatives in Research Animal Use: Scientific Needs and Animal Welfare* (NIH Publication No. 85–2746, 1985), pp. 79–87.

animal research exceeds the level of programmatic proposals and general guidelines. . . .

THE PROBLEM OF ARBITRARY LINES

[A] central issue . . . is the nature of our moral obligation(s), if any, to protect the interests of animals when conducting research. Some influential philosophers have recently argued that there is *no morally relevant difference* between human life and animal life sufficient to justify the claim that *only human life* deserves extensive moral protections. What, they ask, distinguishes the life of a human infant from the life of an adult chimpanzee, so that infants are protected in ways that chimpanzees are not? The idea behind the view that animals do not merit the special protections afforded humans seems to be that animals have a reduced or instrumental value because of their status *as animals*, and this reduced value permits us to value them exclusively, or at least largely, in terms of their value to us. But critics like [Robert] Nozick argue that we need to *justify* our involvement of animals on a rational philosophical basis that takes account of their interests and suffering, and not merely their utility to the human species. Any moral reasons sufficient to forbid certain forms of research on humans, they hold, are also sufficient to forbid research on animals.

From this perspective, there is no consistent way to *draw a line* between human and animal life that will exclude one and include the other in the scope of justified research. It cannot be merely the capacity to feel pleasure and pain that makes the difference, for many animals share that capacity to a significant degree with humans. Nor can it be, for example, that humans have "reason," the "use of language," or "the capacity to interact with the human community" in ways animals do not. In these respects, the retarded, irreversibly comatose, and young infants fall into many relevantly similar categories as animals, or, as Nozick says, chimps may have these same abilities. Wherever the line is drawn between animals and humans, too much will be included or too little excluded in any attempt to extend protections to human subjects alone.

Bernard Rollin contends, correctly I think, that premises built on the idea of there not existing morally relevant differences between humans and animals have served critics of research as "the most powerful tool in the investigation of the moral status of animals." If no morally relevant differences can be defended, it follows logically that the *same* moral concerns extended to humans *must* be extended to animals.[3] However, we have seen and will continue to see many battles over the properties that should count as morally *relevant* differences. It is not a systematically well-formed notion, as we shall now see.

THE APPEAL TO JUSTICE

An argument from principles of justice can be developed from these basic ideas about a lack of morally relevant differences. The so-called "formal principle of justice" asserts that it is impermissible to treat those who are not different differently, but permissible to treat the different differently. (It is *formal* because it states no *particular* respects in which equals ought to be treated the same, or unequals treated unequally.) I shall here assume that this principle is no less applicable to animals than to humans, but I also assume that by itself the principle is powerless to advance the issues over animal research significantly. It is merely an indicator that *whatever* property qualifies humans for moral protection would, *if* possessed by animals, equally qualify the animals for protection.

There are significant philosophical disagreements as to what those properties are, even in the instance of humans. In attempts to *defend* research on animals that could not be carried out on humans, the properties most frequently cited as morally relevant are properties possessed by humans alone. For example, Kant and many others have maintained that only human beings intentionally perform actions that are motivated by *reason* and by *moral rules*. Animals are smart, and perhaps act on reasons; but, they do not act on *moral* reasons or exhibit a *rational will*. Charles Darwin, a classic lover of animals, observed that of the few distinguishing differences between humans and animals, the chief is the capacity to act morally. From this perspective, it might seem a species mistake to treat animals as if they had the same moral status as humans.

However, as Peter Singer has pointed out, this line of argument, if applied to research, also leaves a broad range of *human* subjects unprotected that we would all agree deserve protection.

A difficulty with this argument is that *some* humans come no closer to satisfying the requirement than the animals experimented upon. Mentally retarded human beings, for instance, may be no more rational than a dog; yet we do not consider that they are entirely devoid of rights. . . .

[C]ertain categories of human beings—infants and mentally retarded humans—actually fall below some adult dogs, cats, pigs, or chimpanzees on any test of intelligence, awareness, self-consciousness, moral personality, capacity to communicate, or any other capacity that might be thought to mark humans as superior to other animals. Yet we do not think it legitimate to experiment on these less fortunate humans in the ways in which we experiment on animals.[4]

The formal principle of justice also requires recognition of any *lack* of relevant similarities (i.e., the differences) across classes. Here the possibilities are rich in the case of humans and animals. For example, innumerable differences are only too obvious in comparing humans to rattlesnakes; and thus justice apparently permits treatment of the rattlesnake in at least some quite different ways. . . . [T]he inevitable outcome is that animals do not deserve the *same* scope of rights that humans enjoy, nor will our obligations to animals approximate our obligations to other humans. Any analogy to our obligations to humans or to protections for human subjects of research can easily be carried to absurd extremes if *all* the obligations acknowledged to hold for humans were also under discussion for animals, without taking sufficient account of morally relevant differences. I do not think—and do not think that any fair-minded person thinks—that we have obligations not to deceive animals, obligations to let them vote, and the like. They simply lack the crucial properties that underlie such obligations.

But some humans also lack these properties. A prisoner of war is justifiably denied a great many rights that nonprisoners possess; the POW will lack crucial properties on the basis of which ordinary obligations hold. A prisoner of war, we can rightly say, does not *deserve* such rights. Justice does not demand it, for justice certainly acknowledges the importance of relevant differences such as being a criminal, being a prisoner, being an aggressor, etc. In short, with animals, *as with humans* such as prisoners of war, justice does not demand the full range of rights and obligations, because there are vital—relevant—differences that no analysis can afford to overlook.

Locating the relevant differences in research has proved arduous and contestable, but it is not difficult to spot *some* relevant differences that support research involving animals. Placing fish in (adequately sized) tanks is not a confinement that involves a denial of liberty tantamount to involuntary confinement for (mature, autonomous, and healthy) human subjects. Observational research on the American eagle using video-cameras is not a violation of the eagle's right to privacy. Debeaking chickens to study its effect on their cannibalistic tendencies is painful, but not comparable to cutting a man's nose off to see how it reduces his social aggression. And positive reinforcement of rats and pigeons does not quite seem comparable to Skinner's raising his own daughter in the box. Important differences across the species make such judgments relatively easy.

But, from the fact that there are important differences, it does not follow that there may not also be important similarities that argue against many contemporary research protocols. The most important similarities that come to the fore when we reflect on the use of animals in research stem from capacities for pain and suffering. Jeremy Bentham hammered away at this thesis in the 19th century, yet pain has proved difficult to determine in animals, and suffering even more difficult, partially because of the breadth of the concept of suffering. In the context of animal research, "suffering" is generally used to range over discomfort and disease (as when animals are kept in unsanitary and crowded conditions) as well as tension, anxiety, stress, exhaustion, and fear. Some of the latter categories cannot be easily applied to many animals, but this scarcely suggests that animals do not suffer. Rather, it calls for increased research on these states and the degree of suffering, if any, involved. In any event, this general criterion of pain and suffering provides the reason so many of us resist allowing pregnant baboons to be rammed into walls, rats to be forced to swim until they are exhausted and drown, monkeys to endure severed limbs or bleeding hands, rabbits and cats to suffer raw, swollen and then ruined eyes, and fish to have their eyes enucleated.

Let us now summarize these arguments from justice. *If* some animals share a relatively similar capacity with humans to experience pain and suffering, then we will have to treat them as we would treat humans in order to remain consistent with moral principles that prohibit the causation of pain and suffering. I have isolated the experience of pain and suffering, because I believe intrinsic evil to be the chief concern in the instance of animal research. Others have a similar concern about life itself, and hence would use my same strategy of argument to defend the view that we must treat animals as we would treat humans in order to remain consistent with moral principles that *prohibit the taking of life*. This is not a view I share, although I recognize the force of the claim, its consistency with the formal principle delineated above, and the need to argue against the claim and not merely to assume its mistakenness. That will have to be the subject of another paper.[5] Here I shall set aside questions of permissible killing and bring the discussion in this section to a focus through the following summary argument of the main lines of the argument from justice, which has been advanced by many writers on animal research:[6]

> Treat beings who are similar in the relevant respects the same and treat beings who are different in the relevant respects differently and in direct proportion to the differences between them. (This is the formal principle of justice.)

> Because pain and suffering are undesirable, and because both human and nonhuman animals are capable of pain and suffering, there is at least a *prima facie* case for treating all animals (both human and nonhuman) similarly when the infliction of pain and suffering is involved.

> It follows that, with regard to research that involves pain and suffering, there is a presumption against treating human beings and animals differently unless grounds for a distinction can be shown. That is, if we justifiably treat animals differently from human beings there must be some morally relevant property that one group possesses but the other does not that is relevant to how they should be treated.

> For any property proposed, either some animals possess it or some human beings do not—i.e., there are no morally relevant properties sufficient to justify research that all human beings possess but no animals do.

> Therefore, with regard to research that inflicts pain and suffering, there is no basis for treating *all* human beings one way and *all* animals another. There will always be some human beings on whom it is morally permissible to perform an experiment if it is permissible to perform the experiment on all animals.

> Therefore, if risk of pain and suffering is involved, either it is morally permissible to experiment on certain classes of human beings [without their consent] or it is morally wrong to experiment on at least some animals.

This is a powerful argument that could be applied in a variety of ways. For example, one could use this argument to contend that if the following Proposition I is morally sound, then, as a local matter, so is Proposition II:

> "Human experimentation that involves X level of pain or suffering and that is carried out solely for nontherapeutic, informational purposes is never justified if neither the subjects of the experiment nor a beneficent proxy is able to give informed consent."

> "Animal experimentation that involves X level of pain or suffering and that is carried out solely for nontherapeutic, informational purposes is never justified if neither the subjects of the experiment nor a beneficent proxy is able to give informed consent." . . .

I believe any argument exclusively from justice must lead to this conclusion *if* animals fall under what Tom Regan has called "the postulate of inherent value," according to which all moral agents *and patients*—any creatures who are the *subjects*-of-a-life—are *equal in inherent value*. Using this postulate, Regan rejects all views that humans, having more abundant intellectual, artistic, and moral skills, therefore have more inherent value and thus can justly compel animals to serve human needs and interests.[7] Regan accepts the postulate of inherent value (1) because he views it as *arbitrary* to exclude animals from the realm of creatures with inherent value once we recognize that we have obligations *directly* to the animals and (2) because he believes our considered reflective beliefs to support his contentions.[8]

I think the problem is actually deeper than the arguments he presents acknowledge. We seem here to encounter a metaphysical dispute about the universe of values (and perhaps also one about the acceptability of his views in light of its *implications*). Regan's conviction is that humans and animals "have value of the same kind."[9] The metaphysical problem of whether dogs, chickens, and lizards have less value than humans, and indeed whether there is relatively more or less value across species that reflects our expression "lower on the phylogenetic scale" is not a matter that can be decided by formal justice or equality. As Regan himself observes, it is the other way around: "One's views on the metaphysical question of value will determine one's material principles of justice and equality."[10] While I shall here assume, in disagreement with Regan, that there are different levels of value that attach to creatures in nature, I do so as a presupposition rather than through a process of argument. At the same time, Regan's argument should be met, and thus far the literature has not provided an adequate response.[11] This *may* be because we are here at the level of *absolute presuppositions*, to use R. G. Collingwood's basic category of metaphysical propositions.

THE ANALOGY TO HUMAN SUBJECTS RESEARCH

The above arguments from justice are not designed to prohibit or cripple research with animals, nor would I come close to recommending a moratorium. Some research seems clearly warranted on grounds of the suffering alleviated, which on balance outweighs the suffering caused. But questions remain as to how much suffering, who does the balancing, and whose interests are to be entered into the balancing.

One procedural rule that ought to be resolutely protected is that all research should be subjected to impartial review. To resort again to the history of human subjects research, in the 1950's and early 1960's—and in conformity with a prevailing skepticism about government-imposed standards and a climate conducive to freedom of research—the Public Health Service had been largely content to place sole responsibility for research involving human subjects on the investigator, whose professional judgment was to control the amount and types of information to be disclosed, as well as ethical standards that were to apply. By the mid-1960's, deep concerns would abound both about simple appeals to the moral virtues of investigators and about the lack of Federal regulations with teeth to control the conduct of those who receive Federal grants. Reports of many distressing abuses, together with a substantial increase in funding for research involving human subjects, led officials at NIH to appreciate that federally funded research could be ethically insensitive and could be initiated without adequate peer review or consent procedures.[12]

Actual and potential horrors in animal research are now leading us to similar conclusions, and as a result we will increasingly be pushed in the direction of regulatory initiatives. What I would hope could now be seriously discussed is an increased transference of analogous parts of the IRB apparatus to animal research. The current discussion centering on animal research committees, or ARC's, promises to be just such a development, and I find it a wholly salutary, albeit still underdeveloped initiative. The new emphasis on research and review rather than care (as in the old "animal care committees," which focused on facilities and care) are indications that the idea of a

serious review of the ethical quality of the research has taken hold. Also encouraging is the emphasis mandating lay members on these committees. Again, similar developments occurred in the history of the development of IRB's.

The model of transferring human subjects review will of course have its limits. Certain parts of the IRB apparatus could not be invoked in reviewing animal research without considerable departure from mainline practices in biomedical and behavioral research with human subjects. First-party consent makes no sense for animals, but then it makes no sense in research involving newborn infants either, for a proxy—in the language of the title of this panel—serves as "steward." We will simply have to struggle not to overgeneralize and not to apply moral constraints where they do not fit the context of experimentation with animals.

But I still think it will prove helpful to start with analogous parts of operative or proposed regulations governing certain kinds of research such as fetal research and research involving children. By generalizing from the various provisions and subjecting them to criticism, they could be adapted to regulations governing animals. The following rough rules, for example, could be used as a starting point:

1. All research must be reviewed, and all conflicts of interest (on ARC's or similar bodies) must be avoided.
2. Local review by ARC's should operate pursuant to Federal regulations that establish the composition of and rules for such committees.[13] The committees should also work closely with investigators, ethologists, and veterinarians in improving the ethical quality of the research.
3. The risk of pain and suffering should be minimized, and thresholds of allowable pain and suffering should be established. No research should be carried out if it exceeds the threshold levels. (Thus, "unnecessary suffering" is not the sole or main criterion.)
4. If the threshold in point 3 is not exceeded, benefits of the research can justify the risks and cost involved in using the animals; but the moral costs and the animals' interests must be an integral part of any balancing process.
5. If an animal must be killed, this must be accomplished by a means that is as painless as possible

(e.g., following the procedure established in the American Veterinary Medical Association Panel on Euthanasia).

6. An advocate for the animals should present a case for reduced risk before any review committee (in lieu of consent).

7. An ARC should not only approve all research protocols prior to their submission to a PHS agency, but should monitor the progress of the research and should be empowered to halt the research if it fails to adhere to appropriate standards.

8. There must be sound reasons for performing the research, and it must be based on a sound scientific methodology.

The aforementioned problems of pain and suffering would entail some careful guidelines for investigators and review committees to use in planning and evaluating research, including a grading of research procedures as to their noxious, aversive, or painful properties. This task too will be arduous, but we might begin with the following grading system established by Swedish authorities:[14]

No doubt [these] rules and grading system will not escape controversy. One focus of the discussion is sure to center on whether a threshold of pain and suffering can and should be established. Thus, Rule #3 is likely to be among the most contested of the above rules. The argument against it will be that any threshold proposed will be too restrictive, because some valuable research will have to be foregone merely because of the threshold. That is, the threshold in Rule #3 will on occasion prohibit the kind of balancing of benefits and harms proposed in Rule #4, because a threshold rule trumps a balancing rule. Many will want to see Rule #3 struck, relying entirely on Rule #4. But this, of course, is antithetical to my proposal. Anyone would be saddened by the loss of valuable research, but this is scarcely a sufficient reason for putting animals through terrible pain and suffering. In research with human subjects we insist on such thresholds (at least in nontherapeutic research), and I am simply suggesting that we use this model for animals.

The most important problem, in my judgment, is not *whether* to require a threshold but *where* to draw the line. Of related importance is whether the line will shift across the different animal species, and thus whether the type of permitted research will be species-

Research Techniques, Pain, and Distress

Categories	Examples
1. No pain or only minimal and momentary pain	Injections,* blood samples, tube-feeding,* diet experiments,* breeding studies, behavioral studies without aversive conditioning, routine procedures from small animal veterinary practice
2. Animals painlessly killed or anesthetized animals not allowed to recover	Blood pressure studies, organ and tissue removal, studies on organ survival, perfusion experiments
3. Surgery on anesthetized animals with recovery but where postoperative pain will be minimal	Biopsies, transfusion or vascular studies, cannulation, castration, pituitary removal in rodents using standard techniques, some CNS lesions
4. As above but with considerable postoperative pain	Major surgical operations, burn studies, graft studies
5. Experiments planned on unanesthetized animals expected to become seriously ill from the treatment or to suffer considerable pain or distress	Toxicity testing, radiation, transplants of tumors or infections, stress, shock or burn studies, behavior experiments involving aversive conditioning
6. Experiments on unanesthetized animals (or only local anesthesia) where the animal is curarized or paralyzed	Some physiological or pharmacological studies on CNS

Source: Adapted from Ross, 1978.

*These procedures may produce pathological states (e.g., injection of pathogens, feeding of toxic chemicals) and, if so, would have to be graded differently.

relative. I have no ready solution for these problems and would be the first to agree that the task of determining thresholds will be formidable. But this is no reason for avoiding the task.

Many of us do not have to reach far for starting points in research that has actually been performed and reported in the literature. (One of the major sources of today's detailed regulations involving *human* subjects was Henry Beecher's pioneering use of *published* reports of research which he turned into mini-case studies.) Richard Ryder[15] and others have supplied us with endless lists of such cases, but I cannot pass up the opportunity to report on one case that Edmund Pellegrino brought to my attention: In an attempt to study shock and shock therapy for burn victims, shock was induced in pigs, dogs, and other animals (not, of course, under anesthesia) by means of a blow torch. This example does not provide a ready threshold for our needs, but it gives a clear example of the kind of research that many of us would ban no matter the potential for understanding burns and shock. This, of course, is where the debate will get rough, because, again, many would prefer the suffering of dogs and pigs to be a part of the balancing process in Rule #4, whereas I would invoke Rule #3 and say that we shall simply have to learn about burns and shock from their actual victims.

Rule #5 will also cause resistance among those who fear that research will be dismantled by these rules, but something like this rule must be an integral part of any adequate program. It is possible that an adequate set of provisions for Rule #2 could suffice to replace Rule #5. In particular, if strict rules about lay membership governed the composition of the review committees, it might not be necessary to have advocates. Here we need to study carefully the successes and failures of the Swedish system of review, in which regional review boards are divided into equal numbers of lay members, scientists, and technicians. However, I am skeptical that workable rules governing composition would eventuate in a presentation of the strongest case in defense of the animals, and hence I am reluctant to yield Rule #5. There is reason to suspect that IRB's do not always deliberate with the thoroughness that they should to protect human subjects,[16] and the likelihood of such neglect would dramatically increase in the instance of many animal subjects.

This is likely to prove a particularly sticky matter, because the problem of fair review and advocacy can run in the other direction as well: Militants on a review committee can attempt to block good research for largely irrelevant reasons, or the value of the research may simply be neglected or deflected by other concerns. Again, however, I am skeptical that this will prove to be a major problem. It has not surfaced as an issue in IRB review, and the use of *local* committees seems to me more than an adequate protection against this problem. The more difficult issue, in my judgment, is the related issue raised in Rule #1: avoidance of conflict of interest. A local review committee stacked with animal researchers can provide adequate *peer* review without providing adequate *distance* from the research and without ensuring adequate institutional accountability. The British were onto this problem, when a Royal Commission on cruelty to animals wryly reported in 1876 that "The Inspectors must be persons of such character and position as to command the confidence of the public no less than that of men of science."[17] Since the British system was written to depend strictly on the vigilance and sense of duty of the inspectors, one can imagine the controversy that surrounded their precise credentials, as well as acts that would disqualify them. Proposals for rules to govern both avoidance of conflict of interest and proper institutional "assurances" were then highly controversial, and they are likely to be so today in the United States.

Although I am inclined to defend each rule on the above list of rules, my objective has not been to present fixed necessary and sufficient moral requirements. My main purpose has been to propose a *procedure* for modeling protections for animals on protections for human subjects. The local review process seems to me the most promising mechanism we have, although more detailed rules about conflict of interest, proper representation on the committees, and the like would have to be fashioned in order to avoid further moral complications. But with satisfactory rules of this description in place, I would be willing to accept the outcome of such deliberations no matter the particular recommendation, because conditions of procedural due process have been satisfied. Such institutional procedures will certainly not resolve all conflicts or ambiguities, and will no more satisfy every investigator or protector of animals than IRB's satisfy all parties at present. But such review is nonetheless the best mechanism we have for fair and impartial outcomes once fair and impartial procedures have been established and observed. . . .

I am not prepared to propose a more extensive set of concrete guidelines than Rules 1–8 above, but I do suggest that we will have to develop them if review committees and scholarly examinations of the ethics of animal research are to advance significantly. It is not enough to parade anecdote after anecdote of horrors in crushing the spines of cats or injecting toxic chemicals into the butts of rats. We have learned by now that intuitions are not enough, and indeed are a disaster that breeds both the careless use of animals and considerable and justified enmity by scientists at the ill-informed comments of some critics.

CONCLUSION

I have argued that when we discuss animal rights and human obligations to animals we should be quite specific about the particular right or the particular obligation being defended. To confer a general right to life on animals potentially could have devastating implications for scientific research, and an equally significant impact on those who raise, slaughter, and market animal products. Active opposition to such a general right is consistent with support of an obligation not to cause extreme, undue, or avoidable suffering—a proposition with less devastating implications for human endeavors, but with major significance for animal welfare. The obligation to review research protocols through an impartial committee also has no imperious consequences for scientific research. The point is that—whether we use the language of *rights* or of *obligations*—the acceptability of a moral argument will vary dramatically in accordance with the right or obligation under discussion, and the defense offered in its behalf. I hope that we have moved beyond the dark days when the debate concerned whether we have any obligations to animals whatsoever.[18]

NOTES

1. *The Institutional Guide to DHEW Policy on Protection of Human Subjects* (Washington, D.C.: DHEW Publication No. (NIH) 72–102, December 1, 1971).

2. Jay Katz, ed., *Experimentation with Human Beings* (New York: Russell Sage Foundation, 1972).

3. Bernard E. Rollin, *Animal Rights and Human Morality* (Buffalo, N.Y.: Prometheus Books, 1981), p. 58.

4. Peter Singer, "Animal Experimentation: Philosophical Perspectives," in *The Encyclopedia of Bioethics*, ed. Warren Reich (New York: Free Press, 1978), Vol. I, p. 81. The basic ingredients of this line of argument are all present in Jeremy Bentham's *The Principles of Morals and Legislation* (Oxford, England, 1789), Chap. 17, Sect. 1.

5. The central lines of a solution to this problem were long ago outlined by Bentham (*Principles of Morals and Legislation*): "If the being eaten were all, there is very good reason why we should be suffered to eat such of them as we like to eat: we are the better for it, and they are never the worse. They have none of those long-protracted anticipations of future miseries which we have. The death they suffer in our hands commonly is, and always may be, a speedier, and by that means a less painful one, than that which would await them in the inevitable course of nature. . . . But is there any reason why we should be suffered to torment them? Not any that I can see. Are there any why we should *not* be suffered to torment them? Yes, several. . . ."

6. I am indebted for various parts of the wording in this argument to articles by Tom Regan, Alister Browne, and Louis Katzner. See the earliest published version, Tom Regan, "The Moral Basis of Vegetarianism," *Canadian Journal of Philosophy* 5 (October 1975): 181–214; the latest and most extensive version is Tom Regan, *The Case for Animal Rights* (Berkeley: University of California Press, 1983), Chaps. 7–9, esp. pp. 232f, 239–41, 243–45, 264.

7. Regan, *The Case for Animal Rights*, pp. 236–37.

8. Ibid., pp. 240, 243, 258–61.

9. Tom Regan, "Animal Experimentation: First Thoughts," in his *All That Dwell Therein* (Berkeley: University of California Press, 1982), p. 72.

10. Regan, *The Case for Animal Rights*, p. 248.

11. One of the best and most direct responses is Michael Fox, "'Animal Liberation': A Critique," *Ethics* 88 (January 1978): 106–18, esp. 112–14. (With a Reply by Peter Singer and Tom Regan, and a final Reply by Fox.)

12. In late 1963, after discussions with the Office of U.S. Surgeon General, Director Shannon asked a research resource division at NIH to investigate these problems and make a report with recommendations. An Associate Chief for Program Development, Dr. Robert B. Livingston, issued a report on November 4, 1964: The report warned of "possible repercussions of untoward events which are increasingly likely to occur." It noted the absence of an applicable code of conduct for research and a very uncertain legal context. Surgeon General William H. Stewart ultimately issued a policy statement on February 8, 1966, that would become a landmark. This "Statement of Policy" compelled institutions receiving Federal grant support from PHS to "provide prior review of the judgment of the principle investigator or program director by a committee of his institutional associates." The three topics required to be reviewed were: (1) the rights and welfare of subjects, (2) the appropriateness of methods used to obtain informed consent, and (3) the balance of risks and benefits.

13. This should include the kind of "Animal Welfare Assurance" and "Principles" outlined in "Proposed Public Health Service Policy on Humane Care and Use of Animals by Awardee Institutions" (Bethesda, Md.: NIH, DHHS, Office for Protection from Research Risks, 1984), esp. pp. 1, 5–7, as well as more specific requirements that follow the main lines of the proposals in the several rules I am suggesting. Cf. *Guide for the Care and Use of Laboratory Animals* (Bethesda, Md.: DHEW, DHHS, NIH Publication No. 80–23, revised 1978), first published 1963.

14. Adapted by Rowan, *Of Mice, Models, and Man*, from M. W. Ross, "The Ethics of Animal Experimentation: Control in Practice," *Australian Psychologist* 13 (1978): 375–78.

15. Richard Ryder, *Victims of Science: The Use of Animals in Research* (London: Davis-Poynter, 1975) and his earlier "Experiments on Animals," in S. and R. Godlovitch and J. Harris, eds., *Animals, Men, and Morals* (New York: Taplinger, 1972).

16. See National Commission for the Protection of Human Subjects of Biomedical and Behavioral Research, *Report and Recommendations: Institutional Review Boards*, DHEW Publication No. (OS) 78–0008 (1978); and *Appendix to Report and Recommendations: Institutional Review Boards*, DHEW Publication No. (OS) 78–0009 (1978). See also John A. Robertson, "Taking Consent Seriously: IRB Intervention in the Consent Process," *IRB* 4 (May 1984): 1–5.

17. As quoted in R. S. Vine, "Legislating Against Cruelty," in Paul Turner, ed., *Animals in Scientific Research: An Effective Substitute for Man?* (London: Macmillan, 1983), p. 212.

18. I am indebted to Terry Pinkard for several discussions on these issues and for his permission to rely on a section of an introduction on animal research in our anthology *Ethics and Public Policy*, 2nd ed. (Englewood Cliffs, N.J.: Prentice-Hall, 1983). I am also grateful to Edmund Pellegrino, Ruth Faden, Robert Veatch, and William May for useful criticisms of this paper.

Ethical Review of Research

ROBERT M. VEATCH

Institutional Review Boards: Professional or Representative?

Advisory and review committees have emerged in the last decade as a major force in the scientific enterprise. Critics plead for increasingly stringent and inclusive review mechanisms while researchers see scientific progress grinding to a halt as if "someone had deliberately set out to destroy all major research efforts." Human experimentation committees, now generally referred to as institutional review boards (IRBs), constitute the most significant example. If these committees are to serve the purpose of providing adequate protection of potential research subjects while also furthering important research objectives, it is critical that there be a conscious, carefully worked out understanding of the various proposed models of IRBs so that the best alternative model may be chosen. The aim of this [essay] will be to work toward achieving this end.

Reprinted from Robert M. Veatch, *The Patient as Partner: A Theory of Human Experimentation Ethics* (Bloomington, Ind.: Indiana University Press, 1987), pp. 108–109, 115–120, 122–123, 233.

Since its opening, over 460 multiple assurances and over 4,750 single assurances have been filed for research involving human subjects with the National Institutes of Health, a division of the Department of Health and Human Services (DHHS), not including boards not directly related to the federal government requirements. This makes the sheer size of the movement an important case study.

A second, more theoretical feature of the committees also makes their study important. As an effort to bring interdisciplinary professionals and laypersons into the scientific advisory and review process they are an intermediate case between two models of the review committee. On the one hand is the interdisciplinary professional review model. The national technology assessment panels are examples. Recognizing that scientific policy review and technology assessment are complicated tasks requiring many skills, review committees are not limited to natural scientists. Sociologists, lawyers, clergy and professional philosophers are included.

At the other extreme is what might be called the "jury model." The jury is one of the most potent voices of the ordinary person. Its task is to reflect the common sense of the reasonable person. Expertise relevant to the case at hand is not only not necessary, it often disqualifies one from serving on the jury.

A slight variant on the jury model is what might be called the representative model. As with the jury model the representative model of committee responsibility requires no specific substantive, technical skill. It does, however, require a generalized skill not found in the jury member. The representative ought to be skilled in perceiving and communicating the views of his or her constituents.

Probably no advisory or review committee functions in the ideal type jury model, although paradoxically judicial case law, which is the source of any of the rules of review in groups like IRBs, depends directly on the jury's judgment. The community advisory boards of local hospitals approach the notion of expertise that stands behind the jury or representative models. Diverse, clearly lay representation is expected. To the extent community elections to the committees are based on any concept of expertise at all, the notion of expertise is highly generalized. Elected individuals are expected to be generally wise and skilled in communicating the community's views, not in specific substantive areas like medicine, hospital administration, or law.

IRBs at the moment stand somewhere between the two extremes of the interdisciplinary professional as model and the jury model. Over the last decade they have evolved, broadening their base of representation. Currently they are beginning to look very much like interdisciplinary groups of professionals, but there are clear signs of movement toward the jury or at least the representative model. Behind this shift stands a movement in our understanding of the nature of these committees and the kinds of problems they must solve. . . .

A. GENERAL PURPOSES

At the most general level the purposes of the experimentation committee are fairly clear. The task is to protect human subjects from possible harms and wrongs that they might suffer during the course of biomedical and now behavioral research. It does this by assuring that the risks to subjects are reasonable in relation to anticipated benefits, if any, to subjects and the importance of the knowledge that may reasonably be expected to result, by assuring adequately informed consent, protection of privacy, equitable subject selection, and so forth.

. . . [T]here are some inconsistencies when the DHHS on the one hand uses the committee structure to accomplish these important objectives while at the same time it does not require that *all* research using humans be subject to IRB review. In spite of such inconsistencies, however, the general objectives of the committees are reasonably well defined. What skills are necessary in order to assess risks and welfare, to determine what information is necessary for an adequately informed consent, and to project risks and benefits to the subject and society?

B. SKILLS FOR RESPONSIBLE COMMITTEE REVIEW

While guidelines for committee selection speak freely of necessary competencies, experience, and maturity, no one seems to have given serious attention to exactly what these might be. If it is true that the IRB is an ambiguous case somewhere between the interdisciplinary professional model and the more representative model, we would expect both kinds of skills to be necessary.

1. Professional Skills. From the beginning the committees have done a decent job of accumulating a group with knowledge of the science involved in the research. The committee must judge the benefits of the research, its scientific merit, how much will be learned, and what specific harms might come to the subjects. This is the kind of skill one would expect from a committee set up as a group of the researcher's "institutional associates." His peers should be capable of contributing these skills. Barber found that in four-fifths of the institutions in his study, most of the committee members came from the highest levels including clinical, administrative, and academic hierarchies. At others, the majority came from the intermediate level, but nowhere was the majority from the lower levels of the professional hierarchy.[1]

It is now also recognized that other, non-medical professional skills are essential. There must be knowledge of the law, social science, psychology, and religious traditions if judgments about informed consent, psychological benefits and risks, and rights of subjects are to be made. Knowledge of and ability to analyze the language and structure of arguments has led to adding philosophers to committees as an essential component. Even so, Barber's group found relatively small numbers of these professionals: From personnel within the institution, eighteen percent of the committees had nurses, nine percent lawyers, another nine percent had members of the board and behavioral scientists. From outside the institution four percent had lawyers, five percent behavioral scientists, and four percent clergymen. One institution had a patient representative.[2] It seems likely that members with these non-medical professional skills will remain in a minority of many committees. This, I will argue later, raises some important theoretical problems about the committee's willingness to take risks.

It seems to me that possession of all of these professional skills is essential for the committee to function according to its present mandate. It is naive to believe that laymen can pick up value-relevant scientific facts without professional assistance. Recent studies reported in a professional journal or at a scientific meeting may make the research redundant. Tests may have predictable side effects anticipated only by those knowing in detail the methods used. A new legal decision across the country may place the committee and the researchers in jeopardy if a protocol is approved. Psychological harm may go quite unnoticed to the untrained eye. All of this makes these professional inputs essential.

2. Representative or Jury Skills. The recent recognition that the committees must also have the ability to judge community attitudes, community acceptance, and what the reasonable patient/subject would want to know about the research has complicated the skill requirements tremendously. . . .

The principle of the reasonable person as the proper judge of what is required for an informed consent and the claim that a professional consensus is not an adequate measure of what the reasonable person would want to know have crucial significance for the functioning of the IRB. Professionals are by definition a special class with a special perspective on critical issues in the experimentation situation. As such they are particularly lacking in competence in judging what the reasonable layperson would want to know for his or her consent to be informed. Professionals are unique not only in their socioeconomic status and their ethnic and sex group, but more critically in their occupation. Medical researchers, by definition, have a unique commitment to the value of research. If they are asked to

evaluate the relative harms to the subject in comparison to the benefits to be gained by society from the pursuit of knowledge, they cannot avoid incorporating their conviction that scientific knowledge is valuable.

The problem is not simply one of cronyism. Biases created by the necessity of evaluating the research of one's personal friends and colleagues (occasionally of committee members themselves) produce some difficulties, but, in my opinion, those difficulties are not nearly as critical as the ones created by unique values held in common among a group of professionals committed to common ends—such as the pursuit of knowledge. Obviously the American Civil Liberties Union member, the construction worker, the welfare rights organizer, or the housewife would have very different instincts, but these people—the ones who might serve on a jury to determine reasonableness of the information given for informed consent—very rarely get to serve on experimentation committees. It is the task of the committee to determine how to trade off the welfare and rights of the subject against the benefits to the subject and to society, and to determine how much information is necessary for an informed consent. The determination must logically be influenced by the makeup of the committee. The absence of these "jury" or "representative" skills must influence the outcome of the review. For jury or representative skills the subject would be much better served—at least in theory—by a committee of peers of the subject rather than peers of the researcher.

C. IMPLICATIONS FOR COMMITTEE THEORY

Here then is the dilemma of the IRB: Both the professional skills and the representative or jury skills are essential, yet the two are mutually exclusive. Perhaps by chance some proper combination of professions will be able to represent the views of the reasonable person—that would be fortuitous, but unlikely. Even if that were possible, the egalitarianism and dignity of the layperson would be challenged by the professionalization of the reasonable person. It is a conclusion which saddens me, for practical solutions to the dilemma will be difficult and perhaps sometimes impossible but I believe it an inevitable conclusion which follows logically from the analysis. As one who believes fervently in the good which can come from biomedical and behavioral research, I do not want to see it mired in the continual struggle over an acceptable mechanism for review. But compromises will probably not resolve the dilemma. The theoretical implications are great. A few will be outlined.

1. The Impossibility of Neutralizing Systematic Bias. Recognizing that biomedical scientists have special perspectives, recent mandates for committees have attempted to neutralize bias by adding representatives of other professional disciplines, or even of patient and community groups. The scientist has long recognized that biases are of two types: random and systematic. The professional committee—even in its older, narrower form that included only biomedical scientists—does an excellent job of eliminating random bias. The success-driven researcher with a warped moral perspective is held in check by colleagues with more balanced perspectives. But the systematic value perspectives of the professional group (the use of scientific models, the love of rationality, and most important, the quest for knowledge and scientific progress—these values which all scientists ought to share) in principle cannot be eliminated by the establishment of a committee of those who hold those unique values. What is more, while the addition of other professional groups may eliminate the peculiar scientific value patterns, it almost certainly does not eliminate the wider constellation of values held by the educated, professional class as a whole. Even adding patient or community representatives will only dilute these systematic biases, not eliminate them. As long as one professional is on the "jury," the panel will be skewed from the view of the reasonable layperson.

2. Risk Shift and Its Implications for Experimentation Committees. An interesting phenomenon has been discovered in social psychology research in the last decade that has great potential significance for the experimentation committee. Stoner discovered that the process of decision making by committee in and of itself had a measurable impact on the decision.[3] His initial work led to the conclusion that committees as a whole reach decisions that permit more risky choices than the average of the individual views of the members of the committee would suggest. If this is the case among human experimentation committees, then the committee designed to protect subjects from extravagant risks undertaken by individual researchers will, in

fact, be institutionalizing a decision-making mechanism that systematically increases the willingness to take risks on behalf of the subject. The risk-shift, as the phenomenon has been called, would, of course, still place limits on the most wild, individual risk-takers, but on average, the committee would systematically shift the judgment in favor of taking risks on behalf of the subjects.

There are several theories of why this takes place. One plausible explanation is that many committees have more high-risk takers than low-risk takers. Since, if each were to speak his or her mind, more high-risk taking opinions and arguments would be voiced, then everyone on the committee would shift somewhat in the risk-taking direction. This hypothesis has been tested by forming committees dominated by minimal-risk people, and the predicted anti-risk shift took place.[4]

The implications for experimentation committees are tremendous. If the committee includes a scientist, a clergyman, and maybe a representative of the community as anti-risk takers, in all likelihood they will stand in the minority. Even a feisty member of such a minority will find it extremely difficult to withstand the psychological pressure to cooperate in forming a consensus.

For the normal committee, however, the dominance of the committee by scientific professionals would produce the risk-shift in the direction of the researchers' values—normally in favor of the research. That is not to suggest that the scientific members of the committee are manipulative or even that they fail to exercise utmost caution in attempting to protect subjects and serve their interests—it is simply the nature of the group process. Even if it were the case that those with representative skills stood in the majority and a shift in the committee took place in the direction of those selected to serve as the peers of the subject, the consensus would still be influenced or moderated by the other perspective, thus supporting more risk than those with representative skills were willing to take.

3. Judgments of Scientific Merit. One of the tasks most often thought to require professional, scientific competence is the judgment of scientific merit of the proposal. Some have even proposed division of labor with one committee made up of scientists to judge the scientific merit of the proposal and another, more interdisciplinary or lay, to judge the ethical dimensions. Even here, however, if this analysis is correct, the matter is much more complicated. Merit is an ethical, or at least a value, word. We should be aroused when it is suggested that such value judgments can be made scientifically. We should separate two tasks. First, the protocol must be reviewed to see whether the results sought can theoretically be obtained by the methods, sampling, and design proposed. It seems that evaluation can be most competently carried out by scientists. Second, however, is the task of deciding how valuable the findings would be if the research is worthwhile (another value term). This second judgment will require insight into the possible future uses of the research, which may require great scientific skills, but in the end judgments of worthiness are not scientific. Even the pure science argument that accumulation of knowledge for its own sake with nothing more than a theoretical faith that something good may come out of it justifies the research, is a non-scientific value argument. If risks to subjects are to be evaluated in part in terms of the value of the knowledge to be gained, then certainly the reasonable person's judgment must be the standard-enterprise—unless scientists are used as subjects. . . .

CONCLUSIONS

The human experimentation committee is a fascinating case of an interdisciplinary or lay policy committee in the biomedical enterprise. Unlike both the national technology assessment panels and the community hospital advisory boards, the experimentation committees are clearly more than advisory groups. They have the power to approve or block research. They stand midway between the other two committees on the dimension of whether the committee is an interdisciplinary professional group or a lay group qualified because of the degree to which they represent community attitudes or the "reasonable person."

I have tried to show that both models are important to the experimentation committee and we have not adequately understood how the two tasks are related. I am more and more convinced that the real conflict is not between the scientific committees, which are made up of peers of the researcher (committees of associates) on the one hand, and the broader interdisciplinary professional groups on the other, but rather between the committees made up of professionals (including interdisciplinary professional committees) and those that are truly lay committees chosen because they are either typical reasonable people or because they have skills to represent the typical person.

It appears to me that the trend is clearly in the direction of a broader, more lay membership of these committees. The informed-consent court cases require that the committee be skilled in understanding the reasonable person's perspective. The courts tell us that professionals—at least medical professionals—cannot be presumed to have that perspective.

The move toward committees of half scientists and half laypeople and other professionals is part of this trend, but that cannot be the answer. The consensus of that group in principle cannot approximate the community judgment (unless one hypothesizes that the different professional groups counterbalance one another—and that seems unlikely). Even a committee of half professionals and half laypersons would not meet the objections of the representative or jury model. Two solutions seem possible.

First, the task of experimentation review could be turned over to a group more skilled in representing the community attitudes or the views of the reasonable person. At the moment, the most obvious candidate is the community hospital advisory board in institutions that have such boards. They have been elected or selected for their capacity to represent the layperson, the consumer of the hospital's services. Why these boards have not played a larger role in experimentation review is not clear to me. Certainly if they were to take on this task they would have to be provided with a supporting staff capable of providing the professional skills obviously needed and now obtained through the interdisciplinary professional group.

Second, we might have to resort to dual committees. One would be made up of professionals charged with the professional tasks of determining scientific feasibility and also judging ethical acceptability from their perspective in terms of risks and benefits, informed consent, and the knowledge to be gained. We would not expect that committee to hand down judgments to reflect the reasonable person's standards, but they would provide for the introduction of the professional skills, including judgments of risks knowable only to one with the appropriate training. The second committee would be the community committee, which would have to have, as before, adequate professional staff and would make value judgments of scientific worthiness as well as the more obviously ethical judgments.

I am inclined to think that this is a more practical, fail-safe solution. Exactly what these committees will look like must depend upon our understanding of a theory of their function and structure. It seems to me that we must continue to move in the direction of making the reasonable person the foundation of these committees in what I have called the jury, or representative, model. The professional skills must remain necessary, but the newer skills must be added. I am convinced that resolving this dilemma of providing essential but mutually exclusive skills is both difficult and necessary.

NOTES

    1. Bernard Barber et al., *Research on Human Subjects: Problems of Social Control in Medical Experimentation* (New York: Russell Sage, 1973), p. 152; Bradford H. Gray, *Human Subjects in Medical Experimentation* (New York: Wiley-Interscience, 1975).

    2. Barber et al., *Research on Human Subjects*, p. 153.

    3. J. A. F. Stoner, "A Comparison of Individual and Group Decisions Involving Risk" (Master's thesis, School of Industrial Management, Massachusetts Institute of Technology, 1961).

    4. Colin Fraser et al., "Risky Shifts, Cautious Shifts and Group Polarization," *European Journal of Social Psychology* 1 (1971): 7–30.

P E T E R   C .   W I L L I A M S

Success in Spite of Failure: Why IRBs Falter in Reviewing Risks and Benefits

Institutional Review Boards (IRBs) have been in place for over a decade, long enough for their work to have been carefully reviewed and evaluated. Surprisingly, little systematic study has been reported in the literature. What has appeared suggests a mixed record. There are, for example, questions about the consistency of decisions,[1] complaints either that boards stifle research[2] or are too lenient,[3] and criticisms of their operation.[4] No general conclusions have yet to receive wide empirical confirmation. It is generally agreed, however, that IRBs are much more effective in fulfilling some of their functions than others. In particular, they are rather successful overseeing consent and privacy requirements and relatively unsuccessful in reviewing the balance of risks and benefits of proposed research.

More empirical research would be necessary to confirm the claim that IRBs fail to review adequately

the risks and benefits of research. Nevertheless limited evidence in the public forum supports this conclusion,[5] as does experience I have gained as the chair or a member of various IRBs, and information I have gathered in discussions with members of still other boards. IRBs seldom adequately make the risk/benefit calculations thought necessary to protect subject welfare.

Three factors contribute to the inadequacy of IRB review of the risks and benefits likely to flow from a protocol. The first factor is a bias for approval inherent in the charge given the committees in the Health and Human Services (HHS) guidelines. Second, the composition of IRBs—the populating of committees for those favoring research per se—makes objective evaluation unlikely. Finally, the actual operation of IRBs as committees lessens their effectiveness in balancing risks and benefits.

THE WELFARE CRITERION OF REVIEW

IRBs are asked to apply two broad types of criteria. One type involves norms protecting the welfare of research subjects; the other, norms protecting their

Reprinted from *IRB: A Review of Human Subjects Research* 6 (May/June 1984), pp. 1–4. © 1984, The Hastings Center. Reproduced by permission.

rights. Boards are told that, consistent with effective research, risks to the subject are to be minimized and must be reasonable in relation to anticipated benefits.[6] The second kind of criterion involves protecting certain values irrespective of the probable benefit or harm of the experiment. Autonomy is safeguarded through guidelines on informed consent;[7] privacy is protected through guidelines on confidentiality of research materials;[8] justice is promoted by requiring equity in selection of subjects.[9]

IRBs traditionally are more conscientious about and effective in applying the rights criteria than the welfare ones. The difference arises in part because the harm/benefit guidelines are notoriously ambiguous and contain a marked bias for approval of protocols.

The HHS regulations ask boards to make decisions about degrees of possible harm and possible benefit and then trade them off. "Harm" and "benefit" are wholly undefined. Moreover, boards are asked to compare the impact of research on individuals and on society as a whole; yet boards are given no guidance in how to balance the interests of a particular subject against the interests of the collective. These lacunae in the regulations must be filled on a case-by-case basis by IRB members relying on their own judgment both about what counts as a benefit or danger and how each is to be weighed. Though the lack of guidance in the "guidelines" may protect local autonomy of boards,[10] and concomitantly foster interboard differences,[11] deep intraboard disagreement is also fostered. When the latter occurs, the easiest way to avoid stalemate is to ignore the welfare criteria. There is much less agreement in our society in assigning weights to risks and benefits than there is about the meaning and importance of autonomy, privacy, or justice; hence boards can and do more successfully protect those values.

What is more, to the extent that the regulations give guidance about welfare issues, the deck is stacked in favor of approval. The guidelines seem to allow consideration of the long-range public good that might be derived from the results of research while expressly excluding consideration of possible public harms. Potential immediate ill effects to individuals may be outweighed by long-term benefits society will receive. Potential long-term ill effects to society may not be considered at all! This assymetry decreases the likelihood that committees will find protocols wanting on risk/benefit grounds. The welfare criteria in the regulations, if anything can be said about their clarity, clearly favor approval.

COMMITTEE MEMBERSHIP

HHS regulations properly contain restrictions on the makeup of committees. The basic premise is that a research scientist should not be the sole arbiter of the conflict between the advance of science and the welfare of research subjects. A number of reasons support this conclusion, none of them suggesting that researchers lack morality. Though scientists have little formal training in ethics, most are genuinely concerned with and sensitive to the rights and welfare of their subjects. Nonetheless, professional and institutional pressures tend to impair ethical perceptivity and moral intuitions.

Strong social incentives prompt investigators to do research and publish results; comparable institutional pressure to protect the rights and interests of subjects does not exist.[12] If the person doing research were solely responsible for this protection, it is likely that research efficacy would tend to outweigh subject welfare. This conclusion is supported by now well-known examples of researchers carrying out morally questionable experiments or manufacturing or doctoring experimental results.[13] When one is a judge in his or her own case, mistakes in weighing competing values are more likely.

There is also evidence that peer review also does not adequately ensure the proper weighing of subject welfare.[14] Institutional support for or publication of results of unethical research manifests the tolerance of researchers for the questionable practices of their colleagues. This tolerance is not an expression of ill will or moral turpitude, but of a bias that normally follows the socialization of scientists. In deciding, for example, what psychological experiment should be done or how it should be done, a research physicist has no special insight into the risks or benefits of the proposed research, but does share a constantly reinforced bias for experimentation per se. People who do research should not be the sole decision makers of what research gets done or how it gets done if only because the *potential* for inappropriate overvaluation of benefits over risks is so real.

Through formal constraints on the membership of the committee, there is an attempt to ensure that the rights and welfare of research subjects will be protected and decisions balanced. IRBs must include at least one member whose concerns are in nonscientific areas and at least one member who is not affiliated with the institution under whose auspices the research is being done.[15] HHS stipulations about experience, expertise, diversity, and concerns of board members are designed to help guarantee that fair and wise judgments are reached. These formal requirements, however, cannot themselves provide that guarantee, because there is a preexisting bias in the pool from which members are drawn.

Most IRBs are affiliated with an institution in which research plays a significant role. Consequently the membership on review committees is comprised mainly of fellow researchers or, occasionally, nonresearchers sympathetic to the enterprise of research. It is difficult, for example, to find *anyone* at a university, research institute, medical school, or hospital who does not assign great positive value to research per se.

Might the noninstitutional member balance this bias? It is possible but very unlikely. The smooth operation of the committee and the nature of the noninstitutional members likely to be selected—those who have the interest and background to serve—work to limit selection to those who share the institutional ideology. Even were a committee member not to share the high value placed on the advance of science through research, his or her impact on the committee would be seriously attenuated for reasons discussed later.

The natural bias of committee members reinforces the required reliance on criteria which, as shown above, tend to favor research. The problem of bias is even more troublesome since, for adequate evaluation of a large number of research projects submitted to committees, special scientific knowledge and expertise are required. No committee, unless it becomes cumbersomely large, can be expected to have all the requisite expertise. This need for expertise prompted HHS to allow IRBs to use consultants in their determinations.[16] The consultant is even more likely than the members to favor research in general and often favor it especially in the field being reviewed. The bias for research of committee members is compounded when they rely on experts even more favorably disposed for research in particular areas.

None of these observations is meant to imply that the committees intentionally favor any particular research protocol or are univocal about the value of particular sorts of research. Rather my point is that the committees are populated by those who favor the enterprise of research. This factor further distorts the welfare calculation required of IRBs by presumptive support of the worth of experiments. This bias of committee members compounds an already obvious weighting in favor of research.

COMMITTEE OPERATION

Because of the kind of criteria being applied and the nature of the committees themselves, IRBs are more effective evaluating issues of basic rights than they are at making judgments about welfare. But it is the actual operation of committees that finally explains why serious risk/benefit calculations are so rare. Four problems account for committee (in)action.

1. The Problem of Paternalism. IRB members seem to recognize that it is more justifiable morally for IRBs to oversee subjects' rights—review issues of consent, privacy, and equity—than to oversee subjects' welfare. Resolution of questions about rights are less invasive of the autonomy of the experimenter and subject than are decisions about risks and benefits. The consent requirement is an excellent example. Section 46.116 of the regulations is designed to guarantee that experimental subjects' choices are informed and voluntary. The explicit purpose of the consent provisions of the review process is to facilitate rational decision making on the part of the subject; the implicit task of the risk/benefit analysis is to foreclose that choice.

The HHS guidelines speak of the review committee's making a risk/benefit analysis in order to decide whether, *in its own view*, the risks to the subject are reasonable in relation to the possible benefits to the subject and/or the knowledge pool. If the committee decides the risks are too great, then the protocol can be rejected and the investigator's own evaluation is overridden and the evaluation by potential subjects made impossible. The latter never even see the experiment.

In applying their own risk assessment the committee is being asked to *limit* potential experimental subjects' freedom, to preclude a decision to participate in a protocol. Enforcing the consent requirements, on the other hand, enhances the subjects' freedom by allowing an informed choice to enter or refuse to enter a protocol. It is not difficult to imagine a research subject—perhaps a Barney Clark—who is an especially good samaritan. He or she would be willing to endure significantly greater risk than the reasonable IRB member because of a special concern with the knowledge to be gained or because of a personal weighing of risks and benefits different from that of the committee.

IRBs are more reluctant to act paternalistically by precluding participation than they are to ensure that the good samaritan is fully informed and acts voluntarily. Hence they avoid the former area and focus on the latter.

2. *The Problem of Researcher Competence.* There are special difficulties in weighing risks against benefits that do not arise when evaluating protection of rights. These special difficulties can only be avoided by effectively ignoring the welfare criterion. This problem is more than the genuine difficulties in predicting distant outcomes, selecting which risks and benefits are to count how much, comparing incommensurables, and the like. It is also more than coping with the common and unhappy need to compare infinitesimal potential benefit against miniscule potential risk. Rather committees avoid making risk/benefit assessments because of a more subtle feature of any such assessment, namely, to do so requires a judgment of the competence of the researcher both to do good science and to be morally sensitive.

The potential for benefit or harm depends in part on the capacity of the scientist to design and execute a good protocol. Were committees to involve themselves in a serious risk/benefit analysis, they would be called upon to decide first whether the research design is so poor that no benefit is likely and, second and more important, whether the particular investigator has the capacity to realize the possible benefit and minimize the possible risks.[17] In each of these decisions, but especially the latter, the competence of the investigator *qua* scientist is at issue and those being judged become understandably sensitive.

This poses a serious problem. Only in exceptional instances are IRBs willing to evaluate overtly and objectively the scientific competence of researchers. This is especially true if there is an ongoing professional relationship between the judges and the adjudged. As Robert Levine has pointed out, the experts at an institution most capable of evaluating scientific merit of a protocol and its investigators are likely to be involved in the very protocol under review.[18] Additionally IRB members will have an outside and ongoing relationship, sometimes quite close, with many investigators seeking approval. If, on the other hand, that ongoing relation does not exist, the information necessary to make an evaluation of scientific capability may not be available. The capacity of a person in one field to judge fairly the quality of someone's work in another is questionable and often questioned.

Either way, board members are understandably reluctant to make appraisals of the professional competence of others if they can avoid doing so; and IRB members can. How? By avoiding serious risk/benefit analyses in their deliberations or by simply relying on the determination of others (such as department chairmen, laboratory directors, study sections or grantors), on credentials (such as academic background, prizes, previous grants), or the like. The common strategy of relying on others for judgments of scientific competence of investigators effectively establishes a presumption favoring competence, which reinforces a bias for approving research.

The reluctance to evaluate scientific competence is compounded when it is recognized that a serious risk/benefit analysis would also require boards to evaluate the researcher's ethical competence. A researcher who manufactures or alters data is unlikely to generate experimental benefits. More important but less obvious, an investigator who is morally insensitive—who ignores subjects' privacy or rides roughshod over subjects' autonomy—creates moral "risks" that are serious but difficult to gauge. The inadequacy of IRBs' policing of ongoing research necessitates reliance on the moral integrity of the investigator's implicit promise to follow his or her protocol. Fortunately this reliance is usually justified. Nonetheless boards seldom, if ever, engage in formal assessments of the virtuousness of investigators. A thorough risk/benefit analysis would require that they do so.

In summary, the problem of competence can be recast as a series of disjunctions. Either IRBs avoid serious risk/benefit analyses or they must judge the scientific skills and moral character of the researchers. The latter option poses another choice: they must either rely on their own evaluation of the researcher's capabilities or depend on others to make that evaluation. Either way ignorance or bias is likely to influence the decision. This scenario is so unappealing that IRBs tend to eschew it by avoiding thorough risk/benefit analyses.

3. *The Problem of Remedies.* As in so many decision-making situations the nature of the remedies or solutions available affect the decision procedure. Finding fault with a protocol's consent or privacy provisions yields a quick, discrete remedy. It is relatively easy for a review committee to rewrite a consent

form or build in safeguards for privacy of information; and doing so seldom alters the scientific design. Coming to a negative judgment about the risk/benefit ratio presents, by comparison, an enormous dilemma. Either the committee can reject the experiment outright or the committee can involve itself in redesigning the protocol. Either remedy is unappealing; hence the judgment that would require either is seldom made.

4. *The Problem of Collective Decision Making.* Finally, to the extent that IRBs do undertake comparisons of risks and benefits, the fact that the weighing is done by a committee itself affects the outcome of the deliberations. Decisions made by groups of people differ from those made by individuals. This difference is called the group polarization phenomenon.[19]

In 1961 James Stoner reported research indicating that groups confronted with choices involving risks were willing to take more chances than the average of individuals in the groups.[20] This phenomenon was initially called "risky shift," a term aptly describing the lessening in risk aversion of collectives. Subsequent research has shown that preferences of groups change both toward greater caution as well as greater risk, depending on a number of factors relevant to our topic. It is well confirmed that "the average post group response to risk will tend to be more extreme in the same direction as the average of the pregroup response."[21] In IRBs the change is toward a greater willingness to countenance risks.

The influence of group interaction not only affects risk aversion but also attitudes, for example, about the importance of empirical research,[22] and judgments of facts, for example, about the odds assigned of the occurrence of some consequence of an intervention.[23] Equally important are the findings that the shift of group determinations increases with the initial homogeneity of the group[24] and that a willingness to allow risks increases when the group is making advisory (as opposed to mandatory) decisions.[25]

The significance of these well-established results is obvious. Given the initial preference of most IRB members for allowing risks in and for presuming benefits of research, meeting together to evaluate protocols will reinforce those preferences. Additionally the potential impact of an extra-institutional member will be attenuated. The very structure of the method of review created by the federal regulations reinforces the tendency of boards to avoid rejecting protocols as too risky.

To summarize, the actual operation of IRBs compounds the unlikelihood that welfare criteria will be used to evaluate protocols. All four of the above problems—paternalism, researcher competence, remedies, and collective decision making—further explain why IRBs are reluctant to review protocols according to their risks and benefits, though they may be vigorous in guarding the rights of subjects. Further, to the extent committees do risk/benefit analyses, they will be more likely to view research favorably than unfavorably.

THE VALUE OF IRBs

It is generally conceded—though more empirical research is sorely needed—that IRBs are not effective in reviewing research protocols using the welfare criteria found in the federal regulations. By focusing attention on three aspects of research review—criteria of evaluation, committee composition, and committee operation—I have tried to explain why. They tend to avoid doing the kind of cost/benefit analysis required by the guidelines and, when they do make such an evaluation, tend to be biased in favor of research. IRBs do not work in the ways they were expected to work and, given their structure and the guidelines under which they operate, cannot be expected to.

This conclusion, however troublesome, must be balanced by recognition of some important virtues of IRBs. First the committees will serve a genuine and valuable function in overseeing subjects' rights. This is no small accomplishment. Second and of more importance is the symbolic value of IRBs. In requiring the establishment of the boards, society has stated unequivocally that it is concerned with the ethics of research. This public declaration can guide the actions of present researchers and influence the development of new ones. The final and most important benefit of the committees is educational. Attention of an entire generation of scientists is being turned to the ethics of research. This is a good of inestimable value and itself more than justifies the presence of the boards.

These three combine as a powerful deterrent to the design and execution of improperly risky research. I know of no evidence that unduly dangerous protocols are actually passing committee review. It may be one of the ironies of regulation by bureaucracy that, in spite of the failure of IRBs themselves to review adequately subject welfare, and the likely failure of boards as currently constituted to do so in the future, the very presence of federally sanctioned committees may nonetheless indirectly accomplish the end for which they were designed.

NOTES

1. Goldman, J., Katz, M.: Inconsistency and institutional review boards. *JAMA* 248(2):197–202, 1982; and an editorial response in the same issue by Veatch, R.: Problems with institutional review board inconsistency, pp. 179–180. See also Barber, B., et al., *Research on Human Subjects: Problems of Social Control in Medical Experimentation*. Russell Sage, 1973, pp. 43–44.

2. Gray, B. H., and Cooke, R. A.: The impact of institutional review boards on research. *Hastings Center Report* 10:36–41, February 1980.

3. Barber, B., *op. cit.*, esp. chs. 2–6; Gray, B. H., and Cooke, R. A., *op. cit.*; Susskind, L., and Vandegrift, L.: IRBs and the regulation of social science research. *Human Subjects Research*, R. Greenwald, et al., eds. New York, Plenum Press, 1982, pp. 207–219; and Lewis, P. J.: Drawbacks of research ethics committees. *Journal of Medical Ethics* 8:61–64, 1982. For other research on review boards see Riecken, H. W., and Ravich, R.: Informed consent to biomedical research in Veterans Administration hospitals. *JAMA* 248:344–348, 1982; Allen, P. A., and Waters, W. E.: Development of an ethical committee and its effect on research design. *Lancet* 1(8283):1233–36, May 1982; Gray, B. H., Cooke, R. A., and Tannenbaum, A. S.: Research involving human subjects. *Science* 201:1094–1101, 1978; Gray, B. H.: *Human Subjects in Medical Experimentation*. New York, Wiley-Interscience, 1975.

4. Whether or not articles questioning the operation of IRBs will inspire the needed empirical research is also questionable. In 1975 Robert Veatch introduced some of the points I develop in my analysis and the data needed for firm conclusions are still largely missing in 1983. See Veatch, R. M.: Human experimentation committees: professional or representative? *Hastings Center Report* 5(5):31–40, October 1975.

5. See reference 3.

6. 45 *CFR* 46.111(a)(1–2).

7. 45 *CFR* 46.111(a)(4).

8. 45 *CFR* 46.111(a)(7).

9. 45 *CFR* 46.111(a)(3).

10. The degree to which local autonomy is valuable and necessary is an issue beyond the scope of my analysis. So too is the question of which sorts of considerations are best left to unbridled local determination. Robert Levine has argued that questions of the scientific consequences of research can be evaluated by applying more objective and universal standards than can questions of rights.

See Levine, R. J.: Can (Or Should) the IRB Assume the FDA's Functions at Early Stages of the IND Process? *IRB: A Review of Human Subjects Research* 3(10):5, December 1981. Ironically the guidelines are more specific regarding subject rights.

11. See reference 1.

12. It is interesting to note that in the only major study on IRBs, a study prepared for the National Commission for the Protection of Human Subjects in Biomedical and Behavioral Research (U.S. Government Printing Office, Document #050-003-00556-5, 1978), 28% of the research investigators surveyed felt review procedures then required by the federal funding agencies were "an unwarranted intrusion on an investigator's autonomy. . . ." (p. 1–212) That view was shared by only 6% of the non-scientists surveyed. (p. 1–213)

13. See, for example, the groundbreaking article by Beecher, Henry K.: Ethics and Clinical Research. *NEJM* 274:1354–1360, 1966.

14. Barber et al., *op. cit.*

15. 45 *CFR* 46.107(c–d).

16. 45 *CFR* 46.107(f).

17. These problems are discussed more completely by Robert Levine in *Ethics and Regulation of Clinical Research*. Baltimore, Urban & Schwarzenberg, 1981, esp. 18, and in "Can (Or Should) the IRB Assume the FDA's Functions at Early Stages of the IND Process?"

18. Levine, "Can (Or Should) the IRB Assume the FDA's Functions at Early Stages of the IND Process?"

19. The term originated in writings of Serge Moscovici and his colleagues. Moscovici, S. S., and Zavalloni, M.: The group as a polarizer of attitudes. *Journal of Personality and Social Psychology* 12:125–135, 1969. This aspect of IRB operation was noted by Veatch, *op. cit.* at p. 37.

20. Stoner, J. A. F.: *A comparison of individual and group decisions involving risk*. Unpublished master's thesis, School of industrial management, M.I.T., 1961.

21. Myers, D. G., and Lamm, H.: The group polarization phenomenon. *Psychological Bulletin* 83:602–627, 1976.

22. Moscovici and Zavalloni, *op. cit.*

23. Doise, W.: An apparent exception to the extremization of collective judgments. *European Journal of Social Psychology* 1:511–518, 1971.

24. Myers, D. G., and Bishop, G. D.: Discussion effects on racial attitudes. *Science* 169:778–789, 1970.

25. Myers and Lamm, *op. cit.*, p. 608.

LAWRENCE FINSEN

Institutional Animal Care and Use Committees:
A New Set of Clothes for the Emperor?

I. INTRODUCTION

The last decade has seen a growing concern among philosophers and others about the ethics of our society's manner of using animals for human ends. The activities that have come under scrutinizing eyes have been wide in scope and varied in nature, including everything from the possession of pets to keeping animals in zoological parks, the use of animals in agriculture and in scientific research, blood sports, and the massacre of seals and whales. While elimination of many such activities would imply cultural changes of some significance, it is not hard to imagine a very successful society that refrained from such activities as hunting or blood sports, or prohibited the trapping or ranching of animals for furs.

The issues surrounding the use of animals in scientific research, like some of these other issues, are obviously emotionally charged, involving deeply entrenched assumptions about our dominion over nature. But scientific uses of animals seem to many to be a different matter altogether. The honor ascribed to science is undoubtedly connected to the fact that most people regard the scientific endeavor as perhaps the foremost source of the improvement of the conditions of life in our time. Our fears of deteriorating health in old age, disease, and the hazards we have ourselves placed in the environment, along with compassion for those who suffer such misfortunes, make scientific research seem all the more urgent, a matter of another magnitude of importance than those more frivolous uses of animals. Nonetheless, the ethical concerns about our society's use of animals have not been lim-

ited to the more frivolous uses, for the critical scrutiny has been awakened by a growing sense that the most fundamental assumptions we make about the place of animals in our moral scheme are indefensible. As Peter Singer (1975, ch. 1) has argued, the assumption that the interests of nonhumans need not be given serious consideration in judging what is morally acceptable is indefensible, reflecting irrelevant distinctions between species. Others, such as Tom Regan (1983, pp. 312–315), have argued that such consideration of animals ought to take the form of applying the concept of individual rights to many species other than *homo sapiens*. The case for such an extension of moral consideration and moral rights have been eloquently and convincingly argued at great length elsewhere: I shall not repeat the arguments here. Rather, I shall assume that a strong case does exist for attributing serious moral consideration to the interests of animals, and that in at least some cases this might reasonably be expressed in the language of rights. If this is correct, then clearly the traditional appeal to the benefits accrued by humans as justification for the kind of invasion made daily into the lives of millions of animals in scientific research needs careful reconsideration. . . .

II. THE SELF-REGULATION RESPONSE

One of the ways that advocates of research have responded to concerns about the treatment of animals in research is through development of a system of self-regulation from within institutions that conduct research, modelled partly on the institutional review boards mandated for review of protocols that employ human subjects.[1] The effort to put in place such self-regulation has now emerged as the foremost response of the scientific community to criticisms of animal

Reprinted with permission of the publisher from *The Journal of Medicine and Philosophy* 13 (1988), pp. 145–153, 156–158.

research.[2] It is not hard to see why: surely some, at least, of the criticisms are well-taken and may threaten to bring external restrictions on research. Addressing criticisms through self-regulation appears the wiser route for those who wish to leave research as free as possible to pursue its course. While it is too early to say how well this system is working, in light of its popularity as a response to criticisms it is important to ask what prospects for genuine progress this approach holds.

The effort to regulate research internally has taken the form of local in-house committees whose charge includes discussion and evaluation of the ethical dimension of proposed and ongoing research involving animals. One of the main functions of these committees (and the one I shall address here) is reviewing proposed (and changes in ongoing) uses of animals within their institutions and ultimately approving or disapproving such proposals. Usually any recommendation of disapproval would come only after researchers had the opportunity to revise and resubmit proposals to address any criticisms the committee may have made of the original proposal. Many (but certainly not all) institutions that conduct research have had some such committees, even before the most recent amendment to the Animal Welfare Act made this mandatory for 'research facilities' (however, in the terms of the Act, 'research facility' refers only to institutions that either accept federal money for their animal research, or purchase or transport animals across state lines. Sec. 2132e). In addition, the NIH's revised policy (NIH, 1985) makes use of such a committee a prerequisite for NIH funding. In fact, the NIH concept of such committees is currently providing the most widely recognized model of institutional self-regulation of animal research in the United States, although worthwhile comparisons can be made to Canadian and European systems (Obrink, 1982). In what follows, I shall follow the NIH's practice and refer to such committees as 'Institutional Animal Care and Use Committees' or IACUCs.

The Congressional finding mentioned earlier, which refers to the public concern for laboratory animal care and treatment, points to the importance of meeting this concern in order to assure "that research will continue and progress" (Sec. 2131), and it seems clear that many will see an opportunity to protect research from attack by a system of self-regulation (Fox, 1982, p. 62). Nevertheless, such a system must be judged first and foremost from the point of view of the subjects of research. In this light, the primary aim of such a system is to apply appropriate ethical standards to the question of the acceptability of proposals to use animals. And presumably such ethical standards have the purpose not of protecting institutions from unwanted criticism, but of protecting the subjects of research from unwarranted intrusions. The foremost criterion of the acceptability of such a review system, then, must be potential benefits and protections the research subjects will obtain from it. Otherwise, the endeavor is nothing more than an attempt to shield research from further criticisms.[3]

III. POTENTIAL ADVANTAGES OF THE COMMITTEE SYSTEM

What are the potential advantages such committees could provide? A number of distinct advantages can be identified, provided, of course, that institutions involved give IACUCs the necessary support and the committees take their functions seriously. First, the fact that IACUCs will meet to discuss ethical concerns regarding research may provide a much needed forum within the local institution for expression and adjudication of such concerns. Without such a forum, dissenting voices have nowhere to air concerns except in public, which may not promote the best opportunity for fruitful dialogue between differing points of view. Among other things, those in favor of research may not feel the need to address criticisms, as they undoubtedly maintain the power in this situation. A serious dialogue on these issues would be healthy and might help to sensitize some who would not otherwise concern themselves with the ethical issues, and it might also help to educate where misconceptions about the nature or purpose of research have led to criticism. Of course, dissenters would still be free to take criticisms into the public arena, but a more direct route to influencing institutional policy on such matters would generally be more satisfactory. The larger question of the extent to which IACUCs will actually engage in such a dialogue, and how much this will change matters for animal subjects is difficult to prejudge. I address some of the impediments to this later on.

Second, both the NIH policy and the amended Animal Welfare Act call for inclusion of outsiders on the committee, i.e., at least one individual not affiliated with the institution whose role it is to represent community concerns about the care and treatment of animals. Inclusion on the committees of such outsiders, especially if they are not themselves scientists, could have a number of important results. One of these might be that researchers would have to explain the value of their projects to nonexperts. That may help to avoid acceptance of practices simply because they are standardly accepted within a field. A second advantage might be that fruitful new perspectives on the ethical problems might be introduced. There is nothing like an outsider to reveal the arbitrariness of an assumption that is traditionally treated as axiomatic by insiders.

Third, the discussion of proposed research may have a beneficial effect on the merit of that research, as proposals may receive suggestions for refinement as they go through the review process. The justification of research typically appeals to potential benefits, primarily to humans (Tannenbaum, 1985, pp. 32–43). But poorly designed research cannot fulfill the promise of beneficial research, and so it is never justified. Thus, if IACUCs help to refine the design of research this may increase the chances that only justifiable research is conducted. In conversation, the chair of one university's review committee pointed out that refinement of proposals was an unexpected benefit his committee had achieved.

Whether these advantages will actually secure significant benefits for research animals, however, may still be doubtful. There are a number of questions that need to be asked about such issues as the composition of IACUCs and the scope of the review process.

IV. SCOPE OF THE REVIEW

The most recent revisions to the NIH policy are in part the result of a study conducted by the NIH of ten major research institutions receiving NIH funding. With respect to the committee system in place before the revisions, the study reported that

[S]ite visitors found that the animal care committees were generally not as active as their charters (organizational descriptions) had depicted them: some of the stated responsibilities were not addressed on a regular basis; all or part of the review functions were often delegated to the veterinarian, chairperson, and/or administrative staff, or they were performed in a routine manner . . . animal care committee members (and other scientists within the instutition) sometimes placed too much reliance upon NIH scientific review groups to evaluate research involving laboratory animals ('Site Visits', p. 6).

Given these observations, one would expect that the revised policies would call for regular, non-routine review of proposals; would not permit delegation of review to individuals; and would discourage too great a reliance on the NIH scientific review. In fact, the new guidelines go some way toward these goals. They do permit the IACUCs to review applications in a rather routine way without meeting, much as Institutional Review Boards need not meet in their review of proposals involving human subjects ('Protection', 1983, 45 CFR 46.110). But as all members of the IACUCs will have the pertinent parts of all applications and may call for a full committee review of any of them (NIH, IV.C.2), the routine manner in which the bulk of the applications will be handled may not be a serious shortcoming, though the Swedish approach to this problem of enlarging the committees and allowing subcommittees of three (a scientist, technician, and layman) to discuss proposals may be preferable (Obrink, 1982, p. 56). The new system does improve over the past practice of allowing delegation of review to individuals, and this is given teeth in the requirement that no proposal lacking IACUC approval can be approved by officials of the institution (NIH, IV.C.8). This means that IACUCs serve more than a recommending function: they are a necessary stage in the approval process. These two features are also present in the regulations proposed by the USDA to implement the amendments to the Animal Welfare Act. If the proposed rules are adopted, a quorum would be required for formal actions to be taken by the committee, and no research covered by the regulations could be carried out without prior committee approval of the protocol. The regulations specify a classification of uses of animals that emphasizes the increasing amount of pain or distress likely to be caused (USDA, pp. 10313–10314).

How deeply will this participation in the approval process really go? The NIH regulations state that the IACUCs are to review "those sections of PHS applications or proposals related to the care and use of animals" (NIH, IV.B.5). Again, in discussing the review process, the NIH policy states that "[t]hose sections of applications and proposals that relate to the care and use of animals shall be available to all IACUC members" (IV.C.2). The implication is that there may be portions of such applications that an institution or a researcher need not make available to the members of its IACUC. What portions of such an application might these be? One view is that nonexperts should not be involved in judging the scientific merit of proposals (Mishkin, 1982, p. 36). The NIH policy seems to accept the wisdom of this perspective. The role of IACUC review is to "confirm that the activity will be conducted in accord with the Animal Welfare Act insofar as it applies to the activity, and that the activity is in accord with the *Guide* unless acceptable justification for a departure is presented". The NIH policy goes on to require review to include determination that the activity conforms to a set of standards relating to minimization of pain and discomfort; appropriate uses of sedation, analgesic, etc.; when 'sacrifice' of animals is mandatory, appropriateness of living conditions to species; provision of medical care; qualifications of personnel; and methods of euthanasia (IV.C.1. a–g). Again, the situation is much the same with the committees called for under the amended Animal Welfare Act, which explicitly states that nothing in the Act shall be construed as authorizing the Secretary of Agriculture, who enforces it, to promulgate rules with regard to the design or performance of actual research, or to interfere with it (Sec. 2143a6).

Can an IACUC conduct a coherent review of the moral acceptability of a proposal if it does not consider the scientific merit of the proposal? This depends on our ethical perspective. There are three approaches possible here: one may consider all research (or perhaps all 'invasive' research) morally unjustifiable ('abolitionism'), or one may consider all research justifiable, though there may still be restrictions on treatment of animals, e.g., insisting that it be conducted as 'humanely' as possible ('*laissez faire*'), and finally, one may believe that the truth lies somewhere between: that some, but not all purposes, might justify the use of animals in research (the 'moderate' approach). The abolitionist and *laissez faire* approaches could certainly proceed without considering the merit of the endeavor.[4]

Could moderates proceed in this way? It is often pointed out that nonexperts will be ill equipped to judge the scientific merit of proposals. But if one takes the moderate position—that the justification of research depends on some kind of decision concerning the relative weights of potential benefits of research and the harm of intrusion into the lives of subjects whose consent has not and cannot be obtained—then no decision can reasonably be made in ignorance of the claims made on behalf of the proposed research. And if we accept the principle that outside voices should have a role in this decision-making process, as

the NIH policy clearly does, then researchers and lay committee members will simply have to overcome this hurdle if moderate perspectives are to be considered.

Of course, the funding process involves scientific review at another level, but that review is not primarily (if at all) concerned to ask ethical questions concerning the justification of the proposed research. Further, any research which is not federally funded, but which is conducted in institutions which adopt the NIH model of the IACUCs, would thereby omit any review of scientific merit if they followed this provision of the NIH policy. The point here is not that IACUCs should be responsible to recommend on the scientific merit of proposals, but rather, they must consider the question of the potential importance of the results of the research if they are to form a just assessment of the moral acceptability of the research. This is true no matter how low or high you place the threshold for acceptability, so long as you do not take either an abolitionist or a *laissez faire* position on the acceptability of research.

As mentioned above, the IACUCs are sometimes compared to the committees that review proposals involving human subjects: the IRBs. But the analogy between these two review processes breaks down in an important way here. In the case of research employing human subjects, the difficulties of assessing scientific merit are met by the combination of a number of criteria that IRBs are expected to use in considering proposals ('Protection', 1983, 46.111). First, informed consent is required from the subject or the subject's legal representative; and second, certain kinds of risks are not permitted even where informed consent might be obtained: namely, risks that are unreasonable in relation to anticipated benefits to subjects and to the importance of the knowledge that may reasonably be expected to result. In the case of individuals who are especially vulnerable to coercion or undue influence, the proposals must include additional safeguards to "protect the rights and welfare of those subjects." In other words, while the IRBs may engage in some estimate of the importance of proposed research, this is only employed to decide if the risks are not too great even to accept prospective subjects' consent as sufficient. Thus, the IRB approach explicitly works against the background of a set of assumed rights possessed by potential subjects that research proposals are not permitted to violate.

Nothing comparable to this exists in the IACUC case. The enormous difficulty of nonexperts considering the scientific merit of proposals in fields about which they may know little or nothing is not overcome by a similar specification of a set of principles governing what kinds of intrusion into the lives of prospective experimental subjects are, and what kinds are not permissible. Abolitionism and the *laissez faire* approach both avoid this difficulty because they do specify such principles. But if IACUCs are seriously to consider the moderate position, then they must find ways to deal with this difficulty. One approach, parallel to the IRB approach, might be to define a set of risks to which animal research subjects should not be subjected, though the difficulties here would clearly be significant. Were they overcome, this approach could constitute some real progress on behalf of animals. . . .

VI. CONCLUSION

I must conclude, then, that the IACUC system is at best a mixed blessing. It is possible that greater understanding between some critics of research and researchers will result from the committee experience, and that some research will be refined to assure that it is less objectionable than it may otherwise have been. Further, the structural changes in the revised NIH policy do begin to address the danger that committees will merely go through the motions and rubber stamp proposals. To whatever extent these changes result in improvements for animal subjects, they are welcome.

Nevertheless, it is clear that the IACUC system assumes that the use of animals in research should continue largely as is, and that the role of ethical scrutiny will be focused primarily on assuring that proposed uses of animals conform to the Animal Welfare Act and the NIH's standards. The Animal Welfare Act has in the past been appropriately criticized in many places for such things as its failure to include rodents and to address the conduct of research itself (Rollin, 1981, p. 80). The NIH standards, on the other hand, do address the conduct of research. But these rather broadly stated principles always make clear that any restriction on the conduct of research is contingent on the possibility of conducting the research in another way. Thus, they presuppose that risks to animals are always justified when required by a well designed proposal. In other words, they adopt what I have called the *laissez faire* approach.

Despite the hope that such a system represents some real advance in the open discussion of research ethics, the IACUC system offers little threat to the continued existence of research. To those who fail to see its built-in bias, the misleading impression may be created that the institutions who have IACUCs have engaged in a full and open discussion of the ethical acceptability of their research programs, when in fact certain points of view have probably been excluded from consideration from the start.

IACUCs may still, despite these criticisms, provide the vehicle for some improvements in the living conditions and experimental procedures to which some animals are subjected. These improvements should, of course, be sought. But we should clearly understand the limitations of the system. The hope that IACUCs might provide much greater protection of animals from unwarranted intrusions than is currently provided is unrealistic.

NOTES

* I am indebted to Tom Regan and Susan Finsen for many helpful comments and much encouragement.

1. Advocates of the self-regulation system have occasionally appealed to this similarity as a point in favor of having such committees for animal research. See, for example, Mishkin (1985, pp. 36–37). There are many similarities; but as I argue below . . . the analogy breaks down at a crucial point.

2. See, for example, the recommendations of the First Conference on Scientific Perspectives in Animal Welfare, published in Dodds and Orlans (1982, pp. 123–124). Since publishing this report, the Scientists Center for Animal Welfare has sponsored a number of workshops relating to implementing such committees.

3. Roswell states: "Is the animal welfare issue the result of misconceptions, or is it a real problem? It was generally agreed that there is a problem and that it stems from lack of communication between scientists and the public" [1982, p. 46]. If the *real* problem is public misconception, then the role of committees may well be conceived as educational and promotional.

4. But, of course, abolitionists are standardly excluded from serving on such committees. . . .

REFERENCES

'Animal Welfare Act', 7 U.S.C. sections 2131 et. seq.

Baker, H. J.: 'Responsibilities of institutions for the welfare of experimental animals', in W. J. Dodds and B. Orlans (eds.), *Scientific Perspectives on Animal Welfare*, Academic Press, New York, pp. 49–53.

Fox, J.: 1982, 'Institutional responsibilities: the committee's role', in W. J. Dodds and B. Orlans (eds.), *Scientific Perspectives on Animal Welfare*, Academic Press, New York, pp. 59–62.

Mishkin, B.: 1985, 'On Parallel tracks protecting human Subjects and Animals', *Hastings Center Report* 15, 36–37.

NIH: 1985, 'Public health service policy on humane care and Use of Laboratory animals by awardee institutions', *NIH Guide for Grants and Contracts* 14(8), 1–14.

Obrink, K. J.: 1982, 'Swedish law on laboratory animals', in W. J. Dodds and B. Orlans (eds.), *Scientific Perspectives on Animal Welfare*, Academic Press, New York, pp. 55–58.

'Protection of human subjects', *OPRR Reports*, March 8, 1983, 45 CFR.

Regan, T.: 1983, *The Case for Animal Rights*. University of California Press, Berkeley.

Rollin, B.: 1980, *Animal Rights and Human Morality*, Prometheus Books, Buffalo, New York.

Roswell, H. C.: 1982, 'Summary of workshop on investigator responsibilities', in W. J. Dodds and B. Orlans (eds.), *Scientific Perspectives on Animal Welfare*, Academic Press, New York, pp. 43–46.

Singer, P.: 1975, *Animal Liberation*. New York Review Books, New York.

"Site visits to animal care facilities: a report to the Director of the National Institutes of Health, March, 1984": April 5, 1984, in *NIH Guide for Grants and Contracts*, 13.

Tannenbaum, J., and A. N. Rowan, 'Rethinking the morality of Animal research', *Hastings Center Report* 15, 32–43.

USDA: 1987, 'Animal welfare regulations: Proposed rules', *Federal Register* 52(61), 10313–10314.

SUGGESTED READINGS FOR CHAPTER 9

GENERAL ISSUES

Annas, George J., et al. *Informed Consent to Human Experimentation: The Subject's Dilemma*. Cambridge, Mass.: Ballinger, 1977.

Barber, Bernard. *Informed Consent in Medical Therapy and Research*. New Brunswick, N.J.: Rutgers University Press, 1980.

Barber, Bernard, et al. *Research on Human Subjects: Problems of Social Control in Medical Experimentation*. New York: Russell Sage Foundation, 1973. New Brunswick, N.J.: Transaction Books, 1978.

Beauchamp, Tom L., et al., eds. *Ethical Issues in Social Science Research*. Baltimore, Md.: Johns Hopkins University Press, 1982.

Beecher, Henry K. *Research and the Individual: Human Studies*. Boston: Little, Brown, 1970.

Brieger, Gert H. "Human Experimentation: History." In Reich, Warren T., ed. *Encyclopedia of Bioethics*. New York: Free Press, 1978. Vol. 2, pp. 684–692.

Byar, David P. "Randomized Clinical Trials: Perspectives on Some Recent Ideas." *New England Journal of Medicine* 295 (July 8, 1976), 74–80.

Canada, Medical Research Council. *Ethical Considerations in Research Involving Human Subjects*. Ottawa: Medical Research Council, 1978.

Canada, Medical Research Council. *Guidelines on Research Involving Human Subjects*. Ottawa: Ministry of Supply and Services, 1987.

Capron, Alexander M. "Informed Consent in Catastrophic Disease Research and Treatment." *University of Pennsylvania Law Review* 123 (December 1974), 340–438.

———. "Human Experimentation: Basic Issues." In Reich, Warren T., ed. *Encyclopedia of Bioethics*. New York: Free Press, 1978. Vol. 2, pp. 642–699.

Childress, James F. "Compensating Injured Research Subjects: The Moral Argument." *Hastings Center Report* 6 (December 1976), 21–27.

Freund, Paul, ed. *Experimentation with Human Subjects*. New York: George Braziller, 1970.

Fried, Charles. *Medical Experimentation: Personal Integrity and Social Policy*. New York: American Elsevier, 1974.

———. "Human Experimentation: Philosophical Aspects." In Reich, Warren T., ed. *Encyclopedia of Bioethics*. New York: Free Press, 1978. Vol. 2, pp. 699–702.

Gillmore, Don. *I Swear by Apollo: Dr. Ewen Cameron and the CIA Brainwashing Experiments*. Montreal: Eden Press, 1987.

Gray, Bradford H. *Human Subjects in Medical Experimentation*. New York: Wiley, 1975.

———, et al. "Research Involving Human Subjects." *Science* 201 (September 22, 1978), 1094–1101.

Jones, James H. *Bad Blood: The Tuskegee Syphilis Experiment*. New York: Free Press, 1981.

Katz, Jay, with Capron, Alexander Morgan, and Glass, Eleanor Swift. *Experimentation with Human Beings*. New York: Russell Sage Foundation, 1972.

Levine, Robert J. *Ethics and Regulation of Human Research*, 2nd edition. Baltimore, Md.: Urban & Schwarzenberg, 1986.

Robertson, John A. "Compensating Injured Research Subjects: The Law." *Hastings Center Report* 6 (December 1976), 29–31.

———. "The Law of Institutional Review Boards." *UCLA Law Review* 26 (February 1980), 484–549.

U.S. National Commission for the Protection of Human Subjects. *The Belmont Report: Ethical Principles and Guidelines for the Protection of Human Subjects of Research* and *Appendix*. 3 vols. Washington, D.C.: U.S. Government Printing Office, 1978. [Excerpts published in *Federal Register* 44 (April 18, 1979), 23192–23197.]

———. *Institutional Review Boards: Report and Recommendations* and *Appendix*. 2 vols. Washington, D.C.: U.S. Government Printing Office, 1978. [Excerpts published in *Federal Register* 43 (November 30, 1978), 56174–56198.]

Veatch, Robert M. *Case Studies in Medical Ethics*. Cambridge, Mass.: Harvard University Press, 1977. Chap. 11.

———. "Three Theories of Informed Consent." In U.S. National Commission for the Protection of Human Subjects. *The Belmont Report: . . . Appendix*: Vol. II. Washington, D.C.: U.S. Government Printing Office, 1978, pp. 26–1 to 26–66.

———. *The Patient as Partner: A Theory of Human Experimentation Ethics*. Bloomington, Ind.: Indiana University Press, 1987.

ETHICAL REVIEW OF RESEARCH

Goldman, Jerry, and Katz, Martin D. "Inconsistency and Institutional Review Boards." *Journal of the American Medical Association* 248 (July 1982), 197–202.

Holder, Angela R. "Is This a Job for the IRB? The Case of the ELISA Assay." *IRB: A Review of Human Subjects Research* 7 (November/December 1985), 7–8.

Levine, Carol, and Caplan, Arthur L. "Beyond Localism: A Proposal for a National Research Review Board." *IRB: A Review of Human Subjects Research* 8 (March/April 1986), 7–9.

McCarthy, Charles R. "Experience with Boards and Commissions Concerned with Research Ethics in the United States." In Berg, Kare, and Tranoy, Knut Erik, eds. *Research Ethics*. New York: Alan R. Liss, 1983, 111–122.

Pattulo, E. L. "Institutional Review Boards and the Freedom to Take Risks." *New England Journal of Medicine* 307 (October 1982), 1156–1159.

President's Commission for the Study of Ethical Problems in Biomedical and Behavioral Research. *Implementing Human Research Regulations: Second Biennial Report on the Adequacy and Uniformity of Federal Rules and Policies, and on Their Implementation for the Protection of Human Subjects.* Washington, D.C.: U.S. Government Printing Office, 1983.

Royal College of Physicians. *Guidelines for the Practice of Ethics Committees in Medical Research.* London: Royal College of Physicians, 1984.

Schwartz, Robert L. "Institutional Review of Medical Research: Cost-Benefit, Risk-Benefit Analysis, and the 'Possible Effects of Research on Public Policy,'" *Journal of Legal Medicine* 4 (1983), 143–166.

U.S. Office of Science and Technology Policy. "Proposed Model Policy for Protection of Human Subjects; Response to the First Biennial Report of the President's Commission for the Study of Ethical Problems in Medicine and Biomedical and Behavioral Research." *Federal Register* 56 (June 3, 1986), 20204–20217.

ISSUES IN ANIMAL RESEARCH

Bateson, Patrick. "When to Experiment on Animals." *New Scientist* 109 (February 1986), 30–32.

Cohen, Carl. "The Case for the Use of Animals in Research." *New England Journal of Medicine* 315 (1986), pp. 865–870.

Fox, Michael Allen. *The Case for Animal Experimentation: An Evolutionary and Ethical Perspective.* Berkeley, Calif.: University of California Press, 1986.

Gallup, Gordon, and Suarez, Susan D. "Alternatives to the Use of Animals in Psychological Research." *American Psychologist* 40 (October 1985), 1104–1111.

Great Britain. *The Animals (Scientific Procedures) Act*, 1986.

Jamieson, Dale, and Regan, Tom. "On the Ethics of the Use of Animals in Science." In Regan, Tom, and VanDeVeer, Donald, eds. *And Justice for All.* Totowa, N.J.: Rowman and Littlefield, 1982, pp. 169–196.

Kuhse, Helga. "Interests." *Journal of Medical Ethics* 11 (September 1985), 146–149.

Leader, Robert W., and Stark, Dennis. "The Importance of Animals in Biomedical Research." *Perspectives in Biology and Medicine* Vol. 30, No. 4 (Summer 1987), pp. 470–485.

Rowan, Andrew N. *Of Mice, Models, and Men: A Critical Evaluation of Animal Research.* Albany, N.Y.: State University of New York Press, 1984.

Ryder, Richard. *Victims of Science: The Use of Animals in Research.* Revised edition. London: Anti-Vivisection Society, 1983.

Tannenbaum, Jerry, and Rowan, Andrew N. "Rethinking the Morality of Animal Research." *Hastings Center Report* 15 (October 1985), 32–43.

U.S. Congress, Office of Technology Assessment. *Alternatives to the Use of Animals in Research, Education, and Testing.* Washington, D.C.: OTA, 1984.

U.S. National Institutes of Health. *National Symposium on Imperatives in Research Animal Use: Scientific Needs and Animal Welfare.* Washington, D.C.: U.S. Government Printing Office, 1985.

U.S. National Institutes of Health, Office for Protection from Research Risks. *Public Health Service Policy on Humane Care and Use of Laboratory Animals.* Bethesda, Md.: Office for Protection from Research Risks, 1986.

BIBLIOGRAPHIES

Goldstein, Doris Mueller. *Bioethics: A Guide to Information Sources.* Detroit: Gale Research Company, 1982. See under "Research Involving Human Subjects."

Lineback, Richard H., ed. *Philosopher's Index.* Vols. 1– . Bowling Green, Ohio: Bowling Green State University. Issued quarterly. See under "Animal Experimentation," "Experimentation," and "Research."

Walters, LeRoy, and Kahn, Tamar Joy, eds. *Bibliography of Bioethics.* Vols. 1– . Washington, D.C.: Kennedy Institute of Ethics, Georgetown University. Issued annually. See under "Animal Experimentation" and "Human Experimentation." (The information contained in the annual *Bibliography of Bioethics* can also be retrieved from BIOETHICSLINE, an online database of the National Library of Medicine.)

10.
Frontiers in Biology and Medicine

In most chapters of this book we examine the current status of clinical care or biomedical research. The present chapter examines three facets of biomedical science and technology that have a decidedly futuristic flavor—reproductive technologies and arrangements, genetic technologies, and transplantation technologies. These three types of technological innovation, together with new applications of the neurosciences, are likely to have a decisive impact on the delivery of health care in the twenty-first century.

TECHNOLOGIES AND ARRANGEMENTS IN REPRODUCTION

The birth of Louise Brown in Lancashire, England, in 1978 inaugurated a new era in the history of the reproductive technologies. Louise had not been conceived inside her mother's body but in a petri dish, where eggs removed from her mother had been mixed with sperm from her father, and where fertilization had taken place.

In vitro fertilization (literally, "fertilization in glass") is most often proposed as a technique for overcoming infertility in married couples. The simplest case involves the use of semen from the husband and eggs from the wife. No reproductive cells are donated to the couple, and no "surplus" embryos are produced. All embryos that result from in vitro fertilization (IVF) contain the parents' genes, and all are transferred to the uterus of the wife in the hope that at least one pregnancy will be achieved. In addition, the simplest case involves no freezing and storage of early human embryos.

As the reprinted excerpts from the Warnock Committee report suggest, this relatively straightforward technique for overcoming infertility is surrounded by a series of interesting metaphysical and ethical problems. In a passage reminiscent of the personhood discussion that appeared in Chapter 4 of this book, the committee traces the major stages in early embryonic development and attempts to draw an ethical line on the basis of anatomical data. Where this line is drawn and why will have important implications for the question of research on early human embryos (see Chapter 9). Looking to the future, the committee foresees technical possibilities that seem to be drawn from works of science fiction—interspecies fertilization, the systematic use of embryos for drug testing, extracorporeal gestation, and the genetic modification of early human embryos. In a sketchy and admittedly preliminary way, the Warnock Committee attempts to provide an initial assessment of these new technological possibilities.

In contrast to the new technology of IVF, surrogate parenting involves the combination of a relatively old technology, artificial insemination, with a new social arrangement. The first documented attempt to establish a fee-for-service surrogate motherhood arrangement in the United States occurred in 1976, under the direction of Michigan attorney Noel Keane. According to the terms of such arrangements, which are usually spelled out in written contracts, a woman agrees to become pregnant on behalf of a couple and to deliver the resulting infant to the couple, in exchange for the couple's payment of a fee to the surrogate. In the early years of this new social practice, the technique of artificial insemination donor (AID) was generally employed, using sperm provided by the husband of the future social mother. Thus, the child in the usual or "full" surrogate motherhood arrangement contains genes from the egg of the surrogate mother and the sperm of the would-be social father. However, in 1985 the first instance of surrogate motherhood assisted by IVF occurred. The future social mother was able to produce fertilizable eggs but was medically unable to carry a pregnancy. Her eggs were therefore fertilized in vitro with sperm from her husband, and the resulting embryos were transferred to the uterus of a surrogate mother. In this arrangement, which is sometimes called "partial" surrogacy, the surrogate mother can also be designated a "surrogate carrier" because she makes no genetic contribution to the embryo or infant. (Note that genetic, gestational, and social motherhood can be distinguished in surrogate motherhood arrangements.)

The most celebrated case of surrogate motherhood to date involved Noel Keane as attorney and arranger, Mary Beth Whitehead as surrogate mother, William Stern as intended social father, and an infant, "Baby M," who became the object of an intense and protracted custody dispute. This case eventually came before the New Jersey Supreme Court, which announced its decision in early 1988. The excerpts of the Supreme Court opinion reprinted in this chapter rehearse the facts of the Baby M case and indicate how the court attempted to resolve several of the ethical, legal, and public-policy dilemmas presented by surrogate motherhood arrangements.

Artificial insemination, in vitro fertilization, and surrogate motherhood have made possible an almost dazzling array of new reproductive options. The following chart[1] illustrates sixteen possible modes of reproduction:

Alternative Reproductive Methods

	Source of gametes		Site of fertilization	Site of pregnancy	Notes
	Male	Female			
(1)	H	W	W	W	Customary, AIH
(2)	S	W	W	W	AID
(3)	H	W	L	W	IVF
(4)	S	W	L	W	IVF with donated sperm
(5)	H	S	L	W	IVF with donated egg
(6)	S	S	L	W	IVF with both gametes donated (or donated embryo)
(7)	H	S	S	W	AIH with donor woman plus uterine lavage (semi-donated embryo)
(8)	S	S	S	W	AID with donor woman plus uterine lavage (donated embryo)
(9)	H	W	W	S	
(10)	S	W	W	S	
(11)	H	W	L	S	
(12)	S	W	L	S	Surrogate motherhood
(13)	H	S	L	S	
(14)	S	S	L	S	
(15)	H	S	S	S	
(16)[a]	S	S	S	S	

H = Husband; W = Wife; S = Third party substitute, or surrogate; L = Laboratory.

[a]Planned procreation for placement; traditional adoption is not part of the schematic.

Chart developed by William B. Weil, Jr., and LeRoy Walters.

[1]Reprinted from LeRoy Walters, "Editor's Introduction," *Journal of Medicine and Philosophy* 10 (1985), p. 210.

GENETIC TECHNOLOGIES

There can be no doubt that we live in the golden age of genetics, especially human genetics. Even before the 1950s Gregor Mendel's classic work on various modes of inheritance was available as a framework for understanding how specific traits are transmitted from one generation to the next. However, Watson and Crick's discovery of the molecular structure of DNA in 1953 and the rapid advances made feasible by recombinant DNA techniques in the 1970s and 1980s have opened up entirely new possibilities for genetic diagnosis and therapy.

The genetic structure of human cells is incredibly intricate and complex. Within the nuclei of each human cell there are 46 chromosomes. These chromosomes, in turn, comprise 50,000–100,000 genes plus intervening sequences, the function of which is not yet well understood. The simplest units into which the genes and intervening sequences can be analyzed are individual nucleotides or bases—the familiar A, C, G, and T; two corresponding nucleotides form a base pair. It is estimated that each human cell contains approximately 3 billion base pairs.

Through the remainder of the twentieth century and well into the twenty-first, we will witness an intensive international effort to map and sequence the human genome. The initial fruits of this labor will undoubtedly be diagnostic: Researchers will be able to locate and analyze the "errors" in genetic sequences that cause particular genetic diseases, or even susceptibilities to particular diseases. When tests are developed to identify these errors, new possibilities for prenatal diagnosis, newborn screening, and the counseling of couples considering reproduction will be at hand. Of course, the same tests will also be available for use by insurance companies, employers, or governments seeking to identify individuals who are afflicted with a particular genetic disease or who carry specific deleterious genes.

In the history of medicine, diagnosis is often the necessary prelude to a cure. It thus seems likely that the capacity to identify genetic diseases and susceptibilities will provide new impetus for already existing efforts to develop ways to correct, or at least to compensate for, genetic defects. The general name usually given to these therapeutic initiatives is *gene therapy*, or, more broadly, *genetic intervention*. In the early stages, gene therapy will undoubtedly be focused on relatively simple genetic disorders that involve errors in only a single gene within each cell. Examples of such disorders are cystic fibrosis, sickle-cell anemia, and some types of muscular dystrophy. Later, more complex disorders involving multiple genes may become better understood and may in fact be amenable to gene therapy.

A central distinction in any discussion of gene therapy is the distinction between reproductive and nonreproductive cells, which are often called germ-line and somatic cells, respectively. Somatic cells, like our skin or muscle cells, contain the full complement of 46 chromosomes and cannot transmit genetic information to succeeding generations. Thus, the genetic information contained in somatic cells stops with us and does not pass on to succeeding generations. In contrast, germ-line cells, the egg and sperm cells, contain only 23 chromosomes and are capable of transmitting genetic information to our progeny in the next generation, as well as to their descendants in future generations.

A second important distinction in discussions of human gene therapy is that between the cure or prevention of disease, on the one hand, and the enhancement of human capabilities, on the other. (This distinction is reminiscent of the conceptual analyses included in Chapter 3.) A genetic approach to the treatment of cystic fibrosis would clearly be regarded as gene therapy. On the other hand, the attempt to increase stature or to improve the efficiency of long-term memory would probably be regarded by most observers as an effort to enhance capabilities rather than to cure disease. The two distinctions discussed in this and the preceding paragraph can be arrayed in the following two-by-two matrix:

somatic-cell repair	germ-line repair
somatic-cell enhancement	germ-line enhancement

In the present chapter, several of the ethical questions raised by gene therapy and genetic intervention are discussed. French Anderson outlines the current state of the scientific art and argues against the use of genetic techniques for enhancement purposes. LeRoy Walters surveys ethical issues in somatic-cell and germ-line gene therapy and describes how gene therapy proposals are currently reviewed in the United States. In a more futuristic mode, Jonathan Glover attempts to demolish the traditional arguments against enhancing the capabilities of human beings and opens the way, at least in theory, for highly ambitious and, in his view, creative applications of the new genetic technologies.

TRANSPLANTATION TECHNOLOGIES

Contrary to our expectations, there are strong continuities between somatic-cell gene therapy and transplantation technologies. In somatic-cell therapy as it is currently envisioned, a patient's own bone marrow or liver cells will be removed from the patient's body, and properly functioning genes will be added to the nuclei of as many of the patient's exteriorized cells as possible. The patient will then receive back her or his own cells as a kind of self-transplant, supplemented by the added genes contained in those cells.

In most cases, however, transplantation technologies involve the introduction of "foreign" (that is, non-patient-derived) cells, tissues, or organs into a patient's body with the intention of having the introduced materials become incorporated into the patient's body and persist there, at least for a time. These cells, tissues, or organs may be derived from another human being, living or dead, or from a nonhuman animal, or the material introduced into the patient may be manufactured, as in the case of the artificial heart. The foreign material transplanted can range in volume and complexity from a simple blood transfusion to a heart-lung combination.

For most philosophical and religious traditions (with the notable exception of the Jehovah's Witness community), the introduction of foreign cells, tissues, or organs into the body does not constitute an ethical problem *in principle*, if transplantation is required to restore health or prevent disease. Thus, the image of creating bionic men or women does not generally deter us from using transplantation technologies, even multiple technologies, for the welfare of patients. We have even discovered ways to cope with the previously unthinkable notion of heart transplantation through modifying our definition of death for certain classes of respirator-assisted patients (see Chapter 4). There is, however, a limiting case for transplantation, namely, any hypothetical proposal to perform whole-brain transplants—or perhaps even any proposal to perform cerebral transplants. The identity of human beings is so closely identified with their brains, and particularly with the parts of the brain that are the loci for thinking and remembering, that a whole-brain or cerebral transplant would seem to be a whole-body transplant for the brain or cerebrum rather than a brain transplant for the body.

The essays reprinted in the final section of this chapter do not raise questions about organ transplantation in principle, nor do they deal with speculative issues like brain transplantation. Rather, they treat important ethical questions that surround the current practice of transplantation. Arthur Caplan uses the widely publicized Baby Fae case as the starting point for an analysis of issues involved in the use of animal organs for transplantation into humans (see Chapter 9). Alexander Capron argues against modifying the usual definition of death in an effort to retrieve organs more efficiently from anencephalic infants, that is, infants that lack the parts of the brain necessary for reasoning and remembering (see Chapter 4). According to Albert Jonsen, the dedication of substantial public resources to the artificial heart program would be a misallocation of taxpayers' money and could interfere with efforts to provide access to an adequate level of care for every member of society (see Chapter 11).

L. W.

Technologies and Arrangements in Reproduction

UNITED KINGDOM, DEPARTMENT OF HEALTH AND SOCIAL SECURITY

Report of the Committee of Inquiry into Human Fertilisation and Embryology (The Warnock Committee Report)

THE GENERAL APPROACH

BACKGROUND TO THE INQUIRY

The birth of the first child resulting from the technique of *in vitro*[1] fertilisation in July 1978 was a considerable achievement. The technique, long sought, at last successful, opened up new horizons in the alleviation of infertility and in the science of embryology. It was now possible to observe the very earliest stages of human development, and with these discoveries came the hope of remedying defects at this very early stage. However there were also anxieties. There was a sense that events were moving too fast for their implications to be assimilated. Society's views on the new techniques were divided between pride in the technological achievement, pleasure at the new-found means to relieve, at least for some, the unhappiness of infertility, and unease at the apparently uncontrolled advance of science, bringing with it new possibilities for manipulating the early stages of human development.

Against this background of public excitement and concern, this Inquiry was established in July 1982, with the following terms of reference:

To consider recent and potential developments in medicine and science related to human fertilisation and embryology; to consider what policies and safeguards should be applied, including consideration of the social, ethical

From United Kingdom, Department of Health and Social Security, *Report of the Committee of Inquiry into Human Fertilisation and Embryology* (London: Her Majesty's Stationery Office, 1984), pp. 4, 5, 8, 29, 31–32, 58–62, 66, 70, 71–74.

and legal implications of these developments; and to make recommendations. . . .

. . . While the term "embryo" has been variously defined in considering human embryology, we have taken as our starting point the meeting of egg and sperm at fertilisation. We have regarded the embryonic stage to be the six weeks immediately following fertilisation which usually corresponds with the first eight weeks of gestation counted from the first day of the woman's last menstrual period.

INFERTILITY: THE SCOPE AND ORGANISATION OF SERVICES

In the past, there was considerable public ignorance of the causes and extent of infertility, as well as ignorance of possible remedies. At one time, if a couple were childless, there was very little they could do about it. Generally the cause of infertility was thought to be something in the woman which made her childless; only occasionally was it thought that there might be something wrong with the man. Even today, there is very little factual information about the prevalence of infertility. A commonly quoted figure is that one couple in ten is childless, but accurate statistics are not available, nor is it known what proportion of this figure relates to couples who choose not to have children. In certain religious and cultural traditions, infertility was, and still is, considered sufficient grounds for divorce. In our own society childless couples used to be advised to adopt a child. Now, as a result of improved contraception, the wider availability of legal abortion and changed attitudes towards the single mother, far fewer babies are placed for adoption. . . .

TECHNIQUES FOR THE ALLEVIATION OF INFERTILITY

IN VITRO FERTILISATION

Unlike AID [artificial insemination by donor], *in vitro* fertilisation (IVF) is very much a new development. Of those women who are infertile a small proportion can produce healthy eggs but, although they have a normal uterus, have damaged or diseased fallopian tubes which prevent the egg passing from the ovary to the uterus. A certain proportion of these women can be helped by tubal surgery. Until IVF became a reality, the possibility of achieving a pregnancy for women with tubal problems was not great. IVF may be appro-

priate perhaps for 5% of infertile couples. Recently claims have been made for IVF as a treatment for other forms of infertility including its use in the treatment of oligospermia[2] and unexplained infertility. . . .

ARGUMENTS AGAINST IVF AND RESPONSES

Although many people regard IVF as an exciting new possibility for helping the childless, there are those who are deeply worried by its development. This opposition can be categorised as opposition either based on fundamental principles, or based on the consequences of the practice of IVF. The fundamental arguments against IVF are the same as those against AIH [artificial insemination by husband]—that this practice represents a deviation from normal intercourse and that the unitive and procreative aspects of sexual intercourse should not be separated. Those who hold this view believe that this is an absolute moral principle which must be upheld without exception. This view is sincerely and strongly held. As a question of individual conscience, there will be those who will not wish to receive this form of treatment nor participate in its practice, but we would not rely on those arguments for the formulation of a public policy.

The arguments against IVF based on a consideration of the consequences are more varied; but those who put forward such arguments may take as their starting point the acceptance of IVF as a legitimate form of treatment for infertility. Their reservations start when IVF results in more embryos being brought into existence than will be transferred to the mother's uterus. They argue that it is not acceptable deliberately to produce embryos which have potential for human life when that potential will never be realised. . . . [T]he opinion of the medical profession on the whole is that in the present state of knowledge superovulation is very desirable. But if more embryos are brought into existence than are transferred, it is held to be morally unacceptable to allow them to die.

Another argument against IVF is that which draws an analogy between IVF and heart transplants, or other forms of "high technology" medical care, and asks whether the country can afford such expensive treatment which benefits only a few, and whether money could not be "better" spent, that is, with beneficial effects for more people, elsewhere. While we accept that questions about the uses of resources are proper questions, deserving serious consideration, essentially they relate to the extent of provision, not to whether there should be any provision at all. Further, without some provision of a service there can be no opportunity to evaluate the real costs and benefits of a technique, nor can the technique be refined and developed so as to become more cost-effective. The priorities argument is, in our view, an argument for controlled development, not an argument against the technique itself.

ARGUMENTS FOR IVF

The positive argument in favour of IVF is simple: the technique will increase the chances for some infertile couples to have a child. For some couples this will be the only method by which they may have a child that is genetically entirely theirs.

THE INQUIRY'S VIEW

We have reached the conclusion that IVF is an acceptable means of treating infertility and **we therefore recommend that the service of IVF should continue to be available subject to . . . licensing and inspection. . . .** For the protection and reassurance of the public this recommendation must apply equally to IVF within the NHS [National Health Service] and in the private medical sector. At the present time IVF is available on a limited scale within the NHS and **we recommend that IVF should continue to be available within the NHS**. One member of the Inquiry would not like to see any expansion of NHS IVF services until the results obtained in using this technique are more satisfactory. IVF requires a concentration of skilled medical and scientific expertise, and it is appropriate for only a small proportion of infertile couples. Therefore we would not argue that it should be available at all district general hospitals, or even at all university teaching hospitals. However in order to minimise travelling and other inconvenience to patients, we believe that ultimately NHS centres should be distributed throughout the UK. We recognise that there will be those who will press for at least one in every region. . . .

SCIENTIFIC ISSUES

HUMAN EMBRYOS AND RESEARCH

We now turn to the issues arising from the possible use of human embryos for *scientific research*. The question before the Inquiry was whether such research should be allowed. To answer this we found it necessary to look at the very earliest stages of human embryonic development, described in the following paragraphs.

EARLY HUMAN DEVELOPMENT

At fertilisation the egg and sperm unite to become a single cell. The nucleus of this cell contains the chromosomes derived from both parents. This single cell is totipotential, as from it develop all the different types of tissue and organs that make up the human body, as well as the tissues that become the placenta and foetal membranes during intra-uterine development. *In vivo* fertilisation takes place in the upper portion of the fallopian tube and the fertilised egg then passes down the fallopian tube into the cavity of the uterus over a period of four to five days. At first, when it reaches the cavity of the uterus, it remains free-floating until it begins to attach to the uterine wall at the start of implantation. This is considered to begin on the sixth day following fertilisation. During implantation, which occurs over a period of six to seven days, the embryo enters the endometrium, the lining of the uterus; at the eleventh to thirteenth day after fertilisation, implantation is complete.

While the fertilised egg is still in the upper portion of the fallopian tube, it begins to divide into first two, then four, then eight, then sixteen smaller cells, and so on by a process called cleavage. At the start of cleavage, in a two or four-cell embryo, each cell retains its totipotential capacity. Thus if separation occurs at the two-cell stage, each may develop to form a separate embryo. Such a separation could lead to identical twins.

When sixteen or more cells have resulted from cleavage, the cells hang together in a loosely packed configuration, similar to that of a blackberry, called a morula. The morula stage is reached at about the same time as the embryo *in vivo* reaches the uterine cavity. At about the same time a fluid-filled space begins to form in an eccentric position within the substance of the morula. Once this accumulation of fluid has occurred the embryo is described as a blastocyst. Within the blastocyst a thicker section of the cyst wall becomes identifiable as the inner cell mass; it is within the inner cell mass that the embryo proper, eventually to become the foetus, develops. The remaining cells of the thin walled portion of the blastocyst develop to become part of the placenta and foetal membranes. At about the time that the blastocyst begins to implant, a second fluid-filled space, the amniotic cavity, also appears within the inner cell mass. Between the two cystic spaces within the blastocyst, a plate of cells is formed. This is described as the embryonic disc; within it the first recognisable features of the embryo proper will appear.

The first of these features is the primitive streak, which appears as a heaping-up of cells at one end of the embryonic disc on the fourteenth or fifteenth day after fertilisation. Two primitive streaks may form in a single embryonic disc. This is the latest stage at which identical twins can occur. The primitive streak is the first of several identifiable features which develop in and from the embryonic disc during the succeeding days, a period of very rapid change in the embryonic configuration. By the seventeenth day the neural groove appears and by the twenty-second to twenty-third day this has developed to become the neural folds, which in turn start to fuse and form the recognisable antecedent of the spinal cord.

Once fertilisation has occurred, the subsequent developmental processes follow one another in a systematic and structured order, leading in turn through cleavage, to the morula, the blastocyst, development of the embryonic disc, and then to identifiable features within the embryonic disc such as the primitive streak, neural folds and neural tube. Until the blastocyst stage has been reached the embryo *in vivo* is unattached, floating first in the fallopian tube and then in the uterine cavity. From the sixth to the twelfth or thirteenth day internal development proceeds within the blastocyst while during the same period implantation is taking place. Both the internal and external processes of development are crucial to the future of the embryo. If the inner cell mass does not form within the blastocyst there is no further embryonic development; while if implantation does not occur the blastocyst is lost at or before the next menstrual period.

Identical developmental processes are followed by embryos fertilised *in vitro*. In these, following fertilisation, the first cleavage divisions will occur before the embryo is transferred back to the uterus. Thereafter, where implantation takes place, the developmental process will be identical for both *in vitro* and *in vivo* embryos, but there is a very high wastage rate for both as a result of their frequent failure to implant.

THE STARTING POINT FOR DISCUSSION

It was the development of IVF that, for the first time, gave rise to the possibility that human embryos might be brought into existence which might have no chance to implant because they were not transferred to a uterus and hence no chance to be born as human beings. This inevitably led to an examination of the moral rights of the embryo.

Some people hold that if an embryo is human and alive, it follows that it should not be deprived of a chance for development, and therefore it should not be used for research. They would give moral approval to IVF if, and only if, each embryo produced were to be transferred to a uterus. Others, while in no way denying that human embryos are alive (and they would concede that eggs and sperm are also alive), hold that embryos are not yet human persons and that if it could be decided when an embryo becomes a person, it could also be decided when it might, or might not, be permissible for research to be undertaken. Although the questions of when life or personhood begin appear to be questions of fact susceptible of straightforward answers, we hold that the answers to such questions in fact are complex amalgams of factual and moral judgements. Instead of trying to answer these questions directly we have therefore gone straight to the question of *how it is right to treat the human embryo*. We have considered what status ought to be accorded to the human embryo, and the answer we give must necessarily be in terms of ethical or moral principles.

DEFINING THE LIMITS OF RESEARCH

We have so far simply spoken of research and given little indication of the scope of this term. We believe that a broad division into two categories can be made. The first, which we term pure research, is aimed at increasing and developing knowledge of the very early stages of the human embryo; the second, applied research, is research with direct diagnostic or therapeutic aims for the human embryo, or for the alleviation of infertility in general. Research aimed at improving IVF techniques would come into this second category. We exclude from the concept of research what we have called new and untried treatment, undertaken during the attempt to alleviate the infertility of a particular patient. We recognise that these distinctions are not absolute. The categories may often overlap, but we feel that they have a certain validity.

ARGUMENTS AGAINST THE
USE OF HUMAN EMBRYOS

It is obvious that the central objection to the use of human embryos as research subjects is a fundamental objection, based on moral principles. Put simply, the main argument is that the use of human embryos for research is morally wrong because of the very fact that they are human, and much of the evidence submitted to us strongly supports this. The human embryo is seen as having the same status as a child or an adult, by virtue of its potential for human life. The right to life is held to be the fundamental human right, and the taking of human life on this view is always abhorrent. To take the life of the innocent is an especial moral outrage. The first consequence of this line of argument is that, since an embryo used as a research subject would have no prospect of fulfilling its potential for life, such research should not be permitted.

Everyone agrees that it is completely unacceptable to make use of a child or an adult as the subject of a research procedure which may cause harm or death. For people who hold the views outlined [in the preceding paragraph], research on embryos would fall under the same principle. They proceed to argue that since it is unethical to carry out any research, harmful or otherwise, on humans without first obtaining their informed consent, it must be equally unacceptable to carry out research on a human embryo, which by its very nature, cannot give consent.

In addition to the arguments outlined above, and well represented in the evidence, many people feel an instinctive opposition to research which they see as tampering with the creation of human life. There is widely felt concern at the possibility of unscrupulous scientists meddling with the process of reproduction in order to create hybrids, or to indulge theories of selective breeding and eugenic selection.

Those who are firmly opposed to research on human embryos recognise that a ban on their use may reduce the volume not only of pure research but also research in potentially beneficial areas, such as the detection and prevention of inherited disorders, or the alleviation of infertility, and that in some areas such a ban would halt research completely. However they argue that the moral principle outweighs any such possible benefits.

ARGUMENTS FOR THE USE
OF HUMAN EMBRYOS

The evidence showed that the views of those who support the use of human embryos as research subjects cover a wide range. At one end is the proposition that it is only to *human persons* that respect must be accorded. A human embryo cannot be thought of as a person, or even as a potential person. It is simply a collection of cells which, unless it implants in a human uterine environment, has no potential for development. There is no reason therefore to accord these cells any protected status. If useful results can be obtained from research on embryos, then such research should be permitted. We found that the more generally held position, however, is that though the human embryo is entitled to some added measure of respect beyond that accorded to other animal subjects, that respect cannot be absolute, and may be weighed against the benefits arising from research. Although many research studies in embryology and developmental biology can be carried out on animal subjects, and it is possible in many cases to extrapolate these results and findings to man, in certain situations there is no substitute for the use of human embryos. This particularly applies to the study of disorders occurring only in humans, such as Down's syndrome, or for research into the processes of human fertilisation, or perhaps into the specific effect of drugs or toxic substances on human tissue. . . .

THE INQUIRY'S VIEW

As we have seen, the objection to using human embryos in research is that each one is a potential human being. One reference point in the development of the human individual is the formation of the primitive streak. . . . Most authorities put this at about fifteen days after fertilisation. This marks the beginning of individual development of the embryo. Taking such a time limit is consonant with the views of those who favour the end of the implantation stage as a limit. We have therefore regarded an earlier date than this as a desirable end-point for research. **We accordingly recommend that no live human embryo derived from *in vitro* fertilisation, whether frozen or unfrozen, may be kept alive, if not transferred to a woman, beyond fourteen days after fertilisation, nor may it be used as a research subject beyond fourteen days after fertilisation. This fourteen day period does not include any time during which the embryo may have been frozen. We further recommend that it shall be a criminal offence to handle or to use as a research subject any live human embryo derived from *in vitro* fertilisation beyond that limit. We recommend that no embryo which has been used for research should be transferred to a woman. . . .**

POSSIBLE FUTURE
DEVELOPMENTS IN RESEARCH

There is a number of specific techniques and procedures involving the use of human embryos which have caused much public anxiety. Many of these have not yet reached the stage where they are practical possibilities. We believe that our recommendations for the regulation of research will allay much of that anxiety, as it will be the duty of the proposed licensing body . . . to keep these and other new techniques under constant review; indeed, in some instances our proposals will preclude certain developments altogether. It is important, however, to consider whether further restrictions are required, although it must be borne in mind that we cannot foresee all possible developments. . . .

USE OF HUMAN EMBRYOS
FOR TESTING DRUGS ETC.

It has been suggested that human embryos could be used to test the effects of newly developed drugs or other substances that may possibly be toxic or cause abnormalities. This is an area that causes deep concern because of the possibility of mass production of *in vitro* embryos, perhaps on a commercial basis, for these purposes. We feel very strongly that the routine testing of drugs on human embryos is not an acceptable area of research because this would require the manufacture of large numbers of embryos. We concluded however that there may be very particular circumstances where the testing of such substances on a very small scale may be justifiable.

In our view any research project in this area would have to be subject to very close scrutiny and it would rest with the proposed licensing body . . . to come to a decision according to the merits of each particular research project submitted to it.

ECTOGENESIS

It has been suggested that in the long term further development of current techniques could result in the maintenance of developing embryos in an artificial environment (ectogenesis) for progressively longer periods with the ultimate aim of creating a child entirely *in vitro*. This technique, it is argued, would make it possible to study in detail normal and abnormal human development at the embryonic and foetal stages.

We appreciate why the possibility of such a technique arouses so much anxiety. There are however two points to make about this. First, such developments are well into the future, certainly beyond the time horizon within which this Inquiry feels it can predict. Secondly, our recommendation is that the growing of a human embryo *in vitro* beyond fourteen days should be a criminal offence.

Another cause for concern is the suggestion that a human embryo might be transferred to the uterus of another species for gestation. While the available animal work does not suggest that it is at all likely that human embryos could be nurtured in the uterus of another species, the possibility that such an experiment might be attempted must be recognised. **We recommend that the placing of a human embryo in the uterus of another species for gestation should be a criminal offence.**

PARTHENOGENESIS

This term is used to describe the reproductive process whereby a gamete develops into a new individual without fertilisation. This form of reproduction occurs in some invertebrate species and plants. Although it is known that the application of some substances, for example, alcohol, to an unfertilised mammalian egg can induce the egg to undergo some initial development, we consider that there is no possibility at present of inducing parthenogenesis, or "virgin birth" as it is commonly known, in humans, and indeed we do not believe such a development will take place in the foreseeable future.

CLONING

Cloning is the production of two or more genetically identical individuals. Human identical twins are the result of natural cloning. One method of achieving cloning would be by division of the embryo at a very early stage of development so that identical genetic material is passed on to each of the separate portions. Thus all members of a clone have an identical genetic constitution. This type of cloning has been used successfully on other species but, to the best of our knowledge, has not been carried out artificially on human embryos.

EMBRYONIC BIOPSY

It has been suggested that a similar technique to cloning could be used to investigate the chromosomal structure of embryos fertilised *in vitro* by a couple who have a high chance of procreating an abnormal child. After *in vitro* fertilisation, the embryo would be allowed to develop until it was possible to remove one or more cells without putting at risk the subsequent development of the embryo. This technique is termed embryonic biopsy. The cells of the biopsy would be allowed to continue to develop while the rest of the embryo would be frozen. Once it was possible to determine from the biopsy whether the embryo was free of the abnormality for which it was being tested, a decision could be taken as to whether to thaw the frozen embryo and to transfer it to the mother's uterus.

It is difficult to estimate how likely it is that embryonic biopsy will be developed as a diagnostic technique in the near future. It has the advantage over other techniques such as chorion biopsy . . . that may be used for the early diagnosis of abnormalities, in that it may be carried out before the embryo is transferred and so before there is a pregnancy, thus avoiding the difficult decision for the parents of whether to seek a termination where abnormality is detected. However, it has the disadvantage that it requires the use of IVF. Given the present relatively low success rates for pregnancy following IVF, it is unlikely that embryonic biopsy will become a feasible method of detecting abnormal embryos for some considerable time.

NUCLEUS SUBSTITUTION

Another technique, which has sometimes been referred to as cloning, but which may be more accurately described as nucleus substitution would raise more fundamental questions. These would occur if it became possible to remove the nucleus from a fertilised human egg and, without detriment to its subsequent development, replace it with the nucleus taken from an adult human. This process would open the way for the creation of "carbon copy clones". It has been suggested that one day it might be possible to produce immunologically identical organs for transplantation purposes to replace a diseased organ, for example a kidney. The cloned replacement organ would be grown in an embryo in which the nucleus had been replaced by one taken from the person for whom the replacement organ was intended.

PREVENTION OF GENETIC DEFECTS

If it should become possible to identify at a very early stage of embryonic development certain genetic defects; and to insert a replacement gene which will remedy the defect, a genetically normal embryo could be created. It is argued that this would provide the means to prevent certain genetic diseases.

Public anxiety about these techniques centres, not so much on their possible therapeutic use, but on the idea of the deliberate creation of human beings with specific characteristics. This has overtones of selective breeding. We regard such techniques as purely speculative but believe that any developments in these fields are precluded by the controls we have already recommended. We would however go further. **We recommend that the proposed licensing body promulgate guidance on what types of research, apart from those precluded by law, would be unlikely to be considered ethically acceptable in any circumstances and therefore would not be licensed.** We envisage this guidance being reviewed from time to time to take account of both changes in scientific knowledge and changes in public attitudes.

NOTES

1. This report distinguishes between *in vitro* meaning "in a glass", and *in vivo* meaning "in the body".

2. Oligospermia is the term used to describe semen in which the number of sperm present is reduced or markedly reduced compared with the number of sperm present in normal semen.

NEW JERSEY SUPREME COURT

In the Matter of Baby M

The opinion of the Court was delivered by

WILENTZ, C.J.

In this matter the Court is asked to determine the validity of a contract that purports to provide a new way of bringing children into a family. For a fee of $10,000, a woman agrees to be artificially inseminated with the semen of another woman's husband; she is to conceive a child, carry it to term, and after its birth surrender it to the natural father and his wife. The intent of the contract is that the child's natural mother will thereafter be forever separated from her child. The wife is to adopt the child, and she and the natural father are to be regarded as its parents for all purposes. The contract providing for this is called a "surrogacy contract," the natural mother inappropriately called the "surrogate mother."

We invalidate the surrogacy contract because it conflicts with the law and public policy of this State. While we recognize the depth of the yearning of infertile couples to have their own children, we find the payment of money to a "surrogate" mother illegal, perhaps criminal, and potentially degrading to women. Although in this case we grant custody to the natural father, the evidence having clearly proved such custody to be in the best interests of the infant, we void both the termination of the surrogate mother's parental rights and the adoption of the child by the wife/step-parent. We thus restore the "surrogate" as the mother of the child. We remand the issue of the natural mother's visitation rights to the trial court, since that issue was not reached below and the record before us is not sufficient to permit us to decide it *de novo*.

We find no offense to our present laws where a woman voluntarily and without payment agrees to act as a "surrogate" mother, provided that she is not subject to a binding agreement to surrender her child. Moreover, our holding today does not preclude the Legislature from altering the current statutory scheme, within constitutional limits, so as to permit surrogacy contracts. Under current law, however, the surrogacy agreement before us is illegal and invalid.

I.

FACTS

In February 1985, William Stern and Mary Beth Whitehead entered into a surrogacy contract. It recited that Stern's wife, Elizabeth, was infertile, that they wanted a child, and that Mrs. Whitehead was willing to provide that child as the mother with Mr. Stern as the father.

The contract provided that through artificial insemination using Mr. Stern's sperm, Mrs. Whitehead would become pregnant, carry the child to term, bear it, deliver it to the Sterns, and thereafter do whatever was necessary to terminate her maternal rights so that Mrs. Stern could thereafter adopt the child. Mrs. Whitehead's husband, Richard,[1] was also a party to the contract; Mrs. Stern was not. Mr. Whitehead promised to do all acts necessary to rebut the presumption of paternity under the Parentage Act. *N.J.S.A.* 9:17–43a(1), –44a. Although Mrs. Stern was not a party to the surrogacy agreement, the contract gave her sole custody of the child in the event of Mr. Stern's death. Mrs. Stern's status as a nonparty to the surrogate parenting agreement presumably was to avoid the application of the baby-selling statute to this arrangement. *N.J.S.A.* 9:3–54.

Mr. Stern, on his part, agreed to attempt the artificial insemination and to pay Mrs. Whitehead $10,000 after the child's birth, on its delivery to him. In a

Reprinted from the *Atlantic Reporter*, 537 A.2d 1227, (N.J. 1988).

separate contract, Mr. Stern agreed to pay $7,500 to the Infertility Center of New York ("ICNY"). The Center's advertising campaigns solicit surrogate mothers and encourage infertile couples to consider surrogacy. ICNY arranged for the surrogacy contract by bringing the parties together, explaining the process to them, furnishing the contractual form, and providing legal counsel.

The history of the parties' involvement in this arrangement suggests their good faith. William and Elizabeth Stern were married in July 1974, having met at the University of Michigan, where both were Ph.D. candidates. Due to financial considerations and Mrs. Stern's pursuit of a medical degree and residency, they decided to defer starting a family until 1981. Before then, however, Mrs. Stern learned that she might have multiple sclerosis and that the disease in some cases renders pregnancy a serious health risk. Her anxiety appears to have exceeded the actual risk, which current medical authorities assess as minimal. Nonetheless that anxiety was evidently quite real, Mrs. Stern fearing that pregnancy might precipitate blindness, paraplegia, or other forms of debilitation. Based on the perceived risk, the Sterns decided to forego having their own children. The decision had a special significance for Mr. Stern. Most of his family had been destroyed in the Holocaust. As the family's only survivor, he very much wanted to continue his bloodline.

Initially the Sterns considered adoption, but were discouraged by the substantial delay apparently involved and by the potential problem they saw arising from their age and their differing religious backgrounds. They were most eager for some other means to start a family.

The paths of Mrs. Whitehead and the Sterns to surrogacy were similar. Both responded to advertising by ICNY. The Sterns' response, following their inquiries into adoption, was the result of their long-standing decision to have a child. Mrs. Whitehead's response apparently resulted from her sympathy with family members and others who could have no children (she stated that she wanted to give another couple the "gift of life"); she also wanted the $10,000 to help her family.

Both parties, undoubtedly because of their own self-interest, were less sensitive to the implications of the transaction than they might otherwise have been. Mrs. Whitehead, for instance, appears not to have been concerned about whether the Sterns would make good parents for her child; the Sterns, on their part, while conscious of the obvious possibility that surrendering the child might cause grief to Mrs. Whitehead, overcame their qualms because of their desire for a child. At any rate, both the Sterns and Mrs. Whitehead were committed to the arrangement; both thought it right and constructive.

Mrs. Whitehead had reached her decision concerning surrogacy before the Sterns, and had actually been involved as a potential surrogate mother with another couple. After numerous unsuccessful artificial inseminations, that effort was abandoned. Thereafter, the Sterns learned of the Infertility Center, the possibilities of surrogacy, and of Mary Beth Whitehead. The two couples met to discuss the surrogacy arrangement and decided to go forward. On February 6, 1985, Mr. Stern and Mr. and Mrs. Whitehead executed the surrogate parenting agreement. After several artificial inseminations over a period of months, Mrs. Whitehead became pregnant. The pregnancy was uneventful and on March 27, 1986, Baby M was born.

Not wishing anyone at the hospital to be aware of the surrogacy arrangement, Mr. and Mrs. Whitehead appeared to all as the proud parents of a healthy female child. Her birth certificate indicated her name to be Sara Elizabeth Whitehead and her father to be Richard Whitehead. In accordance with Mrs. Whitehead's request, the Sterns visited the hospital unobtrusively to see the newborn child.

Mrs. Whitehead realized, almost from the moment of birth, that she could not part with this child. She had felt a bond with it even during pregnancy. Some indication of the attachment was conveyed to the Sterns at the hospital when they told Mrs. Whitehead what they were going to name the baby. She apparently broke into tears and indicated that she did not know if she could give up the child. She talked about how the baby looked like her other daughter, and made it clear that she was experiencing great difficulty with the decision.

Nonetheless, Mrs. Whitehead was, for the moment, true to her word. Despite powerful inclinations to the contrary, she turned her child over to the Sterns on March 30 at the Whiteheads' home.

The Sterns were thrilled with their new child. They had planned extensively for its arrival, far beyond the practical furnishing of a room for her. It was a time of joyful celebration—not just for them but for their friends as well. The Sterns looked forward to raising their daughter, whom they named Melissa. While aware by then that Mrs. Whitehead was undergoing an emotional crisis, they were as yet not cognizant of the depth of that crisis and its implications for their newly-enlarged family.

Later in the evening of March 30, Mrs. Whitehead became deeply disturbed, disconsolate, stricken with unbearable sadness. She had to have her child. She could not eat, sleep, or concentrate on anything other than her need for her baby. The next day she went to the Sterns' home and told them how much she was suffering.

The depth of Mrs. Whitehead's despair surprised and frightened the Sterns. She told them that she could not live without her baby, that she must have her, even if only for one week, that thereafter she would surrender her child. The Sterns, concerned that Mrs. Whitehead might indeed commit suicide, not wanting under any circumstances to risk that, and in any event believing that Mrs. Whitehead would keep her word, turned the child over to her. It was not until four months later, after a series of attempts to regain possession of the child, that Melissa was returned to the Sterns, having been forcibly removed from the home where she was then living with Mr. and Mrs. Whitehead, the home in Florida owned by Mary Beth Whitehead's parents.

The struggle over Baby M began when it became apparent that Mrs. Whitehead could not return the child to Mr. Stern. Due to Mrs. Whitehead's refusal to relinquish the baby, Mr. Stern filed a complaint seeking enforcement of the surrogacy contract. He alleged, accurately, that Mrs. Whitehead had not only refused to comply with the surrogacy contract but had threatened to flee from New Jersey with the child in order to avoid even the possibility of his obtaining custody. The court papers asserted that if Mrs. Whitehead were to be given notice of the application for an order requiring her to relinquish custody, she would, prior to the hearing, leave the state with the baby. And that is precisely what she did. After the order was entered, *ex parte*, the process server, aided by the police, in the presence of the Sterns, entered Mrs. Whitehead's home to execute the order. Mr. Whitehead fled with the child, who had been handed to him through a window while those who came to enforce the order were thrown off balance by a dispute over the child's current name.

The Whiteheads immediately fled to Florida with Baby M. They stayed initially with Mrs. Whitehead's parents, where one of Mrs. Whitehead's children had been living. For the next three months, the Whiteheads

and Melissa lived at roughly twenty different hotels, motels, and homes in order to avoid apprehension. From time to time Mrs. Whitehead would call Mr. Stern to discuss the matter; the conversations, recorded by Mr. Stern on advice of counsel, show an escalating dispute about rights, morality, and power, accompanied by threats of Mrs. Whitehead to kill herself, to kill the child, and falsely to accuse Mr. Stern of sexually molesting Mrs. Whitehead's other daughter.

Eventually the Sterns discovered where the Whiteheads were staying, commenced supplementary proceedings in Florida, and obtained an order requiring the Whiteheads to turn over the child. Police in Florida enforced the order, forcibly removing the child from her grandparents' home. She was soon thereafter brought to New Jersey and turned over to the Sterns. The prior order of the court, issued *ex parte*, awarding custody of the child to the Sterns *pendente lite*,* was reaffirmed by the trial court after consideration of the certified representations of the parties (both represented by counsel) concerning the unusual sequence of events that had unfolded. Pending final judgment, Mrs. Whitehead was awarded limited visitation with Baby M.

The Sterns' complaint, in addition to seeking possession and ultimately custody of the child, sought enforcement of the surrogacy contract. Pursuant to the contract, it asked that the child be permanently placed in their custody, that Mrs. Whitehead's parental rights be terminated, and that Mrs. Stern be allowed to adopt the child, *i.e.*, that, for all purposes, Melissa become the Sterns' child.

The trial took thirty-two days over a period of more than two months. It included numerous interlocutory appeals and attempted interlocutory appeals. There were twenty-three witnesses to the facts recited above and fifteen expert witnesses, eleven testifying on the issue of custody and four on the subject of Mrs. Stern's multiple sclerosis; the bulk of the testimony was devoted to determining the parenting arrangement most compatible with the child's best interests. Soon after the conclusion of the trial, the trial court announced its opinion from the bench. 217 *N.J.Super.* 313, 525 *A.*2d 1128 (1987). It held that the surrogacy contract was valid; ordered that Mrs. Whitehead's parental rights be terminated and that sole custody of the child be granted to Mr. Stern; and, after hearing brief testimony from Mrs. Stern, immediately entered an order allow-

---

Ed. note: While litigation was pending.

ing the adoption of Melissa by Mrs. Stern, all in accordance with the surrogacy contract. Pending the outcome of the appeal, we granted a continuation of visitation to Mrs. Whitehead, although slightly more limited than the visitation allowed during the trial.

Although clearly expressing its view that the surrogacy contract was valid, the trial court devoted the major portion of its opinion to the question of the baby's best interests. The inconsistency is apparent. The surrogacy contract calls for the surrender of the child to the Sterns, permanent and sole custody in the Sterns, and termination of Mrs. Whitehead's parental rights, all without qualification, all regardless of any evaluation of the best interests of the child. As a matter of fact the contract recites (even before the child was conceived) that it is in the best interests of the child to be placed with Mr. Stern. In effect, the trial court awarded custody to Mr. Stern, the natural father, based on the same kind of evidence and analysis as might be expected had no surrogacy contract existed. Its rationalization, however, was that while the surrogacy contract was valid, specific performance would not be granted unless that remedy was in the best interests of the child. The factual issues confronted and decided by the trial court were the same as if Mr. Stern and Mrs. Whitehead had had the child out of wedlock, intended or unintended, and then disagreed about custody. The trial court's awareness of the irrelevance of the contract in the court's determination of custody is suggested by its remark that beyond the question of the child's best interests, "[a]ll other concerns raised by counsel constitute commentary." 217 *N.J.Super.* at 323, 525 *A.2d* 1128.

On the question of best interests—and we agree, but for different reasons, that custody was the critical issue—the court's analysis of the testimony was perceptive, demonstrating both its understanding of the case and its considerable experience in these matters. We agree substantially with both its analysis and conclusions on the matter of custody.

The court's review and analysis of the surrogacy contract, however, is not at all in accord with ours. The trial court concluded that the various statutes governing this matter, including those concerning adoption, termination of parental rights, and payment of money in connection with adoptions, do not apply to surrogacy contracts. . . . It reasoned that because the Legislature did not have surrogacy contracts in mind when it passed those laws, those laws were therefore irrelevant. Thus, assuming it was writing on a clean

slate, the trial court analyzed the interests involved and the power of the court to accommodate them. It then held that surrogacy contracts are valid and should be enforced, . . . and furthermore that Mr. Stern's rights under the surrogacy contract were constitutionally protected. . . .

Mrs. Whitehead appealed. This Court granted direct certification. . . . The briefs of the parties on appeal were joined by numerous briefs filed by *amici* expressing various interests and views on surrogacy and on this case. We have found many of them helpful in resolving the issues before us.

Mrs. Whitehead contends that the surrogacy contract, for a variety of reasons, is invalid. She contends that it conflicts with public policy since it guarantees that the child will not have the nurturing of both natural parents—presumably New Jersey's goal for families. She further argues that it deprives the mother of her constitutional right to the companionship of her child, and that it conflicts with statutes concerning termination of parental rights and adoption. With the contract thus void, Mrs. Whitehead claims primary custody (with visitation rights in Mr. Stern) both on a best interests basis (stressing the "tender years" doctrine) as well as on the policy basis of discouraging surrogacy contracts. She maintains that even if custody would ordinarily go to Mr. Stern, here it should be awarded to Mrs. Whitehead to deter future surrogacy arrangements.

In a brief filed after oral argument, counsel for Mrs. Whitehead suggests that the standard for determining best interests where the infant resulted from a surrogacy contract is that the child should be placed with the mother absent a showing of unfitness. All parties agree that no expert testified that Mary Beth Whitehead was unfit as a mother; the trial court expressly found that she was *not* "unfit," that, on the contrary, "she is a good mother for and to her older children," . . . and no one now claims anything to the contrary.

One of the repeated themes put forth by Mrs. Whitehead is that the court's initial *ex parte* order granting custody to the Sterns during the trial was a substantial factor in the ultimate "best interests" determination. That initial order, claimed to be erroneous by Mrs. Whitehead, not only established Melissa as part of the Stern family, but brought enormous pressure on Mrs. Whitehead. The order brought the resulting pressure, Mrs. Whitehead contends, caused her to act in ways that were atypical of her ordinary behavior when not under stress, and to act in ways that were thought to be inimical to the child's best interests in that they demonstrated a failure of character, maturity, and consistency. She claims that any mother who truly loved her child might so respond and that it is doubly unfair to judge her on the basis of her reaction to an extreme situation rarely faced by any mother, where that situation was itself caused by an erroneous order of the court. Therefore, according to Mrs. Whitehead, the erroneous *ex parte* order precipitated a series of events that proved instrumental in the final result.[2]

The Sterns claim that the surrogacy contract is valid and should be enforced, largely for the reasons given by the trial court. They claim a constitutional right of privacy, which includes the right of procreation, and the right of consenting adults to deal with matters of reproduction as they see fit. As for the child's best interests, their position is factual: given all of the circumstances, the child is better off in their custody with no residual parental rights reserved for Mrs. Whitehead.

Of considerable interest in this clash of views is the position of the child's guardian *ad litem*, wisely appointed by the court at the outset of the litigation. As the child's representative, her role in the litigation, as she viewed it, was solely to protect the child's best interests. She therefore took no position on the validity of the surrogacy contract, and instead devoted her energies to obtaining expert testimony uninfluenced by any interest other than the child's. We agree with the guardian's perception of her role in this litigation. She appropriately refrained from taking any position that might have appeared to compromise her role as the child's advocate. She first took the position, based on her experts' testimony, that the Sterns should have primary custody, and that while Mrs. Whitehead's parental rights should not be terminated, no visitation should be allowed for five years. As a result of subsequent developments, mentioned *infra*, her view has changed. She now recommends that no visitation be allowed at least until Baby M reaches maturity.

Although some of the experts' opinions touched on visitation, the major issue they addressed was whether custody should be reposed in the Sterns or in the Whiteheads. The trial court, consistent in this respect with its view that the surrogacy contract was valid, did not deal at all with the question of visitation. Having concluded that the best interests of the child called for custody in the Sterns, the trial court enforced the operative provisions of the surrogacy contract, terminated Mrs. Whitehead's parental rights, and granted an adoption to Mrs. Stern. Explicit in the ruling was the conclusion that the best interests determination removed whatever impediment might have existed in enforcing the surrogacy contract. This Court, therefore, is without guidance from the trial court on the visitation issue, an issue of considerable importance in any event, and especially important in view of our determination that the surrogacy contract is invalid.

II.

INVALIDITY AND UNENFORCEABILITY OF SURROGACY CONTRACT

We have concluded that this surrogacy contract is invalid. Our conclusion has two bases: direct conflict with existing statutes and conflict with the public policies of this State, as expressed in its statutory and decisional law.

One of the surrogacy contract's basic purposes, to achieve the adoption of a child through private placement, though permitted in New Jersey "is very much disfavored." . . . Its use of money for this purpose—and we have no doubt whatsoever that the money is being paid to obtain an adoption and not, as the Sterns argue, for the personal services of Mary Beth Whitehead—is illegal and perhaps criminal. . . . In addition to the inducement of money, there is the coercion of contract: the natural mother's irrevocable agreement, prior to birth, even prior to conception, to surrender the child to the adoptive couple. Such an agreement is totally unenforceable in private placement adoption. . . . Even where the adoption is through an approved agency, the formal agreement to surrender occurs only *after* birth . . . , and then, by regulation, only after the birth mother has been counseled. . . . Integral to these invalid provisions of the surrogacy contract is the related agreement, equally invalid, on the part of the natural mother to cooperate with, and not to contest, proceedings to terminate her parental rights, as well as her contractual concession, in aid of the adoption, that the child's best interests would be served by awarding custody to the natural father and his wife—all of this before she has even conceived, and, in some cases, before she has the slightest idea of what the natural father and adoptive mother are like.

The foregoing provisions not only directly conflict with New Jersey statutes, but also offend long-established State policies. These critical terms, which are at the heart of the contract, are invalid and unenforceable; the conclusion therefore follows, without more, that the entire contract is unenforceable. . . .

III.

TERMINATION

We have already noted that under our laws termination of parental rights cannot be based on contract, but may be granted only on proof of the statutory requirements. That conclusion was one of the bases for invalidating the surrogacy contract. Although excluding the contract as a basis for parental termination, we did not explicitly deal with the question of whether the statutory bases for termination existed. We do so here.

As noted before, if termination of Mrs. Whitehead's parental rights is justified, Mrs. Whitehead will have no further claim either to custody or to visitation, and adoption by Mrs. Stern may proceed pursuant to the private placement adoption statute. . . . If termination is not justified, Mrs. Whitehead remains the legal mother, and even if not entitled to custody, she would ordinarily be expected to have some rights of visitation. . . .

Nothing in this record justifies a finding that would allow a court to terminate Mary Beth Whitehead's parental rights under the statutory standard. It is not simply that obviously there was no "intentional abandonment or very substantial neglect of parental duties without a reasonable expectation of reversal of that conduct in the future," *N.J.S.A.* 9:3–48c(1), quite the contrary, but furthermore that the trial court never found Mrs. Whitehead an unfit mother and indeed affirmatively stated that Mary Beth Whitehead had been a good mother to her other children. . . .

There is simply no basis . . . to warrant termination of Mrs. Whitehead's parental rights. We therefore conclude that the natural mother is entitled to retain her rights as a mother.

IV.

CONSTITUTIONAL ISSUES

Both parties argue that the Constitutions—state and federal—mandate approval of their basic claims. The source of their constitutional arguments is essentially the same: the right of privacy, the right to procreate, the right to the companionship of one's child, those rights flowing either directly from the fourteenth amendment or by its incorporation of the Bill of Rights, or

from the ninth amendment, or through the penumbra surrounding all of the Bill of Rights. They are the rights of personal intimacy, of marriage, of sex, of family, of procreation. Whatever their source, it is clear that they are fundamental rights protected by both the federal and state Constitutions. . . . The right asserted by the Sterns is the right of procreation; that asserted by Mary Beth Whitehead is the right to the companionship of her child. We find that the right of procreation does not extend as far as claimed by the Sterns. As for the right asserted by Mrs. Whitehead, since we uphold it on other grounds (*i.e.*, we have restored her as mother and recognized her right, limited by the child's best interests, to her companionship), we need not decide that constitutional issue, and for reasons set forth below, we should not.

The right to procreate, as protected by the Constitution, has been ruled on directly only once by the United States Supreme Court. *See Skinner v. Oklahoma*, 316 *U.S.* 535, 62 *S.Ct.* 1110, 86 *L.Ed.* 1655 (forced sterilization of habitual criminals violates equal protection clause of fourteenth amendment). Although *Griswold v. Connecticut*, 381 *U.S.* 479, 85 *S.Ct.* 1678, 14 *L.Ed.*2d 510, is obviously of a similar class, strictly speaking it involves the right *not* to procreate. The right to procreate very simply is the right to have natural children, whether through sexual intercourse or artificial insemination. It is no more than that. Mr. Stern has not been deprived of that right. Through artificial insemination of Mrs. Whitehead, Baby M is his child. The custody, care, companionship, and nurturing that follow birth are not parts of the right to procreation; they are rights that may also be constitutionally protected, but that involve many considerations other than the right of procreation. To assert that Mr. Stern's right of procreation gives him the right to the custody of Baby M would be to assert that Mrs. Whitehead's right of procreation does *not* give her the right to the custody of Baby M; it would be to assert that the constitutional right of procreation includes within it a constitutionally protected contractual right to destroy someone else's right of procreation.

We conclude that the right of procreation is best understood and protected if confined to its essentials, and that when dealing with rights concerning the resulting child, different interests come into play. There is nothing in our culture or society that even begins to suggest a fundamental right on the part of the father to the custody of the child as part of his right to procreate weight of the state behind the Sterns' attempt, ultimately successful, to gain possession of the child. The when opposed by the claim of the mother to the same child. We therefore disagree with the trial court: there is no constitutional basis whatsoever requiring that Mr. Stern's claim to the custody of Baby M be sustained. Our conclusion may thus be understood as illustrating that a person's rights of privacy and self-determination are qualified by the effect on innocent third persons of the exercise of those rights.

Mr. Stern also contends that he has been denied equal protection of the laws by the State's statute granting full parental rights to a husband in relation to the child produced, with his consent, by the union of his wife with a sperm donor. . . . The claim really is that of Mrs. Stern. It is that she is in precisely the same position as the husband in the statute: she is presumably infertile, as is the husband in the statute; her spouse by agreement with a third party procreates with the understanding that the child will be the couple's child. The alleged unequal protection is that the understanding is honored in the statute when the husband is the infertile party, but no similar understanding is honored when it is the wife who is infertile.

It is quite obvious that the situations are not parallel. A sperm donor simply cannot be equated with a surrogate mother. The State has more than a sufficient basis to distinguish the two situations—even if the only difference is between the time it takes to provide sperm for artificial insemination and the time invested in a nine-month pregnancy—so as to justify automatically divesting the sperm donor of his parental rights without automatically divesting a surrogate mother. Some basis for an equal protection argument might exist if Mary Beth Whitehead had contributed her egg to be implanted, fertilized or otherwise, in Mrs. Stern, resulting in the latter's pregnancy. That is not the case here, however.

Mrs. Whitehead, on the other hand, asserts a claim that falls within the scope of a recognized fundamental interest protected by the Constitution. As a mother, she claims the right to the companionship of her child. This is a fundamental interest, constitutionally protected. Furthermore, it was taken away from her by the action of the court below. Whether that action under these circumstances would constitute a constitutional deprivation, however, we need not and do not decide. By virtue of our decision Mrs. White-

head's constitutional complaint—that her parental rights have been unconstitutionally terminated—is moot. We have decided that both the statutes and public policy of this state require that that termination be voided and that her parental rights be restored. It therefore becomes unnecessary to decide whether that same result would be required by virtue of the federal or state Constitutions. . . .

V.

CUSTODY

Having decided that the surrogacy contract is illegal and unenforceable, we now must decide the custody question without regard to the provisions of the surrogacy contract that would give Mr. Stern sole and permanent custody. (That does not mean that the existence of the contract and the circumstances under which it was entered may not be considered to the extent deemed relevant to the child's best interests.) With the surrogacy contract disposed of, the legal framework becomes a dispute between two couples over the custody of a child produced by the artificial insemination of one couple's wife by the other's husband. Under the Parentage Act the claims of the natural father and the natural mother are entitled to equal weight, *i.e.*, one is not preferred over the other solely because it is the father or the mother. *N.J.S.A.* 9:17–40.[3] The applicable rule given these circumstances is clear: the child's best interests determine custody. . . .

We are not concerned at this point with the question of termination of parental rights, either those of Mrs. Whitehead or of Mr. Stern. As noted in various places in this opinion, such termination, in the absence of abandonment or a valid surrender, generally depends on a showing that the particular parent is unfit. The question of custody in this case, as in practically all cases, assumes the fitness of both parents, and no serious contention is made in this case that either is unfit. The issue here is which life would be better *for Baby M, one with primary custody in the Whiteheads or one with primary custody in the Sterns.*

The circumstances of this custody dispute are unusual and they have provoked some unusual contentions. The Whiteheads claim that even if the child's best interests would be served by our awarding custody to the Sterns, we should not do so, since that will encourage surrogacy contracts—contracts claimed by the Whiteheads, and we agree, to be violative of important legislatively-stated public policies. Their mother unless she is unfit, regardless of the best interests of the child. We disagree. Our declaration that this surrogacy contract is unenforceable and illegal is sufficient to deter similar agreements. We need not sacrifice the child's interests in order to make that point sharper. . . .

The Whiteheads also contend that the award of custody to the Sterns *pendente lite* was erroneous and that the error should not be allowed to affect the final custody decision. As noted above, at the very commencement of this action the court issued an *ex parte* order requiring Mrs. Whitehead to turn over the baby to the Sterns; Mrs. Whitehead did not comply but rather took the child to Florida. Thereafter, a similar order was enforced by the Florida authorities resulting in the transfer of possession of Baby M to the Sterns. The Sterns retained custody of the child throughout the litigation. The Whiteheads' point, assuming the *pendente* award of custody *was* erroneous, is that most of the factors arguing for awarding permanent custody to the Sterns resulted from that initial *pendente lite* order. Some of Mrs. Whitehead's alleged character failings, as testified to by experts and concurred in by the trial court, were demonstrated by her actions brought on by the custody crisis. For instance, in order to demonstrate her impulsiveness, those experts stressed the Whiteheads' flight to Florida with Baby M; to show her willingness to use her children for her own aims, they noted the telephone threats to kill Baby M and to accuse Mr. Stern of sexual abuse of her daughter; in order to show Mrs. Whitehead's manipulativeness, they pointed to her threat to kill herself; and in order to show her unsettled family life, they noted the innumerable moves from one hotel or motel to another in Florida. Furthermore, the argument continues, one of the most important factors, whether mentioned or not, in favor of custody in the Sterns is their continuing custody during the litigation, now having lasted for one-and-a-half years. The Whiteheads' conclusion is that had the trial court not given initial custody to the Sterns during the litigation, Mrs. Whitehead not only would have demonstrated her perfectly acceptable personality—the general tenor of the opinion of experts was that her personality problems surfaced primarily in crises—but would also have been able to prove better her parental skills along with an even stronger bond than may now exist between her and Baby M. Had she not been limited to custody for four months, position is that in order that surrogacy contracts be deterred, custody should remain in the surrogate

she could have proved all of these things much more persuasively through almost two years of custody.

The argument has considerable force. It is of course possible that the trial court was wrong in its initial award of custody. It is also possible that such error, if that is what it was, may have affected the outcome. We disagree with the premise, however, that in determining custody a court should decide what the child's best interests *would be* if some hypothetical state of facts had existed. Rather, we must look to what those best interests *are*, *today*, even if some of the facts may have resulted in part from legal error. The child's interests come first: we will not punish it for judicial errors, assuming any were made. . . . The custody decision must be based on all circumstances, on everything that *actually* has occurred, on everything that is relevant to the child's best interests. Those circumstances include the trip to Florida, the telephone calls and threats, the substantial period of successful custody with the Sterns, and all other relevant circumstances. . . .

There were eleven experts who testified concerning the child's best interests, either directly or in connection with matters related to that issue. Our reading of the record persuades us that the trial court's decision awarding custody to the Sterns (technically to Mr. Stern) should be affirmed since "its findings . . . could reasonably have been reached on sufficient credible evidence present in the record." . . . More than that, on this record we find little room for any different conclusion. The trial court's treatment of this issue, . . . is both comprehensive and, in most respects, perceptive. We agree substantially with its analysis with but few exceptions that, although important, do not change our ultimate views.

Our custody conclusion is based on strongly persuasive testimony contrasting both the family life of the Whiteheads and the Sterns and the personalities and characters of the individuals. The stability of the Whitehead family life was doubtful at the time of trial. Their finances were in serious trouble (foreclosure by Mrs. Whitehead's sister on a second mortgage was in process). Mr. Whitehead's employment, though relatively steady, was always at risk because of his alcoholism, a condition that he seems not to have been able to confront effectively. Mrs. Whitehead had not worked for quite some time, her last two employments having been part-time. One of the Whiteheads' positive attributes was their ability to bring up two children, and apparently well, even in so vulnerable a household. Yet substantial question was raised even about that aspect of their home life. The expert testimony contained criticism of Mrs. Whitehead's handling of her son's educational difficulties. Certain of the experts noted that Mrs. Whitehead perceived herself as omnipotent and omniscient concerning her children. She knew what they were thinking, what they wanted, and she spoke for them. As to Melissa, Mrs. Whitehead expressed the view that she alone knew what that child's cries and sounds meant. Her inconsistent stories about various things engendered grave doubts about her ability to explain honestly and sensitively to Baby M—and at the right time—the nature of her origin. Although faith in professional counseling is not a *sine qua non* of parenting, several experts believed that Mrs. Whitehead's contempt for professional help, especially professional psychological help, coincided with her feelings of omnipotence in a way that could be devastating to a child who most likely will need such help. In short, while love and affection there would be, Baby M's life with the Whiteheads promised to be too closely controlled by Mrs. Whitehead. The prospects for a wholesome independent psychological growth and development would be at serious risk.

The Sterns have no other children, but all indications are that their household and their personalities promise a much more likely foundation for Melissa to grow and thrive. There *is* a track record of sorts— during the one-and-a-half years of custody Baby M has done very well, and the relationship between both Mr. and Mrs. Stern and the baby has become very strong. The household is stable, and likely to remain so. Their finances are more than adequate, their circle of friends supportive, and their marriage happy. Most important, they are loving, giving, nurturing, and open-minded people. They have demonstrated the wish and ability to nurture and protect Melissa, yet at the same time to encourage her independence. Their lack of experience is more than made up for by a willingness to learn and to listen, a willingness that is enhanced by their professional training, especially Mrs. Stern's experience as a pediatrician. They are honest; they can recognize error, deal with it, and learn from it. They will try to determine rationally the best way to cope with problems in their relationship with Melissa. When the time comes to tell her about her

origins, they will probably have found a means of doing so that accords with the best interests of Baby M. All in all, Melissa's future appears solid, happy, and promising with them.

Based on all of this we have concluded, independent of the trial court's identical conclusion, that Melissa's best interests call for custody in the Sterns. Our above-mentioned disagreements with the trial court do not, as we have noted, in any way diminish our concurrence with its conclusions. We feel, however, that those disagreements are important enough to be stated. They are disagreements about the evaluation of conduct. They also may provide some insight about the potential consequences of surrogacy.

It seems to us that given her predicament, Mrs. Whitehead was rather harshly judged—both by the trial court and by some of the experts. She was guilty of a breach of contract, and indeed, she did break a very important promise, but we think it is expecting something well beyond normal human capabilities to suggest that this mother should have parted with her newly born infant without a struggle. Other than survival, what stronger force is there? We do not know of, and cannot conceive of, any other case where a perfectly fit mother was expected to surrender her newly born infant, perhaps forever, and was then told she was a bad mother because she did not. We know of no authority suggesting that the moral quality of her act in those circumstances should be judged by referring to a contract made before she became pregnant. We do not countenance, and would never countenance, violating a court order as Mrs. Whitehead did, even a court order that is wrong; but her resistance to an order that she surrender her infant, possibly forever, merits a measure of understanding. We do not find it so clear that her efforts to keep her infant, when measured against the Sterns' efforts to take her away, make one, rather than the other, the wrongdoer. The Sterns suffered, but so did she. And if we go beyond suffering to an evaluation of the human stakes involved in the struggle, how much weight should be given to her nine months of pregnancy, the labor of childbirth, the risk to her life, compared to the payment of money, the anticipation of a child and the donation of sperm?

There has emerged a portrait of Mrs. Whitehead, exposing her children to the media, engaging in negotiations to sell a book, granting interviews that seemed helpful to her, whether hurtful to Baby M or not, that suggests a selfish, grasping woman ready to sacrifice the interests of Baby M and her other children for fame and wealth. That portrait is a half-truth, for while it may accurately reflect what ultimately occurred, its implication, that this is what Mary Beth Whitehead wanted, is totally inaccurate, at least insofar as the record before us is concerned. There is not one word in that record to support a claim that had she been allowed to continue her possession of her newly born infant, Mrs. Whitehead would have ever been heard of again; not one word in the record suggests that her change of mind and her subsequent fight for her child was motivated by anything other than love—whatever complex underlying psychological motivations may have existed.

We have a further concern regarding the trial court's emphasis on the Sterns' interest in Melissa's education as compared to the Whiteheads'. That this difference is a legitimate factor to be considered we have no doubt. But it should not be overlooked that a best-interests test is designed to create not a new member of the intelligentsia but rather a well-integrated person who might reasonably be expected to be happy with life. "Best interests" does not contain within it any idealized lifestyle; the question boils down to a judgment, consisting of many factors, about the likely future happiness of a human being. . . . Stability, love, family happiness, tolerance, and, ultimately, support of independence—all rank much higher in predicting future happiness than the likelihood of a college education. We do not mean to suggest that the trial court would disagree. We simply want to dispel any possible misunderstanding on the issue.

Even allowing for these differences, the facts, the experts' opinions, and the trial court's analysis of both argue strongly in favor of custody in the Sterns. Mary Beth Whitehead's family life, into which Baby M would be placed, was anything but secure—the quality Melissa needs most. And today it may be even less so.[4] Furthermore, the evidence and expert opinion based on it reveal personality characteristics, mentioned above, that might threaten the child's best development. The Sterns promise a secure home, with an understanding relationship that allows nurturing and independent growth to develop together. Although there is no substitute for reading the entire record, including the review of every word of each expert's testimony and reports, a summary of their conclusions is revealing. Six experts testified for Mrs. Whitehead: one favored joint custody, clearly unwarranted in this case; one simply rebutted an opposing expert's claim that Mary Beth Whitehead had a recognized person-

ality disorder; one testified to the adverse impact of separation on *Mrs. Whitehead*; one testified about the evils of adoption and, to him, the probable analogous evils of surrogacy; one spoke only on the question of whether Mrs. Whitehead's consent in the surrogacy agreement was "informed consent"; and one spelled out the strong bond between mother and child. None of them unequivocally stated, or even necessarily implied, an opinion that custody in the Whiteheads was in the best interests of Melissa—the ultimate issue. The Sterns' experts, both well qualified—as were the Whiteheads'—concluded that the best interests of Melissa required custody in Mr. Stern. Most convincingly, the three experts chosen by the court-appointed guardian *ad litem* of Baby M, each clearly free of all bias and interest, unanimously and persuasively recommended custody in the Sterns. . . .

VI.

VISITATION

The trial court's decision to terminate Mrs. Whitehead's parental rights precluded it from making any determination on visitation. 217 *N.J.Super.* at 399, 408, 525 *A.*2d 1128. Our reversal of the trial court's order, however, requires delineation of Mrs. Whitehead's rights to visitation. It is apparent to us that this factually sensitive issue, which was never addressed below, should not be determined *de novo* by this Court. We therefore remand the visitation issue to the trial court for an abbreviated hearing and determination as set forth below. . . .

We also note the following for the trial court's consideration: First, this is not a divorce case where visitation is almost invariably granted to the non-custodial spouse. To some extent the facts here resemble cases where the non-custodial spouse has had practically no relationship with the child; . . . but it only "resembles" those cases. In the instant case, Mrs. Whitehead spent the first four months of this child's life as her mother and has regularly visited the child since then. Second, she is not only the natural mother, but also the legal mother, and is not to be penalized one iota because of the surrogacy contract. Mrs. Whitehead, as the mother (indeed, as a mother who nurtured her child for its first four months—unquestionably a relevant consideration), is entitled to have her own interest in visitation considered. Visitation cannot be determined without considering the parents' interests along with those of the child.

In all of this, the trial court should recall the touchstones of visitation: that it is desirable for the child to have contact with both parents; that besides the child's interests, the parents' interests also must be considered; but that when all is said and done, the best interests of the child are paramount.

We have decided that Mrs. Whitehead is entitled to visitation at some point, and that question is not open to the trial court on this remand. The trial court will determine what kind of visitation shall be granted to her, with or without conditions, and when and under what circumstances it should commence. It also should be noted that the guardian's recommendation of a five-year delay is most unusual—one might argue that it begins to border on termination. Nevertheless, if the circumstances as further developed by appropriate proofs or as reconsidered on remand clearly call for that suspension under applicable legal principles of visitation, it should be so ordered.

In order that the matter be determined as expeditiously as possible, we grant to the trial court the broadest powers to reach its determination. A decision shall be rendered in no more than ninety days from the date of this opinion. . . .

CONCLUSION

This case affords some insight into a new reproductive arrangement: the artificial insemination of a surrogate mother. The unfortunate events that have unfolded illustrate that its unregulated use can bring suffering to all involved. Potential victims include the surrogate mother and her family, the natural father and his wife, and most importantly, the child. Although surrogacy has apparently provided positive results for some infertile couples, it can also, as this case demonstrates, cause suffering to participants, here essentially innocent and well-intended.

We have found that our present laws do not permit the surrogacy contract used in this case. Nowhere, however, do we find any legal prohibition against surrogacy when the surrogate mother volunteers, without any payment, to act as a surrogate and is given the right to change her mind and to assert her parental rights. Moreover, the Legislature remains free to deal with this most sensitive issue as it sees fit, subject only to constitutional constraints.

If the Legislature decides to address surrogacy, consideration of this case will highlight many of its potential harms. We do not underestimate the difficulties of legislating on this subject. In addition to the inevitable confrontation with the ethical and moral issues involved, there is the question of the wisdom and effectiveness of regulating a matter so private, yet of such public interest. Legislative consideration of surrogacy may also provide the opportunity to begin to focus on the overall implications of the new reproductive biotechnology—*in vitro* fertilization, preservation of sperm and eggs, embryo implantation and the like. The problem is how to enjoy the benefits of the technology—especially for infertile couples—while minimizing the risk of abuse. The problem can be addressed only when society decides what its values and objectives are in this troubling, yet promising, area.

The judgment is affirmed in part, reversed in part, and remanded for further proceedings consistent with this opinion.

For affirmance in part, reversal in part and remandment—Chief Justice WILENTZ and Justices CLIFFORD, HANDLER, POLLOCK, O'HERN, GARIBALDI and STEIN—7.

Opposed—None.

NOTES

1. Subsequent to the trial court proceedings, Mr. and Mrs. Whitehead were divorced, and soon thereafter Mrs. Whitehead remarried. Nevertheless, in the course of this opinion we will make reference almost exclusively to the facts as they existed at the time of trial, the facts on which the decision we now review was reached. We note moreover that Mr. Whitehead remains a party to this dispute. For these reasons, we continue to refer to appellants as Mr. and Mrs. Whitehead.

2. Another argument advanced by Mrs. Whitehead is that the surrogacy agreement violates state wage regulations, *N.J.S.A.* 34:11–4.7, and the Minimum Wage Standard Act, *N.J.S.A.* 34:11–56a to −56a30. Given our disposition of the matter, we need not reach those issues.

3. At common law the rights of women were so fragile that the husband generally had the paramount right to the custody of children upon separation or divorce. *State v. Baird*, 21 *N.J.Eq.* 384, 388 (E. & A. 1869). In 1860 a statute concerning separation provided that children "within the age of seven years" be placed with the mother "unless said mother shall be of such character and habits as to render her an improper guardian." *L.* 1860, *c.* 167. The inequities of the common-law rule and the 1860 statute were redressed by an 1871 statute, providing that "the rights of both parents, in the absence of misconduct, shall be held to be equal." *L.* 1871, *c.* 48, § 6 (currently

codified at *N.J.S.A.* 9:2–4). Under this statute the father's superior right to the children was abolished and the mother's right to custody of children of tender years was also eliminated. Under the 1871 statute, "the happiness and welfare of the children" were to determine custody, *L.*1871, *c.* 48, § 6, a rule that remains law to this day. *N.J.S.A.* 9:2–4.

4. Subsequent to trial, and by the time of oral argument, Mr. and Mrs. Whitehead had separated, and the representation was that there was no likelihood of change. Thereafter Mrs. Whitehead became pregnant by another man, divorced Mr. Whitehead, and remarried the other man. Both children are living with Mrs. White-head and her new husband. Both the former and present husband continue to assert the desire to have whatever parental relationship with Melissa that the law allows, Mrs. Whitehead continuing to maintain her claim for custody.

We refer to this development only because it suggests less stability in the Whiteheads' lives. It does not necessarily suggest that Mrs. Whitehead's conduct renders her any less a fit parent. In any event, this new development has not affected our decision.

Genetic Technologies

W. FRENCH ANDERSON

Human Gene Therapy: Scientific Considerations

There are four potential levels of the application of genetic engineering for the insertion of a gene into a human being (Anderson, 1982):

(1) Somatic cell gene therapy: this would result in correcting a genetic defect in the somatic (i.e., body) cells of a patient.

(2) Germ line gene therapy: this would require the insertion of the gene into the reproductive tissue of the patient in such a way that the disorder in his or her offspring would also be corrected.

(3) Enhancement genetic engineering: this would involve the insertion of a gene to try to 'enhance' a known characteristic; for example, the placing of an additional growth hormone gene into a normal child.

(4) Eugenic genetic engineering: this is defined as the attempt to alter or 'improve' complex human traits, each of which is coded by a large number of genes; for example, personality, intelligence, character, formation of body organs, and so on.

SOMATIC CELL GENE THERAPY

There are many examples of genes which, when defective, produce serious or lethal disease in a patient. Gene therapy should be beneficial primarily for the replacement of a defective or missing enzyme or protein that must function inside the cell that makes it, or of a deficient circulating protein whose level does not need to be exactly regulated (for example, blood clotting factor VIII which is deficient in hemophilia). Early attempts at gene therapy will almost certainly be done with genes for enzymes that have a simple 'always-on' type of regulation. (For a technical discussion of the state-of-the-art of somatic cell gene therapy, together with extensive references, see Anderson, 1984.)

INITIAL CANDIDATES FOR GENE THERAPY

The most likely genes to be used in the first experiments on human gene therapy are: hypoxanthine-guanine phosphoribosyl transferase (HRPT), the absence of which results in Lesch-Nyhan disease (a severe neurological disorder that includes uncontrollable self-mutilation); adenosine deaminase (ADA), the absence of which results in severe combined immunodeficiency disease (in which children have a greatly weakened resistance to infection and cannot survive the usual childhood diseases); and purine nucleoside phosphorylase (PNP), the absence of which results in another form of severe immunodeficiency disease. For all three, the clinical syndrome is profoundly debilitating. The disorder in each is found in the patient's bone marrow (although the severe central nervous system manifestations of Lesch-Nyhan disease are due to absence of HPRT in brain cells and probably cannot be corrected with current techniques). In all three, there is no, or minimal, detectable enzyme in marrow cells from patients who have no copies of the normal gene. In these patients, the production of a small percentage of the normal enzyme level should be beneficial and a mild overproduction of enzyme should not be harmful. In addition, in the case of all three disorders, the normal gene has been cloned and is available.

Previously, clinical investigators thought that the human genetic diseases most likely to be the initial ones successfully treated by gene therapy would be the hemoglobin abnormalities (specifically, betathalassemia) because these disorders are the most obvious ones carried by blood cells, and bone marrow is the easiest tissue to manipulate outside the body. Regulation of globin synthesis, however, is unusually complicated. Not only are the embryonic, fetal, and adult globin chains carefully regulated during development, but also the subunits of the hemoglobin molecule are coded by genes on two different chromosomes. To understand the regulatory signals that control such a complicated system and to develop means for obtaining controlled expression of an exogenous (i.e., inserted by gene therapy) beta-globin gene will take considerably more research effort.

Severe combined immunodeficiency due to a defect in the ADA gene can be corrected by infusion of normal bone marrow cells from a histocompatible donor. Therefore, selective replication of the normal marrow cells appears to take place. This observation offers hope that defective bone marrow can be removed from a patient, the normal ADA gene inserted into a number of cells through gene therapy, and the treated marrow reimplanted into the patient where it may have a selective growth advantage. There is also evidence that marrow cells containing the normal gene for HPRT may have a selective advantage (in both mice and humans) over cells that do not. If selective growth occurs, elimination of the patient's own marrow would not be necessary. If, however, corrected marrow cells have no growth advantage over endogenous (i.e., the patient's own untreated) cells, then partial or complete marrow destruction (either by irradiation or by other means) may be required in order to allow the corrected marrow cells an environment favorable for expansion. The latter situation would require much greater confidence that the gene therapy procedure would work before a clinical trial should be undertaken. . . .

DELIVERY

At present, the only human tissue that can be used effectively for gene transfer is bone marrow. No other cells (except, perhaps, skin cells) can be extracted from the body, grown in culture to allow insertion of exogenous genes, and then successfully reimplanted into the patient from whom the tissue was taken. In the future, as more is learned about how to package the DNA and to make it tissue-specific, the intravenous route would be the simplest and most desirable. However, attempting to give a foreign gene by injection directly into the bloodstream is not advisable with our present state of knowledge since the procedure would be enormously inefficient and there would be little control over the DNA's fate.

Studies are considerably more advanced with bone marrow than skin cells as a recipient tissue for gene transfer. Bone marrow consists of a heterogeneous population of cells, most of which are committed to differentiate into red blood cells, white blood cells, platelets, and so on. Only a small proportion (0.1 to 0.5 percent) of nucleated bone marrow cells are stem cells (that is, blood-forming cells that have not yet differentiated into specific cell types and which divide as needed to maintain the marrow population). In gene therapy, it would be these rare, unrecognizable stem cells that would be the primary target. Consequently, a delivery system useful for gene therapy must be efficient.

Several techniques for transferring cloned genes into cells have been developed (Anderson, 1984). Each procedure is valuable for certain types of experiments, but none can yet be used to insert a gene into a specific chromosomal site in a target cell. At present the most promising approach for use in humans employs retrovirus-based vectors carrying exogenous genes.

Vectors derived from retroviruses possess several advantages as a gene delivery system. First, up to 100 percent of cells can be infected and can express the integrated viral (and exogenous) genes. Second, as many cells as desired can be infected simultaneously; 10^6 to 10^7 is a convenient number for a simple protocol. Third, under appropriate conditions, the DNA can integrate as a single copy at a single, albeit random, site. Finally, the infection and long-term harboring of a retroviral vector usually does not harm cells. Several retroviral vector systems have been developed; those projected for human use at the present time are constructed from the Moloney murine (mouse) leukemia virus. Evidence obtained from studies with experimental animals and in tissue culture indicates that retroviruses can be used as a reasonably efficient delivery system.

An ideal delivery system would be tissue-specific. When a genetic disorder is in the blood cells, the isolated bone marrow can be treated. But no other tissue (except skin cells) can be removed, treated, and replaced at present. Since many viruses are known to infect only specific tissues (that is, to bind to receptors that are present only on certain cell types), a retroviral particle containing a coat that recognizes only human blood-forming cells would permit the retroviral vector to be given intravenously with little danger that cells other than those in the marrow would be infected. In the future, such specificity could permit the liver and brain, for example, to be treated individually. In addition, the danger of inadvertently infecting germ cells could be eliminated. One problem, however, is that cell replication appears to be necessary for retrovirus integration. It would not be possible to infect nondividing brain cells, for example, so far as we now know.

The optimal system not only would deliver the vector specifically into the cell type of choice, but would also direct the vector to a predetermined chromosomal site. Specific insertion into a selected site on a chromosome can be achieved in lower organisms but has not yet been possible in mammals.

EXPRESSION

In order for gene therapy to be successful, there must be appropriate expression of the new gene in the target cells. Even when a delivery system can transport an exogenous gene into the DNA of the correct cells of an organism, it has been a major problem to get the integrated DNA to function. A vast array of cloned genes have been introduced into a wide range of cells by several gene transfer techniques. 'Normal' expression of exogenous genes is the exception rather than the rule.

Expression of exogenous genes carried by retroviral vectors into intact animals via treated bone marrow cells has been reported by three laboratories. Two studies demonstrated the expression of an antibiotic resistance gene in mice (Joyner et al., 1983; Williams et al., 1984). The most extensive data, however, are from studies with the enzyme HPRT (Miller et al., 1984; Willis et al., 1984). A homozygous Lesch-Nyhan (LN) lymphoblast (white blood cell) line, which lacks a functional HPRT gene, was used to demonstrate that an HPRT$^-$ human blood-forming cell could be corrected by a retroviral vector containing an active HPRT gene. In a corollary study, viral particles containing the HPRT-vector were used to infect mouse bone marrow cells that were then injected into lethally irradiated mice. Both human HPRT protein and chronic production of HPRT-vector particles were detected in the blood-forming tissues of the mice. These data provide hope that vectors can eventually be built with all the regulatory signals necessary to produce correctly controlled expression of exogenous genes in target cells.

SAFETY

Finally, a human gene therapy protocol must be safe. Although retroviruses have many advantages for gene transfer, they also have disadvantages. One problem is that they can rearrange their own structure, as well as exchange sequences with other retroviruses. In the future it might be possible to modify non-infectious retroviral vectors in such a way that they remain stable. At present, however, there is the possibility that a retroviral vector might recombine with an endogenous viral sequence to produce an infectious recombinant virus. Properties that such a recombinant would have are unknown, but there is a potential homology between retroviral vectors and human T-cell leukemia viruses so that the formation of a recombinant that could produce a malignancy is a possibility. There is, however, a built-in safety feature with the mouse retroviral vectors now in use. These mouse structures have a very different sequence from known primate retroviruses, and there appears to be little or no homology between the two. Therefore, it should be possible, with continuing research, to build a safe retroviral vector.

With the present constructs, three types of experiments ought to be carried out before any retrovirus-treated bone marrow is injected into a patient. These protocols, designed to test the safety of the delivery-expression system, are necessary since once treated bone marrow is reinserted into a patient, it and all retroviruses that it contains are irretrievable.

First, studies with human bone marrow in tissue culture are needed. Marrow cultures infected with the therapeutic vector should be tested for a period of time for the production of recombinant viruses. Any infectious virus isolated should be studied for possible pathogenicity.

Second, studies *in vivo* with mice are needed. Treated animals should be followed to determine if genomic rearrangement or the site of chromosomal integration of the retroviral vector has resulted in any pathologic manifestations or the production of any infectious viruses.

Third, studies *in vivo* with primates are needed. A protocol similar to the one planned for human application should be carried out in primates, not just mice, because the endogenous viral sequences in primate, including human, DNA are different from those in mouse DNA. Therefore, the nature of any viral recombinants would be different. Treated bone marrow should be reimplanted into primates, the successful transfer of intact vector DNA into blood-forming cells demonstrated, the expression of at least small amounts of gene product verified, and the existence of infectious recombinant viruses sought.

CONCLUSION

It now appears that effective delivery-expression systems are becoming available that will allow reasonable attempts at somatic cell gene therapy. The first clinical trials will probably be carried out within the next year. The initial protocols will be based on treatment of bone marrow cells with retroviral vectors carrying a normal gene. The safety of the procedures is the remaining major issue. Patients severely debilitated by having no normal copies of the gene that produces the enzyme HPRT, ADA, or PNP are the most likely first candidates for gene therapy.

It is unrealistic to expect a complete cure from the initial attempts at gene therapy. Many patients who suffer from severe genetic diseases, as well as their families, are eager to participate in early clinical trials even if the likelihood is low that the original experiments will alleviate symptoms. However, for the protection of the patients (particularly since those with the most severe diseases and, therefore, the most ethically justifiable first candidates are children), gene therapy trials should not be attempted until there are good animal data to suggest that some amelioration of the biochemical defect is likely. Then it would be necessary to weigh the potential risks to the patient, including the possibility of producing a pathologic virus or a malignancy, against the anticipated benefits to be gained from the functional gene. This risk to benefit determination, a standard procedure for all clinical research protocols, would need to be carried out for each patient.

In summary, Institutional Review Boards and the NIH should carefully evaluate therapeutic protocols to ensure that the delivery system is effective, that sufficient expression can be obtained in bone marrow cultures and in laboratory animals to predict probable benefit, even if small, for the patient, and that safety protocols have demonstrated that the probability is low for the production of either a malignant cell or a harmful infectious retrovirus. Once these criteria are met, I maintain that it would be unethical to delay human trials. Patients with serious genetic diseases have little other hope at present for alleviation of their medical problems. Arguments that genetic engineering might someday be misused do not justify the needless perpetuation of human suffering that would result from an unnecessary delay in the clinical application of this potentially powerful therapeutic procedure.

GERM LINE GENE THERAPY

The second level of a genetic engineering, gene therapy of germ line cells, would require a major advance in our present state of knowledge. It would require that we learn how to insert a gene not only into the appropriate cells of the patient's body, but also how to introduce it into the germ line of the patient in such a way that it would be transmitted to offspring and would be functional in the correct way in the correct cells in the offspring. Based on the small amount of information now available from animal studies, the step from correction of a disorder in somatic cells to correction of the germ line would be difficult.

GERM LINE THERAPY IN ANIMALS

Germ line transmission and expression of inserted genes in mice has been obtained by several laboratories but with a technique that is not acceptable for use in human patients, namely, the physical microinjection of fertilized eggs. Microinjection into tissue culture cells has been used for a number of years and has the advantage of high efficiency (up to one cell in five injected can be permanently transfected). However, the distinct disadvantage is that only one cell at a time can be injected. Transfection of a large number (like 10^6) of blood-forming stem cells is not feasible.

Microinjection has been used with considerable success in transferring genes into mouse zygotes. DNA can be microinjected into one of the two pronuclei of a recently fertilized mouse egg. This egg can then be placed into the oviduct of a pseudopregnant female where it can develop into a normal mouse carrying the exogenous DNA in every cell of its body including its germ cells. Consequently, the injected DNA can be transmitted to offspring in a normal Mendelian manner. Mice carrying an exogenous gene in their genome are called 'transgenic'.

It is this technique that was used to partially correct a mouse with a defect in its growth hormone production (Hammer et al., 1984). By attaching a rat growth hormone gene to an active regulatory sequence (specifically, the promoter that normally directs the synthesis of metallothionein messenger RNA in mice), researchers obtained a recombinant DNA construct that actively produces growth hormone in the genetically defective mouse and in a number of its offspring. Although the level of growth hormone production was inappropriately controlled (that is, influence by signals that normally regulate metallothionein synthesis), these experiments did show that microinjection can be used as a delivery system that can put a gene into every cell of an animal's body, that a genetic disorder can, as a result, be corrected, and that the correction can be passed on to the next generation of animals.

Why is the technique of microinjecting a fertilized egg not acceptable for use for human gene therapy at the present time? First, the procedure has a high failure rate; second, it can produce a deleterious result; and third, it would have limited usefulness. Microinjection

has a high failure rate because the majority of eggs are so damaged by the microinjection and transfer procedures that they do not develop into live offspring. In one recent experiment (Brinster et al., 1983) involving microinjection of an immunoglobulin gene into mouse eggs, 300 eggs were injected, 192 (64 percent) were judged sufficiently healthy to be transferred to surrogate mothers, only 11 (3.7 percent) proceeded to live birth, and just 6 (2 percent) carried the gene. These results are from a highly experienced laboratory in which thousands of identical eggs from the same hybrid cross of inbred mice have been injected over several years. The mice were chosen precisely because they gave the best results for gene transfer by microinjection. Attempts to microinject functional growth hormone genes into livestock eggs met with several major biological and technical problems before being accomplished. Successful gene transfer by microinjection of human eggs, without a long period of trial and error experimentation, is extremely unlikely.

Second, microinjection of eggs can produce deleterious results because there is no control over where the injected DNA will integrate in the genome. For example, the integration of an exogenous rabbit beta-globin gene in transgenic mice can sometimes occur at a chromosomal location that results in expression of the beta-globin gene in an inappropriate tissue, viz., muscle or testis (Lacy et al., 1983). There have also been several cases reported where integration of microinjected DNA has resulted in a pathological condition. Although there is no control over where exogenous DNA will integrate in any gene transfer procedure, the damaging effect caused by a harmful insertion site could be great when it occurs in the egg but may be negligible when it occurs in one or a few of a large number of bone marrow cells.

The third objection to microinjection of eggs is limited usefulness. Not only is it ethically questionable to experiment on human eggs because of the expected losses, but even if 'success' were obtained, it would be applicable primarily when both patients are homozygous for the defect. When the parents are both carriers of a recessive trait, only one fertilized egg out of four would result in an affected child. Since a homozygous defect cannot yet be recognized in early embryos, and since the procedure itself carries such a high risk, it would be improper to attempt any manipulation in this situation. Furthermore, most of the very serious genetic disorders result in infertility (or death before reproductive age) in homozygous patients. Consequently, there would be little use for the procedure even if it were feasible. . . .

ENHANCEMENT GENETIC ENGINEERING

The third level of genetic engineering, enhancement genetic engineering, is considerably different in principle from the first two. This is no longer therapy of a genetic disorder; it is the insertion of an additional normal gene (or a gene modified in a specific way) to produce a change in some characteristic that the individual wants. Enhancement would involve the insertion of a single gene, or a small number of genes, that code for a product (or products) that would produce the desired effect—for example, greater size through the insertion of an additional growth hormone gene into the cells of an infant. Enhancement genetic engineering presents a major additional scientific hurdle, as well as serious new ethical issues. Except under very specific circumstances as detailed below, genetic engineering should not be used for enhancement purposes.

SCIENTIFIC AND ETHICAL CONCERNS

The scientific hurdle to be overcome is a formidable one. Until now, we have considered the correction of a defect, of a 'broken part', if you will. Fix the broken part and the human machine should operate correctly again. Replacing a faulty part is different from trying to add something new to a normally functioning system. To insert a gene in the hope of improving or selectively altering a characteristic might endanger the overall metabolic balance of the individual cells as well as of the entire body. Medicine is a very inexact science. Every year new hormones, new regulators, and new pathways are discovered. There are clearly many more to be discovered. Most impressive is the enormously intricate way that each cell coordinates within itself all of its thousands of pathways. Likewise, the body as a whole carefully monitors and balances a multitude of physiological systems. Much additional research will be required to elucidate the effects of altering one or more major pathways in a cell. To correct a faulty gene is probably not going to be dangerous, but intentionally to insert a gene to make more of one product might adversely affect numerous other biochemical pathways.

We possess insufficient information at present to understand the effects of attempts to alter the genetic machinery of a human. Is it wise, safe, or ethical for parents to give, for example, growth hormone (now that it is available in large amounts) to their normal sons in order to produce very large football or basketball players? Unfortunately, this practice now takes place in this country. But even worse, why would anyone want to insert a growth hormone *gene* into a normal child? Once it is in, there is no way to get it back out. The child's reflexes, coordination, and balance might all be grossly affected. In addition, even more serious questions can be asked: might one alter the regulatory pathways of cells, inadvertently affecting cell division or other properties? In short, we know too little about the human body to chance inserting a gene designed for 'improvement' into a normal healthy person.

AN ACCEPTABLE USE

There is, however, a set of circumstances under which enhancement genetic engineering may be ethical. This is when it could be justified on grounds of preventive medicine. For example, it is well established that heart attacks and stroke are a direct result of atherosclerosis (i.e., hardening of the arteries). The rate of development of atherosclerosis appears to correlate directly with elevated levels of cholesterol in the blood. The level of blood cholesterol is regulated, at least in part, by its rate of clearance from the blood by the low density lipoprotein (LDL) receptors on body cells (Goldstein and Brown, 1983). LDL is the major cholesterol-transport protein in human plasma. If further research should verify that an increased number of LDL receptors on cells would result in lower blood cholesterol levels and, consequently, in a decreased incidence of heart attacks and strokes, then the insertion of an additional LDL receptor gene in 'normal' individuals could significantly decrease the morbidity and mortality caused by atherosclerosis. In this type of situation, the purpose of the intervention would be the prevention of disease, not simply the personal desire of an individual for an altered characteristic. The concerns expressed above about disrupting the regulatory pathways in the body still should be considered, of course. However, since there is a range for the number of receptors on a cell's surface, shifting a person with a "low normal" number of receptors to a "high normal" number may not be disruptive to other physiological or biochemical pathways.

The fourth level is 'eugenic' genetic engineering. This area has received considerable attention in the popular press, with the result that at times unjustified fears have been produced because of claims that scientists might soon be able to re-make human beings. In fact, however, such traits as personality, character, formation of body organs, fertility, intelligence, physical, mental, and emotional characteristics, etc., are enormously complex. Dozens, perhaps hundreds, of unknown genes that interact in totally unknown ways probably contribute to each such trait. Environmental influences also interact with these genetic backgrounds in poorly understood ways. With time, as more is learned about each of these complex traits, individual genes will be discovered that play specific roles. Undoubtedly, disorders will be recognized that are caused by defects in these genes. Then, somatic cell gene therapy could be employed to correct the defect. But the concept of 're-making a human' (i.e., eugenic genetic engineering) is not realistic at present.

Complex polygenic traits may never be influenced in a predictable manner by genetic engineering, but, at a minimum, developing the techniques for producing such changes will take many years. Therefore, there is no point to a scientific discussion of eugenic genetic engineering at present—there is simply no science to discuss. But from a philosophical standpoint, a discussion of the ethics of eugenic genetic engineering is very important. After all, what is it that makes us human? Why are we what we are? Are there genes which are indeed 'human' genes? If we were to alter one of these genes, would we be other than human? These are important questions for us to think about and discuss.

If eugenic genetic engineering were possible today, I would be strongly opposed to its use on philosophical and ethical grounds. Our knowledge of how the human body works is still elementary. Our understanding of how the mind, both conscious and subconscious, functions is even more rudimentary. The genetic basis for instinctual behavior is largely unknown. Our disagreements about what constitutes 'humanhood' are notorious. And our insight into what, and to what extent, genetic components might play a role in what we comprehend as our 'spiritual' side is almost nonexistent. We simply should not meddle in areas where we are so ignorant. Regardless of how fast our technological abilities increase, there should be no attempt to manipulate, for other than therapeutic reasons, the genetic framework (i.e., the genome) of human beings.

CONCLUSION

In summary, somatic cell gene therapy for human genetic disease should be possible in the very near future. The scientific basis on which this new therapeutic approach is founded has been thoroughly documented in a number of publications, as has the ethical justification for its use. Germ line gene therapy is still in the future, but the technical ability to carry it out will almost certainly be developed. Society must determine if this therapeutic option should be used. Enhancement genetic engineering should also be possible and its medical and disturbing ethical implications need continuing discussion. Eugenic genetic engineering, on the other hand, is purely theoretical and will, from a practical standpoint, be impossible for the foreseeable future. The topic is valuable for reflective thinking but not for scientific discussion.

Many of the fears generated by some articles in the popular press that discuss 'gene therapy' or 'genetic engineering' are simply unfounded. Insertion of single functional genes should soon become possible, but claims that new organs, designed personalities, master races, or Frankenstein monsters will be created can be given no credence in the light of what is presently known. Even so, we should be concerned about the possibility that genetic engineering might be misused in the future. The best insurance against possible abuse is a well-informed public. Gene therapy has the potential for producing tremendous good by reducing the suffering and death caused by genetic diseases. We can look forward to the day when, with proper safeguards imposed by society, this powerful new therapeutic procedure is available.

REFERENCES

Anderson, W. F.: 1982, in *Hearings on Human Genetic Engineering Before the Subcommittee on Investigations and Oversight of the Committee on Science and Technology*, 97th Cong. 2d sess., No. 170 (Government Printing Office, Washington, D.C., 1982), pp. 285–292.

Anderson, W. F.: 1984, 'Prospects for human gene therapy', *Science* 226, 401–409.

Brinster, R. L. *et al.*: 1983, 'Expression of a microinjected immunoglobulin gene in the spleen of transgenic mice', *Nature* 306, 332–336.

Goldstein, J. L. and Brown, M. S.: 1983, 'Familial hypercholesterolemia', in J. B. Stanbury *et al.* (eds.), *The Metabolic Basis of Inherited Disease*, 5th edition, McGraw-Hill, New York, pp. 672–712.

Hammer, R. E. *et al.*: 1984, 'Partial correction of murine hereditary growth disorder by germ-line incorporation of a new gene', *Nature* 311, 65–67.

Joyner, A. *et al.*: 1983, 'Retrovirus transfer of a bacterial gene into mouse haematopoietic progenitor cells', *Nature* 305, 556–558.

Lacy, E. *et al.*: 1983, 'A foreign β-globin gene in transgenic mice: integration at abnormal chromosomal positions and expression in inappropriate tissues', *Cell* 34, 343–358.

Miller, A. D. *et al.*: 1984, 'Expression of a retrovirus encoding human HPRT in mice', *Science* 225, 630–632.

Williams, D. A. *et al.*: 1984, 'Introduction of new genetic material into pluripotent haematopoietic stem cells of the mouse', *Nature* 310, 476–480.

Willis, R. C. *et al.*: 1984, 'Partial phenotypic correction of human Lesch-Nyhan (hypoxanthine-guanine phosphoribosyltransferase-deficient) lymphoblasts with a transmissible retroviral vector', *Journal of Biological Chemistry* 259, 7842–7849.

LeROY WALTERS

The Ethics of Human Gene Therapy

Within the next twelve months, it is likely that a proposal to perform gene therapy in humans will be submitted to local and national review bodies in the United States. The proposing research group will be based in one of the eight to ten laboratories in the world now pursuing molecular genetic approaches to the correction of selected inborn errors of metabolism. The hereditary disorders for which gene therapy will initially be attempted are quite rare—adenosine deaminase (ADA) deficiency, which produces severe combined immune deficiency, and Lesch-Nyhan syndrome, which leads to mental retardation and self-mutilation in children.

While gene therapy may sound revolutionary as an approach to human genetic disease, the techniques likely to be used in the near future closely resemble those of conventional medical practice. Thus, gene therapy for ADA deficiency can accurately be described as 'autologous bone marrow transplantation with an extra step'. That extra step will involve not the repair of a malfunctioning gene, but rather, the addition of a properly functioning gene to as many target cells as possible, thereby compensating for the malfunction caused by the defective gene in those cells.

FIRST STEPS

The early attempts at gene therapy will involve only somatic cells, especially the stem cells found in the bone marrow. Molecular genetic modification of germ cells in laboratory animals is still inefficient, and no research groups are currently contemplating the deliberate introduction of genetic alterations into the human germ line. Thus, fears about the transmission to future generations of intentionally induced genetic changes are misplaced, just as they would be after a kidney transplant. For the time being, moreover, only the simplest kinds of genetic defects are considered to be good candidates for gene therapy. These are single-gene defects which are recessively inherited and which result in the lack of an essential enzyme. The production of such enzymes is almost a mechanical function, necessary to be sure, but shared by humans with many other members of the animal kingdom. Thus, any allegation that current gene therapy efforts represent 'tampering' with 'distinctively human characteristics' is simply fallacious.

RISK ASSESSMENT

Ethical questions about gene therapy as now planned are of two kinds, substantive and procedural. The substantive questions can be further subdivided, with some oversimplification, into technical and nontechnical questions. The chief technical questions surrounding gene therapy involve the comparison of potential benefits and harms, or, in contemporary language, risk assessment. The assessment process begins with an evaluation of the genetic disease to be treated. At this stage the central question is: What kinds of morbidity and what mortality rates are associated with the disease? If the disease is severe for the individuals affected by it, one can proceed to consider existing therapies and their effectiveness. If dietary or current medical therapies provide reasonable control for disease victims, the disease may not be a good early candidate for gene therapy. On the other hand, if no effective therapy exists or if the therapy cannot be used with some categories of patients, molecular genetic approaches to treatment may be a reasonable alternative to merely palliative measures.

Like the development of all innovative medical therapies, the pursuit of gene therapy as an alternative therapeutic mode involves preclinical studies in animal models and tissue cultures. At this stage the risk assessment process must seek to determine and evaluate the probable safety and effectiveness of the new technique. Here, researchers attempting to develop gene therapy techniques face a special, but by no means unique, problem: there are few laboratory animal models for the single-gene defects that afflict humans, and, in particular, there are no known non-human models for the enzyme-deficiency diseases which are likely to be judged appropriate early candidates for human gene therapy. Researchers may be able to insert a new gene into appropriate animal cells and monitor the expression of the gene, but they are unlikely to be able to demonstrate a clinical 'cure' in a diseased laboratory animal.

From a safety standpoint, one advantage of a gene therapy approach that uses bone marrow cells is that the cells are treated outside the body, *in vitro*. If a particular experiment goes awry, the cells are simply not returned to the laboratory animal or, in the clinical context, to the patient. But other safety questions are matters of continuing concern. The new genes will probably be carried into the stem cells by carefully designed retroviruses from which much of the native genetic information has been deleted. These defective retroviruses will function as vectors for the new gene. It is possible, but not likely, that the retroviral vectors will recombine with undetected viruses or endogenous DNA sequences in the cells and so become infectious.

It is also possible that the vector/gene combinations, because they integrate randomly into the chromosomes of the cells, will activate previously dormant proto-oncogenes or disrupt essential, properly functioning genes. On the question of efficiency, it is still not clear whether sufficiently high levels of expression can be achieved in primates to offer a reasonable hope of clinical benefit.

OTHER ETHICAL ISSUES

Non-technical questions about human gene therapy, while apparently less amenable to verification by laboratory data, are nonetheless important. These questions derive in part from the recent history of clinical innovation, from renal dialysis in the early 1960s, the first heart transplants in 1967 and recent experience with the artificial heart and xenografting. They are also based on codes of ethics in research published between the late 1940s and the present.

In the early years of renal dialysis, one major issue was the selection of a few patients from among many candidates for life-saving treatment. In Seattle, Washington, a special committee was established to make these decisions. Commentators on the Seattle committee's experience have noted how difficult it is to avoid making judgements about the comparative social worth of patients when not all patients can be offered treatment.[1] With rare genetic diseases, although the potential patient pool will be small, choices will need to be made from among multiple candidates for experimental gene therapy. Thus, fairness in the selection of subjects may be an important issue even in the earliest trials of human gene therapy.

Informed consent will almost certainly also be an important issue. To be adequately informed about their decisions, prospective patients will need to have, or have imparted to them, basic information about bone marrow transplantation and gene therapy techniques. If, as seems likely, parents or guardians are asked to make decisions on behalf of infants or young children, the consent process will be even more complex. Properly informed, potential research subjects or their proxies will be made aware that they are embarking on essentially uncharted territory. This awareness should help to temper their hope—and that of the investigators, also—that they are participating in a major therapeutic breakthrough.

Questions of privacy and confidentiality may also arise. The pioneer recipients of heart transplants and the artificial heart are known to us by name; in contrast, the newborn recipient of a baboon heart, Baby Fae, remained at least partially anonymous until her death in late 1984. With gene therapy, one hopes for a reasonable balance between familial privacy and the desire of the public and the media to know. Researchers will bear the primary responsibility for informing patients and their families of the public interest in gene therapy and for shielding patients from excessive media exposure. If, as seems likely, the earliest patients are infants or young children who are incapable of expressing their own views regarding publicity, they will deserve special protection.

GUIDELINES

In the Declaration of Helsinki and similar codes of ethics in research, biomedical researchers have proposed general standards for human experimentation. The revised Declaration of Helsinki[2], adopted by the World Medical Association in 1975, includes ethical guidelines on research design, risk-benefit analysis, informed consent, privacy and accuracy in reporting research results. In most developed nations, local committees, variously called 'ethics committees' or 'institutional review boards', rely on these international standards and derivative national rules in reviewing individual research protocols. However, when major therapeutic innovations are initially proposed, this carefully evolved approach to the review of proposed human experimentation may need to be supplemented by more specific ethical standards and, possibly, by custom-tailored review mechanisms. *In vitro* fertilization is an example of a new biomedical technology that has been the object of special scrutiny in several countries, including the United Kingdom, Australia and Canada.

During the past two-and-a-half years, a framework for the ethical evaluation of human gene therapy has been developed in the United States. This framework includes a publicly discussed set of questions, called *Points to Consider in the Design and Submission of Human Somatic-Cell Gene Therapy Protocols*[3], and a public national review process. The *Points to Consider* reflect a national and perhaps international consensus on the most important areas of concern surrounding

human gene therapy. Major areas identified in the central section of the document are the following:

(1) Objectives and rationale of the proposed research.

(2) Research design, anticipated risks and benefits: (i) structure and characteristics of the biological system; (ii) preclinical studies; (iii) clinical procedures, including patient monitoring; (iv) public health considerations; (v) qualifications of investigators and adequacy of facilities.

(3) Selection of patients.

(4) Informed consent.

(5) Privacy and confidentiality.

A series of questions is posed about each area of concern, and great latitude is left to investigators in formulating responses to the questions. For example, on the subject of preclinical studies with laboratory animals, investigators are asked: "Has a protocol similar to the one proposed for a clinical trial been carried out in non-human primates and/or other animals? What were the results?".

The *Points to Consider* document was drafted by the Working Group on Human Gene Therapy, an interdisciplinary subcommittee of the NIH Recombinant DNA Advisory Committee (RAC). The Working Group includes three laboratory scientists, three clinicians, three ethicists, three attorneys, two public-policy specialists, and a lay member. The document represents an attempt to distill 15 years of ethical discussion in published articles and books[4-15], at public symposia[16-18], and in government hearings and reports in the United States and Europe[19-22]. *Points to Consider* was published twice for public comment in the United States *Federal Register* and was revised to take into account the suggestions made by respondents.

As a complement to the confidential review of new biological compounds conducted by the federal Food and Drug Administration, a special public review mechanism has also been established to evaluate proposals to perform gene therapy in humans, at least during the early years. This review mechanism was created by the NIH RAC and is modelled after the review process employed by RAC during the early years of recombinant DNA research. After review by local ethics committees, RAC and its subcommittee, the Working Group on Human Gene Therapy, will provide public national review of each gene therapy proposal that is to be supported by NIH funds. All interested persons will therefore have ready access to information about gene therapy proposals, to the review process itself and to its outcome.

When gene therapy has not yet cured a human patient of disease, it may seem premature to discuss questions that may emerge if human gene therapy is successful. Yet, one role of ethics is to provide timely consideration of future questions for public policy. Several issues may arise.

GENETIC DIAGNOSIS

At present, attempts to describe 'the morbid anatomy of the human genome' are outpacing gene therapy by a considerable margin[23]. Within the past year, new markers for several major genetic diseases have been described, among them cystic fibrosis[24-26], polycystic kidney disease[27] and Duchenne muscular dystrophy[28]. At the prenatal stage, early diagnosis of genetic defects presents couples with a decision about selective abortion, but applied to children or adults, the new tests will provide early notice of a tendency to develop a particular disease (such as atherosclerosis[29]) or of the presence of a gene that will cause a late-onset disorder (such as Huntington's disease[30]).

The 'early notice' aspect of the new genetic tests will raise difficult ethical questions in its own right. For example, which children or adults should be tested, and what should they be told about the results of the tests? Moreover, one can anticipate that insurance companies, employers and perhaps even prospective marriage partners, will have a keen interest in securing detailed genetic profiles of particular individuals. The primary implication of these screening techniques for gene therapy is that they may identify additional groups of candidates for curative or pre-emptive intervention.

COMMERCIAL CONSIDERATIONS

Commercially oriented biotechnology companies have been leading participants in the quest for DNA-based diagnostic techniques but seem, at present, relatively uninterested in DNA-mediated approaches to the cure of disease. This lack of interest may reflect the fact that, in the near future at least, human gene therapy will be a labour-intensive procedure, akin to bone marrow transplantation. Each university-based research team involved with gene therapy also seems to be tailoring its own vector/gene combinations to suit its specific purposes. It is possible that there may emerge commercial interest in producing vectors or vector/gene kits for particular diseases, but, given the rarity of the diseases thought to be the likeliest candidates for early attempts at gene therapy, commercial incentives are currently quite weak.

GENE REPLACEMENT

Present approaches to gene therapy can quite literally be described as gene addition. Properly functioning genes, introduced into the appropriate cells, will, it is hoped, compensate for malfunctioning or nonfunctioning genes. This approach holds great promise for the somatic-cell treatment of recessive genetic disorders, but for the treatment of dominant disorders such as Huntington's disease, it may be necessary to inactivate the disease-causing gene or even to remove and replace it with a gene that functions properly. Techniques for this kind of precisely targeted molecular microsurgery have not yet been developed for mammals and will probably not emerge for decades.

GERMLINE THERAPY

No aspect of gene therapy is more highly charged than that of germline or germ-cell therapy; it might seem, therefore, politically prudent to avoid the subject. But what is politically prudent may not be ethically responsible. In fact, timely ethical discussion of this issue, before germline gene therapy in humans is technically feasible, may assist future policy-makers in their deliberations.

The principal rationale for germline human gene therapy, when it becomes a technical possibility, will be a simple argument from efficiency. If somatic-cell therapy becomes a successful cure for single-gene defects of high prevalence, such as cystic fibrosis and sickle-cell anaemia, phenotypically normal patients will grow to adulthood and presumably be capable of reproducing. They will then constitute a new group of homozygous 'carriers' of genetic disease, who can transmit malfunctioning genes to their offspring. Affected offspring could presumably be treated by means of somatic-cell gene therapy in each succeeding generation, but some phenotypically cured patients would probably consider it more efficient to prevent the transmission of specific malfunctioning genes to their offspring, if the option were available.

A second rationale for the germline approach is that some genetic diseases may be treatable only by this method. For example, because of the blood-brain barrier, the brain cells involved in hereditary central nervous system disorders may be inaccessible to somatic-cell gene therapy. Early intervention that affects all the cells of the future organism, including the germ cells, may be the only means available for treating cells or tissues which are not amenable to genetic repair after birth.

Genetic changes have been introduced into the germ lines of several species of laboratory and domestic animals[31-34], but the method for producing such transgenic animals is unlikely to be used with humans. Because the foreign DNA is inserted into the pronuclei of mammalian embryos before the pronuclei fuse and the new genome is established, one would not know in most cases whether a particular embryo were destined to have a genetic disease. A more likely approach in humans is the genetic repair of sperm or egg cells, either *in vivo* or, more probably, *in vitro*. Methods for reliably introducing properly functioning genes into germ cells and for verifying their successful introduction would need to be developed. As simple gene addition would allow the transmission of known malfunctioning genes to future generations, the techniques of gene inactivation or gene replacement would probably be used, if available.

ECONOMIC ISSUES

Given that the first-year costs of cardiac transplantation approximate $90,000 per patient (1983 dollars) in the United States[35], it may reasonably be asked whether gene therapy will be another expensive halfway technology. If employed with bone marrow transplantation, human gene therapy will be labour-intensive and will entail sizeable initial costs. But even if one does not assign an economic value to improvement in the quality of cured patients' lives, the one-time cost for gene therapy may be considerably less than the cost of repeated hospitalization for the treatment of sickle-cell anaemia or cystic fibrosis. In short, for patients suffering from many, if not most, genetic diseases caused by single-gene defects, gene therapy may become a cost-effective method of care.

In the more distant future, the prospects for, and possible approaches to, human gene therapy are not yet clear. But if the link between gene therapy and bone marrow transplantation can be broken, gene therapy may become available to a wider circle of patients. For example, if vectors specific for particular target cells can be developed, vector/gene combinations can perhaps be administered intravenously to outpatients. At that stage, if it is ever reached, medicine will stand at the threshold of a new era in treating the more than 3,000 genetic disorders that afflict our species.

NOTES

1. Ramsey, P. *The Patient as Person*, 239–275 (Yale University Press, New Haven, Connecticut, 1970).

2. World Medical Association *Declaration of Helsinki* revised edn (1975); repr. in *Contemporary Issues in Bioethics* (eds Beauchamp, T. L. & Walters, L.) 511–512 (Wadsworth, Belmont, California, 1982).

3. *Federal Register* 50, 33463 (1985); repr. in *Recomb. DNA Tech. Bull.* 8, 116–122 (1985).

4. Davis, B. D. *Science* 170, 1279–1283 (1970).

5. Friedmann, T. & Roblin, R. *Science* 175, 949–955 (1972).

6. Howard, T. & Rifkin, J. *Who Should Play God?* (Dell, New York, 1977).

7. Shinn, R. in *Encyclopedia of Bioethics* Vol. 2 (ed. Reich, W. T.) 521–527 (Free Press-Macmillan, New York, 1978).

8. Anderson, W. F. & Fletcher, J. C. *New Engl. J. Med.* 303, 1293–1297 (1980).

9. Motulsky, A. *Science* 219, 135–140 (1983).

10. Friedmann, T. *Gene Therapy—Fact and Fiction* (Cold Spring Harbor Laboratory, New York, 1983).

11. Fletcher, J. C. *Virginia Law Rev.* 69, 515–546 (1983).

12. Baskin, Y. *The Gene Doctors* (William Morrow, New York, 1984).

13. Anderson, W. F. *Science* 226, 401–409 (1984).

14. Anderson, W. F. *J. Med. Phil.* 10, 275–291 (1985).

15. Fletcher, J. C. *J. Med. Phil.* 10, 293–309 (1985).

16. Hamilton, M. (ed.) *The New Genetics and the Future of Man*, 109–175 (William B. Erdmans, Grand Rapids, Michigan, 1971).

17. Lappé, M. & Morison, R. S. *Ann. N.Y. Acad. Sci.* 265, 59–65, 141–169 (1976).

18. *Research with Recombinant DNA: An Academy Forum* 7–9 March 1977 (National Academy of Sciences, Washington, DC, 1977).

19. Council of Europe, Parliamentary Assembly, Recommendation 934 (1982) on Genetic Engineering, in *Texts Adopted by the Assembly* (Council of Europe, Strasbourg, 1982).

20. US President's Commission for the Study of Ethical Problems in Medicine and Biomedical and Behavioral Research, *Splicing Life* (US Govt Printing Office, Washington, DC, November 1982).

21. US Congress, House Subcommittee on Investigations and Oversight, *Human Genetic Engineering* (97th Congr., 2nd Sess., 16–18 November 1982).

22. US Congress, Office of Technology Assessment, *Human Gene Therapy: Background Paper* (OTA, Washington, DC, December 1984).

23. McKusick, V. A. *Clin. Genet.* 27, 207–239 (1985).

24. Knowlton, R. G. *et al. Nature* 318, 380–382 (1985).

25. White, R. *et al. Nature* 318, 382–384 (1985).

26. Wainwright, B. J. *et al. Nature* 318, 384–385 (1985).

27. Reeders, S. T. *et al. Nature* 317, 542–544 (1985).

28. Monaco, A. P. *et al. Nature* 316, 842–845 (1985).

29. Joyce, C. *New Scient.* 108, 34 (1985).

30. Gusella, J. F. *et al. Nature* 306, 234–238 (1983).

31. Palmiter, R. D. & Brinster, R. L. *Cell* 41, 343–345 (1985).

32. Hammer, R. E. *et al. Nature* 315, 680–683 (1985).

33. Brinster, R. L., Chen, H. Y., Trumbauer, M. E., Yagel, M. K. & Palmiter, R. D. *Proc. Natn. Acad. Sci. U.S.A.* 82, 4438–4442 (1985).

34. Stout, J. T., Chen, H. Y., Brennand, J., Caskey, C. T. & Brinster, R. L. *Nature* 317, 250–252 (1985).

35. Evans, R. W. *et al. The National Heart Transplantation Study: Final Report* Vol. 3, 28–46 (Battelle Human Affairs Research Center, 1984).

JONATHAN GLOVER

Questions About Some Uses of Genetic Engineering

There is a widespread view that any project for the genetic improvement of the human race ought to be ruled out: that there are fundamental objections of principle. The aim of this discussion is to sort out some of the main objections. It will be argued that our resistance is based on a complex of different values and reasons, none of which is, when examined, adequate to rule out in principle this use of genetic engineering. The debate on human genetic engineering should become like the debate on nuclear power: one in which large possible benefits have to be weighed against big problems and the risk of great disasters. The discussion has not reached this point, partly because the techniques have not yet been developed. But it is also partly because of the blurred vision which fuses together many separate risks and doubts into a fuzzy-outlined opposition in principle.

1. AVOIDING THE DEBATE ABOUT GENES AND THE ENVIRONMENT

In discussing the question of genetic engineering, there is everything to be said for not muddling the issue up with the debate over the relative importance of genes and environment in the development of such characteristics as intelligence. One reason for avoiding

that debate is that it arouses even stronger passions than genetic engineering, and so is filled with as much acrimony as argument. But, apart from this fastidiousness, there are other reasons.

The nature–nurture dispute is generally seen as an argument about the relative weight the two factors have in causing differences within the human species: 'IQ is 80 per cent hereditary and 20 per cent environmental' versus 'IQ is 80 per cent environmental and 20 per cent hereditary'. No doubt there is some approximate truth of this type to be found if we consider variations within a given population at a particular time. But it is highly unlikely that there is any such statement which is simply true of human nature regardless of context. To take the extreme case, if we could iron out all environmental differences, any residual variations would be 100 per cent genetic. It is only if we make the highly artificial assumption that different groups at different times all have an identical spread of relevant environmental differences that we can expect to find statements of this kind applying to human nature in general. To say this is not to argue that studies on the question should not be conducted, or are bound to fail. It may well be possible, and useful, to find out the relative weights of the two kinds of factor for a given characteristic among a certain group at a particular time. The point is that any such conclusions lose relevance, not only when environmental differences are stretched out or compressed, but also when genetic differences are. And this last case is what we are considering.

We can avoid this dispute because of its irrelevance. Suppose the genetic engineering proposal were to try to make people less aggressive. On a superficial view, the proposal might be shown to be unrealistic if there were evidence to show that variation in aggressiveness is hardly genetic at all: that it is 95 per cent environmental. (Let us grant, most implausibly, that such a figure turned out to be true for the whole of humanity, regardless of social context.) But all this would show is that, within our species, the distribution of genes relevant to aggression is very uniform. It would show nothing about the likely effects on aggression if we use genetic engineering to give people a different set of genes from those they now have.

In other words, to take genetic engineering seriously, we need take no stand on the relative importance or unimportance of genetic factors in the explanation of the present range of individual differences found in people. We need only the minimal assumption that different genes could give us different characteristics. To deny *that* assumption you need to be the sort of person who thinks it is only living in kennels which makes dogs different from cats.

2. METHODS OF CHANGING THE GENETIC COMPOSITION OF FUTURE GENERATIONS

There are essentially three ways of altering the genetic composition of future generations. The first is by environmental changes. Discoveries in medicine, the institution of a National Health Service, schemes for poverty relief, agricultural changes, or alterations in the tax position of large families, all alter the selective pressure on genes.[1] It is hard to think of any social change which does not make some difference to who survives or who is born.

The second method is to use eugenic policies aimed at altering breeding patterns or patterns of survival of people with different genes. Eugenic methods are 'environmental' too: the difference is only that the genetic impact is intended. Possible strategies range from various kinds of compulsion (to have more children, fewer children, or no children, or even compulsion over the choice of sexual partner) to the completely voluntary (our present genetic counselling practice of giving prospective parents information about probabilities of their children having various abnormalities).

The third method is genetic engineering: using enzymes to add to or subtract from a stretch of DNA.

Most people are unworried by the fact that a side-effect of an environmental change is to alter the gene pool, at least where the alteration is not for the worse. And even in cases where environmental factors increase the proportion of undesirable genes in the pool, we often accept this. Few people oppose the National Health Service, although setting it up meant that some people with genetic defects, who would have died, have had treatment enabling them to survive and reproduce. On the whole, we accept without qualms that much of what we do has genetic impact. Controversy starts when we think of aiming deliberately at genetic changes, by eugenics or genetic engineering. I want to make some brief remarks about eugenic policies, before suggesting that policies of deliberate intervention are best considered in the context of genetic engineering.

Scepticism has been expressed about whether eugenic policies have any practical chance of success. Medawar has pointed out the importance of genetic polymorphism: the persistence of genetically different types in a population.[2] (Our different blood groups are a familiar example.) For many characteristics, people get a different gene from each parent. So children do not simply repeat parental characteristics. Any simple picture of producing an improved type of person, and then letting the improvement be passed on unchanged, collapses.

But, although polymorphism is a problem for this crudely utopian form of eugenics, it does not show that more modest schemes of improvement must fail. Suppose the best individuals for some quality (say, colour vision) are heterozygous, so that they inherit a gene A from one parent, and a gene B from the other. These ABs will have AAs and BBs among their children, who will be less good than they are. But AAs and BBs may still be better than ACs or ADs, and perhaps much better than CCs or CDs. If this were so, overall improvement could still be brought about by encouraging people whose genes included an A or a B to have more children than those who had only Cs or Ds. The point of taking a quality like colour vision is that it may be genetically fairly simple. Qualities like kindness or intelligence are more likely to depend on the interaction of many genes, but a similar point can be made at a higher level of complexity.

Polymorphism raises a doubt about whether the offspring of the three 'exceptionally intelligent women' fertilized by Dr Shockley or other Nobel prize-winners will have the same IQ as the parents, even apart from environmental variation. But it does not show the inevitable failure of any large-scale attempts to alter human characteristics by varying the relative numbers of children different kinds of people have. Yet any attempt, say, to raise the level of intelligence, would be a very slow affair, taking many generations to make much of an impact. This is one reason for preferring to discuss genetic engineering. For the genetic engineering of human improvements, if it becomes possible, will have an immediate effect, so we will not be guessing which qualities will be desirable dozens of generations later.

There is the view that the genetic-engineering techniques required will not become a practical possibility. Sir MacFarlane Burnet, writing in 1971 about using genetic engineering to cure disorders in people already born, dismissed the possibility of using a virus to carry a new gene to replace a faulty one in cells throughout the body: 'I should be willing to state in any company that the chance of doing this will remain infinitely small to the last syllable of recorded time.'[3] Unless engineering at the stage of sperm cell and egg is easier, this seems a confident dismissal of the topic to be discussed here. More recent work casts doubt on this confidence.[4] So, having mentioned this scepticism, I shall disregard it. We will assume that genetic engineering of people may become possible, and that it is worth discussing. (Sir MacFarlane Burnet's view has not yet been falsified as totally as Rutherford's view about atomic energy. But I hope that the last syllable of recorded time is still some way off.)

The main reason for casting the discussion in terms of genetic engineering rather than eugenics is not a practical one. Many eugenic policies are open to fairly straightforward moral objections, which hide the deeper theoretical issues. Such policies as compulsory sterilization, compulsory abortion, compelling people to pair off in certain ways, or compelling people to have more or fewer children than they would otherwise have, are all open to objection on grounds of overriding people's autonomy. Some are open to objection on grounds of damage to the institution of the family. And the use of discriminatory tax- and child-benefit policies is an intolerable step towards a society of different genetic castes.

Genetic engineering need not involve overriding anyone's autonomy. It need not be forced on parents against their wishes, and the future person being engineered has no views to be overridden. (The view that

despite this, it is still objectionable to have one's genetic characteristics decided by others, will be considered later.) Genetic engineering will not damage the family in the obvious ways that compulsory eugenic policies would. Nor need it be encouraged by incentives which create inequalities. Because it avoids these highly visible moral objections, genetic engineering allows us to focus more clearly on other values that are involved.

(To avoid a possible misunderstanding, one point should be added before leaving the topic of eugenics. Saying that some eugenic policies are open to obvious moral objections does not commit me to disapproval of all eugenic policies. In particular, I do not want to be taken to be opposing two kinds of policy. One is genetic counselling: warning people of risks in having children, and perhaps advising them against having them. The other is the introduction of screening-programmes to detect foetal abnormalities, followed by giving the mother the option of abortion where serious defects emerge.)

Let us now turn to the question of what, if anything, we should do in the field of human genetic engineering.

3. THE POSITIVE–NEGATIVE DISTINCTION

We are not yet able to cure disorders by genetic engineering. But we do sometimes respond to disorders by adopting eugenic policies, at least in voluntary form. Genetic counselling is one instance, as applied to those thought likely to have such disorders as Huntington's chorea. This is a particularly appalling inherited disorder, involving brain degeneration, leading to mental decline and lack of control over movement. It does not normally come on until middle age, by which time many of its victims would in the normal course of things have had children. Huntington's chorea is caused by a dominant gene, so those who find that one of their parents has it have themselves a 50 per cent chance of developing it. If they do have it, each of their children will in turn have a 50 per cent chance of the disease. The risks are so high and the disorder so bad that the potential parents often decide not to have children, and are often given advice to this effect by doctors and others.

Another eugenic response to disorders is involved in screening-programmes for pregnant women. When tests pick up such defects as Down's syndrome (mongolism) or spina bifida, the mother is given the possibility of an abortion. The screening-programmes are eugenic because part of their point is to reduce the incidence of severe genetic abnormality in the population.

These two eugenic policies come in at different stages: before conception and during pregnancy. For this reason the screening-programme is more controversial, because it raises the issue of abortion. Those who are sympathetic to abortion, and who think it would be good to eliminate these disorders will be sympathetic to the programme. Those who think abortion is no different from killing a fully developed human are obviously likely to oppose the programme. But they are likely to feel that elimination of the disorders would be a good thing, even if not an adequate justification for killing. Unless they also disapprove of contraception, they are likely to support the genetic-counselling policy in the case of Huntington's chorea.

Few people object to the use of eugenic policies to eliminate disorders, unless those policies have additional features which are objectionable. Most of us are resistant to the use of compulsion, and those who oppose abortion will object to screening-programmes. But apart from these other moral objections, we do not object to the use of eugenic policies against disease. We do not object to advising those likely to have Huntington's chorea not to have children, as neither compulsion nor killing is involved. Those of us who take this view have no objection to altering the genetic composition of the next generation, where this alteration consists in reducing the incidence of defects.

If it were possible to use genetic engineering to correct defects, say at the foetal stage, it is hard to see how those of us who are prepared to use the eugenic measures just mentioned could object. In both cases, it would be pure gain. The couple, one of whom may develop Huntington's chorea, can have a child if they want, knowing that any abnormality will be eliminated. Those sympathetic to abortion will agree that cure is preferable. And those opposed to abortion prefer babies to be born without handicap. It is hard to think of any objection to using genetic engineering to eliminate defects, and there is a clear and strong case for its use.

But accepting the case for eliminating genetic mistakes does not entail accepting other uses of genetic engineering. The elimination of defects is often called 'negative' genetic engineering. Going beyond this, to bring about improvements in normal people, is by contrast 'positive' engineering. (The same distinction can be made for eugenics.)

The positive–negative distinction is not in all cases completely sharp. Some conditions are genetic disorders whose identification raises little problem. Huntington's chorea or spina bifida are genetic 'mistakes' in a way that cannot seriously be disputed. But with other conditions, the boundary between a defective state and normality may be more blurred. If there is a genetic disposition towards depressive illness, this seems a defect, whose elimination would be part of negative genetic engineering. Suppose the genetic disposition to depression involves the production of lower levels of an enzyme than are produced in normal people. The negative programme is to correct the genetic fault so that the enzyme level is within the range found in normal people. But suppose that within 'normal' people also, there are variations in the enzyme level, which correlate with ordinary differences in tendency to be cheerful or depressed. Is there a sharp boundary between 'clinical' depression and the depression sometimes felt by those diagnosed as 'normal'? Is it clear that a sharp distinction can be drawn between raising someone's enzyme level so that it falls within the normal range and raising someone else's level from the bottom of the normal range to the top?

The positive–negative distinction is sometimes a blurred one, but often we can at least roughly see where it should be drawn. If there is a rough and ready distinction, the question is: how important is it? Should we go on from accepting negative engineering to accepting positive programmes, or should we say that the line between the two is the limit of what is morally acceptable?

There is no doubt that positive programmes arouse the strongest feelings on both sides. On the one hand, many respond to positive genetic engineering or positive eugenics with Professor Tinbergen's thought: 'I find it morally reprehensible and presumptuous for anybody to put himself forward as a judge of the qualities for which we should breed.'

But other people have held just as strongly that positive policies are the way to make the future of mankind better than the past. Many years ago H. J. Muller expressed this hope:

And so we foresee the history of life divided into three main phases. In the long preparatory phase it was the helpless creature of its environment, and natural selection gradually ground it into human shape. In the second—our own short transitional phase—it reaches out at the immediate environment, shaking, shaping and grinding to suit the form, the requirements, the wishes, and the whims of man. And in the long third phase, it will reach down into the secret places of the great universe of its own nature, and by aid of its ever growing intelligence and cooperation, shape itself into an increasingly sublime creation—a being beside which the mythical divinities of the past will seem more and more ridiculous, and which setting its own marvellous inner powers against the brute Goliath of the suns and the planets, challenges them to contest.[5]

The case for positive engineering is not helped by adopting the tones of the mad scientist in a horror film. But behind the rhetoric is a serious point. If we decide on a positive programme to change our nature, this will be a central moment in our history, and the transformation might be beneficial to a degree we can now scarcely imagine. The question is: how are we to weigh this possibility against Tinbergen's objection, and against other objections and doubts?

For the rest of this discussion, I shall assume that, subject to adequate safeguards against things going wrong, negative genetic engineering is acceptable. The issue is positive engineering. I shall also assume that we can ignore problems about whether positive engineering will be technically possible. Suppose we have the power to choose people's genetic characteristics. Once we have eliminated genetic defects, what, if anything, should we do with this power? . . .

4. THE VIEW THAT OVERALL IMPROVEMENT IS UNLIKELY OR IMPOSSIBLE

There is one doubt about the workability of schemes of genetic improvement which is so widespread that it would be perverse to ignore it. This is the view that, in any genetic alteration, there are no gains without compensating losses. On this view, if we bring about a genetically based improvement, such as higher intelligence, we are bound to pay a price somewhere else: perhaps the more intelligent people will have less resistance to disease, or will be less physically agile. If correct, this might so undermine the practicability of applying eugenics or genetic engineering that it would be hardly worth discussing the values involved in such programmes.

This view perhaps depends on some idea that natural selection is so efficient that, in terms of gene survival, we must already be as efficient as it is possible to be. If it were possible to push up intelligence without weakening some other part of the system, natural selection would already have done so. But this is a naive version of evolutionary theory. In real evolu-

tionary theory, far from the genetic status quo always being the best possible for a given environment, some mutations turn out to be advantageous, and this is the origin of evolutionary progress. If natural mutations can be beneficial without a compensating loss, why should artificially induced ones not be so too?

It should also be noticed that there are two different ideas of what counts as a gain or a loss. From the point of view of evolutionary progress, gains and losses are simply advantages and disadvantages from the point of view of gene survival. But we are not compelled to take this view. If we could engineer a genetic change in some people which would have the effect of making them musical prodigies but also sterile, this would be a hopeless gene in terms of survival, but this need not force us, or the musical prodigies themselves, to think of the change as for the worse. It depends on how we rate musical ability as against having children, and evolutionary survival does not dictate priorities here.

The view that gains and losses are tied up with each other need not depend on the dogma that natural selection *must* have created the best of all possible sets of genes. A more cautiously empirical version of the claim says there is a tendency for gains to be accompanied by losses. John Maynard Smith, in his paper on 'Eugenics and Utopia',[6] takes this kind of 'broad balance' view and runs it the other way, suggesting, as an argument in defence of medicine, that any loss of genetic resistance to disease is likely to be a good thing: 'The reason for this is that in evolution, as in other fields, one seldom gets something for nothing. Genes which confer disease-resistance are likely to have harmful effects in other ways: this is certainly true of the gene for sickle-cell anaemia and may be a general rule. If so, absence of selection in favour of disease resistance may be eugenic.'

It is important that different characteristics may turn out to be genetically linked in ways we do not yet realize. In our present state of knowledge, engineering for some improvement might easily bring some unpredicted but genetically linked disadvantage. But we do not have to accept that there will in general be a broad balance, so that there is a presumption that any gain will be accompanied by a compensating loss (or Maynard Smith's version that we can expect a compensating gain for any loss). The reason is that what counts as a gain or loss varies in different contexts. Take Maynard Smith's example of sickle-cell anaemia. The reason why sickle-cell anaemia is widespread in

Africa is that it is genetically linked with resistance to malaria. Those who are heterozygous (who inherit one sickle-cell gene and one normal gene) are resistant to malaria, while those who are homozygous (whose genes are both sickle-cell) get sickle-cell anaemia. If we use genetic engineering to knock out sickle-cell anaemia where malaria is common, we will pay the price of having more malaria. But when we eradicate malaria, the gain will not involve this loss. Because losses are relative to context, any generalization about the impossibility of overall improvements is dubious.

5. THE FAMILY AND OUR DESCENDANTS

Unlike various compulsory eugenic policies, genetic engineering need not involve any interference with decisions by couples to have children together, or with their decisions about how many children to have. And let us suppose that genetically engineered babies grow in the mother's womb in the normal way, so that her relationship to the child is not threatened in the way it might be if the laboratory or the hospital were substituted for the womb. The cruder threats to family relationships are eliminated.

It may be suggested that there is a more subtle threat. Parents like to identify with their children. We are often pleased to see some of our own characteristics in our children. Perhaps this is partly a kind of vanity, and no doubt sometimes we project on to our children similarities that are not really there. But, when the similarities do exist, they help the parents and children to understand and sympathize with each other. If genetic engineering resulted in children fairly different from their parents, this might make their relationship have problems.

There is something to this objection, but it is easy to exaggerate. Obviously, children who were like Midwich cuckoos, or comic-book Martians, would not be easy to identify with. But genetic engineering need not move in such sudden jerks. The changes would have to be detectable to be worth bringing about, but there seems no reason why large changes in appearance, or an unbridgeable psychological gulf, should be created in any one generation. We bring about environmental changes which make children different from their parents, as when the first generation of children in a remote place are given schooling and made literate. This may cause some problems in families, but it is not usually thought a decisive objection. It is not clear that

genetically induced changes of similar magnitude are any more objectionable.

A related objection concerns our attitude to our remoter descendants. We like to think of our descendants stretching on for many generations. Perhaps this is in part an immortality substitute. We hope they will to some extent be like us, and that, if they think of us, they will do so with sympathy and approval. Perhaps these hopes about the future of mankind are relatively unimportant to us. But, even if we mind about them a lot, they are unrealistic in the very long term. Genetic engineering would make our descendants less like us, but this would only speed up the natural rate of change. Natural mutations and selective pressures make it unlikely that in a few million years our descendants will be physically or mentally much like us. So what genetic engineering threatens here is probably doomed anyway. . . .

[6.] RISKS AND MISTAKES

Although mixing different species and cloning are often prominent in people's thoughts about genetic engineering, they are relatively marginal issues. This is partly because there may be no strong reasons in favour of either. Our purposes might be realized more readily by improvements to a single species, whether another or our own, or by the creation of quite new types of organism, than by mixing different species. And it is not clear what advantage cloning batches of people might have, to outweigh the drawbacks. This is not to be dogmatic that species mixing and cloning could never be useful, but to say that the likelihood of other techniques being much more prominent makes it a pity to become fixated on the issues raised by these ones. And some of the most serious objections to positive genetic engineering have wider application than to these rather special cases. One of these wider objections is that serious risks may be involved.

Some of the risks are already part of the public debate because of current work on recombinant DNA. The danger is of producing harmful organisms that would escape from our control. The work obviously should take place, if at all, only with adequate safeguards against such a disaster. The problem is deciding what we should count as adequate safeguards. I have nothing to contribute to this problem here. If it can be dealt with satisfactorily, we will perhaps move on to genetic engineering of people. And this introduces another dimension of risk. We may produce unintended results, either because our techniques turn out to be less finely tuned than we thought, or because different characteristics are found to be genetically linked in unexpected ways.

If we produce a group of people who turn out worse than expected, we will have to live with them. Perhaps we would aim for producing people who were especially imaginative and creative, and only too late find we had produced people who were also very violent and aggressive. This kind of mistake might not only be disastrous, but also very hard to 'correct' in subsequent generations. For when we suggested sterilization to the people we had produced, or else corrective genetic engineering for *their* offspring, we might find them hard to persuade. They might like the way they were, and reject, in characteristically violent fashion, our explanation that they were a mistake.

The possibility of an irreversible disaster is a strong deterrent. It is enough to make some people think we should rule out genetic engineering altogether, and to make others think that, while negative engineering is perhaps acceptable, we should rule out positive engineering. The thought behind this second position is that the benefits from negative engineering are clearer, and that, because its aims are more modest, disastrous mistakes are less likely.

The risk of disasters provides at least a reason for saying that, if we do adopt a policy of human genetic engineering, we ought to do so with extreme caution. We should alter genes only where we have strong reasons for thinking the risk of disaster is very small, and where the benefit is great enough to justify the risk. (The problems of deciding when this is so are familiar from the nuclear power debate.) This 'principle of caution' is less strong than one ruling out all positive engineering, and allows room for the possibility that the dangers may turn out to be very remote, or that greater risks of a different kind are involved in *not* using positive engineering. These possibilities correspond to one view of the facts in the nuclear power debate. Unless with genetic engineering we think we can already rule out such possibilities, the argument from risk provides more justification for the principle of caution than for the stronger ban on all positive engineering. . . .

DECISIONS

Some of the strongest objections to positive engineering are not about specialized applications or about risks. They are about the decisions involved. The

central line of thought is that we should not start playing God by redesigning the human race. The suggestion is that there is no group (such as scientists, doctors, public officials, or politicians) who can be entrusted with decisions about what sort of people there should be. And it is also doubted whether we could have any adequate grounds for basing such decisions on one set of values rather than another. . . .

1. NOT PLAYING GOD

Suppose we could use genetic engineering to raise the average IQ by fifteen points. (I mention, only to ignore, the boring objection that the average IQ is always by definition 100.) Should we do this? Objectors to positive engineering say we should not. This is not because the present average is preferable to a higher one. We do not think that, if it were naturally fifteen points higher, we ought to bring it down to the present level. The objection is to our playing God by deciding what the level should be.

On one view of the world, the objection is relatively straightforward. On this view, there really is a God, who has a plan for the world which will be disrupted if we stray outside the boundaries assigned to us. (It is *relatively* straightforward: there would still be the problem of knowing where the boundaries came. If genetic engineering disrupts the programme, how do we know that medicine and education do not?)

The objection to playing God has a much wider appeal than to those who literally believe in a divine plan. But, outside such a context, it is unclear what the objection comes to. If we have a Darwinian view, according to which features of our nature have been selected for their contribution to gene survival, it is not blasphemous, or obviously disastrous, to start to control the process in the light of our own values. We may value other qualities in people, in preference to those which have been most conducive to gene survival.

The prohibition on playing God is obscure. If it tells us not to interfere with natural selection at all, this rules out medicine, and most other environmental and social changes. If it only forbids interference with natural selection by the direct alteration of genes, this rules out negative as well as positive genetic engineering. If these interpretations are too restrictive, the ban on positive engineering seems to need some explanation. If we can make positive changes at the environmental level, and negative changes at the genetic level, why should we not make positive changes at the genetic level? What makes this policy, but not the others, objectionably God-like?

Perhaps the most plausible reply to these questions rests on a general objection to any group of people trying to plan too closely what human life should be like. Even if it is hard to distinguish in principle between the use of genetic and environmental means, genetic changes are likely to differ in degree from most environmental ones. Genetic alterations may be more drastic or less reversible, and so they can be seen as the extreme case of an objectionably God-like policy by which some people set out to plan the lives of others.

This objection can be reinforced by imagining the possible results of a programme of positive engineering, where the decisions about the desired improvements were taken by scientists. Judging by the literature written by scientists on this topic, great prominence would be given to intelligence. But can we be sure that enough weight would be given to other desirable qualities? And do things seem better if for scientists we substitute doctors, politicians or civil servants? Or some committee containing businessmen, trade unionists, academics, lawyers and a clergyman?

What seems worrying here is the circumscribing of potential human development. The present genetic lottery throws up a vast range of characteristics, good and bad, in all sorts of combinations. The group of people controlling a positive engineering policy would inevitably have limited horizons, and we are right to worry that the limitations of their outlook might become the boundaries of human variety. The drawbacks would be like those of town-planning or dog-breeding, but with more important consequences.

When the objection to playing God is separated from the idea that intervening in this aspect of the natural world is a kind of blasphemy, it is a protest against a particular group of people, necessarily fallible and limited, taking decisions so important to our future. This protest may be on grounds of the bad consequences, such as loss of variety of people, that would come from the imaginative limits of those taking the decisions. Or it may be an expression of opposition to such concentration of power, perhaps with the thought: 'What right have *they* to decide what kinds of people there should be?' Can these problems be side-stepped?

Robert Nozick is critical of the assumption that positive engineering has to involve any centralized decision about desirable qualities: 'Many biologists tend to think the problem is one of *design*, of specifying the best types of persons so that biologists can proceed to produce them. Thus they worry over what sort(s) of person there is to be and who will control this process. They do not tend to think, perhaps because it diminishes the importance of their role, of a system in which they run a "genetic supermarket", meeting the individual specifications (within certain moral limits) of prospective parents. Nor do they think of seeing what limited number of types of persons people's choices would converge upon, if indeed there would be any such convergence. This supermarket system has the great virtue that it involves no centralized decision fixing the future human type(s).'[7]

This idea of letting parents choose their children's characteristics is in many ways an improvement on decisions being taken by some centralized body. It seems less likely to reduce human variety, and could even increase it, if genetic engineering makes new combinations of characteristics available. (But we should be cautious here. Parental choice is not a guarantee of genetic variety, as the influence of fashion or of shared values might make for a small number of types on which choices would converge.)

To those sympathetic to one kind of liberalism, Nozick's proposal will seem more attractive than centralized decisions. On this approach to politics, it is wrong for the authorities to institutionalize any religious or other outlook as the official one of the society. To a liberal of this kind, a good society is one which tolerates and encourages a wide diversity of ideals of the good life. Anyone with these sympathies will be suspicious of centralized decisions about what sort of people should form the next generation. But some parental decisions would be disturbing. If parents chose characteristics likely to make their children unhappy, or likely to reduce their abilities, we might feel that the children should be protected against this. (Imagine parents belonging to some extreme religious sect, who wanted their children to have a religious symbol as a physical mark on their face, and who wanted them to be unable to read, as a protection against their faith being corrupted.) Those of us who support restrictions protecting children from parental harm after birth (laws against cruelty, and compulsion on parents to allow their children to be educated and to have necessary medical treatment) are likely to support protecting children from being harmed by their parents' genetic choices.

No doubt the boundaries here will be difficult to draw. We already find it difficult to strike a satisfactory balance between protection of children and parental freedom to choose the kind of upbringing their children should have. But it is hard to accept that society should set no limits to the genetic choices parents can make for their children. Nozick recognizes this when he says the genetic supermarket should meet the specifications of parents 'within certain moral limits'. So, if the supermarket came into existence, some centralized policy, even if only the restrictive one of ruling out certain choices harmful to the children, should exist. It would be a political decision where the limits should be set.

There may also be a case for other centralized restrictions on parental choice, as well as those aimed at preventing harm to the individual people being designed. The genetic supermarket might have more oblique bad effects. An imbalance in the ratio between the sexes could result. Or parents might think their children would be more successful if they were more thrusting, competitive and selfish. If enough parents acted on this thought, other parents with different values might feel forced into making similar choices to prevent their own children being too greatly disadvantaged. Unregulated individual decisions could lead to shifts of this kind, with outcomes unwanted by most of those who contribute to them. If a majority favour a roughly equal ratio between the sexes, or a population of relatively uncompetitive people, they may feel justified in supporting restrictions on what parents can choose. (This is an application to the case of genetic engineering of a point familiar in other contexts, that unrestricted individual choices can add up to a total outcome which most people think worse than what would result from some regulation.)

Nozick recognizes that there may be cases of this sort. He considers the case of avoiding a sexual imbalance and says that 'a government could require that genetic manipulation be carried on so as to fit a certain ratio'.[8] He clearly prefers to avoid governmental intervention of this kind, and, while admitting that the desired result would be harder to obtain in a purely libertarian system, suggests possible strategies for doing so. He says: 'Either parents would subscribe to an information service monitoring the recent births and so know which sex was in shorter supply (and hence

would be more in demand in later life), thus adjusting their activities, or interested individuals would contribute to a charity that offers bonuses to maintain the ratios, or the ratio would leave 1:1, with new family and social patterns developing.' The proposals for avoiding the sexual imbalance without central regulation are not reassuring. Information about likely prospects for marriage or sexual partnership might not be decisive for parents' choices. And, since those most likely to be 'interested individuals' would be in the age group being genetically engineered, it is not clear that the charity would be given donations adequate for its job.[9]

If the libertarian methods failed, we would have the choice between allowing a sexual imbalance or imposing some system of social regulation. Those who dislike central decisions favouring one sort of person over others might accept regulation here, on the grounds that neither sex is being given preference: the aim is rough equality of numbers.

But what about the other sort of case, where the working of the genetic supermarket leads to a general change unwelcome to those who contribute to it? Can we defend regulation to prevent a shift towards a more selfish and competitive population as merely being the preservation of a certain ratio between characteristics? Or have we crossed the boundary, and allowed a centralized decision favouring some characteristics over others? The location of the boundary is obscure. One view would be that the sex-ratio case is acceptable because the desired ratio is equality of numbers. On another view, the acceptability derives from the fact that the present ratio is to be preserved. (In this second view, preserving altruism would be acceptable, so long as no attempt was made to raise the proportion of altruistic people in the population. But is *this* boundary an easy one to defend?)

If positive genetic engineering does become a reality, we may be unable to avoid some of the decisions being taken at a social level. Or rather, we could avoid this, but only at what seems an unacceptable cost, either to the particular people being designed, or to their generation as a whole. And, even if the social decisions are only restrictive, it is implausible to claim that they are all quite free of any taint of preference for some characteristics over others. But, although this suggests that we should not be doctrinaire in our support of the liberal view, it does not show that the view has to be abandoned altogether. We may still think that social decisions in favour of one type of person rather than another should be few, even if the consequences of excluding them altogether are unacceptable. A genetic supermarket, modified by some central regulation, may still be better than a system of purely central decisions. The liberal value is not obliterated because it may sometimes be compromised for the sake of other things we care about.

3. A MIXED SYSTEM

The genetic supermarket provides a partial answer to the objection about the limited outlook of those who would take the decisions. The choices need not be concentrated in the hands of a small number of people. The genetic supermarket should not operate in a completely unregulated way, and so some centralized decisions would have to be taken about the restrictions that should be imposed. One system that would answer many of the anxieties about centralized decision-making would be to limit the power of the decision-makers to one of veto. They would then only check departures from the natural genetic lottery, and so the power to bring about changes would not be given to them, but spread through the whole population of potential parents. Let us call this combination of parental initiative and central veto a 'mixed system'. If positive genetic engineering does come about, we can imagine the argument between supporters of a mixed system and supporters of other decision-making systems being central to the political theory of the twenty-first century, parallel to the place occupied in the nineteenth and twentieth centuries by the debate over control of the economy.[10]

My own sympathies are with the view that, if positive genetic engineering is introduced, this mixed system is in general likely to be the best one for taking decisions. I do not want to argue for an absolutely inviolable commitment to this, as it could be that some centralized decision for genetic change was the only way of securing a huge benefit or avoiding a great catastrophe. But, subject to this reservation, the dangers of concentrating the decision-making create a strong presumption in favour of a mixed system rather than one in which initiatives come from the centre. And, if a mixed system was introduced, there would have to be a great deal of political argument over what kinds of restrictions on the supermarket should be imposed. Twenty-first-century elections may be about issues rather deeper than economics.

If this mixed system eliminates the anxiety about genetic changes being introduced by a few powerful people with limited horizons, there is a more general unease which it does not remove. May not the limitations of one generation of parents also prove disastrous? And, underlying this, is the problem of what values parents should appeal to in making their choices. How can we be confident that it is better for one sort of person to be born than another?

4. VALUES

The dangers of such decisions, even spread through all prospective parents, seem to me very real. We are swayed by fashion. We do not know the limitations of our own outlook. There are human qualities whose value we may not appreciate. A generation of parents might opt heavily for their children having physical or intellectual abilities and skills. We might leave out a sense of humour. Or we might not notice how important to us is some other quality, such as emotional warmth. So we might not be disturbed in advance by the possible impact of the genetic changes on such a quality. And, without really wanting to do so, we might stumble into producing people with a deep coldness. This possibility seems one of the worst imaginable. It is just one of the many horrors that could be blundered into by our lack of foresight in operating the mixed system. Because such disasters are a real danger, there is a case against positive genetic engineering, even when the changes do not result from centralized decisions. But this case, resting as it does on the risk of disaster, supports a principle of caution rather than a total ban. We have to ask the question whether there are benefits sufficiently great and sufficiently probable to outweigh the risks.

But perhaps the deepest resistance, even to a mixed system, is not based on risks, but on a more general problem about values. Could the parents ever be justified in choosing, according to some set of values, to create one sort of person rather than another?

Is it sometimes better for us to create one sort of person rather than another? We say 'yes' when it is a question of eliminating genetic defects. And we say 'yes' if we think that encouraging some qualities rather than others should be an aim of the upbringing and education we give our children. Any inclination to say 'no' in the context of positive genetic engineering must lay great stress on the two relevant boundaries.

The positive–negative boundary is needed to mark off the supposedly unacceptable positive policies from the acceptable elimination of defects. And the genes–environment boundary is needed to mark off positive engineering from acceptable positive aims of educational policies. But it is not clear that confidence in the importance of these boundaries is justified. . . .

NOTES

1. Chris Graham has suggested to me that it is misleading to say this without emphasizing the painful slowness of this way of changing gene frequencies.

2. *The Future of Man* (The Reith Lectures, 1959), London, 1960, chapter 3; and in 'The Genetic Improvement of Man', in *The Hope of Progress*, London, 1972.

3. *Genes, Dreams and Realities*, London, 1971, p. 81.

4. 'Already they have pushed Cline's results further, obtaining transfer between rabbit and mouse, for example, and good expression of the foreign gene in its new host. Some, by transferring the genes into the developing eggs, have managed to get the new genes into every cell in the mouse, including the sex cells; those mice have fathered offspring who also contain the foreign gene.' Jeremy Cherfas: *Man Made Life*, Oxford, 1982, pp. 229–30.

5. *Out of the Night*, New York, 1935. To find a distinguished geneticist talking like this after the Nazi period is not easy.

6. John Maynard Smith: *On Evolution*, Edinburgh, 1972; the article is reprinted from the issue on 'Utopia' of *Daedalus, Journal of the American Academy of Arts and Sciences*, 1965.

7. *Anarchy, State and Utopia*, New York, 1974, p. 315.

8. Op. cit., p. 315.

9. This kind of unworldly innocence is part of the engaging charm of Nozick's dotty and brilliant book.

10. Decision-taking by a central committee (perhaps of a dozen elderly men) can be thought of as a 'Russian' model. The genetic supermarket (perhaps with genotypes being sold by TV commercials) can be thought of as an 'American' model. The mixed system may appeal to Western European social democrats.

Transplantation Technologies

ARTHUR L. CAPLAN

Ethical Issues Raised by Research Involving Xenografts

On Oct 26, 1984, Dr Leonard Bailey and his associates at the Loma Linda University Medical Center in California implanted a heart from a 7-month-old baboon in a newborn human infant. The child, known publicly as Baby Fae, was afflicted with a fatal congenital abnormality of the heart known as hypoplastic left heart syndrome.[1]

The implant created an enormous controversy both within the medical community and among lay observers of the experiment. The questions it raised and continues to raise concern the competency of the child's mother to give informed consent to the procedure, the morality of killing an animal in order to attempt to save the life of a child, the adequacy of the scientific basis for undertaking this type of transplant in a young child, the competency of the medical team and medical center to undertake the experiment, the adequacy of existing review mechanisms governing human experimentation at Loma Linda University Medical Center, the decision by the university not to disclose various documents pertaining to the implant, such as the informed consent form and research protocol, and the timeliness and accuracy of the information disclosed about the experiment by the university as it proceeded.[2-4]

Reprinted by permission of the author and publisher from *Journal of the American Medical Association* 254 (1985), pp. 3339–3343. © 1985, American Medical Association.

The feasibility of using animals as a source of solid organs for transplantation is a subject that continues to provoke dispute within the medical community. The ongoing severe shortage of solid organs available to both adults and children suffering from renal, cardiac, or liver failure continues to focus the attention of Dr Bailey and other physicians on the possibility of using animals as a source of solid organs. Given the continued interest of physicians at a number of medical centers in xenografting solid organs, it is important that the ethical questions raised by this highly experimental procedure be carefully examined in order that researchers, potential subjects and their families, policymakers, and the general public fully understand the complexities of the moral issues involved in this type of human experimentation.

THE NEED FOR TRANSPLANTABLE SOLID ORGANS

Current research on xenografts is focused on three major organs: kidneys, livers, and hearts. Consideration has been given to the use of other organs such as bowel, pancreas, and lungs, but, for a variety of technical reasons, most physicians interested in xenografts have focused on kidneys, livers, and hearts. There is a demonstrable unmet need for each of these organs among both adults and children.

KIDNEYS

Nearly 80,000 persons are currently receiving dialytic therapy for renal failure in the United States. In 1984 another 6,730 received transplants of kidneys from either cadaver or living related donors.[5] While there is some dispute as to the number of dialysis patients who might benefit from a kidney transplant—partly due to the uncertain medical suitability of the members of this population for surgery, and partly due to uncertainty about the desires of dialysis patients themselves for transplants—there is little doubt that at least 10,000 persons would avail themselves of transplants if a sufficient supply of organs were available.[5] Some experts believe that the pool of potential kidney transplant recipients may be as large as 25,000 patients.[5]

It is difficult to obtain exact figures on the number of newborns and children who might benefit from kidney transplantation. The estimated incidence of end-stage renal disease in children younger than the age of 10 years is 0.3 to 0.4 per million per year.[6] More than 600 children in this age group have received transplants in the United States during the past 20 years.[6] Due to the unavailability of donors, very few of these have been infants or children younger than 1 year of age.

LIVERS

In 1984, three hundred eight liver transplants were performed in the United States, primarily for children and adolescents suffering from congenital defects of this organ.[5] Since there is no means available at present to substitute artificially for the function of the liver, the number of persons actually awaiting transplants at any given time is relatively small—in the neighborhood of 300 individuals, most of whom are infants or children.

However, the need for livers for transplantation may expand rapidly as the technical dimensions of liver transplant surgery are perfected. There are hundreds of children and thousands of adults afflicted with various fatal diseases of the liver who might benefit from a liver transplant were the supply of organs available for this purpose increased.

HEARTS

Approximately 400 heart transplants were performed in the United States in 1984.[5] However, the number of centers capable of attempting this procedure has increased dramatically during the past year. Moreover, the appearance of mechanical hearts that can act as temporary bridges until an organ can be found may significantly increase the number of persons who might benefit from cardiac transplant surgery.

At the present time, there appear to be at least 100 individuals awaiting cardiac transplants at various medical centers around the United States. Recent studies have estimated that at least 12,000 adults might benefit from cardiac tansplantation were a sufficient supply of organs available.[7]

There are also approximately 25,000 infants born each year in the United States with congenital heart disease. Of these, approximately 7,500 of the infants' conditions are considered so serious as to be life threatening. Hypoplastic left heart syndrome, the condition that afflicted Baby Fae, is the fourth most common congenital heart problem, affecting approximately 500 infants each year.[8] The deaths of this group of infants account for nearly one fourth of all cardiac-related mortality occurring during the first week of life.

There are approximately 100,000 fatal accidents in the United States each year. Of this number, most organ procurement specialists believe that between 12,000 and 27,000 might serve as a source of solid organs for transplant.[9,10] The lower estimate is based on the number of brain deaths occurring among those who range in age from 5 to 55 years of age. The higher estimate includes all those suffering brain death from birth to age 65 years.

Stricter suitability criteria, ie, age and comorbidity, are utilized with respect to cardiac and liver donors than are applied to kidney donors. Recent studies indicate that fewer than 1,000 viable donor hearts are available from cadaver sources under existing medical and social policies.[7] A much larger number of those suffering brain death would be suitable donors of kidneys.

The prevailing system for procuring organs, which is based upon voluntary donation by means of written directives in the form of driver's license checkoffs or donor cards or as a result of consent by next of kin when no documentation exists, yields between 10% and 15% of the available cadaver donor pool for kidneys. Between 2,000 and 2,500 persons served as a donor of one or more solid organs in 1984.[11] Approximately one third of all kidneys transplanted in the United States are obtained from living related donors.

The system for obtaining organs from cadaver sources is not marked by a high degree of efficiency. This is particularly true of donations from infants and children. Very few infants who are born anencephalic, or brain dead, are utilized as cadaver donors.

There can be no doubt that a shortfall exists between the available supply of kidneys, livers, and hearts from cadaver sources and the number of persons awaiting transplants of these organs. Moreover, even if the current system of procuring organs from cadaver sources were modified so as to increase the efficiency of cadaver organ procurement, there would still exist a significant shortfall in the number of kidneys, livers, and hearts available for transplantation to children and adults.

THE SCIENTIFIC STATUS OF XENOGRAFTS

CLINICAL TRIALS

Most clinical studies of xenografts were conducted in the early 1960s. These involved attempts to transplant kidneys from chimpanzees or baboons to adults using the then-available forms of immunosuppressive therapy. The vast majority of these grafts failed within two months after surgery.

Three attempts were made during the late 1960s in the United States to transplant livers from animals to human beings. All involved attempts to transplant livers from chimpanzees to young children afflicted with biliary atresia. All three grafts failed within two weeks after the initial surgery.[12,13]

Four attempts have been made to use animal hearts as a means of cardiac substitution. The first involved the transplant of a chimpanzee heart to a 68-year-old man at the University of Mississippi Medical Center in 1964. Two other attempts were made in the late 1970s in South Africa. In these experiments, baboon hearts were used with the intent of facilitating the return of left ventricular function in patients suffering from cardiogenic shock. Both subjects died within four days of the surgery.[14,15]

The fourth case was that of Baby Fae.[1] A baboon heart was used whose blood type did not match that of the recipient (*New York Times*, Oct 17, 1985, p B11). The researchers felt that the ABO barrier would prove surmountable as a result of the recipient's immature immune system when subjected to the newly available immunosuppressive drug cyclosporine. The graft functioned for 20 days.

ANIMAL TRIALS

A relatively small number of researchers have attempted cross-species transplants in various animals over the past 20 years.[16-19] These studies suggest that xenograft rejection resembles allograft rejection with respect to both cellular and humoral factors. There appears to be a powerful correlation between the degree of genetic difference between donor and recipient and the speed with which a xenograft is rejected. A few recent trials involving cyclosporine show improved graft survival in various species.[20-22] Little research has been done to determine which immunosuppressive regimen provides maximal graft survival. Nor has there been much published research involving newborn or very young animals.

THE SCIENTIFIC STATUS OF XENOGRAFTS

The animal and clinical experience obtained to date with respect to the use of animals as a source of solid organs for the replacement or supplementation of the function of human hearts, livers, and kidneys makes it clear that xenografting is a poorly understood, relatively untested, and therefore highly experimental procedure in both children and adults. The research done thus far involving xenografts in human beings might best be understood as approximating the earliest stages in the testing of new cytotoxic drugs.

In clinical pharmacology, phase 1 trials describe the initial introduction of a drug into human beings.[23] Usually, healthy volunteers are used, after extensive animal testing, in an effort to determine the pharmacological activity of new agents and their levels of toxicity. These initial tests involving human subjects are aimed solely at assessing the biological effects of a drug in human beings.

Occasionally, phase 1 trials are undertaken with cytotoxic drugs in terminally ill subjects for whom conventional treatment has failed or does not exist, and when animal studies indicate that a new drug may possess useful therapeutic properties. Such experimentation is permitted only with the full, informed consent of subjects and after the development of a well-designed research protocol that has been closely reviewed by both the National Cancer Institute and the Food and Drug Administration.[23,24]

If human experimentation involving xenografts is closely analogous to phase 1 trials of cytotoxic drugs, then such experimentation must meet the highest ethical and legal standards for the following reasons. (1) The data available concerning clinical trials of xenografts are extremely limited and the outcomes of these trials have been poor. Moreover, the majority of the trials were conducted under scientific and technical circumstances drastically dissimilar to those that now prevail in the field of transplantation, making any generalization from the available data base problematic. (2) The amount of data available in the published, peer-reviewed literature on cross-species transplants among animals, while somewhat promising, is relatively slight. (3) The experience obtained to date with cadaver and living related transplants from human sources indicates that significant problems involving graft rejection, graft-vs-host disease, and other adverse outcomes still exist. (4) Any human subjects involved in future trials would be terminally ill and therefore highly vulnerable. This vulnerable status is particularly apt in describing the status of infants and young children.

The technical, scientific, and psychosocial complexities involved in xenografting hearts, livers, and kidneys to adult human beings are still enormous. The power of newly available immunosuppressive drugs, such as cyclosporine, to counteract graft rejection is poorly understood. Tissue matching capabilities between primates and humans, while much improved in recent years, are still far from perfect.

These problems are, if anything, more daunting where children and infants are concerned. The ability of infants and children to sustain xenografts is a subject of much controversy and dispute among pediatric surgeons.[25] Nor is it known whether or for what period of time animal organs will grow and support normal or near-normal development in newborns and young children.

The obvious questions that arise in considering the ethics of human experimentation involving xenografting are (1) should further research involving xenografts in human subjects be permitted and (2) if so, what ethical standards, regulations, and public policies ought to govern such research?

THE ETHICS OF INITIATING FURTHER RESEARCH INVOLVING HUMAN SUBJECTS AT THE PRESENT TIME

A number of factors must be weighed in evaluating the case for continuing further research involving xenografts in human subjects. Does the demonstrable need for an increase in the supply of organs justify ongoing research involving human beings? Have the medical profession and public officials done all that is reasonably possible to do to maximize the supply of organs that is available to those currently or soon to be in need? What alternatives to xenografts currently exist and what alternatives are likely to exist in the near and long-term future? Are the data available from animal and clinical trials suggestive enough to support further efforts involving human subjects at the present time?

There can be little doubt that a real need exists for developing a viable form of therapy for those persons afflicted with life-threatening forms of organ failure. Many critics of human experimentation involving organ replacement, via both mechanical substitutes and transplants from animal and human sources, note that a greater focus should be placed upon research that might eventuate in strategies for modifying behaviors known to produce irreversible organ failure, such as smoking and alcohol abuse (*Time*, Dec 10, 1984, pp 70–73; *Washington Post*, Nov 14, 1984, p D7). Such strategies could lead to greater decreases in morbidity and mortality at lower cost than might be possible through the development of techniques permitting organ replacements.

But the development of such strategies will do nothing to help those now afflicted or soon to be afflicted with end-stage organ failure. Moreover, preventive measures will do little to benefit those born with congenital defects and dysfunctions of life-sustaining organs. While research on preventive health measures intended to produce modifications in unhealthy life-styles is critical to the reduction of morbidity and mortality in the American population, it offers little hope to those currently or soon to be afflicted with life-threatening organ failure. Nor can those who advocate greater research into public health measures aimed at modifying risk-creating life-styles or unhealthy behaviors guarantee the successful outcome of such inquiries.

It is also true that national public policy has not fully addressed existing deficits in the current system for procuring solid organs from cadaver sources.[11] While it is indisputably true that those in need of transplants are far more likely to receive therapeutic benefit from the receipt of human as opposed to animal organs, it is uncertain whether the general public and its elected representatives are willing to examine carefully the flaws and faults of a system that obtains donations from less than 20% of suitable adult donors and almost none from newborn and infant donors.

The reality facing those now or soon to be afflicted with irreversible end-stage organ failure, their physicians, and the general public is that modifications in existing public policies that might alleviate the existing shortage in human cadaver organs for transplantation are not in the immediate offing. Nor are changes in the setting of basic research priorities, which might lead to reductions in the prevalence of organ failure in the general population as a result of modifications in behavior and life-styles, known to produce life-threatening organ failure. Most importantly, even if organ procurement from human cadaver sources were to become significantly more efficient, there would still remain a gap between the available supply of human organs and the need for them.

End-stage organ failure of the heart, kidney, and liver will continue to take a toll of lives among infants, children, and adults for the foreseeable future. With the exception of end-stage kidney failure, no form of artificial organ replacement is likely to become available in the near future that might serve as a permanent therapeutic option.

At the same time scientific and technical understanding of the biology and immunology of xenografting is, at best, primitive. A great deal of research must be done on cellular and animal models in order to advance present scientific understanding of this procedure.

There would appear to exist a pool of terminally ill persons, both children and adults, for whom no therapeutic alternatives exist or are likely to exist in the near future. Many of these individuals are faced with the prospect of inevitable death or, for some renal patients, a quality of life maintained by artificial means that is lower than they desire and are willing to tolerate.

Given these realities, it would appear ethically defensible to allow research involving xenografting in human subjects to proceed in those areas where no reasonable alternative therapy exists. The plight of those in need, the lack of viable therapeutic options, the low probability that public policy will be modified to enhance access to cadaver organs, and the fact that end-stage organ failure is likely to continue to be a pressing health care problem for the foreseeable future are factors that would appear to weigh heavily against prohibitions, bans, or moratoriums on clinical trials of xenografts at this time. While there are no scientific data that justify the recruitment of potential subjects for the purposes of therapy, the plight of those dying of end-stage organ failure would appear to justify allowing their participation in further clinical trials to advance scientific understanding of the feasibility of xenografting when appropriate ethical and scientific requirements have been met.

KILLING ANIMALS FOR RESEARCH INVOLVING XENOGRAFTS

One factor that might weigh against the continuation of research involving the use of animals as a source of solid organs for humans afflicted with end-stage organ failure is the need to kill animals for this purpose. While it is true that prevailing public policy in the United States allows animals to be killed for a variety of reasons, including general medical research, education, safety and efficacy testing for drugs and commercial products, recreation, and eating, it is also the case that killing animals for the explicit purpose of research intended to develop therapeutic options—which would require the further killing of animals in order to benefit the terminally ill—may raise ethical problems that are unique or specific to xenografting.

In recent years a great deal of effort has been devoted by some members of the general public, the philosophic community, and even the medical and scientific communities to draw attention to questionable practices involving the use and handling of animals for scientific purposes. Some critics of animal experimentation have argued that such practices violate the rights of animal subjects, particularly when they involve significant amounts of pain and suffering for the animals involved.[26]

This is not the place to attempt a review of the pros and cons of the ethics of animal experimentation. However, it is important to note that many of the arguments favoring the continuation of research to develop xenografts are pertinent to the assessment of arguments about the use of animals for this purpose.

If other viable alternative methods existed for generating a sufficient increase in the supply of organs available from cadaver donors, or for making available other therapeutic options for those faced with life-threatening illness or disabilities, then certainly it would be wrong to capture, breed, and kill animals systemically for purposes that might be served in some other manner. Unfortunately, for both scientific and practical reasons, the development of alternative options to benefit those in need are not likely at the present time.

This is not to say that our society is under no obligation to develop such alternatives. Rather, the immediate nonavailability of such options, when combined with a moral point of view that accords greater value to an individual human life than an individual animal life, other things being equal, would appear to justify, at least for the time being, killing animals for the purposes of further research involving xenografts. However, in the long run, serious attention must be given to the morality of killing animals for this purpose if other therapeutic alternatives are possible.

THE REGULATION OF XENOGRAFT RESEARCH INVOLVING HUMAN SUBJECTS

Despite the uncertainty and ignorance that cloud current understanding of the feasibility of using animal organs as a source of transplants for human beings, continued research on cellular, animal, and human subjects would appear to be morally justified. However, the lack of empirical knowledge concerning both biological and psychosocial aspects of this surgery would appear to require that all such research, whether publicly funded or not, be conducted in accordance with strict conformity to existing federal, state, and professional society regulations concerning human experimentation.

Indeed, the vulnerability of the human subjects who might be asked to serve in further clinical trials, particularly those who are infants or children, is so compelling as to demand unusual efforts on the part of researchers and institutional review boards to respect the autonomy, rights, and dignity of potential subjects.[27]

The vulnerability of both healthy and terminally ill human subjects involved in the earliest stages of drug testing has led the federal government to enact strict standards for monitoring research in this area. A similar system of review and monitoring would appear to be appropriate for the regulation of any further attempts involving xenografts. While the Food and Drug Administration has no mandate to extend its regulatory oversight to medical procedures that do not involve drugs or medical devices, it would seem appropriate that such a mandate be granted before further clinical trials are undertaken.

Researchers and the members of institutional review boards are under a strong obligation to make clear to potential subjects, or their surrogates in the case of children or mentally incompetent subjects, the highly experimental nature of all forms of xenografting. Potential subjects or their surrogates must have complete and comprehensible information about the limits of scientific understanding concerning the efficacy of the surgery, their right to terminate participation in the experiment at any time, any other experimental procedures that will be undertaken as part of xenograft surgery, and any and all alternatives to xenografting that are available.[23,24] Researchers interested in pursuing human trials would also appear to be under a strict obligation to inform potential subjects or their surrogates that *nothing* is known as to the long-term viability of xenografts in human beings.

Only those researchers and institutions willing to subject their research protocols and human subject protections to public scrutiny ought to undertake clinical trials of xenografts. Peer review of the competency of researchers and the scientific basis for their research is a sine qua non where terminally ill subjects are concerned. While subject confidentiality and privacy must be fully honored and protected, researchers, institutional review boards, and institutional officials must understand that their primary duty is to protect the autonomy and interests of subjects who are extremely vulnerable to coercion, misunderstandings, and a failure to comprehend the rationale for undertaking a clinical trial. Subjects or their surrogates must understand that the primary goal of research involving xenografts at the present time is to demonstrate the feasibility of such surgery. Only when it is clear to the medical community, regulatory bodies at the local and federal levels, and the general public that both researchers and their subjects or surrogates fully understand that clinical trials involving xenografts have as their primary goal the acquisition of generalizable knowledge should further research be undertaken.

NOTES

1. Bailey LL, Nehlsen-Cannarella SL, Concepcion W, et al: Baboon-to-human cardiac xeno-transplantation in a neonate. *JAMA* 1985; 254:3321–3329.

2. Caplan AL: Good intentions are not enough: The case of Baby Fae. *Transplant Today* 1985; 2:4–7.

3. Annas GJ: Baby Fae: The 'anything goes' school of human experimentation. *Hastings Cent Rep* 1985;15:15–17.

4. Sheldon R: The IRB's responsibility to itself. *Hastings Cent Rep* 1985;15:11–13.

5. *An Update on Organ and Tissue Donation and Transplantation in the United States Today*. Washington, DC, American Council on Transplantation, 1984.

6. Lum CT, Fryd DS, Polta TA, et al: Results of kidney transplantation in the young child. *Transplantation*, 1982;34:167–171.

7. Evans RW, Manninen DL, Overcast TD, et al: *The National Heart Transplantation Study: Final Report*. Seattle, Battelle Human Affairs Research Centers, 1984.

8. Vinocur B: Bailey's answers only provoke more questions. *Med World News*, in press.

9. Guttman FM: Organ transplantation in children. *Pediatr Ann* 1982;11:910–915.

10. Bart KJ, Macon EJ, Humphries AL Jr, et al: Increasing the study of cadaveric kidneys for transplantation. *Transplantation* 1981;31:383–387.

11. Caplan AL: Organ procurement: It's not in the cards. *Hastings Cent Rep* 1984;14:6–9.

12. Starzl TE: Orthotopic heterotransplantation, in *Experience in Hepatic Transplantation*. Philadelphia, WB Saunders Co, 1969, pp. 408–421.

13. Starzl TE, Ishikawa M, Putnam CW, et al: Progress in and deterrents to orthotopic liver transplantation, with special reference to survival, resistance to hyperacute rejection, and biliary duct reconstruction. *Transplant Proc* 1974;6:129–139.

14. Hardy JD, Chavez CM: The first heart transplant in man. *Am J Cardiol* 1968;22:772–781.

15. Barnard CN, Wolpowitz A, Losman JG, et al: Heterotopic cardiac transplantation with a xenograft for assistance of the left heart in cardiogenic shock after cardiopulmonary bypass. *S Afr Med J* 1977;52:1035–1038.

16. Reemtsma K: Heterotransplantation-theoretical considerations. *Transplant Proc* 1971;3:49–57.

17. Perper RJ: Renal heterotransplant rejection. *Transplantation* 1971;12:519–523.

18. Shons AR, Najarian JS: Xenograft rejection in human beings. *Rev Surg* 1975;32:70–91.

19. Chartrand C, et al: Delayed rejection of cardiac xenografts in C6-deficient rabbits. *Immunology* 1979;38:245–249.

20. Danko I, Gebhard C, Scholz S, et al: Transplant aspiration cytology for monitoring of kidney xenograft under cyclosporin-A treatment. *Eur Surg Res* 1983;15:276–283.

21. Hammer C, Chaussy C, Welter H, et al: Exceptionally long survival time in xenogeneic organ transplantation. *Transplant Proc* 1981;13:881–884.

22. Harbin S, Heneghan JB: Growth of dog intestinal mucosa xenografts in nude mice. *Prog Clin Biol Res* 1985;181:467–471.

23. Levine RJ: *Ethics and Regulations of Clinical Research*. Baltimore, Urban & Schwarzenberg, 1981.

24. Barber B: *Informed Consent in Medical Therapy and Research*. New Brunswick, NJ, Rutgers University Press, 1980.

25. Breo DL: Is 'Baby Fae' transplant worth it? Experts mixed. *Am Med News* 1984;27:41–43.

26. Regan T: *The Case for Animal Rights*. Berkeley, University of California Press, 1983.

27. Ackerman TF: Moral duties of investigators toward sick children. *IRB* 1981;3:1–5.

ALEXANDER MORGAN CAPRON

Anencephalic Donors:
Separate the Dead from the Dying

In biomedical ethics, some cases involving individuals present true dilemmas: choosing between two evils (shorter life or longer suffering). Others are perplexing in another way: choosing between two goods (one person's privacy or another's well-being). When biomedical ethics moves to the realm of law and public policy, we face even more complex challenges. Consider, for example, several recent bills that aim to facilitate organ transplantation in infants by allowing organs to be taken from other babies who are born with most of their brains missing. These proposals aim to do good, but they create the possibility of doing great harm.

THE NEED AND THE TECHNOLOGY

In the past few years, medical interest in pediatric organ transplantation has rapidly expanded. Extensive press coverage of developments in immunosuppression and refinement of surgical techniques—particularly cardiac replacement in newborns—has created hope for some patients whose children have otherwise fatal heart, kidney, and liver problems.

Before these transplant procedures move from experimental to therapeutic, they must improve technically. Yet an inadequate supply of usable cadaver organs poses an even more formidable impediment. Cadaver organs for transplantation in older patients come primarily from the victims of accidents, especially automobile and motorcycle collisions. Relatively few newborns and very young children die under

these or other circumstances that would make them suitable organ donors. Present methods of identifying possible donors and receiving permission to harvest their organs provide only a small fraction of the estimated 400 to 500 infant hearts and kidneys and 500 to 1,000 infant livers that are needed in the U.S. each year.

The supply is likely to increase somewhat as transplant techniques are perfected for newborns and infants. And some refinements now underway in the methods for obtaining organs generally—such as the development of a national computerized registry and more intensive local organ procurement efforts—may partially ameliorate the shortage. The chance to make "the gift of life" to another infant may in time become a source of solace commonly offered to the parents of dead infants as it is to relatives of older accident victims.

The present (and perhaps long-range) inadequacy of organ supply for infants has led to proposals that the law be altered to allow organs to be taken from another group of babies—those born with a fatal neurologic condition called anencephaly, the absence of all or most of the cerebral hemispheres. According to Godfrey Oakley of the Centers for Disease Control, approximately 2,000 to 3,000 such babies are born every year. The initiative comes from surgeons who are developing the techniques for infant transplants, but parents of anencephalic infants have also publicly supported the idea, as they search for some meaning and comfort in the face of the death of their newborn.

The legislation takes two forms. The first, illustrated by a proposal made but subsequently withdrawn in the California Senate, is to modify the statutory standards for determining human death set forth in the Uniform Determination of Death Act (UDDA) or simi-

Reprinted by permission of the author and reproduced by permission of the publisher from *Hastings Center Report* 17 (February 1987), pp. 5–9. © The Hastings Center.

lar state laws so that they will encompass anencephalic babies. The second, illustrated by New Jersey Assembly Bill No. 3367, is to permit parents of an anencephalic child to donate its organs even though the child does not meet the requirement set forth in the Uniform Anatomical Gift Act (UAGA) that organs may be removed only after a physician not involved in the transplant procedure determines that the organ donor has died.

Both these attempts are well-meaning but in my view misguided. They would create very substantial problems, as well as undermine the very goal they seek.

AMENDING THE DETERMINATION OF DEATH ACT

For many years, death was "defined" by the law through judicial decisions which, following accepted medical and popular opinion, held that death occurs when all bodily functions, specifically heartbeat and breathing, cease.

With the development of technology to sustain circulation and respiration, medical and popular views diverged. Physicians knew that other functions besides heart and lung activity had to be measured when artificial ventilation and drugs might be causing observable cardiopulmonary activity. By the late 1960s, medical studies had verified that tests detecting the complete absence of brain functions provide an accurate alternative way to establish the *same* physiologic state of death as the heart and lung measurements that are done on persons not on artificial life supports.

Thus, although people frequently speak of new "definitions" of death, what was actually involved was merely an updating of the means for determining death. Beginning with Kansas in 1970, many states gave legal recognition to two standards for determining that death has occurred: the traditional one of irreversible cessation of circulatory and respiratory functions, and the new one—irreversible cessation of all functions of the entire brain, including the brain stem—which is relevant when respirators and other treatments render the traditional standard unreliable.

By the late 1970s, when Congress wrote the mandate for the President's Commission for the Study of Ethical Problems in Medicine and Biomedical and Behavioral Research, a consensus existed among public officials, as well as legal, medical, and ethical commentators, on the need for simple and uniform legislation recognizing the new (brain) standard for determining death alongside the old (heart and lungs).

From the joint efforts of the National Conference of Commissioners on Uniform State Laws, the American Medical Association, the American Bar Association, and the President's Commission, the UDDA emerged in 1982. It has been adopted in sixteen states legislatively, and in two others through explicit judicial recognition; statutes with provisions similar to the UDDA have been enacted in twenty other states, and the highest courts in an additional four states have accepted neurological determinations of death, without explicitly recognizing the UDDA's formulation of the appropriate language to achieve this end.

In February 1986 California Senator Milton Marks introduced Senate Bill 2018. He was apparently moved by an article in the San Francisco *Chronicle* that recounted the frustration of a couple who were unable to donate the organs of their anencephalic baby for transplantation to an infant patient at the University of California Medical Center. As originally proposed, the bill would have amended the UDDA by adding the statement that "an individual born with the condition of anencephaly is dead." Sen. Marks subsequently modified his bill and proposed that a state health advisory board make recommendations about the care of infants with life-threatening conditions, including the "feasibility and necessity" of infant organ transplants, the donation of organs from infants born with anencephaly, and any "necessary changes" in the UAGA or the UDDA.

Adding anencephalics to the category of dead persons would be a radical change, both in the social and medical understanding of what it means to be dead and in the social practices surrounding death. Anencephalic infants may be dying, but they are still alive and breathing. Calling them "dead" will not change physiologic reality or otherwise cause them to resemble those (cold and nonrespirating) bodies that are considered appropriate for post-mortem examinations and burial. The amendment of the UDDA to include anencephalics is therefore unwise, for several reasons.

To begin with, the UDDA provides that determinations of death "must be made in accordance with accepted medical standards." In the case of anencephalics, this provision creates enormous difficulty because physicians do not consider anencephalic infants as dead, but as dying. Their perception is borne out by statistics. One study of liveborn infants with anencephaly, conducted over a thirty-year period, found an equal distribution among males and females. Significantly more males survived the first day of life, but none lived longer than seven days, while female survival was comparable to male after the first day. One female (1.1 percent) survived 14 days:

The results of this study show that over 40 percent of anencephalic infants can be expected to survive longer than 24 hours (51% males; 34% females), and of these, 35 percent will still be alive on the third day and 5 percent on the seventh day.[1]

For most of the infants in this study, anencephaly was the only neural tube defect, and most of these had no anomalies in other organ systems. Among those infants who also had spina bifida or encephalocele (a protrusion of the brain substance through an opening in the skull), one third had defects in another major organ system.

The UDDA's requirement that determinations of death accord with "accepted medical standards" might be read in another way were anencephaly added to the statute. This would hold that the requirement is met if accepted medical standards *for determining anencephaly* are applied. Although the diagnosis is usually made accurately by neurologists, authors of the thirty-year study just mentioned found that in "conducting this study, it became obvious that it is important to verify the diagnosis of anencephaly." They describe several cases of long survival:

One infant initially coded as anencephaly, who survived over 4 months, had hydranencephaly rather than anencephaly, and another who lived for 12 days actually had amniotic band syndrome mimicking anencephaly.

Misdiagnosis by itself would not appear to be a great enough risk to preclude the use of anencephaly as a category to trigger further action (such as declaration of "death"). But the observed relationship to—or even overlapping with—other congenital neurological defects underlines the problems that the proposal would create. For example, hydranencephalics have normal brain development early in gestation; as a result of some event (such as an in utero infection) their cerebral hemispheres are destroyed and replaced with fluid. Like anencephalics, hydranencephalics survive depending upon the extent to which their brain stems are able to regulate vegetative functioning, but they

usually survive somewhat longer because their skulls are intact and thus their brains are not open to infection.

To further complicate the picture, other neurological conditions, such as certain types of microcephaly, are also inconsistent with long-term survival. Microcephaly—literally, a small head—covers a spectrum of problems, including cases in which the hemispheres fail to form. Whatever their clinical differences from anencephalic babies, hydranencephalic and some microcephalic infants are *conceptually* indistinguishable if the characteristic separating anencephalics from normal children is their lethal neurological condition.

Because of the existence of these other diagnostic categories, decision makers will be pressured to expand the "definition" to sweep in other similarly situated "dead" neonates. Indeed, Dr. Alan Shewmon, a pediatric neurologist at UCLA, has pointed out that babies—such as hydranencephalics—who typically live a little longer than anencephalics are actually likely to be *more* attractive sources of organs because of the extra time for development. At present, the regional organ procurement association for California does not accept organs from infants younger than two months of age because of physiologic difficulties (such as the tendency of vessels to clot).

More important, these other diagnostic categories serve as a reminder that the proposals involve a variety of infants who are going to die in a relatively short time. Distinguishing those who will die within a day or two from those (including *some* microcephalics and hydranencephalics as well as the remaining anencephalics) who will die over the following two weeks is inevitably imprecise. The distinctions rest on clinical judgment, not moral principle.

WHAT THE LAW NOW PROVIDES

Amending the UDDA would also open the door to other changes that the proponents of this particular amendment are unlikely to favor. Perhaps those who have proposed the change do not think it involves a major break with existing law because they are confused about what the law now provides.

Part of that confusion can be traced to the use of the term "brain death" to describe the newer standard for determining death. This terminology is misleading because it wrongly suggests that organs rather than organisms die, and because it implies that there are several *kinds* of death, when in fact death is a unitary concept that can be determined by several standards, each appropriate under particular circumstances.

"Defining" anencephalics as dead would place these patients into the same category as patients who lack the capacity to breathe on their own, which has always been taken as a basic sign of life. Perhaps the proponents of this change do not see this as a major alteration because they think the law already lumps together some people who are "more dead" (those whose hearts have stopped) with others who are merely "brain dead." But all persons found to meet the standards of the UDDA are equally dead; it is merely the means of measuring the absence of the integrated functioning of heart, lungs, and brain that differs between those who are and those who are not being treated by methods that can induce breathing and heartbeat.

Defining anencephalics as dead so that they may be used as organ donors could, ironically, actually decrease organ donation. Imagine the effect of the law on the process of seeking organ donations from the relatives of a deceased person. At present, when that situation arises, the person seeking permission can explain that the patient is dead; despite the heaving chest and other appearances of life, if the physicians were to cease the mechanical interventions, it would immediately be apparent that the body is in the same state that we have always recognized as dead. The next-of-kin are told that they do not face a difficult decision over whether to let the patient die; instead they face the reality that their loved one is now a corpse—albeit a corpse with artificially generated heartbeat and breathing—whose organs are still being maintained in a way that would make them useful for transplants. (Remember that only a fraction of persons declared dead on the basis of absence of brain functions are candidates for organ donation.[2])

If anencephalic babies were also regarded as dead bodies suitable for organ donation, this certainty would be lost. For in these cases, decisions about the extent of treatment remain—indeed, some parents may even wish to try heroic or experimental means to lengthen their child's life. The message to those involved in organ transplantation—both as relatives of potential donors and as physicians, nurses, and others seeking permission for donation—is thus likely to introduce new elements of uncertainty. Is *any* particular patient—and not just an anencephalic baby—*really* dead? Or do the physicians mean only that the outlook for the patient's survival is poor, so why not allow the organs to be taken and bring about death in this (useful) fashion?

Alternatively, perhaps some who favor the anencephalic standard for death *do* mean to change the law radically. A few commentators have argued for many years that the statutes on death should move beyond new means for measuring the traditional state of death and should instead declare that persons who have lost only the higher (neocortical) functions of their brains are also dead.[3] These suggestions have been uniformly rejected by legislators across the country—as well as by most medical, ethical, and legal writers. Yet the inclusion of anencephalics in the "definition" of death would amount to the first recognition of a "higher brain" standard—and a first step toward a broader use of this standard—because these babies, despite the massive deficit in their brains, still have some functions (principally at the brain stem level).

To state that such patients are dead would be equivalent to saying that the late Karen Quinlan was "dead" for the more than ten years that she lived after her respirator was removed. Like the anencephalic babies, Ms. Quinlan and other patients in a persistent vegetative state lack the ability to think, to communicate, and probably even to process any sensations of pain and pleasure (at least in the way that we think of these phenomena). Some people may consider such a life as unrewarding, but that does not justify loose use of language about who is "dead." Emotionally, one may be tempted to say that a person in a permanent coma is "as good as dead" because he or she cannot participate in any of the activities that give life meaning. But such a breathing, metabolizing patient does not embody what we mean by dead and is not ready for burial—or organ donation.

A statute that labels anencephalics "dead" is a bad idea because either it will treat differently another group that is identical on the relevant criteria (the permanently comatose, who are dying and lacking consciousness) or it will lead to a further revision in medical and legal standards under which the permanently comatose would also be regarded as "dead" although many of them can survive for years with nothing more than ordinary nursing care.

For many people, the prospect of being in a permanent coma is unacceptable; if that occurred, they would want to be allowed to die without further treatment. But that is a separate problem to which society is already responding in other ways. It would be highly controversial—and, indeed, would be rejected by most people—to call people who are in a coma but who still breathe on their own "dead," especially when the purpose is to allow removal of their vital organs, which *would* then cause their death as that term is now used. This was the nightmarish scenario that took place in the Jefferson Institute in Robin Cook's novel *Coma*.

AMENDING THE ANATOMICAL GIFT ACT

Amending the UDDA would thus open up the possibility of an ever-increasing category of persons who are defined as "dead" because their organs might be useful in a legally sanctioned "Jefferson Institute." Moreover, the change in "definition" would apply far beyond transplantation to all contexts in which death arises, from burials to probate to criminal law. Amending the Anatomical Gift Act to permit organ harvesting from anencephalics might be subject to some of the same pressures for extension to other groups of dying, unconscious patients. But at least such a change in the law would be limited to organ donation and would thus avoid the conceptual problems that arise when dying is confused with death. Certainly, the need for infant organ donors requires serious consideration of proposals such as the one introduced in October 1986 by New Jersey Assemblyman Walter Kern, Jr.

Though the idea of living people choosing to give vital organs (as a better way of dying than simply getting old or sick) has been around for quite a while,[4] it has not been accepted. Anencephalic newborns should not be the opening wedge in such a revision of the organ donor process, for several reasons.

First, if society wants to adopt a policy of sacrificing living patients for their organs, it seems very strange—and a very bad precedent—to start with the most vulnerable patients. Unconsenting, incompetent patients who have never had a chance to express their views about whether, if near death but not yet dead, they would want their bodies cut up for purposes of organ donation, are the *least* suitable source. Moreover, how would one distinguish anencephalics from other possible candidates for involuntary sacrifice for organ donation, such as comatose, demented, or severely retarded patients?

Second, the argument that anencephalics *are* suitable because they are not living *persons* (since they are born with such profound mental defects that they will never be able to establish meaningful human interactions) is a radical redefinition of the accepted criterion

for being considered a person, namely, live birth of the product of a human conception. If an anencephalic is not a living person for purposes of organ removal, what about for purposes of homicide, which might be justified on the same utilitarian grounds as organ removal (a greater benefit to the community) or even on the grounds that the death would be better for the parents or other members of the baby's family?

This concern raises the general issue of the justice of a proposal that would treat one being as a means of achieving a good for other beings (the grieving donor parents, the ailing recipient child). Certainly, one can imagine cases where there would be sufficient justification for sacrificing one child to save the life of another. For example, suppose that Siamese twins were joined by a six-chambered heart and the only chance of saving either one lay in performing an operation in which the twin with just a two-chambered heart was killed. But the agonizing process that would lead to a decision to proceed in such a rare case is very different from establishing a general rule that would be applied (inevitably, not always in such a conscientious fashion) to the thousands of anencephalic children born each year, to say nothing of other potential organ "donors" with other lethal conditions.

Third, even more than other potential involuntary organ "donors," the anencephalic opens the door to manipulation. The diagnosis of anencephaly is now often made prenatally. The parents are usually offered the option of abortion or of normal delivery, after which the child will die. If anencephalics come to be regarded as an attractive source of transplantable organs, women who would otherwise choose abortion may be pressured by physicians or others to carry the fetus to term and then perhaps to deliver by a riskier method (cesarian section) that would optimize the usefulness of the child as a source of organs.

Finally, amending the UAGA to allow organs to be removed from anencephalic babies seems likely to undermine, rather than reinforce, the public's support for, and confidence in, organ transplantation. Indeed, if the UAGA were to be amended in such a fashion, legislators might well insist on many protections. They would want to ensure the absolute reliability of the diagnosis and prognosis, for example, and to guard against any conflicting interests on the part of those seeking organs or consenting to organ removals from anencephalics. This could lead to the misguided addition of such safeguards for organ removal from dead bodies under the existing UAGA, thus undermining public confidence ("With safeguards like this, organ donation must be a bad or risky thing!'') and diminishing the number of donated organs. At the very least it would unnecessarily encumber the process of organ retrieval, increasing its costs and reducing its yield. These would be ironic results for a measure with the well-intentioned purpose of increasing the organs available for transplantation.

Medical ingenuity should be directed toward finding ways to care for dying anencephalic (and other) babies so that when they become brain-dead, they can be organ donors (with their parents' permission). Medicine should not embark on a course of sacrificing living but incompetent patients for the admitted social good of transplanting organs.

NOTES

1. P. A. Baird, and A. D. Sadovnick, "Survival in Infants with Anencephaly," *Clinical Pediatrics* 23 (1984), 268–72.

2. President's Commission for the Study of Ethical Problems in Medicine and Biomedical and Behavioral Research, *Defining Death* (1981), p. 23.

3. See, e.g., Robert M. Veatch, "The Whole-Brain Oriented Concept of Death: An Out-Moded Philosophical Formulation," *Journal of Thanatology* 3 (1975), 13.

4. Belding H. Scribner, "Ethical Problems of Using Artificial Organs to Sustain Human Life," *Transactions of American Society for Artificial Internal Organs* 10 (1964), 209, 211, stating a personal preference, if ill with a fatal disease, to be able to have physician put him to sleep "and any useful organs taken prior to death."

A L B E R T   R .   J O N S E N

The Artificial Heart's Threat to Others

In June, 1972, I received a telephone call from Dr. Theodore Cooper, director of the National Heart and Lung Institute. Dr. Cooper invited me to serve on a ten-member Totally Implantable Artificial Heart Advisory Panel. I had no idea what the Totally Implantable Artificial Heart was, nor had I any idea what advice needed to be given about it. Nevertheless, I accepted.

The Congress had initiated and funded an Artificial Heart Program at the National Heart Institute in 1964. Research was begun, within NIH's own laboratories, and by contract with many others, on the development of a mechanical device that would replace a human heart irreparably damaged by disease.

Soon funded at about $10 million a year, the program expected to have a device ready for clinical testing by 1970. This was, of course, unrealistic. Among the many obstacles was the development of a power source that could replicate the heart's incredible efficiency. Of the various ideas, a nuclear power source was the most attractive; 250 grams of plutonium 238,

implanted with no external connections or impediments in a shielded capsule in the thoracic cavity could supply efficiently more than many lifetimes of energy to propel the artificial pump.

Dr. Cooper charged the panel with an assessment of the social, legal, ethical, and economic implications of a device of this sort. The ethical analysis in the panel's report was rather primitive. In particular, the unique ethical problem that weighed heavily and continuously on the minds of the panelists—the danger posed by the nuclear heart to persons other than the patient—deserved a much sharper analysis than it received. The panel learned that a human being bearing 230 grams of plutonium would be likely to develop lethal blood disease within ten years. Of course, that is a reasonable choice when one is faced with imminent death from heart disease.

But the person whose life had been saved by the nuclear heart would forever be a walking threat to his or her associates. A few would accept this out of love or devotion; most would never know that a secret assassin, who meant them no harm, dwelt among them. Perhaps moved more by impulse, instinct, or insight than by philosophical analysis, the panelists'

Reprinted by permission of the author and reproduced by permission of the publisher from *Hastings Center Report* 16 (February 1986), pp. 9–11. © The Hastings Center.

deliberations inclined them toward a negative judgment about the nuclear power source. (For a fuller account of the panel's deliberations, see my article, "The Totally Implantable Artificial Heart," *Hastings Center Report*, November 1973, pp. 1–4; and Harold P. Green, "Allocation of Resources: The Artificial Heart. An NIH Panel's Early Warnings," *Hastings Center Report*, October 1983, pp. 13–15.)

The National Heart Institute discontinued its support of research into the nuclear power source in 1973 and turned to other energy systems, particularly electrical ones, to provide the power for the implanted artificial pump. I seldom reflected again on this unusual ethical problem. But in June 1983 Dr. Claude L'Enfant, Director of the Institute now titled Heart, Lung and Blood, invited me to participate in a new panel to review the progress of the same program that the 1973 panel had evaluated. This new study would take place in the aftermath of the first clinical implantation of an artificial heart in Dr. Barney Clark at the University of Utah on December 2, 1982.

THE NEW THREAT TO OTHERS

The new advisory group's name, The Working Group on Mechanical Circulatory Support, reflected a major shift in the activities of the NHLBI since the early 1970s. Instead of an almost exclusive attention to replacement of the total heart, that is, a pump with two ventricles that would supplant the natural heart, attention had turned to "partial devices," that is, single ventricle pumps that would supplement, rather than supplant, the natural heart. These devices could be used on a temporary basis—while awaiting a heart transplant, for example—or permanently. They were much less complex and posed fewer bioengineering problems. Thus, the NHLBI was researching and sponsoring broad research in "mechanical circulatory support devices" rather than concentrating exclusively on the total mechanical heart. This difference is important in understanding the Working Group's recommendations.

When the Working Group convened in Bethesda, I was confident that we were dealing with the same ethical problems that are posed by standard medical technologies. Now that the somewhat bizarre concept of a nuclear-powered device had been retired, there seemed to be nothing that made mechanical circulatory support devices radically different from all other

technologies that biomedical science makes possible. But I now think the artificial heart, in particular the total heart, is different and that it shares that difference with the nuclear-powered heart: its existence in the society creates a distinct and direct threat to the health of others. That threat is not in the rads, rems, and curies of radiation—indeed, it is not a threat of physical harm in itself—but it threatens to deprive many persons of access to needed medical care.

The Working Group recommended that the National Heart, Lung and Blood Institute continue its targeted research program into the development of mechanical circulatory support systems. These systems should include the partial and total devices, for temporary and permanent implantation. A careful, though admittedly somewhat speculative, study estimated that between 17,000 and 35,000 persons annually suffer from end-stage cardiac disease and would be suitable candidates for mechanical circulatory support. In the absence of data and experience with these systems, projection of costs and prognoses was based on explicit sets of assumptions. The total cost of a left ventricular assist device, its implantation and maintenance for a projected average survival of 3.5 years might be approximately $150,000 (in 1983 dollars). The gross annual cost to society could fall in the range of $2.5 to $5 billion annually.

The earlier panel had considered the costs and the allocation of the artificial heart, but its reflections were naive. It proposed that the availability of this lifesaving technology should not depend on the ability of individuals to pay for it. It also recommended that "social worth" criteria to select appropriate recipients be avoided in favor of criteria that reflected medical need or, in the case of equal need, a lottery. It then suggested that public financing of medical care would be required if such expensive technologies were to be made available on an equitable basis. These conclusions were colored by the optimism of the early 1970s, when it seemed obvious that some form of national health insurance would be enacted and when the costs of medical care were hardly a cloud on the horizon.

By 1983, that optimism had yielded to a sober realism. Far from moving toward public financing of medical care, the market in medicine has been encouraged and the costs of care are being cut and contained, either to lower government budgets or to gain profits. The Working Group could not assume that the costs of mechanical circulatory support would be met from the public fisc. Indeed, we were vividly reminded that the only current clinical implantations were being done under the auspices of one of the country's largest for-profit hospital chains. Humana had promised to provide the first one hundred implants at no charge to the patient; after the initial phase, that service would presumably carry a price tag for patient and insurers.

Thus, the estimate of a $2.5 to $5 billion annual cost must give pause. Who would pay this bill? How would it affect the costs of medical care generally? The availability of the technology? Other forms of health care? These questions are difficult to answer in the absence of facts about the use of the technology and its desirability to patients; and in a vacuum of information about the political, financial, and scientific interests that the technology might arouse. Yet even a preliminary effort at cost-benefit assessment leads to troubling conclusions.

The Working Group noted that the introduction of mechanical circulatory support devices will not replace any treatment for end-stage cardiac disease that is equally effective and more expensive. Thus, no savings can be expected. Indeed, at present, patients with this condition who might be candidates for cardiac replacement die after relatively short and relatively inexpensive courses of treatment (average life expectancy of several months at a cost of about $22,000). The advent of the artificial heart will, then, add approximately $130,000 to the costs of caring for a patient of this sort.

The Working Group also noted that there are less expensive and more effective means of reducing the incidence of cardiovascular morbidity and mortality. Cigarette smoking provides an example. A smoker's decision to stop smoking, or a youth's decision not to start, is likely to have an impact on that person's prospects for dying of cardiovascular disease many times greater than the ultimate availability of the artificial heart.

To the extent that individuals can be helped to combat their tobacco addiction, the incidence of cardiovascular disease, the need for the artificial heart, and the total cost of cardiovascular disease should all decrease. The case could be made that priority be given to antismoking education and treatment for tobacco addiction.

However, should the technology be perfected, it will undoubtedly save lives. It will rescue individuals from imminent death and give them several years more of life. This prospect is, it seems, more desirable to our society than the economy of allowing the rapid and less expensive demise of these patients under present treatment and more compelling than the saving of statistical lives by prevention. Indeed, this lifesaving function of the artificial heart is precisely what poses the threat to the health of the population.

The threat appears first in the likelihood that public expenditures will be drawn to this technology rather than toward preventive measures that would have, overall, a more beneficial effect on health. Moreover, the possibility exists that a cry will be raised for federal subsidy of clinical implantation of artificial hearts. The sight of individuals doomed to die because they cannot afford an existing lifesaving treatment stimulates the demand for equality: in the face of death, the allocation of a life-saving technology on the basis of an individual's ability to pay seems blatantly discriminatory.

Just as the advent of renal dialysis and transplant thrust Medicare into the significant expenses of the End-Stage Renal Disease Program, so the advent of cardiac replacement will create pressure to finance some portion of the cost of the artificial heart. If this happens, the added burden on publicly financed health care will force certain budgetary reallocations. These are likely to affect less visible, less "urgent" expenses such as those for health education, screening, prevention, community clinics, hospital stay, and so forth. Relatively small restrictions in already underfunded programs may have larger effects on access to care and on the health of the population. In this way, the advent of a new rescue technology can threaten the health of many who depend on public support for their health care. And these are not, it must be noted, only the "underprivileged," but many made poor by age or by heavy medical expenses due to catastrophic illness.

These reflections led the Working Group to a cool and somewhat ambiguous endorsement of a program that is otherwise praiseworthy for its proficiency:

Given the available information, quantitative conclusions cannot be drawn regarding the cost-effectiveness of the artificial heart or its impact on the quality of care in the United States. Such conclusions would require a more formal analysis of other activities that might be more efficient and an exploration of mechanisms for allocating resources according to their efficiency. The Working Group suspects that such an exercise would reveal the existence of more efficient activities and would indicate that a reallocation of health resources, involving not only the artificial heart, could improve the health of our population. Even so, the probability that the artificial heart will be a useful tool for managing terminal cardiovascular disease in patients who have not been helped by other preventive or treatment approaches is judged to be high enough to warrant proceeding with its development ("The Artificial Heart and Assist Devices: Directions, Needs, Costs, Society and Ethical Issues," The Working Group on Mechanical Circulatory Support of the NHLBI, p. 31).

CONTROLLING TECHNOLOGY

This endorsement of the NHLBI program, cool though it was, astonished some observers. Dr. Lawrence Altman wrote,

[This is] probably the single most expensive medical procedure available. . . . Yet, in a report yesterday that could redirect national priorities on one of the boldest experiments in medical history, the Working Group called for a greatly expanded Federal research effort to develop a fully implantable, permanent heart (*New York Times*, May 24, 1985).

However, the Working Group did not endorse "a greatly expanded effort"; it recommended only that the present effort continue. The Working Group did not promote only the "fully implantable, permanent heart," but suggested that a broad program of research on mechanical circulatory support "include the fully implantable, long term total heart." Still, Dr. Altman's wonderment at the positive report is understandable.

Let me explain my agreement with my colleagues in endorsing the NHLBI program. First, the Working Group was convened only to review the NHLBI research program, not the concept of the artificial heart in general. This may seem a specious distinction. However, it is inevitable that the artificial heart in all its forms will be the continued object of commercial interest. The NHLBI research program is a careful, measured one: present schedules call for the first clinical investigations of the left ventricular device in 1988 and the first implantation in a patient of a total heart in 1991. Meanwhile, the many problems that these devices still pose (and which recent clinical experiences have dramatically manifested) will be intensively studied. Electrical and thermodynamic power sources to replace the clumsy pneumatic systems now used will be perfected.

Since commercial development will certainly persist, it seemed important to maintain the paced federal research program as a check on the impetus of private developers. Private developers are inevitably moved by market considerations; the federal program is relatively free of such forces. The federal program can provide performance standards at each phase of development. In the absence of such a control and check, the artificial heart may move (as some think it already has) too rapidly into wide clinical use.

Second, the NHLBI program encompasses all the forms of mechanical circulatory support. In fact, it emphasizes the partial and temporary assist devices rather than the total and permanent ones. Unfortunately, public attention has focused on the more dramatic total, permanent device. It is entirely possible that the partial, temporary ones will be more useful in clinical care. The recent uses of a total heart as a bridge to transplant (which had been tried unsuccessfully several times before) demonstrate a possible utility of the devices that might overshadow the permanent use (although temporary use poses its own problems—see George Annas, "No Cheers for Temporary Artificial Hearts," *Hastings Center Report*, October 1985, pp. 27–28).

Finally, a call to cease and desist from any technological development prior to significant demonstrations of its inefficacy, inefficiency, or danger seems bound to fail in our society. The technological imperative, particularly when linked to marketability, is powerful. We have, in fact, almost no effective means to bring such developments to a halt. FDA controls on development are limited and specific.

Abolition of federal support does not impede private development; refusal to reimburse clinical costs for the needy does not stop the wealthy from purchasing. Foreign developments, as in Japan, will lure patients abroad or spur imports into the American market. It seems necessary that a new device or procedure show itself to be unacceptable before the society will reject it. Thus, a measured and publicly controlled effort to develop and test a new technology as it evolves seems more desirable than a probably vain call for a halt.

The threat is not, I think, so menacing as to stop this and other technological developments—even if they were stoppable—but it is sufficiently real to give pause, to consider how the imperative issued by the President's Commission in its report, *Securing Access to Health Care*, can be realized:

"Society has an ethical obligation to ensure equitable access to an adequate level of health care without the imposition of excessive burdens."

TECHNOLOGIES AND ARRANGEMENTS
IN REPRODUCTION

American Fertility Society, Ethics Committee. "Ethical Statement on In Vitro Fertilization." *Fertility and Sterility* 41 (January 1984), 12.

Andrews, Lori B. *New Conceptions: A Consumer's Guide to the Newest Infertility Treatments Including In Vitro Fertilization, Artificial Insemination, and Surrogate Motherhood*. New York: St. Martin's Press, 1986.

Annas, George J. "The Baby Broker Boom." *Hastings Center Report* 16 (June 1986), 30–31.

Australia, Victoria. *Infertility (Medical Procedures) Act*, No. 10163, 1983.

Bayles, Michael D. *Reproductive Ethics*. Englewood Cliffs, N.J.: Prentice-Hall, 1984.

Brahams, Diana. "Surrogacy, Adoption and Custody." *Lancet* 1 (April 4, 1987), 817.

Cahill, Lisa Sowle. "On the Connection of Sex to Reproduction." In Shelp, Earl, ed. *Sexuality and Medicine. Vol. II: Ethical Viewpoints in Transition*. Boston: D. Reidel, 1987, pp. 39–50.

Cohen, Barbara. "Surrogate Mothers: Whose Baby Is It?" *American Journal of Law and Medicine* 10 (Fall 1984), 243–285.

Elias, Sherman, and Annas, George J. "Social Policy Considerations in Noncoital Reproduction." *Journal of the American Medical Association* 255 (January 1986), 62–68.

Milunsky, Aubrey, and Annas, George J., eds. *Genetics and the Law III*. New York: Plenum Press, 1985.

New Jersey Superior Court, Chancery Division, Family Part, Bergen County. "In the Matter of Baby 'M,' a pseudonym for an actual person." *Atlantic Reporter*, 2d series, March 31, 1987. 525: 1128–1176.

Ontario Law Reform Commission. *Report on Human Artificial Reproduction and Related Matters*. 2 vols. Toronto, Ontario: Ministry of the Attorney General, 1985.

Robertson, John A. "Embryos, Families, and Procreative Liberty: The Legal Structure of the New Reproduction." *Southern California Law Review* 59 (July 1986), 939–1041.

Singer, Peter, and Wells, Deane. *Making Babies: The New Science and Ethics of Conception*. New York: Scribner, 1985.

Uniacke, Suzanne. "In Vitro Fertilization and the Right to Reproduce." *Bioethics* 1 (July 1987), 241–254.

U.S. Congress, Office of Technology Assessment. *Infertility: Medical and Social Choices*. Washington, D.C.: OTA [OTA-BA-358], May 1988.

U.S. Department of Health, Education and Welfare, Ethics Advisory Board. *HEW Support of Research Involving Human In Vitro Fertilization and Embryo Transfer*. Washington, D.C.: U.S. Government Printing Office, 1979.

Walters, LeRoy. "Ethical Issues in Human (In Vitro) Fertilization and Embryo Transfer." In Milunsky, Aubrey, and Annas, George J., eds. *Genetics and the Law III*. New York: Plenum Press, 1985, pp. 215–225.

———. "Ethics and New Reproductive Technologies: An International Review of Committee Statements." *Hastings Center Report* 17 (June 1987), S3–S9.

Australia, National Health and Research Council, Medical Research Ethics Committee. *Ethical Aspects of Research on Human Gene Therapy*. Canberra: Australian Government Printing Office, 1987.

"Biotechnology and the Law: Recombinant DNA and the Control of Scientific Research." *Southern California Law Review* 51 (September 1978), 969–1573. Special issue.

Boone, C. Keith. "Splicing Life, with Scalpel and Scythe." *Hastings Center Report* 13 (April 1983), 8–10.

Culliton, Barbara. "Gene Therapy: Research in Public." *Science* 227 (February 1985), 493–496.

Fletcher, John C. "Ethical Issues in and Beyond Prospective Clinical Trials of Human Gene Therapy." *Journal of Medicine and Philosophy* 10 (August 1985), 293–309.

Grobstein, Clifford. *A Double Image of the Double Helix: The Recombinant-DNA Debate*. San Francisco: W. H. Freeman, 1979.

———. "Human Gene Therapy: Proceed with Caution." *Hastings Center Report* 14 (April 1984), 13–17.

Institute of Medicine. National Academy of Sciences and Eve K. Nichols. *Human Gene Therapy*. Cambridge, Mass.: Harvard University Press, 1988.

Jackson, David A., and Stich, Stephen P., eds. *The Recombinant DNA Debate*. Englewood Cliffs, N.J.: Prentice-Hall, 1979.

Lappé, Marc, and Morison, Robert S., eds. "Ethical and Scientific Issues Posed by Human Uses of Molecular Genetics." *Annals of the New York Academy of Sciences* 265 (1976), 1–208.

Moreno, Jonathan D. "Private Genes and Public Ethics." *Hastings Center Report* 13 (October 1983), 5–6.

President's Commission for the Study of Ethical Problems in Medicine and Biomedical and Behavioral Research. *Splicing Life: A Report on the Social and Ethical Issues of Genetic Engineering with Human Beings*. Washington, D.C.: The Commission, 1982.

"Recombinant DNA and Technology Assessment." *Georgia Law Review* 11 (Summer 1977), 785–878. Special issue.

Research with Recombinant DNA: An Academy Forum, March 7–9, 1977. Washington, D.C.: National Academy of Sciences, 1977.

Richards, John, ed. *Recombinant DNA: Science, Ethics, and Politics*. New York: Academic Press, 1978.

Rose, Steven. "DNA in Medicine: Human Perfectability." *Lancet* 2 (December 1984), 1380–1383.

U.S. Congress, Office of Technology Assessment. *Human Gene Therapy: Background Paper*. Washington, D.C.: OTA, 1984.

———. *Mapping Our Genes*. Washington, D.C.: OTA, 1988.

U.S. National Institutes of Health, Recombinant DNA Advisory Committee, Human Gene Therapy Subcommittee. "Points to Consider in the Design and Submission of Human Somatic-Cell Therapy Protocols." *Recombinant DNA Technical Bulletin* 9 (December 1986), 221–242.

U.S. National Institutes of Health. *Recombinant DNA Research: Documents Relating to "NIH Guidelines for Research Involving Recombinant DNA Molecules."* Multiple volumes. Washington, D.C.: U.S. Government Printing Office, August 1976–

Williamson, Bob. "Gene Therapy." *Nature* 298 (July 1982), 416–418.

GENETIC TECHNOLOGIES

Anderson, W. French. "Prospects for Human Gene Therapy." *Science* 226 (October 1984), 401–409.

TRANSPLANTATION TECHNOLOGIES

American Medical Association, Council on Scientific Affairs, Division of Evaluation and Nomenclature. "Xenografts: Review of the Literature and Current Status." *Journal of the American Medical Association* 254 (December 1985), 3353–3357.

Annas, George J. "Baby Fae: The 'Anything Goes' School of Human Experimentation." *Hastings Center Report* 15 (February 1985), 15–17.

———. "No Cheers for Temporary Artificial Hearts." *Hastings Center Report* 15 (October 1985), 27–28.

Bailey, Leonard L., Nehlsen-Cannarella, Sandra L., Concepcion, Waldo, and Jolley, Weldon B. "Baboon-to-Human Cardiac Xenotransplantation in a Neonate." *Journal of the American Medical Association* 254 (December 1985), 3321–3329.

Caplan, Arthur L. "Should Fetuses Be Used as Organ Donors?" *Bioethics* 1 (April 1987), 119–140.

Capron, Alexander M.; Regan, Tom; Reemtsma, Keith; Sheldon, Richard; McCormick, Richard A., and Gore, Albert. "The Subject Is Baby Fae [six commentaries]." *Hastings Center Report* 15 (February 1985), 8–13.

Cole, Helene M. "Four Years of Replacing Ailing Hearts: Surgeons Assess Data, Questions Remain." *Journal of the American Medical Association* 256 (December 1985), 2921–2930.

Dommell, F. William, et al. "The NIH Report of Its Review of the Baby Fae Case." *IRB: A Review of Human Subjects Research* 8 (March/April 1986), 1–4.

Frey, R. G. "Animal Parts, Human Wholes: On the Use of Animals as a Source of Organs for Human Transplants." In Humber, James M., and Almeder, Robert F., eds. *Biomedical Ethics Reviews: 1987.* Clifton, N.J.: Humana Press, 1987, pp. 89–107.

Gorovitz, Samuel. "The Artificial Heart: Questions to Ask and Not to Ask." *Hastings Center Report* 14 (October 1984), 15–17.

Green, Harold P. "An NIH Panel's Early Warnings." *Hastings Center Report* 14 (October 1984), 13–15.

Harrison, Michael R. "Organ Procurement for Children: The Anencephalic Fetus as Donor." *Lancet* 2 (December 1986), 1383–1386.

Harrison, Michael R., and Meilander, Gilbert. "The Anencephalic Newborn as Organ Donor." *Hastings Center Report* 16 (April 1986), 21–23.

Kushner, Thomasine Kimbrough, and Belliotti, Raymond. "Baby Fae: A Beastly Business." *Journal of Medical Ethics* 11 (December 1985), 178–183.

Lubeck, Deborah P., and Bunker, John P. [Office of Technology Assessment] *The Implications of Cost-Effectiveness Analysis of Medical Technology. Case Study #9: The Artificial Heart: Costs, Risks and Benefits.* Washington, D.C.: U.S. Government Printing Office, May 1982.

Robertson, John A. "Supply and Distribution of Hearts for Transplantation: Legal, Ethical, and Policy Issues." *Circulation* 75 (January 1987), 77–87.

Swazey, Judith P., Watkins, Judith C., and Fox, Renee. "Assessing the Artificial Heart: The Clinical Moratorium Revisited." *International Journal of Technology Assessment in Health Care* 2 (July 1986), 387–410.

U.S. Department of Health and Human Services, Task Force on Organ Transplantation. *Report of the Task Force on Organ Transplantation: Issues and Recommendations.* Washington, D.C.: DHHS, 1986.

BIBLIOGRAPHIES

Goldstein, Doris Mueller. *Bioethics: A Guide to Information Sources.* Detroit: Gale Research Company, 1982. See under "Artificial and Transplanted Organs and Tissues," "Genetic Intervention," and "Reproductive Technologies."

Lineback, Richard H., ed. *Philosopher's Index.* Vols. 1– . Bowling Green, Ohio: Bowling Green State University. Issued quarterly. See under "Genetic Engineering," "In Vitro Fertilization," "Organ Transplants," "Surrogates," "Surrogate Motherhood," and "Transplantation."

Walters, LeRoy, and Kahn, Tamar Joy, eds. *Bibliography of Bioethics.* Vols. 1– . Washington, D.C.: Kennedy Institute of Ethics, Georgetown University. Issued annually. See under "Gene Therapy," "Host Mothers," "In Vitro Fertilization," "Organ Transplantation," and "Reproductive Technologies." (The information contained in the annual *Bibliography of Bioethics* can also be retrieved from BIOETHICSLINE, an online database of the National Library of Medicine.)

11.
The Allocation of Medical Resources

As medicine has expanded its services, the quantity of scarce resources has increased rather than diminished. This scarcity includes expensive equipment, medicine, specialized practitioners, artificial organs, blood for the treatment of hemophilia, donors for organ transplant operations, and research facilities. The basic *economic problem* is how these scarce resources can be efficiently allocated in order to satisfy human needs and desires. The basic *ethical problem* is how these resources can be fairly collected and allocated through schemes of production, contribution, and distribution. These two problems are often intertwined in the formation of public policy, which sometimes disguises the fact that there is both an economic dimension and an ethical dimension to decisions about production and allocation.

These decisions occur at two levels, macroallocation and microallocation. In macroallocation, decisions are made about how much will be expended for medical resources in society, as well as how it will be distributed. These decisions are taken by Congress, state legislatures, health organizations, private foundations, and health insurance companies. At the microallocation level, decisions are taken by particular institutions or health professionals concerning who shall obtain available resources. The problem of macroallocation is emphasized in this chapter, together with related considerations about the right to health care. Discussion of both these topics has recently seen a rise in the language of *rationing* scarce health care resources, a term that suggests financially stringent and possibly emergency circumstances that require social decisions to include some citizens while excluding others. However, some authors in this chapter consider this an unjust approach to the distribution of health care.

Several well-reasoned and systematic answers to these problems have been advanced, all of which are based on an underlying theory of how, consistent with justice, health care goods and services should be distributed. In Chapter 1 we examined general theories of justice and became familiar with the existence of several rival theories (see pages 32–34). The various problems of distribution featured in the present chapter build on this background. The first four articles attempt to answer the question, "Which general system of social and economic organization is most just for the distribution of health care?" The final three articles concern the justification of particular problems in allocation.

Because there is neither a social consensus nor a paramount theory of justice at the present time, it is to be expected that public policies will oscillate, now seizing the premises of one theory, later emphasizing another theory. Such a shift of vision is common in public policy and does not necessarily mean that policies are unjust. But what makes a policy just or unjust?

THE PROBLEM OF MACROALLOCATION

Macroallocation decisions have assumed an increasing significance as federal funds, state funds, and foundation grants have increased in support of ongoing medical research and specialized treatment. Two primary considerations are involved in macroallocation decisions about health care and research: (1) What percentage of the total available resources should be allotted to biomedical research and clinical practice, as they compete for funding with other social projects such as defense, education, transportation, and the like? (2) How much of the amount allotted to biomedicine should go to which specific projects—for example, how much to cancer research, how much to preventive medicine, and how much to the production of expensive machines used in treatment facilities?

An example of the second problem that plays a role in the readings in this chapter is whether allocation for *preventive* medicine should take priority over allocation for *crisis* medicine. From one perspective, the prevention of disease by the alteration of unsanitary environments, by screening programs, and by the provision of health information is cheaper and more efficient in raising health levels and saving lives than is crisis medicine (in the form of kidney dialysis, heart transplantation, intensive care units, and so on). But from another perspective, a concentrated preventive approach is morally unsatisfactory if it leads to the neglect of needy persons who could directly benefit from the resources of crisis medicine—even if the preventive approach is more efficient in the long run in preventing disease and maintaining health.

These problems of macroallocation will be handled differently by competing systems of distribution, and thus we need to decide which are the fairest. Here practical considerations such as whether the poor should receive more medical resources than they now do, whether more hospitals should be located in rural regions, and whether all citizens should have an equal amount of money expended on them each year become practical problems guided by a conception of distributive justice, a topic that was explored in Chapter 1.

REDISTRIBUTING THROUGH DISTRIBUTIVE JUSTICE

One major problem concerning distributive justice and the distribution of health care is whether health care should be distributed at all. Robert Nozick has raised the following profoundly important question about our conception of justice:

The term "distributive justice" is not a neutral one. Hearing the term "distribution," most people presume that some thing or mechanism uses some principle or criterion to give out a supply of things. Into this process of distributing shares some error may have crept. So it is an open question, at least, whether *re*distribution should take place; whether we should do again what has already been done once.[1]

In Chapter 1 we examined the libertarian theory of justice, of which Nozick is a spokesperson. According to this theory, all parties to a contractual social arrangement should be able to freely enter and withdraw from economic arrangements in accordance with their beliefs about their best interests. Libertarian or free-market theorists explicitly reject the conclusion that egalitarian, utilitarian, or socialist patterns of distribution represent a normative ideal for distributing health care. People may be equal in a host of morally significant respects (for example, entitled to equal treatment under the law and equally valued as ends in themselves), but the libertarian contends that it would be a basic violation of *justice* to regard people as deserving of collected and redistributed economic returns such as those involved in funding health care goods and services.

Justice, in this theory, is confined to free and fair exchanges in the marketplace. It has nothing to do with redistribution. Obviously a libertarian prefers a system in which health care insurance is privately and voluntarily purchased by individual initiative, because in this system no one has had his or her property coercively extracted by the state in order to benefit someone else. Because no moral grounds would justify the sacrifice of liberty rights, the libertarian views utilitarianism and egalitarianism as perverted theories of justice that use one set of individuals as means to the end of benefiting another set of individuals.

This form of libertarian theory is defended in this chapter in the article by H. Tristram Engelhardt, Jr., who relies heavily on the principle of respect for autonomy rather than on the development of an independent substantive principle of justice. Engelhardt argues that a theory of justice should work to protect our rights not to be coerced. It should not propound a thesis intended to regulate society through arrangements such as those found in countries in which governments take pronounced steps to redistribute the wealth acquired by individuals acting in accordance with free-market laws. In this theory, use of the tax code to effect social goals such as the alleviation of poverty, saving lives with advanced medical technologies, and the support of the arts are forms of social engineering based on what a majority prefers rather than on what justice demands. Some disadvantages created by ill health, Engelhardt argues, should be viewed as merely *unfortunate*, whereas others (those caused by another person) will be viewed as *unfair*. From this perspective, one will call a halt to the demands of justice where one draws the distinction between the unfair (and therefore obligatory injustice to correct) and the merely unfortunate.

Although the underlying assumptions of libertarianism correspond closely to economic presuppositions in free-market societies, many philosophers, politicians, and health policy experts maintain that, however great the differences between particular people's contributions initially appear to be, all individual contributions shrink to insignificance once the broader context of social production is appreciated. They hold that (1) the alleged contribution that anyone makes simply reflects a diversity of formative influences, including family background, education, and interaction with professional associates, and (2) economic value is generated through an essentially communal process that renders differences between individual contributions morally negligible.

In Chapter 1 we noted that John Rawls's *A Theory of Justice* has been a particularly influential work on social justice. Rawls's central contention is that a social arrangement is a communal effort to advance the good of all who are part of the society. One of Rawls's critical principles rests on the moral viewpoint that because inequalities of birth, historical circumstance, and natural endowment are undeserved, persons in a cooperative society should correct them by making the unequal situation of naturally disadvantaged members more equal. Those who are more fortunate in their social position or naturally endowed with more advantageous properties do not *deserve* those advantaging properties, and hence a just society would seek to nullify the advantages stemming from the accidents of history and biology. As Rawls puts it, these fortuitous advantaging properties seem arbitrary from the moral point of view.

Rawls takes this fair opportunity principle and turns it into a principle of redress: In order to overcome handicapping conditions (whether they arise from biology or society) which are not deserved, his principle compensates those with the handicaps. The goal is to redress the unequal distributions created by undeserved advantage in the direction of greater equality. Evening out handicaps in this way is, Rawls claims, a fundamental part of our shared conception of justice.

Rawls's work on the theory of justice underlies the two rather different approaches advanced in this chapter by Robert Veatch. He accepts and then modifies the general

Rawlsian framework. Veatch begins with the Rawlsian model of justice and proposes two separate applications of egalitarian theory to health care. First, he proposes the "maximin" position, in which those individuals who are worst off in a society (at the minimum level) are guaranteed access to a certain level of medical care and services. In this way, the society maximizes the minimum, increasing the lot of the least fortunate by increasing the minimum level of health care. Veatch draws on egalitarianism to support a theory of health care distribution in which everyone ought to have a chance for the amount of net welfare equal to that available to everyone else in a society.

One need not be a follower of Rawls, of course, to believe in a social system for the distribution of health care resources. Utilitarians, for example, take the view that there is a general moral requirement to perform acts that avoid undesirable consequences. This requirement is not so strong as to require us to constantly produce good consequences, but it does assert that we have an obligation to assist others by preventing evils that might occur to them, such as sickness and threats to health, and we are morally blameworthy if we do nothing at all.

Utilitarians argue that justice is not a principle independent of the principle of utility. Rather, justice is the name for the most paramount and stringent forms of social obligation created by the principle of utility. Justice involves the recognition that each person has an equal claim to happiness and that society must give equal protection to the rights of every individual. In the distribution of health care, utilitarians commonly see justice as involving trade-offs and partial allocations that strike a balance. In devising a system of public funding for health care, we thus must balance public and private benefit, predicted cost savings, the probability of failure, the magnitude of risks, and so on. Many contemporary discussions of just benefits in prepaid health maintenance programs, the justice of programs of care for the mentally retarded, and the burden of payment for national health insurance inescapably involve such trade-offs from a utilitarian perspective.

No author in this chapter is explicitly a defender of the utilitarian system of justice. However, the article by the President's Commission for the Study of Ethical Problems shows a noticeable resemblance to the utilitarian approach. As the commission sees the problem, society has an obligation to ensure equitable access to health care for all, an obligation that rests in the special importance of relieving suffering, preventing premature death, and the like. It sees the act of ensuring equal access as the responsibility of the "collective American community," and it argues that fashioning a system for the distribution of health care involves a balancing of social responsibility, individual responsibility, and social resources. The commission opts for a two-tiered system of health care in which those who wish to purchase more than is provided by the social scheme of insurance are free to do so at their own expense.

THE RIGHT TO HEALTH CARE

One of the more intense debates about distributive justice in recent years has focused on whether nations should have a health policy that confers rights to health care. Under this conception, allocations for health care are not based exclusively on charity, compassion, and benevolence but rather on rights grounded in justice. In this context a "right" is understood as an *entitlement* to some measure of health care, and not simply as a *benefit*. This usage follows traditions in political philosophy, where rights have been understood as entitlements a person possesses to some good, service, or liberty. As entitlements, rights are to be contrasted with mere privileges, ideals, and acts of charity. Rights to Medicaid or to Medicare, for example, are analogous to rights to receive an insurance benefit when required premiums have been paid: Anyone eligible is entitled to receive all services and goods established by the rules of the program.

As noted in Chapter 1, *legal* rights are entitlements supportable by moral systems of rules. In many nations there is a firmly established legal right to health care goods and services for all citizens. The prevailing legal view in the United States, however, seems to be that even if there are solid moral reasons for, and no constitutional constraints against, enactment of a right to health care, there is no *constitutional* right to health care. However, there is also no constitutional obstacle to Congress's providing some types of health care to citizens. Whether there is or ought to be a *moral* right to health care is a more open question and one openly debated in this chapter.

The idea of a right to health care is a relatively recent phenomenon. In 1965 Medicare was passed into law in the United States to provide coverage for health care costs in populations that could not afford adequate coverage, especially the elderly, and it has generally been successful in meeting this goal. Medicare conferred a right to health care on these populations and thereby stimulated discussion as to whether all citizens have, or at least should have, such a right. Recently the discussion has often focused on catastrophic coverage for all citizens, because expenses for those with chronic diseases or those in need of long-term care can still exceed Medicare's provisions (if they are covered at all) and even wipe out a family's assets.

Until Medicare, the United States had largely operated on the libertarian principle that distributions of health care services and goods are best left to charity or to the marketplace, which operates on the material principle of ability to pay. The implications of more egalitarian and utilitarian approaches taken for national health care are far reaching: Each member of society, irrespective of wealth or position, would be provided with some level of health care to which he or she would have a right.

According to the now widely discussed "decent minimum" proposal, which is carefully examined in this chapter by Allen Buchanan, each person has equal access to an adequate (though not maximal) level of health care for all available types of services. The distribution would proceed on the basis of need, and needs would be met by equal access to services. Better services, such as luxury hospital rooms and expensive but optional dental work, might be made available for purchase at personal expense by those who are able to and wish to do so. Yet everyone's health needs would be met at the level of a decent minimum. The President's Commission argues that we have no *right* to this decent minimum of care but that there is a social obligation to provide it. Engelhardt concludes that there is no right and no social obligation, although a society may freely choose to enact such a policy. Buchanan believes there are good theoretical arguments to show that there is both an obligation and a right. Uwe Reinhardt concludes that every citizen, not merely the indigent, should be covered by a national, decent minimum policy.

Others, notably Veatch, hold out for a different conclusion and refuse to use rights and obligations in this way. In Veatch's system there is a right stronger than the right to a decent minimum. He proposes the distribution of health care based on the individual's health care needs, by using the yardstick of an "equal right to health care." The result is that "people have a right to needed health care to provide an opportunity for a level of health equal as far as possible to the health of other people." This application of the principle of justice to health care would result in a health care delivery system with only one class of services available, rather than a two-tiered system. There could not be two tracks—one for the wealthy, one at the minimal level—brought about by unequal social and economic classes competing in the free market.

The decent minimum proposal and Veatch's more demanding theory raise problems of whether one can consistently, fairly, and unambiguously structure a public policy that recognizes a right to exotic and expensive forms of treatment. The problem of justifying such expenses is prominent in each of the final three essays in this chapter, which explore the relationship between economic analysis and distributive justice in an era of both great need and fiscal constraint. The most difficult questions concern which technologies or procedures should be funded. For example, treatment for heart disease would presumably be supported, but would cardiac transplantation be supported as part of the program?

More generally, discussion of the decent minimum carries with it many problems of macroallocation. Two generic issues concern (1) how to establish priorities in the allocation of resources for society at large and within health care and (2) how to understand and design our basic health care institutions. Various approaches to these issues produce different programs for the forms of health care services that will be maintained in society, who will have access to them, who may and should deliver those services, and how the services will be funded and distributed. Each author in this chapter has a vision of how to handle these macro questions. It is not hard to see that each vision, except for the libertarian vision, makes a commitment to the content and scope of the right to health care by further specifying what the program requires in the way of an allocation of resources.

JUST PROCEDURES AND JUST RESULTS

In the literature on distributive justice and health care there also exists an important distinction between just procedures and just results. The term "distribution" may refer to the *procedure used to distribute*, or it may refer to the *result of some system of distribution*. Ideally it is preferable to have just procedures and just results, but it is not always possible to have both. For example, one might achieve a just result in macroallocation by meeting everyone's health care needs, but one might use an unjust procedure, such as undeserved taxation of certain groups in order to achieve it. By contrast, just procedures sometimes eventuate in unjust results, as when a just procedure such as a fair trial reaches unjust results when the innocent are found guilty. In discussions of justice the system itself is often in question, even though those who are criticizing the system may be pointing to unjust results of the system. It is therefore important to be clear on whether the procedures, the results, or both are under consideration.

Many problems of justice and the distribution of health care that we must handle as a cooperative society involve designing a system or set of procedures that provides as much justice as possible. Once we agree on appropriate procedures, then as long as a person is treated according to those procedures, the outcome must be declared just. This is one of the major premises in the theory of justice supported by Engelhardt in this chapter. For example, if we determine that the best procedure in microallocation for heart transplant surgery is a lottery among the medically qualified, then it cannot be said to be unfair if (by chance) all persons selected are wealthy, single males. The result may seem biased and unfair, but the fair procedure makes it a fair outcome. Engelhardt sees decisions about access to intensive care units, as well as all other decisions about access to health care, in this light.

However, because unfortunate (but not necessarily unfair) outcomes are inevitable in purely procedural systems, shifting the issue from results to procedures—as is often done by taking votes in a majoritarian system—will not avoid all ethical controversy. The President's Commission lays strong emphasis on the use of democratic political procedures to make a choice among "just alternatives." But this conclusion requires that we have already delineated a range of just alternatives. Veatch's provocative arguments indicate how difficult this will be and why the controversy will persist. Moreover, the various traditional theories of ethics will likely provide competing theories of criteria of just procedures as well as of just outcomes. Thus, procedural justice may help us with some problems of distributing health care, but it will not resolve them all. No matter how strongly we believe in democracy, consensus, and negotiation, they do not seem capable of handling all questions about the justice of a system of health care distribution.

T. L. B.

NOTES

1. Robert Nozick, *Anarchy, State, and Utopia* (New York: Basic Books, 1974), pp. 149–50.

Just Health Care and the Right to Health Care

PRESIDENT'S COMMISSION FOR THE STUDY OF ETHICAL PROBLEMS IN MEDICINE AND BIOMEDICAL AND BEHAVIORAL RESEARCH

Securing Access to Health Care

. . . The President's Commission was mandated to study the ethical and legal implications of differences in the availability of health services. In this Report to the President and Congress, the Commission sets forth an ethical standard: access for all to an adequate level of care without the imposition of excessive burdens. It believes that this is the standard against which proposals for legislation and regulation in this field ought to be measured. . . .

In both their means and their particular objectives, public programs in health care have varied over the

From *Securing Access to Health Care*, Vol. I. Washington, D.C.: U.S. Government Printing Office, 1983.

years. Some have been aimed at assuring the productivity of the work force, others at protecting particularly vulnerable or deserving groups, still others at manifesting the country's commitment to equality of opportunity. Nonetheless, most programs have rested on a common rationale: to ensure that care be made accessible to a group whose health needs would otherwise not be adequately met.

The consequence of leaving health care solely to market forces—the mechanism by which most things are allocated in American society—is not viewed as acceptable when a significant portion of the population lacks access to health services. Of course, government financing programs, such as Medicare and Medicaid as well as public programs that provide care directly to veterans and the military and through local public hospitals, have greatly improved access to health care. These efforts, coupled with the expanded availability of private health insurance, have resulted in almost 90% of Americans having some form of health insurance coverage. Yet the patchwork of government programs and the uneven availability of private health insurance through the workplace have excluded millions of people. The Surgeon General has stated that "with rising unemployment, the numbers are shifting rapidly. We estimate that from 18 to 25 million Americans—8 to 11 percent of the population—have no health-insurance coverage at all." Many of these people lack effective access to health care, and many more who have some form of insurance are unprotected from the severe financial burdens of sickness. . . .

[W]hile people have some ability—through choice of life-style and through preventive measures—to influence their health status, many health problems are beyond their control and are therefore undeserved. Besides the burdens of genetics, environment, and chance, individuals become ill because of things they do or fail to do—but it is often difficult for an individual to choose to do otherwise or even to know with enough specificity and confidence what he or she ought to do to remain healthy. Finally, the incidence and severity of ill health is distributed very unevenly among people. Basic needs for housing and food are predictable, but even the most hardworking and prudent person may suddenly be faced with overwhelming needs for health care. Together, these considerations lend weight to the belief that health care is different from most other goods and services. In a society concerned not only with fairness and equality of opportunity but also with the redemptive powers of science, there is a felt obligation to ensure that some level of health services is available to all.

There are many ambiguities, however, about the nature of this societal obligation. What share of health costs should individuals be expected to bear, and what responsibility do they have to use health resources prudently? Is it society's responsibility to ensure that every person receives care or services of as high quality and as great extent as any other individual? Does it require that everyone share opportunities to receive all available care or care of any possible benefit? If not, what level of care is "enough"? And does society's obligation include a responsibility to ensure both that care is available and that its costs will not unduly burden the patient?

The resolution of such issues is made more difficult by the spectre of rising health care costs and expenditures. Americans annually spend over 270 million days in hospitals, make over 550 million visits to physicians' offices, and receive tens of millions of X-rays. Expenditures for health care in 1981 totaled $287 billion—an average of over $1225 for every American. Although the finitude of national resources demands that trade-offs be made between health care and other social goods, there is little agreement about which choices are most acceptable from an ethical standpoint. . . . The Commission attempts to lay an ethical foundation for evaluating both current patterns of access to health care and the policies designed to address remaining problems in the distribution of health care resources. . . .

THE CONCEPT OF EQUITABLE ACCESS TO HEALTH CARE

The special nature of health care helps to explain why it ought to be accessible, in a fair fashion, to all. But if this ethical conclusion is to provide a basis for evaluating current patterns of access to health care and proposed health policies, the meaning of fairness or equity in this context must be clarified. The concept of equitable access needs definition in its two main aspects: the level of care that ought to be available to all and the extent to which burdens can be imposed on those who obtain these services.

ACCESS TO WHAT?

"Equitable access" could be interpreted in a number of ways: equality of access, access to whatever an individual needs or would benefit from, or access to an adequate level of care.

Equity as Equality. It has been suggested that equity is achieved either when everyone is assured of receiving an equal quantity of health care dollars or when people enjoy equal health. The most common characterization of equity as equality, however, is as providing everyone with the same level of health care. In this view, it follows that if a given level of care is available to one individual it must be available to all. If the initial standard is set high, by reference to the highest level of care presently received, an enormous drain would result on the resources needed to provide other goods. Alternatively, if the standard is set low in order to avoid an excessive use of resources, some beneficial services would have to be withheld from people who wished to purchase them. In other words, no one would be allowed access to more services or services of higher quality than those available to everyone else, even if he or she were willing to pay for those services from his or her personal resources.

As long as significant inequalities in income and wealth persist, inequalities in the use of health care can be expected beyond those created by differences in need. Given people with the same pattern of preferences and equal health care needs, those with greater financial resources will purchase more health care. Conversely, given equal financial resources, the different patterns of health care preferences that typically exist in any population will result in a different use of health services by people with equal health care needs. Trying to prevent such inequalities would require interfering with people's liberty to use their income to purchase an important good like health care while leaving them free to use it for frivolous or inessential ends. Prohibiting people with higher incomes or stronger preferences for health care from purchasing more care than everyone else gets would not be feasible, and would probably result in a black market for health care.

Equity as Access Solely According to Benefit or Need. Interpreting equitable access to mean that everyone must receive all health care that is of any benefit to them also has unacceptable implications. Unless health is the only good or resources are unlimited, it would be irrational for a society—as for an individual—to make a commitment to provide whatever health care might be beneficial regardless of cost. Although health care is of special importance, it is surely not all that is important to people. . . .

"[N]eed" could be even more expansive in scope than "benefit." Philosophical and economic writings do not provide any clear distinction between "needs" and "wants" or "preferences." Since the term means different things to different people, "access according to need" could become "access to any health service a person wants." Conversely, need could be interpreted very narrowly to encompass only a very minimal level of services—for example, those "necessary to prevent death."

Equity as an Adequate Level of Health Care. Although neither "everything needed" nor "everything beneficial" nor "everything that anyone else is get-

ting" are defensible ways of understanding equitable access, the special nature of health care dictates that everyone have access to *some* level of health care: enough care to achieve sufficient welfare, opportunity, information, and evidence of interpersonal concern to facilitate a reasonably full and satisfying life. That level can be termed "an adequate level of health care." The difficulty of sharpening this amorphous notion into a workable foundation for health policy is a major problem in the United States today. This concept is not new; it is implicit in the public debate over health policy and has manifested itself in the history of public policy in this country. In this chapter, the Commission attempts to demonstrate the value of the concept, to clarify its content, and to apply it to the problems facing health policymakers.

Understanding equitable access to health care to mean that everyone should be able to secure an adequate level of care has several strengths. Because an adequate level of care may be less than "all beneficial care" and because it does not require that all needs be satisfied, it acknowledges the need for setting priorities within health care and signals a clear recognition that society's resources are limited and that there are other goods besides health. Thus, interpreting equity as access to adequate care does not generate an open-ended obligation. One of the chief dangers of interpretations of equity that require virtually unlimited resources for health care is that they encourage the view that equitable access is an impossible ideal. Defining equity as an adequate level of care for all avoids an impossible commitment of resources without falling into the opposite error of abandoning the enterprise of seeking to ensure that health care is in fact available for everyone.

In addition, since providing an adequate level of care is a limited moral requirement, this definition also avoids the unacceptable restriction on individual liberty entailed by the view that equity requires equality. Provided that an adequate level is available to all, those who prefer to use their resources to obtain care that exceeds that level do not offend any ethical principle in doing so. Finally, the concept of adequacy, as the Commission understands it, is society-relative. The content of adequate care will depend upon the overall resources available in a given society, and can take into account a consensus of expectations about what is adequate in a particular society at a particular time in its historical development. This permits the definition of adequacy to be altered as societal resources and expectations change.

It is not enough to focus on the care that individuals receive; attention must be paid to the burdens they must bear in order to obtain it—waiting and travel time, the cost and availability of transport, the financial cost of the care itself. Equity requires not only that adequate care be available to all, but also that these burdens not be excessive.

If individuals must travel unreasonably long distances, wait for unreasonably long hours, or spend most of their financial resources to obtain care, some will be deterred from obtaining adequate care, with adverse effects on their health and well-being. Others may bear the burdens, but only at the expense of their ability to meet other important needs. If one of the main reasons for providing adequate care is that health care increases welfare and opportunity, then a system that required large numbers of individuals to forego food, shelter, or educational advancement in order to obtain care would be self-defeating and irrational.

The concept of acceptable burdens in obtaining care, as opposed to excessive ones, parallels in some respects the concept of adequacy. Just as equity does not require equal access, neither must the burdens of obtaining adequate care be equal for all persons. What is crucial is that the variations in burdens fall within an acceptable range. As in determining an adequate level of care, there is no simple formula for ascertaining when the burdens of obtaining care fall within such a range. . . .

A SOCIETAL OBLIGATION

Society has a moral obligation to ensure that everyone has access to adequate care without being subject to excessive burdens. In speaking of a societal obligation the Commission makes reference to society in the broadest sense—the collective American community. The community is made up of individuals, who are in turn members of many other, overlapping groups, both public and private: local, state, regional, and national units; professional and workplace organizations; religious, educational, and charitable organizations; and family, kinship, and ethnic groups. All these entities play a role in discharging societal obligations.

The Commission believes it is important to distinguish between society, in this inclusive sense, and government as one institution among others in society. Thus the recognition of a collective or societal obligation does not imply that government should be the only or even the primary institution involved in the complex enterprise of making health care available. It is the Commission's view that the societal obligation to ensure equitable access for everyone may best be fulfilled in this country by a pluralistic approach that relies upon the coordinated contributions of actions by both the private and public sectors.

Securing equitable access is a societal rather than a merely private or individual responsibility for several reasons. First, while health is of special importance for human beings, health care—especially scientific health care—is a social product requiring the skills and efforts of many individuals; it is not something that individuals can provide for themselves solely through their own efforts. Second, because the need for health care is both unevenly distributed among persons and highly unpredictable and because the cost of securing care may be great, few individuals could secure adequate care without relying on some social mechanism for sharing the costs. Third, if persons generally deserved their health conditions or if the need for health care were fully within the individual's control, the fact that some lack adequate care would not be viewed as an inequity. But differences in health status, and hence differences in health care needs, are largely undeserved because they are, for the most part, not within the individual's control. . . .

WHO SHOULD ENSURE THAT SOCIETY'S OBLIGATION IS MET?

Although the Commission recognizes the necessity of government involvement in ensuring equity of access, it believes that such activity must be carefully crafted and implemented in order to achieve its intended purpose. Public concern about the inability of the market and of private charity to secure access to health care for all has led to extensive government involvement in the financing and delivery of health care. This involvement has come about largely as a result of ad hoc responses to specific problems; the result has been a patchwork of public initiatives at the local, state, and Federal level. These efforts have done much to make health care more widely available to all citizens, but . . . they have not achieved equity of access.

To a large extent, this is the result of a lack of consensus about the nature of the goal and the proper role of government in pursuing it. But to some degree, it may also be the product of the nature of government activity. In some instances, government programs (of all types, not just health-related) have not been designed well enough to achieve the purposes intended or have been subverted to serve purposes explicitly not intended.

In the case of health care, it is extremely difficult to devise public strategies that, on the one hand, do not encourage the misuse of health services and, on the other hand, are not so restrictive as to unnecessarily or arbitrarily limit available care. There is a growing concern, for example, that government assistance in the form of tax exemptions for the purchase of employment-related health insurance has led to the overuse of many services of only very marginal benefit. Similarly, government programs that pay for health care directly (such as Medicaid) have been subject to fraud and abuse by both beneficiaries and providers. . . .

A RIGHT TO HEALTH CARE?

Often the issue of equitable access to health care is framed in the language of rights. Some who view health care from the perspective of distributive justice argue that the considerations discussed in this [essay] show not only that society has a moral obligation to provide equitable access, but also that every individual has a moral right to such access. The Commission has chosen not to develop the case for achieving equitable access through the assertion of a right to health care. Instead it has sought to frame the issues in terms of the special nature of health care and of a society's moral obligation to achieve equity, without taking a position on whether the term "obligation" should be read as entailing a moral right. The Commission reaches this conclusion for several reasons: first, such a right is not legally or constitutionally recognized at the present time; second, it is not a logical corollary of an ethical obligation of the type the Commission has enunciated; and third, it is not necessary as a foundation for appropriate governmental actions to secure adequate health care for all.

Legal Rights. Neither the Supreme Court nor any appellate court has found a constitutional right to health or to health care. However, most Federal statutes and many state statutes that fund or regulate health care have been interpreted to provide statutory rights in the form of entitlements for the intended beneficiaries of the program or for members of the group protected by the regulatory authority. As a consequence, a host of legal decisions have developed significant legal protections for program beneficiaries. . . .

Moral Obligations and Rights. The relationship between the concept of a moral right and that of a moral obligation is complex. To say that a person has a moral right to something is always to say that it is that person's due, that is, he or she is morally entitled to it. In contrast, the term "obligation" is used in two different senses. All moral rights imply corresponding obligations, but, depending on the sense of the term that is being used, moral obligations may or may not imply corresponding rights. In the broad sense, to say that society has a moral obligation to do something is to say that it ought morally to do that thing and that failure to do it makes society liable to serious moral criticism. This does not, however, mean that there is a corresponding right. For example, a person may have a moral obligation to help those in need, even though the needy cannot, strictly speaking, demand that person's aid as something they are due.

The government's responsibility for seeing that the obligation to achieve equity is met is independent of the existence of a corresponding moral right to health care. There are many forms of government involvement, such as enforcement of traffic rules or taxation to support national defense, to protect the environment, or to promote biomedical research, that do not presuppose corresponding moral rights but that are nonetheless legitimate and almost universally recognized as such. In a democracy, at least, the people may assign to government the responsibility for seeing that important collective obligations are met, provided that doing so does not violate important moral rights.

As long as the debate over the ethical assessment of patterns of access to health care is carried on simply by the assertion and refutation of a "right to health care," the debate will be incapable of guiding policy. At the very least, the nature of the right must be made clear and competing accounts of it compared and evaluated. Moreover, if claims of rights are to guide policy they must be supported by sound ethical reasoning and the connections between various rights must be systematically developed, especially where rights are potentially in conflict with one another. At present, however, there is a great deal of dispute among competing theories of rights, with most theories being so abstract and inadequately developed that their implications for health care are not obvious. Rather than attempt to adjudicate among competing theories of rights, the Commission has chosen to concentrate on what it believes to be the more important part of the question: what is the nature of the societal obligation, which exists whether or not people can claim a corresponding right to health care, and how should this societal obligation be fulfilled?

MEETING THE SOCIETAL OBLIGATION

HOW MUCH CARE IS ENOUGH?

Before the concept of an adequate level of care can be used as a tool to evaluate patterns of access and efforts to improve equity, it must be fleshed out. Since there is no objective formula for doing this, reasonable people can disagree about whether particular patterns and policies meet the demands of adequacy. The Commission does not attempt to spell out in detail what adequate care should include. Rather it frames the terms in which those who discuss or critique health care issues can consider ethics as well as economics, medical science, and other dimensions.

Characteristics of Adequacy. First, the Commission considers it clear that health care can only be judged adequate in relation to an individual's health condition. To begin with a list of techniques or procedures, for example, is not sensible: A CT scan for an accident victim with a serious head injury might be the best way to make a diagnosis essential for the appropriate treatment of that patient; a CT scan for a person with headaches might not be considered essential for adequate care. To focus only on the technique, therefore, rather than on the individual's health and the impact the procedure will have on that individual's welfare and opportunity, would lead to inappropriate policy.

Disagreement will arise about whether the care of some health conditions falls within the demands of adequacy. Most people will agree, however, that some conditions should not be included in the societal obligation to ensure access to adequate care. A relatively uncontroversial example would be changing the shape of a functioning, normal nose or retarding the normal effects of aging (through cosmetic surgery). By the same token, there are some conditions, such as pregnancy, for which care would be regarded as an important component of adequacy. In determining adequacy, it is important to consider how people's welfare, opportunities, and requirements for information and interpersonal caring are affected by their health condition.

Any assessment of adequacy must consider also the types, amounts, and quality of care necessary to respond to each health condition. It is important to emphasize that these questions are implicitly comparative: the standard of adequacy for a condition must reflect the fact that resources used for it will not be available to respond to other conditions. Consequently, the level of care deemed adequate should reflect a reasoned judgment not only about the impact of the condition on the welfare and opportunity of the individual but also about the efficacy and the cost of the care itself in relation to other conditions and the efficacy and cost of the care that is available for them. Since individual cases differ so much, the health care professional and patient must be flexible. Thus adequacy, even in relation to a particular health condition, generally refers to a range of options.

The Relationship of Costs and Benefits. The level of care that is available will be determined by the level of resources devoted to producing it. Such allocation should reflect the benefits and costs of the care provided. It should be emphasized that these "benefits," as well as their "costs," should be interpreted broadly, and not restricted only to effects easily quantifiable in monetary terms. Personal benefits include improvements in individuals' functioning and in their quality of life, and the reassurance from worry and the provision of information that are a product of health care. Broader social benefits should be included as well, such as strengthening the sense of community and the belief that no one in serious need of health care will be left without it. Similarly, costs are not merely the funds spent for a treatment but include other less tangible and quantifiable adverse consequences, such as diverting funds away from other socially desirable endeavors including education, welfare, and other social services.

There is no objectively correct value that these various costs and benefits have or that can be discovered by the tools of cost/benefit analysis. Still, such an analysis, as a recent report of the Office of Technology Assessment noted, "can be very helpful to decision-makers because the process of analysis gives structure to the problem, allows an open consideration of all relevant effects of a decision, and forces the explicit treatment of key assumptions."[1] But the valuation of the various effects of alternative treatments for different conditions rests on people's values and goals, about which individuals will reasonably disagree. In a democracy, the appropriate values to be assigned to the consequences of policies must ultimately be determined by people expressing their values through social and political processes as well as in the marketplace.

Approximating Adequacy. The intention of the Commission is to provide a frame of reference for policymakers, not to resolve these complex questions. Nevertheless, it is possible to raise some of the specific issues that should be considered in determining what constitutes adequate care. It is important, for example, to gather accurate information about and compare the costs and effects, both favorable and unfavorable, of various treatment or management options. The options that better serve the goals that make health care of special importance should be assigned a higher value. As already noted, the assessment of costs must take two factors into account: the cost of a proposed option in relation to alternative forms of care that would achieve the same goal of enhancing the welfare and opportunities of the patient, and the cost of each proposed option in terms of foregone opportunities to apply the same resources to social goals other than that of ensuring equitable access.

Furthermore, a reasonable specification of adequate care must reflect an assessment of the relative importance of many different characteristics of a given form of care for a particular condition. Sometimes the problem is posed as: What *amounts* of care and what *quality* of care? Such a formulation reduces a complex problem to only two dimensions, implying that all care can readily be ranked as better or worse. Because two alternative forms of care may vary along a number of dimensions, there may be no consensus among reasonable and informed individuals about which form is of higher overall quality. It is worth bearing in mind that adequacy does not mean the highest possible level of quality or strictly equal quality any more than it requires equal amounts of care; of course, adequacy does require that everyone receive care that meets standards of sound medical practice.

Any combination of arrangements for achieving adequacy will presumably include some health care delivery settings that mainly serve certain groups, such as the poor or those covered by public programs. The fact that patients receive care in different settings or from different providers does not itself show that some are receiving inadequate care. The Commission believes that there is no moral objection to such a system so long as all receive care that is adequate in amount and quality and all patients are treated with concern and respect. . . .

NOTE

1. Office of Technology Assessment, U.S. Congress, *The Implications of Cost-Effectiveness Analysis of Medical Technology, Summary*, U.S. Government Printing Office, Washington (1980) at 8.

ROBERT M. VEATCH

Justice, the Basic Social Contract, and Health Care

The principle that each person's welfare should count equally is crucial if the community generated is to be a moral community. The moral community is one of impartiality. If the community employed an impartial perspective to draw up the basic principles or practices for the society, the principles would be generated without reference to individual talents, skills, abilities, or good fortune. Another way of formulating this condition is to say that the basic principles or practices established must meet the test of reversibility. That is, they must be acceptable to one standing on either the giving or the receiving end of a transaction.[1] The general notion is that the contractors must take equal account of all persons. It is only by such an abandonment of an egoistic perspective that common social intercourse is possible. As Plato wrote in Book I of the Republic, "the unjust are incapable of common action . . . and [the] utterly unjust, they would have been utterly incapable of action."

The most intriguing contractual theory of ethics that makes this commitment to impartiality or reversibility is that espoused by John Rawls.[2] In his version of social contract theory, Rawls asks us to envision ourselves in what he calls the original position. He does not pretend that such a position exists or ever could exist. Rather, it is a device for making "vivid to ourselves the restrictions that it seems reasonable to impose on arguments for principles of justice, and therefore on these principles themselves."[3] The restrictions on the original position are that no one should be advantaged or disadvantaged in the choice of principles either by natural fortune or social circumstances. Persons in the original position are equal. To help us imagine such a situation, he asks us to impose what he calls a "veil of ignorance," under which "no one knows his place in society, his class position or social status, nor does any one know his fortune in the distribution of natural assets and abilities, his intelligence, strength, and the like."[4]

From that position one can derive impartially a set of principles or practices that provide the moral foundations for a society. Even if we cannot discover a universal basis for ethical decisions, perhaps we can create a community that accepts rules such as respect for freedom and the impartial consideration of interests; that is, one that adopts the moral point of view and thereby provides a common foundation for deciding what is ethical. Those who take this view believe it possible to generate some commonly agreed upon principles or practices for a society. The creation of a contractual framework could then provide a basis for making medical ethical decisions that would be commonly recognized as legitimate. . . .

There is . . . a moral community constituted symbolically by the metaphor of the contract or covenant. There is a convergence between the vision of people coming together to discover a preexisting moral order—an order that takes equally into account the welfare of all—and the vision of people coming together to invent a moral order that as well takes equally into account the welfare of all. The members of the moral community thus generated are bound together by bonds of mutual loyalty and trust. There is a fundamental equality and reciprocity in the relationship, something missing in the philanthropic condescension of professional code ethics. . . .

THE MAXIMIN THEORY

Some say that reasonable people considering alternative policies or principles for a society would not opt to maximize the aggregate benefits that exist in the soci-

From *A Theory of Medical Ethics*. © 1981. Reprinted by permission of the Kennedy Institute of Ethics.

ety. Rather, they say that at least for basic social practices that determine the welfare of members of the moral community, they would opt for a strategy that attempts to assure fundamentally that the least well off person would do as well as possible. . . .

The implication is that those having the greatest burden have some claim on the society independent of whether responding to their needs is the most efficient way of producing the greatest net aggregate benefit. Holders of this view say that the commitment of a principle of justice is to maximize not net aggregate benefit, but the position of the least advantaged members of the society. If the principle of justice is a right-making characteristic of actions, a principle that reasonable people would accept as part of the basic social contract independent of the principle of beneficence, it probably incorporated some moral notion that the distribution of benefits and burdens counts as well well as the aggregate amount of them. One plausible alternative is to concentrate, insofar as we are concerned about justice, on the welfare of the least well off. This is part of those principles of justice defended by Rawls as derived from his version of social contract theory. . . .

Since Rawls's scheme is designed to provide insights into only the basic practices and social institutions, it is very hard to discern what the implications are for specific problems of resource distribution such as the allocation of health care resources. Some have argued that no direct implications can be read from the Rawlsian principles. That seems, however, to overstate the case. At the least, basic social practices and institutional arrangements must be subject to the test of the principles of justice.

It appears, then, that this view will not justify inequalities in the basic health care institutions and practices simply because they produce the greatest net aggregate benefit. Its notion of justice, concentrating on improving the lot of the least advantaged, is much more egalitarian in this sense than the utilitarian system. It would distribute health care resources to the least well off rather than just on the aggregate amount of benefit.

There is no obvious reason why our hypothetical contractors articulating the basic principles for a society would favor a principle that maximized aggregate utility any more than one that maximized minimum utility. Our contract model, as an epistemological device for discovering the basic principles, views them, after all, as committed to the moral point of view, as evaluating equally the welfare of each individual from a veil of ignorance, to use the Rawlsian language. This perspective retains the notion of individuals as identifiable, unique personalities, as noncommensurable human beings, rather than simply as components of an aggregate mass. Faced with a forced choice, it seems plausible that one would opt for maximizing the welfare of individuals, especially the least well-off individuals, rather than maximizing the aggregate.

Nevertheless, the interpretation of justice that attempts to maximize the minimum position in the society (and is hence sometimes called the "maximin" position), still permits inequalities and even labels them as just. What, for example, of basic health care institutional arrangements that systematically single out elites with unique natural talents for developing medical skill and services and gives these individuals high salaries as incentives to serve the interests of the least well off? What if a special health care system were institutionalized to make sure these people were always in the best of health, were cared for first in catastrophes, and were inconvenienced least by the normal bureaucratic nuisances of a health care system?

It is conceivable that such an institutional arrangement would be favored by reasonable people taking the moral point of view. They could justify the special gains that would come to the elites by the improved chances thus created for the rest of the population (who would not have as great a gain as the favored ones, but would at least be better off than if the elite were not so favored). The benefits, in lesser amounts, would trickle down in this plan to the consumers of health care so that all, or at least the least advantaged, would gain. The gap between the elite of the health profession and the masses could potentially increase by such a social arrangement, but at least all would be better off in absolute terms.

So it is conceivable that reasonable people considering equally both the health professionals and the masses would favor such an arrangement, but it is not obvious. Critics of the Rawlsian principles of justice say that in some cases alternative principles of distribution would be preferred. Brian Barry, for example, argues that rational choosers would look not just at the welfare of the least advantaged, but also at the average or aggregate welfare of alternative policies.[5] On the other hand, Barry and many others suggest that in some circumstances, rational choosers might opt for the principle that would maximize equality of outcome.[6] At most, considering the institutionalization of advantages for a health care elite, they would be supported as a prudent sacrifice of the demands of justice in order to serve some other justifiable moral end.

From this perspective, favoring elites with special monetary and social incentives in order to benefit the poor might be a prudent compromise.[7] It might mediate between the demands that see justice as requiring equality of outcome (subject to numerous qualifications) and the demands of the principle of beneficence requiring maximum efficiency in producing good consequences. If that is the case, though, then there is still a fourth interpretation of the principle of justice that must be considered, one that is more radically egalitarian than the maximin strategy.

THE EGALITARIAN THEORY

Those who see the maximin strategy as a compromise between the concern for justice and the concern for efficient production of good consequences must feel that justice requires a stricter focus on equality than the maximin understanding of the principle of justice. The maximin principle is concerned about the distribution of benefits. It justifies inequalities only if they benefit the least well off. But it does justify inequalities—and it does so in the name of justice.

Rawls recognizes that there is an important difference between a right action and a just or a fair action. Fairness is a principle applying to individuals along with beneficence, noninjury, mutual respect, and fidelity. The list is not far removed from the basic principles I have identified. But, given this important difference between what is right in this full, inclusive sense and what is fair, if one is convinced that incentives and advantages for medical elites are justified, why would one claim that the justification is one based on the principle of fairness? One might instead maintain that they are right on balance because they are a necessary compromise with the principle of fairness (or justice) in order to promote efficiently the welfare of a disadvantaged group. It is to be assumed, given the range of basic principles in an ethical system, that conflicts will often emerge so that one principle will be sacrificed, upon occasion, for the sake of another.

The egalitarian understanding of the principle of justice is one that sees justice as requiring (subject to certain important qualifications) equality of net welfare for individuals.[8] . . .

Everyone, according to the principle of egalitarian justice, ought to end up over a lifetime with an equal amount of net welfare (or, as we shall see shortly, a chance for that welfare). Some may have a great deal of benefit offset by large amounts of unhappiness or disutility, while others will have relatively less of both. What we would call "just" under this principle is a basic social practice or policy that contributes to the same extent to greater equality of outcome (subject to restrictions to be discussed). I am suggesting that reasonable people who are committed to a contract model for discovering, inventing, or otherwise articulating the basic principles will want to add to their list the notion that one of the right-making characteristics of a society would be the equality of welfare among the members of the moral community.

The Equality of Persons. The choice of this interpretation of the principle of justice will depend upon how the contractors understand the commitment to the moral point of view—the commitment to impartiality that takes the point of view of all equally into account. We certainly are not asserting the equality of ability or even the equality of the merit of individual claims. . . .

If this is what is meant by the moral point of view, taking into account equally the individuality of each member of the community, then in addition to the right-making characteristics or principles of beneficence, promise keeping, autonomy, truth telling, and avoiding killing, the principle of justice as equality of net welfare must be added to the list. The principle might be articulated as affirming that people have a claim on having the total net welfare in their lives equal insofar as possible to the welfare in the lives of others.

Of course, no reasonable person, even an egalitarian, is going to insist upon or even desire that all the features of people's lives be identical.[9] It seems obvious that the most that anyone would want is that the total net welfare for each person be comparable. . . .

If this egalitarian understanding of the principle of justice would be acceptable to reasonable people taking the moral point of view, it provides a solution to the dilemma of the tension between focusing exclusively on the patient and opening the doors to considerations of social consequences such as in classical utilitarianism. The principle of justice provides another basis for taking into account a limited set of impacts on certain other parties. If the distribution of benefits as well as the aggregate amount is morally relevant, then certain impacts on other parties may be morally more relevant than others. A benefit that accrues to a person who is or predictably will be in a least well-off group would count as a consideration of justice while a benefit of equal size that accrued to other persons not in the least well-off group would not. The hypothetical benefits of a Nazi-type experiment would not accrue to a least well-off group (while the harms of the experiment presumably would). They are thus morally different from, in fact diametrically opposed to, a redistribution scheme that produced benefits for only the least advantaged group.

Equality and Envy. Critics of the egalitarian view of justice have argued that the only way to account for such a position is by attributing it to a psychology of envy.[10] Freud accounted for a sense of justice in this way.[11] They feel the only conceivable reason to strive for equality is the psychological explanation that the less well off envy the better off, and they hold that contractors take that psychological fact into account. Since they believe that envy is not an adequate justification for a commitment to equal outcome, they opt instead for an alternative theory of justice. . . .

The egalitarian holds that there is something fundamentally wrong with gross inequalities, with gross differences in net welfare. The problem is encountered when people of unequal means must interact; say, when representatives of an impoverished community apply to an elite foundation for funds to support a neighborhood health program. There is no way that real communication can take place between the elites of the foundation and the members of the low-income community. It is not simply that the poor envy the foundation executives or that the executives feel resentful of the poor. Rather, as anyone who has been in such a relationship knows, the sense of community is fractured. Not only do the less well off feel that they cannot express themselves with self-respect, but the elites realize that there is no way the messages they receive can be disentangled from the status and welfare differentials. Neither can engage in any true interaction. A moral relationship is virtually impossible. . . .

The Implications of the Egalitarian Formula. It turns out that incorporating health care into this system of total welfare will be extremely difficult. Let us begin, temporarily, therefore, by considering a simpler system dealing only with food, clothing, and shelter. Fairness could mean, according to the egalitarian formula, that each person had to have an equal amount of each of these. No reasonable person, however, would find that necessary or attractive. Rather, what the egalitarian has in mind with his concept of

justice is that the net of welfare, summed across all three of these goods, be as similar as possible. We could arbitrarily fix the amount of resources in each category, but nothing seems wrong with permitting people to trade some food for clothing, or clothing for shelter. If one person preferred a large house and minimal food and could find someone with the opposite tastes, nothing seems wrong with permitting a trade. The assumption is that the need of people for food, clothing, and shelter is about the same in everybody and that marginal utilities in the trades will be about the same. If so, then permitting people to trade around would increase the welfare of each person without radically distorting the equality of net overall welfare. Up to this point, then, the egalitarian principle of justice says that it is just (though not necessarily right) to strive in social practices for equality of net welfare. . . .

For health care and education, however, the situation is much different. Here it is reasonable to assume that human needs vary enormously. Nothing could be more foolish than to distribute health care or even the money for health care equally. The result would be unequal overall well-being for those who were unfortunate in the natural lottery for health, objectively much worse off than others. If the goal of justice is to produce a chance for equal, objective net welfare, then the starting point for consideration of health care distribution should be the need for it. Education (or the resources to buy education) initially would be distributed in the same way. The amount added to the resources for food, clothing, and shelter should then be in proportion to an "unhealthiness status index" plus another amount proportional to an "educational needs index."

However, that proposal raises two additional questions: Should people be permitted to use the resources set aside for health care in some other way? And who should bear the responsibility if people have an opportunity to be healthy and do not take advantage of it?

THE CASE FOR AN EQUAL RIGHT TO HEALTH CARE

Even for the egalitarian it is not obvious why society ought to strive for an equal right to health care. Certainly it ought not to be interested in obtaining the same amount of health care for everyone. To do so would require forcing those in need of great amounts of care to go without or those who have the good fortune to be healthy to consume uselessly. But it is not even obvious that we should end up with a right to health care equal in proportion to need, though that is the conclusion that many, especially egalitarians, are reaching. . . .

Is there any reason to believe that health care is any more basic than, say, food or protection from the elements? All are absolutely essential to human survival, at least up to some minimum for subsistence. All are necessary conditions for the exercise of liberty, self-respect, or any other functioning as part of the human moral community. Furthermore, while the bare minimum of health care is as necessary as food and shelter, in all cases these may not really be "necessities" at the margin. If trades are to be tolerated between marginal food and clothing, is there any reason why someone placing relatively low value on health care should not be permitted to trade, say, his annual checkups for someone else's monthly allotment of steak dinners? Or, if we shall make trading easier by distributing money fairly rather than distributing rations of these specific goods, is there any reason why, based on an "unhealthiness index," we could not distribute a fair portion of funds for health care as well as for other necessities? Individuals could then buy the health care (or health care insurance) that they need, employing individual discretion about where their limit for health care is in comparison with steak dinners. Those at a high health risk would be charged high amounts for health care (or high premiums for insurance), but those costs would be exactly offset by the money supplement based on the index.

Perhaps we cannot make a case for equal access to health care on the basis that it is more fundamental than other goods. There may still be reasons, though, why reasonable people would structure the basic institutions of society to provide a right to equal health care in the sense I am using the term, that is a right equal in proportion to need.

Our response will depend somewhat upon whether we are planning a health care distribution for a just world or one with the present inequities in the distribution of net welfare. . . .

But obviously we do not live in a perfectly just world. The problem becomes more complex. How do we arrange the health care system, which all would agree is fundamental to human well-being at least at some basic level, in order to get as close as possible to equality of welfare as the outcome? Pragmatic consid-

erations may, at this point, override the abstract, theoretical argument allowing trades of health care for other goods even at the margin.

Often defenders of free-market and partial free-market solutions to the allocation of health care resources assume that if fixed in-kind services such as health care are not distributed, money will be. . . .

There is a more subtle case for an equal right to health care (in proportion to need) in an unfair world. Bargaining strengths are likely to be very unequal in a world where resources are distributed unfairly. Those with great resources, perhaps because of natural talents or naturally occurring good health or both, are in an invincible position. The needy, for example those with little earning power because of congenital health problems, may be forced to use what resources they have in order to buy immediate necessities, withholding on health care investment; particularly preventive health care and health insurance, while gambling that they will be able to survive without those services.

It is not clear what our moral response should be to those forced into this position of bargainers from weakness. If the just principle of distribution were Pareto optimality (where bargains were acceptable, regardless of the weaknesses of the parties, provided all gained in the transaction), we would accept the fact that some would bargain from weakness and be forced to trade their long-term health care needs for short-term necessities. If the principle of justice that reasonable people would accept taking the moral point of view, however, is something like the maximin position or the egalitarian position, then perhaps such trades of health care should be prohibited. The answer will depend on how one should behave in planning social policies in an unjust world. The fact that resources are not distributed fairly generates pressures on the least well off (assuming they act rationally) to make choices they would not have to make in a more fair world. If unfairness in the general distribution of resources is a given, we are forced into a choice between two unattractive options: We could opt for the rule that will permit the least well off to maximize their position under the existing conditions or we could pick the rule that would arrange resources as closely as possible to the way they would be arranged in a just world. In our present, unjust society distributing health care equally is a closer approximation to the way it would be distributed in a just society than giving a general resource like money or permitting trades. . . .

I see justice not just as a way to efficiently improve the lot of the least well off by permitting them trades (even though those trades end up increasing the gap between the haves and the have-nots). That might be efficient and might preserve autonomy, but it would not be justice. If I were an original contractor I would cast my vote in favor of the egalitarian principle of justice, applying it so that there would be a right to health care equal in proportion to health care need. The principle of justice for health care could, then, be stated as follows: People have a right to needed health care to provide an opportunity for a level of health equal as far as possible to the health of other people.

The principle of justice for health care is a pragmatic derivative from the general principle of justice requiring equality of objective net welfare. The result would be a uniform health care system with one class of service available for all. Practical problems would still exist, especially at the margins. The principle, for example, does not establish what percentage of total resources would go for health care. The goal would be to arrange resources so that health care needs would, in general, be met about as well as other needs. This means that a society would rather arbitrarily set some fixed amount of the total resources for health care. Every nation currently spends somewhere between five and ten percent of its gross national product (GNP) in this area, with the wealthier societies opting for the higher percentages. Presumably the arbitrary choice would fall in that range.

With such a budget fixed, reasonable people will come together to decide what health care services can be covered under it. The task will not be as great as it seems. The vast majority of services will easily be sorted into or out of the health care system. Only a small percentage at the margin will be the cause of any real debate. The choice will at times be arbitrary, but the standard applied will at least be clear. People should have services necessary to give them a chance to be as close as possible to being as healthy as other people. Those choices will be made while striving to emulate the position of original contractors taking the moral point of view. The decision-making panels will not differ in task greatly from the decision makers who currently sort health care services in and out of insurance coverage lists. However, panels will be committed to a principle of justice and will take the moral point of view, whereas the self-interested insurers try to maximize profits or efficiency or a bargaining position against weak, unorganized consumers.

NOTES

1. Kurt Baier, *The Moral Point of View: A Rational Basis of Ethics* (New York: Random House, 1965), p. 108.

2. John Rawls, *A Theory of Justice* (Cambridge, Mass.: Harvard University Press, 1971).

3. Ibid., p. 18.

4. Ibid., p. 12; cf. pp. 136–42.

5. Brian Barry, *The Liberal Theory of Justice: A Critical Examination of the Principal Doctrines in "A Theory of Justice" by John Rawls* (Oxford: Clarendon Press, 1973), p. 109; see also Robert L. Cunningham, "Justice: Efficiency or Fairness?" *Personalist* 52 (Spring 1971):253–81.

6. Barry, *The Liberal Theory*; idem, "Reflections on 'Justice as Fairness,'" in *Justice and Equality*, ed. H. Bedau (Englewood Cliffs, N.J.: Prentice-Hall, 1971), pp. 103–115; Bernard Williams, "The Idea of Equality," reprinted in Bedau, *Justice and Equality*, pp. 116–37; Christopher Ake, "Justice as Equality," *Philosophy and Public Affairs* 5 (Fall 1975):69–89; Robert M. Veatch, "What Is 'Just' Health Care Delivery?" in *Ethics and Health Policy*, ed. R.M. Veatch and R. Branson (Cambridge, Mass.: Ballinger, 1976), pp. 127–53.

7. Barry, "Reflections," p. 113.

8. See Ake, "Justice as Equality," for a careful development of the notion.

9. Hugo A. Bedau, "Radical Egalitarianism," in *Justice and Equality*, ed. H.A. Bedau, p. 168.

10. Rawls, *A Theory of Justice*, p. 538, note 9.

11. Sigmund Freud, *Group Psychology and the Analysis of the Ego*, rev. ed., trans. James Strachey (London: Hogarth Press, 1959), pp. 51f. (as cited in Rawls, *A Theory of Justice*, p. 439).

ALLEN E. BUCHANAN

The Right to a Decent Minimum of Health Care

THE ASSUMPTION THAT THERE IS
A RIGHT TO A DECENT MINIMUM

A consensus that there is (at least) a right to a decent minimum of health care pervades recent policy debates and much of the philosophical literature on health care. Disagreement centers on two issues. Is there a more extensive right than the right to a decent minimum of health care? What is included in the decent minimum to which there is a right?

PRELIMINARY CLARIFICATION
OF THE CONCEPT

Different theories of distributive justice may yield different answers both to the question 'Is there a right to a decent minimum?' and to the question 'What comprises the decent minimum?' The justification a particular theory provides for the claim that there is a right to a decent minimum must at least cohere with the justifications it provides for other right-claims. Moreover, the character of this justification will determine, at least in part, the way in which the decent minimum is specified, since it will include an account of the nature and significance of health-care needs. To the extent that the concept of a decent minimum is theory-dependent, then, it would be naive to assume that a mere analysis of the concept of a decent minimum would tell us whether there is such a right and what its content is. Nonetheless, before we proceed to an examination of various theoretical attempts to ground and specify a right to a decent minimum, a preliminary analysis will be helpful.

Sometimes the notion of a decent minimum is applied not to health care but to health itself, the claim being that everyone is entitled to some minimal level,

or welfare floor, of health. I shall not explore this variant of the decent minimum idea because I think its implausibility is obvious. The main difficulty is that assuring any significant level of health for all is simply not within the domain of social control. If the alleged right is understood instead as the right to everything which can be done to achieve some significant level of health for all, then the claim that there is such a right becomes implausible simply because it ignores the fact that in circumstances of scarcity the total social expenditure on health must be constrained by the need to allocate resources for other goods.

Though the concept of a right is complex and controversial, for our purposes a partial sketch will do. To say that person A has a right to something, X, is first of all to say that A is entitled to X, that X is due to him or her. This is not equivalent to saying that if A were granted X it would be a good thing, even a morally good thing, or that X is desired by or desirable for A. Second, it is usually held that valid right-claims, at least in the case of basic rights, may be backed by sanctions, including coercion if necessary (unless doing so would produce extremely great disutility or grave moral evil), and that (except in such highly exceptional circumstances) failure of an appropriate authority to apply the needed sanctions is itself an injustice. Recent rights-theorists have also emphasized a third feature of rights, or at least of basic rights or rights in the strict sense: valid right-claims 'trump' appeals to what would maximize utility, whether it be the utility of the right-holder, or social utility. In other words, if A has a right to X, then the mere fact that infringing A's right would maximize overall utility or even A's utility is not itself a sufficient reason for infringing it.[1] Finally, a universal (or general) right is one which applies to all persons, not just to certain individuals or classes because of their involvement in special actions, relationships, or agreements.

The second feature—enforceability—is of crucial importance for those who assume or argue that there is a universal right to a decent minimum of health care. For, once it is granted that there is such a right and that such a right may be enforced (absent any extremely weighty reason against enforcement), the claim that there is a universal right provides the moral basis for using the coercive power of the state to assure a decent minimum for all. Indeed, the surprising absence of attempts to justify a coercively backed decent minimum policy by arguments that do *not* aim at establishing a universal right suggests the following hypothesis: advocates of a coercively backed decent minimum have operated on the assumption that such a policy must be based on a universal right to a decent minimum. The chief aim of this article is to show that this assumption is false.

I think it is fair to say that many who confidently assume there is a (universal) right to a decent minimum of health care have failed to appreciate the significance of the first feature of our sketch of the concept of a right. It is crucial to observe that the claim that there is a right to a decent minimum is much stronger than the claim that everyone *ought* to have access to such a minimum, or that if they did it would be a good thing, or that any society which is capable, without great sacrifice, of providing a decent minimum but fails to do so is deeply morally defective. None of the latter assertions implies the existence of a right, if this is understood as a moral entitlement which ought to be established by the coercive power of the state if necessary. . . .

THE ATTRACTIONS OF THE IDEA
OF A DECENT MINIMUM

There are at least three features widely associated with the idea of a right to a decent minimum which, together with the facile consensus that vagueness promotes, help explain its popularity over competing conceptions of the right to health care. First, it is usually, and quite reasonably, assumed that the idea of a decent minimum is to be understood in a society-relative sense. Surely it is plausible to assume that, as with other rights to goods or services, the content of the right must depend upon the resources available in a given society and perhaps also upon a certain consensus of expectations among its members. So the first advantage of the idea of a decent minimum, as it is usually understood, is that it allows us to adjust the level of services to be provided as a matter of right to

relevant social conditions and also allows for the possibility that as a society becomes more affluent the floor provided by the decent minimum should be raised.

Second, the idea of a decent minimum avoids the excesses of what has been called the strong equal access principle, while still acknowledging a substantive universal right. According to the strong equal access principle, everyone has an equal right to the best health-care services available. Aside from the weakness of the justifications offered in support of it, the most implausible feature of the strong equal access principle is that it forces us to choose between two unpalatable alternatives. We can either set the publicly guaranteed level of health care lower than the level that is technically possible or we can set it as high as is technically possible. In the former case, we shall be committed to the uncomfortable conclusion that no matter how many resources have been expended to guarantee equal access to that level, individuals are forbidden to spend any of their resources for services not available to all. Granted that individuals are allowed to spend their after-tax incomes on more frivolous items, why shouldn't they be allowed to spend it on health? If the answer is that they should be so allowed, as long as this does not interfere with the provision of an adequate package of health-care services for everyone, then we have retreated from the strong equal access principle to something very like the principle of a decent minimum. If, on the other hand, we set the level of services guaranteed for all so high as to eliminate the problem of persons seeking extra care beyond this level, this would produce a huge drain on total resources, foreclosing opportunities for producing important goods other than health care.

So both the recognition that health care must compete with other goods and the conviction that beyond some less than maximal level of publicly guaranteed services individuals should be free to purchase additional services point toward a more limited right than the strong access principle asserts. Thus, the endorsement of a right to a decent minimum may be more of a recognition of the implausibility of the stronger right to equal access than a sign of any definite position on the content of the right to health care.

A third attraction of the idea of a decent minimum is that since the right to health care must be limited in scope (to avoid the consequences of a strong equal access right), it should be limited to the 'most basic' services, those normally 'adequate' for health, or for a 'decent' or 'tolerable' life. However, although this aspect of the idea of a decent minimum is useful because it calls attention to the fact that health-care needs are heterogeneous and must be assigned some order of priority, it does not itself provide any basis for determining which are most important.

THE NEED FOR A SUPPORTING THEORY

In spite of these attractions, the concept of a right to a decent minimum of health care is inadequate as a moral basis for a coercively backed decent minimum policy in the absence of a coherent and defensible theory of justice. Indeed, when taken together they do not even imply that there is a right to a decent minimum. Rather, they only support the weaker conditional claim that if there is a right to health care, then it is one that is more limited than a right of strong equal access, and is one whose content depends upon available resources and some scheme of priorities which shows certain health services to be more basic than others. It appears, then, that a theoretical grounding for the right to a decent minimum of health care is indispensable. . . .

My suggestion is that the combined weight of arguments from special (as opposed to universal) rights to health care, harm-prevention, prudential arguments of the sort used to justify public health measures, and two arguments that show that effective charity shares features of public goods (in the technical sense) is sufficient to do the work of an alleged universal right to a decent minimum of health care.

Arguments from Special Rights. The right-claim we have been examining (and find unsupported) has been a *universal* right-claim: one that attributes the same right to all persons. *Special* right-claims, in contrast, restrict the right in question to certain individuals or groups.

There are at least three types of arguments that can be given for special rights to health care. First, there are arguments from the requirements of rectifying past or present institutional injustices. It can be argued, for example, that American blacks and native Americans are entitled to a certain core set of health-care services owing to their history of unjust treatment by government or other social institutions, on the grounds that these injustices have directly or indirectly had detrimental effects on the health of the groups in question.

Second, there are arguments from the requirements of compensation to those who have suffered unjust harm or who have been unjustly exposed to health risks by the assignable actions of private individuals or corporations—for instance, those who have suffered neurological damage from the effects of chemical pollutants.

Third, a strong moral case can be made for special rights to health care for those who have undergone exceptional sacrifices for the good of society as a whole—in particular those whose health has been adversely affected through military service. The most obvious candidates for such compensatory special rights are soldiers wounded in combat.

Arguments from the Prevention of Harm. The content of the right to a decent minimum is typically understood as being more extensive than those traditional public health services that are usually justified on the grounds that they are required to protect the citizenry from certain harms arising from the interactions of persons living together in large numbers. Yet such services have been a major factor—if not *the* major factor—in reducing morbidity and mortality rates. Examples include sanitation and immunization. The moral justification of such measures, which constitute an important element in a decent minimum of health care, rests upon the widely accepted Harm (Prevention) Principle, not upon a right to health care.

The Harm Prevention argument for traditional public health services, however, may be elaborated in a way that brings them closer to arguments for a universal right to health care. With some plausibility one might contend that once the case has been made for expending public resources on public health measures, there is a moral (and perhaps Constitutional) obligation to achieve some standard of *equal protection* from the harms these measures are designed to prevent. Such an argument, if it could be made out, would imply that the availability of basic public health services should not vary greatly across different racial, ethnic, or geographic groups within the country.

Prudential Arguments. Prudent arguments for health-care services typically emphasize benefits rather than the prevention of harm. It has often been argued, in particular, that the availability of certain basic forms of health care make for a more productive labor force or improve the fitness of the citizenry for national defense. This type of argument, too, does not assume that individuals have moral rights (whether special or universal) to the services in question.

It seems very likely that the combined scope of the various special health-care rights discussed above, when taken together with harm prevention and prudential arguments for basic health services and an argument from equal protection through public health measures, would do a great deal toward satisfying the health-care needs which those who advocate a universal right to a decent minimum are most concerned about. In other words, once the strength of a more pluralistic approach is appreciated, we may come to question the popular dogma that policy initiatives designed to achieve a decent minimum of health care for all must be grounded in a universal moral right to a decent minimum. This suggestion is worth considering because it again brings home the importance of the methodological difficulty encountered earlier. Even if, for instance, there is wide consensus on the considered judgment that the lower health prospects of inner city blacks are not only morally unacceptable but an injustice, it does not follow that this injustice consists of the infringement of a universal right to a decent minimum of health care. Instead, the injustice might lie in the failure to rectify past injustices or in the failure to achieve public health arrangements that meet a reasonable standard of equal protection for all.

Two Arguments for Enforced Beneficence. The pluralistic moral case for a legal entitlement to a decent minimum of health care (in the absence of a universal moral right) may be strengthened further by non-rights-based arguments from the principle of beneficence.[2] The possibility of making out such arguments depends upon the assumption that some principles may be justifiably enforced even if they are not principles specifying valid right-claims. There is at least one widely recognized class of such principles requiring contribution to the production of 'public goods' in the technical sense (for example, tax laws requiring contribution to national defense). It is characteristic of public goods that each individual has an incentive to withhold his contribution to the collective goal even though the net result is that the goal will not be achieved. Enforcement of a principle requiring all individuals to contribute to the goal is necessary to overcome the individual's incentive to withhold contribution by imposing penalties for his own failure to contribute and by assuring him that others will contribute. There is a special subclass of principles whose enforcement is justified not only by the need to overcome the individual's incentive to withhold compliance with the principle but also to ensure that individuals' efforts are appropriately *coordinated*. For example, enforcing the rule of the road to drive only on the right not only ensures a joint effort toward the goal of safe driving but also coordinates individuals' efforts so as to make the attainment of that goal possible. Indeed, in the case of the 'rule of the road' a certain kind of coordinated joint effort is the public good whose attainment justifies enforcement. But regardless of whether the production of a public good requires the solution of a coordination problem or not, there may be no *right* that is the correlative of the coercively backed obligation specified by the principle. There are two arguments for enforced beneficence, and they each depend upon both the idea of coordination and on certain aspects of the concept of a public good.

Both arguments begin with an assumption reasonable libertarians accept: there is a basic moral obligation of charity or beneficence to those in need. In a society that has the resources and technical knowledge to improve health or at least to ameliorate important health defects, the application of this requirement of beneficence includes the provision of resources for at least certain forms of health care. If we are sincere, we will be concerned with the efficacy of our charitable or beneficent impulses. It is all well and good for the libertarian to say that voluntary giving *can* replace the existing array of government entitlement programs, but this *possibility* will be cold comfort to the needy if, for any of several reasons, voluntary giving falters.

Social critics on the left often argue that in a highly competitive acquisitive society such as ours it is naive to think that the sense of beneficence will win out over the urgent promptings of self-interest. One need not argue, however, that voluntary giving fails from weakness of the will. Instead one can argue that even if each individual recognizes a moral duty to contribute to the aid of others and is motivationally capable of acting on that duty, some important forms of beneficence will not be forthcoming because each individual will rationally conclude that he should not contribute.

Many important forms of health care, especially those involving large-scale capital investment for technology, cannot be provided except through the contributions of large numbers of persons. This is also true of the most important forms of medical research. But if so, then the beneficent individual will not be able to act effectively, in isolation. What is needed is a coordinated joint effort.

First argument. There are many ways in which I might help others in need. Granted the importance of health, providing a decent minimum of health care for all, through large-scale collective efforts, will be a more important form of beneficence than the various charitable acts A, B, and C, which I might perform *independently*, that is, whose success does not depend upon the contributions of others. Nonetheless, if I am rationally beneficent I will reason as follows: either enough others will contribute to the decent minimum project to achieve this goal, even if I do not contribute to it; or not enough others will contribute to achieve a decent minimum, even if I do contribute. In either case, my contribution will be wasted. In other words, granted the scale of the investment required and the virtually negligible size of my own contribution, I can disregard the minute possibility that my contribution might make the difference between success and failure. But if so, then the rationally beneficent thing for me to do is not to waste my contribution on the project of ensuring a decent minimum but instead to undertake an independent act of beneficence; A, B, or C—where I know my efforts will be needed and efficacious. But if everyone, or even many people, reason in this way, then what we each recognize as the most effective form of beneficence will not come about. Enforcement of a principle requiring contributions to ensuring a decent minimum is needed.

The first argument is of the same form as standard public goods arguments for enforced contributions to national defense, energy conservation, and many other goods, with this exception. In standard public goods arguments, it is usually assumed that the individual's incentive for not contributing is self-interest and that it is in his interest not to contribute because he will be able to partake of the good, if it is produced, even if he does not contribute. In the case at hand, however, the individual's incentive for not contributing to the joint effort is not self-interest, but rather his desire to maximize the good he can do for others with a given amount of his resources. Thus if he contributes but the goal of achieving a decent minimum for all would have been achieved without his contribution, then he has still failed to use his resources in a maximally beneficent way relative to the options of either contributing or not to the joint project, even though the goal of achieving a decent minimum is attained. The rationally beneficent thing to do, then, is not to contribute, even though

the result of everyone's acting in a rationally beneficent way will be a relatively ineffective patchwork of small-scale individual acts of beneficence rather than a large-scale, coordinated effort.

Second argument. I believe that ensuring a decent minimum of health care for all is more important than projects A, B, or C, and I am willing to contribute to the decent minimum project, but only if I have assurance that enough others will contribute to achieve the threshold of investment necessary for success. Unless I have this assurance, I will conclude that it is less than rational—and perhaps even morally irresponsible—to contribute my resources to the decent minimum project. For my contribution will be wasted if not enough others contribute. If I lack assurance of sufficient contributions by others, the rationally beneficent thing for me to do is to expend my 'beneficence budget' on some less-than-optimal project A, B, or C, whose success does not depend on the contribution of others. But without enforcement, I cannot be assured that enough others will contribute, and if others reason as I do, then what we all believe to be the most effective form of beneficence will not be forthcoming. Others may fail to contribute either because the promptings of self-interest overpower their sense of beneficence, or because they reason as I did in the First Argument, or for some other reason.

Both arguments conclude that an enforced decent minimum principle is needed to achieve coordinated joint effort. However, there is this difference. The Second Argument focuses on the *assurance problem*, while the first does not. In the Second Argument all that is needed is the assumption that rational beneficence requires assurance that enough others will contribute. In the First Argument the individual's reason for not contributing is not that he lacks assurance that enough others will contribute, but rather that it is better for him not to contribute regardless of whether others do or not.

Neither argument depends on an assumption of conflict between the individual's moral motivation of beneficence and his inclination of self-interest. Instead the difficulty is that in the absence of enforcement, individuals who strive to make their beneficence most effective will thereby fail to benefit the needy as much as they might.

A standard response to those paradoxes of rationality known as public goods problems is to introduce a coercive mechanism which attaches penalties to noncontribution and thereby provides each individual with the assurance that enough others will reciprocate so that his contribution will not be wasted and an effective incentive for him to contribute even if he has reason to believe that enough others will contribute to achieve the goal without his contribution. My suggestion is that the same type of argument that is widely accepted as a justification for enforced principles requiring contributions toward familiar public goods provides support for a coercively backed principle specifying a certain list of health programs for the needy and requiring those who possess the needed resources to contribute to the establishment of such programs, even if the needy have no *right* to the services those programs provide. Such an arrangement would serve a dual function: it would coordinate charitable efforts by focusing them on one set of services among the indefinitely large constellation of possible expressions of beneficence, and it would ensure that the decision to allocate resources to these services will become effective. . . .

NOTES

1. Ronald Dworkin, *Taking Rights Seriously* (Cambridge, MA: Harvard University Press, 1977), pp. 184–205.

2. For an exploration of various arguments for a duty of beneficence and an examination of the relationship between justice and beneficence, in general and in health care, see Allen E. Buchanan, "Philosophical Foundations of Beneficence," *Beneficence and Health Care*, ed. Earl E. Shelp (Dordrecht, Holland: Reidel Publishing Co., 1982).

H. TRISTRAM ENGELHARDT, JR.

Rights to Health Care

A basic human right to the delivery of health care, even to the delivery of a decent minimum of health care, does not exist. The difficulty with talking of such rights should be apparent. It is difficult if not impossible both to respect the freedom of all and to achieve their long-range best interests. Rights to health care constitute claims against others for either their services or their goods. Unlike rights to forbearance, which require others to refrain from interfering, rights to beneficence require others to participate actively in a particular understanding of the good life. Rights to health care, unless they are derived from special contractual agreements, depend on the principle of beneficence rather than that of autonomy, and therefore may conflict with the decisions of individuals who may not wish to participate in realizing a particular system of health care. If the resources involved in the provision of health care are not fully communal, private owners of resources may rightly have other uses in mind for their property than public health care. . . . [T]he principles of autonomy and beneficence that lie at the foundations of justice will spawn conflicts within any portrayal of a just allocation of health care resources.

THE LIMITS TO JUSTICE AS BENEFICENCE

These fundamental conflicts between respecting the freedom and achieving the best interests of persons are made worse by commitments to goals that, if pursued without qualification, lead to even more elaborate tensions within any concrete vision of a just health care system. Consider the following four goals that are at loggerheads.

1. The provision of the best possible care for all
2. The provision of equal care for all

From *Foundations of Bioethics* by H. Tristram Engelhardt, Jr. Reprinted by permission of Oxford University Press, 1986.

3. Freedom of choice on the part of health care provider and consumer
4. Containment of health care costs

One cannot provide the best possible health care for all and contain the cost of health care. One cannot provide equal health care for all and maintain freedom in the choice of health care provider and consumer. For that matter, one cannot maintain freedom in the choice of health care services while containing the costs of health care. One also may not be able to provide all with equal health care that is at the same time the very best care because of limits on the resources themselves. These tensions spring not only from a conflict between freedom and beneficence, but from competing views of what it means to pursue and achieve the good in health care (e.g., is it more important to provide equal care to all or the best possible care to the least well-off class?). . . . .

JUSTICE AND INEQUALITY

Interests in justice as beneficence are sustained in part because of inequalities among persons. That some have so little while others have so much properly evokes moral concerns of beneficence to provide help for those in need. . . . . [T]he moral authority to use force to set such inequalities aside is limited. These limitations are in part due to the fact that the resources one could use to aid those in need are often already owned by other people. One is forced to examine the very roots of inequality to determine whether such inequality and need constitute a claim against those in a position to aid.

THE NATURAL LOTTERY

Natural lottery is used here to identify changes in individual fortune that are the result of natural forces, not the actions of persons. It is not used to identify the distribution of natural assets. The natural lottery contrasts with the social lottery, which is used here to identify changes in individual fortune that are not the result of natural forces but the actions of persons. The social lottery is not used to identify the distribution of social assets. The natural and social lotteries together determine the distribution of natural and social assets. The social lottery is termed a lottery, though it is the outcome of personal actions, because of the complex interplay of personal choices. They are both aptly

termed lotteries because of the unpredictable character of their outcomes, which do not conform to an ideal pattern.

All individuals are exposed to the brutal vicissitudes of nature. Some are born healthy and by chance remain so for a long life, free of disease and major suffering. Others are born with serious congenital or genetic diseases, others contract serious crippling fatal illnesses early in life, and yet others are injured and maimed. These natural forces, insofar as they occur outside of human responsibility, can be termed the natural lottery. They bring individuals to good health or disease through no merit or fault of their own or others. Those who win the natural lottery will not be in need of medical care. They will live extraordinarily full lives and die painless and peaceful deaths. Those who lose the natural lottery will be in need of health care to blunt their sufferings and, where possible, to cure their diseases and to restore function. There will be a spectrum of losses, ranging from minor problems such as having bad teeth to major tragedies such as developing childhood leukemia, inheriting Huntington's chorea, or developing amyelotrophic lateral sclerosis.

These tragic outcomes, as the blind deliverances of nature, are acts of God for which no one is responsible (unless, that is, one wishes to impeach divine providence). The fact that individuals are injured by hurricanes, storms, and earthquakes is often simply no one's fault. Since no one is to blame, no one can be charged with the responsibility of making those whole who lose the natural lottery on the ground that they are accountable for the harm. One will need a special argument to show that the readers of this [article] should submit to the forcible distribution of their resources in order to provide health care for the individuals injured. It may very well be unfeeling or unsympathetic not to provide such help, but it is another thing to show that one owes others such help in a way that would morally authorize state force to redistribute resources, as one would collect funds owed in a debt. The natural lottery creates inequalities and places individuals at disadvantage without creating a straightforward obligation on the part of others to aid those in need.

THE SOCIAL LOTTERY

Individuals differ in their resources not simply because of outcomes of the natural lottery, but also due to the actions of others. Some deny themselves immediate pleasures in order to accumulate wealth or to leave inheritances to others. Through a complex web of love, affection, and mutual interest, individuals convey resources, one to another, so that those who are favored prosper, and those who are ignored languish. Some will grow wealthy and others will grow poor, not through anyone's maleficent actions or omissions, but simply because they were not favored by the love, friendship, collegiality, and associations through which fortunes develop and individuals prosper. In such cases there will be no fairness or unfairness, but simply good and bad fortune. In addition, some will be advantaged, disadvantaged, rich, poor, ill, diseased, deformed, or disabled because of the malevolent actions of others. Such will be unfair circumstances, which just and beneficent states should try to prevent and to rectify through retributive justice and forced restitution. Insofar as the injured party has a claim against the injurer to be made whole, not against society, the outcome is unfortunate from the perspective of society's obligations to make the actual restitution. Restitution is owed by the injurer.

When individuals come to purchase health care, some who lose the natural lottery will be able in part at least to compensate for that loss through their winnings at the social lottery. They will be able to afford expensive health care needed to restore health and to regain function. On the other hand, those who lose in both the natural and the social lottery will be in need of health care and without the resources to acquire it.

THE RICH AND THE POOR: DIFFERENCES IN ENTITLEMENTS

If one owns property by virtue of just acquisition or just transfer, then one's title to that property will not be undercut by the needs of others. One will simply own it. On the other hand, if one owns property because such ownership is part of a system that ensures a beneficent distribution of goods (e.g., the greatest balance of benefits over harms for the greatest number, the greatest advantage for the least-well-off class), one's ownership will be affected by the needs of others. [There are] reasons why one should suspect that property is in part privately owned in a strong sense that cannot be undercut by the needs of others. In addition, it would appear that all have a general right to access to the fruits of the earth, if not the universe, which would constitute the basis for a form of taxation as rent in order to provide for fungible payments to individuals, whether or not they are in need. Finally, there are likely to be resources held in common by groups that will need to find reasonable and equitable means for their distribution. The first two forms of entitlements will exist independently of medical or other needs; the last form of entitlement, through the decision of a community, may be conditioned by need.

The existence of any amount of private resources is the basis of an inequality among persons. Insofar as one owns things, one will have a right to them, even if others are in need, and even if the taxation as rent on one's resources is far from excessive or onerous. The test of whether one should transfer one's goods to others will not be whether such a redistribution will prove onerous or excessive for the person subjected to the distribution, but whether the resources belong to that individual. Goal-oriented approaches to the just distribution of resources will need to be restricted to commonly produced and commonly owned goods. Therefore, one must qualify the conclusions of the President's Commission that suggest that excessive burdens should determine the amount of tax persons should pay to sustain an adequate level of health care for those in need.[1] One will need to face a more complicated moral world with three sources of goods for the support of health care.

DRAWING THE LINE BETWEEN THE UNFORTUNATE AND THE UNFAIR

How one regards the moral significance of the natural and social lotteries and the moral force of private ownership will determine how one draws the line between circumstances that are simply unfortunate and those that are unfortunate and in addition unfair in the sense of constituting a claim on the resources of others. Life in general and health care in particular reveal circumstances of enormous tragedy, suffering, and deprivation. The pains of illness and disease and the despair of deformity call upon the sympathy of all to provide aid and give comfort. Injuries and diseases due to the unconsented-to actions of others are unfair. Injuries and diseases due to the forces of nature are unfortunate. As noted, unfortunate outcomes of the unfair actions of others are not necessarily society's fault. The horrible injuries that come every night to the emergency rooms of major hospitals may be someone's fault, even if they are not society's. Such outcomes, though unfair with regard to the relationship of the injured with the injurer, may be simply unfortunate with respect to society. One is thus faced with drawing the difficult line between acts of God and acts of malicious individuals that do not constitute a basis for societal retribution and injuries that provide such a basis. Such a line was drawn by Patricia Harris, the former secretary of the Department of Health, Education, and Welfare, when she ruled that heart transplantations should be considered experimental and therefore not reimbursable through Medicaid.[2] To be in need of a heart transplant and not have the funds available would be an unfortunate circumstance but not unfair. One was not eligible for a heart transplant even if another person had intentionally damaged one's heart. From a moral point of view, things could change if the federal government had in some culpable fashion injured one's heart. So, too, if promises of treatment had been made. For example, to suffer from appendicitis or pneumonia and not receive treatment reimbursable through Medicaid would be unfair, not simply unfortunate.

The line between the unfair and the unfortunate can be drawn because it is difficult if not impossible to translate all needs into claims against the resources of others. First it is hard to distinguish needs from mere desires. Is the request of an individual to have his life extended through a heart transplant at great cost and perhaps only for a few years a desire for an inordinate extension of life, or is it a need to be secure against a premature death? . . . Outside a particular view of the good life, needs do not create rights to the services or goods of others. Finally, there is a certain impracticality in seeing such circumstances as needs that generate claims. Attempts to restore health could indefinitely deplete societal resources in the pursuit of ever-more incremental extensions of life of marginal quality. A relatively limited amount of food and shelter is required to preserve the lives of individuals. But an indefinite amount of resources can be committed to the further preservation of human life. One is forced to draw a line between those needs that constitute claims on the aid of others and those that do not.

BEYOND EQUALITY

The line between the unfortunate and the unfair justifies certain social and economic inequalities. In particular, it justifies inequalities in the distribution of health care resources that are the result of differences in justly acquired resources and privileges. To this one must add that the very notion of equal distribution of health care is itself problematic, a point recognized in *Securing Access to Health Care*, the report of the President's Commission.[3]

1. Though in theory at least one can envisage providing all with equal levels of decent shelter and nutrition, one cannot restore all to or preserve all in an equal state of health. Health needs cannot be satisfied in the same way in which one can address needs for food and shelter.

2. If one provided all with the same amount of funds to purchase health care or the same amount of services, the amount provided would be far too much for many and still insufficient for some who could have always used more investment in treatment and research in the attempt to restore them to a level of function that would ensure equal opportunity.

3. If one attempts to provide equal health care in the sense of allowing individuals to select health care only from a predetermined list of available therapy, which would be provided to all so as to prevent the rich from having access to better health care than the poor, one would have confiscated a portion of the private property of individuals and have restricted the freedom of individuals to join in voluntary relationships. That some are fortunate in having more resources is neither more nor less arbitrary or unfair than some having better health, better looks, or more talents. If significant restrictions were placed on the ability to purchase special treatment with one's resources, one would need not only to anticipate that a black market in health care services would inevitably develop, but also to acknowledge it as a special bastion of liberty and freedom of association. . . .

CONFLICTING MODELS OF JUSTICE

We will [now] turn to a comparison of two radically different understandings of what counts as justice in general and what should count as justice in health care in particular: justice as primarily procedural, a matter of fair negotiation, and justice as primarily structural, a pattern of distributions that is amenable to rational disclosure. As examples of these two contrasting approaches, John Rawls's *A Theory of Justice* and Robert Nozick's *Anarchy, State, and Utopia*, will be briefly examined. Rawls presumes that there is an ahistorical way to discover the proper pattern for the distribution of resources, and therefore presumably for the distribution of health care resources. Moreover, he presumes that societally based entitlements are morally prior to privately based entitlements. Nozick, in contrast, provides a historical account of just distributions. Justice in patterns for the allocation of goods, including health care services, depends on what individual men and women have agreed to do with and for each other. Nozick holds that privately based entitlements are morally prior to societally based entitlements. In contrast with Rawls, who argues that one can discover a proper pattern for the allocation of societal resources, Nozick argues that such a pattern cannot be discovered and that instead one can only identify the characteristics of a just process for fashioning rights to health care. . . .

This contrast between Rawls and Nozick can be appreciated more generally as a contrast between two quite different principles of justice, each of which would have remarkably different implications for the allocation of health care resources.

1. Freedom-based justice is concerned with those distributions of goods made in accord with the notion of the moral community as a peaceable community. It will therefore require the consent of the individuals involved in a historical, cultural nexus of justice-regarding institutions in conformity with the principle of autonomy. The principle of beneficence is pursued within constraints set by the principle of autonomy.

2. Goals-based justice is concerned with the achievement of the good of individuals in society, and where the pursuit of beneficence is not constrained by a strong principle of autonomy. Such justice will vary as one attempts to (a) give each person an equal share; (b) give each person what that person needs; (c) give each person a distribution as a part of a system designed to achieve the greatest balance of benefits over harms for the greatest number of persons; and (d) give each person a distribution as a part of a system designed to maximize the advantage of the least-well-off class within conditions of equal liberty for all and of fair opportunity. . . .

[A] market approach maximizes free choice in the sense of minimizing interventions in the free associations of individuals and in the disposition of private property. In not intervening, it allows individuals to choose as they wish and as they are able what they hold to be best for their health care. It makes no pretense at cost containment. Health care will cost as much and will receive as much commitment of resources as individuals choose. The percentage of the gross national product devoted to health care will rise to a level determined by the free choices of health care providers and consumers. If some element of health care becomes too expensive or not worth as much as a competing possible expenditure, individuals will engage in cost containment through not purchasing such health care, and its price will tend to fall. Finally, there will be no attempt to achieve equality, though there will be considerable room for sympathy and for the loving care of those in need. A free market economy, through maximizing the freedom of those willing and able to participate, may create more resources than any other system and thus in the long run best advantage those most harmed through the natural lottery. By creating a larger middle class, the market may tend to create greater equality at a higher standard of living and of health care than would alternative systems. Further, charity can at least blunt severe losses at the natural and social lotteries.

Whether one accepts a free market approach will depend on one's moral views regarding (1) the rights of individuals to create free associations, as occur in the market with physician–patient contracts; (2) the moral significance of the natural and social lotteries; and (3) the character and scope of private and communal ownership, as well as one's understanding of (4) the factual circumstances, that is, if and to what extent the market is in the long run the best provider of a high standard of living and of health care. If one holds that individuals and society have an obligation to provide a certain level of health care, which conforms to a particular pattern of distribution not achievable through the market and that the obligation overrides rights to free choice and the use of one's property, one will need to abandon market mechanisms either in whole or in part. . . .

A two-tiered system of health care is in many respects a compromise. On the one hand, it provides at least some amount of health care for all, while on the other hand allowing those with resources to purchase additional health care. It can endorse the provision of communal resources for the provision of a decent minimal amount of health care for all, while acknowledging the existence of private resources at the disposal of some individuals to purchase better care. This compromise character of a two-tiered system can find a number of justifications. The utilitarian may in fact find that this approach maximizes the greatest good for the greatest number because it is a compromise. In allowing free choice while providing some health care for all, the system supports two important human goals and sources of satisfaction (i.e., liberty and well-being). A two-tiered system can also be justified in Rawlsian terms insofar as health care is to be treated under the difference principle, that is, to the extent it is to be regarded as justly distributed if the distribution redounds to the benefit of the least-well-off class. One would then allow that amount of additional health care to be purchased by the affluent, which would maximize the quality of care for the least-well-off, or the general status of the least-well-off class.

[My] analyses of the principles of autonomy and beneficence and of entitlements to property support a two-tiered system of health care. Not all property is privately owned. Nations and other social organizations may invest their common resources in insuring their members against losses in the natural and social lotteries. On the other hand, . . . not all property is communal. There are private entitlements, which individuals may freely exchange for the services of others. The existence of a two-tiered system (whether officially or unofficially) in nearly all nations and societies reflects the existence of both communal and private entitlements, of social choice and individual aspiration. A two-tiered system with inequality in health care distribution would appear to be both morally and factually inevitable.

The serious task will be to decide how to create a decent minimum as a floor of support for all members of a society, while allowing money and free choice to fashion a special tier of services for the advantaged members of society. The problem will be to define what will be meant by a "decent minimum" or "minimum adequate amount" of health care. . . .

[T]he concept of adequate care will not be discoverable outside of an appeal to a particular view of the good life and a particular understanding of the charge of medicine. In general, smaller social groups, insofar as they share a common view of the good life, may be able to appeal to such a vision in order to discover what should count as a decent minimum of health care within that understanding. In nations encompassing numerous communities, an understanding of what one will mean by adequate level of health care or a decent

minimum will need to be created through open discussion and fair negotiation. In some communities such as the BaMbuti, there may be little commitment of resources to the endeavors of modern health care. For such communities, a decent level of such care will be no care at all. In nations such as the United Kingdom, the decent minimum of care may not include hemodialysis for individuals over the age of fifty-five or coronary bypass surgery for any but the most promising candidates for surgical treatment (or at least there are informal ways of discouraging such treatment). For many, such a minimal level of investment may not count as a decent level. But one must remember that one creates through negotiation an amount of health care that becomes de facto the decent amount for the community as a whole, though it always remains open to further critique, discussion, and alteration. . . .

Rights are fashioned in terms of the content given to the duty to be beneficent to those in need. It is in terms of such visions of proper beneficent action that communities join together as nations to fashion large-scale webs of entitlements to health care and thus give content to beneficence through a system of rights to health care delivery. As always, however, particular communities may not wish fully to participate or may wish in various ways to have special health care systems with special rights and entitlements of their own (e.g., one might imagine Roman Catholics arguing that the provision of contraceptive, abortion, and sterilization procedures should not be provided through a national health insurance; on the other hand, one can easily imagine other communities wishing to provide such services through their communal insurance plans).

A web of concrete expectations is thus woven through the endorsement and negotiation of the men and women who constitute moral communities and who span moral communities through undertakings such as large-scale nations. In their weaving of patterns of commitment, they include certain goals and exclude others. Particular systems of health care are particular in choosing certain goals but not others, in ranking some goals higher and others lower. That patients in one system will receive care that they would not in another, that patients who would be saved in one system die for lack of care in another, is not necessarily a testimony to moral malfeasance. It may as well be the result of the different choices and visions of different free men and women. As we have seen, there are limits to our capacity as humans to discover correctly what we ought to do together. We humans must instead settle for deciding fairly what we will do together, when we cannot together discover what we ought to do. Even gods and goddesses must choose to create one world rather than another. So, too, must we.

NOTES

1. President's Commission for the Study of Ethical Problems in Medicine and Biomedical and Behavioral Research, *Securing Access to Health Care* (Washington, D.C.: U.S. Government Printing Office, 1983), Vol. 1, pp. 43–6.

2. H. Newman, "Exclusion of Heart Transplantation Procedures from Medicare Coverage," *Federal Register* 45 (Aug. 6, 1980): 52296. See also H. Newman, "Medicare Program: Solicitation of Hospitals and Medical Centers to Participate in a Study of Heart Transplants," *Federal Register* 46 (Jan. 22, 1981): 7072–5.

3. President's Commission, *Securing Access to Health Care*, vol. 1, pp. 18–19.

Problems of Macroallocation and Microallocation

PRESIDENT'S COMMISSION FOR THE STUDY OF ETHICAL PROBLEMS IN MEDICINE AND BIOMEDICAL AND BEHAVIORAL RESEARCH

Ethical Issues in an Era of Contraints

. . . The Commission has found that ethically significant disparities related to income, race, and place of residence still exist both in the adequacy of care received and in the burdens of obtaining it. Although local, state, and Federal efforts have done much to improve access, they have not yet succeeded in making equitable access to health care a reality for all Americans. . . .

CONCERNS ABOUT HEALTH CARE COSTS

The Rise in Health Care Expenditures. The dramatic rise in health care costs during the past 15 years has recently received a great deal of attention. Con-

From *Securing Access to Health Care*, Vol. I. Washington, D.C.: U.S. Government Printing Office, 1983.

cerns have been voiced about the higher total expenditures for health care generally and about the increasing share of government resources devoted to health care. In 1965, Americans spent $42 billion on health care; by 1981 total outlays amounted to $287 billion. The share of the Gross National Product (GNP) devoted to health care rose from 6.0% to 9.8% during this period. Not only has the price of health care goods and services risen at a faster rate than other consumer prices, but the growing share of national wealth devoted to health care has led to understandable concern about the limitations being placed on alternative uses of these resources.

The rise of total spending has been accompanied by a marked shift in the source of financing: government expenditures at the local, state, and Federal levels have accounted for an increasing share of total health care outlays. In 1965, 26% of all national health care expenditures were from public funds; by 1981, that figure reached almost 43%—that is, $123 billion of the $287 billion in total health expenditures that year. . . . [T]hese outlays take several forms, including programs that finance and deliver care for the underserved and the expansion of health care for the total population through the training of health professionals, the construction of hospitals, and research. In addition, the government provides an indirect subsidy for the purchase of employment-related health insurance (although this subsidy is not included in the $123 billion figure).

There is no magical share of the nation's resources that is obviously "correct" for health care. The important question is whether the level of spending reflects the priorities of the American people. Americans have traditionally placed great value on the ready availability of high-quality care. Most would not want to face sharp restrictions in the care available when they or their loved ones are ill. Nevertheless, there seem to be new doubts that the public is receiving sufficient benefits to justify the increased spending. The current preoccupation with rising expenditures may really reflect these doubts rather than dissatisfaction with the level of spending itself.

Eliminating Wasteful Practices. A growing body of expert opinion provides some foundation for this concern about whether Americans are getting their money's worth. Clearly, the availability of medical care has made and will continue to make a tremendous difference to health, for the population as a whole and for individuals with special health problems. Nevertheless, there is evidence that in some cases services could be produced and delivered more inexpensively, and that in other cases fewer services could be provided with little or no effect on a patient's well-being. Indeed, there may be instances when patients would actually be better off with less care. If inefficiencies could be reduced and inappropriate care discouraged, the total savings could be considerable. These savings could be used to improve the distribution of care, so that more people could enjoy the benefits of American medicine without diverting resources from other important social purposes.

Although there is general agreement that savings can be made, there is debate about how large the sav-

ings might be and exactly where they might be found. Information about the magnitude of inefficient and inappropriate care is scarce but the Commission is pleased that physicians and other health professionals, health care institutions, insurers, researchers, and others are now paying increasing attention to this subject and urges that further studies be done.

In addition to questions about the extent of savings, it is often not clear at what point proposed changes will go beyond the elimination of inefficiency in the production and delivery of services and begin also to have unacceptable effects on the quality of care. For example, when surgery is performed on an outpatient rather than an inpatient basis, there may be no change in the risk of complications, or there may be a slightly greater risk that is offset by increased patient convenience as well as lower costs. Thus, the identification of potential savings frequently requires evaluation of the relative importance of the different dimensions of health care.

Even without full consensus on the valuation of costs and benefits, however, there is already sufficient agreement to give credence to the view that the potential savings are substantial. For example, about half the patients treated in hospital emergency rooms are not urgently in need of care; many could receive better care at lower cost in a setting expressly designed for routine ambulatory care. Estimates of the percentage of hospital days that are inappropriate have ranged as high as 20%. Surveys in hospitals have indicated that 50–65% of the antibiotics that are ordered are not indicated at all or are being given incorrectly; one systematic study of ambulatory patients showed that 25–40% of antibiotic injections were unnecessary.

Laboratory tests and X-rays merit particular scrutiny, since the increase in their use has been especially dramatic. Although the automation of laboratory analyses has lowered the cost of individual tests, in some cases reimbursement methods have encouraged hospitals to increase the number of tests done rather than to reduce patients' hospital bills. "Routine orders," for example, for a complete battery of tests for patients entering the hospital are often still written, although many physicians have criticized this practice as wasteful. Furthermore, extra tests increase the probability of "false positive" results, which then lead to further testing and clinical evaluation (and hence additional expenditures) to rule out the apparent new problem. Similarly, studies have revealed that for most adults annual physical examinations provide little more protection than those performed every three to five years. Reports of the Food and Drug Administration suggest that of the 75 million chest X-rays done in 1980, at a cost of nearly $2 billion, nearly one-third were unnecessary because they were unlikely to either detect disease or affect its outcome.

Cardiac pacemakers can make the difference between life and death, but recent studies suggest that their use in inappropriate cases may mean the nation is spending large sums unnecessarily. Many patients now admitted to hospital intensive care units (ICUs) do not require the level of services such units provide. Since costs in these units are two to five times those in other parts of hospitals, a more careful selection of patients could save substantial sums; one estimate is that a 10% reduction in ICU use would save $2 billion and spare many patients the isolation and stress that such units create. It has been estimated that at least 25% of the "respiratory care" (treatments and tests for breathing and oxygen, often involving sophisticated machinery) now given to one in every four hospitalized patients at an annual cost of $5 billion is unneeded. . . .

CONTAINING COSTS IN AN ETHICAL WAY

Medicaid. Traditionally, proposals to trim the increase in Medicaid expenditures have sought to limit government outlays under a particular program rather than attempting to control health care costs through improvements in the functioning of the health care system. [There has been a] dramatic growth in public expenditures under this program: combined Federal and state outlays for Medicaid amounted to $30 billion in 1981, with the Federal government responsible for 55% of all program costs. The states have relied on limiting eligibility, placing limits on the types and amount of services available, and offering low reimbursements to providers in their attempts to contain Medicaid costs. Over half the states limited Medicaid benefits and/or eligibility in 1981.[1]

Considered within the ethical framework discussed [above], these cost-control measures are seen to worsen rather than improve Medicaid's ability to promote equitable access to care. First, . . . many people fall through the cracks of the existing system of mixed public and private insurance coverage. Medicaid eligibility requirements already exclude about half of all poor people, who therefore lack even the limited guarantees provided by that program. Restricting Medic-

aid coverage further will increase their numbers. As pointed out by several foundation executives, who are leading commentators on health policy:

It follows that significant numbers of poor Americans, the elderly and minority citizens may be subtly disenfranchised without us really recognizing that this is occurring by the simple expedient of freezing or dropping Medicaid eligibility requirements. Thus these groups may once again find it difficult to obtain the medical care they need.[2]

Beyond the question of eligibility for services, a second ethical issue concerns the adequacy of care. Arbitrary limits on the scope and amount of Medicaid services already mean that its beneficiaries do not secure adequate care for some health conditions. In some states, for example, the maximum stay in a hospital per year that will be covered is as little as 14 days.[3] This discourages hospitals from admitting Medicaid patients with conditions that may require extended hospitalization. Low reimbursement rates, which are considered inadequate by many providers, lessen their willingness to care for Medicaid patients, making it more difficult for such patients to receive mainstream medical care.

Similarly, the effects of "cost-sharing" on the ethical objective of adequate care deserve attention. Requiring patients to pay a portion of costs out-of-pocket is intended to limit wasteful use. For Medicaid recipients, it is more likely to discourage the use of valuable care (particularly in leading these patients to put off seeking care in a timely fashion). In the past, the requirement of copayment by Medicaid beneficiaries has been accompanied by a notable decline in the use of such services as prenatal care and immunizations—services that are generally regarded as essential for adequate care and as effective in avoiding costlier medical interventions.[4] Moreover, when care is received, even a small out-of-pocket charge can constitute a substantial burden for some Medicaid participants. Thus, these broad-brush devices not only appear undesirable from an ethical standpoint but stand in sharp contrast to cost-containment measures that attempt to distinguish between care that is important to an individual's health and care that offers little benefit (and is thus less critical to the preservation of well-being and the advancement of opportunity).

Third, a reduction in Federal funding of Medicaid would worsen existing inequities in the distribution of the cost of care. Since some of the care will still be provided, payment will simply be shifted to another source. State-supported teaching hospitals and local public hospitals will most likely treat a large share of the former Medicaid beneficiaries; they will pass these added costs on to other patients (and their insurers) or to taxpayers or they will be forced to use funds intended for other purposes, such as teaching and research, to care for these patients. The Health Insurance Association of America estimates that during 1982 hospitals providing a great deal of care to the poor will shift on to patients with commercial insurance $4.8 billion of the costs incurred because of reductions in Medicaid and Medicare. Physicians who do not turn away those low-income patients who are no longer eligible for Medicaid or whose coverage of benefits has been restricted will be forced to absorb the cost of these "charity" patients. Cutbacks in Medicaid thus are likely to transfer a greater share of the burden of caring for these individuals from the Federal level (where it is distributed more evenly) to state and local taxpayers, health care professionals, and privately insured patients.

Paradoxically, some of these cost-control measures may lower Federal outlays in the short run but may actually increase total costs. For example, people who are no longer eligible for Medicaid are likely to seek care in public hospital emergency rooms and outpatient departments rather than in physicians' offices and clinics. Yet hospitals are more expensive settings for routine care and are less likely to provide the information, preventive measures, and follow-up services that could control the need for costly acute care. . . .

Tax Subsidies. Several proposals to reduce the substantial tax subsidies for health-related expenses have recently been considered, and an initial step in this direction was taken in the 1982 Tax Equity and Fiscal Responsibility Act. . . . [H]ealth care expenditures now receive favorable tax treatment in a number of ways.

First, employers' payments of employees' health insurance premiums are not treated as taxable income to the employees. The Federal and state revenues lost as a result of this exclusion are estimated to be $30.7 billion in 1983. If such payments were instead given directly as wages, employees would have to compare the health insurance coverage they wanted with other things they purchase with their ordinary (after-tax) income. The favorable treatment of employer payments of insurance premiums has led employees (especially in collective-bargaining units) to opt for very comprehensive coverage requiring little, if any, out-of-pocket payments. Thus, they have little incentive to take the relative benefits and costs of care into account when seeking care. Many believe that this situation encourages greater use of services that are of only marginal benefit, which unnecessarily inflates aggregate demand for health care. Some employers, who provide extensive insurance coverage for all their employees, have responded by requiring increased cost-sharing of incurred medical expenses.

Several proposals have been made to alleviate this situation. Some have proposed that employer payments of health insurance premiums above a certain level not be tax-deductible to either employer or employee. Others would require employers to offer their employees a choice of health insurance plans and to give a rebate to those who select a lower-cost plan.

Proponents argue that these incentives would encourage workers to choose lower-cost insurance plans that offered fewer benefits and required greater cost-sharing by individual patients. As a result, employees and their families would be expected to become more sensitive not only to the cost of insurance but also to the cost of care, since fewer would probably elect to have very comprehensive, low-or-no-deductible plans.

Reducing the tax exemption would have several ethical implications. First, if properly designed, it is unlikely that such measures would compromise access to adequate health care. It is anticipated that comprehensively insured individuals would be encouraged to use less care that, according to their own priorities, is less beneficial than other uses of their own funds.

Second, this approach to cost containment would not have a disproportionate impact on the most economically vulnerable people who have the greatest difficulty in securing care. Since cuts in the government tax subsidy for employees' health benefits primarily affect middle- and upper-income families, they are likely to reduce total health expenditures by encouraging the people most able to pay for health care to be more selective in their use of services. From an ethical standpoint cost containment should not be aimed chiefly at those for whom access to care is most tenuous.

Third, reductions in the tax exemption would limit the use of public monies to support the purchase of care that is less essential to well-being and opportunity. A fair distribution of cost requires that government funds not finance the receipt of "higher-than-adequate" care for some individuals until access to adequate care for all is ensured. . . .

SETTING SOCIAL PRIORITIES

Society can honor its obligation to secure equitable access to care within the context of finite resources, but in order to do this it must set priorities about how health care dollars should be spent. All health policy embodies ethical principles and values that, although not always explicit, represent very different views about the nature of societal goals and obligations. The Commission's brief discussion of the ethical implications of several cost-containment approaches has focused on how such policies affect the goal of enhancing equitable access to care.

Although the drive to reduce spending on social programs currently holds center stage, the Commission does not accept the position that improvements in access must wait in the wings. Such a view ignores society's moral obligation to achieve equitable access and overlooks the fact that cost-containment efforts are acceptable only if they are compatible with other moral obligations. Improving equity of access to health care need not be inimical to true cost containment—that is, actions that control rising costs through modifications of the delivery and financing of care that affect everyone in the society.

There appears to be a growing acceptance of the position that improvements can be made in the health care system. People are taking greater interest in their health and wish to be more involved in decisions about their care. Moreover, consumers are increasingly indicating a willingness to take account of the financial impact of health care decisions; a survey conducted for the Commission found that two-thirds of the public want physicians to give them more information about the cost of various treatments. People seem generally more willing to address issues related to the financing and organization of health care: private insurers are developing more-efficient delivery systems; coalitions of insurers, care providers, corporations, labor unions, and consumers have been formed to identify ways to reduce duplication and develop alternative delivery systems; attempts by state government to control rising hospital expenditures show a readiness to think in terms of new methods of reimbursement.

These are examples of the serious—and laudable—efforts being made to address many of the economic and political problems in the current health care system. But the ethical aspects of health policy also need analysis of the sort that the Commission has attempted to provide in this Report. Unless these concerns are given explicit attention, society risks establishing policies that take account of economic, political, and scientific factors without giving needed weight to the ethical considerations. The Commission hopes that its efforts will highlight the need for such a process and will provide a framework that is helpful in analyzing the ethical implications of various policies.

NOTES

1. *Recent and Proposed Changes in State Medicaid Programs: A Fifty State Survey*, Intergovernmental Health Policy Project, George Washington University, and State Medicaid Information Center, National Governors' Association, Washington (1982).

2. David E. Rogers, Linda H. Aiken, and Robert J. Blendon, *Personal Medical Care: Its Adaptation to the 1980s*, Institute of Medicine, Washington, mimeo. (1980) at 3.

3. Personal communication, Intergovernmental Health Policy Project, George Washington University, Washington (Dec. 1982).

4. For a review of studies on the barriers to needed care as a result of cost-sharing see Geraldine Dallek and Michael Parks, *Cost-Sharing Revised: Limiting Medical Care to the Poor*, CLEARINGHOUSE REVIEW 1149 (March 1981).

U W E   E .   R E I N H A R D T

An American Paradox

The United States currently finds itself in a situation that would be comical were it not so tragic: Suffering fellow citizens are being denied health care resources of which we have too many! Almost daily, our newspapers bombard us with stories about the physician glut and the surplus of hospital beds. We are also reminded that our nation spends more on health care than does any other nation in the world. And yet we read of a three-year-old comatose girl being denied access to a nearby hospital simply because the child's parents are poor and do not have health insurance,[1] or a woman told, in midlabor, to leave a private hospital for the nearby county hospital, once again because she is uninsured.[2] Anyone interested could easily find fistfuls of similarly distressing vignettes from across the nation.

The denial of urgently needed health services to poor patients within sight of idle resources is a uniquely American phenomenon. It is simply inconceivable, for example, that a Canadian, French, German, or Dutch three-year-old comatose child would ever be denied nearby available health care simply because that child is poor. Similarly, to kick a woman out of the hospital in midlabor just because she is uninsured and poor would be considered completely uncivilized in these civilized nations. Sadly, it can be said that this happens "only in America."

CARING FOR THE UNINSURED

Of course, lack of health insurance in America does not ipso facto imply the denial of health care in times of need. For many years this nation has muddled through with a system that ultimately did make critically needed health care available to the uninsured

who were persistent enough to seek that care and who did not mind approaching the health system literally in the status of health care beggars.

The system worked as follows: For patients covered by health insurance, physicians and hospitals were effectively given the keys to sundry insurance treasuries—including the Medicare treasury—to scoop up whatever financial reward was "usual, customary, and reasonable." Implicit in this open-ended social contract was the understanding that these providers would somehow take care of the nation's uninsured poor. After all, the cost of such indigent care could always be fully recovered from third-party payers and paying patients through a process of "cost shifting." Although much lamented at the time by the commercial insurance industry, cost shifting actually served as a fig leaf over what would otherwise have revealed itself to the world as a national disgrace. It kept us in the club of civilized nations.

Eventually, the ever-escalating cost of that open-ended social contract struck both government and the business community as prohibitive. Since about 1980, these payers have sought to force health care providers into a game of financial musical chairs, otherwise known as the "competitive market." The idea behind this arrangement is that physicians and hospitals should fight for their economic survival by attracting patients through whatever means might do the trick, including price concessions. In a nation that prefers arbitration through market forces to government regulation, the competitive approach to health policy obviously has a certain attraction. On the other hand, it should have been clear to anyone with a basic grasp of economics that, under the rules of a price-competitive market, the providers of health care would have little incentive to sweep off the streets the human debris of society. In such a market the cost of indigent care becomes a bother one likes to transfer to competing providers

From *Health Progress* (November 1986). Reprinted by permission of the Catholic Health Association.

through the practice not of "cost shifting" but of "patient dumping."

Under the old social contract the *cost* of indigent care was the hot potato passed from providers to paying patient. Under the newly emerging contract, the *bodies* of the uninsured poor themselves become the hot potatoes that are being dumped from provider to provider. Politicians ought not to feign surprise at this transformation, nor should they remind physicians of their Hippocratic oath. Indeed, to blame doctors and hospitals for the practice of "patient dumping," all the while refusing to legislate the means of paying for the care rendered to uninsured indigents, strikes me as disingenuous.[3]

POLICY OPTIONS

Americans have debated the issue of health insurance coverage since the end of World War II, only to demonstrate that, in this area at least, the fabled Yankee ingenuity has taken a long leave of absence. The United States now spends close to 11 percent of its gross national product on health care, more than any other industrialized nation in the world. Yet in spite of these enormous outlays, the nation has not succeeded in assuring all its citizens affordable, dignified access to health care—with "dignified" meaning the procurement of health care in a status other than that of a health care beggar who receives care in unpredictable fashion, as an act of noblesse oblige on the part of some kindly provider.

As I have argued at greater length elsewhere,[4] the nation's manifest impotence in this area reflects an inability to agree on the ethical precepts to govern the production and distribution of health care. We have not been able to decide whether health care is intrinsically a private consumption good whose financing should be the primary responsibility of the individual patient or whether it is intrinsically a social good, like elementary education, that should be collectively financed. We have not been able to decide whether the receipt of medically feasible relief from acute pain should or should not be one of an American's basic rights. Finally, we have not been able to decide whether the enforcement of these health care rights should be a federal or a state and local matter. Alternatively put, the question is whether a resident of, say, New Jersey should be at all concerned over what is or is not done for an *American* infant in Florida, and vice versa. Remarkably, this nation's answer to this question so far appears to have been, "The health care of an *American* infant in Florida is not really the New Jer-

seyite's business, and vice versa." The answer betrays a peculiar conception of nationhood.

For public consumption the nation's politicians have long allied themselves with the precepts of an egalitarian distribution of health care, as have the nation's business executives. The public at large, too, has flattered and soothed itself with the notion that ours is a one-tiered health system making the best medical care in the world available to all regardless of ability to pay. But these lofty protestations so far have not been accompanied by adequate funds. In a sense, the nation's poor have been victimized by the very loftiness of our professed goals—as well as by this sentimental nation's uncanny ability to confuse dreams with reality.

The design of a viable health policy for our nation must be firmly based on (1) a clear, unsentimental appreciation of this nation's social ethics and (2) an equally unsentimental understanding of the way in which public policy is legislated and implemented. Let us examine these two facets in turn.

From the vantage point of one who has been reared in the relatively egalitarian social ethics of two other nations, the frequently mouthed proposition that ours is an egalitarian society appears almost ludicrous. While it is true that this nation, probably more than any other, does provide healthy and well-trained individuals wide opportunities to seek economic advantage, it is simply not true that such latitude amounts to "equal opportunity," certainly not for persons born into poverty or ill health. We do not have a one-tiered judicial system, and we do not have a one-tiered educational system.[5]

Under the circumstances, it would be surprising if we truly aspired to a one-tiered health system. Having observed this nation's health policy at close range for the better part of two decades, I am persuaded that the best this nation's poor can ever hope to attain in health care would be a two-tiered or multitiered system in which the poor might be guaranteed unfettered access to critically needed basic care, but in which there would be perceptible differences in at least the amenities accompanying that care, if not also in the clinical quality of that care. To an objective observer with some international experience, that sort of tiering appears as inevitably American as the proverbial apple pie.

The second dimension to be considered in the design of a viable health policy is the political process by which that policy would be implemented. For better or worse, our system of governance is one in which political power grows to a considerable degree out of the power of the purse. Given the wide coverage the media regularly give to moneyed interest groups, it is surely not impudent to suggest that even the best intended health legislation has no chance of survival if it is not countenanced by the moneyed associations of health care providers and insurers who have always dominated and fashioned American health policy. To be viable at all, any policy designed to provide health insurance coverage to the poor must put added funds into the pockets of these associations' members, or at least it must not siphon money away from them.

HEALTH INSURANCE PROGRAM FOR THE POOR

The task at hand, then, will be to fashion a health policy that is attuned to these two particular features of our society: our manifest preference for an *inegalitarian* distribution of basic human services and the *political power of interest groups*. The two features make it unlikely that the United States will soon be able to implement an affordable, operable, universal national health insurance system of the sort now operating in Canada and throughout Europe. Indeed, it is not clear that such a system, if it could be introduced, would be in the nation's best interests because it would require a heavy regulatory superstructure that might stifle our health sector's penchant for innovation—an admirable trait of that sector.

A more viable and potentially humane alternative might be something like the following:

1. As a matter of principle, every American resident should be ipso facto covered by a federal health insurance program that covers a defined set of basic medical benefits. Persons who elect this program—and the bulk of Americans probably would not—would not necessarily enjoy the freedom of choice granted to fellow Americans who elect and can afford private health insurance. Publicly financed patients would have to accept nonemergent care from their choice of a limited number of competing health maintenance organizations. Emergency care could be sought from the nearest provider.

2. The program should be federal, in that a resident in, say, New Jersey should indeed be concerned over what health services are given to an *American* infant or adult in, say, Florida, and vice versa. Ultimate federal responsibility for the program would not preclude active participation by state and local governments in the operation of the program (as has been found useful in most other nations).

3. No U.S. health care provider would ever be asked to render needed health services to patients without a reasonable compensation. This compensation should be negotiated *ex ante* with national associations of the relevant providers. It need not be equal to these providers' *desired* customary charges, but should be high enough that no provider would actually lose economically by having treated publicly covered patients. Although the underlying fee schedules ought to be national in structure, there ought also to be adjustments for regional variations in costs.

4. This national program would be financed on the basis of ability to pay. One approach might be to include on Internal Revenue Service form 1040 a line labeled "Health insurance tax—enter X percent of adjusted gross income." If the taxpayer attached to form 1040 a copy of a private health insurance policy as good as or better than the public policy, then that taxpayer would be excused from paying the X percent tax. Instead, however, that taxpayer would be required to pay a much smaller Y percent toward a fund explicitly earmarked to cover part of the cost of the public insurance program.

5. Added funding might be garnered by eliminating one of the remaining tax shelters in the American tax code: the exclusion of fringe benefits (including employer-paid health insurance) from taxable income. Economists have long argued that this exclusion is not only economically inefficient, but horizontally inequitable as well.

Clearly this program would be a *national* program, but it would not be the type of national health insurance program operated by other nations and rejected by this country, after intensive debate, during the 1970s. It would be a national health insurance program primarily for the nation's lower economic strata, and only this program would be based on ability to pay. The rest of society could continue to seek coverage in the traditional way.

One of the program's political virtues would be that it would not constitute a major inroad into the business base of the private health insurance sector. The tax rate X could be set so as to preserve that industry's role in American health care. To assume that this powerful industry could be legislated out of existence would be unrealistic.

A second virtue of the program would be that it would free health care providers from the increasingly vexing moral obligation to render uncompensated care. Not only that, but it would put added funds into their pockets. Given these providers' current defense of the Medicare program, which they once fought so tenaciously, there is reason to believe that they might have learned from the experience and that they might now support a federal health insurance program for the poor if it offered the prospect of additional revenue.

INDIGENT CARE AND THE FEDERAL DEFICIT

It must be openly conceded that this proposed program would imply an added taxation, unless one were willing to add further to the nation's already indefensibly high federal deficit. Three observations may be registered on this point.

First, the alternative to an explicit, earmarked health insurance tax will inevitably be some other tax, albeit one carefully disguised in the hope that a (presumably) ignorant electorate will not perceive it as a tax or, if it does, will not be able to assess its ultimate incidence.

The hospital-revenue pools now being legislated in some states represent hidden tax systems of this sort. They involve the government's coercive power to divert funds from hospital A to hospital B. Such a diversion is a tax pure and simple.

Even more dubious and economically destructive is a widely proposed hidden tax going by the name "government-mandated employer-paid health insurance." Surely the imposition of such a requirement is a tax, because citizen A is being forced to transfer funds to citizen B. Worse still, the requirement would represent in effect a tax on employment and entrepreneurship, burdening in particular the small business firm and its potential employees—firms that have been the chief source of new jobs in the last two decades.[6]

It is not difficult to understand our politicians' preference for such hidden taxes in the current political climate. These government-coerced transfers among private individuals achieve certain political ends without letting the transferred funds flow through public budgets. The mechanism therefore allows politicians to raise (hidden) taxes, all the while pretending to be avid tax cutters. Furthermore, the device of hidden taxes relieves the legislators imposing them from any accountability for the forced transfers (hidden taxes). In short, such hidden taxes may be politically expedient, but their imposition does not strike me as an honorable form of governance nor, in fact, as an economically efficient one.

A second observation on the nation's current opposition to tax increases is a reminder that ours is actually one of the least-taxed nations in the industrialized world. . . . (1) . . . the U.S. tax burden as a percentage of gross domestic product (GDP) is low by international standards and (2) . . . this burden did not grow much at all from 1970 to 1982, contrary to public belief. Before the decade is over, this nation will have discovered that the only politically acceptable way to bring the federal budget into balance will be a substantial increase in taxes. Neither economic growth nor cuts in government spending will be able to carry the burden of that task by themselves.

To underscore the futility of placing one's hopes on future cuts in spending as a means of controlling the deficit, one merely needs to cite this nation's current policy toward its agricultural sector. In its issue of June 17, 1986, the *Wall Street Journal* observed: "New farm bill raises federal costs and fails to solve big problems. It will shower federal money on prosperous farmers and maintain surpluses." In their usually acerbic editorials, the editors of the *Journal* tend to blame such spending on the venality of members of Congress.[7] Curiously, these editors have kindly overlooked a front-page story in the Aug. 13 issue of the *New York Times* in which President Reagan is standing next to a 14-year-old farmer and a cow, unabashedly claiming credit for having committed record amounts of federal assistance to farmers, and reminding his audience (accurately) that the $26 billion spent on the farm program this year was more than any previous administration spent on the program during its tenure.[8] (By way of contrast, the federal government spent only $21.9 billion on Medicaid in 1985.)

If even this ostensibly budget-conscious president takes pride in spending billions of federal dollars on a program that enriches already well-to-do farmers, that pays farmers for not growing food, that uses tax money to store billions of pounds of unwanted cheese and butter and millions of tons of unwanted grain in government warehouses, and that charges American taxpayers a levy of $15 per ton for every ton of grain sold at this subsidy to the so-called Evil Empire, the Soviet Union—all for the sake of a few votes in the Farm Belt—then surely it would be reckless to expect that the federal deficit will effectively be reduced through future cuts in spending.

Eventually, responsible legislators will vote for the only remedy that will close the federal budget gap: an increase in taxes. With it, perhaps, they will find it in their hearts to legislate also an earmarked health insurance tax designed to alleviate for good the plight of poor fellow Americans (and their children) who cannot afford to pay directly or through health insurance premiums for the marvelous services our health care sector could, in principle, offer them. We shall then be able once more to hold our heads up high at international conferences on health policy.

NOTES

1. "Hospitals in Cost Squeeze 'Dump' More Patients Who Can't Pay Bills," *Wall Street Journal*, March 8, 1985.

2. *National Journal*, Nov. 24, 1984.

3. Some states, for example, have made the dumping of seriously ill patients illegal yet have failed to provide public financing for such care. It makes a thoughtful person lose respect for such legislators.

4. Uwe E. Reinhardt, "Hard Choices in Health Care: A Matter of Ethics," in *Health Care: How to Improve It and Pay for It*, Center for National Policy, Washington, DC, April 1985.

5. Although the leaders of private schools and universities may protest that access to their institutions is based strictly on academic merit, no one working within these institutions could honestly deny that family wealth and lineage act as a partial substitute for academic competence in the admissions process.

6. A lengthier examination of mandated employer-financed health insurance is offered in Uwe E. Reinhardt, "Should All Employers Be Required by Law to Provide Basic Health Insurance Coverage for Their Employees and Dependents?" unpublished paper, April 1986.

7. "How They Do It," *Wall Street Journal*, Aug. 11, 1986.

8. Gerald M. Boyd, "Reagan Pledges His Commitment to Help Farmers Overcome Crisis," *New York Times*, Aug. 13, 1986.

H. TRISTRAM ENGELHARDT, JR. AND MICHAEL A. RIE

Intensive Care Units, Scarce Resources, and Conflicting Principles of Justice

Let us never negotiate out of fear but let us never fear to negotiate.

John F. Kennedy

Humans often have the aspirations of deities, though never the resources. Intensive care units (ICUs) provide an example of the desire to provide an optimal level of care for all who require it, where "optimal" is taken to mean the highest achievable standard of care. However, recent budgetary retrenchments in the provision of funds for health care show that health care is not always an overriding public policy priority. Consequently, as a matter of morality and public policy, it will be necessary to determine at what point undesirable standards of health care are simply unfortunate, but not unfair in the sense of constituting a claim on further resources.

JAMA, March 7, 1986—Vol 255, No. 9. Copyright © 1986, American Medical Association.

We explore the distribution of health care resources by addressing the problem of allocating ICU beds (1) when further admissions to an ICU will jeopardize the standard of health care for all those in the ICU, (2) when those eligible for admission to an ICU (newcomers) appear to show greater promise of benefiting from treatment than those already allocated an ICU bed (early arrivers), or (3) when the investment of resources appears disproportionate given the marginal benefits likely to be obtained. These circumstances raise the issue of the rights of those already receiving ICU care to continue to receive ICU care. The second case raises the complex problem of how to take account of possible comparatively successful treatment responses, including quality of life outcomes, of early arrivers vs newcomers. How ought the merits of an early arriver, whose case is well known and who promises only a dim possibility of survival, and if so with an "unacceptable" quality of life, be compared with those of a newcomer who appears to show great promise of survival, and with an "acceptable" quality of life, but whose circumstances are less well known because he is a newcomer?

THE CARDINAL ROOTS OF INEQUALITY

All social systems for allocating scarce resources suffer from the difficulty that there are unavoidable circumstances leading to considerable inequalities among persons. These obtain even in the absence of any design or attempt directly to disadvantage others. These circumstances can be summarized under the rubrics of natural and social lotteries.[1-3] The term *natural lottery* can be used to indicate that individuals receive, for a variety of reasons, a wide range of talents, abilities, disabilities, deformities, and illnesses. Various forces advantage and disadvantage individuals in ways that either place them at need of health care and social services, or equip them with talents such that they are able to acquire an inadequate or abundant proportion of the primary social goods such as wealth, prestige, and social status.

In addition, there are circumstances that may be referred to as the *social lottery*. For a variety of reasons, some individuals are chosen by individuals or social groups to be the recipients of attention, jobs, love, care, or other benefits, while other individuals are not so chosen. . . .

The moral significance of natural and social lotteries, and the extent to which goods are privately or socially owned, will determine how, with justification, a distinction can be drawn between unfair vs unfortunate outcomes. For example, if losing at the natural and social lotteries does not per se vest any individual with a claim on innocent others for care, and if the goods sought are privately owned, then the fact that individuals in need do not find resources for treatment may be an unfortunate circumstance, not an unfair circumstance.

INSURING AGAINST LOSSES AT THE NATURAL AND SOCIAL LOTTERIES

It is impossible to discover a concrete view of a just system of health care allocation. Rational choice among competing possibilities for the ideal distributions of goods requires an appeal to a particular moral sense. However, there is then the difficulty of establishing to which level of moral sense one ought to appeal. An appeal to a particular moral sense may, in turn, require an appeal to higher moral sense, *ad indefinitum*. At best, moral arguments will be able to establish a range of acceptable models.[4] As a result, a morally justifiable concrete system for providing health care is best secured through common agreement, rather than through rational arguments alone. The recent report *Securing Access to Health Care* by the President's Commission for the Study of Ethical Problems in Medicine and Biomedical and Behavioral Research concurs with this point. As the report states:

> For the purpose of health policy formulation, general theories, as well as ordinary views of equity do not determine a unique solution to defining adequate care, but rather set some broad limits within which that definition should fall. It is reasonable for a society to turn to fair, democratic, political procedures to make a choice among just alternatives. Given the great imprecision in the notion of adequate health care, however, it is especially important that the procedures used to define that level be—and be perceived to be—fair.[5]

As the report indicates, a notion of adequate health care will in part depend on the judgment of health care providers and citizens generally, regarding notions of when expensive health care engenders excessive burdens and when the distribution of costs is unfair.

We propose that an apt metaphor for the elaboration of policy in this area is the choice of insurance policies. In great proportion the building, staffing, and equipping of ICUs and the establishment of guidelines for adequate ICU care, as well as the clarification of the rights of newcomers vs early arrivers in ICUs, reflect particular decisions among alternative means of insuring oneself against losses at the natural and, to some extent, the social lotteries. A certain amount of funds are invested in order to have services available should problems develop that would benefit incrementally from the availability of ICU care. Beyond that, insofar as ICU care is provided independently of the patient's ability to pay, individuals are insured against losses of the social lottery as well. The insurance metaphor also reminds us that resources for such expensive endeavors as ICUs must be provided in advance. It is not possible to take out fire insurance while the house is burning.

The development of a policy for the distribution of health care in general, and of ICU care in particular, represents the societal creation of an insurance policy that determines what will count as unfair vs unfortunate outcomes. . . . Fairness or unfairness will be determined by (1) the provision of that level of health care to which there has been agreement (eg, ICU care);

(2) the provision of health care under the circumstances to which there has been agreement (eg, in accord with the rules for the rights of newcomers vs early arrivers); (3) the opportunity for those who sustain the costs of care to determine its scope (eg, the nonprovision of ICU care to individuals with permanent loss of consciousness); and (4) the securing of general publicity regarding what services will be provided.

THE INTENSIVE CARE UNIVERSE

Intensive care units exist to provide close monitoring and frequent therapeutic interventions to patients who manifest or are at risk of physiological instability. Rapid application of labor-intensive high technology is expected to provide qualitatively superior health care outcomes with less comorbidity than routine hospital care. These benefits are purchased at great economic cost. . . . [I]n 1978 through 1979 at Massachusetts General Hospital, Boston, the entire hospital allocation for all ICUs resulted in an 18% budget allocation for approximately 7% of the total hospital patient days that year. These figures are consistent with the general observation of others.[6,7]

In this setting, patients arrive at varying intervals with a wide range of medical conditions. In some ICUs it is possible to maintain control over the balance between bed availability and new admissions by virtue of their point of origin. Such a situation might apply, for example, in surgical units where those who require care will need it by virtue of elective surgery, such that it may be feasible to delay operations when ICU beds are filled with patients deemed to be requiring and benefiting from the care. On the other hand, most ICUs in small and large hospitals admit patients from both the community and the inhospital populations who become physiologically unstable with little warning. In some locations, these ICUs may be the only available resource. In such circumstances, the health care system may operate on a stated policy that all in need of care (regardless of the likelihood of benefit from such resource allocation) will receive it; yet when the number of identifiable individuals in need of care in a given ICU or hospital exceeds the capacity of the facility to care for the identified patients within the usual standard of care, then a dilemmatic choice exists for the system either to raise the census (and thereby lower the established standard of care) or to look critically at the entitlement claims of both ICU early arrivers and newcomers to receive such services.

While the first alternative might seem morally acceptable to some, . . . such an option may constitute legally negligent behavior, particularly when the failure to meet established standards of care results in an uninformed exposure to risk and injury to an individual who would have benefited from the usual standard of care. . . .

CRITERIA FOR ADMISSION AND CRITERIA FOR EXPEDITED DISCHARGE

To direct the use of resources in cases such as the *Von Stetina* case[8] in a manner consistent with the proposed insurance metaphor, it will be necessary to develop general criteria for admission to, and continued treatment in, and discharge from an ICU. To frame such criteria, it will be necessary to determine indexes of likelihood for success, indexes of quality of success, and indexes of length of survival. The more considerable the benefits likely to be achieved and the more likely their attainment, the more appealing, all else being equal, will the investment in ICU treatment appear. However, all is not likely to be equal. Different patient circumstances will require different levels of investment of resources in order to pursue a benefit that is available at a particular probability. By judiciously balancing these considerations, one appeals either explicitly or implicitly to what may be termed an *ICU treatment entitlement index* (ICU-EI). The concept of such an index facilitates the development of explicit resource allocation policies and signals the circumstances under which it is prudent to provide ICU treatment as a part of the general societal covenant and society's insurance against losses at the natural and social lotteries.

Such an index will need to mark the permissible investment limits of costly treatments and technologies. Cost alone can defeat the reasonableness of a policy to treat. If societal resources indeed are finite, there may not be sufficient funds to treat all "needy" citizens at a cost of $6 million per person (even if the chances of success were 100% with an unimpaired quality of life) while maintaining at our disposal sufficient funds to support those enterprises that make survival worthwhile. Quality of life and cost may also lead to policy considerations prohibiting expenditure of funds. For instance, Karen Quinlan and Paul Brophy may come to mind who if they have no sentience can in no sense be the beneficiaries of treatment. Under such circumstances an individual can neither enjoy nor suffer from the actions of others. The worth of treating would then approach zero. The likelihood and degree of success must be considered in framing a societal policy. One would not be obliged to invest considerable funds with little likelihood of benefit, even if the benefit (were it achievable) would be full quality of life. It is not reasonable to regularly invest considerable resources in endeavors that are unlikely to be successful, even if occasional investments of such resources may have a symbolic value.[9] These considerations can be expressed in the following equation:

$$\text{ICU-EI} = \frac{PQL}{C}$$

where P indicates the probability of the successful outcome; Q, quality of success; L, length of life remaining; and C, costs required to achieve therapeutic success. As the costs increase and the quality and quantity of success decrease, the reasonableness of the investment (and therefore of the duty to invest) diminishes. The significance of the costs can, in part, be appreciated by comparing them with non-ICU care costs so as to indicate that the incremental value of ICU care is not justified by the additional costs. These reflections have a general significance and can be used to suggest when even modest costs will no longer be justified by the benefits they will realize (eg, providing a consideration in favor of writing "do not resuscitate" orders).

Also, there will be some score level cutoff above which it may be agreed that all should be treated. When more patients above such a cutoff level are in need of ICU care than there are ICU beds available, and they cannot be safely transferred to another hospital, then there may be moral grounds for overadmitting. To choose any particular ICU-EI as the threshold for the decision to treat is to commit a society to a particular investment of resources in ICUs rather than in other communal undertakings. Such choices, we have argued, should be understood as society investing in advance in a particular insurance policy for its members against possible losses of natural and social lotteries. Individuals who wished to purchase greater ICU care entitlement than that offered under the general societal covenant should have the option of purchasing private insurance to pay for the direct and indirect costs (excluding capital costs) not supported by the general insurance system, should a facility be willing to provide such services.

It is unlikely that societies will quantify quality of success in terms of expected periods of survival, other than to take cognizance of very short periods of survival. Thus, if a good quality of life can be achieved only for a few days at a high cost, then society may be able to agree that such a possibility of survival will not merit a major investment of resources for its realization. Societies will likely retreat from comparing the relative merits of different expected periods of survival once they become fairly considerable (eg, more than six months). Nor is it likely that complex comparisons of quality of outcomes will be made, though distinctions may be drawn between a survival with the capacity to perform the activities of daily living and survival without those capacities with a consequent need for long-term nursing home care. The point remains that some calculation of an index for treatment is better than no such calculation. Only through such an index, however informally drawn, will one be able to provide a basis for creating a societally endorsed and implementable policy regarding the use of scarce resources in general, and ICU resources in particular.

CLINICAL APPLICATION OF THE ICU-EI

Uncertainty of prognosis is nearly universal in individual cases and is argued by physicians to be the primary reason favoring treatment in ICUs so as to err on the side of possibly saving the patient's life. Such arguments are supported by data showing ranges of individual outcome in patient categories considered to carry varying prognoses.[10] These studies in medical and surgical settings tend to support the importance of underlying health status as well as the degree of physiologic end-organ dysfunction in predicting the effectiveness of ICU care.[11] Despite the prognostic insensitivity inherent in currently available scoring scales of illness severity,[12] the following fictive cases have heuristic value for the development of ICU-EI weightings.

CASE EXAMPLES

Case 1.—A 60-year-old woman, Mrs A, suffering with diabetes mellitus since the age of 15 years, has been admitted to the hospital from a nursing home for care of a gangrenous decubitus ulcer of the foot. Severe and poorly controlled hypertension preceded bilateral intracerebral hemorrhagic infarcts two years prior to admission. Mrs A has been severely demented since that time, requiring continuous nursing care. A devoted daughter visits her daily in the hospital. Mrs A has undergone uneventful amputation of her foot. One week postoperatively the patient is found slumped over in bed with a mouthful of gastric contents, cyanotic, with a pulse rate of 40 beats per minute. Endotracheal intubation and cardiopulmonary resuscitation are successful and mechanical ventilatory support is started with a dopamine infusion required for blood pressure support. Her daughter, who witnesses the event, insists that she be transferred to the ICU. The ICU, with a capacity of ten, has a census of nine.

Case 2.—Mr B is a 55-year-old man with adenocarcinoma of the colon diagnosed at colectomy one year prior to this admission. Liver metastases were documented at surgery and have failed to respond to chemotherapy, including selective hepatic arterial infusion chemotherapy. The patient is now admitted to the hospital with a three-day history of dyspnea and a temperature to 39.5°C (103°F). After five days of appropriate antibiotic therapy for documented bacterial pathogens in the sputum culture, the patient has developed impending respiratory failure. He is fully awake without pain, deeply cyanotic, and has an arterial oxygen partial pressure of 40 mm Hg on face-mask oxygen therapy. His physician requests transfer to the ICU in anticipation of endotracheal intubation and mechanical ventilation. His wife is insistent that he receive all the potential benefits of intensive care. The ICU (whose census is ten beds) is currently filled with seven patients and three additional beds are promised for three patients who are currently undergoing surgery with good to excellent surgical prognoses that should lead to a high quality of life. Mr B is a well-documented chemotherapy failure with a life expectancy of three to six months.

Case 3.—Mrs C is a 60-year-old widow with persistent hip pain following an unsuccessful placement of a right total hip prosthesis two years prior to hospital admission. Her respiratory function is severely impaired by chronic bronchiectasis and allergic airways disease. She is severely disabled due to her pulmonary condition and requires nearly total homemaker assistance. She is, however, alert and desires relief of pain that is intolerable. She consulted an orthopedic surgeon who declined to offer surgical replacement of her hip prosthesis, given the underlying pulmonary condition. Another orthopedic surgeon consented to perform the surgery and, in conjunction with a pulmonologist, informed her that the procedure would carry a 40% probability of death. Admission to the

ICU was requested and approved in advance of surgery. Surgery was complicated by severe intraoperative bronchospasm and profuse but anticipated surgical bleeding. The patient was admitted to the ICU from surgery and developed rapidly progressive pneumonia despite intensive antibiotic therapy, mechanical ventilation, and chest physiotherapy. Bilateral tension pneumothoraces required thoracostomy drainage, and ventilation was barely adequate due to the bronchopleural fistulas. By the 21st post-surgical day the patient's renal function has declined to total anuria, but dialysis is not yet thought to be necessary. The patient is intermittently awake but confused. The patient's brother and sister desire that all possible ICU care be provided. However, the ICU is currently at full capacity and the emergency room has called to inform the ICU that a 45-year-old man with multiple abdominal and thoracic gunshot wounds will need admission after emergency surgery. It appears that this patient's prognosis is favorable. All other ICU patients are thought to be salvageable, with good life expectancies and quality of life. However, interhospital transfer of these other ICU patients is not thought to be appropriate. It is also considered inadvisable to transfer either the man with the gunshot wounds or Mrs C. Mrs C is anticipated to die with full ICU support within one to four weeks. Transfer of Mrs C to a general ward may lead to an earlier death with a higher rate of complication.

These three cases offer a range from a lower to a higher ICU-EI. In the first case, Mrs A has a prospect of short life expectancy with very low quality. Though the costs involved in treating Mrs A will not be dramatic, a policy decision to treat such individuals would in the long run commit society to considerable costs. In this particular case, with this particular ICU, there is, in fact, one bed available and its use would not in and of itself produce inordinate costs, since the staffing and capital resources have already been invested whether or not this bed is used. However, a policy of admitting such individuals to ICUs will increase the daily census, causing such ICUs to be more often overadmitted. The long-range policy accommodation to that circumstance may then be to invest money in further expansion of ICUs and in securing an expanded staff. We, therefore, conclude that cases such as this should not be admitted for ICU care.

We draw this conclusion as a moral point on the basis of the insurance metaphor that we have previously introduced. We find it to be unlikely that reasonable and prudent individuals would expend resources in advance to acquire an insurance policy that would give them the privilege of having a few weeks or months more of life extension while severely demented. In short, we take this case as a clear example of when there should be unconditional nonentitlement to ICU treatment. Therefore, we recommend that public policy reflect what we take to be a prudent choice for the use of disposable resources: Government and third-party insurance programs should explicitly state that funds will not be made available for ICU coverage under such circumstances. As we have argued, such policies will need to be announced in advance to avoid confusion. The daughter ought to be able to be assured that it is the settled judgment of the participants in the insurance scheme that such coverage is not worth the investment.

Mr B, however, represents an instance of a class of individuals who should be acknowledged as possessing conditional entitlement to ICU treatment. His quantity and quality of life are marginal. Moreover, the prospects of a lengthy extension of life expectancy are close to nil. It is unclear how many individuals would indeed wish to invest resources in the purchase of an insurance policy to prolong their lives under the circumstances in which Mr B finds himself. His conditions of life are not pleasant. The circumstances, however, give some prospect of being able to treat him in the ICU and to return him to his pre-ICU admission status for a period of weeks to months. We, therefore, offer him as an example of a class of intermediate cases in which treatment should be offered if beds are available. However, one should not admit Mr B, even in an emergency circumstance, if this would lead to exceeding the census limit of the ICU.

Overadmitting in extreme circumstances might be considered . . . if all of the individuals to be admitted have a high probability of being saved and restored to a good quality of life and transfer to another institution is not possible. But Mr B would not qualify. Indeed, Mr B may need to be transferred from the ICU, should there be a need to admit individuals with a higher probability of being saved and restored to a good quality of life.

The third case, that of Mrs C, offers an instance of a class of individuals whose conditions, after admittance, may worsen, so that further ICU care is no longer warranted. We take her to be a case in which entitlement to ICU treatment should be withdrawn. When the initial commitment to provide ICU treatment was made, there were good prospects of being

able to offer Mrs C a considerable quantity of life at good quality. However, subsequent to her surgical procedure and during her ICU care, the facts of the matter have changed. It is no longer plausible, given her multiple serious organ dysfunctions, to expect a significant chance of offering an appreciable extension of life. To continue her treatment in an ICU with such dim prospects of success would be to invite the long-range expansion of ICU beds with consequent increases in costs. We find it plausible that individuals, in contemplating their investments for insurance coverage, would not see as a prudent investment the purchase of insurance that would provide ICU care in order to extend their process of dying for a week to a few months at most. This is not to say that in the passion of the moment they may not seek a few extra days' life, just as the person seeing his house on fire may wish he had purchased the most complete fire policy. But decisions regarding the investment of resources to meet various possible contingencies must be made in advance, considering that range of possibilities before any one of them is realized. Planning in advance for contingencies is exactly planning prior to any of the contingencies obtaining in actuality.

CONCLUSION

There will be a divergence of opinion concerning proper public policy regarding the provision of ICU care. Insofar as policies involve the common investment of resources, they may be resolved only by a communal decision. The proposal articulated here is offered as a policy alternative that would be embraced by most men and women if they approached the fashioning of public policy in this area as they would the purchase of an insurance policy against possible losses at the natural and social lotteries. The incremental contribution of benefits from ICU care will often not justify the acquisition of "insurance" for the unconditional provision of ICU care.

NOTES

1. Engelhardt HT Jr: Shattuck Lecture—Allocation of scarce medical resources and the availability of organ transplantation: Some moral presuppositions. *N Engl J Med* 1984;311:66–71.

2. Rawls J: *A Theory of Justice*. Cambridge, Mass, Belknap Press, 1971.

3. Nozick R: *Anarchy, State, and Utopia*. New York, Basic Books Inc, Publishers, 1974.

4. Engelhardt HT Jr: *The Foundations of Bioethics*. New York, Oxford University Press, 1985.

5. *Securing Access to Health Care*. President's Commission for the Study of Ethical Problems in Medicine and Biomedical and Behavior Research, 1983, p 42.

6. Russel LB: The role of technology assessment in cost control, in McNeil BJ, Cravalho EG (eds): *Critical Issues in Medical Technology*. Boston, Auburn House, 1982, pp 129–138.

7. *Intensive Care Units (ICUs): Clinical Outcomes, Cost and Decision Making; Health Technology Case Study 28*. Office of Technology Assessment, 1984.

8. *Von Stetina v Florida Medical Center*, 2 Fla Supp 2d 55 (Fla 17th Cir 1982), 436 So Rptr 2d 1022 (1983), 10 Florida Law Weekly 286 (Fla May 24, 1985).

9. Calabresi G: Reflection on medical experimentation in humans, in Freund PA (ed): *Experimentation in Human Subjects*. New York, George Braziller Publishers, 1969, pp 178–196.

10. Scheffler RM, Knaus WA, Wagner DP, et al: Severity of illness and the relationship between intensive care and survival. *Am J Public Health* 1982;72:449–460.

11. Knaus WA, Draper EA, Wagner DP: The use of intensive care: New research initiatives and their implications for national health policy. *Milbank Mem Fund Q* 1983;61:561–583.

12. Knaus WA, Zimmerman JE, Wagner DP, et al: APACHE—acute physiology and chronic health evaluation: A physiologically based classification system. *Crit Care Med* 1981;9:591–597.

SUGGESTED READINGS FOR CHAPTER 11

Battin, Margaret P. "Age Rationing and the Just Distribution of Health Care: Is There a Duty to Die?" *Ethics* 97 (January 1987), 317–340.

Bayles, Michael D. "National Health Insurance and Non-Covered Services." *Journal of Health Politics, Policy and Law* 2 (Fall 1977), 335–348.

Beauchamp, Tom L., and Childress, James F. *Principles of Biomedical Ethics*. 3rd edition. New York: Oxford University Press, 1989. Chap. 6.

Blank, Robert. *Rationing Medicine*. New York: Columbia University Press, 1988.

Brody, Baruch. "Health Care for the Haves and Have-Nots: Toward a Just Basis of Distribution." In Shelp, E. E., ed. *Justice and Health Care*. Boston, Mass.: D. Reidel, 1981, pp. 151–159.

Buchanan, Allen. "Justice: A Philosophical Review." In Shelp, Earl, ed. *Justice and Health Care*. Boston, Mass.: D. Reidel, 1981, pp. 3–21.

Callahan, Daniel. *Setting Limits: Medical Goals in an Aging Society*. New York: Simon & Schuster, 1987.

Childress, James F. "A Right to Health Care?" *Journal of Medicine and Philosophy* 4 (June 1979), 132–147.

———. "Ensuring Care, Respect, and Fairness for the Elderly." *Hastings Center Report* 14 (October 1984), 27–31.

———. "Rights to Health Care in a Democratic Society." In Humber, James, and Almeder, Robert, eds. *Biomedical Ethics Reviews 1984*. Clifton, N.J.: Humana Press, 1984, pp. 47–70.

Churchill, Larry M. *Rationing Health Care in America: Perceptions and Principles of Justice*. Notre Dame, Ind.: University of Notre Dame Press, 1987.

Daniels, Norman. "A Reply to Some Stern Criticisms and a Remark on Health Care Rights." *Journal of Medicine and Philosophy* 8 (November 1983), 363–371.

———. *Just Health Care*. New York: Cambridge University Press, 1985.

———. "Why Saying No to Patients in the United States Is So Hard: Cost Containment, Justice, and Provider Autonomy." *New England Journal of Medicine* 314 (May 22, 1986), 1380–1383.

"Due Process in the Allocation of Scarce Life-Saving Medical Resources." *Yale Law Journal* 84 (July 1975), 1734–1749.

Engelhardt, H. Tristram, Jr. "Shattuck Lecture—Allocating Scarce Medical Resources and the Availability of Organ Transplantation: Some Moral Presuppositions." *New England Journal of Medicine* 311 (July 5, 1984), 66–71.

Fein, Rashi. "But, on the Other Hand: High Blood Pressure, Economics, and Equity." *New England Journal of Medicine* 296 (March 31, 1977), 751–753.

Feldstein, Paul J. "National Health Insurance: An Approach to the Redistribution of Medical Care." *Health Care Economics*. New York: Wiley, 1979. Chap. 19.

Freedman, Benjamin. "The Case for Medical Care: Inefficient or Not." *Hastings Center Report* 7 (April 1977), 31–39.

Fried, Charles. "Rights and Health Care—Beyond Equity and Efficiency." *New England Journal of Medicine* 293 (July 31, 1975), 241–245.

———. "Equality and Rights in Medical Care." *Hastings Center Report* 6 (February 1976), 29–34.

Green, Ronald M. "Health Care and Justice in Contract Theory Perspective." In Veatch, Robert M., and Branson, Roy, eds. *Ethics and Health Policy*. Cambridge, Mass.: Ballinger, 1976, pp. 111–126.

———. "The Priority of Health Care." *Journal of Medicine and Philosophy* 8 (November 1983), 373–380.

Havighurst, Clark C. "The Ethics of Cost Control in Medical Care." *Soundings* 60 (Spring 1977), 22–39.

Hiatt, Howard H. *America's Health in the Balance: Choice or Chance?* New York: Harper & Row, 1987.

Jennings, Bruce, Callahan, Daniel, and Caplan, Arthur. "Ethical Challenges of Chronic Illness." *Hastings Center Report* 18 (March 1988). Special supplement, 1–16.

Jones, Gary E. "The Right to Health Care and the State." *Philosophical Quarterly* 33 (1983), 278–287.

Jonsen, Albert R. "Health-Care: Right to Health-Care Services." In Reich, Warren T., ed. *Encyclopedia of Bioethics*. New York: Free Press, 1978. Vol. 2, pp. 623–630.

Journal of Medicine and Philosophy 4 (1979). Special issue on "The Right to Health Care."

Journal of Medicine and Philosophy 13 (1988). Special issue on "Justice Between Generations and Health Care for the Elderly."

Lomasky, Loren E. "Medical Progress and National Health Care." *Philosophy and Public Affairs* 10 (Winter 1981), 65–88.

Mechanic, David. *From Advocacy to Allocation: The Evolving American Health Care System*. New York: Free Press, 1986.

Menzel, Paul T. *Medical Costs, Moral Choices*. New Haven, Conn.: Yale University Press, 1983.

Moskop, John C. "Rawlsian Justice and a Human Right to Health Care." *Journal of Medicine and Philosophy* 8 (November 1983), 329–338.

President's Commission for the Study of Ethical Problems in Medicine and Biomedical and Behavioral Research. *Securing Access* _to Health Care._ Vols. I–III. Washington: U.S. Government Printing Office, 1983.

Ramsey, Paul. _The Patient as Person._ New Haven, Conn.: Yale University Press, 1970. Chap. 7.

Reinhardt, Uwe E. "Health Insurance and Health Policy in the Federal Republic of Germany." _Health Care Financing Review_ 3 (December 1981), 1–14.

Relman, Arnold S. "The Allocation of Medical Resources by Physicians." _Journal of Medical Education_ 55 (February 1980), 99–104.

Sade, R. "Medical Care as a Right: A Refutation." _New England Journal of Medicine_ 285 (December 2, 1975), 1288–1292.

Sass, Hans-Martin. "Justice, Beneficence, or Common Sense?: The President's Commission's Report on Access to Health Care." _Journal of Medicine and Philosophy_ 8 (November 1983), 381–388.

"Scarce Medical Resources." _Columbia Law Review_ (April 1969), 620–692.

Shelp, Earl, ed. _Justice and Health Care._ Boston: D. Reidel, 1981.

Smeeding, Timothy M., ed. _Should Medical Care Be Rationed by Age?_ Totowa, N.J.: Rowman and Littlefield, 1987.

Veatch, Robert M. "Ethical Aspects of the Right to Health Care." In Hiller, Marc D., ed. _Medical Ethics and the Law: Implications for Public Policy._ Cambridge, Mass.: Ballinger, 1981, pp. 53–72.

———. "The Ethics of Resource Allocation in Critical Care." _Critical Care Clinics_ 2 (1986), 73–89.

———. _The Foundations of Justice: Why the Retarded and the Rest of Us Have Claims to Equality._ New York: Oxford University Press, 1986.

Veatch, Robert M., and Branson, Roy, eds. _Ethics and Health Policy._ Cambridge, Mass.: Ballinger, 1975.

Weinstein, Milton C., and Stason, William B. "Allocating Resources: The Case of Hypertension." _Hastings Center Report_ 7 (October 1977), 24–29.

Winslow, Gerald R. _Triage and Justice._ Berkeley, Calif.: University of California Press, 1982.

BIBLIOGRAPHIES

Goldstein, Doris Mueller. _Bioethics: A Guide to Information Sources._ Detroit: Gale Research Company, 1982. See under "Allocation of Scarce Medical Resources," "Equality and Rights in Health Care," and "Health Care for Particular Groups."

Lineback, Richard H., ed. _Philosopher's Index._ Vols. 1– . Bowling Green, Ohio: Philosophy Documentation Center, Bowling Green State University. Issued quarterly. See under "Allocation," "Cost-Benefit Analysis," "Distributive Justice," "Health Care," "Human Rights," "Medicine," "Resources," and "Rights."

Walters, LeRoy, and Kahn, Tamar Joy, eds. _Bibliography of Bioethics._ Vols. 1– . New York: Free Press. Issued annually. See under "Health Care," "Resource Allocation," and "Selection for Treatment." (The information contained in the annual _Bibliography of Bioethics_ can also be retrieved from BIOETHICS-LINE, an online database of the National Library of Medicine.)

12.
Health Policy

We are generally agreed as a society that government is constituted to protect citizens against risk from the environment, risk from external invasion, risk from crime, risk from fire, risk from highway accidents, and the like. It seems a natural extension that government is obligated to protect citizens against risks to health and safety, and health policies have often been fashioned to this end. As a matter of justice, many have argued that we should allocate funds to eradicate or at least reduce infectious disease, environmental pollution, automobile hazards that produce injuries and deaths, tobacco use, alcohol use, drugs that induce deaths and disabilities, hazards of the workplace, and the ineffective distribution of medical care.

Testing, screening, preventive measures, health education, and policy development are costly, however, and it has been objected that in many cases the costs are more than we can or should bear. These allocational questions resemble the problems of justice encountered in Chapter 11. But questions of liberty and autonomy are no less insistent in health policy. These questions range from freedom from burdensome taxation to the right to control personal information (issues of privacy and confidentiality).

A major part of this question concerns the extent to which government should restrain or encourage competitive, free-market activities in the interest of health, safety, and the environment—a matter about which we do not seem, as a society, to have settled convictions. For example, although almost everyone now agrees that the primary responsibilities for risk reduction and disclosure of information about risk in the workplace are those of employers rather than government, there is no consensus regarding the actual role of government in effecting the process. There are also a number of questions about whether government should stimulate competition in the health care industry, especially by encouraging for-profit health care. Finally, there is substantial controversy about the *methods* that may be used to develop policies to protect the public, workers, and the environment. These methods include disclosure of information about risks as well as risk-reduction and cost-reduction techniques. In this chapter these topics in health policy are under active debate.

COST/BENEFIT ANALYSIS

Cost/benefit analysis (CBA) is one of the most controversial tools for deciding which programs should be encouraged or funded. This technique has become widely used in both government and industry as a systematic, analytical framework that can serve as the basis for developing health policies and evaluating medical technologies. Cost/benefit analysis has been presented as a device for the clarification of the overt and covert trade-offs often made in public-policy decisions. These are trade-offs, for example, between lives that will be lost and money expended on new technology that might save them, between environmental quality and factory productivity, and between the quality of gasoline and the quality of the health of those who produce it.

The simple idea behind these sometimes complicated procedures in cost/benefit analysis is that the analyst should measure costs and benefits by some acceptable device, at the same time identifying uncertainties and possible trade-offs, in order to present policy makers with specific, relevant information on the basis of which a decision can be reached. "Costs" is a broad term, as used here, covering any consequence that is disvalued and any depletion of resources required to bring about a benefit. These may be opportunity costs, financial costs, health costs, and so on. However, cost/benefit analysis concentrates on costs expressed in monetary terms, using quantitative measurements of these costs—for example, number of accidents, statistical deaths, dollars expended, and number of workers fired. The analyst then attempts to convert and express these seemingly incommensurable units of measurement into a common monetary unit, so that competitive costs and benefits can be directly compared. This form of monetary conversion is not essential to a cousin of cost/benefit analysis known as *cost-effectiveness* analysis, which simply displays which of a number of alternatives either maximizes the consequences, given a fixed set of resources (dollars, say), or minimizes the costs in order to achieve a desired consequence. Thus, cost-effectiveness analysis offers a bottom line such as "cost per year of life saved," while CBA offers analyses in terms of a benefit-cost ratio stated in monetary figures only.

Perhaps the main argument favoring use of both cost/benefit and cost-effectiveness analyses is that without a systematic evaluative system for discussing the costs of health care programs we may stand condemned to the arbitrary preferences of those who emerge in society as the makers of policy. Their decisions might be based on paternalism, on self-interest, or on an idiosyncratic sense of justice. For example, policy makers need to be able to ascertain in a systematic manner whether the cost of decreasing a risk is worthwhile when the risk is one of death; they must also be able to make that decision when expenditures to combat the risk dictate that resources be severely limited in other areas where there are also risks of death. The reduction of intuitive weighing and the avoidance of purely political calculations in making decisions offer the greatest promise in the cost/benefit approach.

The cost/benefit method contains weaknesses, however, as its proponents are quick to agree. There are difficulties in making commensurable all the units it is desirable to compare, and this problem can lead to arbitrary decision making. Cost/benefit methods have also proved difficult to implement. Economists have generally discussed how such analyses can be carried out in theory rather than providing practical examples, and those who might wish to structure such an analysis have sometimes been left without a proper means for reducing all trade-off variables to a single form. Another significant objection to cost/benefit analysis concerns whose values are to count and how many values can be counted in the weighing and assessment of harms and benefits. The old and the young weigh priorities differently, and some but not all persons rank the absence of suffering over the promotion of happiness—to take two examples. Some costs—such as the costs of making a patient insecure—may also be so difficult to quantify that they are lost in the shuffle. Assessments may also be subject to biased judgment and ad hoc specifications of "the method" to be used.

In this chapter Michael Baram presents a series of criticisms of cost/benefit analysis, and Herman Leonard and Richard Zeckhauser defend the methodology. The latter do not deny that there are ethical pitfalls in these analyses, but they believe the problems are not insurmountable. Their view is widely held: The cost/benefit approach continues to be viewed in influential policy circles as holding out great promise as a rational and ethically justified methodology for public policy analysis. But can that view find an adequate philosophical basis?

ACCEPTABLE RISK

Another important form of policy analysis closely related to cost/benefit analysis is referred to as risk assessment. The objective is to identify risks, provide estimates of their probability, and evaluate the significance of the risk. There has been a growing concern in recent years that the approaches we have traditionally used to determine acceptable risk are outdated and in need of revision. For example, we do not have an adequate grasp of the risks inherent in thousands of toxic chemicals, foods, drugs, sources of energy, machines, and environmental emissions—some of which may have serious and irreversible consequences. Intractable problems seem to confront our demands for scientific evidence, testing for side effects, and risk assessments. The *probability* of exposure to a risk may be known with some precision, while virtually nothing is known about the *magnitude* of harm; or the magnitude may be precisely expressible, while the probability is too indefinite to be calculated accurately. In many cases "wild guess" may best describe the accuracy with which risks of physical and chemical hazards may be determined—especially for life-long risks such as the risk of smoking or the risk of a worker who constantly changes locations, who works with multiple substances, and whose physical condition is in part attributable to factors independent of the workplace.

Because risk assessment is now a major factor in decisions about whether or not to permit substances in a workplace, to produce a new technology, or to evaluate environmental impact, the concept of risk and the scope of the risks under consideration should be made clear. The term "risk" is used to refer to a possible future harm, and statements of risk are usually probabilistic estimates of such harms. However, the *probability* of a harm's occurrence is only one way of expressing a risk and should be distinguished from the *magnitude* of the possible harm—a second way of expressing risk. When such vague expressions as "minimal risk" or "high risk" are used, they commonly refer to an aggregation of the chance of suffering a harm (probability) and the severity of the harm (magnitude) if suffered. Uncertainty may, of course, be present in formal assessments of either the probability or the magnitude of harm, and commonly major uncertainties exist in health policy. For example, in the workplace there is uncertainty as to the dangers of chemicals and how to predict health consequences.

One major question in risk assessment concerns what counts as minimal risk, sometimes called *de minimus* risk. For example, one might define a risk of getting skin cancer from sunbathing as minimal if it is less than one in a million for certain kinds of exposures. Any risk above that figure would be above minimal risk. However, there is no general consensus on what level of probability of a serious harm constitutes a risk high enough to demand steps to reduce or eliminate the risk or to require that information be provided to those affected. Only rather speculative (perhaps intuitive) guidelines have been suggested. For example, it has been held that risks (expressing probabilities of death per year of an individual's exposure to a given risk) below 1 in 1 million are acts of God too infrequent to merit attempts at control; that risks in the vicinity of 1 in 100,000 may be sufficient to justify issuing warnings; that risks of 1 in 10,000 merit public subsidies in an attempt to eliminate or reduce the risk; and that risks of serious harm greater than 1 in 1,000 are unacceptable.[1]

With the exception of situations of minimal or de minimus risk, most risks will be viewed as "acceptable" only in relation to the benefits realized by undertaking the risks. No one wants to take the risk of being exposed to a carcinogenic chemical unless there is a compensating benefit. For this reason risk/benefit assessments, rather than simply risk assessments, turn out to be the crucial instruments for health policy. Naturally, individuals vary appreciably in the amount of risk they are willing to assume, and this too complicates the development of health policy.

OCCUPATIONAL RISKS

Health policies are often gauged to protect against risks in the workplace. For example, the following kinds of hazards and associated health problems have all been the focus of sustained policy discussion:

Benzene (leukemia)

Asbestos (asbestosis)

Lead (destruction of reproductive capacities)

Microwaves (cataractogenic effects, decreased sperm count)

Petrochemicals (brain tumors, sterility)

Machines (ear damage from noises)

Construction (injury due to accident)

Cotton textiles (byssinosis)

Coal dust (black lung)

Hydrocarbons (childhood cancer in offspring)

Although the Occupational Safety and Health Act of 1970 sought to assure safety in the workplace, there have been no significant declines in injury and fatality rates since the act was passed. Government statistics show that there are approximately 6,000 fatal accidents and 5 million nonfatal accidents in the workplace each year in the United States. Disease statistics are either unknown or too unreliably gathered to be meaningful.

Relatively little is known at present about the knowledge and comprehension of workers, but there is evidence that in at least some industries ignorance is a causal factor in occupational illness or injury. A detailed study was done, for example, of the Hurley Reduction Works—a smelter owned by Kennecott Copper. It concluded that "the smelter's work force has little or no understanding of occupational health hazards, their evaluation, or prevention"—especially regarding airborne arsenic, sulfur dioxide, and copper dust, all of which appear in high to very high levels in the reverberators and converter areas.[2] The simple solution to such problems is, of course, to ban hazardous products from use. But to do so would entail shutting down many industrial manufacturing plants. Many of these products are valuable and there is no alternative product that can be substituted. For example, for more than 2,500 products that use asbestos there is no desirable substitute.

The main goal in regulating risks in the workplace has always been and probably always will be to determine an objective level of acceptable risk and then to ban or limit conditions of exposure above that level. However, this goal of safety is not the primary justification for *disclosures* of risk. Individuals need the information upon which the objective standard is based in order to determine whether the risk it declares acceptable is *acceptable to them*. Here, we might say, a subjective standard of acceptable risk seems more appropriate than an objective standard established by "experts." Choosing a risk generally seems a right that workers should possess, especially if it cannot be adequately decided by health and safety standards established for aggregated groups of workers. Even with objective standards, a situation of substantial ambiguity commonly prevails, where the risks are uncertain by the assessment of the most informed expert, and the dosage levels at which there is concern for health and safety can be made no clearer.

There seem to be problems about both the strategy of information disclosure and the strategy of protection, if either is used in isolation. There are often no meaningful figures defining the relationship between the acceptability of a risk and the ease with which the risk can be eliminated or controlled. There also may be no consensus on which levels of probability of serious harm, such as death, constitute risks sufficiently high that steps ought to be taken to reduce or eliminate the risk or to provide information to those affected. Moreover, the trade-offs involved—such as those between control of health hazards and increased production costs or between cessation of production and negative employment effects—are assessed differently by different parties. Worker representatives and management generally disagree about acceptable levels of risk, about appropriate epidemiological evidence, and about acceptable increases in corporate costs to control or eliminate risk. Workers' assessments can also differ markedly from those of government.

In one essay in this chapter, June Fessenden-Raden and Bernard Gert try to show how to reduce areas of disagreement, eliminate irrelevant considerations from the decision-making process, and provide an impartial procedure for reasoning about problems of hazards in the workplace. This procedure considers the costs, risks, and benefits of proposals and in addition demands universalizing rules in order to control for biased reasoning. The next essay, by Ruth Faden and Tom Beauchamp, appeals to the principle of respect for autonomy to support a standard of information disclosure and standards for determining whether a refusal to work or a safety walkout is justified.

TESTING AND SCREENING PROGRAMS

The capacity to test and to screen for diseases and disease traits on a mass, public health basis has increased dramatically in recent years. There is every reason to suspect that we will continue to enlarge the class of diseases for which screening is possible and that the number and kinds of mass screening programs will continue to increase as well. But these programs have moral problems that merit as much attention as their benefits.

A central moral problem for all screening programs is whether participation in the program ought to be compulsory or merely voluntary. "Voluntary" here means that every individual is free to decide whether to participate in the program and also free to refuse participation. For example, the state of Maryland has a law that compels hospitals to offer newborn screening for PKU (phenylketonuria)[3] and other metabolic disorders to all women immediately following childbirth and to obtain the informed consent of all women who decide to participate. Thus, participation in this newborn screening program is voluntary for patients but not for health care providers, in the sense that health care providers are obligated by law to offer screening.

The most widely discussed problem of screening in recent years derives from the spread of AIDS. This problem suggests a strong public health response, but presumably one consistent with confidentiality, liberty, and privacy for AIDS patients. Almost every dimension of the public health response to AIDS carries moral problems. Questions of justice include who should pay for AIDS victims, the effect on insurance policies, and the cost of and access to new treatments. Questions focusing on liberty rights—in cases where public health allegedly is in conflict with the individual—include discussions of quarantine, the right to work, the right to attend public schools, and laws requiring reports on AIDS patients. But the most difficult issue, and the one predominantly treated in this chapter, concerns HIV testing for mass populations.

The lack of an available vaccine or therapeutic treatment for AIDS has led to suggestions that traditional infection control techniques be used. Proposals specifically include the use of compulsory testing and screening of targeted, high-risk populations in order to identify individuals who have been infected with the AIDS virus. Questions have arisen about the accuracy of these tests, about the appropriateness of requiring participation, and about the role of medical confidentiality. We need, then, a set of general standards for the justifiability of compulsory (and also of voluntary) testing and screening programs. In this chapter Richard D. Mohr argues that civil liberties and discrimination are more threatened in the AIDS case than at any time since the internments of Japanese-Americans in World War II. He proposes a policy that allows a maximal level of freedom for the individual, and he also argues for a different way of framing the problem. In particular, he characterizes the present situation as one involving social discrimination and pleads for a premium to be placed on the rights of individuals rather than on general welfare and social ideals. In the following selection, Ronald Bayer, Carol Levine, and Susan Wolf argue in favor of a balanced approach that stresses the voluntary cooperation of those at risk. In this scheme, voluntary participation, research, health education, and counseling play a more important role than legal requirements.

FOR-PROFIT HEALTH CARE

In the last decade public policy has encouraged a competitive environment in health care, and with it has come a sharp rise in investor-owned health care facilities such as hospitals that operate to maximize profit, just as businesses do. Although the terms "competition" and "for-profit" are far from synonymous, a health policy oriented toward competition in a capitalist system is bound to eventuate in increased numbers of stockholder-controlled, for-profit corporations.

These policies and for-profit corporations have come under heavy criticism in recent years. For example, the following criticisms have all been voiced:

(1) The for-profit movement has created a medical-industrial alliance of such power that collectively it can control the course of public policy—for example, by blocking all attempts at national health insurance.
(2) Medicine is becoming a business rather than a profession, and therefore health care is becoming a commodity rather than a right.
(3) The for-profit motive works to block the indigent from access to health care centers while the rich are enabled to have luxury care and facilities, creating a privileged class with special forms of access and care.
(4) Competition and profit inevitably combine to cut back costs as sharply as possible, which will cause all close trade-off decisions (and perhaps non-trade-off situations) to be decided against the best interests of patients.
(5) The for-profit motive introduces a host of problems of conflict of interest, especially for physicians who own part or all of a facility and also practice medicine in the facility. Here the patient's best interest is squarely in conflict with the physician's financial interests.
(6) Medical research that has no immediate profit potential and medical education are both undermined by for-profit institutions.

Several of these criticisms are considered in the present chapter by Dan W. Brock and Allen Buchanan, who are fundamentally sympathetic to for-profit arrangements. They maintain that some criticisms of for-profit arrangements could turn out to be valid but that thus far the objections have been poorly formulated and are filled with questionable assumptions. However, they caution that this relatively new orientation of for-profit health care does have a significant potential for damaging the physician-patient relationship— especially its dimensions of commitment and trust—and for reducing the quality of care.

A sharp critique of for-profit hospitals is found in the next essay by Mark Yarborough. He argues that for-profit health care institutions are morally inappropriate for the delivery of health care. His argument begins from a premise about the commitment of a physician to a patient: The basic obligation of the physician is to restore the patient's autonomy insofar as it has been affected by illness and suffering. Hospitals have the goal of facilitating this objective, but for-profits will be tempted to forsake this goal in the interests of returning profits to investors. From Yarborough's perspective, they have every motive to do so, because their primary obligation is to stockholders rather than to either patients or physicians. This arrangement encourages the institution to exploit both physicians and patients while failing to facilitate their relationship.

The underlying problem in these discussions is not whether for-profit arrangements should be allowed. The profit motive has always played an important role in the fee-for-service system of paying for physicians' services, and also in purchasing pharmaceutical products and medical devices. The major questions are whether we should continue to develop policies that offer incentives to for-profit institutions such as hospitals and treatment centers and whether a just allocation of health care resources can be achieved under a for-profit health care system.

T.L.B.

NOTES

1. *Royal Commission on Environmental Pollution*, 6th Report, Cmnd 6618 (London: HMSO, 1976.).
2. Manuel Gomez et al., "Kennecott/Hurley," in Vol. 3 of *At Work in Copper: Occupational Health and Safety in Copper Smelting* (New York: Inform, 1979), p. 132.
3. An inborn error of metabolism that, if untreated, can lead to mental retardation.

HERMAN B. LEONARD
AND RICHARD J. ZECKHAUSER

Cost-Benefit Analysis Applied to Risks:
Its Philosophy and Legitimacy

Cost-benefit analysis, particularly as applied to public decisions involving risks to life and health, has not been notably popular. A number of setbacks—Three Mile Island is perhaps the most memorable—called into question the reliability of analytic approaches to risk issues, as well as the competence of public regulators and decision-makers. The public does not always believe that cost-benefit analyses employ its values, or that analysis is conducted dispassionately on its behalf.

In this chapter we examine the basis for this mistrust. Why does cost-benefit analysis not enjoy greater public acceptance and a better general reputation? We shall focus on the philosophical principles underlying cost-benefit analysis. On what bases can they be supported? We shall also examine problems of implementation. How can cost-benefit analysis be expected to perform in practice?

We shall not attempt a systematic review of the use of cost-benefit techniques. Any technique employed in the political process may be distorted to suit parochial ends and particular interest groups. Cost-benefit analysis can be an advocacy weapon, and it can be used by knaves. But it does not create knaves, and to some extent it may even police their behavior. The critical question is whether it is more or less subject to manipulation than alternative decision processes. Our claim is that its ultimate grounding in analytic disciplines affords some protection. It is widely (though not universally) agreed that cost-benefit analyses should be subjected to scrutiny and debate, and that the expressed preferences of the citizenry are the appropriate

reference in making value judgments. Risks to lives or property, for example, should be assigned the same value by government decision-makers that the individuals at risk themselves would apply. We do not believe that cost-benefit analysis is inherently easier to abuse than any other system used to guide decisions.

The misuse charge is not, however, the primary objection to cost-benefit analysis. Most of those who claim that it is misused in practice would not be satisfied if, for example, a science court were made responsible for objective use of the discipline. Many observers contend that the fundamental moral and ethical underpinnings of cost-benefit analysis are at variance with our ordinary moral judgments. This is the argument we will address. . . .

Risks to life, health, and property present a complex of troubling decision problems. Risks are especially difficult to deal with for three reasons. First, they are hard to measure; we do not generally know what "quantity" of risk is transferred or created in any given transaction. Even in private transactions like the purchase of an airline ticket, an individual will not generally know how much risk he is accepting. Second, people are generally unsophisticated in their treatment of risks. Even if fully informed about risk levels, they would have a difficult time interpreting them and making self-interested decisions about them. Third, people do not generally have property rights in risk levels to which they are exposed. Risks may be imposed or removed without compensation or charge. Quite frequently they are imposed by one individual on others: A drunk driver creates risks for others on the road; a nuclear-power plant may impose a risk on all individuals in its geographic area. In the language of

From *Values at Risk*, Douglas MacLean, ed., 1986. Reprinted by permission of Rowman and Littlefield.

economics, risks frequently involve public goods and externalities.

None of these problems would be particularly troubling if we could appropriately compensate injured parties after the fact. If we could costlessly identify the responsible party and measure the damage done, a system of *ex post* liability would lead to an economically efficient outcome. Only the creator of the risk would need to measure the risk level, and because compensation for damages would be guaranteed, no individual would care if risk(s) were imposed on him. Obviously, such a perfect system of *ex post* compensation is impossible. Many losses associated with risks—death is the most telling example—are not compensable after the fact. Even if they were, it is frequently difficult to identify the cause of an unfortunate outcome. Did the individual contract liver cancer from exposure to toxic chemicals or from his own voluntary use of alcohol? If there is joint causality, how should we divide the responsibility?

Since fully efficient *ex post* compensation cannot generally be arranged, society must devise institutionally feasible and morally defensible procedures for determining *ex ante* which risks should be imposed. This [essay] concerns the use of cost-benefit analysis as a potentially defensible social mechanism for risk allocation. We consider the method both in principle (its philosophical foundations) and in practice (the features that have made risk analysis so controversial).

The central principle on which all of the following discussion rests is that if risks could be conveyed in voluntary exchanges as private goods, informed and competent individuals should be allowed to accept or decline them. We extrapolate from this basic principle to guidelines for decisions when voluntary exchange is not feasible. Since our analysis is complex, it is worth stating our basic argument briefly here.

Since many important risks cannot be exchanged on a voluntary basis, it is essential to have a centralized decision process that will regulate or determine their levels. In choosing among alternative projects that create different levels of risk, the government (or other responsible decision-makers) should seek the outcomes that fully informed individuals would choose for themselves if voluntary exchange were feasible. Risks are not different in principle from other commodities, such as park services, public transit, or housing.

In many public decisions, it is not feasible to compensate those who would have preferred an alternative outcome. In such circumstances, assuming that the changes wrought by the decision are not extremely large relative to an individual's wealth position, we use "hypothetical consent" as a guideline for government action. Our test for a proposed public decision consists of two questions. First, are the net benefits of the action positive? Second, did those favored by the decision gain enough that they would have a net benefit even if they compensated those hurt by the decision? If so, our principle of hypothetical compensation calls for acceptance of the decision. It would of course be preferable to carry out the compensation, but that is often not possible. (We will discuss the distributional concerns raised by this proposal.)

Cost-benefit analysis, which begins by totaling the gains and losses of each party, is the appropriate way to determine which public decisions affecting risk levels would gain the hypothetical consent of the citizenry. We know of no other mechanism for making such choices that has an ethical underpinning.

Basically, we are taking what might be thought of as a constitutional approach to the morality issue. What mechanism for making decisions would individuals choose if they had to contract before they knew their identities in society or the kinds of problems they would confront? Our answer is that, on an expected-value basis, cost-benefit analysis would serve them best and hence would be chosen.

Two strong objections to this approach can be raised. First, one can argue that it is never morally acceptable to take property, which obviously includes imposing bodily risks, without compensation. Some would even reject the notion of compensation determined by a legislature or a court, for there can be no guarantee that such compensation would be sufficient to obtain voluntary assent. We cannot defeat this argument on moral grounds. Speaking pragmatically, however, we would observe that requiring voluntary assent for every government action would essentially paralyze the government. A second major objection to the cost-benefit approach is that, while acceptable in theory, in practice it leads to the usurpation of private decision-making power, the growth of government influence in society, and ultimately the loss of freedom.

The first of these arguments might be labeled the libertarian objection, and the second the slippery-slope objection. We believe that, interestingly enough, neither of these views would be espoused by the most vocal critics of cost-benefit analysis, who tend to believe that it hinders government action and the free flow of the political process.

Cost-benefit analysis is unpopular, particularly when used in applications involving the determination of risk levels. We will point out some problems that we believe explain the method's poor acceptance to date and argue that efforts should be made to win wider support for it. Cost-benefit analysis is *especially* important where risks are involved because less formal methods, which may be used for more routine decision problems, are not adequate for handling decision problems involving risk. Without cost-benefit analysis, we would be forced to rely on an unpredictable political process. That process frequently leads to stalemate and reliance on the status quo; at other times it careens in response to popular perceptions and whims of the moment. The government thus has an important role to play in regulating risks by finding, developing, and legitimating methods for making centralized decisions.

We are not arguing that cost-benefit analysis is a perfect representation of an idealized collective decision process. Rather, we feel that it is both the most practical of ethically defensible methods and the most ethical of practically usable methods for conducting public decision-making. It cannot substitute for—nor can it adequately encompass, analyze, or consider— the application of sensitive social values. Thus it cannot be made the sole or final arbiter of public decisions. But it does add a useful structure to public debate, and it does enable us to quantify some of the quantifiable aspects of public decisions. Our defense parallels Winston Churchill's argument for democracy: it is not perfect, but it is better than the alternatives. . . .

DISTRIBUTION

Distributional considerations are closely related to the issue of how and whether compensation should be paid or required of the decision criterion for public choices. Two distinct types of distributional issues are relevant in cost-benefit analysis. First, we can be concerned about the losers in a particular decision, whoever they may be. Second, we can be concerned with the transfers between income classes engendered by a given project. If costs are imposed differentially on groups that are generally disadvantaged, should the decision criterion include special consideration of their interests? Should the public decision process weight the interests of each individual in society equally, or should more weight be given to the interests of the disadvantaged or the losers? This question is closely intertwined with the issue of compensation, because it is often alleged that the uncompensated costs of projects

evaluated by cost-benefit criteria frequently fall on those who are disadvantaged to start with.

The distributional issue is particularly prominent when risks to lives are concerned, as in the debate over the volunteer army. Despite the evident advantages of the volunteer military in terms of economic efficiency, many people are disturbed that the sons of the rich do not have to serve. Two of their objections appear to have logical support. (1) If the sons of the rich are not involved, we will enter more wars. Those who think that our nation is too bellicose may thus object on strategic grounds to having a volunteer army. (2) There may be an externality among members of a society that pertains to the social classes of its warriors. For example, if we as a society care more about the life risks members of the poorer classes take than about the financial compensation they receive, then we may judge that the poor may have suffered from the advent of the all-volunteer force.

This raises the natural question of whether lives or risks to lives are different from other goods in the way they affect our concerns about distribution. Would the same class of arguments apply if we were worried about excessively arduous jobs? Should this lead us to ban cigarettes, perhaps because the poor smoke them disproportionately and we care less about each other's smoking pleasure than about each other's health?

Accept for the moment that risks to lives are in some sense different from other risks. Is the critical factor the existence of different income groups within society? Or would we have the same attitudes if income were distributed equally? If we would feel differently with an equal income distribution, then we must recognize that we are hurting the poor if we deny them opportunities that they would take for themselves. Differences in medical care or health condition convey much stronger impressions of inequality and inequity than differences in income or wealth. Surely that is part of the reason that so much of society's aid to the poor is given through in-kind transfers, in particular of medical care. It may even be efficient if the middle class likes to make transfers in this fashion. But if it tends to cloud perceptions of income inequality, such a pattern of transfers may be a bad strategic choice by the poor or their representatives.

The question of whether and how cost-benefit analysis should embody distributional concerns is difficult to resolve in principle. At the risk of appearing to take inconsistent positions on this issue, we would argue that (1) it is theoretically quite possible to build such concerns into cost-benefit analysis, but (2) there are good reasons for not doing so.

We see no reason why any widely agreed upon notion of equity, or weighting of different individuals' interests, cannot in principle be built into any cost-benefit-decision framework. This amounts merely to defining carefully what is meant by a benefit or a cost. If, in society's view, benefits (or costs) to some individuals are more valuable (or more costly) than those to others, this can be reflected in the construction of the decision criterion. It may be difficult in practice for the community to agree on what the weights should be, and it will nearly always be difficult to implement such schemes, but it is hardly fair to criticize the method because the problem is difficult—unless we can propose some more effective way of coping with it.

Although distribution concerns could be systematically included in cost-benefit analyses, it is not always, or even generally, a good idea to do so. We should first make it clear that we regard decisions about the appropriate income distribution as one of the central legitimating functions of collective political organisms. It does not obviously follow, however, that questions about how the income distribution should be modified should be raised with each project a government undertakes. For several reasons, distributional issues should not be included in every public deliberation or indeed in any deliberations that do not significantly alter that distribution. Taxes and direct expenditures represent a far more efficient means of effecting redistribution than virtually any other public program. We would strongly prefer to rely on one consistent comprehensive tax and expenditure package for redistribution than on attempts to redistribute within every project.

The first reason for not considering distributional issues in every public decision is that they may be handled more consistently through a specialized function than if treated piecemeal. If distributional issues are considered everywhere, this is likely to mean that they will be adequately, carefully, and correctly treated nowhere. Assuming a given social propensity to redistribute, we suspect that the more diffused the redistribution process is, the less will be accomplished in total. Many critics of cost-benefit analysis believe that project-based distributional analysis would constitute a net *addition* to society's total redistributional effort; we suggest that it might instead be only an inefficient substitution. It therefore seems unwise, from the perspective of the very individuals whose welfare is at stake, to ask each separate public decision to carry part of the burden of income redistribution.

Second, treating distributional concerns within each project can only lead to transfers within the group affected by a project, often only a small subset of the community. Why should the larger society not share the burden of redistribution? It is unrealistic to expect project-based cost-benefit analysis to result in a fully equitable distribution of welfare across parties affected by the project. Cost-benefit analysis for a particular project should reflect distributional considerations only *within the confines of the project*. If we observe, for example, that those construction workers who bear the greatest risks in building public projects are also the poorest, some might want to weight costs imposed upon or benefits given to them more heavily. We should not, however, expect that doing so will correct basic underlying inequities in the distribution of income.

Third, the view that distributional considerations should be treated project by project appears to reflect a presumption that on average they do not balance out— that is, that some groups systematically lose more often than others and that transfers should be directed toward those groups rather than away from them. Minorities are a commonly cited example. If it were found that some groups were severely and systematically disadvantaged by the application of cost-benefit analyses that ignore distributional concerns, we would certainly favor redressing the imbalance. We do not believe this is generally the case, however. The systematically uncompensated impacts of public projects are typically fairly small. If it is clear that one group will be substantially affected by a project, some form of compensation is usually offered. This implies that the biases among the remaining, smaller, uncompensated costs imposed must be severe indeed to constitute a serious inequity on balance. If identified groups are systematically found to be uncompensated losers—or winners not required to pay for the benefits they receive—we would support general redistribution toward (or away) from them rather than piecemeal consideration of their interests in every decision, and we would propose to carry it out through the explicit tax and expenditure system.

In spite of our general view that distributional concerns should be handled separately, we can see one important practical reason for including them in the project decision process. The usefulness of cost-benefit analysis depends very much on whether the public regards it as a legitimate decision criterion. If the use of distributional weights contributes to legitimacy, it may well be a trade-off worth making.

In summary, we would characterize our views about project-based distributional considerations as follows:

1. It is generally undesirable to include them in project analysis.
2. They can be included if it *is* desirable (or desired).
3. The uncompensated transfers engendered by public projects are generally small and largely random.
4. When there are large and systematic transfers as a result of public projects, we should—and generally we do—arrange compensation for them.
5. The principal argument in favor of including distributional considerations in project analysis is that it may improve public legitimacy, which is ultimately a crucial component of successful application of this approach.

CONSISTENCY WITH SENSITIVE SOCIAL VALUES

. . . Cost-benefit analysis, it is frequently alleged, does a disservice to society because it does not and cannot treat important social values with appropriate sensitivity. We believe that this view does a disservice to society by unduly constraining the use of a reasonable and helpful method for organizing the debate about public decisions. This does not mean that every important social value can be represented effectively within the confines of cost-benefit analysis. Some social values will never fit in a cost-benefit framework and will have to be treated as "additional considerations" in coming to a final decision. Some, such as the non-sacrifice of human life, may be binding constraints. We cannot make a cost-benefit-analysis decision concerning which values should be included and which should be treated separately. This decision will always have to be handled in an ad hoc manner.

Obviously, we have to be extremely careful to give social values an appropriate role, neither too wide nor too narrow. Widely held and vitally important social values will act as a "trump" to cost-benefit analysis. Many of these values are "brittle": They cannot be bent without breaking. Suppose, for example, that a town would like to take several houses by eminent domain in order to complete a highway extension that is justified on a cost-benefit basis, but it does not have sufficient funds to offer owners the compensation required by law. The social value of following the law is

likely to outweigh the cost-benefit analysis for that project. We cannot bend the standard of law easily, nor should we seek to, for if we do, we challenge the whole rule of law in society. We are willing to give up considerable short-run economic efficiency to retain this widely held value. Indeed, doing so will preserve efficiency in the long run, for it means that our basic operating rules are secure. Without this assurance, the economy will surely falter. We fully accept the role of "untouchable" values as overriding considerations in public decision-making. They do not invalidate cost-benefit analyses; they merely illustrate that more is at stake than just costs and benefits. . . .

ETHICS AND RISK ANALYSIS

Even those who accept the ethical propriety of cost-benefit analysis of decisions involving transfers of money or other tangible economic costs and benefits sometimes feel that the same principles do not extend to analyzing decisions involving the imposition of risks. We believe that such applications constitute a *particularly* important area in which cost-benefit analysis can be of value. The very difficulties of reaching appropriate decisions where risks are involved make it all the more vital to employ the soundest methods available, both ethically and practically.

Historically, cost-benefit analysis has been applied widely to the imposition and regulation of risks, in particular to risks of health loss or bodily harm. There are good reasons for this. Few health risks can be exchanged on a voluntary basis. Their magnitude is difficult to measure. Even if they could be accurately measured, individuals have difficulty interpreting probabilities or gauging how they would feel should the harm eventuate. Complementing these problems of valuation are difficulties in contract. Risks are rarely conveyed singly between one individual and another. Commonly, risks are a public bad, as when a factory pollutes the air. If voluntary acceptance of risk were sought, it would be essential to deal with thousands of individuals. This would not be an insurmountable problem if the dollar magnitude of the risk imposed on each were substantial, but frequently it is not. A decision that potentially imposes a risk valued at five dollars on each of 100,000 people is a consequential decision, but it would hardly be worthwhile to spend ten dollars to draw up a contract with each "participant." Even if transactions costs were low, the "land assembly" problem would still remain. Given that the risk cannot be conveyed in a manner that excludes a few persons who do not wish to join, individuals will always have the incentive to demand far more than true valuations. Technologies rarely allow some individuals to be excluded from a risk at a relatively low cost.

The problem of risks conveyed in the absence of contractual approval is not a new one and has been addressed for centuries through the common law and specifically the law of torts, which is designed to provide compensation after a harm has been received. If only a low-probability risk is involved, it is often efficient to wait to see whether a harm occurs, for in the overwhelming majority of circumstances transactions costs can be avoided. This approach also limits debate over the magnitude of a potential harm that has not yet eventuated. The creator of the risk has the incentive to gauge accurately, for he is the one who must pay if harm does occur. . . .

ETHICAL FOUNDATIONS OF COST-BENEFIT ANALYSIS

The critical choice of a standard for public decisions is between actual consent and what we have defined as hypothetical consent—the cost-benefit criterion in the absence of required compensation. The ethical foundations of actual consent are unimpeachable, but it poses insuperable practical problems. Hypothetical consent provides an ethically acceptable and practically superior alternative. It is not perfect ethically— elemental theories of property rights would reject it outright—but it seems to be at least tenable ethically. It may sometimes engender uncompensated transfers among individuals, but we suspect that most individuals, in forming their social contracts, would accept a public decision process with this drawback in order to permit making any public decisions at all.

This accommodation—trading off ethical purity for practicality—is not a fully comfortable one, for we are left endorsing a system that is less than ideal ethically and yet not obviously highly practical. How practical the system is depends crucially on our definition of practicality. If we take it to mean the ability to make a decision that we do not know is wrong, then many decision methods are practical, and cost-benefit decisions are no more so than a variety of others. We take practicality to mean something more: that the process is *workable* but still has a strong tendency toward the appropriate decision. With this definition both actual consent and an unfettered political process are relatively impractical. We would rate the three decision processes on three criteria:

	Ethics	Practicality	Legitimacy
Actual Consent	A+	D	A
Hypothetical Consent	A−	B	Unclear
Pure Politics	B	B−	A−

While actual consent is fully ethical and therefore clearly legitimate politically, its impracticality rules it out: It is simply unworkable. Unfettered politics, on the other hand, although politically legitimated, has an unsound ethical basis: It provides no guarantee that it will seek efficiency or pay attention to general welfare. It is also impractical, not in the sense that it cannot get things done, but in the sense that it may not take advantage of the best available information. By contrast, hypothetical consent is only a bit less ethical than actual consent, but it is considerably more workable. Its practicality is a combination of being workable and of systematically considering at least some of the more important issues involved in any decision. It shows some promise of being able to get at least some decisions "right," as well as some ability to ensure that the decisions that are wrong will not be wrong by much.

We have left for future discussion the issue of the public legitimacy of the cost-benefit criterion. Obviously, we believe that it should be politically acceptable and legitimated on the basis of its claim to a reasonable ethical foundation and its relative practicality. It is apparent, however, that it has not yet attained that stature in the community at large.

MICHAEL S. BARAM

Cost-Benefit Analysis: An Inadequate Basis for Health, Safety, and Environmental Regulatory Decision Making

INTRODUCTION

The use of cost-benefit analysis in agency decision making has been hailed as the cure for numerous dissatisfactions with governmental regulation. Using this form of economic analysis arguably promotes rational decision making and prevents health, safety, and environmental regulations from having inflationary and other adverse economic impacts. Closer analysis, however, reveals that the cost-benefit approach to regulatory decision making suffers from major methodological limitations and institutional abuses. In practice, regulatory uses of cost-benefit analysis stifle and obstruct the achievement of legislated health, safety, and environmental goals.

This article critically reviews the methodological limitations of cost-benefit analysis, current agency uses of cost-benefit analysis under statutory requirements, the impact of recent Executive orders mandating economic balancing analyses for all major regulatory agency decisions, and agency efforts to structure their discretion in the use of cost-benefit analysis. The article concludes that if the health, safety, and environmental regulators continue to use cost-benefit analysis, procedural reforms are needed to promote greater accountability and public participation in the decision-making process. Further, to the extent that economic factors are permissible considerations under enabling statutes, agencies should conduct cost-effectiveness analysis, which aids in determining the least costly means to designated goals, rather than cost-benefit analysis, which improperly determines regulatory ends as well as means.

From *Ecology Law Quarterly* 8 (1980), 473–475, 477–492. Reprinted with permission of the author.

COST-BENEFIT ANALYSIS AS A MEANS TO STRUCTURE AGENCY DISCRETION

DELEGATION OF AUTHORITY TO ACHIEVE MULTIPLE OBJECTIVES

In response to increasing concerns about risks to health, safety, and environmental quality, Congress has enacted several statutes providing new schemes for agency decision making. These statutes specify the problems to be addressed and the procedures to be followed, but provide little guidance on the analytical processes the federal agency should use in reaching regulatory decisions.

The statutes typically prescribe a variety of general policy objectives, decisional criteria, and legislative findings to guide the agency in dealing with the substantive aspects of its decision making. These factors usually fall into two competing categories: (1) the reduction of certain risks to health, safety, or environmental quality; and (2) the minimization of adverse economic effects on regulated entities, their employees, and consumers. In addition, an agency may be required to consider using the best practicable or available technology to reduce risks, promote energy conservation or national security, protect the small business sector, or encourage innovation.

Agencies must also consider the additional, and often inconsistent, objectives and requirements imposed by other statutes. Operating with limited resources and conflicting objectives, federal agencies must therefore "make policy when Congress could make none" and afford "a fair degree of predictability of decision in the great majority of cases and of intelligibility in all."[1]

USE OF COST-BENEFIT ANALYSIS

Defining Cost-Benefit Analysis. Cost-benefit analysis derives from simple profit and loss accounting traditionally practiced by business organizations.[2] Cost-benefit analysis

involves translating the attribute performances of alternatives into dollar quantities. The favorable attribute performances are added together to become the benefits. The sum of the unfavorable attribute performances is the cost. Thus, the cost-benefit analysis can be viewed as a process of deriving dollar values for each entry in a performance matrix and aggregating all of the performances into one attribute, either net benefits (benefit minus cost) or a benefit to cost ratio.[3]

A decision is justifiable when net benefit is positive or a benefit-to-cost ratio is greater than one.

Policy analysts have broadened the meaning of cost-benefit analysis to encompass virtually any analytical method that organizes information on alternative courses of action or displays possible tradeoff opportunities, thereby structuring decision making. Thus, the cost-benefit rubric encompasses many different types of analyses. Some of these analyses simply adopt a previously determined objective, leaving only the "cost" side of the balance sheet to be developed. For example, in establishing an emission standard for the discharge of ionizing radiation from a nuclear reactor, an analyst may be "given" a preexisting standard for the ambient level of radiation necessary to protect human health near the reactor. This standard represents a conclusive determination of the degree of social benefit to be achieved and reduces the analyst's task to finding the most cost-effective method to meet the ambient standard. Hence, the analysis in this truncated format is a simpler task of cost-effectiveness analysis. *Cost-benefit analysis*, then, is used by the decision maker to establish societal goals as well as the means for achieving these goals, whereas *cost-effectiveness analysis* only compares alternative means for achieving "given" goals. This article focuses on cost-benefit analysis.

Adoption of Cost-Benefit Analysis by Federal Agencies. The continuing efforts of regulatory agencies to balance competing considerations, such as public health and economic feasibility, are beset by a number of special problems. The technical problems include an ever-expanding, but limited and generally inconclusive data base, disagreement among experts on methods for using data, lack of consensus as to findings and their applicability to problems at hand, and unquantifiable attributes. Regulators must also value low-probability, high-cost events while taking into consideration the diverse and changing values of our pluralistic society. Moreover, an atmosphere of "crisis management" is promoted by statutory time limitations and pressures from various interests.

Mandated by statutes and recent Executive orders to conduct complex "balancing analyses" to reach decisions, regulatory agencies are under considerable pressure to adopt cost-benefit analysis.[4] The use of cost-benefit analysis in regulatory decision processes has been promoted by economic consultants and advisory committees to the agencies drawn from the scientific and engineering communities, including the National Academy of Sciences. In addition, regulated industries have urged agencies to use cost-benefit analysis in considering the economic impacts of regulations.

• • •

METHODOLOGICAL ISSUES IN REGULATORY USES OF COST-BENEFIT ANALYSIS

Many studies have identified the methodological limitations in the use of cost-benefit analysis as a basis for governmental decision making. Nevertheless, regulatory agencies continue to use cost-benefit analysis on many questions that present significant difficulties. The problems discussed in this section are not uniquely attributable to the analytical restraints of cost-benefit analysis, but stem from estimates based on scanty technical facts and the consideration of diverse values. Furthermore, many of the cost-benefit analysis problems are fundamental problems of the regulatory process itself, including good faith objectivity, effective citizen participation, and agency accountability. Other problems arise from unresolved constitutional problems, including the congressional delegation of broad and unguided authority to agencies and presidential intervention to promote consideration of economic factors conflicting with statutory requirements that stress health, safety, or environmental considerations. The following discussion briefly inventories methodological issues raised by the use of cost-benefit analysis in regulatory agency decision making.

One of the first steps in cost-benefit analysis is identifying the implications of regulatory options. Forecasting techniques notoriously fail to identify the possible primary, secondary, and tertiary consequences of a proposed action—particularly if that action sets a standard with diffuse health or environmental consequences that extend geographically and temporally. For example, analysts have great difficulty estimating the specific social and economic costs and benefits of regulatory options for controlling carcinogens. Cost-benefit analysis "offers no protection against historically bad assumptions. . . . [F]oolproof techniques for forecasting unforeseen consequences are by definition nonexistent."

The problem of inadequate or impossible measurement of attributes is related to the deficiencies of forecasting techniques. For instance, the "skimpy science" of toxicity is an acknowledged problem for regulatory officials seeking to measure costs and benefits of possible regulatory options for the control of toxic substances. Without the knowledge, techniques, trained personnel, and funds to measure these factors adequately, gross error in estimation may result. Similarly, many environmental effects, such as changes in ecosystems, cannot be estimated with confidence because no acceptable method exists to measure these attributes.

Furthermore, characterization of attributes may be problematic. An attribute deemed a benefit by an agency official may pose the problem of beneficiaries who do not desire the benefit or who do not even consider the attribute to be a benefit. For example, "cheap energy" is normally characterized as a benefit in a proceeding considering the construction of an energy facility. It may, however, be immaterial to those who have enough energy, or may be viewed as a cost to proponents of resource conservation.

Even if costs and benefits are identified, they may not be included in subsequent analysis for pragmatic reasons. Attributes may be too costly or too complex to measure. Exclusion may be based on a tenuous causal connection between the planned action and the possible attribute, as with the predicted probabilities of secondary or tertiary effects of a proposed agency action. Identified attributes also may be excluded for self-serving reasons. For example, if consideration of a possible disastrous consequence of a regulatory decision would tilt the outcome of the analysis against a favored agency action, it might be omitted from the final balancing process.

QUANTIFYING THE VALUE OF HUMAN LIFE AND OTHER TRADITIONALLY UNQUANTIFIABLE ATTRIBUTES

Cost-benefit analysis works best when (1) a socially accepted method, such as market pricing, is available to measure the costs and benefits, and (2) the measurement can be expressed in dollars or some other commensurable unit. Regulatory agencies using cost-benefit analysis face a critical problem when confronted with attributes that defy traditional economic valuation.

Analysts are well aware of these problems. Some refrain from placing their own values on immeasurable attributes and redirect their analyses. More typically, analysts recommend cautious use of cost-benefit analysis. Inconclusive analyses of valuation difficulties in cost-benefit literature reflect the hope that the problem will fade or be forgotten. For instance, although Stokey and Zeckhauser maintain that the complexity and importance of measuring intangible costs and benefits should not be underestimated, they ultimately conclude that perhaps quantification should be consciously postponed.

In some cases, it may be best to avoid quantifying some intangibles as long as possible, carrying them along instead in the form of a written paragraph of description. Maybe we will find that the intangible considerations point toward the same decision as the more easily quantified attributes. Maybe one or a few of them can be adequately handled by a decision-maker without resort to quantification. We will find no escape from the numbers. . . . Ultimately the final decision will implicitly quantify a host of intangibles; there are no incommensurables when decisions are made in the real world.[5]

This use of cost-benefit analysis is morally and intellectually irresponsible.

Today, a number of agencies assign monetary values to human life. The Nuclear Regulatory Commission (NRC) uses a value of $1,000 per whole-body rem in its cost-benefit analysis. This figure, multiplied by the number of rems capable of producing different types of deaths, provides dollar values for human life. The Environmental Protection Agency's Office of

Radiation Programs establishes its environmental radiation standards at levels that will not cost more than $500,000 for each life to be saved. The Consumer Product Safety Commission uses values ranging from $200,000 to $2,000,000 per life in its analyses.

But the fundamental issue is whether cost-benefit analysis is appropriate at all. Without an answer to this question from Congress or the courts, consideration turns to lesser issues: the proper method of valuation, the substantive basis for valuation (possibly relying on insurance statistics, jury awards, or potential lifetime earnings), and the extent agencies should articulate these issues and provide procedures for participation in the valuation process.

To date, agencies have expressed surprisingly little concern about these unresolved problems associated with cost-benefit analysis. Although officials deny valuing unquantifiable factors, these valuations are implicit in any cost-benefit based policy decision involving risks to human life. Responsible decision making demands that implicit valuations be acknowledged and addressed explicitly.

• • •

IMPROPER DISTRIBUTION OF COSTS AND BENEFITS

Every regulatory decision on health, safety, or environmental problems results in costs and benefits that will be distributed in some pattern across different population sectors, and in many cases, over several generations. For example, a decision to allow the commercial distribution of a toxic substance may result in economic benefits to the industrial users, their shareholders and employees, and consumers. It may also result, however, in adverse health effects and property damage to plant employees and those living near the plant. In addition, future generations may suffer mutagenic health effects or the depletion or pollution of natural resources.

Analysts and decision makers using cost-benefit analysis recognize these implications. Nonetheless, in the absence of public policy directives, analysts frequently apply personal assumptions about the allocation of costs and benefits while calling for objective "fairness" in dealing with distributional problems. Thus according to Stokey and Zeckhauser:

1. A program should be adopted when it will yield benefits to one group that are greater than the losses of another group, provided that the two groups are in roughly equivalent circumstances and the changes in welfare are not of great magnitude. . . .
2. If the benefits of a proposed policy are greater for one group than the costs for another group, and if it redresses the discriminatory effects of earlier policy choices, that policy should be undertaken. . . .
3. It is not so clear whether policies should be undertaken if they will benefit some groups only by imposing significant costs on others. It is sometimes proposed that a policy change should be adopted if and only if it passes a two-part test: (a) it yields positive net benefits, and (b) the redistributional effects of the change are beneficial. . . .[6]

Such earnest analytical approaches to determining fair distributions of costs and benefits ignore constitutional precepts underlying public sector decision making. Constitutional guarantees of due process, equal protection, property rights, and representative government should carry greater weight in solving the distributional problem than assumptions about fairness developed by economists and analysts.

Issues of temporal distribution, involving the allocation of costs and benefits for future generations, transcend even these constitutional values. Future generations possess neither present interests nor designated representatives to advance those interests. Our laws and values favor current benefits to those that accrue later. Cost-benefit analysis also reflects a preference for current benefits over future ones. Distribution over time, therefore, like the discount rate, is essentially an ethical issue for the nation. The assumptions that analysts must make about temporal distributions in using cost-benefit analysis are inadequate precisely because analysts, and not society, have made them.

PROMOTING SELF-INTEREST AND OTHER ANALYTICAL TEMPTATIONS

Users of cost-benefit analysis can easily play a "numbers game" to arrive at decisions that promote or justify agency actions reached on other grounds. The purportedly objective framework of cost-benefit analysis can be used to promote rather than to analyze options by manipulating the discount rate, assigning arbitrary values to identified costs and benefits, excluding costs that would tilt the outcome against the preferred option, and using self-serving assumptions about distributional fairness. Indeed, the very use of cost-benefit analysis leads some observers to conclude that the action under consideration is scheduled for approval. Even self-corrective measures are suspect. For example, the use of safety factors ostensibly chosen to avoid certain effects may prove to be a facile solution that does not alter the preferred analytical result if these factors are determined only *after* completing a preliminary analysis. Furthermore, these factors are usually based on technical estimates and do not properly consider the value-laden aspects of large, irreversible risks.

In addition, the "technology-forcing function" of regulatory programs can be stifled by limited technical and economic information. Governmental officials must often rely on the regulated industry for news of recent technological developments. Industry information is likely to be unduly pessimistic about the costs, reliability, and availability of new techniques. Thus, cost-benefit analysis based upon industrial information may become a mechanism for economically convenient regulation that tends to perpetuate the technological status quo. This result is particularly predictable when regulatory agencies have not defined their objectives. If such objectives were established initially, they would "drive" the regulatory process and more readily force development of new technology.

SPECIAL PROBLEMS OF ACCOUNTABILITY

The use of cost-benefit analysis raises new issues in addition to the usual problems of ensuring agency accountability to the courts, Congress, the President, and the public. Certainly the jargon, presumably objective numbers, and analytical complexities of cost-benefit analysis obscure the subjective assumptions, uncertain data, and arbitrary distributions and valuations of the decision-making process, thereby preventing meaningful review of agency activity. Agency uses of cost-benefit analysis tend to promote the role of experts and diminish the participatory and review roles of nonexperts.

Senator Muskie has voiced his concern about agencies including "questionable benefits" that can make projects appear "economically sound."[7] He has called for evaluating projects at different stages of completion "to find if the validity of benefits claimed at project authorization can be reaffirmed during and after construction."[8] No governmental agency has adopted this approach despite its obvious value in improving subsequent uses of cost-benefit analysis.

In its cost-benefit analysis of nuclear reactor licensing decisions, NRC estimates the population that will live near the reactor site in the future. Yet neither NRC nor any other governmental body attempts to control actual population growth in the areas surrounding nuclear plants. Thus the estimated cost-benefit basis for approving a proposed activity is not used as a planning tool for maintaining predicted costs and benefits once the activity is undertaken. The actual costs and benefits consequently may vary considerably from those projected in the analysis.

Additionally, the combination of fragmented regulatory jurisdiction over pervasive problems and increased agency reliance on cost-benefit analysis ultimately leads to increased societal risk. For example, a trace metal such as mercury constitutes a health and environmental quality hazard. It is regulated by several agencies, including the Environmental Protection Agency (EPA), Occupational Safety and Health Administration (OSHA), Consumer Product Safety Commission (CPSC), and Food and Drug Administration (FDA). Each agency may permit some activity introducing an additional incremental amount of the pollutant into the environment because the minor amount of calculable human exposure or environmental harm in each instance is offset by a broad range of postulated societal benefits. Even though each agency may be making careful and objective decisions, without overall interagency accounting for the increasing risk to the general population and the environment from these many small decisions, the total societal risk will continue to aggregate.

The above taxonomy of methodological problems reveals the need for a "best efforts" approach, fostered by Congress and the President, and administered by the agencies and the courts, to exclude the use of cost-benefit analysis under certain conditions and to resolve rational and humanistic concerns. This best efforts approach should focus on: (1) improving the technical and objective quality of cost-benefit analysis; (2) establishing the limits and societal implications of cost-benefit analysis; (3) improving public participation; and (4) designing more effective measures for congressional and executive oversight of agency practices.

NOTES

1. Friendly, *The Federal Administrative Agencies: The Need for a Better Definition of Standards*, 75 Harv. L. Rev. 873, 874 (1962).

2. See E. J. Mishan, *Cost-Benefit Analysis* 6 (1973).

3. Battelle Pacific Northwest Labs, Review of Decision Methodologies for Evaluating Regulatory Actions Affecting Public Health and Safety (December 1976), p. 53. See also E. Stokey and R. Zeckhauser, *A Primer for Policy Analysis* (N.Y.: Norton, 1978), pp. 136–137.

4. However, the courts have given the regulatory agencies a relatively free hand to establish procedures for conducting cost-benefit analysis. *See* Vermont Yankee Nuclear Power Corp. v. Natural Resources Defense Council, Inc., 435 U.S. 519 (1978). In that case, the NRDC challenged an AEC rulemaking procedure dealing with spent fuel from a reactor and the use of the rule in cost-benefit analysis for licensing Vermont Yankee's light water reactor. The District of Columbia Court of Appeals overturned the rulemaking because of the AEC's failure to employ certain procedural devices beyond the statutory minima. The Supreme Court held that the circuit court had improperly intruded into the AEC's rulemaking authority and remanded the case.

5. Stokey and Zeckhauser, *supra* note 3, p. 153.

6. *Ibid.*, pp. 281–282.

7. Letter from Senator Edmund Muskie to Comptroller General Elmer Staats (August 5, 1977), reprinted in General Accounting Office, *Improved Formulation and Presentation of Water Resources Project Alternatives Provide a Basis for Better Management Decisions* 18 (February 1, 1978), p. 19.

8. *Ibid.*

Occupational Safety and Health

JUNE FESSENDEN-RADEN AND BERNARD GERT

A Philosophical Approach to the Management of Occupational Health Hazards

It has been estimated that all workers at some time in their employment life encounter toxic material—most often without ever knowing about the hazard or the risks—with over 55,000,000 persons exposed on a regular basis. Although clearly there needs to be increased support for research in the area of occupational health, we cannot do nothing while we wait for more data. Even given this scientific uncertainty and disagreement, the appropriate role of government, employers, and employees in dealing with occupational health problems must be delineated now. The reduction of occupational health hazards by an agreed upon disciplined approach to these problems, an approach that goes beyond the traditional cost (risk) benefit analysis currently in vogue, is needed. Equally important is the question of what should be done when no exposure standards exist or the risks cannot be prevented.

This paper presents an analytical procedure based on a moral theory that can be used by government officials, employers, and employees when faced with analysis of an occupational health problem. The proposed philosophical-based analytical procedure will assist in determining the relevant facts and justifying the subsequent decision. While this approach will not provide unique answers in every case, we will show that it can (1) reduce the areas of disagreement, (2) eliminate irrelevant facts and reasonings from intruding into the decision-making process, and (3) provide a precise and objective procedure for reasoning about values and facts. . . .

Reprinted by permission of the Social Philosophy and Policy Center.

Many occupational-related maladies take 10, 20, even 40 years to develop, or may manifest themselves only in the next generation. The long lag time, the lack of exposure information and medical documentation, plus the impact of an individual's lifestyle, all serve to confuse and even mask the relationship between employment conditions and chronic diseases, birth defects, and reproductive maladies. Statistical inferences from retrospective epidemiological studies are notoriously unreliable. The true scope of employment-related health problems is just not known.

. . . Chemicals, natural and synthetic, are vital to our high quality of life and the U.S. economy. Also, it is known that most chemicals when used under normal conditions will not cause harm to the average healthy adult. In the workplace, unfortunately, conditions of exposure are not "normal"; that is, the concentration of the hazardous substance is often much higher than under so-called "normal" conditions.

Cardiovascular diseases and preventable deaths were found to be abnormally high among workers exposed to carbon monoxide, such as those employed in the veracose rayon industry. Blood and neurological disorders are associated with exposure to such chemicals as solvents (e.g. benzene, carbontetrachloride, and toluene) and heavy metals (e.g. lead, mercury, cadmium, beryllium) and are estimated to affect in excess of 500,000 workers.[1] Exposure to cotton dust has put nearly a million workers at risk of developing byssinosis (brown lung).[2] Hypersensitivity lung diseases, such as asthmas and allergic alveolitis caused by inhalation of chemical gases or fumes, occur not only among miners and factory workers, but are seen in high numbers among quite diverse groups such as artists, firefighters, and meat wrappers.[3] . . .

Six million workers are estimated to have been exposed to known or suspected carcinogens. It is variously estimated that from 5 to 20 percent of all cancers are occupationally related, with many of these concentrated among specific industries (e.g. those having asbestos and pesticide).[4] Using the American Cancer Society estimates of 835,000 new cancer cases for 1982,[5] that would mean from 41,750 to 167,000 new cancer cases are job-related and potentially preventable.

The U.S. Public Health Service in 1975 estimated that 390,000 new cases of occupational disease appear annually with as many as 100,000 deaths having been occupationally induced each year.[6] In excess of 800,000 cases of job-related skin disorders are diagnosed annually: the result of exposure to hazardous substances. It is also known that low levels of hazardous substances can cause subclinical changes, thus making some workers more susceptible to other illnesses. The true dimension of the occupational health problem is not known. And it will not be known until employees, employers, the medical profession, and the government are able to work cooperatively to recognize and correlate specific maladies to employment activities. Many occupational health specialists suggest that the workers most closely involved with an activity can often suggest the most practical ways of reducing the hazard. Paradoxically, in some cases, it is these employees that have not been made aware of the hazards. . . .

AN ANALYTICAL APPROACH BASED ON IMPARTIAL RATIONALITY

Since it is very difficult, often impossible, to prove that a health problem, especially if chronic, is the result of an employment-related exposure to a hazardous substance, and given the different self-interests, some procedure(s) must be available to justify the respective responsibilities of employees, employers, and government. This section presents and uses a morally-based analytical procedure that could be agreed upon and used to resolve disagreements, including determining the appropriate kinds and limits of government intervention as well as determining the responsibilities of employers and employees.

To morally justify breaking a moral rule (e.g. deprive of freedom or opportunity), it is first required that one determine[s] what facts are morally relevant to the specific violation. The first part of our proposed approach consists of four questions that provide a guideline for determining the morally relevant facts in each situation. These questions are:

1. What is (are) the moral rule(s) being violated?;
2. What is the amount of harm (its probability + severity) caused by the violation?;
3. What is the amount of harm avoided or prevented by the violation?; and
4. What are the rational desires of those toward whom the moral rule is being violated?

Once one has the answers to these four questions, one knows all of the morally relevant facts and can proceed to determine whether or not one regards that violation of a moral rule as morally justified.

The second part of the proposed procedure insures impartiality by requiring that a rational person use all, but only, the morally relevant facts determined as outlined in the four questions above, and then decide if the action described by these facts could be publicly advocated. If the rational desires of those toward whom the moral rule is being violated give their valid consent to the violation, this in itself provides moral justification for the violation, because all rational persons would agree to such a violation. But when people do not want the rule violated, we must consider whether at least some rational persons, given just these relevant facts provided by the answers to questions 2 and 3, would agree that the evil prevented by universally allowing the violation significantly outweighs the evil caused by such a universal violation. If no rational person would agree to the violation it is not morally justified. If some would, it is at least weakly justified. If all rational persons would agree to the violation, then the action is strongly justified and it would be morally wrong not to break the rule. While this procedure allows for moral disagreement, it should be able to reduce the points of disagreement and make clearer whether there is a disagreement on the facts of the case or on the ranking of the different evils.

When considering government intervention to regulate a hazardous substance, the procedure would be to first ask the four questions to determine the morally relevant facts, that is, to determine what counts as the same violation. Then one would decide if the regulation could be morally justified and determine if the violation could be publicly advocated (rationality is assumed). The four questions would be responded to as follows:

1. Regulations break the moral rule "Don't deprive of freedom or opportunity."
2. The amount of harm that regulation inflicts on both the employers and employees would be considered.
3. The amount of worker death, disability, and pain prevented by the regulation would be considered. Employer harm avoided, usually in terms of economic costs of worker absenteeism, medical and disability insurance, etc., would also be relevant.
4. The rational desires of those who are being deprived of freedom and opportunity (i.e. the regulated employers) would be considered.

. . . Recently several national management groups, as well as several unions, successfully convinced OSHA to reinstate a federal directive requiring a uniform hazard communication standard. The current plan would require labelling of over 300 hazardous chemicals, preparation of Material Data Sheets (MDS), and training programs. The unions supported the regulation as a means of informing workers. Some management groups desired such regulations even though they lost some freedom, because to have had separate states enacting different labelling and/or 'right-to-know' laws would have entailed complying with several different laws, resulting in a greater cost.

Employers who are conscious of the degradation of the environment by industrial pollution and who have diminished their own pollution output would be expected to favor certain clean water and clean air legislation. Without some federal mandate any pollution-conscious company could be put at a competitive disadvantage by an unconcerned company. Also, if there were only state regulations that differed from state to state, a given company would be disadvantaged or advantaged depending on the specific regulations of the state in which the company operated. Thus, concerned companies and/or companies operating in several states would be expected to support national legislation. In these examples, that of setting speed limits, pollution containment measures, and the labelling of hazardous chemicals, the primary justification is that considerably more harm is prevented than is caused. However, it is also true in these cases that most of the persons affected by the regulations have a rational desire to have their freedom curtailed in order to gain the greater benefits of such limitations.

The procedure we have been discussing may seem to be the familiar cost-benefit analysis with risk assessment tacked on. It is, however, important to distinguish it from (1) standard utilitarian cost-benefit analysis, which attempts to convert all factors to common negotiable tender, and (2) risk assessment, which considers only facts relevant to risks. Both of these procedures share a common problem in that they do not take into account the distribution of goods and evils, the fairness of risk, or justice. Although cost-benefit analysis and risk assessment play a role in determining the relevant facts, our proposed procedure differs from both in that it claims that more facts are relevant (e.g. it regards as essential the determination of who pays what cost, who takes what risk, and who receives what benefit). When the same person or group receives the benefits and pays the costs or takes the risks, a simple balancing of benefits and costs or risks would result in the same conclusion as the procedure proposed above. There is, however, an insidious nature to traditional cost-benefit analysis that could allow a few to suffer great harm to benefit many others in some small way. Rational persons would hardly consent to such a risk for themselves unless coerced in some manner, and it would be immoral to subject anyone to such a risk for such a gain without his/her consent. It is essential, therefore, that any prescribed procedure not have this fault.

Our proposed analytical procedure does not merely consider the costs, risks, and benefits of a particular violation, but what would be the costs, risks, and benefits if this kind of violation were to be universally allowed, that is, if one publicly advocated this kind of violation? Universalizing increases impartially by moving from the particular to the general, which counterbalances the fallibility of people. It seems quite natural for people to expect that one specific violation will not do much harm, but from past experiences it is known that people consistently underestimate the harm they cause and overestimate the harm they prevent. By requiring that all cases of the "same kind" be considered, rather than only one particular action, a decision-maker is forced to think about and describe a given case in more general terms, since "same kind" is determined completely by the general factors given in answer to the four questions discussed above. The universalizing further supports impartiality by forcing one to take more seriously the fact that the harm prevented is only probable while some of the harm caused by a violation is certain. . . .

APPLICATION OF THE ANALYTICAL APPROACH

. . . Given the magnitude of current and future harms, nearly everyone would agree that exposure to asbestos should be controlled and that government intervention to establish exposure standards is justified. Intuitively, most of us would reject allowing such a potentially significant harm to continue unabated and feel government intervention to limit exposure justified. But is it?

Using our analytical approach to determine if regulation of worker exposure to asbestos is justified, we would first determine the relevant facts by answering the four questions:

1. What moral rule is being broken? As with all regulations, there is some deprivation of freedom.

2. What harms will the regulation cause? There will be increased economic costs for the employers to bring their workplaces within established worker exposure limits. For the employees, there is inconvenience when they must wear personal protection equipment and clothing.

3. What harms will the regulation prevent? The benefits are both economic—a lowering of future employer costs (e.g. insurance), and health-related—the prevention of significant pain, disability and premature death (e.g. asbestosis, cancer).

4. What are the rational desires of the employees and employers? The employees would be expected to be willing to give up some freedom for better health. It is also plausible to assume that given the magnitude of the asbestos-related maladies and the compensation costs, some employers would be willing to give up some freedom, although they may prefer voluntary guidelines.

Given the above facts, some level of enforceable regulation would be universally advocated by all impartial rational persons for all cases of this kind. It is, therefore, clearly morally justified for the government to intervene and provide the legal force to ensure that the employers do what is morally required (i.e. not to harm). . . .

PERMISSIBLE EXPOSURE LIMITS (PEL)

While employers and employees will probably agree that some type of government regulation of asbestos is justified, they would be expected to disagree on the specifics of that regulation. Employees would want a regulation that set their health risks as low as possible; that is, they would advocate immediate implementation of an exposure standard for asbestos fibers that represented the lowest technically possible exposure level with minimal employee inconvenience (e.g. being required to wear special equipment). Employers would be expected to prefer an exposure guideline with the standard set at a level that would not require great technological retooling. Also they would want as much time as possible in which to comply with the standard. Once it has been determined that some exposure level regulation is justified, one can determine the justification of a specific exposure standard using the same procedure and answering the same four questions.

It is essential to know if available technology can lower the workplace asbestos concentration to the desired level or, if it is not available, what the feasibility of its development is, and over how long a period of time.

To fully understand the future harm prevented or avoided, unbiased scientific risk assessments must be available for each of the exposure conditions under consideration. For example, in determining what size asbestos particles should be excluded from the workplace, one would need to know that a majority of the asbestos fibers found at autopsy in human lungs were more than 5 μm in length. Moreover, seldom were fibers found more than 200 μm in length. The diameter of the fibers ranged from about 0.5 μm to 3.3 μm. Data have shown that fibers in these ranges of length and width can cause cancer and asbestosis. Applying our proposed procedure utilizing all available and relevant information, including uncertain information, one would opt for a regulatory standard rather than a guideline. Also the PEL fiber size selected would be the one to provide the maximum feasible protection from available technology within a reasonable time. . . .

The restriction on employer freedom by government regulatory intervention is justified when the evil(s) to be avoided or ameliorated are very great, much greater than the loss of freedom, and are such that it would be irrational for any impartial person not to favor the restriction of freedom in order to avoid the evil(s); though as noted above there can be legitimate disagreement on the extent of the restriction.

Unfortunately, not all regulatory determinations are ever this clear-cut; most involve some disagreement. Policy decisions often must be made where there is scientific uncertainty and disagreement on the interpretation of the data which lead to disagreement on the solution. It is with these cases that the analytical approach we have suggested could be helpful in establishing the relevant facts needed to propose a specific action (e.g. regulation). Once the irrelevant facts are excluded, we then ask, "Could that action be one that is advocated for all similar cases all of the time?" This, however, does not guarantee agreement on the specific solution, only that each proposed standard is one that could be justified given what was known at the time it was proposed. . . .

Utilizing this same approach there would be a general consensus that those substances with no known or suspected toxic properties, or only weakly toxic properties (e.g. sodium chloride), should be free from all regulation. Many other chemicals such as the approximately 400 listed by NIOSH/OSHA in the "Occupational Health Guidelines for Chemical Hazards",[7] will justifiably have guideline standards or strict governmental control. Most of the 40,000 substances listed in the NIOSH "Registry of Toxic Effects of Chemical Substances" will, however, fit into neither the control nor the no-control category.[8] For most of these substances, there will be considerable disagreement about their toxicity due to a limited amount of unbiased data, scientific uncertainty, or scientific disagreement. There are also thousands of chemicals that are not listed by NIOSH because no toxicity data exist, but which, nevertheless, may be toxic or hazardous in some other way (e.g. explosive or flammable), or for which only minimal data exist. To control these chemicals would unduly restrict freedom and cannot be justified.

The prevention of workplace health problems requires more than voluntary control programs and controlling employee exposure. Standards in and of themselves are not sufficient to prevent harm to some workers, therefore the actual and potential harms of any workplace must be made known to the workers, and this requirement must be [e]nforced by OSHA. . . .

SHARED RESPONSIBILITY

It is now recognized that informed employees and their supervisors are sometimes in a much better position than the government to solve many of the hazardous substances exposure problems. Both employers and employees have certain morally required responsibilities. Employers, because of their positions of management and control, are expected to assume the major share of the responsibility for providing a safe and healthful workplace.

ROLE OF THE EMPLOYER

The moral requirement not to harm imposes a duty on employers to (1) eliminate, wherever feasible, hazardous substances from the workplace; and whenever elimination is not feasible, to (2) control all hazardous substances so as to minimize worker exposure, (3) provide information to all employees, and (4) train employees so that they understand and appreciate the information provided. In this way no worker will ever be exposed to a hazardous substance without his/her valid consent. . . .

Learning what is harmful is helpful for avoiding harm. Thus, employee education and training should be a part of any job requirement. It is recognized that employees will not be uniformly interested in acquiring information, training, or understanding. However, employees cannot neglect the duties associated with their employment in order to be "macho" and show their fearlessness, or because the personal protective equipment is awkward and uncomfortable, or because they do not want to learn about, understand, or face the possible health hazards. The job requirement should be used to enforce what is morally required. The requirement not to harm imposes a responsibility on employees to act on relevant health hazard information in such a way that they will not cause harm to others. Employees cannot arbitrarily decide to ignore a prescribed procedure for handling a toxic substance and thereby expose another employee to an increased risk of cancer. That would clearly be causing harm and be immoral and punishable.

Employees must follow established health and safety procedures in their work practices even if they would seem to be the only ones who would be harmed if the procedures were not followed. First, it is very unlikely that the employee would be the only one placed at increased risk. Second, even if it were possible to directly harm no one else, every accident or illness, death, or disability, affects the employer's insurance and compensation costs. Indirectly, other workers, consumers of the goods or services, and taxpayers may be adversely affected by such actions: this justifies imposing a duty on employees to follow all health and safety regulations. . . .

Employees or prospective employees who refuse the information provided or cannot demonstrate that they understand the information (e.g. pass an informal test) could be considered incompetent for that job and justifiably be fired or not hired. Such employees would legitimately be considered unqualified for the job.

Those who fail to follow the procedures would be appropriately considered negligent. Further, employees should be encouraged to actively seek information whenever they have questions or concerns or suspect a possible hazard, to support proper monitoring and enforcement of health and safety practices and standards, and to suggest possible ways of better controlling a hazardous substance. . . .

. . . As people become better educated they will be more able to make valid decisions about risks to themselves and their families. It would, therefore, seem to be a most opportune time in which to give legal standing to what is already morally required.

NOTES

1. NIOSH, National Occupational Hazard Survey, Vol. III, Survey Analysis and Supplemental Tables. Cincinnati: USHEW NIOSH Publ. No. 78–114, 1977.

2. Gemmill, Daphne, De J. and Edward C. Prest, "Occupational Lung Disease—We're Seeing Only the Tip of the Iceberg." *Amer. Lung Assoc. Bull.* 63 (August 1977): 12–16.

3. Anderson, J. Marion, "Prevention of Job-Related Lung Diseases." *Amer. Lung Assoc. Bull.* 65 (January 1979): 10–13.

4. "German Research." Jan. 11, 1982, as reported in *Occupational Safety and Health Letter* 12 (4): 5. Washington, D.C.: Environews, Inc., 1982.

5. Silverberg, Edwin, "Cancer Statistics, 1982." *CA-A Cancer J. for Clinicians* 32 (1982): 15–31.

6. Ashford, Nicholas A., *Crisis in the Workplace: Occupational Disease and Injury*. Cambridge: MIT Press, 1976: 10.

7. Mackean, F. W., R. S. Stricoff, and L. J. Partridge, Jr. (eds.), *Occupational Health Guidelines for Chemical Hazards*, 3 volumes. Washington, D.C.: USDHHS and U.S. Dept. of Labor, NIOSH Publ. No. 81–123, 1981.

8. Lewis, R. J., Sr., and R. L. Tathen (eds.), *The Registry of Toxic Effects of Chemical Substances*, 2 volumes. Cincinnati: USHHS, NIOSH Publ. No. 80–111, 1981.

RUTH R. FADEN AND TOM L. BEAUCHAMP

The Right to Risk Information and the Right to Refuse Health Hazards in the Workplace

In recent years, the right of employees to know about health hazards in the workplace has emerged as a major issue in occupational health policy.[1] This paper focuses on several philosophical and policy-oriented problems about the right to know and correlative duties to disclose. Also addressed are related rights, such as the right to refuse hazardous work and the right of workers to contribute to the development of safety standards in the workplace.

I

A general consensus has gradually evolved in government and industry that there is a right to know, and correlatively that there is both a moral and legal obligation to disclose relevant information to workers. The National Institute for Occupational Safety and Health (NIOSH) and other U.S. federal agencies informed the U.S. Senate as early as July 1977 that "workers have the right to know whether or not they are exposed to hazardous chemical and physical agents regulated by the Federal Government."[2] The Occupational Safety and Health Administration (OSHA) promulgated regulations guaranteeing workers access to medical and exposure records in 1980,[3] and then developed regulations in 1983 and 1986 pertaining to the right to know about hazardous chemicals and requiring right-to-know training programs in many industries.[4] Legislation has also passed in numerous states and municipalities that is often more stringent than federal requirements.[5] For example, one of the earliest state bills, in New York, declared that employees and their representatives have a right to "*all* information relating to toxic substances"—a right that cannot be "waived as a condition of employment."[6] Many corporations—including Monsanto, DuPont, and Hercules—have also initiated right-to-know programs.

Although the general view that workers have some form of right to information about health hazards is now well established under law, there is no consensus about the nature and extent of an employer's moral or legal obligation to disclose such information. Considerable ambiguity also attends the nature and scope of the right—that is, which protections and actions the right entails and to whom the right applies.[7] For example, there is often a failure to distinguish among disclosing already available information, seeking information through literature searches or new research, and communicating about hazards through educational or other training programs. It is also often unclear whether there exists an affirmative duty to disclose information about health hazards to workers or merely a duty to honor worker-initiated or physician-initiated requests for access to records. What corporations owe their workers over and above the demands of federal and state requirements is likewise little discussed in the literature.

II

The belief that citizens and communities in general (and sometimes workers in particular) have a right to know about significant risks is reflected in a diverse set of recent laws and federal regulations in the United States. These include the Freedom of Information Act;

the Federal Insecticide, Fungucide, and Rodenticide Amendments and Regulations; the Motor Vehicle and School Bus Safety Amendments; the Truth-in-Lending Act; the Pension Reform Act; the Real Estate Settlement Procedures Act; the Federal Food, Drug, and Cosmetic Act; the Consumer Product Safety Act; and the Toxic Substances Control Act. Taken together, the implicit message of this corpus of legislation is that manufacturers and other businesses have a moral (and in some cases a legal) obligation to disclose information without which individuals could not adequately decide about matters of participation, usage, employment, or enrollment.[8]

Recent legal developments in the right to know in the workplace have been consistent with this general trend toward disclosure and have included a more sweeping notion of corporate responsibility to provide adequate information to workers than previously prevailed. These developments could have a pervasive and revolutionary effect on major American corporations. Until the 1983 final OSHA Hazard Communication Standard went into effect in 1986,[9] workers did not routinely receive extensive information from many employers. Now some corporations are beginning to establish model programs. For example, the Monsanto Company has a right-to-know program in which it distributes information on hazardous chemicals at its fifty-three plants, screens its employees, and both notifies and monitors past and current employees exposed to carcinogenic chemicals. Hercules has training sessions using videotapes with frank discussions of workers' anxieties. The tapes include depictions of dangers and of on-the-job accidents. Those employees who have seen the Hercules film are then instructed in how to read safety data and how to protect themselves.[10]

That such programs are needed in many corporations is evident from the sobering statistics on worker exposure and injury and on dangerous chemicals in the workplace. The annual Registry of Toxic Effects of Chemical Substances lists over 25,000 hazardous chemicals, at least 8,000 of which are present in the workplace. As OSHA pointed out in the preamble to its final Hazard Communication Standard, an estimated 25 million largely uninformed workers in North America (one in four workers) are exposed to toxic substances regulated by the federal government. About 6,000 American workers die from workplace injuries each year, and perhaps as many as 100,000 deaths annually are caused in some measure by workplace exposure and consequent disease. One percent of the labor force is exposed to known carcinogens, and over 44,000 U.S. workers are exposed *full time* to OSHA-regulated carcinogens.[11]

III

The most developed models of general disclosure obligations and the right to know are presently found in the extensive literature on informed consent, which also deals with informed refusal. This literature developed largely from contexts of fiduciary relationships between physicians and patients, where there are broadly recognized moral and legal obligations to disclose known risks (and benefits) associated with a proposed treatment or research maneuver. No parallel obligation has traditionally been recognized in nonfiduciary relationships, such as between management and workers. Risks in this environment were largely handled by workmen's compensation laws, which were originally designed for problems of accident in instances of immediately assessable damage. Duties to warn or to disclose are irrelevant under the "no-fault" conception operative in workmen's compensation, and thus these duties went undeveloped.

However, needs for information in clinical medicine and in the workplace have become more similar in light of recent knowledge about occupational disease—in particular, knowledge about the serious long-term risks of injury, disease, and death from exposure to toxic substances. In comparison to traditional accident and safety issues, these recently discovered risks to health in the workplace carry with them increased need for information on the basis of which a person may wish to take various actions. These include choosing to forego employment completely, to refuse certain work environments within a place of employment, to request improved protective devices, or to request lowered levels of exposure.

Employee-employer relationships—unlike physician-patient relationships—are often confrontational, with few goals shared in common and therefore with undisclosed risk to workers a constant danger. This danger of harm to employees and their relative powerlessness in the employer-employee relationship may not be sufficient to justify employer disclosure obligations in *all* industries, but few would deny that placing relevant information in the hands of workers is morally appropriate in at least some cases. By what criteria, then, shall such disclosure obligations be determined?

One plausible argument is the following: Because large employers, unions, and government agencies must deal with multiple employees and complicated causal conditions, no standard should be *more* demanding than the so-called objective reasonable person standard. This is the standard of what a fair and informed member of the relevant community believes is needed. Under this standard, no employer, union, or other party should be held responsible for disclosing information beyond that needed to make an informed choice about the adequacy of safety precautions, industrial hygiene, long-term hazards, and the like, as determined by what the reasonable person in the community would judge to be the worker's need for information material to a decision about employment or working conditions.

It does not follow, however, that this general standard of disclosure is adequate for all individual disclosures. At least in the case of serious hazards—such as those involved in short-term but concentrated doses of radiation—a *subjective* standard may be more appropriate.[12] In cases where disclosures to individual workers may be expected to have significant subjective impact that varies with each individual, the reasonable person standard should perhaps be supplemented by a standard that takes account of each worker's personal informational needs. A viable alternative might be to include the following as a component of all general disclosures under the reasonable person standard: "If you are concerned about the possible effect of hazards on your individual health, and you seek clarification or personal information, a company physician may be consulted by making an appointment." Perhaps the most satisfactory solution to the problem of a general standard is a compromise between a reasonable person and a subjective standard: Whatever a reasonable person would judge material to the decision-making process should be disclosed, and in addition any remaining information that is material to an individual worker should be provided through a process of asking whether he or she has any additional or special concerns.[13]

This standard is indifferent as to *which* groups of workers will be included. Former workers, for example, often have as much or even more need for the information than do presently employed workers. The federal government has the names of approximately 250,000 former workers whose risk of cancer, heart disease, and lung disease has been increased by exposure to asbestos, polyvinyl chloride, benzene, arsenic, betanaphthyalamine, and dozens of other chemicals. Employers have the names of several million such workers. Legislation has been in and out of the U.S. Congress to notify workers at greatest risk so that checkups and diagnoses of disease can be made before an advanced stage.[14] At this writing, neither industry nor the government has developed a systematic program, claiming that the expense of notification would be enormous, that many workers would be unduly alarmed, and that existing screening and surveillance programs should prove adequate to the task of monitoring and treating disease. Critics charge, however, that existing programs are far from adequate and that, in any event, there are duties to inform workers so that they can pursue potential problems on their own initiative.[15]

IV

Despite the apparent consensus about the appropriateness of having *some* form of right to know in the workplace, there are reasons why it will prove difficult to implement this right. There are, for example, complicated questions about the kinds of information to be disclosed, by whom, to whom, and under what conditions. Trade secrets have also been a long-standing thorn in the side of progress, because companies resist disclosing information about an ingredient or process that they claim is a trade secret.[16] There is also the problem of what to do if workers are inhibited from taking actions they otherwise would take because of economic or other constraints. For example, in industries where ten people stand in line for every available position, bargaining for increased protection is an unlikely event.

However, we must set most of these problems aside here in order to consider perhaps the most perplexing difficulty about the right to know in the workplace: the right to refuse hazardous work assignments and to have effective mechanisms for workers to reduce the risks they face. In a limited range of cases, it is possible for informed workers to reject employment because they regard health and safety conditions as unacceptable. This decision is most likely to be reached in a job market where workers have alternative employment opportunities or where a worker is being offered a new assignment with the option of remaining in his or her current job. More commonly, however, workers are not in a position to respond to information about health hazards by seeking employment elsewhere. For the information to be useful, it must be possible for workers to effect changes on the job.

The United States Occupational Safety and Health Act of 1970 (OSH Act)[17] confers a series of rights on employees which appear to give increased significance to the duty to disclose hazards in the workplace. Specifically, the OSH Act grants workers the right to request an OSHA inspection if they believe an OSHA standard has been violated or an imminent hazard exists. Under the act, employees also have the right to "walk around," that is, to participate in OSHA inspections of the worksite and to consult freely with the inspection officer. Most importantly, the OSH Act expressly protects employees who request an inspection or otherwise exercise their rights from discharge or any discriminatory treatment in retaliation for legitimate safety and health complaints.[18]

While these worker rights under the OSH Act are important, they are not sufficiently strong to assure that all workers have effective mechanisms for initiating inspections of suspected health hazards. Small businesses (less than ten workers) and federal, state, and municipal employees are not covered by the OSH Act. There are also questions about the ability of the Occupational Safety and Health Administration (OSHA) to enforce these provisions. If workers are to make effective use of disclosed information about health hazards, they must have access to an effective and efficient regulatory system.

It is also essential that workers have an adequately protected right to refuse unsafe work. It is difficult to determine the extent to which this right is legally protected at the present time. Although the OSH Act does not grant a general right to refuse unsafe work,[19] provisions to this effect exist in some state occupational safety laws. In addition, the Secretary of Labor has issued a regulation that interprets the OSH Act as including a limited right to refuse unsafe work, a right that was upheld by the U.S. Supreme Court in 1980.[20] A limited right of refusal is also protected in the Labor-Management Relations Act (LMRA) and implicitly in the National Labor Relation Act (NLRA).[21]

Unfortunately, these statutory protections vary significantly in the conditions under which they grant a right to refuse and in the consequences they permit to follow from such refusals. For example, the OSHA regulation allows workers to walk off the job where there is a "real danger of death or serious injury," while the LMRA permits refusals only under "abnormally dangerous conditions."[22] Thus, under the LMRA, the nature of the occupation determines the extent of danger justifying refusal, while under OSHA the character of the threat, or so-called "imminent

danger," is determinative. By contrast, under the NLRA a walkout by two or more workers may be justified for even minimal safety problems, as long as the action can be construed as a "concerted activity" for mutual aid and protection and a no-strike clause does not exist in any collective bargaining agreements.[23] Although the NLRA would appear to provide the broadest protection to workers, employees refusing to work under the NLRA may lose the right to be reinstated in their positions if permanent replacements can be found.[24]

The relative merits of the different statutes are further confused by questions of overlapping authority, called "preemption." It is not always clear (1) whether a worker is eligible to claim protection under a given law, (2) which law affords a worker maximum protections or remedies in a particular circumstance, and (3) whether or under what conditions a worker can seek relief under another law or through the courts, once a claim under a given law has not prevailed.

The current legal situation concerning the right to refuse hazardous work leaves many other questions unresolved as well. Consider, for example, whether a meaningful right to refuse hazardous work entails an obligation to continue to pay nonworking employees, or to award the employees back pay if the issue is resolved in their favor. On the one hand, workers without union strike benefits or other income protections would be unable to exercise their right to refuse unsafe work because of economic pressures. On the other hand, to permit such workers to draw a paycheck is to legitimate a strike with pay, a practice generally considered unacceptable by management and by Congress. Also unresolved is whether the right to refuse unsafe work should be restricted to cases of obvious, imminent, and serious risks to health or life (the current OSHA and LMRA position) or should be expanded to include lesser risks and uncertain risks—for example, exposure to suspected toxic or carcinogenic substances that, although not immediate threats, may prove more dangerous over time. If "the right to know" is to lead to meaningful worker action, workers must be able to remove themselves from exposure to *suspected* hazards as well as obvious or known hazards.

Related to this issue is the question of the proper standard for determining whether a safety walkout is justified. At least three different standards have been applied in the past: a good-faith subjective standard, which requires only a determination that the worker honestly believes that the health hazard exists;

a reasonable person standard, which requires that the belief be reasonable under the circumstances as well as sincerely held; and an objective standard, which requires evidence—generally established by expert witnesses—that the threat actually exists. Although the possibility of worker abuse of the right to refuse has been a major factor in a current trend to reject the good-faith standard, recent commentary has argued that this trend raises serious equity issues in the proper balancing of this concern with the needs of workers confronted with basic self-preservation issues.[25]

No less important is whether the right to refuse hazardous work should be protected only until a formal review of the situation is initiated (at which time the worker must return to the job) or whether the walkout should be permitted until the alleged hazard is at least temporarily removed. As long as the hazards covered under a right to refuse are restricted to risks that are obvious in the environment and that are easily established as health hazards, this issue is relatively easy to resolve. However, if the nature of the risk is less apparent, a major function of any meaningful right to refuse will be to call attention to an alleged hazard and to compel regulatory action. If this chain of events is set in motion, requirements that workers continue to be exposed while the OSHA or the NLRB conduct investigations may be unacceptable to workers and certainly will be unacceptable if the magnitude of potential harm is perceived to be significant. However, compelling employers to remove suspected hazards during the evaluation period may also result in intolerable economic burdens. We therefore need a delineation of the conditions under which workers may be compelled to return to work while an alleged hazard is being evaluated and the conditions under which employers must be compelled to remove immediately alleged hazards.

V

Legal rights will be of no practical consequence if workers remain ignorant of their options. It is doubtful that many workers, particularly nonunion workers, are aware that they have a legally protected right to refuse hazardous work, let alone that there are at least three statutory provisions protecting that right.[26] Even if workers were aware of such a right, it is unlikely that they could weave their way through the maze of legal options unaided. If there is to be a meaningful right

to know in the workplace, there will also have to be an adequate program to educate workers about their rights and how to exercise them, as well as adequate legal protection of this and related worker rights.

It is to be hoped that many corporations will follow the model guidelines and programs established by Monsanto and Hercules on the right to know and will make these rights as meaningful as possible by confirming a right to (at least temporarily) refuse work under unduly hazardous conditions. Potentially effective programs of information and training in hazards are as important for managers as for the workers they manage. In several recent court cases, for example, executives of corporations have been tried—and in some cases convicted—for murder because of negligence in causing the deaths of workers by failing to warn them of hazards. The Los Angeles District Attorney has announced that he will investigate all occupational deaths as possible homicides, and similar cases of criminal action have been prosecuted in Chicago.[27] A better system of corporate responsibility in disclosing risks thus stands to benefit management no less than employees.

NOTES

1. For developments in this area, see *Protecting Workplace Secrets, A Manager's Guide to Workplace Confidentiality*, Joseph P. O'Reilly Executive Enterprises, N.Y., 1985; Elihu D. Richter, "The Worker's Right to Know: Obstacles, Ambiguities, and Loopholes," *Journal of Health Politics, Policy and Law* 6 (1981), p. 340.

2. NIOSH, et al., "The Right to Know: Practical Problems and Policy Issues Arising from Exposures to Hazardous Chemical and Physical Agents in the Workplace," a report prepared at the request of the Subcommittee on Labor and Committee on Human Resources, U.S. Senate (Washington, D.C.: July 1977), pp. 1 and 5.

3. Occupational Safety and Health Administration, "Access to Employee Exposure and Medical Records—Final Rules," *Federal Register*, May 23, 1980, pp. 35212–35277. (Hereafter referred to as OSHA Access regulations.)

4. OSHA, Regulations 29 CFR 1910.1200 et seq; printed in 48 FR 53, 278 (1983) and (1986). See also *United Steelworkers* v. *Auchter*, No. 83–3554 et al.; 763 F2d 728 (3rd Cir.) (1985).

5. See Barry Meier, "Use of Right-to-Know Rules Increasing," *The Wall Street Journal*, May 23, 1986, p. 10; Vilma R. Hunt, "Perspective on Ethical Issues in Occupational Health," in J. Humber and R. Almeder, eds., *Biomedical Ethics Reviews 1984* (Clifton, N.J.: Humana Press, 1984), p. 194; and "Bhopal Has Americans Demanding the Right to Know," *Business Week*, February 18, 1985.

6. State of New York, 1979–1980 Regular Sessions, 7103-D, Article 28, Para. 880.

7. 762 F2d 728.

8. Cf. Harold J. Magnuson, "The Right to Know," *Archives of Environmental Health* 32 (1977), pp. 40–44.

9. 29 CFRs 1910. 1200; 48 FR 53, 280 (1983). See also Mary Melville, "Risks on the Job: The Worker's Right to Know," *Environment* 23 (1981), pp. 12–20, 42–45.

10. Laurie Hays, "New Rules on Workplace Hazards Prompt Intensified On the Job Training Programs," *The Wall Street Journal*, July 8, 1986, p. 31; Cathy Trost, "Plans to Alert Workers," *The Wall Street Journal*, March 28, 1986, p. 15.

11. See 48 CFR 53, 282 (1983), Office of Technology Assessment, *Preventing Illness and Injury in the Workplace* (Washington, D.C.: U.S. Government Printing Office, 1985); "Suit Challenges OSHA Limits on Worker's Right to Know Standards," *The Nation's Health* (July 1984), p. 1; U.S. Department of Labor, *An Interim Report to Congress on Occupational Disease* (Washington, D.C.: U.S. Government Printing Office, 1980), pp. 1–2; NIOSH, et al., "The Right to Know," pp. 3–9.

12. For an account that in effect demands a subjective standard for carcinogens, see Andrea Hricko, "The Right to Know," in Thomas P. Vogl, ed., *Public Information in the Prevention of Occupational Cancer: Proceedings of a Symposium*, December 2–3, 1976 (Washington, D.C.: National Academy of Science, 1977), especially p. 72.

13. As more and more data are gathered regarding the effects of workplace hazards on particular predisposing conditions, the need for disclosure of such information can be identified through pre-employment physical examinations without the worker's needing to ask questions.

14. High Risk Occupational Disease Notification and Prevention Act, HR 1309.

15. See Cathy Trost, "Plans to Alert Workers to Health Risks Stir Fears of Lawsuits and High Costs," *The Wall Street Journal*, March 28, 1986, p. 15; Peter Perl, "Workers Unwarned," *The Washington Post*, January 14, 1985, pp. A-1, A-6.

16. OSHA initially asserted that by requiring the "worst" areas of illness, it had "preempted" (or replaced) state "right-to-know" laws when it promulgated OSHA's Hazard Communication Standard. OSHA also claimed that its broad definition of trade secret exemptions for employers superseded state trade secret laws. Connecticut, New York, and New Jersey joined with several other states and challenged both of these assertions in *United Steelworkers* v. *Auchter*, 763 F2d 728 (3rd Cir.) (1985). The Steelworkers court held that the OSH Act enabled the Secretary of Labor to promulgate minimum standards to protect workers but that in the absence of coverage, states remain free to "fill the void" (between the need for regulation and actual hazards) with valid state laws. Consequently, insofar as OSHA's standard does not cover workers, there can be no "preemption" of state laws.

17. 29 USC S 651–658 (1970).

18. OSH Act 29 USC S 661 (c). *Note*: if the health or safety complaint is not determined to be legitimate, there are no worker protections.

19. Susan Preston, "A Right Under OSHA to Refuse Unsafe Work or a Hobson's Choice of Safety or Job?," *University of Baltimore Law Review* 8 (Spring 1979), pp. 519–550.

20. The Secretary of Labor's interpretation of the OSH Act was upheld by the Supreme Court on February 26, 1980. *Whirlpool* v. *Marshall* 445 US 1 (1980).

21. Susasn Preston, "A Right Under OSHA to Refuse Unsafe Work or a Hobson's Choice of Safety or Job?," pp. 519–550.

22. 29 USC S 143 (1976), and 29 CFR S 1977.12 (1978).

23. Nicholas Ashford and Judith P. Katz, "Unsafe Working Conditions: Employee Rights Under the Labor-Management Relations Act and the Occupational Safety and Health Act," *Notre Dame Lawyer* 52 (June 1977), pp. 802–837.

24. Susan Preston, "A Right Under OSHA to Refuse Unsafe Work or a Hobson's Choice of Safety or Job?," p. 543.

25. Nancy K. Frank, "A Question of Equity: Workers' Right to Refuse Under OSHA Compared to the Criminal Necessity Defense," *Labor Law Journal* 31 (October 1980), pp. 617–626.

26. In most states, these rights are not extended to public employees or domestic workers.

27. See *Illinois* v. *Chicago Magnet Wire Corporation*, No. 86–114, *Amicus Curiae* for the American Federation of Labor and Congress of Industrial Organizations; Jonathan Tasini, "The Clamor to Make Punishment Fit the Corporate Crime," *Business Week*, February 10, 1986, p. 73.

RICHARD D. MOHR

AIDS, Gays, and State Coercion

ALARUMS AND EXCURSIONS

Of those dead and dying from AIDS three-quarters are gay men. Government funding for AIDS research was at best sluggish till the disease appeared to the dominant non-gay culture as a threat. That perceived threat has spawned state-mandated discrimination against groups at risk for AIDS in employment and access to services, allegedly on medical grounds but in pointed contradiction to the judgments of the very medical institutions to which society has entrusted the determination of such grounds (the US Department of Health and Human Services, the Centers for Disease Control, and the National Institutes of Health).[1]

Government's disregard for medical opinion and for the lives of gays strongly suggests that prejudicial forces are at work. There is of course nothing new in this, but the stakes here are high. The armed forces have already established quarantines of those at risk for AIDS on some bases (*The Washington Post*, 19 October 1985, A12; *The Advocate*, #442, 18 March 1986, p. 14). With state-mandated discriminations installed and calls for civilian quarantines circulating, it is clear that the AIDS crisis is going to test the country's mettle. Not since the Supreme Court affirmed the internments of Japanese-Americans in World War II has so live a danger existed to America's traditional commitment to civil liberties. And again the danger is created by hysteria and not a reasoned necessity.

The hysteria, when not simply an expression of old anti-gay prejudices, is based on the presumption that the disease is spread indiscriminately. This presumption permitted Jeane Kirkpatrick to begin a syndicated column by using AIDS as a metaphor for international terrorism—'it can affect anyone'—in the serene belief that her audience, educated America, already thought this about AIDS and might even be ready for extreme measures (*The Washington Post*, 13 October 1985, B8).

ALLEGED HARMS TO OTHERS

For public policy purposes, the most important fact about AIDS is not that it is deadly but that it, like hepatitis B, is caused by a blood-transmitted virus. For the disease to spread, bodily fluids of someone with the virus must *directly enter the bloodstream of another*; 'It appears that, in order to infect, this virus must be virtually injected into the blood stream.'[2] But not just any bodily fluid will do. Only blood and semen have been implicated in the transmission of the virus (*MMWR* 34:45, p. 682).

That the virus is blood transmitted means first and foremost that, in countries with reasonable sanitation, groups at risk for the disease are clearly definable— more so than for virtually any other disease known— with 96 per cent of cases having clearly demarcated modes of transmission and cause. And now that blood supplies are screened with a test for antibodies to the AIDS virus, the number of these groups is indeed dropping. Hemophiliacs not already exposed and blood transfusion recipients are now no longer groups at risk. . . .

The July 1985 cover of *Life* informed the nation in three-inch red letters that 'NOW NO ONE IS SAFE FROM AIDS.' The magazine used as its allegedly compelling example a seemingly typical Pennsylvania family all but one of whose members has the disease. But it turns out that all those members with the disease were indeed in high risk groups. The father was a hemophiliac, his wife had sex with him, and she conveyed the virus to a child in the process of giving birth. No one got the disease either mysteriously or through casual contact. The family example in fact was evidence *against* the article's generic contagion thesis.

Reprinted by permission of the author.

Equally irresponsible journalists, lobbyists, and elected officials have compared AIDS to air-borne viral diseases like influenza and the common cold.

The case for general contagion cannot be made. In consequence government policy which is based on that fear is unwarranted. The extraordinary measures—including the suspension of civil liberties—which government might justifiably take, as in war, to prevent wholesale slaughter simply do not apply here. In particular, quarantining the class of AIDS-exposed persons in order to protect society from indiscriminate harm is unwarranted.

HARM TO SELF

The disease's mode of contagion assures that those at risk are those whose actions contribute to their risk of infection, chiefly through intimate sexual contact and shared hypodermic needles. In the transmission of AIDS, it is the general feature of self-exposure to contagion that makes direct coercive acts by government—like bathhouse closings—particularly inappropriate as efforts to abate the disease.

If independence—the ability to guide one's life by one's own lights to an extent compatible with a like ability on the part of others—is, as it is, a major value, one cannot respect that value while preventing people from putting themselves at risk through voluntary associations. Voluntary associations are star cases of people acting in accordance with the principle of independence, for mutual consent guarantees that the 'compatible extent' proviso of the principle is fulfilled. But the state and even the courts have not been very sensitive to the distinction between one harming oneself and one harming another—nor has the medical establishment.[3] It appears to all of them that a harm is a harm, a disease a disease, however caused or described. The moral difference, however, is enormous. Preventing a person from harming another is required by the principle of independence, but preventing someone from harming himself is incompatible with it. While no further justification is needed for the state to protect a person from others, a rather powerful justification is needed if the state is to be warranted in protecting a person from himself.

In the absence of such a justification, the state sometimes tries to split the moral difference and argues that state coercion *may* be used when the harm to others is remote and indirect. Such an argument from indirect harms runs to the effect that state-coerced use of, say, seatbelts and motorcycle helmets is warranted, for helmetless motorcycle crashes and seatbeltless car accidents harm even those not involved in the accidents, by raising everyone's insurance costs and burdening the public purse when victims end up in county hospitals. Here state coercion comes in through the backdoor.

This line of argument has been used with increasing frequency even by self-described liberals like New York's Governor Cuomo, and it is beginning to be heard in AIDS discussions. This is not surprising, for the cost of AIDS patient care from diagnosis to death is somewhere between $35,000 and $150,000. Private funds are often quickly exhausted, and the patient ends up on the dole—harming everyone, and so allegedly warranting state coercion of the means of possible AIDS transmission.

J. S. Mill's rule-of-thumb for appraising such appeals to indirect harms is exactly on target: an indirect harm counts toward justifying state coercion only when the harm grows large enough to be considered a violation of another person's right. This understanding of harm to others is necessary so that independence is not rendered nugatory and, *as a right*, is only outweighed by something comparable to it. Now, while it is nice if products (like insurance) are cheap and taxes low, the considered opinion of our society is not that one's rights have been violated when taxes or the price of milk goes up. Indeed, in the case of taxes, the considered opinion is cast as a Constitutional provision. So arguments that smuggle coercion in through the backdoor of indirect harms are not successful. . . .

STATE PATERNALISM CONSIDERED

The important question remains whether AIDS warrants paternalistic state coercion to prevent those not-exposed from harming themselves, through banning or highly regulating the means of possible viral transmission. Usually paternalistic arguments cannot be made sensible and consistent. For example: federal AIDS funding for FY 1986 in the House came with a paternalistic rider giving the surgeon general a power he already has—to close bathhouses, gay social institutions, if they are determined to facilitate the transmission or spread of the disease, which indeed they do. (So do parks and bedrooms.) The sponsor of the rider argued that it was 'a small step to help those who are unable or unwilling to help themselves' (*The Washington Blade*, 4 October 1985, p. 1). Cast *so* baldly, the argument simply denies independence as a value. For it is consistent with the presumption that the majority gets to determine both what the good life is and to enforce it coercively. The argument could as well be used to justify compulsory religious conversion—those who are unable or unwilling to see the light are helped to see it. . . .

PUBLIC HEALTH AND TOTALITARIANISM

Arguments offered so far by the medical community against quarantines and bathhouse closings have largely adopted the terms of mere practicality, appealing to such facts as the large number of people involved, the permanence of the virus in those exposed, and the possibility that the sexual arena may simply shift away from bathhouses where some educational efforts may be possible. I have suggested to the contrary that quarantines and closings should be opposed, not because they are impractical (though they may be), but because they are immoral.

Doctors tend to hold their unrefined view that health policy is merely a matter of strategy because they, not surprisingly, tend to see health itself as a trumping good, second to none in importance. This is a dangerous view, especially when coupled with their idea that health is an undifferentiated good. They fail to distinguish between my harming my health and my harming your health. Behind this oversight lies the further (sometimes unarticulated) presumption that you and I both are absorbed into and subordinated under something called the public health—a concept that tends to be analyzed in inverse proportion to the frequency with which it is used when trying to justify coercive acts.

No literal sense exists in which there could be such thing as a public health. To say the public has a health is like saying the number seven has a color: such a thing cannot have such a property. You have health or you lack it and I have health or lack it, because we each have a body with organs that function or do not function. But the public, an aggregate of persons similarly disposed as persons, has no such body of organs with functions which work or fail. There are, however, two frequently used metaphoric senses of public health that do have a reference: one, is a legitimate use but largely inapplicable to the AIDS crisis; the other, when used normatively, is the pathway to totalitarianism.

The legitimate sense places public health in the same conceptual scheme as national defense and water purification. These are types of public goods in a technical sense—not what most people want and thus what democratic governments give them nor what tend to maximize by state means some type of good (pleasure, happiness, beauty), but what everyone wants but cannot get or get efficiently through voluntary arrangements and which thus require coercive coordinations from the state, so that *each* person gets what he wants. Thus, the private or voluntary arrangements of the market system do not seem likely to provide adequate national security, because a defense system that protects those who pay for it will also protect those who do not; everyone (reasonably enough) will tend to wait for someone else to pay for it, so that national security ends up not being purchased at all, or at least far less of it is purchased than everyone would agree to pay for if there were some means to manifest that agreement. The coercive actions of the state through taxation are then required to achieve the public good of national defense.

For exactly the same reason, the state is warranted in using coercive measures to drain swamps and provide vaccines against air-borne viruses. But the state is not warranted by appeal to the public good in coercing people to take the vaccine once it is freely available, for then *each* person is capable on his own—without further state coercion—of getting the protection from the disease he wants. The mode of AIDS contagion makes it relevantly like this latter case. Each person on his own—without state coercion—can get the protection from the disease that he wants through his own actions, and indeed can get it by doing himself what he might be tempted to try to get the state to force upon others, say, avoiding bathhouses. As far as the good of protection is concerned, it can be achieved with no state coercion.

Is there a public good involved simply in reducing the size of the pool of AIDS-exposed people? I see just one, the one I argued for—the ability to have a robust sex life, without fear of death. But this good does not permit every form of state coercion. Not every public good motivates every form of coercion. The public goods mentioned so far could all be achieved by *equitable* coercion (e.g., universal conscription, taxation, compensated taking of property). When equitable coercion is the means, the public good can be quite slight and still be justified (as in government support for the arts). But when the coercion is inequitably dispersed, the public good served must be considerably more compelling than the means are intrusive. Thus, dispersed coercion against select individuals that involves restricted motion and physical suffering is warranted only by unqualifiedly necessary ends: when the individuals coerced have harmed others (as in punishment) or when it is necessary to the very existence of the country (as a partial military draft may be for a nation at defensive war). And thus too, the substantial good of civil rights protections is advanced only through the considerably weak intrusion of barring the desire of employers to indulge in whimsical and arbitrary hiring practices. The public good of an unencumbered sex life however fails this weighted ends-to-means test if the means are a dispersedly coerced sex life. For the intrusion and the good are on a par—on the one hand encumbered sex, on the other unencumbered sex. And so it appears that only equitably coercive means are available to achieve the end of reducing the pool of AIDS-exposures—taxation for preventive measures like vaccine development, but not coercive measures that effect some but not others, like closing bathhouses or banning or regulating sex practices selectively.

Those who do not find the possibility of carefree sex a public good—probably the bulk of those actually calling for state coercion—will find no legitimate help in the notion of public health for state coercion here. Those who do will find it justifies only equitable measures.

The other metaphoric sense of public health takes the medical model of the healthy body and unwittingly transfers it to society—the body politic. But this transfer (when it has any content at all) bears hidden and extremely dangerous assumptions. Plato in the *Republic* was the first thinker systematically to press the analogy of the good society to the healthy body. The state stands to the citizenry and its good, as a doctor stands to the body and its health. Society, so it is claimed, is an organism in which people are mere functional parts, ones that are morally good and emotionally well-off only insofar as they act for the sake of the organism. The analogy is alive and well today and calling out for extreme measures now: 'Much as a physician treating one organ must consider the effects on the entire organism, a public official has the community as the patient and must attend to all factors in seeking the greatest overall good' (Silverman and Silverman, p. 22). On this view, the individual however harmed cannot fulfill his role. A damaged organ, the spleen for example, can be, to continue the analogy, simply cut out. By comparison, quarantines and coerced sex lives might appear as mild remedies on this analogy. But something has been lost here—persons.

The medical model of society is the conceptual engine of totalitarianism. It presumes not that the goods of individuals are final goods but that individuals are good only as they serve some good beyond themselves, that of the state or body politic. The state exists not for the sake of individuals—to protect and enhance their prospects as rational agents—but rather individuals exist for the state and are subordinated to society as a whole, the worth of which is to be determined only from the perspective of the whole. The individual, thus, is not an end in himself but exists for some social good—whether that good be some hoped-for overall happiness or some social ideal—like, purity, wholesomeness, decency, or 'traditional values'. Unconscious obedient servicing is dressed up as virtue.

The worst political consequence of the AIDS crisis would not be simply the further degradation of gays. Gay internments would not be anything new to this century. In the European internment camps of World War II, gypsies wore brown triangle identifying badges, Jehovah's Witnesses purple, political prisoners red, race defilers black, and gays pink triangles. Worse than the further degradation of gays in America would be a general, and not easily reversed, shift in the nation's center of gravity toward the medical model and away from the position, acknowledged in America's Constitutional tradition, that individuals have broad yet determinate claims against both general welfare and social ideals. The consequence of such a shift would be that people would come to be treated essentially as resources, sometimes expendable—a determination no less frightening when made by a combined father, colonel, and doctor than by a fearful mob.

NOTES

1. See particularly the CDC's guidelines for preventing transmission in the workplace, 'Recommendations for Preventing Transmission of Infection with Human T-Lymphotrophic Virus Type III/Lymphadenopathy-Associated Virus in the Workplace,' *Morbidity and Mortality Weekly Report* (*MMWR*), 15 November 1985, 34:45, 682–95.

2. Krim, Mathilde. 1985. 'AIDS: The Challenge to Science and Medicine'. *AIDS: The Emerging Ethical Dilemmas, A Hastings Center Report Special Supplement*, p. 4.

3. For instance, Mervyn F. Silverman, former Director of Health for San Francisco, shows no cognizance of the distinction in his argument for his unsuccessful 1984 attempt to close that city's bathhouses: Silverman, Mervyn F. and Silverman, Deborah B. 'AIDS and the Threat to Public Health,' *Special Supplement* (see n. 2 above), pp. 21–2.

RONALD BAYER,
CAROL LEVINE, AND
SUSAN M. WOLF

HIV Antibody Screening: An Ethical Framework for Evaluating Proposed Programs

The acquired immunodeficiency syndrome (AIDS) poses a compelling ethical challenge to medicine, science, public health, the legal system, and our political democracy. This report focuses on one aspect of that challenge: the use of blood tests to identify individuals who have been infected with the retrovirus human immunodeficiency virus (HIV). In this article we follow the terminology recently proposed by the International Committee on the Taxonomy of Viruses; that is, we use the term *human immunodeficiency virus*. This replaces the more cumbersome dual terminology of human T-cell lymphotropic virus type III/lymphadenopathy-associated virus (HTLV-III/LAV).

The issue is urgent: the tests are already in use and plans to implement them much more broadly are being proposed.[1] The issue is also complex: at stake is a potential conflict between the community's interests in stopping the spread of a devastating disease and in preserving important values of individual liberty and equal rights. . . .

The reported cases of AIDS represent what is commonly called the "tip of the iceberg." Using the Centers for Disease Control's projections of ten cases of AIDS-related complex (ARC) (not a reportable condition) for every case of AIDS, the concealed portion includes an estimated 210,000 cases of ARC, many more cases of minor illness, and up to 1.5 million people who have been infected with the virus but who show no clinical signs of disease.[2,3]

Because HIV is a retrovirus whose genome becomes permanently integrated into its host's genetic material, all people infected can be presumed to be infected for life. Experts disagree on how many infected individuals will go on to develop disease. Early estimates of 5% to 10% were optimistic. Some now suggest that as many as 45% will develop AIDS or ARC within five years. How many will do so over more extended periods of time is at present not known. However, it must now also be assumed that all infected individuals can transmit the virus to others because the naturally produced antibodies do not completely neutralize the virus.[4] Although the virus has been isolated in nearly all body fluids, it is most concentrated in blood.[5] . . .

SCREENING FOR HIV ANTIBODIES

The test now being used to detect the presence of antibodies elicited by HIV viral antigens is an enzyme-linked immunosorbent assay—the ELISA (or EIA) test. Because the ELISA test was developed to protect the blood supply, the cutoff between reactive and nonreactive values was set very low to capture all true-positives. The price of such sensitivity is a loss of specificity. In high-risk populations there will be comparatively few false-positives. In low-risk populations, however, as many as 90% of the small number of initially reactive results will be false-positives. To distinguish true-positives, it is necessary to repeat the ELISA and to use an independent, supplemental test such as the Western blot.[6]

In addition to the false-positives, there may be

false-negatives; that is, the tests may fail to detect antibodies, or there may be none, even though the person is infected. The problem of false-negatives is only partly a characteristic of the test; it also reflects the latency period (on rare occasions as long as six months) between infection with the HIV virus and the development of antibodies.

Despite these problems, the ELISA test has served its initial purpose—screening blood donations—satisfactorily. The antibody test also enables clinicians to monitor the infection status of their patients. . . .

PRINCIPLES AND PREREQUISITES FOR EVALUATING A SCREENING PROGRAM

To evaluate the ethical acceptability of a proposed screening program, we recommend an analysis based on seven prerequisites. The prerequisites are based on the principle of respect for persons, the harm principle, beneficence, and justice. These four widely accepted ethical principles are derived from secular, religious, and constitutional traditions and are commonly applied to medicine, research, and public health.[7,8] . . .

PREREQUISITES FOR SCREENING

The following seven prerequisites constitute the threshold requirements for ethical acceptability, but as we will discuss later, they do not cover all the ethical problems that may arise.

1. *The purpose of the screening must be ethically acceptable.* There is at present one acceptable purpose for screening to stop the spread of AIDS. This purpose draws on the principle of beneficence—our duty to protect the welfare of those who might become infected with HIV. The use of medical tests and the public health power of the state is justifiable to protect the health of the community. However, to use these resources merely to express social disapproval of sexual orientation or drug use violates the principles of justice and respect for persons. If a therapy or vaccine becomes available, screening may be justified to benefit those at risk.

2. *The means to be used in the screening program and the intended use of the information must be appropriate for accomplishing the purpose.* If a screening program is intended to stop the spread of HIV infection, but designed in a way that precludes achieving that end, it is unjustifiable. It would involve an invasion of privacy without any public health benefit. For example, screening all food handlers is not justifiable, since there is no evidence that the disease is spread through food.

3. *High-quality laboratory services must be used.* Given the importance of interpreting not just one but a series of tests to arrive at a confirmed positive result, the availability of highly qualified technicians and laboratory services is essential. Beneficence requires that persons not be subjected to any risk—whether social, psychological, or medical—if the information about them to be generated in screening does not meet the current standard levels of accuracy. The need for confirmatory testing applies to both low- and high-risk populations.

4. *Individuals must be notified that screening will take place.* Respect for persons requires that individuals be notified that they are or may be the subjects of screening. In some cases individuals may choose not to participate in the activity for which screening is required (for example, they may choose not to donate blood or semen). In other cases, they may not have that option, but they should, nevertheless, be notified to protect their autonomy; they should also be made aware that highly sensitive data about them will be generated, with the associated psychological burdens and risks of breaches of confidentiality. Physicians who contemplate testing an individual on the basis of membership in a risk group should notify the person and should seek consent. This prerequisite does not preclude the use, without notification, of blood or other samples unlinked to personal identifiers in Institutional Review Board-approved research.

5. *Individuals who are screened have a right to be informed about the results.* There is no ethical justification for withholding test results. Certainly that information may be profoundly disturbing—not just to the individual but to the health care provider who has to convey it—but both respect for persons and beneficence support notification.

The converse—whether individuals have a "right not to know"—is a disputed question. We believe that persons who are screened and whose seropositivity is confirmed have a moral obligation to learn that information; that is, we reject the "right not to know" in this case.[9]

The most important potential benefit of the knowledge of a positive test result to an individual is the motivation to change behavior that puts others at risk.

A person at low risk (for example, a blood donor who has no knowledge of a sexual partner's drug abuse) has no reason to suspect that he or she is infected and, therefore, has no reason to change behavior. To protect others, that person must know the fact of potential infectiousness.

This conclusion is generally accepted; the major controversy concerns the right of individuals at high risk not to know. The claim is made that as long as such an individual acts as though he or she were seropositive and avoids high-risk behavior, there is no need for knowledge of seropositivity. Moreover, the argument continues, such information may be so psychologically devastating that the individual will suffer greatly without any benefits to himself or herself or additional benefits to others.

We acknowledge the potential burden of such information. We also recognize that there is insufficient evidence to determine whether notification will in fact motivate behavioral change or whether it will lead to enormous distress with no compensating benefits. However, there are two problems with the arguments in favor of a "right not to know." First, they underestimate the power of denial and the difficulty of sustaining behavioral change in the absence of specific information. Second, there is no way to discern in advance who of the infected people will modify their behavior without notification and who will not, much less who will be consistent in these changes.

Therefore, we conclude that given the disastrous consequences of HIV infection and the imperative of the harm principle, those who are infected have an obligation to know their antibody status, to inform their sexual partners, and to modify their behavior. We urge immediate research into both the positive and negative consequences of notification.

6. *Sensitive and supportive counseling programs must be available before and after screening to interpret the results, whether they are positive or negative.* Individuals should be counseled about the test before screening, told the significance of both positive and negative results, and informed about the availability of future counseling. A confirmed positive test result should not be conveyed by letter. It should be provided by personal contact in the context of, or with referral to, competent counseling services. Referral to a person's private physician may not be adequate, since many physicians in general practice, particularly those in low-incidence areas, have little experience with interpreting HIV antibody test results.

7. *The confidentiality of screened individuals must be protected.* Respect for the privacy of those who undergo therapeutic and diagnostic procedures demands that the results of such procedures be kept confidential. In the case of HIV antibody testing, where the inadvertent or unwarranted disclosure of positive test results could have disastrous social consequences for individuals, the importance of preserving confidentiality is especially critical.

However, there are a few circumstances in which public health reasons could provide a justification for the breach of confidentiality. For example, if it were known that a seropositive individual had recently donated blood, notifying the blood collection agency would be appropriate on grounds of benefiting blood recipients. However, that agency would then have the obligation to protect the confidentiality of the information received.

Appropriate legislation or administrative regulations should be designed to protect the confidentiality of antibody test results. Whenever disclosure is to occur, individuals must be informed that a breach of confidentiality will take place and why it is necessary. Under no circumstances should test results be used in ways that bear no relationship to legitimate public health concerns.

MASS SCREENING AND SCREENING IN SPECIAL SETTINGS: APPLYING THE ETHICAL PREREQUISITES

Using the framework we have established in the previous sections, we now turn to the specific application of the principles and prerequisites to the current policy debates.

SHOULD UNIVERSAL MANDATORY SCREENING BE UNDERTAKEN?

Universal mandatory screening can be justified on the basis of beneficence when a therapeutic intervention is available or when an infectious state puts others at risk merely by casual contact. However, neither is the case with AIDS. Thus, there is no demonstrable public health benefit that justifies universal mandatory screening, given the invasion of privacy involved.

At the most extreme, advocates of universal mandatory screening suggest it be a prelude to isolation.[10] This would entail a sweeping deprivation of civil and human rights—the segregation of a million or more people for life on the assumption that they will behave in ways that spread disease. Such a drastic measure cannot be justified, particularly when less intrusive measures are available. Isolation would probably increase the incidence of disease because those who were segregated would become a closed community, with the prospect of repeated reinfection.

Others justify mandatory screening less drastically. They see it as a way of making each individual learn his or her antibody status, hoping it will prompt behavioral change. However, long-term behavioral modification is a complex process that is less likely to be achieved under circumstances of coercion, where long-term follow-up and support are nearly impossible to provide on a mass scale. Even in this case, universal mandatory screening would require the creation of an enormous and costly apparatus. Since screening would have to be periodically repeated, it would be necessary to trace each individual's whereabouts to preclude avoidance of the test. Even were such screening feasible, it would require an extraordinary and repeated intrusion into the privacy of all Americans for little probable benefit. Therefore, on grounds of beneficence, it would be unacceptable.

SHOULD MANDATORY SCREENING BE IMPLEMENTED IN SPECIAL SETTINGS?

There are limited circumstances in which mandatory screening is appropriate—only where it can be shown, under stringent standards of scientific evidence, to reduce certain dangers. The mandatory screening of all blood donations has aroused virtually no opposition because everyone has an interest in a blood supply that is free of HIV. For similar reasons there should be routine screening of semen donors for artificial insemination and organ donations for transplant purposes under conditions consistent with our ethical prerequisites.[11] In blood, semen, or live organ donations, individuals can avoid screening by avoiding the activity; these activities may be desired but are not central to a person's life plans.

Screening all applicants for marriage licenses presents quite a different situation. Marriage, unlike donating blood, is central to an individual's freedoms. The likelihood of detecting a significant number of true-positives, a goal that might be defended on grounds of beneficence, is exceedingly small in relation to the economic costs and ethical dangers of invasions of privacy and potential curbs on individual liberties in instituting a screening program. Those at risk for con-

tracting AIDS are not likely to be the ones applying for marriage licenses. Moreover, neither sex nor childbearing is dependent on marriage in our society.

The state has an interest in stopping the spread of AIDS, but any bar to marriage for a seropositive individual would pose serious legal and ethical problems. Seropositive heterosexuals, like gay men in long-term relationships, can practice "safer sex" and take their antibody status into account in making childbearing plans. Individuals who are at high risk, or who are concerned about their own or their partner's antibody status, may voluntarily take the test before marriage, with appropriate counseling.

General workplace screening is unjustifiable under our ethical prerequisites because the usefulness of such screening for the protection of others is unsupported by epidemiologic or clinical evidence.[12] In some cases the protection of the public health is the stated purpose for workplace screening, while the underlying reason is the desire to avoid the economic burden of providing health care benefits for people who might become ill with AIDS. The economic costs of AIDS are a matter of serious concern and ought to be addressed directly so that equitable mechanisms for sharing the burden can be developed. However, to disguise these concerns as matters of public health serves neither purpose well.

But are there circumstances that fall between the extremes of blood screening and general employment screening where mandatory screening might be ethically acceptable?

Employment Settings. Since casual contact is not a route of transmission of HIV, the only employment settings in which mandatory screening might be justified are, first, health care involving the open wounds of others and, second, prostitution. Careful investigation of the potential of HIV transmission from infected workers and professionals to patients indicates no evidence of such transmission when standard infection control precautions are taken.[13] Since the risks are, therefore, only theoretical, there are no grounds at present for instituting routine screening of health care workers, including dentists. Prudence, however, dictates that health care personnel at high risk for AIDS, whether or not they know their antibody status, take all precautions when they come into a situation where contact might pose a hazard to others.

A strong public health argument can be made for screening prostitutes. First, male and female prostitutes may have significant rates of seropositivity, either because of drug use, because of a greater risk of infection due to their large numbers of sexual contacts, or because of high-risk sexual practices in which they may engage. Second, seropositive prostitutes can potentially infect large numbers of people. Because the great majority of infected persons in this country are male, and because male-to-male transmission of HIV is most common, it is likely that male prostitutes constitute a greater threat to their clients than do female prostitutes at this time. Finally, prostitutes' motivation to practice "safer sex" or to stop prostitution may be questionable; even if they are so motivated, the pressures to maintain their current behavioral patterns are probably considerable.

As a practical matter, however, only where prostitutes are licensed and subject to periodic health examinations could such screening, when used in conjunction with license revocation, interrupt the transmission of HIV without creating enormous problems. Nevada has recently introduced such screening.[14] Where prostitution is illegal, screening can occur only as an adjunct to arrest. Those prostitutes who are seropositive would have to be threatened with rearrest and perhaps isolation if they continued to engage in prostitution. Effective and consistent enforcement would raise difficult logistical and legal questions.

These practical difficulties, and the moral issues raised by singling out one group for a regimen of screening, arrest, and isolation, warrant immediate attention. Although moving incrementally is morally permissible, targeting a specific population requires particular justification to prevent invidious discrimination. There is an urgent need for educating prostitutes and their clients. It is also important to examine possible ways to reduce the spread of HIV that take account of the social realities of prostitution.

Since the only ethical justification for workplace screening is based on beneficence—reducing the risk of infection to others—the Department of Defense's routine screening of all recruits and active duty personnel is troubling. Communal living does not result in the transmission of HIV. The Department of Defense publicly justifies its policy with the claim that each member of the armed services is a potential blood donor and that in a battlefield emergency there would

be no time to screen blood.[15] However, it is not at all clear that soldier-to-soldier battlefield transfusions are in fact standard practice today. Moreover, the rejection of seropositive recruits cannot be justified on such grounds if seropositive active duty personnel are not also being discharged. Even if all seropositive individuals were discharged, one-time screening would not suffice to protect the military donor pool over time. Given the social costs associated with repeated screening, it would be more appropriate to ensure alternatives to battlefield soldier-to-soldier transfusion.

More plausible is the justification that screening identifies those whose compromised immune system might lead to adverse reactions to live-virus vaccines routinely given to recruits. But even this paternalistic justification is weak. The HIV tests are not the only way to identify these individuals.

As in general employment screening, other factors may be concealed under the guise of public health: the military's policies against homosexuality and drug use, relations with foreign governments concerned about the exportation of AIDS by American servicemen, and the desire to avoid the economic burden of AIDS. Here, too, we urge direct discussion of these concerns, not masking them as purported public health issues. . . .

ALTERNATIVES TO SCREENING: THE PROMISE OF VOLUNTARISM

We believe that those at high risk for developing AIDS have a moral obligation to take all possible steps to prevent harm to others, including taking the antibody test. This moral obligation should not, however, be translated into legal coercion. Mandating universal screening, as we have explained, would violate norms of beneficence and respect for persons and might drive the HIV infection underground, thus subverting public health goals. . . .

Given the risks associated with AIDS and the uncertainty about what will in fact modify high-risk behavior, there is a strong community interest in encouraging voluntary testing. Public health authorities and clinicians should encourage the use of such tests, to be taken anonymously or with strict confidentiality protections.

In addition, there is a moral obligation for antibody-positive individuals to notify their sexual partners, especially when their partners have no reason to suspect that they have had contact with an individual at risk for HIV infection. Counselors have a professional duty to encourage such notification.

We recognize that sexual contact tracing by public health officials might be considered the next logical step because some individuals may refuse to notify their sexual partners directly. This is an issue that needs further discussion, to consider both whether this is an appropriate strategy at this time and what kinds of protection would be needed. Sexual contact tracing might be justified in low-risk groups and low-incidence areas, for example, but not in other settings.[16] . . .

The most serious threat to the widespread use of voluntary testing comes from proposals or already enacted regulations that require reporting the names of those who are antibody positive to state public health officials. The arguments for such reporting are like those that are used to justify the mandatory reporting of AIDS itself—now universally required in the United States—as well as other venereal diseases and infectious conditions. It has been asserted that epidemiologic study, sexual contact tracing, and future therapeutic interventions all require mandatory reporting by private physicians as well as all health care facilities.

In fact mandatory reporting by name rather than code may deter rather than encourage voluntary testing. The knowledge that names will be given to public health authorities, even when those authorities affirm their commitment to confidentiality, is not conducive to voluntary testing. Some have even suggested that mandatory reporting may encourage anonymous sexual activity, so that individuals could not be named as sexual partners if contact tracing were implemented.

Testing should be widely available, not only in alternative test sites, but also in clinics established for the treatment of sexually transmitted diseases, drug treatment facilities, and prenatal clinics. Information in these settings should describe the services available in alternative test sites under conditions of anonymity as well.

Moreover, under the principle of justice, voluntary testing should be publicly funded. Many individuals at high risk, especially those who are intravenous drug users, do not have the resources to pay the cost of testing. The cost of widely available testing programs will be substantial, especially when the requisite services of counselors are considered. But to the extent that significant public health benefits might be achieved, these costs should not be a barrier to the creation of testing centers throughout the United States. Further-

more, since the primary purpose of testing is the protection of other individuals, including potential offspring, the burden of paying for testing ought to be borne by the public.

SUMMARY

We believe that the greatest hope for stopping the spread of HIV infection lies in the voluntary cooperation of those at higher risk—their willingness to undergo testing and to alter their personal behavior and goals in the interests of the community. But we can expect this voluntary cooperation—in some cases, sacrifice—only if the legitimate interests of these groups and individuals in being protected from discrimination are heeded by legislators, professionals, and the public. Yet voluntary testing is not enough. We must proceed with vigorous research and educational efforts to eliminate both the scourge of AIDS and the social havoc that has accompanied it.

REFERENCES

1. Additional recommendations to reduce sexual and drug abuse-related transmissions of human T-lymphotropic virus type III/lymphadenopathy-associated virus. *MMWR* 1986;35:152–155.

2. Public Health Service plan for the prevention and control of AIDS and the AIDS virus. Read before the Coolfront Planning Conference, Berkeley Springs, WVa, June 4–6, 1986.

3. Curran JW, Morgan WM: Acquired immunodeficiency syndrome: The beginning, the present, and the future, in Cole HM, Lundberg GD (eds): *AIDS from the Beginning*. Chicago, American Medical Association, 1986, p 23.

4. Landesman SH, Ginzburg HM, Weiss SH: The AIDS epidemic. *N Engl J Med* 1981;253:221–225.

5. An evaluation of acquired immunodeficiency syndrome (AIDS) reported in health-care personnel—United States. *MMWR* 1983;32:358–360.

6. Weiss SH, Goedart JJ, Sarngadharan MG, et al: Screening test for HTLV-III (AIDS agent) antibodies: Specificity, sensitivity, and applications. *JAMA* 1985;253:221–225.

7. National Commission for the Protection of Human Subjects of Biomedical and Behavioral Research: *The Belmont Report: Ethical Principles and Guidelines for the Protections of Human Subjects of Research*, publication (OS) 78–0013. US Dept of Health, Education, and Welfare, 1978.

8. Beauchamp TL, Childress JF: *Principles of Biomedical Ethics*. New York, Oxford University Press, 1979, pp. 97–126.

9. Provisional public health service interagency recommendations for screening donated blood and plasma for antibody to the virus causing acquired immunodeficiency syndrome. *MMWR* 1985; 34:1–5.

10. Grutsch J, Robertson AD: The coming of AIDS: It didn't start with homosexuals and it won't end with them. *Am Spectator* 1986;19:12–15.

11. Testing donors of organs, tissues, and semen for antibody to human T-lymphotropic virus type-III/lymphadenopathy-associated virus. *MMWR* 1985;34:294.

12. Recommendations for preventing transmission of infection with human T-lymphotropic virus type III/lymphadenopathy-associated virus in the workplace. *MMWR* 1985;34:681–686, 691–695.

13. Update: Evaluation of human T-lymphotropic virus type III/lymphadenopathy-associated virus infection in health-care personnel—United States. *MMWR* 1985;34:575–578.

14. Prostitutes to undergo HTLV-III testing. *Am Med News* 1986;29:30.

15. Norman C: Military AIDS testing offers research bonus. *Science* 1986;232:818–820.

16. Mills M, Wofsey CB, Mills J: Special report: The acquired immunodeficiency syndrome. *N Engl J Med* 1986;314:931–936.

Competition and Profit in Health Care

DAN W. BROCK AND
ALLEN BUCHANAN

Ethical Issues in For-Profit Health Care

The American health care system is undergoing a rapid socioeconomic revolution. Within a general environment of heightening competition, the number of investor-owned for-profit hospitals has more than doubled in the past 10 years, while the number of independent proprietary for-profit hospitals has declined by half. Investor-owned for-profit corporations are controlled ultimately by stockholders who appropriate surplus revenues either in the form of stock dividends or increased stock values. Independent proprietary institutions are for-profit entities owned by an individual, a partnership, or a corporation, but which are not controlled by stockholders. Nonprofit corporations are tax-exempt and are controlled ultimately by boards of trustees who are prohibited by law from appropriating surplus revenues after expenses (including salaries)

are paid. Although the increase in investor-owned hospitals has been most dramatic and publicized, a rise in investor-owned health care facilities of other types, from dialysis clinics to outpatient surgery and "urgent care" centers has also occurred. . . .

This essay will focus primarily on the ethical implications of the growth of for-profit health care institutions in the legal sense. However, although the ethical problems we shall explore have been brought to public attention by the rapid rise of for-profit institutions (in the legal sense), it would be a mistake to assume that they are all peculiar to institutions that have this legal form.

In what follows, "for-profit" will be used only to denote a distinctive legal status and not as a vague reference to "commercial" motivation or decision making and organizational structure, or as a synonym for the equally nebulous concept of "competitive health care." . . .

Reprinted by permission of National Academy Press.

This criticism of for-profits can be interpreted in either of two different ways. The first understands it as a charge . . . that for-profits skim the cream and gain a competitive advantage over nonprofits by failing to discharge their institutional obligations to bear their fair share of the costs of providing care for indigents and those with unprofitable diseases. But the metaphor of cream-skimming suggests another possible aspect of the charge of unfair competition that it is worth saying a little more about. This is that besides not taking a fair share of the "bad" (unprofitable) patients, the for-profits also take more than their share of the "good" (profitable) patients. . . .

[I]f no one is *entitled* to the profitable patients, it is unclear why seeking to get as many as possible of them is unfair. Nor is it clear that the nonprofits do not also seek as many as possible of the profitable patients. If the for-profits get a disproportionate share of the profitable patients, which may be true at some places but not others, why would that be? Since paying patients have a choice about where and from whom they receive care, their choice of for-profits must in significant part reflect their view that for-profits offer a more attractive product: for example, more convenient location, more modern and higher quality facilities, additional amenities, cost-saving efficiencies, and so forth. It is difficult to see why getting a disproportionate share of the profitable patients simply because one offered a better product is unfair. Of course, when for-profits get more of the profitable patients because of factors such as tie-in arrangements with physicians, this may constitute unfair competition, but nonprofits may engage in such anticompetitive practices as well.

According to the second interpretation of the unfair competition charge, nonprofit health care institutions make a distinctive and valuable social contribution—one that is so important that they ought to be protected from the threat of extinction through competition with for-profits. Three main arguments can be given in favor of perpetuating the nonprofit legal status for health care institutions and, hence, for social policies that are designed to protect them from destructive competition from for-profits. First, nonprofit health care institutions are properly described as charitable institutions. As such they help nurture and perpetuate the virtue of charity among members of our otherwise highly self-interested society, and this virtue is of great value. The nonprofit legal form stimulates charity by

exempting charitable institutions from taxes. Because it also ensures that those who administer charitable funds do not appropriate revenue surpluses, the nonprofit legal form encourages charity by providing potential donors with the assurance that they will not be taken advantage of and that their donations will be used for the purposes for which they were given. This assurance is especially vital in the case of donations for health care because donors usually lack the knowledge and expertise to determine whether the providers they support are using their resources properly.

Second, nonprofit health care institutions both function as and are perceived to be an important community resource, serving the entire community, rather than a commercial enterprise ultimately serving its shareholders and restricted to "paying customers." Like the virtue of charity, the sense of community is an important though fragile value in modern American society, and institutions that contribute significantly to it should not be lightly discarded.

Third, nonprofit health care institutions nurture a professional ethos that is more likely to keep the patient's interest at center stage than do for-profit institutions, in which the commercial spirit is given freer rein. Hence nonprofits are valuable because they protect quality of care. The quality-of-care argument will be examined in detail later.

The first argument above assumes that most nonprofit health care institutions are properly described as charitable institutions in the sense that a substantial portion of their financial resources comes from donations. At present, however, most nonprofit hospitals are not charitable institutions in this sense; they are "commercial" rather than "donative" institutions insofar as the major portion of their resources comes from selling services rather than from donations.[1] The more closely nonprofit health care institutions approximate the purely "commercial" nondonative type, which is becoming the dominant form among nonprofit hospitals, the weaker the value of charity appears as a justification for perpetuating the nonprofit legal status. Nevertheless, even if only a small portion of most nonprofits' revenues comes from charitable donations and is in turn used for unpaid care, nonprofits may still be properly regarded as "charitable" *if* they do in fact serve as the provider of last resort for those who are unable to pay for their care and who are not covered by any insurance or government program to fund their care. Even if such care represents only a small portion of a hospital's overall revenues, it may still be perceived as an important charitable activity and thereby reinforce altruistic and charitable motivations.

It should be clear that the charity and community arguments are not unrelated. It is partly because non-profits stand ready to provide unpaid health care to the poor (if they do) that they are seen to be a community resource available to the entire community. They can serve to symbolize a shared community commitment that no member of the community should be denied access to an adequate level of health care. This commitment is especially important in the mission of public hospitals. Moreover, control of nonprofits will commonly rest with a board of trustees composed of members of the local community, rather than with a board of directors of a large national or multinational chain. This effect of nonprofits on the sense of community as shared by members of the community is somewhat intangible and difficult to measure. It is also certainly true that nonprofit hospitals are not the only institutions supporting this sense of community, or even the only means of supporting it within health care, and that for-profit hospitals can often contribute to it as well. Nevertheless, we believe the nonprofits are in general more likely than the for-profits to promote this significant value of community. . . .

FOR-PROFITS DAMAGE THE PHYSICIAN/ PATIENT RELATIONSHIP, ERODE TRUST, CREATE NEW CONFLICTS OF INTEREST, AND DIMINISH QUALITY OF CARE

It is undeniable that for-profit health care involves potential conflicts between the interests of providers (physicians, managers, administrators, and stockholders) and those of patients. In the most general terms, the conflict is simply this: an institution with a strong if not an overriding commitment to maximizing profit may sometimes find that the best way to do this is not to act in its patients' best interests.

This fundamental potential conflict of interest is said to be of special concern in health care, not only because health care interests are so important, but also because the "consumer" of health care, unlike the consumer of most other goods and services provided by profit-seeking firms, is in an especially vulnerable position for two reasons. First, he will often lack the special knowledge and expertise needed for judging whether a particular health service is necessary or would be beneficial, whether it is being rendered in an appropriate way, and even in some cases whether it has been successful. Second, because illness or injury can result in anxiety and loss of self-confidence, the patient may find it difficult to engage in the sort of self-protective bargaining behavior expressed in the admonition "caveat emptor."

Whether this conflict of interest will damage the physician/patient relationship will depend on the extent that it also exists outside for-profit settings. And it is quite clear that this fundamental potential for conflict of interest is not peculiar to for-profit health care. A health care institution may exhibit a strong commitment to maximizing profit, and this commitment may result in practices that are not in patients' best interests, even if the institution is of nonprofit form. When we ask whether an institution's or an individual's pursuit of profits is prejudicial to the patient's interests, the appropriate sense of the phrase "pursuit of profits" is quite broad, not the narrower legal sense in which nonprofit institutions do not by definition pursue profits. After all, the issue is whether the opportunities for attaining *benefits* for themselves provide incentives that influence behavior on the part of providers that is not in patients' best interest. Whatever form these incentives take and whatever kinds of benefits are pursued, they may all run counter to the patient's interests.

In any form of medical practice operating under a fee-for-service system, under any system of prepayment (as in health maintenance organizations [HMOs]), and under any system of capitation, where physicians are paid a salary determined by the number of patients they treat (as in independent practice associations [IPAs]), a basic conflict of interest will exist, regardless of whether the organization is for-profit or nonprofit. In a fee-for-service system, the conflict is obvious: physicians have an incentive to overutilize services because their financial return will thereby be increased. The incentive for overutilization of services can conflict with the patient's interest in three distinct ways: it can lead physicians to (1) provide services whose *medical costs* to the patient outweigh their *medical benefits* (as in the case of surgery or X-rays that actually do more medical harm than good), (2) impose financial costs on the patient that exceed the medical benefits provided (greater out-of-pocket expenses for the patient), and (3) contribute to higher health care costs (including higher insurance premiums) for everyone.

In prepayment or capitation systems, providers are subject to conflicts of interest because of incentives to underutilize care. In HMOs, providers have an incentive to limit care because the overall financial well-being of the organization requires it and because salary increases and year-end bonuses as well as new personnel, new equipment, and new services are all financed by these savings. In IPAs and other organizations that operate on a capitation system, conflicts of interest due to the incentive for underutilization are equally clear: spending less time and using fewer scarce resources enable physicians to handle a larger number of patients, and this results in a larger salary. Whether, or to what extent, these incentives actually result in reduced quality of care is an extremely difficult question. But what is clear is that they create conflicts of interest, in both for-profit and nonprofit settings.

Some analysts have recognized that the preceding sorts of conflicts of interest are unavoidable because they result from two features that will be found in any form of health care institution or organization: (1) the patient's special vulnerability and (2) the need to provide some form of incentive for providers that is related in some fashion to the amount and kind of services they provide. They have then gone on to argue that what makes conflicts of interest especially serious in for-profits is that for-profits provide physicians with opportunities for *secondary income*. This secondary income may come either from charges for services, which they themselves do not provide but which they recommend or which are provided by others under their supervision, or from being a shareholder in the for-profit health care corporation.

Secondary income, however, and the conflict of interest it involves, is also neither a new phenomenon in health care nor peculiar to for-profits. Several forms of "fee splitting" are practiced by physicians working in nonprofit settings. One of the most common is an arrangement whereby a physician receives a percentage of the fee charged for X-rays, laboratory tests, other diagnostic procedures, physical therapy, or drug or alcohol counseling that he recommends but which are performed by people he employs or supervises. In some cases, licensing and certification laws and reimbursement eligibility requirements for Medicare, Medicaid, and private insurance require nonphysician health care professionals to be supervised by a physician, thus creating a dependence which makes it possible for physicians to reap this secondary income. Physicians may also charge fees for interpreting diag-

nostic tests, such as electrocardiograms, that they recommend and which are performed by others even if they do not split the fee for the procedure itself.

It may still be the case that the opportunities for secondary income and other conflicts of interest tend to be *greater* in most for-profit institutions than in most nonprofit institutions. At present, however, neither the extent of these differences, nor, more importantly, the extent to which they are taken advantage of in ways that reduce quality of care, increase costs, or otherwise compromise patients' interests is documented. It may also be the case that even though serious conflicts of interest, from secondary income and other sources, already exist in nonprofit health care, the continued growth of for-profits, both in their own activities and the influence they have on the behavior of nonprofits, will result in a significant worsening of the problem. Our current lack of data, however, makes it premature to predict that this will happen or when it will happen. . . .

[I]n the fee-for-service, third-party payment system in nonprofit as well as for-profit settings the cumulative result of many physicians acting on the desire to do what is best for the individual patient can result in overutilization that is contrary to all patients' best interest. Some critics of for-profits suggest that we must either pay the price of this overutilization or cope with it by methods that do not undermine physicians' commitments to doing what is best for their individual patients. They then conclude that even if it could be shown that the growth of for-profits would restrain overutilization by introducing greater price competition into health care, the price would be too high to pay because the physician's all-important commitment to do his best for each patient would eventually be eroded by the increasing "commercialization" of health care that is being accelerated if not caused by the growth of for-profits.

The force of this objection to for-profits depends, of course, not only upon the correctness of the prediction that the growth of for-profits will in fact contribute to a weakening of the physician's commitment to do the best he can for each patient; it also depends upon the assumption that under the current system that commitment has been a dominant force in physician behavior. This last point may be cast in a slightly different way. How concerned we should be about the tendency for the behavior of physicians to become more like that of businessmen depends upon how great the difference in behavior of the two groups is and has been. If one assumes that as a group physicians have been significantly more altruistic than businessmen and if one also assumes that altruism is the only effective safeguard against exploitation of the patient's special vulnerability, then one will oppose any development, including the growth of for-profit health care, which can be expected to make physicians more like businessmen.

Those who make the first assumption tend to overlook two points which call it into question. First, our society does in fact expect, and in some cases enforces by the power of the law, significant restrictions on the pursuit of profit by "mere businessmen." In fact, it can be argued that the moral obligations of businessmen to their customers are not significantly less demanding than those of physicians toward their patients *when equally important interests are at stake*. Robert Veatch has observed that if a physician becomes aware that another physician is acting on misinformation or performing a procedure incorrectly, then the first physician is under an obligation to bring this to the attention of the second and perhaps to help him remedy the defect.[2]

Veatch then goes on to say that a businessman who learns that a competitor is acting on misinformation or using sloppy production techniques is under no obligation to point this out to the competitor. Veatch's contrast between the moral obligations of physicians and businessmen, however, is overdrawn if not outright mistaken. It is not clear that a physician has a moral obligation to inform another physician that he is misinformed or even that his technique is deficient unless significant patient interests are at stake. It may be true, however, that important interests are more frequently potentially at stake in health care than in ordinary business transactions.

Yet surely a businessman has a moral obligation to inform a competitor that he is unwittingly endangering people's lives even if in giving his competitor this information he prevents his competitor from ruining himself and, thereby, foregoes a chance to eliminate the competition. Moreover, if a businessman lies to or defrauds a customer, we conclude not only that he has done something illegal but that he has acted immorally. . . .

In assessing these questions of conflict of interest, we think it is helpful to distinguish the behavior of physicians acting as an organized profession addressing matters of health policy from the behavior of individual physicians toward individual patients. As we have noted above, much behavior of medicine as an organized profession (as reflected for example in the political role the American Medical Association (AMA) has played in seeking to maintain physician dominance in the health care profession) to protect and enhance physician incomes, and so forth, has served the self-interest of physicians. Controversial is the extent to which the self-interested function of the motivation for supporting such practices as medical licensure is manifest or latent, explicit or implicit. In considering the conduct of professional trade associations such as the AMA, we believe that forwarding the economic and other interests of the members of the profession is often the explicit and conscious intent of the representatives of the profession. To the extent that the profession has been successful in forwarding its members' interests, we would expect to find an institutional, organizational, and legal structure shaping the practice of medicine that serves the economic and other interests of members of the profession. Moreover, it would be hard to look back over the evolution in this century of the position and structure of the medical profession without concluding that the profession has had considerable success in promoting its interests. . . .

Despite the extent that the profession has forwarded its members' interests and that individual members have not been self-sacrificing in addressing the most serious deficiencies in the health care system, we believe it would be a serious mistake to conclude that the patient-centered ethic that has defined the traditional physician/patient relationship is mere sham and rhetoric, a thin guise overlaying the physician's self-interest.

An alternative, and we believe more plausible, perspective is that in part just because the medical profession has been exceptionally successful in promoting and protecting an institutional and organizational setting that well serves physicians' economic and other interests, individual physicians have thereby been freed to follow the traditional patient-centered ethic in their relations with their individual patients. Put oversimply, a physician whose overall practice structure assures him a high income need not weigh economic benefits to himself when considering treatment recommendations for his individual patients. . . .

Either perspective is by itself stubbornly one-sided in its view of physicians simply as self-interested economic accumulators or as devoted altruists. We favor a view which recognizes that these two perspectives are *not* incompatible and accepts the elements of truth in each of them. . . .

What, more specifically, is the worry about the erosion of the physician/patient relationship by the rise of for-profit health care institutions? We think that worry can be most pointedly brought out by initially overstating the possible effect. The traditional account of the patient-centered ethic makes the physician the agent of the patient, whose "highest commitment is the patient."[3] The physician is to seek to determine together with the patient that course of treatment which will best promote the patient's well-being, setting aside effects on others, including effects on the physician, the patient's family, or society.

This commitment to the patient's well-being responds to the various respects discussed above in which patients are in a very poor position to determine for themselves what health care, if any, they need. Because the patient is unusually dependent on the physician, it is especially important to the success of their partnership in the service of the patient's well-being that the patient believe that the physician will be guided in his recommendations solely by the patient's best interests. Patients have compelling reasons to want the physician/patient relationship to be one in which this trust is warranted, quite apart from the putative therapeutic benefits of such trust.

Suppose the rise of for-profit health care so eroded this traditional relationship, and in its place substituted a commercial relationship, that patients came to view their physicians as they commonly now view used car salesmen. We emphasize that such a radical shift in view is not to be expected. We use this "worst-case" example of a caveat emptor commercial relationship only because it focuses most pointedly the worry about the effect on the physician/patient relationship of the commercialization of health care. Many factors will inhibit such a shift from actually taking place in patients' views of their physicians, including traditional codes of ethics in medicine, requirements of informed consent, fiduciary obligations of physicians, as well as powerful traditions of professionalism in medicine. Recognizing that the stereotype of the used car salesman substantially overstates what there is any reason to expect in medicine, nevertheless what would a shift in this direction do to the physician/patient relationship?

Most obviously and perhaps also most importantly, it would undermine the trust that many patients are prepared to place in their physicians' commitment to seek their (the patients') best interests. In general, there is no such trust of a used car salesman, but rather his claims and advice are commonly greeted with a cool skepticism. He is viewed as pursuing his own economic interests, with no commitment to the customer's welfare. It is the rare (and probably in the end sorry) consumer who places himself in the hands of the car salesman. Anything like the fiduciary relationship in which a patient trusts the physician's commitment first to the patient's interest is quite absent with the used car salesman. . . .

The realistic worry, concerning which the data are not yet in, is . . . that over time the increased importance of investor-owned for-profit institutions may permit considerations of economic self-interest increasingly to invade the heretofore somewhat protected sphere of the physician/patient relationship, and thereby weaken the patient-centered ethic on which that relationship has traditionally depended. . . .

The most obvious worry, then, is that the increasing prominence of for-profits may contribute to a shift in physicians' patient-oriented behavior, which may in turn affect the patient trust important to a well-functioning physician/patient relationship. The test of that hypothesis would then be the extent to which physician behavior is actually different within for-profit settings. But it is important to realize that patient trust may be eroded, and so the physician/patient relationship adversely affected, even in the absence of any actual shift toward more self-interested behavior by physicians. Even if outward behavior does not change, a change in the motivations of the behavior, and in turn of perceptions by others of those motivations, may be important. If physicians are increasingly perceived by patients as motivated by self-interest rather than by a commitment to serving their patient, then even in the absence of a change in physicians' behavior, it is reasonable to expect an erosion in patient *trust* that physicians will act for their patients' best interests. Part of what is important to patients in health care is the reassurance that the professional *cares* about them and their plight. (This is one respect in which other health care professionals, for example nurses, are often more important than physicians in patient care.) A change in a physician's motivations, or even in the patient's perceptions of those motivations, may be enough to affect the patient's belief about whether the physician "really cares" about him. This point should give pause to those who propose to test the effects of for-profits on the physician/patient relationship and on patient trust by looking only at changes in physician behavior. . . .

FOR-PROFITS AND THE POLITICAL POWER OF THE MEDICAL-INDUSTRIAL COMPLEX

The widespread view that the medical profession's dominance in the U.S. health care system is waning has already been noted. One important aspect of the weakening of professional dominance is said to be the decreasing effectiveness of organized medicine's lobbying efforts in recent years. Whether or not one greets this development with enthusiasm or regret will depend, of course, upon the extent to which one believes that these efforts to influence public policy have promoted or impeded the public interest. However, both the supporters and the critics of professional dominance have voiced a concern that it may be replaced by the dominance of a few extremely wealthy—and politically powerful—giant health care corporations forming a medical-industrial complex.[4] The fear is that a handful of the largest corporations might "capture" the regulators, molding public policy to their own needs through lobbying, campaign contributions, and use of the media to sway the electorate.

The real concern here should be the political effects of highly concentrated *corporate* power in health care—not simply the power of *for-profit* health care corporations. While it is true that the hospital "industry" is becoming increasingly concentrated, it is important to point out that some of the largest hospital chains are owned or operated by large nonprofit corporations. Further, there is nothing to prevent large nonprofit corporations from using their wealth and power to influence public policy and little reason to believe that they will in general be less willing to do so than large for-profit corporations. At present, however, it is difficult to predict how concentrated the health care sector will become or to what extent the disparate interest groups within and across health care institutions can be welded together under corporate leadership to function as a unified influence on public policy.

The issue, then, is whether it may become necessary in the future to utilize regulation or some other form of societal control to neutralize or minimize the political effects of the economic power wielded by large health care corporations, whether nonprofit or for-profit. Some possible, even if not politically likely, controls include limitations on campaign contributions and on political advertisements in the media, special laws designed to disqualify legislators or regulators with conflicts of interest, or limitations on the maximum size of corporations.

It has often been remarked that it is a hallmark of a profession to be self-regulating. In the case of the medical profession, the idea that the physician/patient relationship is fiduciary along with the belief that medicine is a service for healing and comfort rather than simply one commercial enterprise among others have buttressed the profession's claim that it can be trusted to regulate itself.

Until recently it was widely assumed not only that the medical profession should regulate itself, but that it should also be chiefly responsible for regulating health care in general. This position rested on three main premises: (1) physicians and only physicians have the technical training and knowledge needed for informed control of their own professional activities, (2) physicians' professional activities are largely autonomous from other activities in health care, (3) the activities of other health care professionals are almost exclusively dependent upon physicians' decision making. The recognition that some of the most perplexing decisions concerning the use of medical treatments require complex moral, social, and legal judgments has undermined the first premise. (Decisions to forgo life-sustaining treatments for terminally ill or comatose patients are only the most obvious cases where medical judgment is not sufficient for guiding the physicians' own professional activities. These decisions require moral judgments because they rest on assumptions about the nature of individuals' rights and the quality and value of life.) The second and third premises also become dubious once it is seen that physicians' professional activities are increasingly dependent, not only upon decisions of other types of health care professionals (such as biomedical engineers and laboratory and radiology technicians) who sometimes possess specialized knowledge which physicians lack, but also upon a complex web of institutional functions, including planning, investment, and allocation of resources.

Some of the same reasons that make it implausible to leave regulation of health care to physicians make it equally implausible to entrust it to corporations or groups of corporations. In particular, the vast commitment of public resources to health care grounds a legitimate public concern that the resources be used efficiently and fairly, and the growing list of ethical dilemmas concerning the uses of medical technology is no more amenable to the administrative expertise of the corporate manager than to the professional judgment of the physician. There is, however, one reason why the public is perhaps even less likely to tolerate self-regulation by health care corporations than by the medical profession. If health care is perceived to be controlled by corporations—whether for-profit or nonprofit—that are in many respects indistinguishable from other commercial enterprises, then the presumption in favor of self-regulation, which flourished under professional dominance, will erode. For if the key decision makers in health care are perceived to be businessmen rather than fiduciaries committed to healing and comfort, an important barrier to societal regulation of all forms of health care will have fallen. Whether new forms of regulation will be needed to constrain the political influence of large health care corporations can only be determined after careful study not only of the impact that these organizations have on public policy, but also of the expected effectiveness of proposed regulations. . . .

NOTES

1. Hansmann, Henry D. (1980) The role of nonprofit enterprise. *Yale Law Journal* 89(5):835–901.

2. Veatch, R. (1983) Ethical dilemmas of for-profit enterprise in health care, B. H. Gray, ed., *The New Health Care for Profit* (Washington, D.C.: National Academy Press), pp. 145–146.

3. *American College of Physicians Ethics Manual* (1984) p. 7.

4. The term "medical-industrial complex" is borrowed from an article by Relman, A. (1980) The new medical-industrial complex, *The New England Journal of Medicine*, 303(17):963–970. Relman expresses a number of the concerns about the for-profits analyzed in the present essay, including the fear that large for-profit corporations may exert undue influence on public policy.

MARK YARBOROUGH

Patients and Profits

INTRODUCTION

An alarming and growing trend has been identified in health care.[1-2] That trend is the move toward for-profit health care institutions. Of course, there is nothing new about profit and medicine in the United States. As long as there has been the fee-for-service system, physicians have profited from health care, as have pharmaceutical and medical supply corporations. But one segment of the health care field, for the most part, was excluded from this profit motive. That segment was the hospital. Most hospitals, until the past decade or so, were seen as community resources. They were established to help serve the health care needs of the community by facilitating the administration of care.

While the physician who administered care there, or the pharmacist who dispensed drugs there, or the company that provided medical supplies there, did so at least in part to make a profit from the association, the hospital itself by and large did not. Whatever profit it generated was usually given back to the community in the form of new services, better facilities, or better quality of care. This is quickly changing, though. Now hospitals provide facilities to remove a patient's appendix not only to relieve suffering but to reward stockholders for their investments as well. This raises an obvious moral concern. Are profit-making health care institutions more prone to misuse or mistreat patients due to their profit-making survival needs than are not-for-profit institutions?

While this misuse and mistreatment does not necessarily occur, both the possibility and the likelihood of its occurrence is morally sufficient to argue against the trend of for-profit health care institutions. In order to show this, several types of issues need to be addressed. First, various conceptual issues need to be examined. These are the institutional nature of medicine and health care, the role of the hospital, and the nature of the doctor/patient relationship. Then the purported economic virtues of For Profit Hospitals will be examined. These issues will be discussed in order to lay the groundwork for the moral argument that is presented. The moral issue to be discussed is that the advent of For Profit Hospitals unduly violates the moral foundations of the doctor/patient relationship. Let us begin with the conceptual issues.

THE NATURE OF MEDICINE AND HEALTH CARE

First of all, medicine and health care are public goods, not private commodities to be bought and sold. Health care, simply stated, is the attempt to cure illness and provide comfort for the suffering. I assume that the motivation underlying this attempt stems from the belief that health is good as a means in that it enables one to realize the end of being self-directive. Health allows one to exert control over one's body and life plans within the boundaries set by social and political institutions. Hence, health care is valued as a means to both preserving and restoring this self-directive capacity known as autonomy. This care is made possible by public funding for education, training, and research and the collective distribution of the results and achievements of the funded activities. The procedures and medicines administered to patients are developed by physicians and researchers who discover and test these various administrations over a period of time and who share their results with one another and with the society at large. Most of the research takes place at state supported hospitals and universities. Consequently, the results which ensue from these endeavors are made possible by and large from public funding. Also, given that the advancements are made in an academic setting, the results are shared collectively with that community so that all practitioners, and thus patients as well, can share in the results. Medicine is a collective institution which has the goal and mission of serving the public. Of course, I am making the empirical assumption that our present health care system has developed, at least in part, from meritorious obliga-

tions. While I cannot substantiate this claim, I think it is a safe one to make in light of the fact that medicine is a discipline dedicated to healing.[3]

THE ROLE OF THE HOSPITAL

The same can be said of the hospital as well. The presence of a hospital in a community is symbolic of perhaps the most basic moral value we have, the value of beneficence. As was previously stated, we collectively recognize the need to alleviate human suffering in the guise of illness. The modern hospital is the edifice we have constructed and peopled in order to act on this beneficent motive. While, as was mentioned, the individuals who administered care in the hospital may have done so in part out of economic motives, the institution's motive, with the exception of teaching and research hospitals, was wholly beneficent. Hospitals were erected to take care of the sick and dying. They were charitable institutions. As such, they were a community resource, there to serve the community (not be served by it, which is what For Profit Hospitals seek to do). Furthermore, the presence of the hospital expresses a commitment of assistance to the community to help those who are ill regain their health.[4] In providing this assistance, the hospital is subject to the same basic obligations that a physician is, viz., provide competent care, "act in the patient's interest, never do deliberate harm, protect confidentiality, and treat the patient honestly, considerately, and personally."[5] These obligations and the more general obligation of beneficence held by the hospital correspond with the expectations of patients. Those who suffer from pain and illness expect to receive therapeutic and palliative measures in the hospital. Furthermore, they expect that no other institutional needs or motives will interfere with the provision of these measures. In short, they expect the hospital to do that which is necessary to enable the physician and nurse to practice and administer medicine. Hence the earlier description of the hospital as a facilitator. As I will argue later, the emergence of For Profit Hospitals is changing this historical beneficent relationship between hospitals and patients into a self-gratifying capitalistic relationship for the benefit of the hospital's investors, possibly at the expense of patients.

THE ROLE OF THE PHYSICIAN

Now that we have addressed the role of the hospital, let us turn to the role of the physician. Specifically, I will address the basic moral characteristics of the physician/patient relationship. Paul Ramsey describes the relationship as one involving a 'canon of loyalty'.[6] Medicine is a 'co-operative enterprise'[7] between a professional and a client in which the client must at all times be treated as a 'personal subject'[8] and not merely as a scientific object. These guarantees are met through the requirement of informed consent. "Consent lies at the heart of medical care",[9] and it is the key to sustaining the loyalty and trust between patient and physician.

We see from this that a patient approaches a physician in an attitude of trust. Not only does he trust the physician's medical expertise, but he also trusts the physician's commitment to respect the personhood of the patient. Thus, there is a covenant of faithfulness between the two. The physician is expected to be faithful to the needs and welfare of the patient. This covenant of faithfulness precludes the physician from treating the patient in ways that lay outside the needs and interests of the patient unless the patient gives a free and informed consent. In other words, the covenant demands that the patient is treated as an end at all times. And he is treated as a means only in the sense that he is, in part, the physician's means to making a living. The patient is aware that the physician profits from the services he provides. But these profits, if the covenant of faithfulness is maintained, in no way conflict with the needs, interests, and expectations of the patient. So, we see from a moral point of view that the relationship between patient and physician is one characterized by trust, loyalty, and faithfulness. The role of the physician in this relationship is to operate within the constraints that these impose in the attempt to provide a cure if possible. If it is not, the role is to provide comfort.

FOR PROFIT HOSPITALS

Thus far we have addressed the nature of medicine and health care as well as the roles of the hospital and physician. Now let us turn to some claims that are often advanced in favor of For Profit Hospitals. Proponents contend that there are sufficient economic reasons for allowing the increasing numbers of For Profit Hospitals. We are all familiar with the skyrocketing costs of health care. Costs for several years have increased more than inflation has increased. There are too many physicians, as a rule, in our large urban centers just as there are too many hospital beds. More expensive diagnostic tests are continually introduced, often without replacing other diagnostic tests. Hence, the result is that technological advances tend to make health care more expensive, but not always more efficient. Perhaps most importantly, the present reimbursement system provides incentives for *generating* expenditures, not *decreasing* them, since the present system, excluding Medicare charges, provides reimbursement for each performed procedure. Hence, the incentive is to perform more rather than fewer procedures. As a result we hear that the present health care system is simply out of control. In light of this, some contend that the way to provide the much needed control is to return health care to the marketplace. If there are too many hospitals generating too much cost, what is needed is competition. Competition will insure that the most efficient institutions will continue to provide health care while the wasteful institutions will not be able to survive. Administrators and physicians will become accountable to the market, and thus to the society at large, rather than merely to themselves and their patient's interests.

This argument could take various forms, but the ideological basis for it is that the marketplace is best suited to provide the discipline and incentives necessary to make the health care system more cost efficient. The first fault with this argument is that it begs the most obvious question. It assumes from the outset that cost efficiency should be the most important attribute of our health care system. It will be argued later that it should not since this position potentially compromises the basic tenet of the doctor/patient relationship. There are two other issues in the argument to be addressed at this point though. First, it will be shown that For Profit Hospitals are not necessarily more cost efficient than are Not For Profit Hospitals. Second, it will be shown that the 'marketplace' for health care is not the typical marketplace. Hence, the argument uses the wrong model to base its remedies on.

Recent statistical evidence disputes the claim that For Profit Hospitals are more or equally cost-efficient than are Not For Profit Hospitals.[10] Studies show that charges in For Profit Hospitals range anywhere from 15–24% higher than they do in Not For Profit Hospitals. Collections range from 10–12% higher. No one should really be surprised by these figures. After all, For Profit Hospitals exist in order to make money. It is easier with the fee-for-service system to make more money by charging more, not less. Thus, the hope that For Profit Hospitals will be more cost efficient and less expensive in the long run seems ill-fated at the outset.

Given the present reimbursement system, each admission, each diagnostic test, and each medical supply generates charges to the payer. Since For Profit Hospitals hope to maximize the return on investment, it comes as no surprise that For Profit Hospitals usually have more tests done on patients and use more medical supplies per admission than do Not For Profit Hospitals. This at least suggests that For Profit Hospitals are willing to sacrifice patient comfort and well-being in the interests of profit since diagnostic tests as a rule are not completely benign.

One might contend that this is the fault of the reimbursement system more than the For Profit Hospitals. But, if this were totally true one would expect the charges in For Profit Hospitals to be only somewhat higher than Not For Profit Hospitals since the For Profit Hospitals have no tax exempt status and receive no charitable contributions. Yet their charges are considerably higher. So the present reimbursement system can not bear all the blame. The results of the studies previously referred to also suggest that the discrepancies would remain even if the reimbursement system changed. For Profit Hospitals have an institutional incentive to spend as little as possible on patients yet collect as much as possible. Thus, it seems they will always generate the highest charges that they can collect. There is no reason for them to do otherwise.

Furthermore, there is no reason to believe that the existence of For Profit Hospitals increases the cost of health care in general and not just hospital costs. Many individual physicians now work for For Profit Hospitals. Given the high costs of office space and equipment, lab fees, recordkeeping and personnel, physicians find it more and more difficult to maintain a solo practice. For Profit Hospitals seize this present economic condition as an opportunity for drawing physicians under their corporate umbrella. They provide the aforementioned services and facilities for a much lower charge and require in return only that the physician send patients to the hospital for lab work, diagnostic tests, admissions and the like.

Physicians who are cost and pain conscious for their patients are the least suitable physicians for these hospitals though. Since they generate fewer charges due to less utilization of hospital services and due to fewer tests and admissions, they run the risk of not having their leases renewed.[11] Of course, the physician who orders many tests and generates many admissions runs no such risk. Overutilization is a virtue and underutilization is a vice in the world of corporate health care. Yet this hardly reflects the attitudes of the patient/consumer.

And it must be noted that a patient is not a typical consumer in the fullest sense of the term. The patient does not play the same role in the health care marketplace as the normal consumer does in the typical marketplace. This is so because there is no textbook market as such for health care. Theoretically, consumers make purchases in light of how the cost of a product corresponds to the product's perceived value. But of course this is not true of the patient consumer. For a patient, cost is a secondary concern.[12] If the patient is ill enough, cost may be no concern at all. Health care consumers, as Arnold S. Relman states, simply "do not have the usual incentives to be prudent, discriminating purchasers".[13] So patients are not just consumers who purchase products. Instead, as I stated earlier, they are self-directive agents seeking either the preservation or restoration of their self-directive capacities. Illness and suffering above all else jeopardizes our ability to function as physiologically free, unrestrained agents. Thus, a patient in need of health care is usually not an optional consumer-purchaser. Instead, he or she is a compelled user of the health care system. These cases are so atypical of the theoretical consumer that it simply makes no sense to treat a patient as a typical consumer.

First of all, then, we see that a patient is not a voluntary seeker of an economic product. Instead, he is compelled to seek assistance. He enlists an advocate to obtain this assistance from the health care system, viz., a physician. Indeed, a patient cannot 'purchase' anything from the hospital without the physician's permission. This underscores the second major distinction that separates patients from typical consumers. A patient can make fully informed choices only with the aid of the physician. The physician is the one who instructs the patient as to what his medical needs and ways of satisfying those needs are.[14] In this role, the patient has historically assumed, except in cases where an acute shortage of a scarce resource is involved, that only two parties have a vested self-interest. These two parties were the patient and the physician. If a third party is involved, damage is done to the physician's ability to function as the informed advocate of the patient. In this role, the patient is informed by the physician as to the availability of treatment options and his expert advice as to which option is medically best. The patient is then free to decide which option best suits his needs and life plan. Of course, it has always been possible for the physician to push a particular treatment in order to further his own economic interests and patients should be alerted to this possibility.

MORAL ASSESSMENT

But the advent of investor-owned For Profit Hospitals could very well further compromise the physician's ability to function in the role of the informed advocate. As I mentioned previously, For Profit Hospitals could put pressure on a physician to order expensive tests and treatments in lieu of less expensive alternatives. This would change the patient/physician relationship from a two party relationship into a three party relationship where the physician would lack the decision-making autonomy with respect to the availability of treatment plans that he once enjoyed. So, the advent of For Profit Hospitals fundamentally alters the patient/physician relationship. Historically, the physician was serving directly his own and the patient's interests and was only indirectly serving the hospital's interest in providing competent medical care to the community. Now, the physician must serve directly not only his and his patients' interests, but he must serve directly the economic interests of the hospital as well. Those economic interests consist primarily of the necessity of the hospital to provide investors with a return, and it best be a healthy return, on their invested capital. To borrow from Marx, the 'naked self-interest' of the hospital is there at the bedside of each and every patient. But how can the economic interests of the hospital be allowed to compete with the moral interests the patient has in pursuing the restoration or preservation of his ability to function autonomously?

Even though these economic interests should not compete, they most likely do when one considers the nature of the For Profit Hospital itself. It is primarily a corporation designed to make a profit by providing health care services to a community. Investors give capital to these institutions in good faith, expecting the institution to use this capital in such a way that there will be a financial return to the investor. If such a return is not made, eventually investors will look elsewhere for investment opportunities. Thus, the institution's survival in the long-run depends on its ability to provide a return on investment. This is the major purpose for its existence. The treatment of patients is the way this return on investment is provided. But of course the hospital can not treat patients. It must depend on physicians for this.

But the hospital is not simply a passive partner. The hospital places certain expectations on the physician. He or she must generate a sufficient balance of income received over costs incurred. If not, the hospital will have no reason to provide a physician with admitting privileges. This is the crux of the moral issue. Instead of being a mere facilitator like the community Not-For-Profit hospital, the For-Profit hospital represents an interest in its own right that places certain self-interested demands on the physician and thus the patient as well.

It is possible and very likely, I think, that the patient/physician relationship in the for-profit setting will become a three party relationship wherein the hospital seeks to maximize profit to generate capital for its investors. Hence, you have the physicians serving the interests of an anonymous investor as well as those of the identified patient. This is clearly contrary to the obligation of faithfulness inherent in the doctor/patient relationship. A patient enters into such a relationship with every expectation that his therapeutic interests and the physician's interest in making a living are co-present. However, there is no expectation that a third party's interest in achieving financial affluence is present as well.

One might contend that the alteration of the doctor/patient relationship caused by For Profit Hospitals is more of a theoretical rather than a practical concern. I think the previously cited statistics dispute this claim. For Profit Hospitals generate more charges than do their counterparts. These charges are generated by touches on the patient's body. Unnecessary touches are clearly in violation of the covenant that should hold between doctor and patient. But is this covenant sufficiently strong enough to protect the patient? I think it will prove insufficient for the following reasons.

First of all, as was stated, in order to survive, For Profit Hospitals must be profitable for their investors. In order to be profitable they must be competitive in the health care arena. Since there is a present glut of hospital beds in most communities, competition will likely be fierce. This in turn could threaten the professional autonomy of physicians. As hospitals become threatened, admitting privileges may become more and more difficult both to obtain and maintain. Thus, hospitals will be in a position to dictate treatment standards to physicians. For Profit Hospitals will have every reason to dictate standards that will prove to be as profitable as possible. If the physician does not abide by these standards, his or her ability to practice the profession of medicine will be jeopardized. Abusing the therapeutic interests of patients may be necessary in order to protect the self-interests of the physician. Thus, the financial interests of investors will dictate standards of medical care in possible violation of the professional interests of the physician and the therapeutic interests of the patient.

These considerations demonstrate the moral deficiency of For Profit Hospitals. Despite any competitive or economic virtues For Profit Hospitals may provide, their existence threatens the very nature of the doctor/patient relationship that serves as the moral foundation for the practice of medicine. That relationship is altered from a two party fiduciary relationship into a three way relationship designed ultimately to obtain monetary gain for outside investors. This alteration adds insult to injury. Patients presently endure the injury of illness in terms of suffering and diminished autonomy. For Profit health care institutions compound these by adding economic exploitation to the process.

CONCLUSION

In conclusion, let me hasten to add that the foregoing should be taken only as an indictment of For Profit Hospitals and nothing more. It certainly should not be taken as a full endorsement of the present health care system apart from profit-making institutions. There is sufficient economic waste and patient-exploitation in the present system to justify withholding unqualified support. However, in my view the advent of For Profit Hospitals will only exacerbate these current problems. Regardless of the reforms and changes to be made in our health care system, one thing need not be reformed. That is our understanding of the physician/patient relationship. The covenant of faithfulness between doctor and patient must be maintained if the administration of health care is to respect personal autonomy. Thus, any changes and reforms in our health care system must be consistent with the dictates of this covenant. For Profit Hospitals clearly contain many institutional incentives and priorities that are inconsistent with the covenant. Thus, we tolerate the presence of them in our health care system at the expense of the covenant that protects patient welfare.

NOTES

1. Relman, A. S., 'The new medical industrial complex', *N. Eng. J. Med.* 303 (1980), 963–970.

2. Wohl, S., *The Medical Industrial Complex*, New York, Harmony Books, 1984.

3. Pellegrino, E. D. and Thomasma, D. C., *A Philosophical Basis of Medical Practice*, New York, Oxford University Press, 1981, p. 65.

4. Pellegrino, E. D., *Humanism and the Physician*, Knoxville, University of Tennessee Press, 1970, p. 145.

5. Ibid.

6. Ramsey, P., *The Patient as Person*, New Haven, Yale University Press, 1970, p. 2.

7. Ibid., p. 6.

8. Ibid., p. 5.

9. Ibid., p. 11.

10. Relman, A. S., 'Investor-owned hospitals and health-costs', *N. Eng. J. Med.* 309 (1983), 370.

11. Wohl, S., *The Medical Industrial Complex*, New York, Harmony Books, 1984, p. 4.

12. Relman, A. S., 'The new medical-industrial complex', *N. Eng. J. Med.* 303 (1980), 966.

13. Ibid.

14. Ibid., p. 967. Relman claims the physician acts as a trustee.

SUGGESTED READINGS FOR CHAPTER 12

COST AND RISK ASSESSMENT

Doubilet, Peter, Weinstein, Milton C., and McNeil, Barbara J. "Use and Misuse of the Term 'Cost Effective' in Medicine." *New England Journal of Medicine* 314 (January 23, 1986), 253–256.

Fischoff, B., et al. *Acceptable Risk.* Cambridge: Cambridge University Press, 1981.

Humber, James M., and Almeder, Robert F., eds. *Quantitative Risk Assessment. Biomedical Ethics Reviews 1986.* Clifton, N.J.: Humana Press, 1987.

Lave, Lester B. "Health and Safety Risk Analyses: Information for Better Decisions." *Science* 236 (April 17, 1987), 292–293.

MacLean, D., ed. *Values at Risk.* Totowa, N.J.: Rowman and Littlefield, 1986.

Rescher, Nicholas. *Risk.* Washington, D.C.: University Press of America, 1983.

Sagoff, Mark. *Risk-Benefit Analysis in Decisions Concerning Public Safety and Health.* Dubuque, Iowa: Kendall/Hunt, 1985.

U.S. Congress, Office of Technology Assessment. *The Implications of Cost-Effectiveness Analysis of Medical Technology.* Washington, D.C.: U.S. Government Printing Office, August 1980. See especially the Appendix.

Warner, Kenneth E., and Luce, Bryan R. *Cost-Benefit and Cost-Effectiveness Analysis in Health Care.* Ann Arbor, Mich.: Health Administration Press, 1982.

OCCUPATIONAL SAFETY AND HEALTH

American Public Health Association. "Increasing Worker and Community Awareness of Toxic Hazards in the Workplace." *American Journal of Public Health* 75 (March 1985), 305–308.

Ashford, Nicholas A., and Caldart, Charles C. "The 'Right to Know': Toxics Information Transfer in the Workplace." In Breslow, Lester, et al., eds. *Annual Review of Public Health.* Palo Alto, Calif.: Annual Reviews, 1984. Vol. 6, pp. 383–401.

Bayer, Ronald. "Notifying Workers at Risk: The Politics of the Right-to-Know." *American Journal of Public Health* 76 (November 1986), 1352–1356.

Daniels, Norman. *Just Health Care*. Cambridge: Cambridge University Press, 1985. Chap. 7.

Hunt, Vilma R. "Perspective on Ethical Issues in Occupational Health." In Humber, James M., and Almeder, Robert F., eds. *Biomedical Ethics Reviews*. Clifton, N.J.: Humana Press, 1984, pp. 175–201.

Lappé, Marc. "Ethical Issues in Testing for Differential Sensitivity to Occupational Hazards." *Journal of Occupational Medicine* 25 (November 1983), 797–808.

McElveen, Junius C. "Reproductive Hazards in the Workplace: Some Legal Considerations." *Journal of Occupational Medicine* 28 (February 1986), 103–109.

Murray, Thomas H., and Bayer, Ronald. "Ethical Issues in Occupational Health." In Humber, James M., and Almeder, Robert F., eds. *Biomedical Ethics Reviews 1984*. Clifton, N.J.: Humana Press, 1984, pp. 153–173.

Shrader-Frechette, Kristin. "Occupational Risk and the Theory of Compensating Wage Differential." In *Risk Analysis and Scientific Method*. Dordrecht: D. Reidel, 1985, pp. 97–124.

U.S. Congress, Office of Technology Assessment. *Reproductive Hazards in the Workplace*. Washington, D.C.: U.S. Government Printing Office, December 1985.

SCREENING

"AIDS: Public Health and Civil Liberties." *The Hastings Center Report* 16 (December 1986), 1–36. Special supplement.

Capron, Alexander Morgan. "Current Issues in Genetic Screening." In Humber, James M., and Almeder, Robert F., eds. *Biomedical Ethics Reviews 1984*. Clifton, N.J.: Humana Press, 1984, pp. 121–149.

Faden, Ruth R., et al. "What Participants Understand About a Maternal Serum Alpha-Fetoprotein Screening Program." *American Journal of Public Health* 75 (December 1985), 1381–1384.

Gostin, Lawrence O., Curran, William J., and Clark, Mary E. "The Case Against Compulsory Casefinding in Controlling AIDS—Testing, Screening and Reporting." *American Journal of Law and Medicine* 12 (1987), 17–53.

Hubbard, Ruth, and Henifin, Mary Sue. "Genetic Screening of Prospective Parents and of Workers: Some Scientific and Social Issues." In Humber, James M., and Almeder, Robert F., eds. *Biomedical Ethics Reviews*. Clifton, N.J.: Humana Press, 1984, pp. 73–120.

Kopelman, Loretta. "Genetic Screening in Newborns: Voluntary or Compulsory?" *Perspectives in Biology and Medicine* 22 (Autumn 1978), 83–89.

Law, Medicine, and Health Care 15 (Summer 1987). Special issue on "AIDS: Law and Policy."

Miller, David, et al. "HTLV-III: Should Testing Ever Be Routine?" *British Medical Journal* 292 (April 5, 1986), 941–943.

Oppenheimer, Gerald M., and Padgug, Robert A. "AIDS: The Risks to Insurers, the Threat to Equity." *Hastings Center Report* 16 (October 1986), 18–22.

U.S. Congress, Office of Technology Assessment. *The Role of Genetic Testing in the Prevention of Occupational Disease*. Washington, D.C.: U.S. Government Printing Office, April 1983.

Walters, LeRoy. "Ethical Issues in the Prevention and Treatment of HIV Infection and AIDS." *Science* 239 (February 5, 1988), 597–603.

COMPETITION AND PROFIT IN HEALTH CARE

Brody, Baruch A. "Justice and Competitive Markets." *Journal of Medicine and Philosophy* 12 (February 1987), 37–50.

Daniels, Norman. "Why Saying No to Patients in the United States Is So Hard: Cost Containment, Justice, and Provider Autonomy." *New England Journal of Medicine* 314 (May 22, 1986), 1380–1383.

Eisenberg, Leon. "Health Care: For Patients or for Profits?" *American Journal of Psychiatry* 143 (August 1986), 1015–1019.

Goldworth, Amnon, and Lomasky, Loren. Symposium: "Who Should Profit from the Business of Science?" *Hastings Center Report* 17 (June 1987), 5–10.

Graham, Gordon. "The Doctor, the Rich, and the Indigent." *Journal of Medicine and Philosophy* 12 (February 1987), 51–61.

Gray, Bradford, ed. *For-Profit Hospital Care: Who Profits? Who Cares?* Washington, D.C.: National Council of Senior Citizens, 1986.

Gray, Bradford H., ed. Institute of Medicine, Committee on Implications of For-Profit Enterprise in Health Care. *For-Profit Enterprise in Health Care*. Washington, D.C.: National Academy Press, 1986.

Menzel, Paul T. "Economic Competition in Health Care: A Moral Assessment." *Journal of Medicine and Philosophy* 12 (February 1987), 63–84.

Pellegrino, Edmund. "Competition: New Moral Dilemmas for Physicians, Hospitals." *Hospital Progress* 64 (1983), 8, 10, 22–25.

Rainbolt, George W. "Competition and the Patient-Centered Ethic." *Journal of Medicine and Philosophy* 12 (February 1987), 85–99.

BIBLIOGRAPHIES

Goldstein, Doris Mueller. *Bioethics: A Guide to Information Sources*. Detroit: Gale Research Company, 1982. See under "Genetic Counseling and Screening" and "Treatment for Defective Newborns and Infanticide."

Lineback, Richard H., ed. *Philosopher's Index*. Vols. 1– . Bowling Green, Ohio: Philosophy Documentation Center, Bowling Green State University. Issued quarterly. See under "Birth Control," "Birth Defects," "Cost-Benefit Analysis," "Genetic Engineering," "Liberty," "Medicine," "Mentally Retarded," "Public Policy," "Quality of Life," "Risk(s)," and "Social Control."

Walters, LeRoy, and Kahn, Tamar Joy, eds. *Bibliography of Bioethics*. Vols. 1– . New York: Free Press. Issued annually. See under "Eugenics," "Genetic Screening," and "Occupational Medicine." (The information contained in the annual *Bibliography of Bioethics* can also be retrieved from BIOETHICSLINE, an on-line database of the National Library of Medicine.)

About the Authors

W. FRENCH ANDERSON is Chief of the Laboratory of Molecular Hematology at the National Heart, Lung, and Blood Institute, National Institutes of Health.

GEORGE J. ANNAS is Utley Professor of Health Law and Chief of the Health Law Section at Boston University School of Public Health.

MICHAEL S. BARAM directs the Program in Law and Technology at Boston University Law School, teaches health law at Boston University School of Public Health, and practices law with the firm of Bracker and Baram.

RONALD BAYER is Associate Professor of Public Health at the School of Public Health, Columbia University, New York.

TOM L. BEAUCHAMP is a Professor in the Department of Philosophy and a Senior Research Scholar at the Kennedy Institute of Ethics, Georgetown University.

CHRISTOPHER BOORSE is Professor of Philosophy at the University of Delaware.

DAN W. BROCK is a professor in the Department of Philosophy and Professor of Human Values in Medicine within the Program in Medicine at Brown University.

BARUCH BRODY is Leon Jaworski Professor of Biomedical Ethics, Director of the Center for Ethics, Medicine, and Public Issues, and Professor of Medicine and Community Medicine at Baylor College of Medicine in Houston, Texas.

ALLEN BUCHANAN is Professor of Philosophy at the University of Arizona.

DANIEL CALLAHAN is a philosopher and the Director of the Hastings Center, Briarcliff Manor, New York.

ARTHUR L. CAPLAN is Director of the Center for Biomedical Ethics and Professor in the Departments of Philosophy and Surgery at the University of Minnesota.

ALEXANDER MORGAN CAPRON holds the Norman Topping Chair in Law, Medicine and Public Policy at the University of Southern California, where he teaches in both the law and medical schools.

JAMES F. CHILDRESS is Edwin B. Kyle Professor of Religious Studies and Professor of Medical Education at the University of Virginia. He is also Chairman of the Department of Religious Studies and Principal of the Monroe Hill Residential College.

PAUL CHODOFF is a physician and Clinical Professor of Psychiatry at George Washington University School of Medicine.

K. DANNER CLOUSER is a Professor in the Department of Humanities at the Pennsylvania State University College of Medicine in Hershey.

RONALD CRANFORD is Director of the Neurological Intensive Care Unit and Cochairperson of the Biomedical Ethics Committee at the Hennepin County Medical Center, Minneapolis, and Associate Professor of Neurology at the University of Minnesota.

LEON EISENBERG is the Maude Lillian Presley Professor of Psychiatry at Harvard Medical School and holds a clinical appointment at the Children's Hospital Medical Center in Boston.

H. TRISTRAM ENGELHARDT, JR., is Professor of Medicine and Community Medicine and a Member of the Center for Ethics, Medicine, and Public Issues at Baylor College of Medicine, Houston, Texas.

RUTH R. FADEN is a Professor in the Department of Health Policy and Management at the School of Hygiene and Public Health, Johns Hopkins University. She is also a Senior Research Scholar at the Kennedy Institute of Ethics, Georgetown University.

JUNE FESSENDEN-RADEN is Associate Professor of Biochemistry and Biology and Society, a Member of the Program on Science, Technology and Society, and a Member of the Institute for Comparative and Environmental Toxicology at Cornell University.

JOEL FEINBERG is Professor of Philosophy at the University of Arizona.

LAWRENCE FINSEN is Associate Professor of Philosophy at the University of Redlands, California.

MICHAEL J. FLOWER is Assistant Research Biologist in the Department of Biology and the Program in Science, Technology, and Public Affairs at the University of California, San Diego.

NORMAN FOST is a Professor in the Department of Pediatrics and Director of the Program in Medical Ethics at the University of Wisconsin School of Medicine.

BERNARD GERT is the Stone Professor of Intellectual and Moral Philosophy and Codirector of the Institute for the Study of Applied and Professional Ethics at Dartmouth College. He is also Adjunct Professor of Psychiatry at Dartmouth Medical School.

RAANAN GILLON is Director of Imperial College Health Service, Department Director of the Institute of Medical Ethics in London, Senior Fellow at the Center for Medical Law and Ethics in London, and Editor of the *Journal of Medical Ethics*.

LEONARD H. GLANTZ is Professor of Health Law at Boston University School of Public Health.

JONATHAN GLOVER is Fellow and Tutor in Philosophy, New College, Oxford University.

ALEXANDER Z. GUIORA is Professor Emeritus of Psychiatry and Psychology at the University of Michigan.

JAMES M. GUSTAFSON is University Professor of Theological Ethics and a faculty member in the Committee on Social Thought and the Divinity School at the University of Chicago.

ANDRÉ E. HELLEGERS (d. 1979) was the founder and first Director of the Kennedy Institute of Ethics at Georgetown University.

WORTHINGTON HOOKER, M.D. (1806–1867) was Professor of the Theory and Practice of Medicine at Yale College.

HANS JONAS is Professor Emeritus of Philosophy at the New School for Social Research in New York City.

ALBERT R. JONSEN is Professor and Chairman in the Department of Medical History and Ethics at the University of Washington.

JAY KATZ is a psychiatrist and Professor of Law and Psychiatry at Yale University Law School.

HERMAN B. LEONARD is Associate Professor of Public Policy at the John F. Kennedy School of Government, Harvard University.

CAROL LEVINE is Executive Director of the Citizens' Commission on AIDS for New York City and Northern New Jersey, Managing Editor for *IRB: A Review of Human Subjects Research*, and Adjunct Associate at the Hastings Center.

MICHAEL LOCKWOOD is Staff Tutor in Philosophy in the Department of External Studies at Oxford University.

JOANNE LYNN is Associate Professor of Medicine at the George Washington University School of Medicine and Medical Director of the Washington, D.C. Home and Hospice.

RUTH MACKLIN is Professor of Bioethics at Albert Einsten College of Medicine, New York City.

H. J. McCLOSKY is Professor of Philosophy at La Trobe University in Victoria, Australia.

LAURENCE B. McCULLOUGH is Professor of Medicine and Community Medicine and a Member of the Center for Ethics, Medicine, and Public Issues at Baylor College of Medicine in Houston, Texas.

KEN MARTYN is a former member of the *UCLA Law Review*.

RICHARD D. MOHR is Associate Professor of Philosophy at the University of Illinois.

JOHN C. MOSKOP is Associate Professor in the Department of Medical Humanities at the East Carolina School of Medicine, Greenville, North Carolina.

JOHN T. NOONAN, JR. is Judge, United States Court of Appeals, Ninth Circuit, California.

EDMUND D. PELLEGRINO is Director of the Kennedy Institute of Ethics, Georgetown University, and John Carroll Professor of Medicine and Medical Humanities at the Georgetown University School of Medicine.

JAMES RACHELS is Professor of Philosophy at the University of Alabama at Birmingham.

TOM REGAN is Professor of Philosophy at North Carolina State University in Raleigh.

UWE E. REINHARDT is James Madison Professor of Political Economy at the Woodrow Wilson School of Public and International Affairs, Princeton University.

ARNOLD S. RELMAN is Editor of the *New England Journal of Medicine*.

MICHAEL RUSE is Professor of History and Philosophy at the University of Guelph, Ontario.

RITA L. SALADANHA is a neonatologist at Brookdale Hospital in Brooklyn, New York.

ARTHUR SCHAFER is Associate Professor of Philosophy at the University of Manitoba, Winnipeg.

HENRY SIDGWICK (1838–1900) was the Knightsbridge Professor of Moral Philosophy at Cambridge University.

MARK SIEGLER is Professor of Medicine and Director of the Center for Clinical Medical Ethics at the Pritzker School of Medicine, University of Chicago.

PEGGY STINSON is a part-time school teacher and holds a graduate degree in German language and literature.

ROBERT STINSON is Associate Professor of History at Moravian College, Pennsylvania.

THOMAS SZASZ is a physician and Professor of Psychiatry at the State University of New York Health Sciences Center in Syracuse.

JUDITH JARVIS THOMSON is Professor of Philosophy at the Massachusetts Institute of Technology.

STEPHEN E. TOULMIN is Professor of Philosophy at Northwestern University, Evanston, Illinois.

ROBERT M. VEATCH is Professor of Medical Ethics at the Kennedy Institute of Ethics, Georgetown University.

LeROY WALTERS is Director of the Center for Bioethics at the Kennedy Institute of Ethics and Associate Professor in the Department of Philosophy, Georgetown University.

MARY ANNE WARREN is Professor of Philosophy at San Francisco State University.

PETER C. WILLIAMS is an attorney and philosopher who teaches in the Department of Community and Preventive Medicine at the State University of New York at Stony Brook.

GERALD R. WINSLOW is Professor of Christian Ethics at Loma Linda University in Loma Linda, California.

SUSAN M. WOLF is Associate for Law at the Hastings Center, Briarcliff Manor, New York, and Adjunct Associate Professor at New York University School of Law.

MARK YARBOROUGH is Assistant Professor of Philosophy at the University of Colorado, Denver.

RICHARD J. ZECKHAUSER is Professor of Political Economy at the John F. Kennedy School of Government, Harvard University.